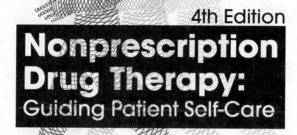

4th Edition

Nonprescription Drug Therapy:
Guiding Patient Self-Care

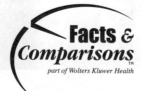

Facts &
Comparisons™
part of Wolters Kluwer Health

Nonprescription Drug Therapy™: Guiding Patient Self-Care,
Fourth Edition

© **2005 Wolters Kluwer Health, Inc.**

Indexed by Coughlin Indexing Services, Inc., Annapolis, Maryland.

ISBN 1-57439-223-9

Printed in the United States of America

The information contained in this publication is intended to supplement the knowledge of health care professionals regarding appropriate nonprescription treatment of certain conditions. This information is advisory only and is not intended to replace sound clinical judgment or individualized patient care in the delivery of health care services. The information published is derived from literature research and is subject to review and approval by the Editor and the Editorial Review Panel. However, Wolters Kluwer Health, Inc. disclaims all warranties, whether express or implied, including any warranty as to the quality, accuracy, or stability of this information for any particular purpose.

The content contained in *Nonprescription Drug Therapy™: Guiding Patient Self-Care* is available for licensing as source data. For more information on data licensing, please call 1-800-223-0554.

Facts & Comparisons®
part of Wolters Kluwer Health
77 Westport Plaza, Suite 450
St. Louis, Missouri 63146-3125
www.drugfacts.com
314/216-2100 • 800/223-0554

NONPRESCRIPTION DRUG THERAPY™
GUIDING PATIENT SELF-CARE

EDITOR
Tim R. Covington, MS, PharmD
Birmingham, Alabama

FACTS & COMPARISONS® PUBLISHING GROUP

CEO, Clinical Tools	Kenneth H. Killion
Vice President and Publisher	Cathy H. Reilly
Senior Managing Editor, Content Development	Renée M. Wickersham
Senior Managing Editor, Quality Control and Production	Julie A. Scott
Managing Editor	Angela J. Schwalm
Associate Editors	Jennifer A. Guimaraes Joseph R. Horenkamp Nicholas R. Weber
Assistant Editor	Carolee Ann Corrigan
Senior Quality Control Editor	Susan H. Sunderman
Composition Specialist	Jennifer M. Reed
Senior SGML Specialist	Linda M. Jones
Purchasing Specialist	Heather L. Broad
Clinical Director	Renée Rivard, PharmD
Clinical Manager	Cathy A. Meives, PharmD
Director, Referential Product Management	Teri H. Burnham

NONPRESCRIPTION DRUG THERAPY™
EDITORIAL REVIEW PANEL

EDITOR

Tim R. Covington, MS, PharmD
Bruno Professor of Pharmacy
Director, Managed Care Institute
McWhorter School of Pharmacy
Samford University
Birmingham, Alabama

FACTS & COMPARISONS®
EDITORIAL ADVISORY PANEL

Louis Almekinders, MD
Associate Professor
Department of Orthopedic
  Surgery
University of North Carolina
  School of Medicine
Chapel Hill, North Carolina

Jerome M. Aronberg, MD
Assistant Professor of
  Dermatology
Washington University
School of Medicine
St. Louis, Missouri

Karim A. Calis, PharmD, MPH
Clinical Specialist, Endocrinology
  & Women's Health
Coordinator, Drug Information
  Services
National Institutes of Health
Warren G. Magnuson Clinical
  Center
Department of Pharmacy
Bethesda, Maryland

Edwina Chan, PharmD
Assistant Professor
Department of Pharmacy Practice
McWhorter School of Pharmacy
Samford University
Birmingham, Alabama

**Bruce D. Clayton, BS, PharmD,
RPh**
Professor of Pharmacy Practice
College of Pharmacy and Health
  Sciences
Butler University
Indianapolis, Indiana

Tim R. Covington, MS, PharmD
Bruno Professor of Pharmacy
Director, Managed Care Institute
McWhorter School of Pharmacy
Samford University
Birmingham, Alabama

Donald Fagan, PharmD
Assistant Director of Pharmacy,
  Clinical Services
St. Joseph Hospital Pharmacy
Omaha, Nebraska

Amy L. Friedman, PharmD
Product Support Specialist
HCMO Pharmaceutical Services
Mutual of Omaha Insurance
  Company
United of Omaha Life Insurance
  Company
Mutual and United South
Omaha, Nebraska

Rex Ghormley, OD, FAAO
Private Practitioner
Contact Lens Consultants
St. Louis, Missouri

Ellen Hamburg, PharmD
Associate Professor of Clinical
  Pharmacy
Arnold and Marie Schwartz
  College of Pharmacy and Health
Long Island University
Brooklyn, New York

Steven K. Hebel, RPh
Director of Pharmacy
Corum Health Services, Inc.
St. Louis, Missouri

Amy Heck, PharmD
Specialized Resident in Drug
  Information Practice and
  Pharmacotherapy
Drug Information Service
Warren G. Magnuson Clinical
  Center
National Institutes of Health
Bethesda, Maryland

Anne Hoffmeister, PharmD
Philadelphia College of Pharmacy
  and Science
Philadelphia, Pennsylvania

**Kristine E. Keplar, BS, PharmD,
RPh**
Assistant Professor of Pharmacy
  Practice
College of Pharmacy and Health
  Sciences
Butler University
Richard L. Roudebush VA
  Medical Center
Indianapolis, Indiana

Mary Gail Kwiecinski, DPM
Private Practice Podiatrist
Libertyville, Illinois

Ann Macro, BS, RPh
Director of Pharmacy Services
Stephens Memorial Hospital
Norway, Maine

**Elizabeth C. McGuffey, BS
  Pharm, PhD**
Retail Pharmacist
Kroger, Inc.
Durham, North Carolina

Wendy Munroe, PharmD
President
MedOutcomes, Inc.
Richmond, Virginia

Anita Murdock, PharmD
Fellow in Managed Care
  Pharmacy
Managed Care Institute
McWhorter School of Pharmacy
Samford University
Birmingham, Alabama

Betsy Naeger, RN
Enteral Stomal Therapy
  Consultant
Medical West
St. Louis, Missouri

Omudhome Ogbru, PharmD
Assistant Professor of Pharmacy
  Practice, Regional Coordinator
University of the Pacific
School of Pharmacy and Health
  Sciences
Stockton, California

Jeffrey T. Reed, MD
Private Practitioner
Dermatology and Cutaneous
  Surgery, Inc.
St. Louis, Missouri

Mary Beth Rhomberg, OD
University of Missouri – St. Louis
School of Optometry
St. Louis, Missouri

Leo Semes, OD
Associate Professor
School of Optometry
The University of Alabama at
  Birmingham
Birmingham, Alabama

Condit Steil, PharmD, CDE
Associate Professor and Director
Center for Pharmaceutical Care
  Development in Community
  Practice
School of Pharmacy
Samford University
Birmingham, Alabama

Burgunda V. Sweet, PharmD
Director, Drug Information and
  Investigational Drug Services
Clinical Associate Professor of
  Pharmacy
University of Michigan Health
  System and College of Pharmacy
Ann Arbor, Michigan

David S. Tatro, PharmD
Drug Information Analyst
San Carlos, California

Karen J. Tietze, PharmD
Assistant Professor of Clinical
  Pharmacy
Philadelphia College of Pharmacy
  and Science
Philadelphia, Pennsylvania

Candy Tsourounis, PharmD
Assistant Clinical Professor
Drug Information Analysis
  Service
School of Pharmacy
University of California, San
  Francisco
San Francisco, California

**Katie von Oldenburg, RD,
  CNSD, LMNT**
Clinical Dietitian
Department of Case Management
St. Joseph Hospital
Omaha, Nebraska

Eric Wittbrodt, PharmD
Assistant Professor of Clinical
  Pharmacy
University of the Sciences in
  Philadelphia
Philadelphia, Pennsylvania

**Nicholas Zacharczenko, DDS,
  RPh**
Private Practice Prosthodontist
Clifton Park, New York

CONTRIBUTING REVIEWERS

Jerome M. Aronberg, MD
Assistant Professor of Dermatology
Washington University
School of Medicine
St. Louis, Missouri

Daphne B. Bernard, PharmD, CACP
Assistant Professor
Howard University School of
Pharmacy
Washington, DC

Karim Calis, PharmD, MPH
Clinical Specialist, Endocrinology &
Women's Health
Coordinator, Drug Information
Services
National Institutes of Health
Warren G. Magnuson Clinical Center
Department of Pharmacy
Bethesda, Maryland

Michael Cirigliano, MD, FACP
Associate Professor of Medicine
University of Pennsylvania
School of Medicine
Philadelphia, Pennsylvania

Tim R. Covington, MS, PharmD
Executive Director
Managed Care Institute
Bruno Professor of Pharmacy
McWhorter School of Pharmacy
Samford University
Birmingham, Alabama

Julia Elenbaas, PharmD
Shawnee Mission, Kansas

Constance Grauds, RPh
President, Association of Natural
Medicine Pharmacists
San Rafael, California

Nancy de Guire, PharmD
Assistant Professor of Pharmacy
Practice
Coordinator, Introductory Practical
Experience Program
University of the Pacific
School of Pharmacy and Health
Sciences
Stockton, California

Berit Gundersen, PharmD
Associate Professor
University of the Pacific
School of Pharmacy and Health
Sciences
Stockton, California

Zora S. Hanko, DMD
Private Practitioner
St. Louis, Missouri

Amy Heck, PharmD
Specialized Resident in Drug
Information Practice and
Pharmacotherapy
Drug Information Service
Warren G. Magnuson Clinical Center
National Institutes of Health
Bethesda, Maryland

William J. Keller, PhD
Secretary
American Society of Pharmacognosy
Professor and Chair
Department of Pharmaceutical
Sciences
McWhorter School of Pharmacy
Samford University
Birmingham, Alabama

Julio Lopez, PharmD
Assistant Professor
University of the Pacific
Assistant Clinical Professor
School of Pharmacy
University of California, San Francisco
Chief, Pharmacy Service
VA Northern California Health Care
System
Martinez, California

Ann Macro, BS, RPh
Director of Pharmacy Services
Stephens Memorial Hospital
Norway, Maine

Maryam R. Mohassel, PharmD
Specialized Resident in Drug
Information Practice and
Pharmacotherapy
Drug Information Service
Warren G. Magnuson Clinical Center
National Institutes of Health
Bethesda, Maryland

Gail D. Newton, PhD, RPh
Associate Professor
Department of Pharmacy Practice
School of Pharmacy and Pharmacal
Sciences
Purdue University
West Lafayette, Indiana

Omudhome Ogbru, PharmD
Assistant Professor of Pharmacy
Practice, Regional Coordinator
University of the Pacific
School of Pharmacy and Health
Sciences
Stockton, California

Bernie R. Olin, PharmD
Associate Clinical Professor and
Director
Drug Information and Learning
Resource Center
Harrison School of Pharmacy
Auburn University
Auburn, Alabama

Jeffrey T. Reed, MD
Private Practitioner
Dermatology and Cutaneous Surgery,
Inc.
St. Louis, Missouri

Irv Reich, BS Pharm
Instructor, Department of Pharmacy
Practice, Pharmacy Administration
Manager, Professional Laboratories
Philadelphia College of Pharmacy and
Science
Philadelphia, Pennsylvania

Mary Beth Shirk, PharmD, RPh
Specialty Practice Pharmacist in
Critical Care and Pain Management
The Ohio State University Medical
Center
Clinical Assistant Professor
The Ohio State University College of
Pharmacy
Columbus, Ohio

Frank Simo, MD
Private Practice, Facial Plastic and
Reconstructive Surgery
Assistant Clinical Professor of
Otolaryngology
Saint Louis University School of
Medicine
Saint Louis, Missouri

Burgunda V. Sweet, PharmD
Director, Drug Information
Clinical Associate Professor of
Pharmacy
University of Michigan
Ann Arbor, Michigan

Candy Tsourounis, PharmD
Assistant Clinical Professor
Drug Information Analysis Service
School of Pharmacy
University of California,
San Francisco
San Francisco, California

Alan Wickenhauser, DMD
Private Practice, General Dentistry
Bethalto, Illinois

Nicholas Zacharczenko, DDS, RPh
Private Practice Prosthodontist
Clifton Park, New York

NONPRESCRIPTION DRUG THERAPY™
TABLE OF CONTENTS

■ ■ ■

III. GI/GU CONDITIONS

IV. MUSCULOSKELETAL CONDITIONS

VIII. OTIC CONDITIONS

IX. PODIATRIC CONDITIONS

X. RESPIRATORY CONDITIONS

XI. WOMEN'S HEALTH

XII. DIABETES MANAGEMENT

XII. HOME DIAGNOSTICS/DEVICES

XIII. COMPLEMENTARY THERAPIES

XIV. APPENDIX

XV. INDEX

INTRODUCTION

Nonprescription Drug Therapy™ *(NDT): Guiding Patient Self-Care* is a timely, comprehensive, and authoritative publication that is carefully designed to serve the informational needs of pharmacists, physicians, other health care providers, and the self-medicating consumer. When used properly, NDT will foster value-based, patient-focused, pharmaceutical care that is driven toward the attainment of optimal health outcomes in patients taking nonprescription drugs.

The publisher, editors, and scores of authors and reviewers of NDT have defined the following primary goals for this publication:

- Foster the safe, appropriate, effective, and economical use of nonprescription drugs in treating and mitigating symptoms of a wide variety of commonly occurring, self-treatable medical conditions.
- Serve the best interests of the public health by providing pharmacists, other health care providers, and consumers with in-depth, comprehensive, current information on nonprescription drug therapy in a logical and practical format.

NDT is complementary to other Facts & Comparisons® publications but is unique among them in its exclusive focus on nonprescription drug therapy. This publication is the definitive, applied reference source addressing nonprescription pharmacotherapy and is a cornerstone of drug information designed to assist in the mitigation of symptoms and management of illness.

The format of NDT fosters a logical thought process that begins with a presentation of the medical condition to be treated (eg, definition, etiology, incidence, pathophysiology, signs and symptoms). The monograph then progresses to the diagnostic process by presenting focused assessment parameters that can be determined through clinical observation and interview. Each monograph culminates with a thorough review of appropriate pharmacotherapeutic management (eg, drug selections, drug use, patient education, product information).

The configuration of the NDT content is similar to that of a standard medical text and supports the universal recognition that one cannot adequately treat a patient or that patients cannot appropriately treat themselves unless there is full understanding and appreciation of the medical condition the drug therapy is designed to treat. One may then assess the symptom or symptom complex and determine whether the patient should be triaged to a physician or other health care provider or if the patient should self-treat with one or more nonprescription drugs.

The tone of the work is resolute, the language is crisp, the sequencing is logical, and the content is rational and relevant, preventing readers from getting lost in extraneous and inapplicable narrative. NDT is designed to remain up-to-date. The current drug information "explosion" in the information age in which we live virtually requires this level of currency if patient health interests are to be properly served.

Powerful market forces support the value of and need for this publication. These forces are societal, cultural, economic, and medical-management based. Nonprescription drug therapy is a major component of modern health care. Individual consumers are increasingly expressing the desire and demonstrating the will to self-medicate and increase ownership of their own health care. Further, millions of informed consumers demonstrate their ability to successfully self-treat themselves every day. Nonprescription drugs, vitamins, nutritionals, and herbal products represent a $35 billion annual health care expenditure. More than half of all pharmaceutical dosage forms consumed per year are nonprescription drugs. Approximately 30% of the nation's total drug expenditure is for nonprescription drug therapy. Pharmacists are disproportionately influential in assisting patients with nonprescription pharmacotherapy and are well qualified to do so. The US Food and Drug Administration remains committed to moving more prescription drugs to nonprescription status if safety and efficacy can be reasonably assured.

Today, individual consumers are increasingly "self-diagnosing" their medical condition(s) and "prescribing" their own nonprescription drug therapies. Some would argue that package labeling adequately addresses patient information needs relative to nonprescription pharmacotherapy. That argument loses validity when considering the inability of package labeling to adequately address the complexity of pharmacotherapy and a near-infinite combination of comorbidities and coexisting prescription and nonprescription drug regimens (polypharmacy).

There is no substitute for educated consumers, pharmacists, and other health care providers who are informed in nonprescription drug selection, use, and monitoring. Further, there is no substitute for a comprehensive and current database devoted to nonprescription drug therapy and optimal management of the medical conditions these drugs are indicated to treat.

The publisher, editors, editorial board, reviewers, and advisers are pleased to serve the market with *Nonprescription Drug Therapy*™: *Guiding Patient Self-Care*. Reader feedback and suggestions are earnestly sought, encouraged, and appreciated.

Timothy R. Covington, MS, PharmD
Editor

PUBLISHER'S PREFACE

Nonprescription Drug Therapy™ *(NDT): Guiding Patient Self-Care* is a reference source we are proud to publish. As patient self-care continues to grow, we feel a responsibility to provide health care professionals and consumers with a publication that will aid them in making appropriate and well-informed decisions in the treatment of their conditions. This book is designed to help accomplish this goal.

In an approach that is unique for Facts & Comparisons®, NDT discusses the treatment options from a condition perspective. Patients develop a condition or a series of symptoms and want to know the best available therapies to help alleviate the problem. The chapters of this book are, for the most part, divided by body system, allowing the health care professional or consumer to easily locate the conditions based on the patient's signs and symptoms. A detailed index will also help locate the appropriate section.

Over 100 frequently occuring health conditions potentially treatable by nonprescription drugs are discussed succinctly, including information on etiology, incidence, and signs and symptoms of the condition. A physical assessment section also is included, which contains general information on diagnosing the condition and an interview section that provides a list of topics to discuss with the patient or for patients themselves to consider. These sections provide information to help the patient determine available treatment options that include: a) nondrug therapy, b) nonprescription drug therapy, or c) referral to a physician. If OTC therapy is selected, detailed information on the drug therapy is provided along with a quick-reference product table listing the major brands available, followed by a patient counseling section. Monographs also have detailed graphics, when applicable, to aid the health care professional or consumer in understanding the source/location of the condition.

This publication was developed and will be updated under the editorial direction of Tim R. Covington, MS, PharmD, a nationally known expert in the field of nonprescription drug therapy and patient care. Dr. Covington, along with a distinguished panel of health care professionals including pharmacists, physicians, and dentists, and the dedicated publishing staff has developed the premier publication in the area of patient self-care and nonprescription drug therapy.

As health care changes and evolves, we are changing and evolving to provide reference sources that will continue to serve the information needs of health care providers and consumers. Comments and suggestions are always encouraged.

The Publisher

HOW TO USE NONPRESCRIPTION DRUG THERAPY™

This unique reference book has been designed to help health care professionals assist patients with common, noncritical, medical conditions where, in certain cases, self-treatment with OTC agents may be appropriate. While every effort is made to ensure the data provided herein is complete and up-to-date, readers must bear in mind that this book is **not** intended to replace sound clinical judgment. Keep the following in mind to ease navigation through the book:

Nonprescription Drug Therapy™ (NDT): *Guiding Patient Self-Care* is organized into chapters that describe conditions related to particular body systems (eg, CNS, GI). Throughout each chapter, readers will encounter the sections described below. Each section plays a role in helping the health care professional identify and, when appropriate, recommend treatment (in the form of nondrug therapy or OTC agents) or physician referral.

Definition: Explains what the condition is and provides commonly used names.

Etiology: Describes the origin of the condition.

Incidence: Presents incidence and prevalence data, when known.

Pathophysiology: Describes how the condition develops and affects the body.

Signs/Symptoms: Lists physical or psychological symptoms.

Diagnostic Parameters/Physical Assessment: Describes additional clues to the nature of disease. Also includes an "Interview" section, which provides discussion topics to help ensure the proper diagnosis and treatment. "Nondrug Therapy" and "Pharmacotherapy" subsections provide details of treatment options; the "Pharmacotherapy" section indicates when physician or specialist referral is warranted and includes complete drug monographs for appropriate OTC agents. Product listings, which follow each drug monograph, include a representative group of products available OTC.

In addition to the condition-related monographs, *NDT* includes the following:

Appendices - Includes Treatment of Acute Hypersensitivity Reactions and Treatment of Acute Overdosage, Administration Techniques, and common abbreviations and calculations.

Index - Includes names of conditions, drug agents, and trade names.

Wolters Kluwer Health, Inc. strives to provide health care professionals with accurate, reliable, and useful information in an up-to-date and easy-to-use format. It is our intent to help you help your patients. As readers, you are the most important critics of this book; to help us best meet your needs, please send comments to:

Facts & Comparisons®
part of Wolters Kluwer Health
77 Westport Plaza, Suite 450
St. Louis, Missouri, 63146-3125

CNS
CONDITIONS

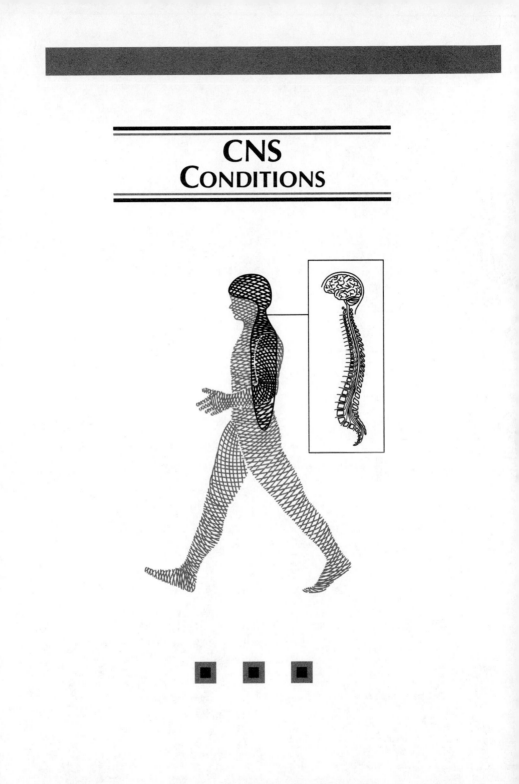

NONPRESCRIPTION DRUG THERAPY
TABLE OF CONTENTS

■ ■ ■

CNS CONDITIONS

INTRODUCTION

The central nervous system (CNS) consists of the brain and spinal cord. Disorders that can manifest in the CNS include fever, headaches, sleep disorders, motion disturbances, chemical dependencies, and obesity. Agents acting on the CNS can selectively reduce fever, relieve pain, induce sleep or arousal, alleviate the tendency to vomit, abate nicotine dependency, or suppress the desire to eat. The use of over-the-counter (OTC) medications is highly prevalent among the general population, particularly in the treatment of CNS disorders that adversely affect daily functioning. Pharmacists are confronted with numerous therapeutic options when caring for patients with CNS disorders. These pharmacotherapeutic approaches to the prevention, reversal, or treatment of these disorders are often confounded by an incomplete knowledge of the physiology, anatomy, and chemistry of the CNS. Often an assessment of these disorders discloses an underlying cause that must be initially addressed, such as concurrent medical conditions or the use of substances (eg, alcohol, caffeine). Therefore, it is important to obtain a thorough evaluation of the patient's condition and consider general issues of safety, such as pregnancy and renal or hepatic impairment, prior to recommending both pharmacologic and nonpharmacologic therapy.

As the trend toward self-medicating is increasing and more prescription drugs are switching to OTC status, it is important that health care providers and patients are aware of the potential benefits and hazards of self-treatment. The benefits of self-medicating enable consumers to assume a greater role in the management of their own health and to decrease health care expenditures, but only if they are well informed and administer the medications responsibly. The risks involved with self-medicating include inappropriate use, overuse, rebound phenomenon, drug interactions, toxicity, and overdose. It is the pharmacist's role to emphasize the importance of adhering to the recommended dosing schedule and not to exceed the recommended maximum dose. Acetaminophen, present in many over-the-counter preparations for fever and headaches, is one of the most frequent causes of poisonings and deaths associated with a pharmaceutical agent. In addition, the ubiquitous attributes of salicylates have resulted in both acute and chronic poisonings, particularly in young children and the elderly.

Many of these CNS medications have undesirable adverse effects. In light of research indicating that patients do not read OTC labeling closely, it is the pharmacist's duty to warn patients of adverse events. As of October 1998, the Food and Drug Administration announced that all OTC pain relievers and fever reducers must carry warning labels advising people to consult their physicians if three or more alcoholic beverages are consumed per day. This includes OTC products containing aspirin, other salicylates, acetaminophen, ibuprofen, naproxen, or ketoprofen. Warn chronic alcohol users of the possibility of increased risk of hepatic damage or GI bleeding when using these drugs.

Antihistamines and anticholinergics approved for motion sickness serve as alternatives to prescription sedative-hypnotics for mild insomnia. Despite the fact that these agents can induce drowsiness, daytime sedation, psychomotor impairment, and anticholinergic effects, they continue to have widespread use. Failure of a pharmacist to point out potential hazards may result in liability issues if an accident occurs.

Natural products are currently marketed as dietary supplements and do not undergo the regulations applied to prescription and OTC medications. However, melatonin has demonstrated symptomatic improvement of insomnia and jet lag. Although well-designed clinical trials have not been conducted on this hormone, pharmacists must not neglect their role in providing patient counseling. Because of limited information on product labeling, pharmacists are in a prime position to offer patient counseling on proper dosing, potential adverse effects, drug interactions, and contraindications.

The availability of OTC nicotine replacement therapy provides the opportunity and responsibility for pharmacists to practice pharmaceutical care. Pharmacists can actively promote smoking cessation as well as identify smokers who are candidates to quit. Pharmacists can encourage the use of nicotine replacement therapy when appropriate, help select these products, provide counseling through the process, and arrange follow-up therapy.

Pharmacists can play an important role in the management of obesity because they are a readily accessible source of information on the appropriate use of weight control agents and other weight loss strategies. Pharmacists must be aware of remarks suggesting that a patient is looking for information or trying to ascertain whether a weight loss approach is likely to be successful. Be aware of the misuse of medications, and warn patients of potential dependence, adverse events, drug interactions, and therapeutic failure. Tolerance to the medication may occur; therefore, advise patients not to increase the dosage without medical supervision.

Over-the-counter preparations are not always appropriate for disorders of the CNS. It is important to tell the patient that many drugs are a temporary solution, and behavioral adjustments are just as important in alleviating most of these problems, except for fever or motion disturbances. In cases where symptoms are recurrent, persistent, or severe, a physician referral is highly recommended.

DROWSINESS/LETHARGY

DEFINITION

Drowsiness is a state of decreased mental alertness that normally precedes sleep. A person usually complains of drowsiness when it occurs during daytime hours. Lethargy, fatigue, and lack of energy are complaints associated with drowsiness.

ETIOLOGY

Sleep is a physiological state that allows the body to rest, replenish, and reenergize. Individuals typically feel fully rested and alert during daytime hours when they receive the quantity and quality of sleep their bodies require. The quantity of sleep needed varies among individuals and averages approximately 8 hours per day for adults. Quality of sleep is based on the individual's biological clock, which regulates the daily rhythm of sleep and wakefulness during a 24-hour period.

Drowsiness is often caused by a decrease in the quantity of sleep or a deviation from the usual sleep/wake rhythm. Prolonged wake cycles because of work or societal demands contribute to drowsiness in adults. Late partying or long study sessions before examinations can cause drowsiness in young adults. Sleep disorders of the sleep/wake cycle (eg, insomnia, sleep apnea, narcolepsy) cause daytime drowsiness. Medical conditions, such as respiratory or cardiac disorders, can cause brief periods of poor oxygenation during sleep, that disrupt the sleep pattern and result in daytime drowsiness. Drugs (eg, narcotics, anxiolytics, alcohol) and diseases (eg, hypothyroidism, depression, anemia) can also cause drowsiness. Overexertion or increased physical activity by a person who is not physically fit results in an increased need for rest and can also cause drowsiness.

INCIDENCE

Everyone experiences drowsiness at some time. Millions of Americans experience daytime drowsiness because the increased demands of employment and family schedules result in inadequate sleep. Young adults are particularly affected because sleep requirements increase during the adolescent growth phase but are often not met because of school and social pressures. While most cases of lethargy are due to inadequate sleep or alterations of the circadian rhythm, 18% of reported cases are due to a preexisting medical condition. Drowsiness and lethargy not only affect productivity levels at home and work, but also decrease mental and physical alertness, which cause an estimated 200,000 auto accidents each year.

SIGNS/SYMPTOMS

Heavy eyelids and sluggish motor responses are common indicators of drowsiness. Other symptoms of drowsiness and lethargy include irritability, loss of concentration, and indifference. Lethargic and drowsy people may also drift into a sleep state but will be easily aroused and respond appropriately when spoken to in normal voice tones.

DIAGNOSTIC PARAMETERS/PHYSICAL ASSESSMENT

Interview: Clinical observation may not reveal drowsiness or lethargy. The patient may have generalized complaints of fatigue or of being unusually tired. Therefore, open-ended questions are crucial when determining whether symptoms are related to lifestyle changes or underlying pathology. Patients describing symptoms of prolonged lethargy or daytime drowsiness that significantly impact their daily functioning should be referred to a physician. It may be useful to inquire about the following:

- Lifestyle (ie, diet, exercise, sleep patterns).
- Occupational/academic status.
- Severity, duration, and frequency of symptoms.
- Diagnosed medical conditions.
- Medications (prescription and nonprescription) and dietary or natural product supplements.
- Other symptoms that accompany drowsiness and lethargy.
- Alcohol and nicotine consumption.
- Whether the problem can be resolved with sleep or rest.

TREATMENT

Approaches to therapy: Identifying and eliminating the factors that cause drowsiness is the ideal approach to therapy. However, when disease or underlying pathology is suspected, as observed with prolonged lethargic states, refer the patient to a physician.

Nondrug therapy: Lifestyle modifications are perhaps the best approach to combatting daytime drowsiness resulting from decreased sleep periods or overexertion during daily activities. Advise patients to obtain an appropriate amount of sleep and to maintain a regular sleep schedule that has the least effect on the body's circadian rhythm. They should avoid caffeine-containing products and sympathomimetic decongestants at bedtime because these agents may adversely affect sleep. The amount of sleep required for each individual varies. Researchers define adequate sleep as the amount needed to wake up without an alarm. The increasing demands of the workplace and family may not allow one to ideally incorporate this practice. Therefore, other modifications may help patients achieve a more invigorated lifestyle. Proper nutritional habits, avoidance of overeating, and daily aerobic exercise often help people feel more energized and alert.

Pharmacotherapy: Caffeine, one of the world's most popular drugs, is the only nonprescription CNS stimulant to receive FDA approval for the management of drowsiness or lethargy. Before recommending a stimulant for mental alertness, interview the patient and address why the product may be needed. The decision to recommend nonprescription stimulants should be individualized for each situation.

CAFFEINE

▶ **Actions**

Caffeine's effects vary and depend on the amount and frequency of ingestion, and on individual metabolism and sensitivity to the agent. Caffeine directly stimulates the CNS at all levels; however, the exact mechanism of action is unknown. Proposed mechanisms involve phosphodiesterase inhibition and adenosine receptor antagonism.

When taken prior to bedtime, caffeine can delay sleep onset, decrease total sleep, increase motor activity, and allow easy arousal.

Caffeine also increases physical endurance, which most likely occurs via the agent's effects on striated muscle.

▶ **Indications**

Caffeine may be used for preventing or relieving lethargy or drowsiness. Caffeine's actions on the cortex of the brain reverse signs of exhaustion and restore mental alertness. Caffeine intake does not improve performance in those who are rested and awake.

▶ **Warnings**

Anxiety or panic disorders: Caffeine may aggravate CNS conditions/disorders because of its stimulatory effects.

Cardiac disease: Use caffeine with caution in patients who have hypertension, angina, or cardiac arrhythmias. Caffeine may increase heart rate, stimulate the force of contractions, increase the myocardial oxygen requirement, and produce transient elevations in blood pressure. Patients who have suffered a recent heart attack should not use caffeine.

Diabetes mellitus: Patients with diabetes should use caffeine with caution; caffeine use may result in hyperglycemia, thus disrupting glycemic control.

GI disorders (eg, GERD, gastric acid disorders): Caffeine decreases lower esophageal sphincter tone and increases gastric acid secretion. Caffeine use may exacerbate duodenal ulcers and may cause diarrhea in patients with irritable bowel syndrome.

Hepatic disease: Caffeine is partially metabolized by the liver. Moderate-to-severe hepatic disease or insufficiency may produce caffeine toxicity.

Hyperthyroidism: The stimulatory effects of caffeine may be additive with increased thyroid hormone levels.

Withdrawal: Daily intake of 350 mg or more of caffeine produces physical dependence on the agent; however, dependence may occur with daily doses as low as 100 mg. The most commonly cited withdrawal symptom is headache, which may be severe. Other symptoms of caffeine withdrawal include irritability, lethargy, and drowsiness. Symptoms generally occur within 12 to 24 hours after abrupt discontinuation and may persist for 4 to 7 days following cessation. Resuming caffeine intake usually relieves symptoms and is the most commonly reported reason for chronic caffeine ingestion.

Pregnancy: Category B. Safety for use in pregnancy has not been determined. Caffeine crosses the placenta; fetal and maternal blood and tissue concentrations achieve similar levels. Increased fetal loss, low birth weight, and premature births have been associated with excessive caffeine intake (more than 600 mg/day) during pregnancy.

Lactation: Caffeine is excreted in the breast milk of nursing mothers. Use with caution, if at all, during lactation.

▶ **Drug Interactions**

CNS stimulants or psychostimulants: When combined with other CNS stimulants, caffeine may cause nervousness, jitteriness, excitability, irritability, insomnia, tachycardia, and cardiac arrhythmias. Caffeine in combination with phenylpropanolamine has been associated with markedly elevated blood pressure and stroke.

Fluconazole, quinolone antibiotics (eg, ciprofloxacin, norfloxacin, enoxacin), cimetidine: Hepatic metabolism may be impaired, resulting in decreased caffeine clearance. Increased caffeine levels may cause excessive cardiovascular and CNS effects.

Drug-food interactions:

Grapefruit juice – Limited data suggest that the serum concentration and duration of action of caffeine may be increased with concomitant administration of grapefruit juice. The proposed mechanism for this interaction is the inhibition of cytochrome P450 hepatic enzymes caused by a component of grapefruit juice.

Caution patients about using caffeine-containing stimulants while ingesting caffeine from dietary sources. When caffeine has been added to foods or beverages, the FDA requires the presence of caffeine to be indicated on the ingredient list. The FDA allows up to 6 mg/ounce of caffeine to be added to beverage products.

Dietary Sources of Caffeine	
Products	**mg/8 fl oz**
Coffee	
Starbucks	250
Drip, regular	140-250
Instant	70-110
Tea	
Brewed, US brands	32-128
Iced	45-50
Instant	35-58
Carbonated Beverages	
Jolt	47.5
Mr. Pibb (sugar free)	39.2
Pepsi One	37
Mountain Dew (regular and diet)	36.6
Mello Yello	35.2
Surge	34
Coca-Cola (regular and diet)	30.4
Shasta (regular, diet, and cherry)	29.6
Mr. Pibb	27.2
Sunkist Orange	26.7
Dr. Pepper	26.4
Pepsi (regular and diet)	24.8
Canada Dry Cola	20
Barq's Root Beer	15.3
A & W Root Beer	0
Chocolate	
Hot chocolate	2.5-10.5
Chocolate milk	10
Chocolate ice cream	4
Chocolate candy bar	5-60 mg/50 g bar
Milk chocolate	5-10 mg/ounce
Baking chocolate (unsweetened)	35-60 mg/ounce
Baking chocolate (sweet and semi-sweet)	10-20 mg/ounce

▶ **Adverse Reactions**

Cardiovascular: Palpitations; sinus tachycardia; cardiac rhythm disturbances; angina (with preexisting ischemic heart disease); hypertension.

CNS: Anxiety; irritability; jitteriness; headache; insomnia; tremor and muscle twitches; excitement; tinnitus; dizziness; sweating; talkativeness.

GI: Nausea; vomiting; diarrhea; abdominal pain.

Miscellaneous: Frequent urination; hyperglycemia; hypersensitivity reactions (eg, dermatitis).

▶ **Administration and Dosage**

Drowsiness/Lethargy (adults): 100 to 200 mg may be given orally every 3 to 4 hours as needed.

Total daily dose (24-hour period) generally should not exceed 600 mg and should never be greater than 1000 mg within a 24-hour period.

These products are not recommended for children younger than 12 years of age.

CAFFEINE PRODUCTS	
Trade name	**Doseform**
357 Magnum Maximum Strength	**Tablets**: 200 mg
Caffedrine	**Tablets**: 200 mg. Lactose.
Keep Alert	**Tablets** : 200 mg. Sugar.
NoDoz	**Tablets** : 200 mg. Sucrose.
Stay Alert Extra Strength	**Tablets**: 200 mg
Stay Awake	**Tablets**: 200 mg. Dextrose
Vivarin	**Tablets**: 200 mg. Dextrose.
NoDoz	**Tablets, chewable** 100 mg. 15 mg phenylalanine, mannitol. Spearmint flavor.
Snapback	**Powder**: 200 mg. Mannitol
Enerjets	**Lozenges**: 75 mg. Sugar. Mocha mint, butterscotch, and coffee flavors.

Products listed are representative of currently available and widely distributed brands. Similar products, including regional and private label brands, may also exist.

PATIENT INFORMATION
Caffeine

- These products should not be used as a substitute for sleep.
- Do not take caffeine products at bedtime.
- Use with caution in the presence of a medically confirmed anxiety disorder, cardiovascular disease (eg, hypertension, ischemic heart disease, cardiac rhythm disturbance), diabetes, peptic ulcer disease, gastroesophageal reflux disease, and hepatic disease.
- Nonprescription CNS stimulants are for occasional use only. These products should not be taken on a daily basis. The need for chronic CNS stimulation with caffeine stimulants beyond 5 to 7 consecutive days requires medical evaluation.
- Abrupt discontinuation may produce withdrawal symptoms (eg, fatigue, headache, decreased performance).
- Discontinue use or decrease dosage if adverse effects occur.

FEVER

DEFINITION

Fever is defined as an increase in body temperature greater than that seen in normal daily body temperature variations. Fever has long been recognized as a common manifestation of illness, particularly with infection. The occurrence of fever is widespread throughout the animal kingdom, which suggests that it is an adaptive response.

Febrile seizures are the most common convulsive disorder among young children and may be considered focal or generalized events; they occur in children from 3 months to 5 years of age who do not have any underlying neurologic disease or other identifiable cause. There are 2 types of febrile seizures: simple febrile seizures last 15 minutes or less, are generalized with no recurrence, and have a short postictal state; complex seizures last longer than 15 minutes, occur more than once within 24 hours, and are focal.

ETIOLOGY

Fever may be related to infectious or noninfectious conditions (eg, autoimmune disorders, drugs [hypersensitivity], malignancies, inflammatory events), with infection being the most common cause of acute fever. Fever is caused by either exogenous or endogenous pyrogens. Exogenous pyrogens (eg, microbial pathogens or their products/toxins) cause fever by inducing the release of endogenous pyrogens. Endogenous pyrogens (eg, IL-1, TNF, IL-6, IFN-alpha) cause fever by initiating metabolic changes in the hypothalamic thermoregulatory center.

Febrile seizures occur in approximately 2% to 4% of all children between 3 months and 5 years of age. Onset is most common during the second year. Eighty percent of febrile seizures are simple, while 20% are complex. Among children who experience 1 febrile seizure, approximately 33% will have a second occurrence, and 9% will have 3 or more febrile seizures. Seventy-five percent of recurrences happen within 6 to 12 months of the first seizure. If there is no recurrence within 1 year, the chance of another decreases to 10% to 15%.

PATHOPHYSIOLOGY

Normal body temperature is between 96.5°F (35.8°C) and 99°F (37.2°C). It is usually lowest in the early morning hours (between 2 AM and 4 AM) and highest later in the day (between 6 PM and 10 PM). Fever raises the hypothalamic set point for body temperature. This results in heat conservation through peripheral vasoconstriction and heat generation through shivering. Increasing body temperature by a few degrees is thought to improve the killing efficiency of macrophages and impair the ability of many microorganisms to replicate. Once a fever breaks, the hypothalamic set point is adjusted downward, resulting in heat loss through sweating and vasodilation.

Most febrile seizures are due to common infections, such as viral upper respiratory tract infections, bacterial pnemonia, gastroenteritis, otitis media, and tonsillitis. The human herpesvirus-6 has been associated with 30% of febrile seizures. Other viruses associated with febrile seizures include adenovirus, influenza type A and B, and parainfluenza type 2. Diphtheria, pertussis, tetanus (DPT) vaccine has been associated with febrile seizures, usually occurring within 48 hours after immunization. Measles, mumps, rubella (MMR) vaccine has also been associated with febrile seizures, usually occurring 7 to 10 days after immunization. In these cases, the seizures are not an allergic reaction and future immunizations are not contraindicated.

SIGNS/SYMPTOMS

The primary sign of fever is an elevation in body temperature to more than 100°F (37.8°C) orally or 100.8°F (38.2°C) rectally. There may also be an increase in neutrophils (including an increase in immature circulating neutrophils), anemia, tachycardia, and hyperventilation.

Seizures usually occur early in the course of a febrile illness, often as the first sign. The seizures may be of any type but are most commonly tonic-clonic. The child may cry and then lose consciousness and muscular rigidity. There may be apnea and incontinence during the tonic phase. This is followed by the clonic phase, which includes repetitive, rhythmic jerking movements, then postictal lethargy or sleep. Other types of seizure manifestations include staring accompanied by stiffness or limpness, jerking movements without prior stiffening, or focal stiffness or jerking.

DIAGNOSTIC PARAMETERS/PHYSICAL ASSESSMENT

Clinical Observation: Temperature can be measured by oral, rectal, axillary, or otic methods. Oral temperatures generally measure 0.4°F less than blood temperature and axillary temperatures measure 1°F less than blood temperature. When evaluating a fever, it is important to get an accurate history from the patient of similar symptoms that may have recently been seen in family members or coworkers. Evaluate new drug therapies to rule out drug-induced fever. For complete instructions on taking children's temperatures, refer to Appendix D, Administration Techniques.

Interview: To assist patients with proper treatment of or physician referral for a fever, it may be beneficial to ask about the following:

- Duration of fever.
- Method used to measure fever (eg, location on the body, type of thermometer used).
- Range of fever temperatures.
- Any other significant symptoms.
- Presence of rash.
- Time of day temperature was taken.
- Use of nonprescription and prescription medication.

TREATMENT

Approaches to therapy: The need to control low-grade fevers is a topic of much debate because the host defense mechanisms are enhanced with increased temperatures. This is especially pertinent for parents who tend to administer acetaminophen or ibuprofen to their children at the first sign of an increased temperature. Low-grade fevers should be controlled when the patient is uncomfortable or if the patient has severely compromised cardiac function or dementia. **Contact physician if a very high temperature (over 102°F [38.8°C]) exists or if a fever is sustained for 24 hours or more.**

Febrile seizures – Routine prophylaxis to prevent recurrence of febrile seizures is not recommended. Give parents the following advice:

1.) Remain calm.
2.) Loosen the child's clothing, especially around the neck.
3.) If the child is unconscious, place him/her in the supine position. Keep the head lower than the body and turn the head sideways. Wipe off any vomit or discharge around the mouth and nose with gauze. **Do not insert anything into the mouth.**
4.) Take the child's temperature (use the axillary method; avoid the oral route) and observe and record the length of time and features of the seizure.
5.) Do not give the child any drugs or fluid orally.
6.) Stay near the patient until the seizure has subsided.

Parents should take the child to the hospital if any of the following occur:

• The seizure lasts longer than 10 minutes.
• Frequent short-term seizures occur with loss of consciousness in between.
• Only 1 part of the body is affected (local seizure) or the seizure is focused in one part of the body, although the entire body appears to be involved (partial seizures).
• The seizure is the child's first (at any age, but especially in children younger than 6 months of age).
• The seizure and fever are accompanied by neurolgical symptoms (eg, loss of consciousness, postictal paralysis).

Advise parents that although febrile seizures are frightening, they do not cause brain damage. There is a risk for more febrile seizures during the current or subsequent febrile illnesses. Seizures may occur as the first sign of a febrile illness.

Nondrug therapy: When presenting with a fever, a patient should moderate daily activities to provide additional rest, eat light meals, and avoid strenuous or tiring tasks. Maintain hydration, especially in children and the elderly. A bath or sponging with tepid (not cold) water may be soothing but will not have a significant effect on body temperature. Do not use alcohol sponge baths.

Pharmacotherapy: Drugs that are effective for lowering fever include aspirin, acetaminophen, and nonsteroidal anti-inflammatory drugs (NSAIDs). **Do not use aspirin and other salicylates in children and adolescents for chicken pox or influenza symptoms (including fever) because of the risk of Reye syndrome, a rare but serious illness.**

SALICYLATES

► **Actions**

Salicylates have analgesic, antipyretic, anti-inflammatory, and antirheumatic effects. These agents lower body temperature through vasodilation of peripheral vessels, thus enhancing dissipation of excess heat. Of the salicylates, only aspirin significantly inhibits platelet aggregation.

► **Indications**

For the treatment of mild to moderate pain and fever. These agents have other labeled indications as well.

► **Contraindications**

Hypersensitivity to salicylates or nonsteroidal anti-inflammatory drugs (NSAIDs). Use with extreme caution in patients with a history of adverse reactions to salicylates. Cross-sensitivity may exist between aspirin and other NSAIDs and between aspirin and tartrazine. Aspirin cross-sensitivity does not appear to occur with sodium salicylate, salicylamide, or choline salicylate. Aspirin hypersensitivity is more prevalent in those with asthma, nasal polyposis, or chronic urticaria.

Also contraindicated in patients with hemophilia or bleeding ulcers or those in hemorrhagic states.

► **Warnings**

Concurrent medications: Many other medications, specifically multi-ingredient cough and cold products, also contain aspirin or acetaminophen. It is important to advise patients of this possibility and to inquire about other medications they might be taking before recommending an analgesic in order to avoid exceeding the maximum daily dose.

Otic effects: Discontinue use if dizziness, ringing in ears (tinnitus), or impaired hearing occurs. Tinnitus probably represents blood salicylate levels reaching or exceeding the upper limit of the therapeutic range; therefore, it is a helpful guide to toxicity. Temporary hearing loss disappears gradually upon discontinuation of the drug.

Hypersensitivity: Do not use if there is a history of sensitivity to aspirin or NSAIDs.

Aspirin intolerance, manifested by acute bronchospasm, generalized urticaria/angioedema, severe rhinitis, or shock occurs in 4% to 19% of asthmatic patients. Symptoms occur within 3 hours after ingestion.

Foods may contribute to a reaction. Some foods with high salicylate content include curry powder, paprika, licorice, Benedictine liqueur, prunes, raisins, tea, and gherkins. A typical American diet contains 10 to 200 mg/day of salicylate.

Hepatic function impairment: Use with caution in patients with liver damage, preexisting hypoprothrombinemia, and vitamin K deficiency.

GI effects: Use with caution in patients who are intolerant to salicylates because of GI irritation, and in those with gastric ulcers, peptic ulcers, diabetes, gout, erosive gastritis, esophagitis, or bleeding tendencies.

Hematologic effects: Aspirin interferes with hemostasis. Avoid use in patients with severe anemia, a history of blood coagulation defects, or those who take anticoagulants.

Pregnancy: Category D (aspirin); Category C (salsalate, magnesium salicylate, other salicylates). Aspirin may produce adverse effects in the mother, such as anemia, ante- or postpartum hemorrhage, or prolonged gestation and labor. Salicylates readily cross the placenta. By inhibiting prostaglandin synthesis, salicylates may cause constriction of ductus arteriosus and possibly other untoward fetal effects. Maternal aspirin use during later stages of pregnancy may cause adverse fetal effects, such as low birth weight, increased incidence of intracranial hemorrhage in premature infants, stillbirth, or neonatal death. Salicylates may be teratogenic. Avoid use during pregnancy, especially in the third trimester.

Lactation: Salicylates are excreted in breast milk in low concentrations. Adverse effects on platelet function in the nursing infant are a potential risk. The American Academy of Pediatrics recommends that aspirin be used cautiously in nursing mothers.

Children: Administration of aspirin to children (including teenagers) with acute febrile illness has been associated with the development of Reye syndrome. Do not use in children and adolescents.

► **Drug Interactions**

Salicylate Drug Interactions		
Precipitant drug	**Object drug***	**Description**
Charcoal, activated	Aspirin ↓	Coadministration decreases aspirin absorption, depending on charcoal dose and interval between ingestion.
Urinary acidifiers	Salicylates ↑	Ammonium chloride, ascorbic acid, and methionine decrease salicylate excretion.
Antacids, urinary alkalinizers	Salicylates ↓	Decreased pharmacologic effects of salicylates may occur. The magnitude of the antacid interaction depends on the agent, dose, and pretreatment urine pH.
Carbonic anhydrase inhibitors	Salicylates ↔	Salicylate intoxication has occurred after coadministration of these agents. However, salicylic acid renal elimination may be increased by these drugs if urine is kept alkaline. Conversely, salicylates may displace acetazolamide from protein-binding sites, resulting in toxicity. Further study is needed.
Corticosteroids	Salicylates ↓	Corticosteroids increase salicylate clearance and decrease salicylate serum levels.
Nizatidine	Salicylates ↑	Increased serum salicylate levels have occurred in patients receiving high doses (3.9 g/day) of aspirin and concurrent nizatidine.
Salicylates	Alcohol ↑	The risk of GI ulceration increases when salicylates are given concomitantly. Ingestion of alcohol during salicylate therapy may also prolong bleeding time.
Salicylates	Angiotensin-converting enzyme inhibitors ↓	Antihypertensive effectiveness of these agents may be decreased by concurrent salicylate administration, possibly because of prostaglandin inhibition. Consider discontinuing salicylates if problems occur.
Aspirin	Heparin ↓	Aspirin can increase the risk of bleeding in heparin-anticoagulated patients.
Salicylates	Loop diuretics ↓	Loop diuretics may be less effective when given with salicylates in patients with compromised renal function or with cirrhosis with ascites; however, data conflict.
Salicylates	Methotrexate ↑	Salicylates increase drug levels, causing toxicity by interfering with protein binding and renal elimination of the antimetabolite.

Salicylate Drug Interactions			
Precipitant drug	**Object drug***		**Description**
Aspirin	Nitroglycerin	↑	Nitroglycerin, when taken with aspirin, may result in unexpected hypotension. Data is limited. If hypotension occurs, reduce the nitroglycerin dose.
Aspirin	NSAIDs	↓	Aspirin may decrease NSAID serum concentrations. Avoid concomitant use; it offers no therapeutic advantage and may significantly increase incidence of GI effects.
Salicylates	Probenecid, sulfinpyrazone	↔	Salicylates antagonize the uricosuric effect. While salicylates in large doses (more than 3 g/day) have a uricosuric effect, smaller amounts may reduce the uricosuric effect of these agents.
Salicylates	Spironolactone	↓	Salicylates may inhibit the diuretic effects; antihypertensive action does not appear altered. Effects depend on the dose of spironolactone.
Salicylates	Sulfonylureas, exogenous insulin	↑	Salicylates in doses more than 2 g/day have a hypoglycemic action, perhaps by altering pancreatic beta-cell function. They may potentiate the glucose-lowering effect of these drugs.
Aspirin	Valproic acid	↑	Aspirin displaces valproic acid from its protein-binding sites and may decrease its total body clearance, thus increasing the pharmacologic effects.

* ↑ = Object drug increased. ↓ = Object drug decreased. ↔ = Undetermined clinical effect.

▶ **Adverse Reactions**

Adverse reactions can be seen in the following body systems: GI (nausea, dyspepsia, heartburn, epigastric discomfort), hematologic (prolonged bleeding time, leukopenia, thrombocytopenia, purpura, decreased plasma iron concentration, shortened erythrocyte survival time), and dermatologic (rash, hives, and angioedema may occur, especially in patients suffering from chronic urticaria). Additional miscellaneous adverse reactions that have occurred include fever, thirst, and dimness of vision.

Allergic and anaphylactic reactions have been noted when hypersensitive individuals took aspirin. Fatal anaphylactic shock, while not common, has been reported.

Aspirin has an irreversible effect on platelet aggregation for the life of the platelet (approximately 7 days).

▶ **Overdosage**

Symptoms: The acute lethal dose for adults is approximately 10 to 30 g, and for children, approximately 4 g. Respiratory alkalosis is seen initially in acute salicylate ingestions. Hyperpnea and tachypnea occur as a result of increased CO_2 production and a direct stimulatory effect of salicylate on the respiratory center. Other symptoms may include nausea, vomiting, hypokalemia, tinnitus, neurologic abnormalities (eg, disorientation, irritability, hallucinations, lethargy, stupor, coma, seizures), dehydration, hyperthermia, hyperventilation, hyperactivity, thrombocytopenia, platelet dysfunction, hypoprothrombinemia, increased capillary fragility, and other hematologic abnormalities. Symptoms may progress quickly to depression, coma, respiratory failure, and collapse. Chronic salicylate toxicity may occur when more than 100 mg/kg/day is ingested for 2 days or more. It is more difficult to recognize than acute overdosage and is associated with increased morbidity and mortality. Compared with acute poisoning, hyperventilation, dehydration, systemic acidosis, and severe CNS manifestations occur more frequently.

Treatment: Initial treatment includes induction of emesis or gastric lavage to remove any unabsorbed drug from the stomach. Activated charcoal diminishes salicylate absorption most effectively if given within 2 hours after ingestion. It is important to contact a local poison control center or emergency room if overdosage is suspected.

ASPIRIN

▶ Administration and Dosage

Adults: 325 to 650 mg orally every 4 hours as needed. Some extra-strength products recommend dosages of 500 mg every 3 hours or 1000 mg every 6 hours.

Children: The analgesic/antipyretic dosage is 10 to 15 mg/kg/dose every 4 hours as needed (see table), up to 60 to 80 mg/kg/day. Do not use in children or teenagers with chicken pox or flu symptoms because of the possibility of Reye syndrome. Dosage recommendations by age and weight are as follows:

Recommended Aspirin Dosage in Children					
Age (years)	Weight		Dosage (mg every 4 hours)	No. of 81 mg tablets (every 4 hours)	No. of 325 mg tablets (every 4 hours)
	lbs	kg			
2-3	24-35	10.6-15.9	162	2	½
4-5	36-47	16-21.4	243	3	N/A
6-8	48-59	21.5-26.8	324	4	1
9-10	60-71	26.9-32.3	405	5	N/A
11	72-95	32.4-43.2	486	6	1½
12-14	≥ 96	≥ 43.3	648	8	2

ASPIRIN PRODUCTS	
Trade name	Doseform
Genuine Bayer Aspirin	**Tablets, Caplets**: 325 mg
	Gelcaps: 325 mg. Parabens.
Extra Strength Bayer Aspirin	**Caplets**: 500 mg
	Gelcaps: 500 mg. Parabens.
Adult Low Strength Ecotrin	**Tablets, enteric coated**: 81 mg
Halfprin 81	**Tablets, enteric coated**: 81 mg. Lactose.
Halfprin 162	**Tablets, enteric coated**: 162 mg. Lactose.
Ecotrin Regular Strength, Regular Strength Ascriptin	**Tablets, enteric coated**: 325 mg
Bayer Children's Chewable Aspirin	**Tablets, chewable**: 81 mg. Dextrose, saccharin. Orange and cherry flavors.
BUFFERED ASPIRIN PRODUCTS	
Regular Strength Ascriptin	**Tablets, enteric coated**: 325 mg with alumina-magnesia and calcium carbonate.
Arthritis Pain Ascriptin	**Tablets**: 325 mg with alumina-magnesia and calcium carbonate. Sugar, sorbitol, and saccharin.
Extra Strength Bayer Plus	**Tablets**: 500 mg with 250 mg calcium carbonate.
Maximum Strength Ascriptin	**Tablets**: 500 mg with alumina-magnesia and calcium carbonate. Sugar, sorbitol, and saccharin.
Adprin-B	**Tablets, coated**: 325 mg with calcium carbonate, magnesium carbonate, and magnesium oxide.

Products listed are representative of currently available and widely distributed brands. Similar products, including regional and private label brands, may also exist.

PATIENT INFORMATION
Aspirin

- High or prolonged fever may indicate a serious illness; consult a physician.
- Patient instructions accompany each product. Read these instructions carefully before use, preferably before leaving the pharmacy, in case you have any questions.
- May cause GI upset; take with food or after meals. Enteric-coated products may prevent or reduce stomach/GI distress.
- Take with a full glass of water (240 mL) to reduce the risk of the medication lodging in the esophagus.
- Avoid taking antacids within 2 hours of taking enteric-coated tablets.
- Patients allergic to tartrazine dye should avoid aspirin.
- Notify physician if persistent pain, rash, difficult breathing, ringing in the ears, or persistent GI pain occurs. Internal bleeding may occur with no GI symptoms and may be indicated by bloody or black stools.
- Do not use aspirin if it has a strong vinegar-like odor. This suggests deterioration of aspirin and loss of potency.
- Do not use in children or adolescents because of the potential risk of Reye syndrome.
- Inform physician or dentist of aspirin use before surgery or dental care.
- Be aware of other OTC (eg, combination products for pain, cold, cough, allergy) and prescription medications that contain aspirin.

ACETAMINOPHEN (APAP)

▶ Actions

Acetaminophen reduces fever by a direct action on the hypothalamic heat-regulating centers, which increases dissipation of body heat via vasodilation and sweating. The action of endogenous pyrogen on heat-regulating centers is inhibited.

Generally, the antipyretic and analgesic effects of APAP and aspirin are comparable. The site and mechanism of the analgesic effect of acetaminophen is unclear.

▶ Indications

For the treatment of mild to moderate pain and fever. Also used as an analgesic/antipyretic in the presence of aspirin allergy, in patients with blood coagulation disorders who are being treated with oral anticoagulants, and in patients with bleeding diatheses (eg, hemophilia), upper GI disease (eg, ulcer, gastritis, hiatal hernia), and gouty arthritis. This agent has other labeled indications as well.

▶ Contraindications

Hypersensitivity to acetaminophen.

▶ Warnings

Concurrent medications: Many other medications, specifically multi-ingredient cough and cold products, also contain aspirin or acetaminophen. It is important to advise patients of this possibility and to inquire about other medications they might be taking before recommending an analgesic.

Hepatotoxicity: Hepatotoxicity and severe hepatic failure have occurred in patients with chronic alcoholism following therapeutic doses. This hepatotoxicity may be caused by induction of hepatic microsomal enzymes, resulting in an increase in toxic metabolites, or by the reduced amount of glutathione responsible for conjugating toxic metabolites. A safe dose for chronic alcohol abusers has not been determined, and they should be cautioned to limit acetaminophen intake to 2 g/day or less.

Overdosage: Taking more than the recommended daily dosage can result in death. Unintentional overuse of acetaminophen has occurred. Advise patients not to take more than the recommended daily dose, take another dose before the appropiate time interval has passed, exceed the maximum recommended doses in a 24-hour peroid, or take more than one product containing the ingredient.

Pregnancy: Category B. Acetaminophen crosses the placenta, but has been used routinely in all stages of pregnancy; when used in therapeutic doses, it appears safe for short-term use.

Lactation: Acetaminophen is excreted in low amounts, but no adverse effects have been reported. The American Academy of Pediatrics considers acetaminophen to be compatible with breastfeeding.

Children: Consult a physician before using in children younger than 3 years of age, or for use for longer than 3 days (adults and children) for fever reduction.

▶ **Drug Interactions**

Acetaminophen Drug Interactions			
Precipitant drug	**Object drug***		**Description**
Alcohol, ethyl	APAP	↑	Hepatotoxicity has occurred in patients with chronic alcoholism following various dose levels (moderate to excessive) of acetaminophen.
Anticholinergics	APAP	↔	The onset of acetaminophen effect may be delayed or decreased slightly, but the ultimate pharmacologic effect is not significantly affected by anticholinergics.
Beta blockers, propranolol	APAP	↑	Propranolol appears to inhibit the enzyme systems responsible for glucuronidation and oxidation of APAP. Therefore, the pharmacologic effects of acetaminophen may be increased.
Charcoal, activated	APAP	↓	Charcoal reduces acetaminophen absorption when administered as soon as possible after overdose.
Contraceptives, oral	APAP	↓	Oral contraceptives increase glucuronidation, resulting in increased plasma clearance and a decreased half-life of acetaminophen.
Probenecid	APAP	↑	Probenecid may increase the therapeutic effectiveness of acetaminophen slightly.
APAP	Lamotrigine	↓	Serum lamotrigine concentrations may be reduced, producing a decrease in therapeutic effects.
APAP	Loop diuretics	↓	The effects of loop diuretics may be decreased because APAP may decrease renal prostaglandin excretion and decrease plasma renin activity.
APAP	Zidovudine	↓	The pharmacologic effects of zidovudine may be decreased because of enhanced nonhepatic or renal clearance of zidovudine.

* ↑ = Object drug increased. ↓ = Object drug decreased. ↔ = Undetermined clinical effect.

The potential for hepatotoxicity caused by acetaminophen may be increased by large doses or long-term administration of barbiturates, carbamazepine, hydantoins, rifampin, and sulfinpyrazone. The therapeutic effects of acetaminophen may also be decreased.

► **Adverse Reactions**

When used as directed, acetaminophen rarely causes severe toxicity or side effects. However, the following adverse reactions have been reported:

Hematologic: Hemolytic anemia; neutropenia; leukopenia; pancytopenia; thrombocytopenia.

Hepatic: Jaundice.

Metabolic: Hypoglycemia.

Hypersensitivity: Skin rash; fever.

► **Overdosage**

Symptoms: Acute poisoning may be manifested by nausea, vomiting, drowsiness, confusion, liver tenderness, low blood pressure, cardiac arrhythmias, jaundice, and acute hepatic and renal failure. These occur within the first 24 hours and may persist for 1 week or longer. Death has occurred because of liver necrosis. Acute renal failure may also occur. However, there are often no specific early signs or symptoms. The course of acetaminophen poisoning is divided into 4 stages (postingestion time):

Stage 1 (12 to 24 hours) – Nausea; vomiting; diaphoresis; anorexia.

Stage 2 (24 to 48 hours) – Clinically improved; angiotensin sensitivity test (AST), bilirubin, and prothrombin levels begin to rise.

Stage 3 (72 to 96 hours) – Peak hepatotoxicity; AST of 20,000 not unusual.

Stage 4 (7 to 8 days) – Recovery.

Hepatotoxicity may result. The minimal toxic dose is 10 g (140 mg/kg), but liver damage has occurred with a single 5.85 g dose; doses of at least 20 to 25 g are potentially fatal. Children appear less susceptible to toxicity than adults because they have less capacity for glucuronidation metabolism. Initial signs of toxicity may include nausea, vomiting, anorexia, malaise, diaphoresis, abdominal pain, and diarrhea. Hepatotoxicity is usually not apparent for 48 to 72 hours. Hepatic failure may lead to encephalopathy, coma, and death.

Plasma acetaminophen levels of more than 300 mcg/mL at 4 hours postingestion were associated with hepatic damage in 90% of patients; minimal hepatic damage is anticipated if plasma levels at 4 hours are less than 120 mcg/mL or less than 30 mcg/mL at 12 hours after ingestion.

Chronic excessive use (more than 4 g/day) may lead to transient hepatotoxicity. The kidneys may undergo tubular necrosis; the myocardium may be damaged.

Treatment: Perform gastric lavage in all cases, preferably within 4 hours of ingestion. Refer also to General Management of Acute Overdosage. It is important to contact a local poison control center or emergency room if overdosage is suspected.

► **Administration and Dosage**

Adults: 325 to 650 mg every 4 hours, or 1 g three to four times daily as needed; do not exceed 4 g daily for all formulations containing acetaminophen.

Children: The usual dose is 10 mg/kg/dose, which may be repeated 4 to 5 times daily. Do not exceed 5 doses in 24 hours.

Acetaminophen Dosages for Children			
Weight	Dosage (mg)	Weight	Dosage (mg)
6-11 lbs	40	48-59 lbs	320
12-17 lbs	80	60-71 lbs	400
18-23 lbs	120	72-95 lbs	480
24-35 lbs	160	> 95 lbs	640
36-47 lbs	240		

Rectal suppositories:

Adults – 650 mg every 4 to 6 hours as needed; do not exceed 4 g in 24 hours.

Children (3 to 11 months) – 80 mg every 6 hours as needed.

(1 to 3 years) – 80 mg every 4 hours as needed; maximum of 400 mg in 24 hours.

(4 to 6 years) – 120 to 125 mg every 4 to 6 hours as needed; do not exceed 720 mg in 24 hours.

(7 to 12 years) – 325 mg every 4 to 6 hours as needed; do not exceed 2.6 g in 24 hours.

Storage: Store suppositories below 27°C (80°F) or refrigerate. Store tablets and oral solutions at 15° to 30°C (59° to 86°F).

ACETAMINOPHEN PRODUCTS	
Trade name	Doseform
Children's Tylenol	**Tablets, chewable:** 80 mg. Aspartame. Grape[1], fruit[1], and bubble gum[2] flavors.
Junior Strength Tylenol	**Tablets, chewable:** 160 mg. Aspartame, 6 mg phenylalanine. Fruit and grape flavors.
Regular Strength Tylenol	**Tablets:** 325 mg
Aspirin Free Anacin Extra Strength	**Tablets:** 500 mg
Extra Strength Tylenol	**Tablets, caplets:** 500 mg
	Gelcaps, geltabs: 500 mg. Parabens, EDTA.
Tylenol Arthritis Pain Extended Relief	**Caplets:** 650 mg
Infants' FeverAll	**Suppositories:** 80 mg
Children's FeverAll	**Suppositories:** 120 mg
Acephen	**Suppositories:** 120 mg
Junior Strength FeverAll, Acephen	**Suppositories:** 325 mg
Adults FeverAll, Acephen	**Suppositories:** 650 mg
Children's Silapap	**Elixir:** 80 mg/2.5 mL. Alcohol and sugar free.
Children's Tylenol	**Elixir:** 80 mg/2.5 mL. Alcohol free. Sorbitol, sucrose, butylparaben
Aceta	**Elixir:** 120 mg/5 mL
Infants' Silapap Drops	**Drops:** 80 mg/0.8 mL. Alcohol free. Methylparaben, saccharin.
Children's Tylenol Liquid	**Suspension:** 160 mg/5 mL. Butylparaben, corn syrup, sorbitol. Cherry, grape, and bubble gum flavors.
Infants' Tylenol Concentrated Drops	**Drops:** 160 mg/1.6 mL. Sorbitol, butylparaben, corn syrup. Cherry and grape flavors.

Products listed are representative of currently available and widely distributed brands. Similar products, including regional and private label brands, may also exist.

[1] Contains 3 mg phenylalanine per tablet.
[2] Contains 6 mg phenylalanine per tablet.

PATIENT INFORMATION

Acetaminophen

- High or prolonged fever may indicate a serious illness; consult a physician.
- Patient instructions accompany each product. Read these instructions carefully before use, preferably before leaving the pharmacy, in case you have any questions.
- Do not exceed the recommended dosage. Do not exceed a total dose of 4 g/day of acetaminophen in all formulations consumed.
- Be aware of other OTC (eg, combination products for pain, cold, cough, or allergy) and prescription medications that contain acetaminophen.
- Do not use in children younger than 2 years of age without consulting a physician.
- Do not take acetaminophen for more than 3 days for fever. If symptoms persist, worsen, or if new symptoms develop, contact a physician.
- Avoid alcohol consumption and aspirin while taking this drug.

NONSTEROIDAL ANTI-INFLAMMATORY DRUGS

▶ **Actions**

Nonsteroidal anti-inflammatory drugs (NSAIDs) have analgesic and antipyretic activities. Their exact mode of action is unknown. The major mechanism of action for NSAIDs is believed to be inhibition of cyclooxygenase activity and prostaglandin synthesis. Other mechanisms, such as inhibition of lipoxygenase, leukotriene synthesis, lysosomal enzyme release, neutrophil aggregation, and various cell-membrane functions, may exist as well.

NSAIDs are capable of inhibiting the enzyme cyclooxygenase (COX). COX allows the conversion of arachidonic acid into prostaglandins, which are mediators of the inflammatory response. Prostaglandin inhibition peripherally at the site of injury can decrease the inflammatory response and pain. Prostaglandin inhibition centrally can also result in analgesia similar to other centrally acting drugs such as acetaminophen. NSAIDs may also have a direct inhibiting effect on inflammatory cells.

▶ **Indications**

For the treatment of mild to moderate pain and fever. These agents have other labeled indications as well.

▶ **Contraindications**

NSAID hypersensitivity: Because of potential cross-sensitivity to other NSAIDs, do not give these agents to patients in whom aspirin, iodides, or other NSAIDs have induced symptoms of asthma, rhinitis, urticaria, nasal polyps, angioedema, bronchospasm, or other symptoms of allergic or anaphylactoid reactions.

▶ **Warnings**

Acute renal insufficiency: Patients with preexisting renal disease or compromised renal perfusion are at greatest risk for acute renal insufficiency. A form of renal toxicity seen in patients with prerenal conditions leads to reduced renal blood flow or blood volume. NSAID use may cause a dose-dependent reduction in prostaglandin formation and precipitate overt renal decompensation. Patients at greatest risk are the elderly, premature infants, those with heart failure, renal or hepatic dysfunction, systemic lupus erythematosus (SLE), chronic glomerulonephritis, dehydration, diabetes mellitus, impaired renal function, septicemia, pyelonephritis, those taking ACE inhibitors, concomitant use of any nephrotoxic drug, extracellular volume depletion from any cause, and those receiving diuretics. Recovery usually follows discontinuation.

Hypersensitivity: Because of potential cross-sensitivity to other NSAIDs, do not give these agents to patients in whom aspirin or other NSAIDs have induced symptoms of asthma, rhinitis, urticaria, nasal polyps, angioedema, bronchospasm, and other symptoms of allergic or anaphylactoid reactions. Severe, rarely fatal anaphylactic-like and asthmatic reactions have been reported in such patients receiving NSAIDs.

Anaphylactoid reactions: Anaphylactoid reactions have occured in patients with aspirin hypersensitivity.

Renal function impairment: NSAID metabolites are eliminated primarily by the kidneys. Use with caution in those with impaired renal function. Reduce dosage to avoid excessive accumulation.

Hepatic function impairment: Naproxen may exhibit an increase in unbound fraction and a reduced clearance of free drug in cirrhotic liver patients, suggesting an increased potential for toxicity in this group; consider reducing the dose.

Platelet aggregation: NSAIDs can inhibit platelet aggregation; the effect is quantitatively less and of shorter duration than that seen with aspirin. These agents prolong bleeding time (within normal range) in healthy subjects. This may be exaggerated in patients with underlying hemostatic defects; use with caution in persons with intrinsic coagulation defects and in those on anticoagulant therapy.

Cardiovascular effects: May cause fluid retention and peripheral edema. Use caution in compromised cardiac function, hypertension, patients on chronic diuretic therapy, or other conditions predisposing to fluid retention. NSAIDs may be associated with significant deterioration of circulatory hemodynamics in severe heart failure and hyponatremia, presumably because of inhibition of prostaglandin-dependent compensatory mechanisms.

Infection: NSAIDs may mask the usual signs of infection. Use with extra care in the presence of existing controlled infection.

Photosensitivity: Photosensitivity may occur; caution patients to take protective measures (eg, sunscreens, protective clothing) against UV or sunlight until tolerance is determined.

GI effects: GI toxicity (including NSAID-induced ulcers and GI bleeding disorders) can occur with or without warning with chronic use of NSAIDs. High-dose NSAIDs probably carry a greater risk of causing GI adverse effects, although clinical trials generally do not reflect this. Studies have shown patients with a history of peptic ulcer disease or GI bleeding who use NSAIDs have a greater than 10-fold risk of developing GI bleed than patients with neither of these risk factors. Have patients with a history of GI lesions consult a physician before using these products. In addition, treatment with oral corticosteroids or anticoagulants, longer duration of NSAID therapy, smoking, alcoholism, older age, and poor general health status contribute to an increased risk for a GI bleed.

Ibuprofen: Do not take for more than 3 days for fever or more than 10 days for pain. If symptoms persist, worsen, or if new symptoms develop, contact a physician.

Pregnancy: Category B; third trimester *Category D*. Safety for use during pregnancy has not been established; use is not recommended. There are no adequate, well-controlled studies in pregnant women. An increased incidence of dystocia, postimplantation loss, and delayed parturition has occurred in animals. Agents that inhibit prostaglandin synthesis may cause closure of the ductus arteriosus and other unto-ward effects in the fetus. GI tract toxicity is increased in pregnant women in the last trimester. Some NSAIDs may prolong pregnancy if given before onset of labor. Avoid use during pregnancy, especially during the third trimester.

Lactation: Most NSAIDs are excreted in breast milk in low concentrations. The American Academy of Pediatrics considers ibuprofen and naproxen to be compatible with breastfeeding. Data on the use of ketoprofen during nursing are lacking.

Children: Use of ibuprofen is not recommended in infants younger than 6 months of age. The use of naproxen is not recommended in children younger than 12 years of age unless directed by a physician. Ketoprofen is not recommended for use in children younger than 16 years of age.

Elderly: Age appears to increase the possibility of adverse reactions to NSAIDs. The risk of serious ulcer disease is increased in elderly patients (older than 65 years of age) taking NSAIDs; this risk appears to increase with dose. Use with greater care in the elderly and begin with reduced dosages.

▶ Drug Interactions

NSAID Drug Interactions			
Precipitant drug	**Object drug***		**Description**
NSAIDs	ACE inhibitors	↓	Reports suggest that NSAIDs may diminish the antihypertensive effect of ACE inhibitors.
NSAIDs	Anticoagulants	↑	Coadministration may prolong prothrombin time (PT). Also consider the effects NSAIDs have on platelet function and gastric mucosa. Monitor PT and patients closely, and instruct patients to watch for signs and symptoms of bleeding.
NSAIDs	Beta blockers	↓	The antihypertensive effect of beta blockers may be impaired, possibly because of NSAID inhibi-tion of renal prostaglandin synthesis, thereby allowing unopposed pressor systems to produce hypertension. Avoid using this combination if possible. Monitor blood pressure and adjust beta blocker doses as needed. Consider using a nonin-teracting NSAID (eg, sulindac).
NSAIDs	Cyclosporine	↑	Nephrotoxicity of both agents may be increased.
NSAIDs	Digoxin	↑	Ibuprofen may increase digoxin serum levels.
NSAIDs	Diuretics	↓	Effects of diuretics may be decreased.
NSAIDs	Hydantoins	↑	Serum phenytoin levels may be increased, result-ing in an increase in pharmacologic and toxic effects of phenytoin.
NSAIDs	Lithium	↑	Serum lithium levels may be increased.
NSAIDs	Methotrexate	↑	The risks of methotrexate toxicity (eg, stomatitis, bone marrow suppression, nephrotoxicity) may be increased.
NSAIDs	Thiazide diuretics	↔	Decreased antihypertensive and diuretic action of thiazides may occur with concurrent naproxen.
Bisphosphonates	NSAIDs	↑	Risk of gastric ulceration may be increased. Use cautiously.
Cholestyramine	NSAIDs	↓	The effects of NSAIDs may be decreased.
Cimetidine	NSAIDs	↔	NSAID plasma concentrations may be increased or decreased by cimetidine; some studies report no effect.

NSAID Drug Interactions			
Precipitant drug	**Object drug***		**Description**
Probenecid	NSAIDs	↑	Probenecid may increase the concentrations and possibly the toxicity of NSAIDs.
Salicylates	NSAIDs	↓	Plasma concentrations of NSAIDs may be decreased by salicylates. Avoid concurrent use because it offers no therapeutic advantage and may significantly increase the incidence of GI effects.

* ↑ = Object drug increased.   ↓ = Object drug decreased.   ⟷ = Undetermined clinical effect.

▶ **Adverse Reactions**

Cardiovascular: Edema; congestive heart failure; palpitations.

CNS: Dizziness; drowsiness; headache; light-headedness; vertigo.

Dermatologic: Erythema; pruritus; rash; increased sweating.

GI: Bleeding; diarrhea; dyspepsia; heartburn; nausea; vomiting; abdominal pain; cramps; constipation; flatulence.

Miscellaneous: Muscle cramps; thirst; edema; dyspnea; tinnitus; visual disturbances/changes.

IBUPROFEN

▶ **Administration and Dosage**

Adults: 200 mg every 4 to 6 hours as needed while symptoms persist. If fever does not respond to 200 mg, 400 mg may be used. Do not exceed 1.2 g in 24 hours. Do not take for fever for more than 3 days unless directed by physician. Use the smallest effective dose.

Children (6 months to 12 years of age): Adjust dosage on the basis of the initial temperature level. If baseline temperature is 102.5°F (39.2°C) or lower, the recommended dose is 5 mg/kg. For fevers higher than 102.5°F (39.2°C), the recommended dose is 10 mg/kg. The duration of fever reduction is usually 6 to 8 hours. Maximum daily dose is 40 mg/kg.

IBUPROFEN PRODUCTS	
Trade name	**Doseform**
Children's Motrin	**Tablets, chewable**: 50 mg. 1.4 mg phenylalanine, aspartame. Orange flavor.
Children's Advil	**Tablets, chewable**: 50 mg. 2.1 mg phenylalanine, aspartame. Fruit and grape flavors.
Junior Strength Advil	**Tablets, chewable**: 100 mg. Parabens, sucrose.
Junior Strength Motrin	**Tablets, chewable**: 100 mg. Aspartame, 2.8 mg phenylalanine. Orange and grape flavors.
	Caplets: 100 mg
Maximum Strength Midol Cramp	**Tablets**: 200 mg
Advil	**Tablets, caplets**: 200 mg. Parabens, sucrose.
	Gelcaps: 200 mg
Motrin IB	**Tablets, caplets**: 200 mg
	Gelcaps: 200 mg. Parabens, EDTA, benzyl alcohol.
Advil Liqui-Gels	**Gelcaps**: 200 mg. Sorbitol.
Infants' Motrin Concentrated Drops	**Liquid**: 50 mg/1.25 mL. Sorbitol, sucrose. Berry and dye-free berry flavors.

IBUPROFEN PRODUCTS	
Trade name	**Doseform**
Children's Advil	**Suspension**: 100 mg/5 mL. EDTA, sorbitol, sucrose. Fruit, grape, and blue-raspberry flavors.
Children's Motrin	**Suspension**: 100 mg/5 mL. Sucrose. Berry, grape, bubble gum, and dye-free berry flavors.
Infants' Advil	**Concentrated drops**: 50 mg/1.25 mL. EDTA, sorbitol, sucrose. Fruit and grape flavors.

Products listed are representative of currently available and widely distributed brands. Similar products, including regional and private label brands, may also exist.

PATIENT INFORMATION
Ibuprofen

- High or prolonged fever may indicate a serious illness; consult a physician.
- Patient instructions accompany each product. Read instructions carefully before use, preferably before leaving the pharmacy, in case you have any questions.
- Because of possible drug interactions, patients are encouraged not to take any OTC or prescription medications without consulting a physician or pharmacist.
- Take with a full glass of water (240 mL) to reduce the risk of the medication lodging in the esophagus.
- May cause GI upset; take with food or after meals.
- Notify physician if rash, itching, visual disturbances, edema, black stools (melena), or persistent headache occur.
- Do not take OTC NSAIDs for more than 3 days for fever. If symptoms persist, worsen, or if new symptoms develop, contact a physician.
- Avoid alcohol consumption and aspirin while taking this medication.

KETOPROFEN

▶ Administration and Dosage

Adults: 12.5 mg with a full glass of liquid every 4 to 6 hours as needed. If fever persists after 1 hour, follow with 12.5 mg. With experience, some patients may find an initial dose of 25 mg will give better relief. Do not exceed 25 mg in a 4- to 6-hour period or 75 mg in a 24-hour period. Use the smallest effective dose.

Children: Do not give to children younger than 16 years of age unless directed by a physician.

KETOPROFEN PRODUCTS	
Trade name	**Doseform**
Orudis KT	**Tablets**: 12.5 mg. Sugar, tartrazine.

Products listed are representative of currently available and widely distributed brands. Similar products, including regional and private label brands, may also exist.

PATIENT INFORMATION
Ketoprofen

- High or prolonged fever may indicate a serious illness; consult a physician.
- Patient instructions accompany each product. Read instructions carefully before use, preferably before leaving the pharmacy, in case you have any questions.
- Because of possible drug interactions, patients are encouraged not to take any OTC or prescription medications without consulting a physician or pharmacist.
- Take with a full glass of water (240 mL) to reduce the risk of the medication lodging in the esophagus.
- May cause GI upset; take with food or after meals.
- Notify physician if rash, itching, visual disturbances, edema, black stools (melena), or persistent headache occur.
- Do not take OTC NSAIDs for more than 3 days for fever. If symptoms persist, worsen, or if new symptoms develop, contact a physician.
- Avoid alcohol consumption and aspirin while taking this medication.

NAPROXEN

► Administration and Dosage

Adults (younger than 65 years of age): 200 mg with a full glass of water every 8 to 12 hours while symptoms persist. With experience, some patients may find an initial dose of 400 mg followed by 200 mg 12 hours later, if necessary, will give better relief. Do not exceed 600 mg in 24 hours, unless otherwise directed. Use the smallest effective dose. Patients consuming 3 or more alcohol-containing drinks per day should consult their doctor for advice on when and how to take naproxen and other pain relievers.

Elderly (older than 65 years of age): Do not take more than 200 mg every 12 hours.

Children: Do not give to children younger than 12 years of age unless under the advice and supervision of a physician.

NAPROXEN PRODUCTS	
Trade name	Doseform
Aleve	Tablets, caplets, and gelcaps[1]: 200 mg (220 mg naproxen sodium)

Products listed are representative of currently available and widely distributed brands. Similar products, including regional and private label brands, may also exist.

[1] Contains EDTA.

PATIENT INFORMATION
Naproxen
- High or prolonged fever may indicate a serious illness; consult a physician.
- Patient instructions accompany each product. Read these instructions carefully before use, preferably before leaving the pharmacy, in case you have any questions.
- Because of possible drug interactions, patients are encouraged not to take any OTC or prescription medications without consulting a physician or pharmacist.
- Take with a full glass of water (240 mL) to reduce the risk of the medication lodging in the esophagus.
- May cause GI upset; take with food or after meals.
- Notify physician if skin rash, itching, visual disturbances, edema, black stools (melena), or persistent headache occur.
- Do not take OTC NSAIDs for more than 3 days for fever. If symptoms persist, worsen, or if new symptoms develop, contact a physician.
- Avoid alcohol consumption and aspirin while taking this medication.

HEADACHE
(Cephalalgia)

DEFINITION

Headache is a diffuse pain in various parts of the head. The International Headache Society has developed and published criteria for classification of headaches, as follows: Headaches may be divided into two major categories, primary and secondary headache disorders. Primary headaches consist of tension-type, migraine (with and without aura), cluster headaches, and rebound headaches. Secondary headaches are symptoms of underlying disease (eg, vascular defect, sinus, influenza-related), or situational (eg, alcohol consumption [hangover], cold-induced [ice-cream headache]).

ETIOLOGY

The etiology of primary headaches is often unknown. However, primary headaches (comprising approximately 90% of all headaches) are frequently associated with depression, anxiety, and analgesic overuse (rebound headache). In approximately 10% of women over age 40, menopause may trigger the onset of migraine. Secondary headaches are symptoms of an underlying disease. These types of headaches may be associated with head trauma, emotional states (eg, tension, stress, fatigue, depression), neurologic symptoms (eg, visual disturbance), infection (eg, meningitis), cardiovascular disease (eg, hypertension), or an underlying lesion (eg, brain tumor, subarachnoid hemorrhage). The cause of cluster headaches is unknown but may relate to a vascular disorder or a serotonergic disturbance. However, most headaches are self-limiting and are not accompanied by underlying pathology.

INCIDENCE

The exact incidence of headache is difficult to determine, because in many cases only patients who experience severe headaches that do not respond to over-the-counter (OTC) treatment seek medical consultation. Headaches account for 18 million outpatient visits and nearly 640 million days of lost work per year. Tension-type headaches are the most common type of headache, occurring in nearly 70% of men and 90% of women. Self-medication with OTC drugs usually occurs with tension-type headaches. In patients reporting headaches, the frequency decreases with advancing age, as does severity in women but not men.

Migraine headaches are responsible for 80% to 85% of all vascular headaches. This type of headache is most common in individuals between the ages of 12 to 40 and occurs more frequently in women than in men. Attacks tend to decrease in frequency and severity with age. Migraine attacks may subside or be triggered by menopause. For more information on migraines, see the Migraine monograph. Cluster headaches are not familial and occur 5 times more frequently in men than in women. The incidence of cluster headaches is less than tension-type or migraine headaches, occurring at a rate of 0.01% to 1.5% in various populations.

PATHOPHYSIOLOGY

In general, the pathogenesis of headaches is theoretical. Underlying symptoms frequently determine the selection of treatment. The brain is insensitive to pain; however, other head structures (eg, skin, muscles) are sensitive to pain. Peripheral pain transmission is believed to be caused by the neurotransmitters substance P and excitatory amino acids. Pain transmission in the spinal cord is attributed to enkephalins and γ-aminobutyric acid (GABA). Pain is transmitted in the CNS partly by the serotonergic and adrenergic systems.

SIGNS/SYMPTOMS

Signs and symptoms that may accompany headaches are usually vague and nonspecific and may be associated with underlying symptoms of other conditions, including tension, depression, and anxiety.

Tension-type headaches: As a result of stress, patients with tension-type headaches may experience prolonged contractions of head and neck muscles, which may produce headache secondary to compression of the cranial artery. Tension-type headaches are usually bilateral and occur at the back of the head, in the forehead, or at the temples (the "hatband" distribution) and can change location during the attack. Duration of headache pain can persist from 30 minutes to several days. The pain is mild-to-moderate and may be described as a steady, dull ache or vise-like constriction around the head. Some patients may experience neck or jaw discomfort, with tender spots and sharply localized nodules in the cervical or pericranial muscles. Tension-type headaches are not associated with nausea or vomiting and are not aggravated by routine physical activity.

Migraine headaches: Migraine headaches are episodic and vary in intensity. They may or may not be accompanied by an aura. Migraines with an aura are preceded by neurologic symptoms, including numbness, dizziness, and visual symptoms (eg, flashing lights, scintillating scotomata), which last approximately 60 minutes. Duration of the migraine can be 4 to 72 hours. Additional symptoms include nausea, vomiting, and photophobia. Daily activities may aggravate an attack.

Cluster headaches: Cluster headaches are characterized by severe unilateral orbital, supraorbital, or temporal pain that lasts 15 minutes to several hours when untreated and are associated with at least one of the following signs: Conjunctival injection, lacrimation, nasal congestion, rhinorrhea, forehead and facial sweating, miosis, ptosis, and eyelid edema. Attacks occur daily for periods of several weeks to months, followed by periods of remission for several months to years. Vomiting is rare and daily activities may aggravate an attack.

DIAGNOSTIC PARAMETERS/PHYSICAL ASSESSMENT

Clinical Observation: An essential factor in the diagnosis of headaches is the patient interview. Physical examination (eg, funduscopic assessment) and laboratory and diagnostic tests performed by a physician may be useful in ruling out an underlying cause in cases of severe refractory headaches.

Interview: To help the patient determine if physician referral or self-treatment is warranted, it is beneficial to ask about the following:

- Family history of headaches.
- Age at onset of headaches.
- Time of day or seasonality of occurrences.
- Site of pain (eg, temporal, unilateral).
- Intensity of pain.
- Duration of headache.
- Headache frequency.
- Accompanying symptoms (eg, visual, neurological, psychological, fever, nausea, vomiting).
- Precipitating factors, including air pollution, alcohol, diet (eg, caffeine, wine, cheese, chocolate, monosodium glutamate), fatigue, hypoglycemia, medications (eg, analgesic overuse, antidepressants [SSRIs], estrogens, H_2 antagonists, nifedipine, nitrates), oversleeping, perfumes.
- Response of headaches to previous medical treatment.
- Other medical conditions.

TREATMENT

Approaches to therapy: Evaluate patients using the above diagnostic parameters. Depending on various factors (eg, symptoms, duration, recurrence, severity), health care providers may recommend either (1) a non-drug approach, (2) appropriate pharmacotherapy, or (3) immediate referral to a physician for medical evaluation. In cases of severe, refractory, or frequent headaches, physician referral is appropriate.

Nondrug therapy: Techniques utilizing non-drug therapy have been successful in relief of migraine and tension-type headache pain in 50% to 70% of patients. Techniques include decreasing sensory stimuli, reducing stress exposure, application of cool compresses or ice packs to the area most severely affected, physical therapy, relaxation techniques, biofeedback, dietary modification, psychotherapy, hypnosis, and acupuncture.

Pharmacotherapy: Once it is determined that drug treatment is necessary, several OTC medications are available, including acetaminophen, aspirin and other salicylates, nonsteroidal anti-inflammatory drugs (NSAIDs), and caffeine. Self-medication with OTC medications usually occurs in patients with tension-type headaches and migraines. When treatment with a drug is started or if an existing medication is discontinued, caution patients to inform their physician or pharmacist of other medications they are taking so that possible drug interactions and overdoses may be discussed.

ACETAMINOPHEN (APAP)

▶ **Actions**

Acetaminophen's mechanism of action as an analgesic is unclear. However, acetaminophen inhibits prostaglandin synthetase in the CNS and reduces fever by direct action on the hypothalamic heat-regulating center.

Generally, the antipyretic (fever reducing) and analgesic (pain relieving) effects of APAP and aspirin are comparable.

▶ **Indications**

For the treatment of mild to moderate pain and fever. Also used as an analgesic-antipyretic in the presence of aspirin allergy, in patients with blood coagulation disorders who are being treated with oral anticoagulants, in bleeding diatheses (eg, hemophilia), in upper GI disease (eg, ulcer, gastritis, hiatal hernia), and gouty arthritis; a variety of arthritic and rheumatic conditions involving musculoskeletal pain, as well as in other painful disorders; headache; pain associated with earache, teething, tonsillectomy, menstruation; toothache; diseases accompanied by discomfort and fever such as the common cold, "flu," and other bacterial or viral infections.

▶ **Contraindications**

Hypersensitivity to acetaminophen.

▶ **Warnings**

Concurrent medications: Many other medications, specifically multi-ingredient cough and cold products, also contain aspirin or acetaminophen. It is important to advise patients of this possibility and to inquire about other medications they may be taking before recommending an analgesic.

Hepatotoxicity: Hepatotoxicity and severe hepatic failure have occurred in chronic alcoholics following therapeutic doses. This hepatotoxicity may be caused by induction of hepatic microsomal enzymes, resulting in an increase in toxic metabolites, or by the reduced amount of glutathione responsible for conjugating toxic metabolites. A safe dose for chronic alcohol abusers has not been determined. Caution chronic alcoholics and heavy drinkers to limit acetaminophen intake to no more than 2 g/day.

Pregnancy: Category B. Acetaminophen crosses the placenta, but has been used routinely in all stages of pregnancy; when used in therapeutic doses, it appears safe for short-term use.

Lactation: Excreted in low amounts, but no adverse effects have been reported. The American Academy of Pediatrics considers acetaminophen to be compatible with breastfeeding.

Children: Consult a physician before using in children under 3 years of age, or for use for more than 3 days (adults and children) for fever reduction.

▶ **Drug Interactions**

Acetaminophen Drug Interactions			
Precipitant drug	**Object drug***		**Description**
Alcohol, ethyl	APAP	↑	Hepatotoxicity has occurred in chronic alcoholics following various dose levels (moderate-to-excessive) of acetaminophen.
Anticholinergics	APAP	↔	The onset of acetaminophen effect may be delayed or decreased slightly, but the ultimate pharmacological effect is not significantly affected by anticholinergics.

Acetaminophen Drug Interactions			
Precipitant drug	Object drug*		Description
Beta blockers, propranolol	APAP	↑	Propranolol appears to inhibit the enzyme systems responsible for the glucuronidation and oxidation of APAP. Therefore, the pharmacologic effects of acetaminophen may be increased.
Charcoal, activated	APAP	↓	Charcoal reduces acetaminophen absorption when administered as soon as possible after overdose.
Contraceptives, oral	APAP	↓	Oral contraceptives increase glucuronidation, resulting in increased plasma clearance and a decreased half-life of acetaminophen.
Probenecid	APAP	↑	Probenecid may slightly increase the therapeutic effectiveness of acetaminophen.
APAP	Lamotrigine	↓	Serum lamotrigine concentrations may be reduced, producing a decrease in therapeutic effects.
APAP	Loop diuretics	↓	The effects of loop diuretics may be decreased because APAP may decrease renal prostaglandin excretion and decrease plasma renin activity.
APAP	Zidovudine	↓	The pharmacologic effects of zidovudine may be decreased because of enhanced nonhepatic or renal clearance of zidovudine

* ↑ = Object drug increased. ↓ = Object drug decreased. ↔ = Undetermined clinical effect.

The potential for hepatotoxicity caused by acetaminophen may be increased by large doses or long-term administration of barbiturates, carbamazepine, hydantoins, rifampin, and sulfinpyrazone. The therapeutic effects of acetaminophen may also be decreased.

▶ **Adverse Reactions**

When used as directed, acetaminophen rarely causes severe toxicity or side effects. However, the following adverse reactions have been reported:

Hematologic: Hemolytic anemia; neutropenia; leukopenia; pancytopenia; thrombocytopenia.

Hepatic: Jaundice.

Metabolic: Hypoglycemia.

Hypersensitivity: Rash; fever.

▶ **Overdosage**

Symptoms: Acute poisoning may be manifested by nausea, vomiting, drowsiness, confusion, liver tenderness, hypotension, cardiac arrhythmias, jaundice, and acute hepatic and renal failure. These occur within the first 24 hours and may persist for 1 week or longer. Death has occurred because of liver necrosis. Acute renal failure may also occur. However, there may be no specific early signs or symptoms. The course of acetaminophen poisoning is divided into 4 stages (postingestion time):

Stage 1 (12 to 24 hours) – Nausea; vomiting; diaphoresis; anorexia.

Stage 2 (24 to 48 hours) – Clinically improved; AST, bilirubin, and prothrombin levels begin to rise.

Stage 3 (72 to 96 hours) – Peak hepatotoxicity; AST of 20,000 not unusual.

Stage 4 (7 to 8 days) – Recovery.

Hepatotoxicity may result. The minimum toxic dose is 10 g (140 mg/kg), but liver damage has occurred with a single 5.85 g dose; doses greater than or equal to 20 to 25 g are potentially fatal. Children appear less susceptible to toxicity than adults because they have less capacity for glucuronidation metabolism. Initial signs of toxicity may include nausea, vomiting, anorexia, malaise, diaphoresis, abdominal pain, and diarrhea. Hepatotoxicity is usually not apparent for 48 to 72 hours. Hepatic failure may lead to encephalopathy, coma, and death.

Plasma acetaminophen levels greater than 300 mcg/mL at 4 hours postingestion were associated with hepatic damage in 90% of patients; minimal hepatic damage is anticipated if plasma levels at 4 hours are lower than 120 mcg/mL, or lower than 30 mcg/mL at 12 hours after ingestion.

Chronic excessive use (more than 4 g/day) may lead to transient hepatotoxicity. The kidneys may undergo tubular necrosis; the myocardium may be damaged.

Treatment: Perform gastric lavage in all cases, preferably within 4 hours of ingestion. Refer also to General Management of Acute Overdosage. It is important to contact a local poison control center (1-800-222-1222) or emergency room if overdosage is suspected.

▶ **Administration and Dosage**

Adults: 325 to 650 mg every 4 to 6 hours as needed, or 1 g 3 to 4 times daily as needed; do not exceed 4 g daily for all formulations containing acetaminophen.

Children: The usual dose is 10 mg/kg/dose, which may be repeated 4 to 5 times daily as needed. Do not exceed 5 doses in 24 hours. Do not use in children under 3 years of age without consulting a physician.

Acetaminophen Dosages for Children			
Age	Dosage (mg)	Age	Dosage (mg)
0-3 months	40	6-8 years	320
4-11 months	80	9-10 years	400
1-2 years	120	11 years	480
2-3 years	160	12-14 years	640
4-5 years	240	> 14 years	650

Rectal suppositories:

Adults – 650 mg every 4 to 6 hours as needed; do not exceed 4 g in 24 hours.

Children (3 to 11 months) – 80 mg every 6 hours as needed.

(1 to 3 years) – 80 mg every 4 hours.

(3 to 6 years) – 120 to 125 mg every 4 to 6 hours as needed; do not exceed 720 mg in 24 hours.

(6 to 12 years) – 325 mg every 4 to 6 hours as needed; do not exceed 2.6 g in 24 hours.

Storage: Store suppositories below 27°C (80°F) or refrigerate. Store tablets and oral solutions at 15° to 30°C (59° to 86°F).

ACETAMINOPHEN PRODUCTS	
Trade name	**Doseform**
Regular Strength Tylenol, Genapap, APAP	**Tablets**: 325 mg
Aspirin Free Anacin Extra Strength, Extra Strength Tylenol, APAP Extra Strength	**Tablets**: 500 mg. (*Extra Strength Tylenol* tablets are gelatin coated.)
Children's Tylenol	**Tablets, chewable**: 80 mg
Junior Strength Tylenol	**Tablets, chewable**: 160 mg
Meda-Cap	**Capsules**: 500 mg
Extra Strength Genapap	**Caplets**: 500 mg
Extra Strength Tylenol	**Caplets, gelcaps, and geltabs**: 500 mg
Tylenol Arthritis Pain Extended Relief	**Caplets**: 650 mg
Infants' FeverAll	**Suppositories**: 80 mg
Children's FeverAll	**Suppositories**: 120 mg
Junior Strength FeverAll	**Suppositories**: 325 mg
Acephen	**Suppositories**: 120 mg, 325 mg, 650 mg
FeverAll	**Suppositories**: 650 mg
Children's Silapap, Dolono Elixir	**Elixir**: 80 mg/2.5 mL. Alcohol free.
Infants' Tylenol Concentrated Drops	**Liquid**: 80 mg/0.8 mL. Alcohol free. Saccharin, butylparaben, sorbitol.
Extra Strength Tylenol	**Liquid**: 500 mg/15 mL
Infants' Silapap Drops	**Solution**: 80 mg/0.8 mL. Alcohol free.
Children's Tylenol Liquid	**Suspension**: 160 mg/5 mL

Products listed are representative of currently available and widely distributed brands. Similar products, including regional and private label brands, may also exist.

PATIENT INFORMATION

Acetaminophen

- Patient instructions accompany each product. Read these instructions carefully before use, preferably before leaving the pharmacy, in case you have any questions.
- Do not exceed the recommended dosage. Do not exceed a total adult dose of 4 g/day of acetaminophen in all formulations consumed.
- Be aware of other OTC (eg, combination products for pain, cold, cough, or allergy) and prescription medications that contain acetaminophen.
- If pain persists for more than 5 days, consult physician.
- Do not use in children under 3 years of age without consulting a physician.
- For pain, do not use for longer than 5 days in children or more than 10 days in adults without consulting a physician.
- Avoid alcohol and aspirin while taking this drug.

SALICYLATES

► **Actions**

These products produce analgesia by inhibiting prostaglandin synthesis, reduce fever (by vasodilation), and have anti-inflammatory effects. In addition, of the salicylates, only aspirin significantly inhibits platelet aggregation.

► **Indications**

Relief of mild to moderate pain; fever; various inflammatory conditions (eg, rheumatic fever). These agents have other labeled indications as well.

▶ **Contraindications**

Hypersensitivity to salicylates or NSAIDs. Use with extreme caution in patients with a history of adverse reactions to salicylates. Cross-sensitivity may exist between aspirin and other NSAIDs and between aspirin and tartrazine. Aspirin cross-sensitivity does not appear to occur with sodium salicylate, salicylamide, or choline salicylate. Aspirin hypersensitivity is more prevalent in those with asthma, nasal polyposis, or chronic urticaria.

Also contraindicated in patients with hemophilia or bleeding ulcers or those in hemorrhagic states.

▶ **Warnings**

Concurrent medications: Many other medications, specifically multi-ingredient cough and cold products, also contain aspirin or acetaminophen. Advise patients of this possibility and inquire about other medications they might be taking before recommending an analgesic.

Otic effects: Discontinue use if dizziness, ringing in ears (tinnitus), or impaired hearing occurs. Tinnitus may represent blood salicylate levels reaching or exceeding the upper limit of the therapeutic range; therefore, it is a helpful guide to toxicity. Temporary hearing loss disappears gradually upon discontinuation of the drug.

Hypersensitivity: Do not use if there is a history of sensitivity to aspirin or NSAIDs.

Aspirin intolerance, manifested by acute bronchospasm, generalized urticaria/angioedema, severe rhinitis, or shock occurs in 4% to 19% of asthmatics. Symptoms occur within 3 hours of ingestion.

Foods may contribute to a reaction. Foods with high salicylate content include curry powder, paprika, licorice, Benedictine liqueur, prunes, raisins, tea, and gherkins. A typical American diet contains 10 to 200 mg/day of salicylate.

Hepatic function impairment: Use caution in patients with liver damage, preexisting hypoprothrombinemia, and vitamin K deficiency.

GI effects: Use with caution in patients intolerant of salicylates because of GI irritation, and in those with gastric or peptic ulcers, diabetes, gout, erosive gastritis, or bleeding tendencies.

Hematologic effects: Aspirin interferes with hemostasis. Avoid use in patients with severe anemia, a history of blood coagulation defects, or who take anticoagulants until you have dismissed aspirin use with your doctor.

Pregnancy: Category D (aspirin); *Category C* (salsalate, magnesium salicylate, other salicylates). Aspirin may produce adverse effects in the mother, such as anemia, ante- or postpartum hemorrhage, or prolonged gestation and labor. Salicylates readily cross the placenta. By inhibiting prostaglandin synthesis, salicylates may cause constriction of ductus arteriosus and, possibly, other untoward fetal effects. Maternal aspirin use during later stages of pregnancy may cause adverse fetal effects, such as low birth weight, increased incidence of intracranial hemorrhage in premature infants, stillbirth, or neonatal death. Salicylates may be teratogenic. Avoid use during pregnancy, especially in the third trimester.

Lactation: Salicylates are excreted in breast milk in low concentrations. Adverse effects on platelet function in the nursing infant are a potential risk. The American Academy of Pediatrics recommends that aspirin be used cautiously in nursing mothers.

Children: Administration of aspirin to children (including teenagers) with acute febrile illness has been associated with Reye syndrome. Do not use in children and adolescents.

▶ Drug Interactions

Salicylate Drug Interactions			
Precipitant Drug	**Object Drug***		**Description**
Charcoal, activated	Aspirin	↓	Coadministration decreases aspirin absorption, depending on charcoal dose and interval between ingestion.
Urinary acidifiers	Salicylates	↑	Ammonium chloride, ascorbic acid, and methionine decrease salicylate excretion.
Antacids, urinary alkalinizers	Salicylates	↓	Decreased pharmacologic effects of salicylates. The magnitude of the antacid interaction depends on the agent, dose, and pretreatment urine pH.
Carbonic anhydrase inhibitors	Salicylates	⟷	Salicylate intoxication has occurred after coadministration of these agents. However, salicylic acid renal elimination may be increased by these drugs if urine is kept alkaline. Conversely, salicylates may displace acetazolamide from protein binding sites, resulting in toxicity. Further study is needed.
Corticosteroids	Salicylates	↓	Corticosteroids increase salicylate clearance and decrease salicylate serum levels.
Nizatidine	Salicylates	↑	Increased serum salicylate levels have occurred in patients receiving high doses (3.9 g/day) of aspirin and concurrent nizatidine.
Alcohol	Salicylates	↑	The risk of GI ulceration increases when salicylates are given concomitantly. Ingestion of alcohol during salicylate therapy may also prolong bleeding time.
Salicylates	Angiotensin-converting enzyme inhibitors	↓	The antihypertensive effectiveness of these agents may be decreased by concurrent salicylate administration, possibly because of prostaglandin inhibition. Consider discontinuing salicylates if problems occur.
Aspirin	Heparin	↑	Aspirin can increase the risk of bleeding in heparin-anticoagulated patients.
Salicylates	Loop diuretics	↓	Loop diuretics may be less effective when given with salicylates in patients with compromised renal function or with cirrhosis with ascites; however, data conflict.
Salicylates	Methotrexate	↑	Salicylates increase drug levels, causing toxicity by interfering with protein binding and renal elimination of the antimetabolite.
Aspirin	Nitroglycerin	↑	Nitroglycerin, when taken with aspirin, may result in unexpected hypotension. Data are limited. If hypotension occurs, reduce the nitroglycerin dose.
Aspirin	NSAIDs	↓	Aspirin may decrease NSAID serum concentrations. Avoid concomitant use; it offers no therapeutic advantage and may significantly increase incidence of GI adverse effects.
Salicylates	Probenecid, Sulfinpyrazone	⟷	Salicylates antagonize the uricosuric effect. While salicylates in large doses (more than 3 g/day) have a uricosuric effect, smaller amounts may reduce the uricosuric effect of these agents.

Salicylate Drug Interactions			
Precipitant Drug	**Object Drug***		**Description**
Salicylates	Spironolactone	↓	Salicylates may inhibit the diuretic effects; antihypertensive action does not appear altered. Effects depend on the dose of spironolactone.
Salicylates	Sulfonylureas, exogenous insulin	↑	Salicylates in doses greater than 2 g/day have a hypoglycemic action, perhaps by altering pancreatic beta-cell function. They may potentiate the glucose-lowering effect of these drugs.
Aspirin	Valproic acid	↑	Aspirin displaces valproic acid from its plasma protein binding sites and may decrease its total body clearance, thus increasing the pharmacologic effects.

* ↑ = Object drug increased. ↓ = Object drug decreased. ↔ = Undetermined clinical effect.

▶ **Adverse Reactions**

Adverse reactions can be seen in the following body systems: GI (nausea, dyspepsia, heartburn, epigastric discomfort), hematologic (prolonged bleeding time, leukopenia, thrombocytopenia, purpura, decreased plasma iron concentration, shortened erythrocyte survival time), and dermatologic (rash, hives, and angioedema may occur, especially in patients suffering from chronic urticaria). Additional miscellaneous adverse reactions that have occurred include fever, thirst, and dimming of vision.

Allergic and anaphylactic reactions have been noted when hypersensitive individuals took aspirin. Fatal anaphylactic shock, while not common, has been reported.

Aspirin has an irreversible effect on platelet aggregation for the life of the platelet (approximately 7 days).

▶ **Overdosage**

Symptoms: The acute lethal dose for adults is approximately 10 to 30 g, and for children, approximately 4 g. Respiratory alkalosis is seen initially in acute salicylate ingestions. Hyperpnea and tachypnea occur as a result of increased CO_2 production and a direct stimulatory effect of salicylate on the respiratory center. Other symptoms may include nausea, vomiting, hypokalemia, tinnitus, neurologic abnormalities (eg, disorientation, irritability, hallucinations, lethargy, stupor, coma, seizures), dehydration, hyperthermia, hyperventilation, hyperactivity, thrombocytopenia, platelet dysfunction, hypoprothrombinemia, increased capillary fragility, and other hematologic abnormalities. Symptoms may progress quickly to depression, coma, respiratory failure, and collapse. Chronic salicylate toxicity may occur when more than 100 mg/kg/day is ingested for 2 or more days. It is more difficult to recognize than acute overdosage and is associated with increased morbidity and mortality. Compared with acute poisoning, hyperventilation, dehydration, systemic acidosis, and severe CNS manifestations occur more frequently.

Treatment: Initial treatment includes induction of emesis or gastric lavage to remove any unabsorbed drug from the stomach. Activated charcoal diminishes salicylate absorption most effectively if given within 2 hours after ingestion. Contact a local poison control center (1-800-222-1222) or emergency room if overdosage is suspected.

ASPIRIN

▶ Administration and Dosage

Adults: 325 to 650 mg orally every 4 hours as needed. Some extra-strength products recommend dosages of 500 mg every 3 hours or 1000 mg every 6 hours as needed.

Children: The analgesic/antipyretic dosage is 10 to 15 mg/kg/dose every 4 hours as needed (see table), up to 60 to 80 mg/kg/day. Do not use in children or teenagers with chicken pox or "flu" symptoms because of the possibility of Reye syndrome. Dosage recommendations by age and weight are as follows:

Recommended Aspirin Dosage in Children					
Age (years)	Weight		Dosage (mg every 4 hours)	No. of 81 mg tablets (every 4 hours)	No. of 325 mg tablets (every 4 hours)
	lbs	kg			
2-3	24-35	10.6-15.9	162	2	½
4-5	36-47	16-21.4	243	3	N/A
6-8	48-59	21.5-26.8	324	4	1
9-10	60-71	26.9-32.3	405	5	N/A
11	72-95	32.4-43.2	486	6	1½
12-14	≥ 96	≥ 43.3	648	8	2

ASPIRIN PRODUCTS	
Trade name	Doseform
Adult Low Strength Aspirin Regimen Bayer	**Tablets, coated:** 81 mg
Original Bayer Aspirin	**Tablets, caplets, and gelcaps:** 325 mg
Aspirin	**Tablets, coated:** 325 mg
Extra Strength Bayer Aspirin	**Caplets and gelcaps:** 500 mg
Bayer Children's Chewable Aspirin	**Tablets, chewable:** 81 mg
Adult Low Strength Ecotrin	**Tablets, enteric coated:** 81 mg
Ecotrin Regular Strength, Regular Strength Aspirin Regimen Bayer	**Tablets, enteric coated:** 325 mg
Ecotrin Maximum Strength	**Tablets, enteric coated:** 500 mg
Original Alka-Seltzer	**Tablets, effervescent:** 325 mg, 1000 mg citric acid, 1916 mg sodium bicarbonate
Aspergum	**Gum:** 227 mg
BUFFERED ASPIRIN PRODUCTS	
Medique Tri-Buffered Aspirin	**Tablets:** 325 mg buffered with calcium carbonate, magnesium carbonate, magnesium oxide
Bufferin	**Tablets, coated:** 325 mg
Extra Strength Bufferin, Arthritis Strength Bufferin	**Tablets, coated:** 500 mg buffered with calcium carbonate, magnesium carbonate, magnesium oxide
Arthritis Pain Ascriptin	**Caplets, coated:** 325 mg, buffered with 75 mg aluminum hydroxide, 75 mg magnesium hydroxide, calcium carbonate
Extra Strength Bayer Plus	**Caplets:** 500 mg with calcium carbonate
Maximum Strength Ascriptin	**Caplets, coated:** 500 mg with 80 mg magnesium hydroxide, 80 mg aluminum hydroxide, calcium carbonate

Products listed are representative of currently available and widely distributed brands. Similar products, including regional and private label brands, may also exist.

PATIENT INFORMATION
Aspirin

- Patient instructions accompany each product. Read these instructions carefully before use, preferably before leaving the pharmacy, in case you have any questions.
- May cause GI upset; take with food or after meals. Enteric-coated products may prevent or reduce stomach/GI distress.
- Take with a full glass of water (240 mL) to reduce the risk of the medication lodging in the esophagus.
- Avoid taking antacids within 2 hours of taking enteric-coated tablets.
- Patients allergic to tartrazine dye should avoid aspirin.
- Notify physician if persistent pain, rash, difficult breathing, ringing in the ears, or persistent GI pain occurs. Internal bleeding may occur with no GI symptoms and may be indicated by bloody or black stools.
- Do not use aspirin if it has a strong vinegar-like odor. This suggests deterioration of aspirin and loss of potency.
- Do not use in children or adolescents with chicken pox or flu-like symptoms because of the potential development of Reye syndrome.
- Inform physician or dentist of prior aspirin use before surgery or dental care.
- Be aware of other OTC (eg, combination products for pain, cold, cough, or allergy) and prescription medications that contain aspirin.

MAGNESIUM SALICYLATE

▶ **Actions**

Magnesium salicylate has fewer GI side effects than aspirin.

▶ **Administration and Dosage**

Adults and children (over 12 years of age): 404 mg or 808 mg every 4 hours as needed; maximum 10 tablets/day.

MAGNESIUM SALICYLATE PRODUCTS	
Trade name	Doseform
Mobigesic	**Tablets**: 404 mg, 30 mg phenyltoloxamine citrate

Products listed are representative of currently available and widely distributed brands. Similar products, including regional and private label brands, may also exist.

PATIENT INFORMATION
Magnesium Salicylate

- Patient instructions accompany each product. Read these instructions carefully before use, preferably before leaving the pharmacy, in case you have any questions.
- May cause GI upset; take with food or after meals.
- Do not use in children or adolescents with chicken pox or flu-like symptoms because of the potential development of Reye syndrome.
- Notify physician if persistent pain, rash, difficult breathing, ringing in the ears, or persistent GI pain occurs. Internal bleeding may occur with no GI symptoms and may be indicated by bloody or black stools.

ANALGESIC COMBINATIONS

▶ **Actions**

Caffeine: Caffeine, a traditional component of many analgesic formulations, may be beneficial in certain vascular headaches.

Antacids: Antacids are included as ingredients in some products to minimize gastric upset by salicylates.

▶ **Administration and Dosage**

The average adult dose is 1 or 2 capsules or tablets or 1 powder packet, every 2 to 6 hours as needed for pain. Check individual product labeling for guidelines.

ANALGESIC COMBINATION PRODUCTS	
Trade name	**Doseform**
Pain Relief	**Tablets, film coated**: 110 mg acetaminophen, 162 mg aspirin, 152 mg salicylamide, 32.4 mg caffeine
Saleto	**Tablets, film coated**: 115 mg acetaminophen, 210 mg aspirin, 16 mg caffeine anhydrous, 65 mg salicylamide
Extra Strength Excedrin, Excedrin Migraine	**Tablets, caplets, & geltabs**: 250 mg acetaminophen, 250 mg aspirin, 65 mg caffeine
Pain-Off	**Tablets, film coated**: 250 mg acetaminophen, 250 mg aspirin, 65 mg caffeine
Percogesic	**Tablets, coated**: 325 mg acetaminophen, phenyltoloxamine citrate
Aspirin Free Bayer Select Maximum Strength Headache	**Tablets**: 500 mg acetaminophen, 65 mg caffeine
Excedrin PM	**Tablets, caplets & gelatabs**: 500 mg acetaminophen, 38 mg diphenhydramine citrate
Anacin	**Tablets, coated**: 400 mg aspirin, 32 mg caffeine
Cope	**Tablets**: 421 mg aspirin, 32 mg caffeine
Extra Strength Anacin	**Tablets, coated**: 500 mg aspirin, 32 mg caffeine
Aspirin Free Excedrin Extra Strength	**Caplets & geltabs**: 500 mg acetaminophen, 65 mg caffeine.
Motrin Sinus/Headache	**Caplets**: 200 mg ibuprofen, 30 mg pseudoephedrine HCl
Goody's Extra Strength Headache Powders	**Powder**: 260 mg acetaminophen, 520 mg aspirin, 32.5 mg caffeine

Products listed are representative of currently available and widely distributed brands. Similar products, including regional and private label brands, may also exist.

PATIENT INFORMATION

Analgesic Combination Products

- Patient instructions accompany each product. Read these instructions carefully before use, preferably before leaving the pharmacy, in case you have any questions.
- Take with food or after meals.
- Take with a full glass of water (240 mL) to reduce the risk of the medication lodging in the esophagus.
- Do not use if allergic to tartrazine dye.
- Notify physician if persistent pain, rash, difficult breathing, ringing in the ears, or persistent GI pain occurs. Internal bleeding may occur with no GI symptoms and may be indicated by bloody or black stools.
- Avoid taking antacids within 2 hours of taking enteric-coated tablets.
- Do not use the product if it has a strong vinegar-like odor. This suggests deterioration of the product and loss of potency.
- Do not give to children or teenagers with chicken pox or flu-like symptoms without consulting physician because of the potential development of Reye syndrome.
- Inform physician or dentist of use before surgery or dental care.
- Be aware of other OTC (eg, combination products for pain, cold, cough, or allergy) and prescription medications that contain acetaminophen or aspirin.

NONSTEROIDAL ANTI-INFLAMMATORY DRUGS

▶ **Actions**

Nonsteroidal anti-inflammatory drugs (NSAIDs) have analgesic (pain relieving) and antipyretic (fever reducing) activities. Their exact mode of action is unknown. The major mechanism of action of NSAIDs is believed to be inhibition of cyclooxygenase activity and prostaglandin synthesis. Other mechanisms, such as inhibition of lipoxygenase, leukotriene synthesis, lysosomal enzyme release, neutrophil aggregation, and various cell-membrane functions, may exist as well.

NSAIDs are capable of inhibiting the enzyme cyclooxygenase (COX). COX allows conversion of arachidonic acid into prostaglandins, which mediate inflammatory response. Prostaglandin inhibition peripherally at the site of injury can decrease the inflammatory response and pain. Prostaglandin inhibition can result in analgesia similar to other centrally acting drugs such as acetaminophen. NSAIDs may also have a direct inhibiting effect on inflammatory cells.

▶ **Indications**

Relief of mild to moderate pain, fever, and various inflammatory conditions.

▶ **Contraindications**

NSAID hypersensitivity: Because of potential cross-sensitivity to other NSAIDs, do not give these agents to patients in whom aspirin, iodides, or other NSAIDs have induced symptoms of asthma, rhinitis, urticaria, nasal polyps, angioedema, bronchospasm, and other symptoms of allergic or anaphylactoid reactions.

▶ **Warnings**

Acute renal insufficiency: Patients with preexisting renal disease or compromised renal perfusion are at greatest risk for acute renal insufficiency. A form of renal toxicity seen in patients with prerenal conditions leads to reduced renal blood flow or blood volume. NSAID use may cause a dose-dependent reduction in prostaglandin formation and precipitate overt renal decompensation. Patients at greatest risk are the elderly, premature infants, those with heart failure, renal or hepatic dysfunction, systemic lupus erythematosus (SLE), chronic glomerulonephritis, dehydration, diabetes mellitus, impaired renal function, septicemia, pyelonephritis, those taking ACE inhibitors, concomitant use of any nephrotoxic drug, extracellular volume depletion from any cause, and those receiving diuretics. Recovery usually follows discontinuation.

Hypersensitivity: Because of potential cross-sensitivity to other NSAIDs, do not give these agents to patients in whom aspirin or other NSAIDs have induced symptoms of asthma, rhinitis, urticaria, nasal polyps, angioedema, bronchospasm, and other symptoms of allergic or anaphylactoid reactions. Severe, rarely fatal anaphylactic-like and asthmatic reactions have been reported in such patients receiving NSAIDs.

Anaphylactoid reactions: Anaphylactoid reactions have occured in patients with aspirin hypersensitivity.

Renal function impairment: NSAID metabolites are eliminated primarily by the kidneys; use with caution in patients with significantly impaired renal function. Reduce dosage to avoid excessive accumulation.

Hepatic function impairment: Naproxen may exhibit an increase in unbound fraction and a reduced clearance of free drug in cirrhotic liver patients, suggesting an increased potential for toxicity in this group; consider reducing the dose.

Platelet aggregation: NSAIDs can inhibit platelet aggregation; the effect is quantitatively less and of shorter duration than that seen with aspirin. These agents prolong bleeding time (within normal range) in healthy subjects. This may be exaggerated in patients with underlying hemostatic defects; use with caution in persons with intrinsic coagulation defects and in those on anticoagulant therapy.

Cardiovascular effects: May cause fluid retention and peripheral edema. Use caution in compromised cardiac function, hypertension, patients on chronic diuretic therapy, or other conditions predisposing to fluid retention. NSAIDs may be associated with significant deterioration of circulatory hemodynamics in severe heart failure and hyponatremia, presumably because of inhibition of prostaglandin-dependent compensatory mechanisms.

Infection: NSAIDs may mask the usual signs of infection. Use with extra care in the presence of existing controlled infection.

Photosensitivity: Photosensitivity may occur; caution patients to take protective measures (ie, sunscreens, protective clothing) against UV or sunlight until tolerance is determined.

GI effects: GI toxicity (including NSAID-induced ulcers and GI bleeding disorders) can occur with or without warning with chronic use of NSAIDs. High-dose NSAIDs probably carry a greater risk of causing GI adverse effects, although clinical trials generally do not reflect this. Studies have have shown patients with a history of peptic ulcer disease or GI bleeding who use NSAIDs have a greater than 10-fold risk of developing GI bleed than patients with neither of these risk factors. Have patients with a history of GI lesions consult a physician before using these products. In addition, treatment with oral corticosteroids or anticoagulants, longer duration of NSAID therapy, smoking, alcoholism, older age, and poor general health status contribute to an increased risk for a GI bleed.

Ibuprofen: Do not take for more than 3 days for fever or more than 10 days for pain. If symptoms persist, worsen, or if new symptoms develop, contact a physician.

Pregnancy: Category B; Category D in third trimester. Safety for use during pregnancy has not been established; use is not recommended. There are no adequate, well-controlled studies in pregnant women. An increased incidence of dystocia, increased post-implantation loss, and delayed parturition has occurred in animals. Agents that inhibit prostaglandin synthesis may cause closure of the ductus arteriosus and other untoward effects in the fetus. GI tract toxicity is increased in pregnant women in the last trimester. Some NSAIDs may prolong pregnancy if given before onset of labor. Avoid use during pregnancy, especially during the third trimester.

Lactation: Most NSAIDs are excreted in breast milk in low concentrations. The American Academy of Pediatrics considers ibuprofen and naproxen to be compatible with breastfeeding. Data on the use of ketoprofen during nursing are lacking.

Children: Use of ibuprofen is not recommended in infants younger than 6 months of age. The use of naproxen is not recommended n children younger than 12 years of age unless directed by a physician. Ketoprofen is not recommended for use in children younger than 16 years of age.

Elderly: Age appears to increase the possibility of adverse reactions to NSAIDs. The risk of serious NSAID-induced ulcer disease is increased in elderly patients (older than 65 years of age); this risk appears to increase with dose and duration of therapy. Use with greater care in the elderly and begin with reduced dosages.

► **Drug Interactions**

NSAID Drug Interactions			
Precipitant drug	**Object drug***		**Description**
NSAIDs	ACE inhibitors	↓	Reports suggest that NSAIDs may diminish the antihypertensive effect of ACE inhibitors.
NSAIDs	Anticoagulants	↑	Coadministration may prolong prothrombin time (PT). Also consider the effects NSAIDs have on platelet function and gastric mucosa. Monitor PT and patients closely, and instruct patients to watch for signs and symptoms of bleeding.
NSAIDs	Beta blockers	↓	The antihypertensive effect of beta blockers may be impaired, possibly because of NSAID inhibition of renal prostaglandin synthesis, thereby allowing unopposed pressor systems to produce hypertension. Avoid using this combination if possible. Monitor blood pressure and adjust beta blocker doses as needed. Consider using a noninteracting NSAID (eg, sulindac).
NSAIDs	Cyclosporine	↑	Nephrotoxicity of both agents may be increased.
NSAIDs	Digoxin	↑	Ibuprofen may increase digoxin serum levels.
NSAIDs	Diuretics	↓	Effects of diuretics may be decreased.
NSAIDs	Hydantoins	↑	Serum phenytoin levels may be increased, resulting in an increase in pharmacologic and toxic effects of phenytoin.
NSAIDs	Lithium	↑	Serum lithium levels may be increased.
NSAIDs	Methotrexate	↑	The risks of methotrexate toxicity (eg, stomatitis, bone marrow suppression, nephrotoxicity) may be increased.
NSAIDs	Thiazide diuretics	↔	Decreased antihypertensive and diuretic action of thiazides may occur with concurrent naproxen.

NSAID Drug Interactions			
Precipitant drug	**Object drug***		**Description**
Bisphosphonates	NSAIDs	↑	Risk of gastric ulceration may be increased. Use cautiously.
Cholestyramine	NSAIDs	↓	The effects of NSAIDs may be decreased.
Cimetidine	NSAIDs	↔	NSAID plasma concentrations may be increased or decreased by cimetidine; some studies report no effect.
Probenecid	NSAIDs	↑	Probenecid may increase the concentrations and possibly the toxicity of NSAIDs.
Salicylates	NSAIDs	↓	Plasma concentrations of NSAIDs may be decreased by salicylates. Avoid concurrent use because it offers no therapeutic advantage and may significantly increase the incidence of GI effects.

* ↑ = Object drug increased.   ↓ = Object drug decreased.   ↔ = Undetermined clinical effect.

► **Adverse Reactions**

Cardiovascular: Edema; congestive heart failure; palpitations.

CNS: Dizziness; drowsiness; headache; light-headedness; vertigo.

Dermatologic: Erythema; pruritus; rash; increased sweating.

GI: Bleeding; diarrhea; dyspepsia; heartburn; nausea; vomiting; abdominal pain; cramps; constipation; flatulence.

Miscellaneous: Muscle cramps; thirst; edema; dyspnea; tinnitus; visual disturbances/changes.

IBUPROFEN

► **Administration and Dosage**

Adults: 200 mg every 4 to 6 hours as needed while symptoms persist. If pain or fever does not respond adequately to 200 mg, 400 mg may be used. Do not exceed 1.2 g (6 tablets) in 24 hours. Do not take for pain for more than 10 days unless directed by physician. If GI upset occurs, take with meals or milk.

Children (3 to 12 years of age): 4 to 10 mg/kg/dose every 6 to 8 hours as needed.

Children (younger than 3 years of age): Do not use for headache unless directed by physician.

For migraine pain: 200 to 400 mg with a glass of water. Do not exceed 400 mg in 24 hours, unless directed by physician.

For patients under 18 years of age, contact a physician.

IBUPROFEN PRODUCTS	
Trade name	**Doseform**
Junior Strength Advil	**Tablets, coated**: 100 mg
Advil[1], Maximum Strength Midol, Motrin IB, Haltran, Iprin	**Tablets**: 200 mg
Children's Motrin	**Tablets, chewable**: 50 mg
Junior Strength Motrin	**Tablets and caplets, chewable**: 100 mg
Junior Strength Motrin	**Caplets**: 100 mg
Motrin Migraine Pain	**Caplets**: 200 mg
Advil Migraine	**Capsules, liquid-filled**: 200 mg
Advil Liqui-Gels, Motrin IB[2]	**Gelcaps**: 200 mg

IBUPROFEN PRODUCTS	
Trade name	Doseform
Infants' Motrin Concentrated Drops	**Liquid**: 50 mg/1.25 mL
Advil Pediatric Drops	**Liquid**: 100 mg/2.5 mL
Children's Advil³, Children's Motrin	**Suspension**: 100 mg/5 mL. Sucrose.

Products listed are representative of currently available and widely distributed brands. Similar products, including regional and private label brands, may also exist.

[1] Contains sucrose.
[2] Contains parabens.
[3] Contains sorbitol.

PATIENT INFORMATION
Ibuprofen

- *Adults:* Do not exceed 1.2 g/day (6 tablets) for pain, or 400 mg/day for migraine pain, unless directed by a physician.
- Patient instructions accompany each product. Read instructions carefully before use, preferably before leaving the pharmacy, in case you have any questions.
- Because of possible drug interactions, patients are encouraged not to take any OTC or prescription medications without first consulting a physician or pharmacist.
- Take with a full glass of water (8 oz; 240 mL).
- May cause GI upset; if GI upset occurs with use, take with food or after meals.
- Notify physician if rash, itching, difficulty breathing, visual disturbances, edema, black stools (melena), or persistent headache occurs.
- Do not take for more than 10 days for pain or more than 3 days for fever. If symptoms persist, worsen, or if new symptoms develop, notify a physician.
- Avoid alcohol and aspirin while taking this medication.

KETOPROFEN

► Administration and Dosage

Adults: 12.5 mg with a full glass of liquid every 4 to 6 hours as needed for pain. If pain persists after 1 hour, follow with 12.5 mg. Some patients may find an initial dose of 25 mg (2 tablets) will give better relief. Do not exceed 25 mg in a 4- to 6-hour period or 75 mg in a 24-hour period. Use the smallest effective dose.

Children: Do not give to children under 16 years of age unless directed by a physician.

KETOPROFEN PRODUCTS	
Trade name	Doseform
Orudis KT	**Tablets, coated**: 12.5 mg. Tartrazine, sugar

Products listed are representative of currently available and widely distributed brands. Similar products, including regional and private label brands, may also exist.

PATIENT INFORMATION
Ketoprofen

- Do not exceed 75 mg/day (6 tablets) for pain, unless directed by a physician.
- Patient instructions accompany each product. Read instructions carefully before use, preferably before leaving the pharmacy, in case you have any questions.
- Because of possible drug interactions, patients are encouraged not to take any OTC or prescription medications without consulting a physician or pharmacist.
- Take with a full glass of water (8 oz; 240 mL).
- May cause GI upset; if GI upset occurs with use, take with food or after meals.
- Notify physician if rash, itching, visual disturbances, edema, black stools (melena), or persistent headache occurs.
- Do not take for longer than 10 days for pain or longer than 3 days for fever. If symptoms persist, worsen, or if new symptoms develop, notify a physician.
- Avoid alcohol and aspirin while taking this medication.

NAPROXEN

► Administration and Dosage

Adults (under 65 years of age): 200 mg with a full glass of liquid every 8 to 12 hours as needed while symptoms persist. Some patients may find an initial dose of 400 mg (2 dosage units) followed by 200 mg every 12 hours, if necessary, will give better relief. Do not exceed 600 mg in 24 hours unless directed by a physician. Use the smallest effective dose.

Adults (65 years of age or older): Do not take more than 200 mg every 12 hours.

Children: Do not give to children under 12 years of age unless directed by a physician.

NAPROXEN PRODUCTS	
Trade name	Doseform
Aleve	Tablets, caplets, and gelcaps[1]: 200 mg. Sodium.

Products listed are representative of currently available and widely distributed brands. Similar products, including regional and private label brands, may also exist.

[1] Contains EDTA.

PATIENT INFORMATION

Naproxen

- Do not exceed 60 mg/day (3 tablets), unless directed by a physician.
- Patient instructions accompany each product. Read these instructions carefully before use, preferably before leaving the pharmacy, in case you have any questions.
- Because of possible drug interactions, patients are encouraged not to take any OTC or prescription medications without consulting a physician or pharmacist.
- Take with a full glass of water (8 oz; 240 mL) to reduce the risk of the medication lodging in the esophagus.
- May cause GI upset; if GI upset occurs with use, take with food or after meals.
- Notify physician if rash, itching, visual disturbances, edema, black stools (melena), or persistent headache occurs.
- Do not take for more than 10 days for pain or more than 3 days for fever. If symptoms persist, worsen, or if new symptoms develop, notify a physician.
- Avoid alcohol and aspirin while taking this medication.

MIGRAINE

DEFINITION

Migraine is a recurring headache disorder of moderate to severe intensity that is frequently associated with gastrointestinal (nausea and vomiting) and neurologic (photophobia, numbness, dizziness, and visual symptoms) dysfunction. The International Headache Society (IHS) has developed and published criteria classification as migraine without aura (formerly called common migraine) or migraine with aura based on the presence of focal neurologic symptoms prior to the onset of headache (formerly called classical migraine). The IHS will publish updated migraine criteria in 2003.

Migraine with aura is subclassified into migraine with typical aura (aura lasting less than 1 hour), migraine with prolonged aura (aura lasting longer than 1 hour but less than 1 week), familial hemiplegic migraine (hemiplegia accompanies migraine attack), basilar migraine (aura implicates the brainstem or cerebellum), migraine aura without headache, and migraine with acute onset aura.

Additional migraine types include ophthalmoplegic migraine, retinal migraine, childhood periodic syndromes, status migrainosus, and migrainous infarction.

ETIOLOGY

The etiology of migraine is unknown. However, several precipitants of migraine headaches have been identified and include: air pollution, alcohol, cheese, chocolate, fatigue, hypoglycemia, monosodium glutamate (MSG), oversleeping, perfumes, and drugs (eg, estrogens, nifedipine, nitrates). In approximately 10% of women over 40 years of age, menopause may trigger the onset of migraine.

INCIDENCE

Migraine headaches are 3 times more prevalent in women (18%) than men (6%). The average age of onset is 15 to 35 years of age, with the highest prevalence occurring between 30 and 49 years of age. While the frequency of migraine attacks varies among patients, approximately half experience 1 to 3 headaches per month.

The direct cost to treat migraine pain is exceeded by the indirect costs of migraine-related disability, which total approximately $5.6 to $17.2 billion annually. Approximately 49% of migraine sufferers are treated with OTC medications only, 23% with prescription medication only, 23% with both, and 5% receive no treatment.

PATHOPHYSIOLOGY

The vascular hypothesis of migraines theorizes that the aura of a migraine is caused by intracerebral vasoconstriction followed by extracranial vasodilation resulting in headache pain. While unsupported by blood flow studies, the aura may be related to cerebral blood flow changes. A neuronal dysfunction hypothesis is now the currently accepted cause of migraine pain. Activity within the trigeminovascular system initiates and promotes tissue inflammation, that produces a hyperanalgesic state to prolong headache pain. In addition, activation of unmyelinated C fibers stimulate pain neurons that are regulated by noradrenergic and serotonergic neurons (specifically 5-HT$_2$ receptors). Due to unstable serotonergic neurotransmission in the dorsal raphe neurons of the brainstem, migraine patients may have a lowered biologic threshold for headache. This trigeminovascular system is stimulated in response to emotion or stress, excessive afferent stimulation (eg, glare, noise, smells), or changes in the internal clock or environment.

SIGNS/SYMPTOMS

Migraine headaches are episodic and vary in intensity. They may or may not be accompanied by an aura. Migraines with an aura are preceded by neurologic symptoms, including numbness, dizziness, and visual symptoms (eg, flashing lights, scintillating scotomata), which last approximately 60 minutes. Duration of the migraine can be exhibited 4 to 72 hours. Additional symptoms include nausea, vomiting, and photophobia. Daily activities may aggravate an attack.

Symptoms: Signs and symptoms of a migraine headache are divided into the prodrome, aura, headache, and postdromal phases. The prodrome phase occurs hours or days prior to the headache and includes psychologic (eg, depression, fatigue, irritability), neurologic (eg, photophobia, phonophobia), and autonomic (eg, stiff neck, cold feeling, food cravings) symptoms. The aura phase precedes or accompanies the headache, affects approximately 10% to 20% of migraine suffers, lasts less than 1 hour, and consists of visual or sensory symptoms. The headache phase usually lasts 4 to 72 hours and is unilateral and pulsating, throbbing, or pulsing in nature. Additional symptoms include nausea, vomiting, and photophobia. Following the headache phase, patients may experience a postdromal phase characterized by irritability, impaired concentration, or mood changes.

DIAGNOSTIC PARAMETERS/PHYSICAL ASSESSMENT

Clinical Observation: An essential factor in the diagnosis of headaches is the patient interview. General physical (eg, fundoscopy) and neurologic (eg, cranial nerve deficit) exams and laboratory tests (eg, erythrocyte sedimentation rate) are useful to exclude systemic causes of a migraine.

Interview: The following questions are used to assist in establishing a migraine diagnosis:

Headache history
- Family history
- Age at onset
- Location, radiation, onset, and severity of pain
- Frequency and duration of attacks

- Time of day when attacks occur
- Precipitating factors
- Aura description
- Accompanying symptoms (eg, fever, nausea, vomiting)
- Significance of the attack to the patient
- Previous medical treatment
- A headache diary (includes nature, severity, and frequency of headache symptoms) should be encouraged

TREATMENT

Approaches to therapy: While medication is the primary treatment for migraine headaches, some patients benefit from behavioral or nondrug interventions.

Nondrug therapy: Techniques utilizing nondrug therapy have been successful in relief of migraine and tension-type headache pain in 50% to 70% of patients. Techniques include decreasing sensory stimuli, reducing stress exposure, application of cool compresses or ice packs to the area most severely affected, physical therapy, relaxation techniques, biofeedback, dietary modification, psychotherapy, hypnosis, and acupuncture.

Utilizing behavioral interventions to reduce and eliminate headache triggers may reduce the need for medication in up to 25% of patients. Key triggers include:

- Lifestyle (eg, stress, fatigue, skipping meals)
- Diet (eg, alcohol, caffeine, MSG, tyramine-containing foods and beverages)
- Hormonal (eg, menstruation, menopause)
- Environmental (eg, changes in weather, high altitude, loud noise, bright or flickering lights, glare, smoke)
- Medications (eg, estrogen, H_2 blockers such as cimetidine, indomethacin, nicotine, oral contraceptives)
- Psychological (eg, anxiety, depression)

Additional nondrug therapies include relaxation and cognitive therapy, biofeedback techniques, and operant behavior therapy.

Pharmacotherapy: Once it is determined that drug treatment is necessary, several OTC medications are available, including acetaminophen, aspirin, and other salicylates, non-steroidal anti-inflammatory drugs (NSAIDs), and caffeine. Relief is best achieved when medication is given early during an acute migraine before the attack has fully developed. Nonsteroidal anti-inflammatory drugs may also be beneficial to reduce the frequency and severity of future migraines. Prophylactic therapy should be considered if migraine attacks occur more than twice a month, result in severe impairment, or are predictable in nature. Preventive medication should be continued while treating yourself for an acute attack.

ACETAMINOPHEN (APAP)

▶ **Administration and Dosage**

Adults: 650 mg to 1000 mg every 4 hours as necessary; up to 4 daily.

For product and patient information, see the Headache monograph.

SALICYLATES

▶ **Actions**

For a full discussion of salicylates, see Headache monograph.

ASPIRIN

▶ **Administration and Dosage**

Treatment: 650 mg to 1000 mg every 4 hours as needed; up to 4 g daily.

Prophylaxis: 1300 mg daily, divided into 4 doses.

For product and patient information, see the Headache monograph.

PATIENT INFORMATION

Aspirin

- Patient instructions accompany each product. Read these instructions carefully before use, preferably before leaving the pharmacy, in case you have any questions.
- May cause GI upset; take with food or after meals. Enteric-coated products may prevent or reduce stomach/GI distress.
- Take with a full glass of water (240 mL) to reduce the risk of the medication lodging in the esophagus.
- Avoid taking antacids within 2 hours of taking enteric-coated tablets.
- Patients allergic to tartrazine dye should avoid aspirin.
- Notify physician if persistent pain, rash, difficult breathing, ringing in the ears, or persistent GI pain occurs. Internal bleeding may occur with no GI symptoms and may be indicated by bloody or black stools.
- Do not use aspirin if it has a strong vinegar-like odor. This suggests deterioration of aspirin and loss of potency.
- Do not use in children or adolescents with chicken pox or flu-like symptoms because of the potential development of Reye syndrome.
- Inform physician or dentist of prior aspirin use before surgery or dental care.
- Be aware of other OTC (eg, combination products for pain, cold, cough, or allergy) and prescription medications that contain aspirin.

ANALGESIC COMBINATION PRODUCTS

► **Actions**

For a full discussion of analgesic combination products, see Headache monograph.

PATIENT INFORMATION

Analgesic Combination Products

- Patient instructions accompany each product. Read these instructions carefully before use, preferably before leaving the pharmacy, in case you have any questions.
- Take with a glass of water (8 oz; 240 mL).
- Limit the use of caffeine-containing medications, foods, or beverages while taking this product, because too much caffeine may cause nervousness, irritability, sleeplessness, and, occasionally, rapid heartbeat.
- Notify your physician if you consume 3 or more alcoholic drinks every day.
- Stop using this medicine and notify your physician if your migraine is not relieved or worsens after the first dose, new or unexpected symptoms occur, or you experience ringing in the ears or loss of hearing.
- Be aware of other OTC (eg, combination products for pain, cold, cough, or allergy) and prescription medications that contain acetaminophen or aspirin.

NONSTEROIDAL ANTI-INFLAMMATORY DRUGS

► **Indications**

For a full discussion of NSAIDs, see Headache monograph.

IBUPROFEN

► **Actions**

Inhibition of prostaglandin synthesis by NSAIDs may relieve migraine pain by preventing inflammation in the trigeminovascular system.

► **Indications**

Migraines that occur before, during, or after menstruation may respond well to NSAIDs.

► **Administration and Dosage**

400 mg to 600 mg at onset; repeat in 1 to 2 hours.

See product table in the Headache monograph.

PATIENT INFORMATION
Ibuprofen

- Patient instructions accompany each product. Read these instructions carefully before use, preferably before leaving the pharmacy, in case you have any questions.
- Take with a glass of water (8 oz; 240 mL).
- Use the smallest effective dose.
- Consult your physician if symptoms persist or worsen.
- Notify your physician if you consume 3 or more alcoholic drinks every day.
- Stop using this medicine and notify your physician if your migraine is not relieved or worsens after the first dose, new or unexpected symptoms occur, or if you experience stomach pain or upset stomach that gets worse or lasts.

KETOPROFEN

▶ Administration and Dosage

Prophylaxis: 150 mg daily, divided into 3 doses.

For product and patient information, see the Headache monograph.

PATIENT INFORMATION
Ketoprofen

- Do not exceed 75 mg/day (6 tablets) for pain, unless directed by a physician.
- Patient instructions accompany each product. Read instructions carefully before use, preferably before leaving the pharmacy, in case you have any questions.
- Because of possible drug interactions, patients are encouraged not to take any OTC or prescription medications without consulting a physician or pharmacist.
- Take with a full glass of water (8 oz; 240 mL).
- May cause GI upset; if GI upset occurs with use, take with food or after meals.
- Notify physician if rash, itching, visual disturbances, edema, black stools (melena), or persistent headache occurs.
- Do not take for more than 10 days for pain or more than 3 days for fever. If symptoms persist, worsen, or if new symptoms develop, notify a physician.
- Avoid alcohol and aspirin while taking this medication.

NAPROXEN

▶ Administration and Dosage

Treatment: 500 mg to 750 mg at onset; 250 mg as needed; up to 1375 mg/day.

Prophylaxis: 550 mg to 1100 mg daily, divided into 2 or 3 doses.

For product and patient information, see the Headache monograph.

PATIENT INFORMATION
Naproxen

- Patient instructions accompany each product. Read these instructions carefully before use, preferably before leaving the pharmacy, in case you have any questions.
- Because of possible drug interactions, patients are encouraged not to take any OTC or prescription medications without consulting a physician or pharmacist.
- Take with a full glass of water (8 oz; 240 mL) to reduce the risk of the medication lodging in the esophagus.
- May cause GI upset; if GI upset occurs with use, take with food or after meals.
- Notify physician if rash, itching, visual disturbances, edema, black stools (melena), or persistent headache occurs.
- Do not take for more than 10 days for pain or more than 3 days for fever. If symptoms persist, worsen, or if new symptoms develop, notify a physician.
- Avoid alcohol and aspirin while taking this medication.

INSOMNIA

DEFINITION

Insomnia is a subjective symptom defined as difficulty falling asleep, difficulty maintaining sleep, or a lack of restful sleep despite sufficient opportunity for sleep. As classified in the DSM-IV guidelines, insomnia is associated with complaints about the quantity, quality, or timing of sleep at least 3 times a week for at least 1 month.

ETIOLOGY

Insomnia is generally classified into primary and secondary insomnia.

Primary: Primary (ie, psychophysiological insomnia) is considered when medical and psychiatric disorders have been ruled out and is categorized by intense worry and self-defeating behaviors relating to not being able to sleep on schedule. Primary insomnia is generally longstanding with little relationship to immediate somatic or psychic events. Patients with psychophysiologic insomnia fall asleep more easily at unscheduled times (when not trying) or outside the home environment. Chronic primary insomnia is defined as difficulty in initiating or maintaining sleep or the presence for at least 1 month of nonrestorative sleep that causes marked distress or impairment in social, occupational, or other important areas of functioning.

Secondary: Secondary insomnia (ie, extrinsic insomnia) is generally due to physiological (eg, pain, drug/alcohol withdrawal) or psychological (eg, anxiety, depression) factors and may be described in terms of length and onset. Transient insomnia, lasting only a few days, is often a result of acute stress, acute medical illness, jet lag, or self-medication. An example of a transient extrinsic sleep disorder resolving within 2 to 3 weeks includes transient situational insomnia, which results from a change in sleeping environment or a significant life event (eg, bereavement). Transient insomnia may progress to short-term insomnia, which is usually characterized as lasting up to 3 weeks. Insomnia lasting longer than 3 weeks is considered chronic insomnia and usually has different causes.

Other subtypes of extrinsic insomnia include altitude insomnia, drug/alcohol-induced insomnia, environmental insomnia, and inadequate sleep hygiene.

Identifying the nature of the sleep disruption aids in the selection of appropriate treatment. Insomnia is subdivided as: difficulty falling asleep (sleep onset insomnia), frequent or sustained awakenings (sleep maintenance insomnia), early morning awakenings (sleep offset insomnia), or persistent sleepiness despite sleep of adequate duration (nonrestorative sleep).

Drugs may either produce the side effect of insomnia during use or produce insomnia during withdrawal. It is important to note that although alcohol can increase drowsiness and shorten sleep latency, even moderate amounts of alcohol increase awakenings after sleep onset by interfering with the ability of the brain to maintain sleep.

Drugs that may cause insomnia: alcohol, antichlonergics (eg, ipratropium bromide), antidepressants (eg, buproprion, fluoxetine, monoamine oxidase inhibitors, tricyclic antidepressants), antihypertensives (eg, atenolol, clonidine, methyldopa, pindolol, propranolol, reserpine), antineoplastics (eg, medroxyprogesterone, leuprolide acetate, goserelin acetate, pentostatin, daunorubicin, interferon alfa), CNS stimulants (eg, methylphenidate), hormones (eg, oral contraceptives, thyroid preparations, cortisone, progesterone), hypnotics, nicotine, sympathomimetics (amphetamines, appetite suppressants, β-adrenergic agonists, albuterol, caffeine, metaproterenol, phenylephrine, pseudophedrine, salmeterol, terbutaline, theophylline), miscellaneous (corticosteriods, levodopa, methysergide, phenytoin, quinidine).

Drugs that may cause withdrawal insomnia: alcohol, antihistamines, barbiturates, benzodiazepines, hypnotics (eg, bromides, chloral hydrate, ethchlorvynol, glutethimide), monoamine oxidase inhibitors, tricyclic antidepressants, miscellaneous (eg, amphetamines, cocaine, marijuana, opiates, phencyclidine).

INCIDENCE

Thirty-three percent of the population currently suffers from some type of insomnia. In addition, it is estimated that 50% of the population will experience insomnia in one form or another within their lifetime. Reports of insomnia tend to increase with age and are more prevalent among the elderly.

SIGNS/SYMPTOMS

The symptoms of insomnia may also be accompanied by complaints of daytime fatigue, difficulty concentrating, difficulty coping with minor irritations, and memory problems.

DIAGNOSTIC PARAMETERS/PHYSICAL ASSESSMENT

Interview: Interviewing the patient and obtaining a proper history is crucial when deciding on a recommended course of action.

Ask open-ended questions about the following:
- Duration, onset, and frequency of insomnia.
- Characteristics of insomnia (eg, does the patient wake up too early, wake up frequently, or have trouble falling asleep when going to bed?).
- Sleep hygiene habits.
- History of previous treatments.
- Family history of sleep disorders.
- Underlying psychiatric causes (depression, anxiety, or panic).
- Underlying medical causes (arthritis, hyperthyroidism, congestive heart failure, obstructive sleep apnea, or pulmonary disease).
- Underlying pharmacologic causes (caffeine, alcohol, hypnotic withdrawal, akathesias secondary to psychotropics, or antidepressants).
- Recent events in patient's life (eg, unusually stressful situations).

- As appropriate, ask the bed partner if the patient snores loudly, behaves abnormally during sleep, or is excessively sleepy during the day.

As appropriate, refer the patient to a physician if treatable causes of insomnia exist such as depression, anxiety, reflux esophagitis, or painful states.

TREATMENT

Approaches to therapy: After identifying and relieving any precipitating factors of insomnia such as medical or psychiatric problems, primary goals for treatment include preventing progression of transient to chronic insomnia and improving the patient's quality of life. Achieving these goals involves education, as well as behavioral, and often pharmacologic, interventions. Using a long-term approach to the management of chronic insomnia and working through insomnia complaints systematically helps achieve successful therapy.

Nondrug therapy:
1.) Eliminate the precipitating factors, if any.
2.) Sleep hygiene.
   a.) Obtain regular daytime exercise.
   b.) Avoid large meals at night.
   c.) Avoid caffeine, tobacco, and alcohol.
   d.) Reduce evening fluid intake.
   e.) Avoid bright lights (including television and illuminated clocks), noise, and temperature extremes during the evening.
3.) Stimulus control recommendations.
   a.) Stabilize sleep-wake schedules (temporal control) by establishing a regular time to wake up and go to sleep (including weekends).
   b.) Maintain a consistent wake up time regardless of how much sleep is received the previous night.
   c.) Sleep only as long as necessary to feel rested.
   d.) Avoid long periods of wakefulness in bed by limiting the use of the bedroom to sleep and sex/intimacy. Do not watch television or read in bed.
   e.) Avoid trying to force sleep. If you do not fall asleep within 20 to 30 minutes, leave the bedroom and perform a relaxing activity (eg, read, listen to music) until drowsy; repeat as often as necessary.
   f.) Avoid or limit daytime napping.
4.) Develop relaxation techniques (eg, breathing exercises) to reduce stress.

Pharmacotherapy: When nondrug therapy and good sleep hygiene techniques fail, pharmacologic treatment for insomnia may be appropriate. General guidelines for pharmacologic management of insomnia include:

- Use the lowest effective dose of medications.
- Use intermittent dosing (2 to 4 times weekly).
- Prescribe medication for short-term use (regular use for no more than 3 to 4 weeks).
- Discontinue medication gradually and be alert for rebound insomnia following discontinuation.
- For patients with both insomnia and pain, a combination product (eg, diphenhydramine, acetaminophen, and aspirin) has been proven significantly more effective than an analgesic or sedative alone.

- Refer patients with chronic or long-term insomnia to a physician for further evaluation of potential underlying medical disorders.

Antihistamines – Antihistamines have been employed as adjuncts in the management of insomnia. Both diphenhydramine and doxylamine are members of the ethanolamine group of antihistamines most likely affecting sleep due to their affinity for histamine and muscarinic receptors. A variety of products used to treat the symptoms of the "common cold," for example, may contain a sedating antihistamine or an "at bedtime" dose to foster a more restful sleep. Antihistamines should **not** be viewed and used as sleep aids for serious, long-term sleep disorders. Overuse can lead to daytime sedation, impaired coordination, decreased physical dexterity, delayed reaction time, and mental clouding. Always evaluate OTC antihistamines with significant sedative properties for their anticholinergic activity as well. Anticholinergic adverse effects may not be well tolerated by patients with comorbid conditions (eg, prostatic hypertrophy, glaucoma, angina, any cardiac rhythm disturbance).

Melatonin – Sold in the US as a dietary supplement, melatonin is a hormone secreted by the pineal gland known to shift the circadian clock and induce drowsiness. Although well-designed clinical studies are limited, melatonin may be effective for jet lag and for elderly patients with insomnia and low melatonin levels. Melatonin's ability to shorten sleep latency may suggest its role in patients with initial insomnia.

Valerian – Valerian root extract is considered a dietary supplement with documented effectiveness as a sleep aid.

L-tryptophan – L-tryptophan has been used in the past to treat insomnia, but evidence of its efficacy is lacking. Use is strongly discouraged because of evidence of severe and potentially life-threatening adverse reactions (primarily eosinophilia-myalgia syndrome). Products containing L-tryptophan were pulled from the market in 1990, but some protein supplements and enteral nutrition products may still contain it.

ANTIHISTAMINES

► **Actions**

Antihistamines cause significant drowsiness and the potential for sedation.

► **Indications**

Diphenhydramine is indicated for allergy relief, prevention and treatment of motion sickness, as an antiparkinsonism agent, as an antitussive, and for minor (short-term, episodic) sleep disorders. Doxylamine is indicated as a sleep aid.

► **Contraindications**

Asthma, narrow- or closed-angle glaucoma, prostate gland enlargement (unless under physician supervision).

► **Warnings**

Do not use for longer than 2 weeks. Do not use doxylamine during pregnancy, while breastfeeding, or in children younger than 12 years of age. Diphenhydramine is a Pregnancy *Category B* agent but is contraindicated during breastfeeding because of limited evidence documenting the excretion of the drug into breast milk and the sensitivity of infants to antihistamines. Both agents can cause drowsiness. Practice caution when mental concentration is necessary. Use with extreme caution in patients with cardiovascular disease (eg, angina, cardiac dysrhythmia).

▶ **Drug Interactions**

Both medications can potentiate the sedative effects of other CNS depressants, including alcohol. An increase in anticholinergic side effects is seen when used in combination with MAO inhibitors.

▶ **Adverse Reactions**

Drowsiness and sedation are the most common adverse reactions. Anticholinergic side effects such as dry mouth, urinary retention, and constipation can confound the use of antihistamines to treat minor sleep disorders. Other less common side effects include nervousness, paradoxical insomnia, and excitement. Hypotension and palpitations also have occurred rarely. These agents are often associated with a "hangover" effect. They decrease the sleep latency time but do not help promote restful sleep and can often have the opposite effect. Pediatric and geriatric patients are particularly prone to paradoxical stimulation. Antihistamines may markedly impair cognitive ability in elderly patients.

▶ **Administration and Dosage**

As a sleeping aid, 25 to 50 mg diphenhydramine or 25 mg doxylamine before bedtime may be utilized by adults. Combination products are available with both an antihistamine and analgesic when sleeplessness accompanies pain.

DOXYLAMINE

▶ **Administration and Dosage**

Adults: 25 mg doxylamine before bedtime.

DOXYLAMINE PRODUCTS	
Trade name	**Doseform**
Unisom Nighttime Sleep Aid	**Tablets**: 25 mg doxylamine succinate

Products listed are representative of currently available and widely distributed brands. Similar products, including regional and private label brands, may also exist.

DIPHENHYDRAMINE

▶ **Administration and Dosage**

Adults: 50 mg diphenhydramine HCl or 76 mg diphenhydramine citrate before bedtime.

DIPHENHYDRAMINE PRODUCTS	
Trade name	**Doseform**
Nytol[1], Sominex	**Tablets**: 25 mg diphenhydramine HCl
Sominex Pain Relief Formula	**Tablets**: 25 mg diphenhydramine HCl, 500 mg acetaminophen
Aspirin Free Excedrin PM	**Tablets, Caplets, and Geltabs**: 38 mg diphenhydramine citrate, 500 mg acetaminophen. Methylparaben, propylparaben, mineral oil.
Alka-Seltzer PM	**Effervescent tablets**: 38 mg diphenhydramine citrate, 325 mg aspirin. Aspartame.
Nytol QuickCaps[1], Simply Sleep	**Caplets**: 25 mg diphenhydramine HCl

DIPHENHYDRAMINE PRODUCTS	
Trade name	**Doseform**
Extra Strength Bayer PM	**Caplets:** 25 mg diphenhydramine HCl, 500 mg aspirin
Compoz Nighttime Sleep Aid Maximum Strength[1], Sominex, Twilite[1]	**Caplets:** 50 mg diphenhydramine HCl
Legatrin PM	**Caplets:** 50 mg diphenhydramine HCl, 500 mg acetaminophen. Talc.
Extra Strength Tylenol PM	**Caplets, Gelcaps, and Geltabs:** 25 mg diphenhydramine HCl, 500 mg acetaminophen
Dormin	**Capsules:** 25 mg diphenhydramine HCl
Compoz Nighttime Sleep Aid Maximum Strength Gel Liquid Capsules, Maximum Strength Nytol Quick Gels, Maximum Strength Sleepinal[1]	**Capsules:** 50 mg diphenhydramine HCl
Maximum Strength Sleepinal[1], Maximum Strength Unisom SleepGels	**Softgels:** 50 mg diphenhydramine HCl

Products listed are representative of currently available and widely distributed brands. Similar products, including regional and private label brands, may also exist.

[1] Contains lactose.

PATIENT INFORMATION
Antihistamines

- Patient instructions accompany each product. Read these instructions carefully before use, preferably before leaving the pharmacy, in case you have any questions.
- Avoid alcoholic beverages while taking these products.
- Do not take these products if you are taking sedatives or tranquilizers without first consulting a physician.
- May cause drowsiness; observe caution while driving or performing other tasks requiring alertness, coordination, or physical dexterity.
- Do not use if you have asthma, narrow- or closed-angle glaucoma, emphysema, chronic pulmonary disease, shortness of breath, difficulty breathing, coronary artery disease, a cardiac rhythm disturbance, or difficulty urinating caused by prostate enlargement, unless directed by a physician.
- Do not take for longer than 2 weeks.

MELATONIN

▶ **Actions**

Melatonin (N-acetyl-5-methoxytryptamine) is a hormone produced by the pineal gland, which controls the natural circadian sleep-wake cycle. Production is stimulated during darkness and inhibited by light. The exact mechanism of action of melatonin for insomnia is unknown. Research has suggested melatonin may work by inducing a hypnotic effect or by a direct effect on circadian rhythm resynchronization.

▶ **Indications**

Currently, melatonin is marketed and sold as a dietary supplement. As such, it is not regulated as closely as prescription or OTC medications. Because melatonin is not regulated by the FDA, it does not have an FDA-approved indication for insomnia. However, studies have been conducted on the use of melatonin in the treatment of insomnia, shift-work circadian sleep-wake disturbances, seasonal affective disorder, tinnitus, depression, bipolar disorder, and in the prevention of jet lag.

▶ Contraindications

Melatonin is not appropriate for everyone; patients should check with their physician or pharmacist before self-medicating. Melatonin is produced in abundant amounts in children: There is limited information as to the safety of exogenous melatonin in children. Until more information is available, the use of melatonin in children is not recommended. Pregnant women and breastfeeding mothers should avoid using melatonin because it has been shown to have contraceptive effects at high doses (300 mg/day and higher) and may increase prolactin levels. Because melatonin may stimulate the immune system, patients with severe allergies and autoimmune system disorders (eg, systemic lupus erythematosis, rheumatoid arthritis) should avoid taking melatonin until more information is known about its effects.

▶ Warnings

Avoid performing tasks that require attention and motor skills for 4 to 5 hours after taking a dose.

Various formulations of melatonin are currently available as nutritional supplements. To avoid potential adverse effects, melatonin made from a synthetic source is desired. Animal-derived products carry a greater risk for allergies, contamination, and possible viral transmission than synthetically derived products.

Melatonin is not FDA-approved for use in preventing or treating insomnia.

▶ Drug Interactions

Drug interactions with exogenous melatonin supplementation have not been thoroughly evaluated. However, endogenous melatonin levels may increase when taken with MAOIs and SSRI antidepressants (eg, fluoxetine [eg, *Prozac*], sertraline [*Zoloft*], paroxetine [*Paxil*]). Some beta blockers (ie, atenolol, propranolol) inhibit nocturnal secretion. Melatonin may interfere with the antihypertensive effects of nifedipine.

▶ Adverse Reactions

Melatonin, even in low "doses," has caused drowsiness, depression, hypothermia, and headache. Long-term adverse effects have not been systematically studied and are currently unknown. One short-term study has shown that exogenous melatonin administration did not alter endogenous production once therapy was stopped.

▶ Administration and Dosage

No conclusions can be drawn as to the most effective melatonin regimen because of conflicting data on dose and administration times. Doses of melatonin employed in clinical trials have included 0.3, 1, and 5 mg/day.

Refer to the labeling of specific products for dosing and administration.

Melatonin is not FDA-approved for use in preventing or treating insomnia.

MELATONIN PRODUCTS	
Trade name	Doseform
Melatonex	**Tablets**: 3 mg with vitamin B_6
Melatonin	**Tablets**: 1 mg
Melatonin	**Tablets**: 3 mg with calcium

Products listed are representative of currently available and widely distributed brands. Similar products, including regional and private label brands, may also exist.

PATIENT INFORMATION
Melatonin

- Products containing melatonin are considered dietary supplements and are **not** FDA-approved for medical use. Products containing this agent should be considered **complementary** therapies and not **alternative** therapies. Standard medical care and prescribed therapy should not be abandoned, nor should appropriate medical attention be delayed. Such practices can be dangerous.
- Notify your health care provider(s) that you are taking melatonin.
- Do not use this drug if you are pregnant or breastfeeding.
- Do not administer this drug to prepubescent children.
- Do not take more than the recommended amount.
- Melatonin may interact with other medications; let your health care provider(s) know what medications you are taking, if you are taking any new medications, or if you are taking over-the-counter medicines.
- Avoid driving or performing tasks that require your full attention for 4 to 5 hours after taking melatonin, because it may impair coordination, slow reaction time, and adversely affect digital dexterity.
- Avoid alcohol when taking melatonin.

VALERIAN

▶ **Actions**

Valerian (*Valeriana officinalis*) is a malodorous root from a pink-flowered perennial popular for its calming and sleep-promoting effects. Valerian causes CNS depression and muscle relaxation partly by inhibiting the breakdown of GABA. Controlled clinical trials have demonstrated significantly improved sleep quality and decreased sleep latency in 2 randomized, blind, placebo-controlled, crossover trials. Valerian is classified as GRAS (generally recognized as safe) in the United States for use as a flavoring agent for foods and beverages such as root beer.

▶ **Indications**

Valerian is commonly used for its anxiolytic, antispasmodic, and sleep-promoting properties.

▶ **Warnings**

Products containing valerian are considered dietary supplements and are not FDA-approved for medical use. Do not use valerian if you are pregnant or breastfeeding. Valerian should not be used by children younger than 2 years of age. Do not use valerian before driving or in other situations when alertness is required.

▶ **Drug Interactions**

Avoid concomitant use with alcohol or other central nervous system depressants due to the potential for excessive sedation from concomitant use.

▶ **Adverse Reactions**

Side effects include headache, excitability, cardiac disturbances, drowsiness, blurred vision, restlessness, palpitations, and insomnia. Cardiac complications and delirium have been reported during valerian-root withdrawal. Fatigue, crampy abdominal pain, chest tightness, tremors, and lightheadedness have been reported during an overdose of 18.8 to 23.5 mg of valerian root.

▶ **Administration and Dosage**

Significant sedative effects of 400 to 900 mg valerian extract 30 to 60 minutes before retiring to sleep have been demonstrated in controlled trials. The German Commission E recommends 2 to 3 g of the dried root 1 or more times a day for "restlessness and nervous disturbance of sleep."

VALERIAN PRODUCTS	
Trade name	Doseform
Alluna Sleep	**Tablets**: 500 mg valerian extract, 120 mg hops extract. Hydrogenated castor oil.

Products listed are representative of currently available and widely distributed brands. Similar products, including regional and private label brands, may also exist.

PATIENT INFORMATION

Valerian

- Products containing valerian are considered dietary supplements and are **not** FDA-approved for medical use. Products containing this agent should be considered **complementary** therapies and not **alternative** therapies. Standard medical care and prescribed therapy should not be abandoned, nor should appropriate medical attention be delayed. Such practices can be dangerous.
- Has been used for the treatment of restlessness and sleep disorders. Valerian is classified as GRAS (generally recognized as safe) in the US for food use.
- May interact adversely with a variety of prescribed and OTC drugs that have sedation as a side effect.
- Notify your health care provider(s) that you are taking valerian.
- Do not use this drug if you are pregnant or breastfeeding.
- Do not take more than the recommended amount.
- Avoid alcohol when taking valerian.

JET LAG
(Rapid Time Zone Change)

DEFINITION

Jet lag is the symptomatology associated with an abrupt shift in the sleep-wake cycle that occurs after rapid transmeridian travel involving the crossing of 3 or more time zones.

ETIOLOGY

Jet lag results from a mismatch between the external time (local time in the new time zone) and a traveler's 24-hour internal time. This intrinsic biological clock, also termed the circadian clock, contributes to the daily rhythms of sleep and wakefulness; body temperature; cardiovascular, endocrine and metabolic, gastrointestinal, and respiratory functions. Following long distance air travel, the alignment of the circadian clock from the home time zone to the new external time occurs slowly, averaging approximately 60 minutes per day for eastbound flights and 90 minutes per day for westbound flights. Therefore, several days may be required to fully adjust to a new time zone.

INCIDENCE

Frequent long distance travelers such as flight crews and international business travelers are affected the most.

PATHOPHYSIOLOGY

The intrinsic biological or circadian clock is located in the suprachiasmatic nucleus (SCN) of the hypothalamus. Synchronization to the 24-hour day is achieved through zeitgebers, which are cues for the biological clock resulting directly or indirectly from the environment.

Light is a potent zeitgeber and the time of exposure has the potential to shift the phase of the circadian clock. Bright light during the **first** half of the normal dark period (westbound travel) causes phase delays characterized by difficulty remaining asleep in the morning and tiredness in the afternoon and evening. Westbound travel is associated with evening drowsiness. Bright light during the **second** half of the normal dark period (eastbound travel) causes phase advances characterized by difficulty falling asleep in the new nighttime and tiredness in the morning. Eastbound travel is associated with greater insomnia and daytime sleepiness.

In addition to light, the pineal hormone melatonin, a zeitgeber, is involved in the synchronization process. Melatonin secretion is regulated by light acting through the SCN. Exposure to light inhibits secretion. Conversely, endogenous melatonin is synthesized and secreted at night, with serum concentrations rising immediately at the onset of darkness and peaking around midnight.

Another possible zeitgeber is diet. A high-protein breakfast may promote the synthesis of norepinephrine and dopamine, which activate the arousal system of the body. In addition, a high-carbohydrate dinner promotes the synthesis of serotonin, which plays an important role in sleep regulation and is a precursor of melatonin. However, this theory has limited support.

SIGNS/SYMPTOMS

Patients who develop jet lag suffer from daytime sleepiness, insomnia, fatigue, "fuzzy thinking," irritability, GI disturbances, and frequent awakenings. The symptoms are transient in nature and typically resolve within 2 to 14 days. The duration of symptoms depends on the number of time zones crossed and the direction of travel. Eastbound travel results in greater insomnia and daytime sleepiness, whereas evening drowsiness is more common with westward travel. The patient's age may also play a role in the ability to compensate for these changes.

DIAGNOSTIC PARAMETERS/PHYSICAL ASSESSMENT

Clinical Observation: Generally, the patient will complain of increased insomnia and daytime sleepiness after eastbound travel or early morning rising and evening drowsiness after westbound travel.

Interview: To help determine if symptomatology is related to jet lag, it is important to obtain an accurate patient history. It may be beneficial to ask about the following:

- Description and duration of sleep disorder or other symptoms
- Use of prescription and over-the-counter medications
- Concomitant disease states possibly contributing to sleep disruption
- Changes in social habits or psychosocial issues

TREATMENT

Approaches to therapy: Depending on the severity and duration of symptoms, health care providers may recommend a nondrug approach or appropriate pharmacotherapy. Usually, time to adjust to the new time zone and proper sleep hygiene is the only treatment necessary.

Nondrug therapy: Adaptation to the new time zone can be enhanced through nondrug therapy. Tell patients to adopt the new local hours of sleep and wakefulness despite fatigue. They should start the day with moderate exercise and avoid prolonged napping. Maximizing exposure to daylight readjusts the pattern of light and dark stimulation and helps patients recover sooner than staying indoors. Patients should restrict the intake of alcohol, caffeine, and nicotine 4 to 5 hours prior to bedtime and increase water consumption. At bedtime, they should rest in a dark, quiet, and comfortable bedroom.

Light therapy – The use of bright light therapy to alleviate symptoms of jet lag has produced conflicting results. Some unsettled issues include timing of therapy (pre- or post-flight), duration, and intensity of exposure. Although effects of phototherapy are not fully known, reported adverse effects include headaches and eyestrain.

The jet lag diet – The theory of this diet applies the effects of food constituents on the sleep-wake cycle. However, a study revealed that subjects experienced reduced sleep efficiency possibly because of caffeine consumption close to bedtime. In addition, the rate of circadian rhythm alignment to local time was not increased.

Pharmacotherapy: Currently, there is no FDA-approved drug product for the prevention or treatment of jet lag. Melatonin, sold in the US as a dietary supplement, is a hormone that has been studied in the prevention of symptoms associated with jet lag. Although well-designed clinical studies have not been conducted on this hormone, patients have reported symptom improvements. Subjective improvements in jet lag symptoms have been seen, including decreased daytime fatigue, improved mood, and shortened recovery time. Not all patients will respond the same way, and an optimal dosing regimen has not been determined.

MELATONIN

▶ Actions

Melatonin is a hormone that is produced by the pineal gland, which controls the natural circadian sleep-wake cycle. Production is stimulated during darkness and is inhibited by light. The exact mechanism of action of melatonin for managing jet lag is unknown. Research has suggested melatonin may work by inducing an hypnotic effect or by a direct effect on circadian rhythm resynchronization.

▶ Indications

Currently, melatonin is marketed and sold as a dietary supplement only. As such, it is not regulated as closely as prescription or OTC medications. Because melatonin is not regulated by the FDA, it does not have an FDA-approved indication for preventing or treating jet lag. In fact, the FDA warns that melatonin users take it "without any assurance that it is safe or that it will have any beneficial effect." However, studies have been conducted on the use of melatonin in the prevention of jet lag and the treatment of insomnia, shift work, circadian sleep-wake disturbances, seasonal affective disorder, depression, and bipolar disorder. Results varied.

▶ Contraindications

Melatonin is not for everyone with jet lag; patients should check with their doctor or pharmacist before self-medicating.

Melatonin is produced in abundant amounts in children, and there is limited information on the safety of exogenous melatonin in children. Until more information is available, the use of melatonin in children is not recommended.

Pregnant women and nursing mothers should avoid using melatonin because it has been shown to have contraceptive effects at high doses (300 mg/day and higher) and may increase prolactin levels.

Because melatonin may stimulate the immune system, patients with severe allergies and autoimmune system disorders (eg, systemic lupus erythematosis, rheumatoid arthritis) should avoid taking melatonin until more information on its effects is known.

▶ Warnings

Melatonin is not FDA-approved for use in preventing or treating jet lag.

Avoid performing tasks that require attention and motor skills for 4 to 5 hours after taking.

Various formulations of melatonin are currently available as nutritional supplements. To avoid potential adverse effects, melatonin made from a synthetic source is desired. Animal-derived products carry a greater risk for allergies, contamination, and possible viral transmission than synthetically derived products.

▶ **Drug Interactions**

Drug interactions with exogenous melatonin supplementation have not been evaluated. However, endogenous melatonin levels may increase when taken with monoamine oxidase inhibitors (MAOIs) and selective serotonin reuptake inhibitor (SSRI) antidepressants. On the other hand, some beta blockers (eg, atenolol, propranolol) inhibit nocturnal secretion.

▶ **Adverse Reactions**

Melatonin, even in low "doses," has caused drowsiness, tachycardia, pruritus, depression, and headache. Long-term adverse effects have not been systematically studied. One short-term study has shown that exogenous melatonin administration did not alter endogenous production once therapy was stopped.

▶ **Administration and Dosage**

No conclusions can be drawn as to the most effective melatonin regimen because of conflicting data on "dose" and administration times. Most experts recommend taking 1 to 3 mg of melatonin approximately 20 minutes before bedtime. However, doses of melatonin employed in clinical trials have included 5, 8, and 10 mg daily.

The optimal dose and timing of melatonin ingestion appears to depend on the direction of travel and number of time zones crossed. One study involving 474 patients describes administering melatonin between 6 and 7 pm on the day of departure and between 10 and 11 pm local time for 4 days after arrival when traveling east. For westbound flights, melatonin has been administered after arrival between 10 and 11 pm local time for 4 days. The importance of preflight melatonin is controversial for eastbound flights.

Refer to the labeling of specific products for "dosing and administration."

Melatonin is not FDA-approved for use in preventing or treating jet lag.

MELATONIN PRODUCTS	
Trade name	**Doseform**
Natrol	**Tablets**: 1 mg with 28 mg calcium
Melagesic PM	**Tablets (caplets)**: 1.5 mg with 500 mg acetaminophen
Nature Made, Nature's Bounty	**Tablets**: 3 mg
Melatonin	**Tablets**: 3 mg with 22 mg calcium
GNC A-Z Melatonin 3	**Tablets**: 3 mg with 2 mg vitamin B_6
Natrol	**Tablets**: 3 mg with 10 mg vitamin B_6, 63 mg calcium
GNC A-Z Melatonin 1	**Tablets, sublingual**: 1 mg
GNC A-Z Melatonin 3	**Tablets, timed-release**: 3 mg
Natrol	**Tablets, timed-release**: 3 mg with 63 mg calcium
Melatonex	**Tablets, timed-release**: 3 mg with 10 mg vitamin B_6, 31 mg calcium, 1 mg iron

MELATONIN PRODUCTS	
Trade name	Doseform
Melatonin	**Capsules**: 2.5 mg
Nature's Way	**Lozenges, sublingual**: 500 mcg
Natrol	**Liquid**: 0.25 mg/mL
GNC A-Z Liquid Melatonin	**Liquid**: 2.5 mg/mL

Products listed are representative of currently available and widely distributed brands. Similar products, including regional and private label brands, may also exist.

PATIENT INFORMATION
Melatonin

- Notify your health care provider(s) that you are taking melatonin.
- Do not use this drug if you are pregnant or lactating.
- Do not administer this drug to prepubescent children.
- The first dose should be taken on the evening of departure and for no more than 3 days after arriving at your destination.
- Do not take more than the recommended amount on the package labeling.
- Melatonin may interact with other medications; let your health care provider(s) know what medications you are taking, if you are taking any new medications, or if you are taking over-the-counter medicines.
- Do not share melatonin with others.
- Avoid driving or performing tasks that require your full attention for 4 to 5 hours after taking melatonin because it may make you sleepy, impair coordination, slow reaction time, and adversely affect digital dexterity.
- When taking melatonin, avoid alcohol or other medications that may make you feel drowsy or tired.

MOTION SICKNESS

DEFINITION

Motion sickness is a normal response to an abnormal situation. It is not a true sickness, but rather a disorder of normal physiological function.

ETIOLOGY

The primary cause of motion sickness is excessive stimulation of the vestibular apparatus by motion.

PATHOPHYSIOLOGY

For motion sickness to occur there must be an intact vestibular system. While individual susceptibilities vary greatly, it can occur in most individuals given the right conditions. The sensory conflict theory is most commonly used to describe motion sickness. According to this theory, motion sickness occurs when the brain receives conflicting information about body motion from visual and vestibular receptors and proprioceptors.

SIGNS/SYMPTOMS

The symptoms of motion sickness vary among patients, but within the same person the symptoms are usually consistent. The most common symptom of motion sickness is nausea. Other symptoms include pallor of the perioral area, cold sweats, yawning, hypersalivation, hyperventilation, frontal headache, drowsiness, and malaise. Vomiting is often present and can become a concern if it is severe enough to cause dehydration and hypotension. Vertigo is usually not present. With prolonged exposure to motion, patients often adapt and return to a normal state.

DIAGNOSTIC PARAMETERS/PHYSICAL ASSESSMENT

Clinical Observation: Generally, patients will be familiar with their symptoms of motion sickness as well as specific situations that result in these symptoms. However, it may be beneficial to inquire about these situations. If the symptoms reported by the patient do not coincide with scenarios that are likely to cause motion sickness (eg, average day-to-day activities), it may be prudent to refer the patient to a physician for further observation.

Interview: To ensure the proper diagnosis and treatment, it may be beneficial to ask about the following:

• Symptoms.
• Specific situations that result in motion sickness.

TREATMENT

Approaches to therapy: Prevention of motion sickness is easier than treatment. The mainstays of therapy involve the use of anticholinergic agents and antihistamines.

Nondrug therapy: Patients who are susceptible to motion sickness should minimize their travel and exposure to motion. If travel is unavoidable, they should travel in a supine or semirecumbent position with their head braced. Patients should be advised to avoid reading while traveling, keep their vision focus at 45° above the horizon, and remain in a well ventilated area. Avoid alcohol and dietary excesses prior to traveling. When traveling for short distances, avoid food and drink. For longer trips, consume small amounts of fluid and simple foods often.

Pharmacotherapy: The only OTC medications available for managing motion sickness are antihistamines. Transdermal scopolamine patches, a popular therapy, are available by prescription only.

ANTIHISTAMINES

▶ Actions

These agents have anticholinergic, antihistaminic, and antiemetic properties. They also reduce the sensitivity of the labyrinthine apparatus.

▶ Indications

Prevention and treatment of nausea, vomiting, and dizziness from motion sickness. These agents have other labeled indications as well.

▶ Contraindications

Hypersensitivity to the drug or any of its components; narrow-angle glaucoma; symptomatic prostatic hypertrophy; MAO inhibitor use. Dimenhydrinate is contraindicated in neonates.

▶ Warnings

Pregnancy: Category B.

Lactation: Safety for use in the nursing mother has not been established.

Children: Use with caution and according to package label instructions in children younger than 12 years of age. Dimenhydrinate is not indicated for use in children younger than 2 years of age unless directed by a physician.

▶ Drug Interactions

Concomitant use of alcohol or other CNS depressants with antihistamines may have an additive effect. MAOIs may prolong and intensify the anticholinergic effects of antihistamines.

▶ Adverse Reactions

Adverse reactions can be seen in the CNS (drowsiness, irritability, restlessness, blurred vision), GI system (dry mouth, constipation, anorexia), GU system (urinary retention), and cardiovascular system (hypotension, palpitations, tachycardia).

CYCLIZINE

▶ Administration and Dosage

Adults: 50 mg taken 30 minutes before departure and repeated every 4 to 6 hours. Do not exceed 200 mg daily.

Children (6 to 12 years of age): 25 mg up to 3 times daily.

CYCLIZINE PRODUCTS	
Trade name	Doseform
Marezine	Tablets: 50 mg (as HCl)

Products listed are representative of currently available and widely distributed brands. Similar products, including regional and private label brands, may also exist.

PATIENT INFORMATION

Cyclizine

- Patient instructions accompany each product. Read these instructions carefully before use, preferably before leaving the pharmacy, in case you have any questions.
- Keep out of reach of children.
- These agents may cause drowsiness; observe caution while driving or performing other tasks requiring alertness, coordination, or physical dexterity.
- Avoid concurrent use of alcohol or other CNS depressants.
- Inform physician of a history of glaucoma, peptic ulcer disease, urinary retention, or pregnancy before starting this medication.
- May cause nervousness, insomnia, and dry mouth, loss of appetite, and constipation.

DIMENHYDRINATE

▶ **Administration and Dosage**

Adults: 50 to 100 mg every 4 to 6 hours, not to exceed 400 mg daily.

Children 6 to 12 years of age: 25 to 50 mg every 6 to 8 hours, not to exceed 150 mg daily.

Children 2 to 6 years of age: 12.5 to 25 mg every 6 to 8 hours, not to exceed 75 mg daily.

DIMENHYDRINATE PRODUCTS	
Trade name	Doseform
Dramamine, Motion Sickness Relief, Triptone	Tablets: 50 mg
Dramamine	Tablets, chewable: 50 mg. With aspartame and sorbitol.
Children's Dramamine	Liquid: 12.5 mg/5 mL. 5% alcohol.

Products listed are representative of currently available and widely distributed brands. Similar products, including regional and private label brands, may also exist.

PATIENT INFORMATION
Dimenhydrinate

- Patient instructions accompany each product. Read these instructions carefully before use, preferably before leaving the pharmacy, in case you have any questions.
- Keep out of reach of children.
- These agents may cause drowsiness; observe caution while driving or performing other tasks requiring alertness, coordination, or physical dexterity.
- Avoid concurrent use of alcohol or other CNS depressants.
- Inform physician of a history of glaucoma, peptic ulcer disease, urinary retention, or pregnancy before starting this medication.
- May cause nervousness, insomnia, and dry mouth, loss of appetite, and constipation.

DIPHENHYDRAMINE

▶ Administration and Dosage

Adults: 25 to 50 mg 3 or 4 times daily given 30 minutes before departure and repeated before meals and at bedtime for the duration of travel.

Children more than 20 lb (9.1 kg): 12.5 to 25 mg 3 or 4 times daily.

DIPHENHYDRAMINE PRODUCTS	
Trade name	**Doseform**
Banophen, Benadryl Allergy, Benadryl Allergy Ultratabs	**Tablets**: 25 mg
AllerMax Caplets	**Tablets**: 50 mg. With lactose.
Benadryl Allergy	**Tablets, chewable**: 12.5 mg. With aspartame and 4.2 mg phenylalanine.
Banophen	**Capsules**: 25 mg. With lactose and parabens.
Benadryl Dye-Free Allergy Liqui-Gels	**Capsules, soft gels**: 25 mg. With sorbitol.
Diphenhydramine 50	**Capsules**: 50 mg
AllerMax Allergy & Cough Formula, Benadryl Dye-Free Allergy, Diphen AF, Genahist, Scot-Tussin Allergy DM	**Liquid**: 12.5 mg/5 mL. *AllerMax* contains 0.5% alcohol. *Benadryl Dye-Free Allergy* contains saccharin and sorbitol. *Diphen AF* contains saccharin and sugar. *Genahist* contains 14% alcohol. *Scot-Tussin Allergy DM* contains parabens.
Diphenhist	**Solution**: 12.5 mg/5 mL. With saccharin and sucrose.
Siladryl	**Elixir**: 12.5 mg/5 mL. With 5.6% alcohol.
Diphen Cough	**Syrup**: 12.5 mg/5 mL. With 5.1% alcohol, sucrose, and parabens.

Products listed are representative of currently available and widely distributed brands. Similar products, including regional and private label brands, may also exist.

PATIENT INFORMATION
Diphenhydramine

- Patient instructions accompany each product. Read these instructions carefully before use, preferably before leaving the pharmacy, in case you have any questions.
- Keep out of reach of children.
- These agents may cause drowsiness; observe caution while driving or performing other tasks requiring alertness, coordination, or physical dexterity.
- Avoid concurrent use of alcohol or other CNS depressants.
- Inform physician of a history of glaucoma, peptic ulcer disease, urinary retention, or pregnancy before starting this medication.
- May cause nervousness, insomnia, and dry mouth, loss of appetite, and constipation.

MECLIZINE

▶ Administration and Dosage

25 to 50 mg taken 1 hour before departure; dose may be repeated every 24 hours for the duration of travel.

MECLIZINE PRODUCTS	
Trade name	Doseform
Dramamine Less Drowsy Formula	Tablets: 25 mg
Bonine	Tablets, chewable: 25 mg. With lactose.

Products listed are representative of currently available and widely distributed brands. Similar products, including regional and private label brands, may also exist.

PATIENT INFORMATION
Meclizine

- Patient instructions accompany each product. Read these instructions carefully before use, preferably before leaving the pharmacy, in case you have any questions.
- Keep out of reach of children.
- These agents may cause drowsiness; observe caution while driving or performing other tasks requiring alertness, coordination, or physical dexterity.
- Avoid concurrent use of alcohol or other CNS depressants.
- Inform physician of a history of glaucoma, peptic ulcer disease, urinary retention, or pregnancy before starting this medication.
- May cause nervousness, insomnia, and dry mouth, loss of appetite, and constipation.

Tobacco Use and Smoking Cessation

DEFINITION

Tobacco use is a learned behavior that can result in physical and psychological dependence. Nicotine, the physically addictive component of tobacco, yields dependence characterized by tolerance (the need for progressively larger doses to produce the same effects) and a withdrawal syndrome when the drug is removed. Withdrawal is characterized by irritability, restlessness, dysphoric mood, and an intense sense of craving cigarettes. Psychological dependence on nicotine is a state of mind in which the desire to experience pleasure or avoid discomfort becomes motivation for using the drug or causes cravings for the drug. More Americans die each year from smoking-related diseases (more than 430,000) than die from AIDS, drug abuse, car accidents, and homicide combined. Smoking tobacco is the most preventable cause of illness and death in our society. Chewing/Dipping tobacco is another form of tobacco use that results in dependence; however, this monograph will concentrate on smoking tobacco.

ETIOLOGY

Most people smoke to fill a certain need, and most smokers (approximately 80%) are addicted by 18 years of age. Whether it is peer acceptance, passage into adulthood, or other psychological or social factors, this learned behavior is practiced and strengthened and eventually becomes associated with daily activities (eg, finishing a meal, drinking coffee or alcohol, talking on the phone, driving, stressful situations). These situations begin to serve as cues for smoking, transforming it into a triggered behavior that is reinforced with each positive experience. After years of practice and reinforcement, this learned behavior becomes automatic, a habit no longer associated with any specific reason or trigger.

INCIDENCE

Approximately 25% of adult Americans smoke tobacco. More than 70% of adolescents have experimented with smoking tobacco, and 33% are regular smokers. Data from the US Public Health Service indicate that each day more than 3000 people younger than 18 years of age become tobacco users. The incidence of smoking is higher among men than women (28% vs 23%), higher in Americans with a high school education than a college education (38% vs 12%), and higher for individuals living below the poverty level than those living at or above the poverty level (35% vs 24%). The highest incidence overall of cigarette smoking is among male American Indians (54%). The lowest incidence is among female Asian-Americans (7.5%).

PATHOPHYSIOLOGY

Smoking is associated with, and contributes to, the progression of coronary heart disease, hypertension, arteriosclerotic peripheral vascular disease, chronic bronchitis, chronic obstructive pulmonary disease, stroke, and cerebrovascular disease. Smoking is the cause of 87% of lung cancers and accounts for 30% of all cancer deaths. Leukemia, as well as cancers of the mouth, pharynx, larynx, esophagus, pancreas, cervix, kidney, and bladder are associated with smoking. Smoking also impairs fertility in women and possibly in men, retards fetal growth, and increases the risk of spontaneous abortion, preterm delivery, low birth weight, perinatal mortality, and Sudden Infant Death Syndrome (SIDS).

Cigarette smoke contains more than 4,000 chemical compounds, including carbon monoxide, acetaldehyde, benzene, hydrogen cyanide, and at least 43 known carcinogens. Statistical evidence over the last 30 years has implicated smoking as a cause of lung cancer, but not until recently have studies provided evidence for a direct cause of cancer at the molecular level. The carcinogen benzo(a)pyrene found in cigarette smoke has been shown in vitro to bind to and damage a tumor-suppressor gene known as P53. The result is unregulated cell division and tumor growth.

Nicotine is a potent and addictive CNS stimulant that binds to nicotinic-cholinergic receptors in several organs of the body, including the brain. The effects of nicotine include central and peripheral nervous system stimulation and depression, skeletal muscle relaxation, catecholamine release by the adrenal medulla, and peripheral vasoconstriction causing increased blood pressure, heart rate, cardiac output, and oxygen consumption. Nicotine promotes platelet aggregation and hypercoagulability and stimulates lipolysis to produce an atherogenic lipid profile.

Smoking has been shown to increase the rate of bone loss in postmenopausal women and in older men, leading to decreased bone mineral density and an increased risk of age-related fractures. This effect is thought to be related to the negative effect smoking has on the synthesis of estrogen and other steroid hormones. Furthermore, women who smoke and take estrogen-containing birth control pills are at higher risk of thromboembolic disease. This is particularly true for women older than 35 years of age who smoke more than 15 cigarettes/day.

The effects of cigarette smoking on the body are directly proportional to the number of cigarettes smoked per day, the duration of smoking behavior, and the amount of smoke inhaled.

SIGNS/SYMPTOMS

CNS stimulation by nicotine in naive tobacco users can produce nausea, vomiting, and dysphoria. With continued use, behavior-reinforcing properties develop, including relaxation, increased alertness, decreased fatigue, improved cognitive performance, and a "reward" effect. Many of these effects are dose-dependent. At low doses, stimulation of the cerebral cortex results in increased alertness and cognitive performance, while the reward effect, mediated by the limbic system, occurs at high doses. Nicotine has also been associated with loss of body weight.

Cardiovascular symptoms of nicotine consumption include an initial increase in blood pressure, coronary vasoconstriction, and tachycardia, possibly followed by hypotension, dizziness, and bradycardia, depending on the amount of nicotine ingested.

Musculoskeletal effects may produce an increase in hand tremor, skeletal muscle relaxation, and a decrease in deep tendon reflexes.

Withdrawal symptoms of physical dependence on nicotine become evident within 24 hours after abrupt removal of nicotine from the system and can last several days or weeks.

Signs and Symptoms of Nicotine Withdrawal:
- Anger, hostility, frustration
- Anxiety
- Depression
- Drowsiness, fatigue
- Impaired concentration
- Impatience, irritability
- Nervousness, restlessness
- Craving for cigarettes
- Decreased heart rate
- GI disturbances
- Headache
- Increased appetite, weight gain
- Insomnia
- Myalgia

Nicotine toxicity presents similarly to nicotine withdrawal but is usually differentiated by the presence of palpitations, nausea, and sweating. Withdrawal is more likely to be represented by anxiety, nervousness, and irritability. Other toxic symptoms include vomiting, abdominal pain, diarrhea, flushing, dizziness, hypersalivation, hearing and visual disturbances, confusion, weakness, altered respirations, and hypotension.

DIAGNOSTIC PARAMETERS/PHYSICAL ASSESSMENT

Clinical Observation: Other than observing a tobacco product physically present in a patient's mouth, assessment and intervention is based on systematically screening patients for tobacco use.

Interview: The Agency for Healthcare Research and Quality (AHRQ) has developed the following model for tobacco-cessation intervention for health professionals based on the evidence derived from its review and analysis of the literature.

The following 5 strategies (referred to as "The 5 As") are recommended:

1.) **Ask** - Systematically screen all patients at every visit to identify all tobacco users.
2.) **Advise** - Strongly urge all smokers to quit.
3.) **Assess** and identify smokers willing to attempt to quit.
4.) **Assist** the patient in quitting.
5.) **Arrange** - Schedule follow-up contact.

TREATMENT

Approaches to therapy: Approximately 16 million smokers attempt to quit each year; only approximately 1.5 million (9.4%) are successful. Tobacco cessation interventions that utilize behavioral modification techniques, social support, and nicotine-replacement therapy are the most effective in achieving cessation and preventing relapse. These interventions are applicable to users of both smokeless and smoked tobacco products and should be offered to all patients who use tobacco.

Nicotine replacement therapy has variable efficacy. Smoking cessation success rates as high as 54% have been reported for short terms (up to 7 weeks). However, abstinence tends to decrease over time.

Nondrug therapy: Behavioral modification strategies that couple problem-solving skills with behavior alternatives are an effective means to facilitate smoking cessation by helping the self-motivated tobacco user identify and take control of the habit. Common elements of behavioral modification include, (1) recognition of triggers or high-risk situations thought to increase the risk of smoking or relapse, (2) development of coping skills that will reduce stress, control weight, improve health and quality of life, or produce pleasure, and (3) provision of basic information about smoking and successful quitting. Cessation rates increase when these techniques are used in conjunction with social support, whether it is individual or group counseling.

Several other types of nondrug interventions including hypnosis, acupuncture, and cue exposure (repeated exposure to smoking cues without the opportunity to smoke) are described in the literature, but insufficient evidence exists to evaluate their efficacy.

Pharmacotherapy: The decision to initiate pharmacologic therapy should be made after weighing the risks associated with continued smoking and estimating the likelihood of success in quitting, with or without pharmacologic therapy. Nicotine replacement therapy reduces nicotine withdrawal symptoms and improves rates of smoking cessation. It is recommended as a primary pharmacotherapy for smoking cessation. Except in the presence of serious medical precautions, nicotine replacement should be encouraged.

Failure at an initial attempt at smoking cessation using nicotine replacement therapy should be evaluated. Additional psychosocial support may be indicated during a second course of nicotine replacement therapy. Alternatively, some experts believe that referral to a physician for bupropion therapy is indicated at this point. Sustained-release bupropion (*Zyban*) is indicated specifically for smoking cessation and is the only nonnicotine, first-line pharmacological agent used for smoking cessation therapy. This prescription-only drug is believed to reduce cravings. Its exact role in smoking cessation, whether first-line or second-line, is still evolving.

NICOTINE REPLACEMENT THERAPY

► **Actions**

Two forms of nicotine replacement therapy are currently available OTC: Nicotine polacrilex (chewing gum and lozenge) and nicotine transdermal systems (patches). Nicotine from these products has the same pharmacologic effects as nicotine from tobacco, but doses are lower and smokeless.

► **Indications**

Approved as a smoking cessation aid for the relief of nicotine withdrawal symptoms, including nicotine craving, preferably in conjunction with behavior modification therapy.

► **Contraindications**

Nonsmokers; patients with known hypersensitivity or allergy to nicotine or any component of product formulations (including menthol); those who continue to smoke, chew tobacco, or use snuff.

► **Warnings**

General: Urge the patient to stop smoking completely when initiating nicotine replacement therapy. Inform patients that if they continue to smoke while using the product, they may experience serious adverse effects.

Cardiovascular: Generally, do not use during the immediate post-MI (heart attack) period, with serious arrhythmias, or with severe or worsening angina pectoris. Have patients with coronary heart disease, cardiovascular disease not controlled by medication, cardiac arrhythmias, or vasospastic diseases evaluated by their physician before nicotine replacement therapy is recommended. Occasional reports of tachycardia have been associated with nicotine replacement therapy; discontinue the drug if cardiovascular symptoms occur. Nicotine should be used in hypertensive patients only when the benefits of such a deterrent outweigh the risks.

Endocrine: Use with caution in patients with hyperthyroidism, pheochromocytoma, or insulin-dependent diabetes because of nicotine's effect on the adrenal medulla, which results in catecholamine release.

Renal/Hepatic Impairment: Nicotine metabolism and clearance are dependent on hepatic blood flow; decreased hepatic function could result in reduced nicotine clearance. Only severe renal impairment should affect clearance of nicotine or its metabolites from circulation.

Fertility Impairment: Fertility may be reduced in female smokers. Sperm motility, quality, and quantity may be decreased in male smokers, however more studies are needed to confirm these effects.

Oral/GI: Because nicotine delays healing in peptic ulcer disease, use in patients with active or inactive peptic ulcer only when benefits of including nicotine in a smoking cessation program outweigh risks. Use with caution in patients who suffer frequent heartburn or GERD.

Dental: When used over an extended period of time, nicotine gum may cause severe occlusal stress due to its heavier viscosity than ordinary chewing gum. Nicotine gum may cause loosening of inlays or fillings, can stick to dentures, and can damage oral mucosa and natural teeth. Hard, sugarless candy between doses of gum is recommended to help provide the oral stimulation required by some patients. Temporomandibular joint (TMJ) dysfunction and pain also have been reported with excessive chewing.

Abuse and Dependence: Transferral of dependence on nicotine in tobacco to nicotine in replacement systems is a possibility. However, nicotine replacement therapies lack carcinogens and other toxic constituents found in cigarette smoke.

Pregnancy: Category D (transdermal patch); *Category C* (gum, lozenge). Nicotine may cause fetal harm or harm to the newborn infant when used by a pregnant woman. Maternal smoking is associated with low birth weight, increased risk of spontaneous abortion, perinatal mortality, and SIDS.

Lactation: Nicotine is secreted significantly into breast milk. Infants who are breast-fed by mothers who smoke have a higher frequency of bronchitis, pneumonia, and otitis media in the first year of life than do breastfed children of nonsmoking mothers. Breastfeeding mothers who smoke are more likely to stop breastfeeding earlier than nonsmoking mothers. It is believed that nicotine may reduce the prolactin levels in breastfeeding mothers.

Decide whether to discontinue nursing or to discontinue the drug, weighing the risk of exposure of the infant to nicotine from replacement therapy against the risks associated with the infant's exposure to nicotine from continued smoking by the mother and from nicotine therapy alone or in combination with continued smoking.

Children: Safety and efficacy in children or adolescents younger than 18 years of age who smoke have not been thoroughly evaluated.

► **Drug Interactions**

Smoking cessation, with or without nicotine substitutes, may alter response to concomitant medication in ex-smokers.

Cigarette smoking is an inducer of CYP1A2 enzymes, the primary mechanism for drug interactions. For drugs whose metabolism is stimulated by enzyme inducers, the dose may need to be increased upon initiation of inducer (smoking) therapy and decreased when the inducer (smoking) is discontinued.

Smoking Drug Interactions			
Precipitant drug	**Object drug***		**Description**
Smoking	Alcohol	↓	May decrease the rate of absorption and peak serum concentrations.
Smoking	Benzodiazepines (diazepam, chlordiaze-poxide)	↓	Smoking may decrease sedation and drowsiness probably by CNS stimulation.
Smoking	Beta adrenergic blockers	↓	Sympathetic activation by nicotine may decrease end organ responsiveness. Beta blockers may be less effective for blood pressure and heart rate control in smokers.
Smoking	Caffeine Clozapine Fluvoxamine Olanzapine Tacrine Theophylline	↓	Smoking is an inducer of CYP1A2 enzymes. It can increase clearance and decrease AUC, mean plasma concentration, half-life, and volume of distribution.
Smoking	Clorazepate Lidocaine (oral)	↓	Smoking can decrease AUC.

Smoking Drug Interactions			
Precipitant drug	Object drug*		Description
Smoking	Estradiol	↓	Smoking can increase 2-hydroxylation with possible antiestrogenic effects.
Smoking	Flecanide Imipramine	↓	Smoking can increase clearance and decrease serum concentrations.
Smoking	Heparin	↓	Smoking can increase clearance and decrease half-life. The smoker may require higher doses of heparin.
Smoking	Insulin	↓	Smoking can cause decreased SC absorption resulting in higher insulin requirements for smokers.
Smoking	Mexiletine	↓	Smoking may increase oral clearance and decrease half-life.
Smoking	Opioids (propoxyphene, pentazocine)	↓	Smoking can decrease the analgesic effect; therefore smokers may require higher doses for analgesia.
Smoking	Propranolol	↓	Smoking can increase oral clearance.
Smoking Nicotine	Catecholamines Cortisol	↑	Smoking and nicotine can increase circulating cortisol and catecholamines. Therapy with adrenergic agonists or adrenergic blockers may need to be adjusted upon changes in nicotine therapy or smoking status.

* ↑ – Object drug increased. ↓ = Object drug decreased.

Drug-food interactions: Effective absorption of nicotine polacrilex is dependent upon mildly alkaline saliva; do not eat or drink within 15 minutes or during use of nicotine gum.

▶ Adverse Reactions

Nicotine polacrilex gum/lozenge: Injury to mouth, teeth, or dental work; belching; increased salivation; mild jaw muscle ache; sore mouth or throat.

Transdermal nicotine: Redness, itching, and/or burning at the application site.

▶ Overdosage

Symptoms: Signs and symptoms of acute nicotine overdose include the following: pallor, cold sweat, nausea, salivation, vomiting, abdominal pain, diarrhea, heartburn, headache, dizziness, rapid heartbeat, disturbed hearing and vision, tremor, mental confusion, weakness. Prostration, hypotension, and respiratory failure may occur with large overdoses. Lethal doses quickly produce convulsions and death as a result of peripheral or central respiratory paralysis, or less frequently, cardiac failure. The oral minimum acute lethal dose for nicotine in adult humans is reported to be 40 to 60 mg.

Treatment: Large oral nicotine ingestions cause vomiting, and the consequences of an overdose will vary. Institute gastric lavage and/or activated charcoal (with protected airway) when appropriate. Avoid syrup of ipecac.

Other supportive measures include diazepam or barbiturates for seizures, atropine for excessive bronchial secretions or diarrhea, respiratory support for respiratory failure, and vigorous fluid support for hypotension and cardiovascular collapse.

Transdermal: Remove patch, flush the skin with water, and dry. Do not use soap, which may increase nicotine absorption. If the patch has been ingested, administer activated charcoal. In an unconscious patient, secure an airway before administering activated charcoal via a nasogastric tube. As long as the patch remains in the GI tract, repeated doses of activated charcoal should be administered because the patch will continue to release nicotine. A saline cathartic or sorbitol may be added to the first dose of activated charcoal to enhance passage of the patch.

▶ Administration and Dosage

The daily dosage of nonprescription nicotine replacement should follow the FDA-approved administration and dosage guidelines on the package label. Little research is available on the use of these products in light smokers (fewer than 10 to 15 cigarettes/day); therefore, consider lower starting doses in these patients. Patients who smoke soon after awakening, smoke when ill, smoke more in the morning, or find the first cigarette of the day the most difficult to do without, have a particularly difficult time quitting smoking.

NICOTINE TRANSDERMAL SYSTEMS

▶ Administration and Dosage

FDA-approved dosing for transdermal delivery systems should be followed (see table). However, some patients may use nicotine replacement therapy for longer periods, which is preferable to a relapse. Individualize treatment based on specific patient characteristics, such as previous experience with the patch, amount smoked, degree of addiction, etc (eg, patients weighing more than 100 pounds or who smoke more than 10 to 15 cigarettes/day might benefit from starting with the 21 mg patches).

Nicotine Transdermal Systems (Patches)	
Brand/strength	FDA-approved regimen
Habitrol[1]	
21 mg/day	4 weeks, then...
14 mg/day	2 weeks, then...
7 mg/day	last 2 weeks
Nicoderm[1]	
21 mg/day	6 weeks, then...
14 mg/day	2 weeks, then...
7 mg/day	last 2 weeks
Nicotrol	
15 mg/16 hours	6 weeks, then...
10 mg/16 hours	2 weeks, then...
5 mg/16 hours	last 2 weeks

[1] Start with 14 mg/day for 6 weeks for patients who smoke less than 10 cigarettes/day. Decrease dose to 7 mg/day for the final 2 weeks.

The transdermal patch has been medically shown to be a safe and effective way to quit smoking. However, the patch is not appropriate for everyone. Advise patients to consult their doctor before using the patch if they are younger than 18 years of age, are pregnant or nursing, have heart disease (eg, coronary artery disease, hypertension, cardiac rhythm disturbance, peripheral vascular disease, vasospastic disease), have had a recent heart attack or irregular heartbeat, have high blood pressure not controlled with medication, take prescription medicine for depression or asthma, are diabetic (insulin-dependent), are allergic to adhesive tape, or have skin problems. Be sure to read all the information accompanying the product for this and other important warning information.

Advise patients not to use the patch if they continue to smoke, chew tobacco, use snuff, use a nicotine gum or other nicotine-containing products, or take *Zyban*. Advise patients to stop using the patch and see their doctor if skin redness caused by the patch does not go away after 4 days or if their skin swells or a rash develops. Also have patients stop if they develop irregular heartbeats or palpitations or symptoms of nicotine overdose such as nausea, vomiting, dizziness, weakness, headache, diarrhea, and rapid heartbeat.

Application: Apply the system promptly upon its removal from the protective pouch. Apply only once a day to a hairless, clean, dry skin site on upper body or upper arm or hip. Hold for 10 seconds. Wash hands thoroughly after application. Do not wear more than one patch at a time. Do not cut patch in half or into smaller pieces.

Habitrol, Nicoderm CQ – After 24 hours, remove the used system and apply a new sytem to an alternate skin site. Do not leave patch on for more than 24 hours because it may irritate the skin, and it loses strength after 24 hours. Apply at the same time each day. Do not use the patch for longer than 8 weeks (*Habitrol*) or 10 weeks (*Nicoderm CQ*). If patients have vivid dreams or other sleep disturbances, they may remove the patch at bedtime and apply a new one in the moring.

Nicotrol – Each day, apply a new system upon waking and remove at bedtime. If the patient forgets to remove the patch at bedtime, that person may have vivid dreams or other sleep disruptions. Do not wear the patch longer than 16 consecutive hours. Refer to the table for length of therapy.

Disposal: When the used system is removed from the skin, fold it over and place in the protective pouch that contained the new system. Immediately dispose of the used system to prevent its access by children or pets.

NICOTINE TRANSDERMAL SYSTEMS		
Trade name	**Doseform**	**Duration**
Nicotine Transdermal System	**Patch**: 21 mg nicotine over 24 hours	Weeks 1 through 4
	Patch: 14 mg nicotine over 24 hours	Weeks 5 through 6
	Patch: 7 mg nicotine over 24 hours	Weeks 7 through 8
Habitrol	**Patch**: 21 mg nicotine over 24 hours	Weeks 1 through 4
	Patch: 14 mg nicotine over 24 hours	Weeks 5 through 6
	Patch: 7 mg nicotine over 24 hours	Weeks 7 through 8
Nicoderm CQ[1]	**Patch**: 21 mg nicotine over 24 hours	Weeks 1 through 6
	Patch: 14 mg nicotine over 24 hours	Weeks 7 through 8
	Patch: 7 mg nicotine over 24 hours	Weeks 9 through 10
	Step 1 Kit: 7 (or 14) 21 mg patches, User's Guide, audiocassette, Committed Quitters Program enrollment	
	Step 2 Kit: 7 (or 14) 14 mg patches, User's Guide, audiocassette, Committed Quitters Program enrollment	
Nicotrol	**Patch**: 15 mg nicotine over 16 hours	Weeks 1 through 6
	Patch: 10 mg nicotine over 16 hours	Weeks 7 through 8
	Patch: 5 mg nicotine over 16 hours	Weeks 9 through 10
	Starter Kit: 7 (15 mg) patches, audiotape, Taking Action Booklet, Tips Card	

Products listed are representative of currently available and widely distributed brands. Similar products, including regional and private label brands, may also exist.

[1] Available in original and clear patches.

NICOTINE POLACRILEX

▶ Administration and Dosage

Gum/Lozenge: Advise patient to stop smoking completely when beginning to use the gum or lozenge. Clinical experience suggests that abstinence rates may be higher when patients use nicotine gum or lozenge on a fixed schedule than as needed. Research supports tailoring the duration of therapy to fit the patient's needs. If the patient smokes less than 25 cigarettes/day or smokes the first cigarette more than 30 minutes after waking, start with the 2 mg nicotine gum or lozenge. Use of 4 mg gum or lozenge is recommended for highly dependent smokers who smoke 25 or more cigarettes/day or within 30 minutes of waking, patients with severe withdrawal symptoms, and those whose therapy failed with the 2 mg strength. Use the gum or lozenge according to the following 12-week schedule:

Nicotine Polacrilex Dosing Schedule (Gum and Lozenge)		
Weeks 1 to 6	Weeks 7 to 9	Weeks 10 to 12
1 piece every 1 to 2 hours	1 piece every 2 to 4 hours	1 piece every 4 to 8 hours

Gum: Instruct patient to chew the gum (2 mg or 4 mg) slowly until it tingles, then park it between the cheek and gum. When the tingle is gone, instruct the patient to begin chewing again until the tingle returns. Repeat the process until most of the tingle is gone (approximately 30 minutes).

Advise patient not to eat or drink for 15 minutes before chewing the gum or while chewing a piece. To improve the chances of quitting, use at least 9 pieces/day for the first 6 weeks. If there are strong and frequent cravings, use a second piece within the hour. However, do not use more than one piece at a time or continuously use one piece after another because this may cause hiccoughs, heartburn, nausea, rapid heart rate, or other side effects.

Do not use more than 24 pieces/day. Stop using the nicotine gum at the end of 12 weeks. If there is still a need to use nicotine gum, have the patient contact a physician.

Lozenge: Place the 2 mg or 4 mg lozenge in your mouth and allow the lozenge to slowly dissolve (approximately 20 to 30 minutes). Minimize swallowing. Do not chew or swallow the lozenge. A warm or tingling sensation may occur. Occasionally, move the lozenge from one side of the mouth to the other until completely dissolved (approximately 20 to 30 minutes).

Advise patients not to eat or drink for 15 minutes before using a lozenge or while the lozenge is in their mouth. To improve the chances of quitting, use at least 9 lozenges/day for the first 6 weeks. Do not use more than 1 lozenge at a time or continuously use 1 lozenge after another because this may cause hiccoughs, heartburn, nausea, rapid heart rate, or other side effects.

Do not use more than 5 lozenges in 6 hours, or more than 20 lozenges/day. Stop using the nicotine lozenge at the end of 12 weeks. If there is still a need to use nicotine lozenges, have the patient contact a physician.

Disposal:

Gum – Place used chewing pieces in a wrapper and dispose of in such a way to prevent access by children or pets. Pieces of nicotine gum may have enough nicotine to make children or pets sick. In case of overdose, contact a physician or a Poison Control Center.

Lozenge – Store lozenges in a safe, secure area to prevent access by children or pets. In case of overdose, contact a physician or a Poison Control Center.

NICOTINE POLACRILEX PRODUCTS	
Trade name	**Doseform**
Nicotine Gum, *Nicorette*[1]	**Chewing gum**: 2 mg nicotine (as polacrilex)/square
	Chewing gum: 4 mg nicotine (as polacrilex)/square
Commit[2]	**Lozenge**: 2 mg nicotine (as polacrilex)/lozenge. Phenylalanine 3.4 mg, aspartame.
	Lozenge: 4 mg nicotine (as polacrilex)/lozenge. Phenylalanine 3.4 mg, aspartame.

Products listed are representative of currently available and widely distributed brands. Similar products, including regional and private label brands, may also exist.

[1] In orange, mint, and original flavors.
[2] Light mint flavor.

PATIENT INFORMATION
Smoking Cessation Products

- Patient instructions containing important information regarding proper use of nicotine replacement therapy and disposal of used patches, gum, or lozenges are enclosed with each product. Read instructions carefully before use, preferably before leaving the pharmacy in case you have any questions.
- Do not smoke while using nicotine replacement therapy because of increased risk of nicotine toxicity.
- *Patches* — Apply daily to a hairless, clean, dry skin site on the upper body or upper, outer arm. Remove 24-hour systems prior to the application of a new patch; remove 16-hour systems at bedtime. Alternate skin sites with each application; do not reuse skin sites for at least 1 week.
- *Gum* — Chew gum slowly until a "peppery" taste emerges, then "park" between cheek and gum to facilitate nicotine absorption through the oral mucosa. Slowly and intermittently "chew and park" gum for about 30 minutes. Do not eat or drink anything during or 15 minutes before chewing the gum.
- *Lozenge* — Place the lozenge in the mouth and allow to dissolve over 20 to 30 minutes. Do not chew or swallow the lozenge. Move lozenge from one side of the mouth to the other until completely dissolved. Do not eat or drink anything for 15 minutes before using the lozenge or while the lozenge is in the mouth.

WEIGHT MANAGEMENT

DEFINITION

Obesity and overweight are conditions of excess body fat associated with increased health risks. Being *overweight* is defined as having a body mass index (BMI) of 25 to 29.9 kg/m^2; being *obese* is defined as having a BMI of 30 kg/m^2 or more. Being overweight is not always synonymous with being obese. For example, a body builder may weigh more than the height-derived ideal but may have a very low percentage of body fat. The accumulation of excess body fat associated with overweight and obesity is linked to increased morbidity and mortality.

The tables below, released by the National Institutes of Health, were developed by the National Heart, Lung, and Blood Institute with cooperation from the National Institute of Diabetes and Digestive and Kidney Diseases. They provide BMI calculations and categorizations by height. BMIs of 19 to 40 kg/m^2 are provided for adults from 58 to 76 inches tall and 91 to 328 lbs.

BMI Calculations	
Metric conversion formula = Weight (kg)/Height (m^2)	Non-metric conversion formula = Weight (lbs)/height (inches^2) $\times$ 703

BMI Units for Specific Heights													
	Body Mass Index (kg/m^2)												
Height (inches)	19	20	21	22	23	24	25	26	27	28	29	30	35	40
	Body Weight (lbs)												
58	91	96	100	105	110	115	119	124	129	134	138	143	167	191
59	94	99	104	109	114	119	124	128	133	138	143	148	173	198
60	97	102	107	112	118	123	128	133	138	143	148	153	179	204
61	100	106	111	116	122	127	132	137	143	148	153	158	185	211
62	104	109	115	120	126	131	136	142	147	153	158	164	191	218
63	107	113	118	124	130	135	141	146	152	158	163	169	197	225
64	110	116	122	128	134	140	145	151	157	163	169	174	204	232
65	114	120	126	132	138	144	150	156	162	168	174	180	210	240
66	118	124	130	136	142	148	155	161	167	173	179	186	216	247
67	121	127	134	140	146	153	159	166	172	178	185	191	223	255
68	125	131	138	144	151	158	164	171	177	184	190	197	230	262
69	128	135	142	149	155	162	169	176	182	189	196	203	236	270
70	132	139	146	153	160	167	172	181	188	195	202	207	243	278
71	136	143	150	157	165	172	179	186	193	200	208	215	250	286
72	140	147	154	162	169	177	184	191	199	206	213	221	258	294
73	144	151	159	166	174	182	189	197	204	212	219	227	265	302
74	148	155	163	171	179	186	194	202	210	218	225	233	272	311
75	152	160	168	176	184	192	200	208	216	224	232	240	279	319
76	156	164	172	180	189	197	205	213	221	230	238	246	287	328

ETIOLOGY

Weight gain and accumulation of excessive body fat occur when energy intake exceeds energy expenditure. The etiology of obesity is clearly multifactorial, involving genetic, metabolic, biochemical, psychological, and physiological factors that contribute to obesity.

A number of factors, including cellular, molecular, metabolic, behavioral, social, and physiological influences, may influence weight and obesity. Genetic factors are thought to account for 40% to 70% of the variability in measures of obesity. In mice, an inherited defective gene (the *ob* gene) is associated with obesity and type 2 diabetes; a similar correlation is likely to exist in humans. The *ob* gene codes for the hormone involved in satiation; however, animals with a defective *ob* gene fail to produce adequate levels of the protein leptin, which signals the hypothalamus (the body's controller of satiety). Thus, the brains of these animals are never given a strong signal to stop eating and they become obese. Another mutation of the beta-3 adrenergic gene in humans and mice is thought to impede the ability to burn fat. Studies demonstrate that genetic factors influence weight by affecting both the amount of food consumed and the metabolism of fat. Environmental factors also clearly play an important role in the etiology of obesity; these factors are primarily related to levels of physical activity and food intake. In the US, mechanization (eg, cars, remote controls, computers, electrical equipment, etc.) has decreased the necessity of physical activity, making sedentary lifestyles more prevalent. (It is unclear whether reduced physical activity causes obesity or whether obesity causes reduced physical activity, but either way, a vicious cycle results.) Furthermore, many Americans have the opportunity to enjoy an abundance of high-calorie foods, and, in many cases, overeating is encouraged at social functions and during stressful times.

The increased prevalence of obesity can be attributed to a number of additional factors, including reduced cigarette smoking and decreased motivation for physical activity. All of these powerful influences make it increasingly difficult to reduce caloric intake and to increase energy expenditure on a long-term basis.

INCIDENCE

An estimated ⅓ to ½ of American adults meet the criterion for obesity or overweight, (eg, having a BMI 25 kg/m^2 or higher). African-American and Mexican-American women experience a higher prevalence of obesity and overweight than either white Americans or men. Approximately 25% of adult men and 45% of adult women are reportedly trying to lose weight at any point in time. The annual US expenditure for weight loss products and services exceeds $33 billion.

In spite of the obsession with thinness and the large monetary output to manage obesity, an obesity epidemic continues to flourish. Although the proportion of dietary fat has declined, total caloric intake has increased since 1979.

It has been estimated that only ⅕ of the population gets enough exercise to affect health and weight positively.

The cost of obesity-related illness is estimated to be $70 billion annually in direct health care expenditures and indirect costs due to lost occupational productivity. Obesity-related complications claim over 300,000 lives each year, second only to smoking-related illness.

PATHOPHYSIOLOGY

Obesity is a metabolic disease that has significant sequelae that profoundly affect a number of physiological processes. Hyperinsulinemia, a common feature of obesity, results in insulin resistance, which is thought to be due to a reduced number of insulin receptors or to a postreceptor defect in insulin sensitivity. The majority of type 2 diabetic patients are obese, and obesity clearly contributes to insulin resistance.

Dyslipidemias are another consequence of obesity. Although a modest correlation exists between obesity and circulating levels of low density lipoproteins (LDL), triglycerides are much more likely to be elevated in obese than in nonobese patients. High density lipoprotein (HDL) levels are often low in obese patients, perhaps because of reduced physical activity. In addition, cholesterol turnover may be increased, leading to increased biliary excretion of cholesterol and an increased incidence of gallstone formation.

The incidence and severity of hypertension is increased in obese patients. But it should be noted that the use of a normal sized blood pressure cuff in a grossly obese patient may yield an erroneously high reading. A large-sized blood pressure cuff should be used.

The combination of hypertension and hypertriglyceridemia is a deadly one, increasing risk of coronary heart disease, cardiovascular disease, stroke, and MI in obese patients.

Other disorders associated with obesity include hypoventilation syndrome, gastroesophageal reflux disease (GERD), osteoarthritis (especially of the hips and knees), varicose veins, ventral and hiatal hernias, and thromboembolism. Obesity can also increase the risk of prostate cancer, colorectal cancer, and in postmenopausal women, breast and endometrial cancer. There are no advantages to obesity.

In spite of the multitude of serious adverse effects associated with obesity, an initial reduction of only 5% to 10% of body weight can have substantial health benefits. Health benefits of weight management include reduced blood pressure, improved glycemic control and insulin sensitivity in type 2 diabetic patients, lowered LDL and triglycerides, increased HDL, and improved sleep apnea and osteoarthritis. However, rapid and large loss of body weight has been associated with gallstone formation and loss of lean body mass.

DIAGNOSTIC PARAMETERS/PHYSICAL ASSESSMENT

Clinical Observation: In the past, obesity has been defined as a body weight of more than 20% over one's ideal body weight, based on weight-height charts from the Metropolitan Life Insurance Company, dating back to 1959. Today obesity is more commonly measured by body mass index (BMI), which is weight (in kg) divided by height (in meters) squared.

A BMI of 25 to 29.9 kg/m^2 is considered overweight, and a BMI of 30 or higher indicates frank obesity. The following table shows an overweight/obesity classification based on BMI.

BMI and Overweight/Obesity Classifications		
Weight Classification	Obesity Classification	BMI (kg/m^2)
Underweight		< 18.5
Normal		18.5-24.9
Overweight		25-29.9
Obesity	I	30-34.9
	II	35-39.9
Extreme Obesity	III	≥ 40

Weight charts may indicate sex or body type (eg, lean or muscular), but rarely consider age. It is widely accepted that modest body weight increases that occur with age are not necessarily associated with increased risk to health. However, higher BMIs have been linked to increased morbidity associated with type 2 diabetes, coronary heart disease, hypertension, stroke, and certain types of cancer. Respiratory disorders, sleep apnea, pregnancy complications, and psychological problems have also been associated with overweight and obesity.

Waist circumference is correlated with abdominal fat content out of proportion to total body fat, which is a predictor of obesity-related risk factors and morbidity. Adults at high risk for developing obesity-related disease are classified as those with a BMI of greater than 25 kg/m^2, men with a waist circumference greater than 40 inches, and women with a waist circumference greater than 35 inches.

The waist-to-hip ratio can also help predict increased health risk. Men and postmenopausal women tend to store fat in the abdominal area, referred to as the "apple" distribution of fat, whereas premenopausal women tend to have more of a "pear" shape with fat deposited primarily in the hips, buttocks, and thighs. A waist-to-hip ratio greater than 1.0 in men and 0.8 in women has been linked to increased risk of hypertension, hyperlipidemia, coronary heart disease, and type 2 diabetes. Waist circumference, however, is usually considered a better indicator of increased risk than waist-to-hip ratio.

Interview: To determine the cause of obesity, it may be beneficial to ask the patient about the following:

- Medical history. (Specifically, history of heart disease, elevated lipid levels, diabetes, glaucoma, kidney disease, thyroid disease, or enlarged prostate.
- Diet.

- Weight, height, and history of overweight (including any history of eating disorders).
- Family history of obesity.
- Current medications.
- Level of physical activity or exercise.
- Recent reduction in cigarette smoking.
- Past weight loss treatments or weight management practices (eg, diet, exercise, prescription or OTC drugs).

TREATMENT

Approaches to therapy: Treatment for overweight and obese patients is recommended based on evidence linking this condition with increased risk factors for other disease, as well as increased morbidity and mortality. In overweight and obese patients, weight loss has been shown to reduce blood pressure, serum triglycerides, LDL- and total cholesterol, and blood glucose levels, and to increase HDL-cholesterol. The American Dietetic Association has refocused the goal of obesity treatment from weight loss to weight management, which means achieving the best weight possible in the context of overall health. "Weight management" is defined as the adoption of healthful and sustainable eating and exercise behaviors indicated for reduced disease risk and improved feelings of energy and well-being.

All weight management programs should include training in lifestyle modification to achieve the following goals:

- Gradual change to healthful eating style with increased intake of whole grains, fruits, and vegetables.
- Nonrestrictive approach to eating based on hunger and satiety
- Gradual increase in enjoyable physical activity of 30 minutes duration at least 3 times per week.

The single most important component of any weight management plan is an individualized plan with realistic goals and sustainable eating and exercising behavior.

Patient counseling efforts should be focused on increasing awareness of the caloric and fat content of food. A patient who has an accurate conception of food content and portion size can make informed decisions about food selection and consumption. Even though it is not feasible to expect complete avoidance of fast food, educating patients to be aware of caloric and fat content enables them to make smarter food selections, even in a fast food context. Authoritative consumer self-help references on food content are good, inexpensive supplementary resources for pharmacies or individual patients.

Counseling efforts should emphasize that even modest reductions in body weight can result in significant clinical improvement in blood pressure, glycemic, and cholesterol control. Setting realistic weight management goals empowers patients to take control in the maintenance of their own health. Having control of one's health encourages self-sufficiency and well-being and engenders compliance with a weight management plan.

Further, patients should better realize the benefit of increasing physical activity. The term "physical activity" rather than "exercise" may be preferable and less threatening to non-active people. The usual exercise prescription of 30 minutes of aerobic activity at 60% to 80% of the maximum heart rate at least 3 times a week is encouraged, but not realistic for most sedentary individuals. Any exercise is better than none. It is also important to help patients select exercise that is enjoyable and likely to be sustainable.

Pharmacists are well positioned to help patients choose a moderate plan for weight management. The plan should include strategies to gradually reduce caloric intake and increase physical activity. All recommendations should be focused on individually based, realistic goals.

Pharmacotherapy: As a weight management strategy, pharmacotherapy should be considered secondary therapy that is effective only when used with a proper diet and exercise routine. Despite OTC diet aids available, few products have any scientific basis of efficacy in suppressing appetite. No controlled studies have shown weight loss with OTC products alone.

For decades, many OTC products contained phenylpropanolamine (PPA). In November 2000 the Food and Drug Administration (FDA) issued a public health advisory regarding PPA asking manufacturers of products containing PPA to voluntarily discontinue marketing any drug products containing PPA, or to reformulate to remove PPA, if applicable. This was based on recommendations of the FDA's Nonprescription Drugs Advisory Committee and a Yale University School of Medicine Study that suggested PPA increased the risk of hemorrhagic stroke.

The FDA plans to initiate rulemaking to classify PPA as nonmonograph (not generally recognized as safe and effective) for OTC use and to remove it from prescription drug products.

Somewhat more misleading for consumers are products referred to as "fat burners," which contain amino acids, vitamins, and minerals and claim to have a "lipotropic effect on the excessive accumulation of fats." Most of the "fat-burner" products contain chromium picolinate. There is no evidence that chromium picolinate has a beneficial effect in reducing body fat. "Fat burners," combined with aerobic exercise and a well-balanced low-fat diet, claim to be significant to any body sculpting program.

Many other weight loss/appetite suppressant products are available over-the-counter; however, the vast majority of these products have not been shown to be effective; some may even be considered dangerous. (For example, ma huang, an ephedra product used for weight loss, has been associated with serious adverse reactions and death). Among the active ingredients in some of the nonprescription weight loss products currently available are ephedra, L-Arginine, guarana, guar gum, and green tea. For more complete information, see the individual monograph in the **Complementary Therapies** chapter.

While most OTC weight loss products should be used for no longer than 12 weeks, several agents may be prescribed by physicians as longer-term weight loss drugs. Such agents may be appropriate for patients who are severely obese (eg, those with a BMI greater than 30 with no concomitant obesity-related risk factors or with a BMI of 27 or more with obesity-related risk factors). Weight loss drugs should be used with lifestyle modifications, including dietary therapy and physical activity. While dexfenfluramine and fenfluramine were withdrawn from the market in 1997 for safety reasons, sibutramine (*Meridia*) is FDA-approved and has been shown to be effective for treatment of obesity for up to 1 year. Another anti-obesity agent, orlistat (*Xenical*), was approved by the FDA in 1999 and has been shown to be safe and effective for up to 2 years.

WEIGHT MANAGEMENT PRODUCTS

▶ Administration and Dosage

These products have not been evaluated by the Food and Drug Administration. Dosage varies, follow instructions supplied with individual products.

WEIGHT MANAGEMENT PRODUCTS	
Trade Name	**Doseform**
Acutrim Natural A.M.	**Tablets**: 100 mg niacin; 100 mg bitter orange extract; 300 mg guarana extract; 25 mg polygonum cuspidatum; 450 mg L-arginine HCl; 200 mg guar gum; 50 mg citrus pectin
Acutrim Natural P.M.	**Tablets**: 180 mg niacin; 450 mg L-arginine HCl; 30 mg polygonum cuspidatum; 100 mg inositol hexanicotinate; 40 mg L-glutamine; 250 mg guar gum; 50 mg citrus pectin
Dexatrim Natural Ephedrine Free Formula	**Caplets**: 83 mcg chromium; 120 mg bitter orange peel; 340 mg proprietary blend of siberian ginseng, green tea leaf with caffeine, kola nut with caffeine, ginger root, licorice root, vanadium amino acid chelate
Dexatrim Natural Green Tea Formula	**Caplets**: 250 mcg chromium; 70 mg calcium; 30 mcg iodine; 100 mcg vanadium; 200 mg green tea leaf; 150 mg proprietary blend of panax ginseng extract, licorice root, cinnamon bark, ginger root, kelp
Dexatrim Natural No Caffeine Formula	**Caplets**: 250 mcg chromium; 100 mcg vanadium; 120 mg heartleaf extract (equiv. to 12 mg ephedrine); 100 mg proprietary blend of steatite, atractylode rhizome, baikal skullcap root, balloon-flower root, licorice root, terra alaba, da huang root, mirabilite, dong quai root, mint leaf, forsythia fruit, gardenia fruit, ginger root, lovage root, *schizonepeta tenufolia* stem, siler root, peony root

Products listed are representative of currently available and widely distributed brands. Similar products, including regional and private label brands, may also exist.

DERMATOLOGICAL CONDITIONS

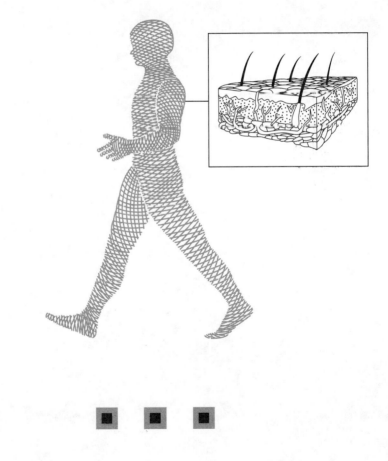

NONPRESCRIPTION DRUG THERAPY
TABLE OF CONTENTS
■ ■ ■

DERMATOLOGICAL CONDITIONS

INTRODUCTION

Dermatology is the study of skin function and disease. The skin is the largest organ in the body. A unique feature of skin in comparison to other organs is the visibility of skin disease to the patient and the physician. In some cases, patients may not experience any symptoms except visible changes or abnormalities of their skin, prompting them to treat the condition or seek medical advice. Diseases of the skin are extremely common. It is estimated that 1 in 3 people in the US has a skin disorder each year.

Skin disease is a serious medical condition. While some skin conditions are merely cosmetic, affecting one's appearance with no associated symptoms, many can cause suffering, resulting in disability, discomfort, or disfigurement with significant economic loss, particularly if the condition is not treated. Because of the visibility of the skin, certain skin conditions cannot be hidden; this may result in patient anxiety and self-consciousness. Additionally, the importance of skin disease to all physicians cannot be overlooked. The skin may provide visible evidence of otherwise invisible internal disease. The skin is often referred to as the "window to internal disease."

The management of skin disorders centers around prevention and medical treatment. Patient education is the key to treating and preventing skin disease. As nonmelanoma skin cancer is the most common of cancers, education about sun exposure and sun protection is the first step in reducing skin cancer. Similarly, educating patients about self-skin exams and mole checks with evaluation of changing moles can help reduce the ever-increasing incidence of potentially deadly melanomas.

Treatment of skin disease can be accomplished primarily on 3 levels: Patient-self-treatment, primary care physicians, and dermatologists. The most common and accessible of these 3 options is self-treatment with over-the-counter (OTC) medications. Patients are faced with the daunting task of determining which of the many OTC products to select for their condition, be it acne, psoriasis, or eczema. Thus the pharmacist plays a vital role in assisting with their decisions. For this reason, it is important that pharmacists be familiar with common skin disorders, OTC treatments, and the need for physician/dermatologist evaluation. The purpose of this chapter is to provide pharmacists with easily accessible information that will allow them to assist patients with proper care of their skin disease. Pharmacists should remember to inform patients that if their skin condition does not improve with OTC medications, physician evaluation is warranted.

Primary care physicians must also recognize their role in the evaluation and treatment of skin disease. With the changes in health care, an emphasis is placed on the role of the "gatekeeper" primary care physician. However, it is often economically wise to refer the patient directly to a dermatologist – the skin specialist. Ultimately, the most cost-effective approach to skin disease starts with patient education and public awareness, followed by physician evaluation and management if necessary. This chapter is intended to help the pharmacist participate in educating patients on self-treatment with OTC medications.

ACNE VULGARIS

DEFINITION

Acne is a disorder of the pilosebaceous follicles, often androgen-driven, usually involving eruptions on the face, neck, chest, and back of comedones, papules, pustules, nodules, and cysts. Usually, the disease is self-limited.

ETIOLOGY

Although the actual cause for acne is unknown, much of what does occur with acne is known. The epithelium of the pilosebaceous unit in the skin becomes disordered. Sebaceous material (eg, sebum, bacteria, keratin) then escapes from within the follicle into the dermis, causing a marked inflammatory response that clinically becomes either a papulopustule or a cyst. If the material stays within the follicle and distends it, a noninflammatory comedone develops.

The type of bacteria within the sebaceous material is generally *Propionibacterium acnes*, an anaerobe. These bacteria release chemicals that irritate the follicular wall, causing disruption of the wall and attracting inflammatory cells that release enzymes that help destroy local tissue. Further, *P. acnes* converts the noninflammatory esterified fatty acids in normal sebum to lipase-mediated, inflammatory free fatty acids.

The development of enlarged sebaceous glands is under the influence of testosterone (which is converted to dihydrotestosterone by a local enzyme, 5-alpha reductase). It is the enlarged pilosebaceous unit that supports the greater number of *P. acnes* organisms; the subsequent chain reaction leads to the development of an acne lesion.

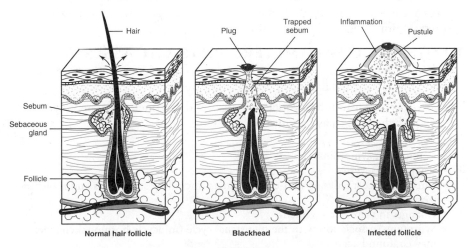

Figure 1. Development of an Acne Lesion

INCIDENCE

Acne, the most common of skin conditions, generally occurs during adolescence but can occur any time during the third or fourth decade of life, affecting 80% to 90% of the population at some time with varying degrees of severity. Approximately 17 to 20 million Americans use acne treatment at any point in time. The peak of acne severity occurs between 15 to 17 years of age in females and 16 to 18 years of age in males. It is more common in males, with the severity of the disease being familial.

SIGNS/SYMPTOMS

Acne is characterized by the development of different types of lesions:

- *Comedones* (open and closed) – Noninflammatory, slightly raised follicular impaction of keratin and lipid. Open comedones are known as "blackheads." Closed comedones are known as "whiteheads."
- *Papules* – Small (less than 5 mm) inflamed, raised bumps.
- *Pustules* – Papules (inflamed) with obvious core of pus within.
- *Nodules* – Large (more than 5 mm) inflamed bumps within the skin.
- *Cysts* – Large (more than 1 cm) inflamed nodules with liquid or semi-solid centers contained within their walls.

Lesions generally occur on the face, neck, chest, and back, but may also occur on the arms, buttocks, and legs. The comedones may persist, but the inflammatory lesions usually subside spontaneously within 2 to 3 weeks. Depending upon the depth of the inflammation (if any), scarring may result.

Signs and symptoms may be confounded by a variety of factors, such as drugs (eg, androgenic/anabolic steroids, progestin-dominant oral contraceptives, lithium, phenytoin, azathioprine), excessive humidity, prolonged perspiration, poor hygiene, local irritation, friction, physical or emotional stress, oily or greasy cosmetics or hair dressings, and chronic exposure to volatilized lipids (grease), for example, by fry cooks, etc.

DIAGNOSTIC PARAMETERS/PHYSICAL ASSESSMENT

Clinical Observation: Usually, the disorder is self-evident, with the patient knowing the correct diagnosis and seeking treatment.

Interview: To ensure the proper diagnosis and treatment of acne vulgaris, it may be beneficial to ask about the following:

- Age.
- Duration of symptoms.
- Changes in severity.
- The type of cosmetics or skin-care products (including sunscreens and moisturizers) used.
- Changes in skin-care regimen.
- Symptoms' association with the menstrual cycle (midcycle hormonal changes may confound acne).
- Treatment with acne-fighting agents.
- Sensitivity to these agents.

- Current medication regimen. Some drugs (eg, corticosteroids, androgenic/anabolic steroids, phenobarbital, phenytoin, progestin-dominant oral contraceptives, bromides, iodides, some cytoxics, isoniazid, PUVA therapy, lithium, danazol, penicillins, cephalosporins) may cause or aggravate acne.

Referral to a physician for treatment is necessary if the disease is of such severity that scarring is inevitable or if OTC therapy is unsuccessful. It is important to find out if the patient has done anything that would hamper the exodus of the sebaceous material (eg, using heavy moisturizers or oily products [sunscreens or non-oil-free makeup preparations]), or works in an environment that could contribute to the problem.

TREATMENT

Approaches to therapy: Treatment of acne vulgaris is multifactorial. A broad-based approach to management should include nondrug and drug therapy measures as appropriate. It should be appreciated that acne may produce significant physical, psychological, and social discomfort, particularly in adolescents. Efforts should be made to remove excess sebum, unblock and prevent closure of the pilosebaceous duct, and minimize conditions conducive to the development of acne.

Nondrug therapy: Washing with a mild, nonmoisturizing soap (such as *Purpose* or *Dial*) a minimum of twice daily will generally remove excess sebum. A soft wash cloth is essential. For mild acne, salicylic soap may help dislodge superficial hyperkeratotic debris. If the patient has sensitive skin, use a mild, water-washable soap. Astringent cleansing pads may be used between washings. Avoid abrasive cleansers (and vigorous scrubbing) because they do not remove the clogged keratinous material and they irritate, and consequently swell, the skin. In addition, control of diet, stress, and other confounding factors should be a part of acne therapy.

Pharmacotherapy: Benzoyl peroxide is the most effective nonprescription product available today for the treatment of mild to moderate acne. Several different concentrations (2.5% to 10%) and vehicle bases (eg, lotions, gels, solutions, creams) are available. Because benzoyl peroxide is an irritant, it is necessary to use the lowest concentration that is beneficial and a vehicle base that is mild and allows for penetration of the skin by the active chemical. Many patients prefer the astringent (drying) effect of the gel vehicle.

BENZOYL PEROXIDE

▶ **Actions**

The efficacy of benzoyl peroxide is primarily attributable to its keratolytic and antibacterial activity, especially against *P. acnes*, the predominant organism in sebaceous follicles and comedones. The keratolytic actions foster skin sloughing (desquamation) and re-epithelization. The antibacterial activity presumably is caused by the release of active or free radicals of oxygen capable of oxidizing bacterial proteins and killing bacteria. Resolution of the acne (ie, reduction in comedones and acne lesions) usually coincides with reduction in the levels of *P. acnes* and of lipids and irritating free fatty acids in the follicle. This is aided by a drying action, removal of excess sebum, mild desquamation (drying and peeling), and sebostatic effects.

▶ **Indications**

For the treatment of mild to moderate acne vulgaris and oily skin. May be used in more severe cases as an adjunct in therapeutic regimens including benzoyl peroxide gels, antibiotics (topical and systemic), retinoic acid products, and sulfur/salicylic acid-containing preparations. Improvement of the condition depends on degree and type of acne, frequency of product use, and nature of other therapies.

▶ **Contraindications**

Hypersensitivity to benzoyl peroxide. Cross-sensitivity may occur with benzoic acid derivatives.

▶ **Warnings**

Carcinogenesis: The FDA downgraded benzoyl peroxide from Category I (safe and effective) to Category III (data insufficient to permit classification) in the tentative final monograph for OTC topical anti-acne drugs based on reports that the drug was a tumor promoter in rodents. There is no evidence that the drug is carcinogenic in humans. It will remain on the market while additional tests are conducted in animals.

Irritation: The rule in initiating therapy with benzoyl peroxide is to start at lower concentrations and move to higher concentrations incrementally as clinically needed. If severe irritation develops, discontinue use and institute appropriate therapy. After the reaction clears, treatment may often be resumed with a lower concentration, less frequent application, or shorter exposure time. The hypersensitivity rate to benzoyl peroxide is approximately 1% to 3%. Because the drug is photosensitizing, protect skin from ultraviolet (UV) exposure from natural sunlight or tanning beds while product is on skin.

For external use only: Keep away from eyes, eyelids, mouth, inside of nose, and mucous membranes. If contact occurs, rinse thoroughly with water. May bleach hair and clothing.

Pregnancy: Category C. Topical administration is generally considered safe for use during pregnancy. Use in pregnant women only if clearly needed.

Lactation: It is not known whether this drug is excreted in breast milk. Administer with caution to nursing mothers.

Children: Safety and efficacy in children younger than 12 years of age have not been established.

Sulfite sensitivity: Some products contain sulfites, which may cause allergic-type reactions including anaphylactic symptoms and asthmatic episodes in susceptible patients. The overall prevalence in the general population is unknown and probably quite low. Such reactions are seen more frequently in asthmatic patients.

▶ **Drug Interactions**

Concomitant use with tretinoin (*Retin-A*) may cause significant skin irritation.

Cross-sensitization with benzoic acid derivatives (eg, cinnamon and certain topical anesthetics) may occur.

▶ **Adverse Reactions**

Excessive drying, manifested by marked peeling, erythema, and possible edema (approximately 4%); allergic contact sensitization/dermatitis (1% to 3%).

► **Overdosage**

Symptoms: Excessive dryness and scaling, erythema, or edema.

Treatment: Discontinue use. If reaction is caused by excessive use and not allergy, cautiously reinstate at reduced dosage after signs and symptoms subside. To hasten resolution of adverse effects, use emollients, cool compresses, or topical corticosteroids (eg, 1% hydrocortisone cream).

► **Administration and Dosage**

Cleansers: Wash once or twice daily. Wet skin areas to be treated prior to administration. Rinse thoroughly and pat dry. Control amount of drying or peeling by modifying dose frequency or concentration.

Other doseforms: Apply once daily; start with a low concentration (eg, 2.5%, 4%, 5% benzoyl peroxide) and gradually increase concentration and frequency of application and time on skin as tolerance permits. After cleansing the skin, smooth a small amount over the affected area. Expect modest warmth, stinging, dryness, and eventual sloughing when applied. If bothersome dryness or peeling occurs, reduce the dosage. If excessive stinging or burning occurs after any single application, remove with mild soap and water; resume use the next day. Leave the initial application on the skin for only 15 minutes. Exposure time should be increased in 15-minute increments as tolerance allows. Once tolerated for 2 hours, it can be left on the skin overnight. One application per day (usually evening) may be all that is required. A morning dose may also be applied if tolerated. Advise patients that it may take 2 to 6 weeks of regular daily use to achieve full therapeutic effect.

BENZOYL PEROXIDE PRODUCTS	
Trade name	Doseform
PanOxyl-5	**Bar**: 5% benzoyl peroxide
PanOxyl Maximum Strength	**Bar**: 10% benzoyl peroxide
Neutrogena Acne Mask	**Mask**: 5% benzoyl peroxide
Clearasil Maximum Strength Tinted, Clearasil Maximum Strength Vanishing	**Cream**: 10% benzoyl peroxide
Oxy Balance Emergency Spot Treatment	**Gel**: 5% benzoyl peroxide
Clean & Clear Persa-Gel 10, Essential Care Acne Treatment, Fostex 10% Vanishing, Oxy 10 Balance Emergency Spot Treatment	**Gel**: 10% benzoyl peroxide
Benzoyl Peroxide Wash	**Liquid**: 5% benzoyl peroxide
Benzoyl Peroxide Wash, Fostex 10% Wash, Oxy 10 Balance Wash	**Liquid**: 10% benzoyl peroxide
Brevoxyl Cleansing	**Lotion**: 4% benzoyl peroxide
Loroxide	**Lotion**: 5.5% benzoyl peroxide
Brevoxyl-8 Cleansing	**Lotion**: 8% benzoyl peroxide
Benoxyl 10	**Lotion**: 10% benzoyl peroxide

Products listed are representative of currently available and widely distributed brands. Similar products, including regional and private label brands, may also exist.

PATIENT INFORMATION

Benzoyl Peroxide

- For external use only. Avoid contact with eye, eyelids, lips, mucous membranes, and highly inflamed or damaged skin. If accidental contact occurs, rinse thoroughly with water.
- Start with low concentrations and increase exposure time and concentration as tolerated or as the clinical condition requires.
- Benzoyl peroxide is an oxidizing agent; avoid contact with hair and colored fabric as it may bleach the area.
- Some products may contain sulfites, which may cause allergic-type reactions in susceptible people.
- Avoid excessive exposure to all sources of UV radiation (eg, sunlight, tanning beds, sun lamps) due to risk of a photosensitivity reaction in area of application.
- Advise patient that 2 to 6 weeks of regular use may be required to achieve a full therapeutic effect.
- Advise patients that a transient feeling of warmth or stinging, skin dryness, and some skin sloughing is normal.
- If severe irritation develops, discontinue use and institute appropriate therapy. After the reaction clears, treatment may often be resumed with less frequent application, lower concentration, or shorter exposure time.
- If excessive inflammation occurs, recommend cool compresses and short-term (24 to 48 hours) use of an OTC topical steroid cream (eg, 1% hydrocortisone).
- Avoid other sources of skin irritation (eg, sunlight, sun lamps, other topical acne medications) unless directed by a physician.
- Use with PABA-containing sunscreens may cause transient skin discoloration.
- Normal use of water-based cosmetics is permissible.

SULFUR PREPARATIONS

▶ **Actions**

Sulfur, a keratolytic, provides skin sloughing and a drying action. Although it may help to resolve comedones, it may also promote the development of new ones by increasing horny cell adhesion.

▶ **Indications**

For secondary use as an aid in the treatment of mild acne and oily skin in concentrations of 3% to 10%.

▶ **Warnings**

For external use only. Avoid contact with eyes, eyelids, and mucous membranes. Certain individuals may be sensitive to 1 or more components. If undue skin irritation develops or increases, discontinue use and consult a physician.

▶ **Administration and Dosage**

Apply a thin layer. Use 1 to 3 times daily. For best results, wash skin thoroughly with a mild cleanser prior to application.

SULFUR PRODUCTS	
Trade name	**Doseform**
Zapzyt	**Bar**: 3% sulfur
Sulpho-Lac Acne Medication	**Cream**: 5% sulfur
Liquimat	**Lotion**: 4% sulfur
Essential Care Sulfur Acne Treatment Masque	**Mask**: 6.4% sulfur
Sulmasque	**Mask**: 6.4% sulfur
Sulpho-Lac	**Soap**: 5% sulfur

Products listed are representative of currently available and widely distributed brands. Similar products, including regional and private label brands, may also exist.

PATIENT INFORMATION

Sulfur Preparations

• Keep away from eyes, eyelids, and mucous membranes.

• May cause skin irritation; discontinue use and notify physician if this occurs.

MISCELLANEOUS ACNE PRODUCTS

▶ **Actions**

The products listed below contain keratolytics and astringents to aid in removing keratin and to dry the skin. Many products also have hydroalcoholic or organic solvent bases to aid in removal of sebum. Individual components and their actions include:

Benzalkonium chloride, ethanol, isopropyl alcohol, triclosan, sulfur, acetone: Weak antiseptic properties.

Zinc oxide: Astringent.

Salicylic acid, resorcinol, sulfur: Keratolyic properties. (Note: Only concentrations of salicylic acid in the 0.5% to 2% range are FDA-approved for use in acne management. Only concentrations of sulfur of 3% to 10% are FDA-approved for use in acne management. The most effective concentrations of resorcinol in acne management are 2% to 3%.)

Titanium dioxide, zinc oxide: Protectives and adsorbants.

MISCELLANEOUS ACNE PRODUCTS	
Trade name	**Doseform**
Acnotex	**Lotion**: 8% sulfur, 2% resorcinol, 20% isopropyl alcohol
Fostril	**Lotion**: Sulfur, zinc oxide, parabens, EDTA
RA	**Lotion**: 3% resorcinol, 43% alcohol, 6% calamine
Rezamid	**Lotion**: 5% sulfur, 2% resorcinol, 28% alcohol
Sebasorb	**Lotion**: 2% salicylic acid, attapulgite
Sulforcin	**Lotion**: 5% sulfur, 2% resorcinol, 11.65% SD alcohol 40, methylparaben
Essential Care Flesh Tinted Acne Treatment Lotion	**Lotion**: 8% sulfur, 2% resorcinol
Acnomel	**Cream**: 8% sulfur, 2% resorcinol, 15% alcohol
Bensulfoid	**Cream**: 8% sulfur, 2% resorcinol, 12% alcohol
Clearasil Tinted AdultCare	**Cream**: Sulfur, resorcinol

MISCELLANEOUS ACNE PRODUCTS	
Trade name	Doseform
Stridex Body Focus Shower Gel	**Gel**: 2% salicylic acid, glycerin, parabens, witch hazel
Clearasil Clearstick Maximum Strength	**Stick**: 2% salicylic acid, 39% alcohol, menthol, EDTA
Clearasil StayClear Zone Control Clearstick	**Stick**: 2% salicylic acid, EDTA, menthol
Clean & Clear Overnight Acne Patches	**Patch**: 2% salicylic acid, glycerin
MEDICATED BAR CLEANSERS	
Clearasil Antibacterial Soap	**Bar**: Triclosan
Fostex Acne Medication Cleansing	**Bar**: 2% salicylic acid, EDTA, boric acid, lactic acid
SAStid Soap	**Bar**: 10% precipitated sulfur, EDTA
Sulfur Soap	**Bar**: 10% precipitated sulfur, EDTA
Cuticura Dry Skin Medicated Antibacterial, Cuticura Oily Skin Medicated Antibacterial, Cuticura Original Formula Medicated Antibacterial	**Bar**: 1.5% triclocarban
ABRASIVE CLEANSERS	
Brasivol	**Cleanser**: Aluminum oxide particles in a surfactant cleansing base
Pernox Scrub for Oily Skin	**Cleanser**: Sulfur, salicylic acid, EDTA
Ionax Scrub	**Scrub**: Benzalkonium chloride, SD alcohol 40
Seba-Nil Cleansing Mask	**Scrub**: SD alcohol 40, castor oil, methylparaben, titanium dioxide, bentonite
LIQUID CLEANSERS	
Clearasil Stay Clear Deep Clean Astringent	**Liquid**: 2% salicylic acid, SD alcohol 40, menthol, EDTA
Clearasil Stay Clear Acne Defense Cleanser	**Liquid**: 2% salicylic acid, glycerin, stearyl alcohol, cetyl alcohol, behenyl alcohol, menthol, EDTA
SalAc Cleanser	**Liquid**: 2% salicylic acid, benzyl alcohol, glyceryl cocoate
Essential Care Medicated Acne Treatment Cleanser	**Liquid**: 2% salicylic acid
Essential Care Exfoliating Astringent for Oily Skin	**Liquid**: 2% salicylic acid, 40% alcohol
Oxy Balance Facial Cleansing Wash	**Liquid**: 2% salicylic acid, EDTA, glycerin
Ionax Astringent Cleanser	**Liquid**: Salicylic acid, EDTA, isopropyl alcohol, acetone
Seba-Nil Oily Skin Cleanser	**Liquid**: SD alcohol 40, acetone
Tyrosum Cleanser	**Liquid**: 50% isopropanol, 10% acetone, 2% polysorbate 80
Neutrogena Oil-Free Acne Wash	**Liquid**: 2% salicylic acid
Stri-Dex Anti-Bacterial Foaming Wash	**Liquid**: 1% triclosan, aloe vera gel, glycerin, menthol, parabens, witch hazel
Neutrogena Alcohol-Free Antiseptic Cleanser	**Liquid**: 0.14% benzethonium chloride, butylene glycol, methylparaben, menthol, peppermint oil, eucalyptus oil, rosemary oil, witch hazel extract, camphor
MISCELLANEOUS CLEANSING PADS	
Stridex Facewipes to Go	**Liquid**: 0.5% salicylic acid, menthol, 28% SD alcohol 40
Clearasil StayClear Pads	**Liquid**: 2% salicylic acid, aloe barbadensis gel, SD alcohol 40, EDTA

MISCELLANEOUS ACNE PRODUCTS	
Trade name	**Doseform**
MISCELLANEOUS CLEANSING PADS	
Stri-Dex Pads	**Liquid, regular strength**: 0.5% salicylic acid, citric acid, menthol, EDTA
	Liquid, maximum strength: 2% salicylic acid, citric acid, menthol, EDTA
	Liquid, sensitive skin: 0.5% salicylic acid, citric acid, menthol, aloe barbadensis gel, EDTA, witch hazel extract
	Liquid, triple action super scrub: 2% salicylic acid, menthol, citric acid, EDTA
Oxy Balance Medicated Cleanser and Pads	**Maximum strength pads**: 2% salicylic acid, 50% alcohol, citric acid, menthol, glycerin
	Gentle pads: 0.5% salicylic acid, 22% alcohol, menthol, EDTA, glycerin
	Regular strength pads: 0.5% salicylic acid, 43% alcohol, citric acid, glycerin, menthol
	Normal skin daily cleansing pads: 0.5% salicylic acid, 34% alcohol, EDTA

Products listed are representative of currently available and widely distributed brands. Similar products, including regional and private label brands, may also exist.

PATIENT INFORMATION

Miscellaneous Acne Products

- *Note*: Rx agents may be required to assist in the management of moderate to severe acne. These may include the following: Tretinoin (*Retin-A*); topical tetracycline, erythromycin, or clindamycin; oral tetracycline, doxycyline, or minocycline; or isotretinoin (*Accutane*) for the most severe, recalcitrant forms of nodulocystic acne most likely to produce permanent scarring if not aggressively treated.

BLISTERS
(Vesicles; Bulla)

DEFINITION

A blister is a fluid-filled space under the epidermis (subepidermal) or within the epidermis (intraepidermal). If the blister is smaller than 0.5 cm, it is referred to as a vesicle. If it is larger than 0.5 cm, it is called a bulla.

ETIOLOGY

Blisters result from disturbances of intraepidermal cohesion or dermal/epidermal adhesion that are either caused or followed by influx of fluid. The list of causes for blisters is extensive, and a detailed discussion is beyond the scope of this text. A simplistic approach is to place the causes in broad categories, as follows:

Immunologic diseases (eg, dermatitis herpetiformis), poorly defined immunologic disorders (eg, erythema multiforme, minor and major), spongiosis (eg, reactions to insect bites), toxin-related disorders (eg, porphyria cutanea tarda), infections (eg, herpes zoster, impetigo, inflammatory tinea), trauma processes (eg, friction blisters), and mechanical defects (eg, epidermolysis bullosa simplex).

INCIDENCE

Traumatic blisters are exceedingly common, particularly in areas having thick, horny layers, such as the palms of the hands or soles of the feet. The incidence rates of blisters, in general, are unknown.

PATHOPHYSIOLOGY

Fluid influx into the skin is typically the end result of a sequence of pathogenic events. Impairment or loss of skin cohesion may be the primary event with resulting cleavage of the skin. Various causes may impair skin cohesion: Genetic or acquired structural defects of epidermal cells or the dermal fibrillar apparatus, neoplastic transformations, various chemical agents, immunologic reactions, and cell lysis. Traumatic blisters typically result from repetitive friction from excessive or prolonged rubbing. This results in shearing forces within the epidermis, which disrupt cell cohesion, resulting in inflammation and separation within the epidermis. Fluid influx then fills this space, causing a clinically distinguishable blister.

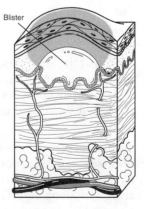

Figure 1. Blister Formation

SIGNS/SYMPTOMS

A blister will appear as a fluid-filled elevated lesion. Intact blisters may appear tense and intact or flaccid and partly ruptured, depending on the level of the cleavage within the skin. Traumatic or friction blisters typically occur on the hands and feet over bony prominences. They appear as tense, painful, non-inflammatory vesicles or bullae.

DIAGNOSTIC PARAMETERS/PHYSICAL ASSESSMENT

Clinical Observation: Blisters are diagnosed by history, clinical presentation, and, in some cases, histopathologic examination of biopsy specimens. Through observation of the signs and symptoms described above and key history points, health professionals should be able to diagnose traumatic blisters. Other causes of blisters may require further laboratory studies for diagnosis.

Interview: For a patient suspected of having a traumatic blister, inquire about the following:

- Blister location, duration, and severity.
- Precipitating events leading to blister formation.
- Patient's occupation and hobbies, including type and amount of exercise.
- Associated or additional symptoms.
- Underlying conditions (eg, diabetes, arthritis) that can exacerbate problems from blisters.

TREATMENT

Approaches to therapy: Treatment modalities will depend upon the etiology of the blistering disorder. Most traumatic blisters can be treated conservatively with non-drug and pharmacotherapeutic approaches. Nontraumatic blisters should be evaluated by a physician; their treatment is beyond the scope of this monograph.

Nondrug therapy: Prevention of traumatic blisters can be accomplished by first eliminating the source of friction or trauma. If this is not possible, then protection of the area is essential. For feet, wearing absorbent stockings reduces the moist hot environment that contributes to friction blisters. Wearing acrylic socks or 2 pairs of socks of different fabric, using foot powders, wearing properly fitted shoes, and trimming calluses may also help prevent blister formation.

To protect areas of chronic foot blistering, *Moleskin* and adhesive tape have been advocated by sports medicine professionals. Application of these adhesives on potential blister sites reduces the frictional effects on the skin by creating a frictional interface with the surface of the sock. Hydrocolloid dressings, such as *Duoderm* and *Spenco Second Skin*, are postulated to prevent blisters by cushioning the shearing forces. Benzoin tincture may decrease blisters, but contact dermatitis may occur in some patients. Initially, petroleum jelly may decrease shearing forces when locally applied; however, shearing forces may increase with prolonged activity.

To prevent forefoot blisters, toe glides have been used after taping for an athletic event. The toe glides, made of coated paper, mold to the foot through
metabolic heat and are worn over the forefoot and under the shoe counter to
decrease friction. Similarly, protection of the hands with leather gloves or
tape can be beneficial.

Treat friction blisters by leaving the epidermal roof intact so as to act as a protective membrane. Painful blisters can be drained through small punctures
at the blister edge up to 3 times in the first 24 hours. Unroofed blisters are best
treated with a hydrocolloid dressing or frequent application of an antibacterial ointment.

Pharmacotherapy: If the top of the blister is almost completely torn off, remove
it. For unroofed friction blisters, treat as an open wound; the only pharmaceutical therapy needed is a topical antibiotic ointment. If the wound appears
to be infected (ie, warm, red, and tender with pus), refer the patient to a physician, who will likely prescribe systemic antibiotic therapy.

ANTI-INFECTIVES, TOPICAL

▶ Actions

OTC topical anti-infectives may be bactericidal or bacteriostatic. Most inhibit protein synthesis. Bacitracin inhibits cell-wall synthesis. Bacitracin is most effective
against gram-positive organisms, polymyxin is more effective against gram-negative
organisms, and neomycin has both gram-positive and gram-negative antimicrobial
activity.

▶ Indications

These antibiotic preparations are used for mixed infection treatment or prophylaxis
in minor cuts, wounds, burns, and skin abrasions, as an aid to healing, and for the
treatment of superficial skin infections caused by susceptible organisms amenable to
local treatment.

▶ Contraindications

Hypersensitivity to any component of the product; ophthalmic use.

▶ Warnings

For external use only: Do not use in or near the eyes, nose, mouth, or any mucous membrane.

Systemic therapy: Deeper cutaneous infections may require systemic antibiotic therapy
in addition to local treatment. Use caution when applying over large areas of the
body or for deep puncture wounds, animal bites, or serious burns.

Neomycin toxicity: Because of the potential nephrotoxicity and ototoxicity of neomycin, use with care in treating extensive burns, trophic ulceration, or other extensive conditions where absorption is possible. Do not apply more than once daily in
burn cases where more than 20% of BSA is affected, especially if the patient has
impaired renal function or is receiving another aminoglycoside antibiotic concurrently
via a parenteral route.

Neomycin hypersensitivity: Chronic application of neomycin sulfate to inflamed skin
of individuals with allergic contact dermatitis and chronic dermatoses (eg, chronic otitis externa, stasis dermatitis) increases the possibility of sensitization. Low-grade reddening with swelling, dry scaling, and itching or a failure to heal usually are

manifestations of this hypersensitivity. During long-term use of neomycin-containing products, perform periodic examinations and discontinue use if symptoms appear. Symptoms regress upon withdrawal of medication, but avoid neomycin-containing products thereafter. Patients sensitive to neomycin generally can be treated with topical prescription gentamicin.

Superinfection: Prolonged use of topical antibiotics may result in overgrowth of non-susceptible organisms, particularly fungi. Such overgrowth may lead to a secondary infection. Discontinue the drug and take appropriate measures if superinfection occurs.

Children: Safety and effectiveness have not been established.

▶ **Adverse Reactions**

Bacitracin ointment: Allergic contact dermatitis has occurred.

Neomycin: Ototoxicity and nephrotoxicity have occurred (see Warnings) but are highly unlikely with short-term topical use.

MISCELLANEOUS ANTI-INFECTIVE PRODUCTS	
Trade name	Doseform
Baciguent	**Ointment**: 500 units bacitracin/g. Mineral oil, white petrolatum.
Neosporin	**Ointment**: 5000 units polymyxin B sulfate, 3.5 mg neomycin, 400 units bacitracin/g. White petrolatum, cottonseed oil, olive oil.
Betadine First Aid Antibiotics + Moisturizer, Polysporin	**Ointment**: 10,000 units polymyxin B sulfate, 500 units bacitracin/g. White petrolatum.
Lanabiotic Maximum Strength First Aid & Pain Relief	**Ointment**: 10,000 units polymyxin B sulfate, 5 mg neomycin, 500 units bacitracin, 40 mg lidocaine/g. Aloe, lanolin, mineral oil, petrolatum.
Betadine Plus First Aid Antibiotics + Pain Reliever	**Ointment**: 10,000 units polymyxin B sulfate, 500 units bacitracin, 10 mg pramoxine HCl/g
Maximum Strength Neosporin + Pain Relief, Spectrocin Plus	**Ointment**: 10,000 units polymyxin B sulfate, 3.5 mg neomycin, 500 units bacitracin, 10 mg pramoxine/g. White petrolatum.
Maximum Strength Neosporin + Pain Relief	**Cream**:10,000 units polymyxin B sulfate, 3.5 mg neomycin, 10 mg pramoxine/g. Methylparaben, mineral oil, white petrolatum.

Products listed are representative of currently available and widely distributed brands. Similar products, including regional and private label brands, may also exist.

PATIENT INFORMATION
Miscellaneous Anti-Infectives, Topical
- For external use only. Cleanse affected area of skin prior to application (unless directed otherwise).
- Do not use in or near the eyes.
- Apply a small amount of drug in a thin layer on the affected area 1 to 2 times daily.
- Deeper skin infections may require oral or injectable antibiotic therapy in addition to topical treatment.
- If rash or irritation develops or worsens where the antibiotic is applied, contact a physician.

BURNS

DEFINITION

A burn is defined as skin damage caused by intense heat or other physical stimuli (eg, chemical, radiation, electrical).

ETIOLOGY

Physical stimuli that can cause a burn include thermal energy (eg, fire, hot iron, stove), electricity, microwave, ultraviolet, and medical radiation, and caustic chemicals (acids and alkalis).

INCIDENCE

Recent statistics indicate that more than 2 million burns require medical attention each year in the United States, with many more unreported, but self-treated, burns.

PATHOPHYSIOLOGY

The severity of a burn is determined by temperature, duration of exposure, and extent of tissue damage or destruction.

Thermal burns: In thermal burns, the greatest damage usually is central, with coagulation necrosis of the epidermis and dermis accompanied by disruption or thrombosis of the blood vessels, a rapid loss of intravascular fluid and protein, and cell destruction. Surrounding this zone is a zone of sluggish capillary blood flow. A final surrounding zone is hyperemia caused by dilated and congested superficial blood vessels, which represent the usual inflammatory response of healthy tissue to nonlethal injury. Mild thermal burns exhibit only hyperemia.

Electrical burns: Electrical burns are caused by heat and direct injury by electricity. The severity of the injury depends on the current voltage, thickness and wetness of the skin, and duration of contact. Cell and tissue damage occurs in internal organs along the path of the electrical current.

Acidic chemicals: Acidic chemicals produce burns by causing coagulation necrosis, whereas alkalis form proteinates and saponify fats. The depth of necrosis depends on the concentration, duration of contact, and time before treatment is instituted.

Microwave radiation: Microwave radiation is nonionizing, high-frequency, and short-wavelength and can cause burns by its effect on water molecules and generation of heat. Internal tissue damage often occurs with burns from microwave radiation.

SIGNS/SYMPTOMS

Changes in skin because of burns are classified into three degrees, with a fourth degree classification representing damage beyond the skin (see Figure 1):

- **First-degree** burns only involve the epidermis. The skin is erythematous and sensitive to touch. Epidermal desquamation occurs as the skin heals. The pain and increased surface heat may be severe, and constitutional symptoms may develop if a large area is involved.

- **Second-degree** burns involve the epidermis and dermis. Serum transudation from the capillaries results in edema of the superficial tissues. Vesicles and bullae (ie, blisters) develop beneath the outer layers of the epidermis.

- **Third-degree** burns result in actual loss of the full thickness of the skin and, sometimes, subcutaneous tissues. Skin structures, such as hair follicles and sweat glands, also are destroyed. An ulcerating wound is produced and may have a pearly translucent or a brown and dry appearance.

- **Fourth-degree** burns are defined as the destruction of the entire skin, subcutaneous fat, and underlying tendons. All **third-** and **fourth-degree** burns are followed by constitutional symptoms and sometimes shock and toxemia. Complications from extensive, severe burns include infection, irregularities in electrolytes and fluid balance, loss of serum proteins, and death.

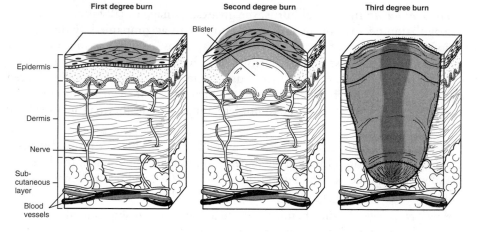

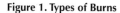

Figure 1. Types of Burns

DIAGNOSTIC PARAMETERS/PHYSICAL ASSESSMENT

Clinical Observation: Thermal burns are diagnosed primarily by the clinical presentation. The extent and severity of electrical, chemical, and radiation burns may not be readily apparent.

Interview: It is important to determine the etiology and timing of burns. Additionally, assessing thickness (degree) and extent of the burn as well as the patient's age may determine management and outcome. Any extensive or third- to fourth-degree burn is considered a medical emergency and should be evaluated promptly by a physician.

To determine the proper treatment of burns, it may be beneficial to ask about the following:

- Cause(s) of burn: Immediately refer an electrical, chemical, or radiation burn to a physician or hospital. Refer thermal burns that are extensive or third- or fourth-degree. First-degree and second-degree thermal burns involving limited areas of the body often can be self-treated.
- Size of burn: The need for medical attention for burns often is determined by the percent of body surface area (BSA) affected. A quick estimate of BSA can be made by using the patient's palm size to represent approximately 1% BSA. Immediately refer third- and fourth-degree burns of any size to a physician or hospital. Second-degree burns of less than 1% BSA and first-degree burns of any size can be self-treated. However, if these patients have constitutional symptoms (eg, fever, nausea) or signs of complications (eg, infection), physician referral is warranted.
- Location of burn: Regardless of the burn size, refer the patient to a physician if it involves the hands, face, eyes, ears, feet, or perineum, as functional or cosmetic impairment may result.
- Age of the patient: Young and elderly patients have thinner skin layers and should be referred to a physician.
- Coexisting medical conditions: Patients with compromised healing, such as those with diabetes mellitus or immune deficiency, require extra medical attention. Patients with obesity, alcoholism, or cardiovascular disease also may be more susceptible to complications.
- Duration of healing: First-degree burns usually heal within a week, and second-degree burns usually heal in 2 to 3 weeks. Delayed healing may suggest an underlying problem or infection that should be referred to a physician.

TREATMENT

Approaches to therapy: Treatment modalities depend on the extent and severity of the burn. For extensive and destructive third- and fourth-degree burns, hospital treatment will be necessary. However, small second-degree burns and most first-degree burns can be managed at home and will heal without scarring.

Nondrug therapy: Immediate treatment for minor thermal burns consists of prompt, cold applications (eg, ice water) that are continued until pain does not return. Do not open vesicles or bullae of second-degree burns unless they become tense and painful. Then, the fluid may be evacuated under aseptic conditions by needle puncture or aspiration.

Immediate, early treatment of most electrical burns and microwave radiation burns is similar to thermal burns. However, quickly refer all chemical, electrical, and microwave burns to a physician or hospital.

For significant thermal burns, use dressings to provide a mechanical barrier to extrinsic infection. Such dressings usually consist of a nonadherent inner layer, an absorptive layer, and a conforming outer bandage. Change the dressing when exudate seeps through.

For full-thickness burns (third- or fourth-degree) of less than 10% BSA, early excision and grafting usually is required.

Initial treatment of chemical burns consists of copious washing or flooding of the exposed skin with water and removal of contaminated clothing.

Moisturizing lotions may soothe itchiness that occurs with epidermal desquamation during healing of first-degree burns. For further information about moisturizers, see the Dry Skin monograph in the Dermatological Conditions chapter.

Pharmacotherapy: For mild (first-degree) burns, topical corticosteroids and oral analgesics or NSAIDs can be helpful. For further information about analgesics and NSAIDs, refer to the Aches and Pains monograph in the CNS Conditions chapter.

Small second-degree burns may be treated with a broad-spectrum, topical anti-infective ointment (except for cream) to minimize bacterial growth and keep the lesion moist while reepithelialization occurs.

Severe burns, which should be managed in the hospital, are treated with prescription antimicrobial agents to prevent bacterial colonization from developing into cellulitis or septicemia. The most widely used prescription agent is silver sulfadiazine; others include silver nitrate aqueous solution, mafenide (currently has orphan drug status), and chlorhexidine. If soft tissue infection or septicemia is suspected or confirmed, the patient is treated with appropriate systemic antibiotics administered orally or parenterally.

CORTICOSTEROIDS, TOPICAL

▶ Actions

The primary therapeutic effect of topical corticosteroids is their anti-inflammatory activity, which is nonspecific (ie, they act against most causes of inflammation, including mechanical, chemical, microbiological, and immunological).

By suppressing DNA synthesis, topical corticosteroids decrease the rate of epidermal cell formation. This property is useful in treating proliferative disorders such as psoriasis, but also can be demonstrated in normal skin.

The amount of corticosteroid absorbed from the skin depends on the intrinsic properties of the drug itself, the vehicle used, the duration of exposure, and the surface area and condition of the skin to which it is applied. In general, absorption is enhanced by increased skin temperature, hydration, application to inflamed or denuded skin, intertriginous areas (eg, eyelids, groin, axilla), or skin surfaces with a thin stratum corneum layer (eg, face, scrotum). Palms, soles, and crusted skin surfaces are less permeable. Occlusive dressings greatly enhance skin penetration, and therefore increase drug absorption.

Infants and children have a higher total body surface-to-body weight ratio that decreases with age. Therefore, proportionately more of any topical medication will be absorbed systemically in this population, which puts infants and children at a greater risk for systemic effects.

Vehicles: Ointments are more greasy and occlusive and are preferred for dry, scaly lesions. Therefore, use creams on oozing lesions or in intertriginous areas where the occlusive effects of ointments may cause maceration and folliculitis. Creams often are preferred by patients for aesthetic reasons, although their water content makes them more drying than ointments. Gels, aerosols, lotions, and solutions are useful on hairy areas. Urea enhances the penetration of hydrocortisone and selected steroids by hydrating the skin. As a general rule, ointments and gels are slightly more potent than creams or lotions. However, optimized vehicles that have been formulated for some products have demonstrated equal potency in cream, gel, and ointment forms. Steroid impregnated tapes are useful for occlusive therapy in small areas.

Occlusive dressings: Occlusive dressings, such as a plastic wrap, increase skin penetration approximately 10-fold by increasing the moisture content of the stratum corneum. Occlusion can be beneficial in resistant cases, but it also may lead to sweat retention and increased bacterial and fungal infections. Additionally, increased absorption of corticosteroids may produce systemic side effects. Therefore, do not use occlusive dressings for longer than 12 hours/day or when using very potent topical corticosteroids or unless directed to do so by a physician.

Relative potency: The relative potency of a product depends on several factors, including the characteristics and concentrations of the drug and the vehicle used.

▶ Indications

Relief of inflammatory and pruritic manifestations of a variety of corticosteroid-responsive dermatoses (eg, contact dermatoses, contact dermatitis, rash, pruritus, minor skin inflammation).

Topical corticosteroids are indicated for alternative/adjunctive treatment of psoriasis. More specifically, nonprescription hydrocortisone preparations are indicated for temporary relief of itching or inflammation caused by psoriasis.

▶ Contraindications

Hypersensitivity to any component of the product; treatment of rosacea, perioral dermatitis, or acne; use on the face, groin, or axilla (very high or high-potency agents); ophthalmic use (prolonged ocular exposure may cause steroid-induced glaucoma and cataracts).

▶ Warnings

Systemic effects: Systemic absorption of chronically applied topical corticosteroids, particularly the high-potency prescription products, has produced reversible hypothalamic-pituitary-adrenal (HPA) axis suppression, Cushing syndrome, hyperglycemia, and glycosuria. Conditions that augment systemic absorption include the application of more potent steroids, use over large surface areas, prolonged use, and the use of occlusive dressings.

As a general rule, little effect on the HPA axis will occur with use of an OTC or prescription topical corticosteroid in amounts of less than 50 g weekly for an adult and 15 g weekly for a small child, without occlusion. To cover the adult body 1 time requires 12 to 26 g.

Local irritation: If local irritation develops, discontinue use and wash affected area with mild soap and water. Medications containing alcohol may produce dry skin or burning sensations/irritation in open lesions. Allergic contact dermatitis usually is diagnosed by observing the failure to heal rather than noting clinical exacerbation, as with most topical products that do not contain corticosteroids.

Skin atrophy – Skin atrophy is common and may be clinically significant after 3 to 4 weeks of regular use of potent prescription preparations. Atrophy occurs most readily at sites where percutaneous absorption is high.

Patients should exercise caution when using around the eye or in the genital area. The use of high-potency prescription formulations on the face and in intertriginous areas should be avoided because of resulting striae.

Psoriasis: Do not use nonprescription or prescription topical corticosteroids as the sole form of therapy in patients with widespread plaque.

In rare instances, treatment (or withdrawal of treatment) of psoriasis with corticosteroids is thought to have provoked the pustular form of the disease.

Atrophic changes: Certain areas of the body, such as the face, groin, and axillae, are more prone to atrophic changes than other areas of the body following chronic treatment with topical corticosteroids. Frequent observation of the patient is important if these areas are to be treated.

Infections: In the presence of an infection, institute appropriate therapy. If a favorable response does not occur promptly, discontinue the corticosteroid until the infection has been controlled. Treating skin infections with topical corticosteroids can worsen the infection.

For external use only: Avoid ingestion, contact with the eyes, or the inhalation of steroid-containing aerosols.

Vehicles: Many topical corticosteroids are in specially formulated bases designed to maximize their release and potency. Mixing these formulations with other bases or vehicles may affect the potency of the drug far beyond what would normally be expected from the dilution. Exercise caution before mixing; if necessary, contact the manufacturer to determine if there may be an incompatibility.

Occlusive therapy: Discontinue the use of occlusive dressings if infection develops, and institute appropriate therapy.

Pregnancy: Category C. Corticosteroids are teratogenic in animals when administered systemically at relatively low doses. The more potent corticosteroids are teratogenic after dermal application in animals. There are no adequate and well-controlled studies in pregnant women. Therefore, use during pregnancy only if the potential benefits outweigh the potential hazards to the fetus. In pregnant patients, do not use in large amounts or for prolonged periods of time.

Lactation: It is not known whether topical corticosteroid application could result in sufficient systemic absorption to produce detectable quantities in breast milk. Systemic corticosteroids are secreted into breast milk in quantities not likely to have a deleterious effect on the infant. Nevertheless, exercise caution when administering topical corticosteroids to a nursing mother.

Children: Children may be more susceptible to topical corticosteroid-induced HPA axis suppression and Cushing syndrome than adults because of their larger skin surface area-to-body weight ratio.

Hypothalamic-pituitary axis suppression, Cushing syndrome, and intracranial hypertension have occurred in children receiving topical corticosteroids. Manifestations of adrenal suppression include linear growth retardation, delayed weight gain, low plasma cortisol levels, and absence of response to adrenocorticotropic hormone (ACTH) stimulation.

Limit administration to the least amount compatible with effective therapy. Chronic corticosteroid therapy may interfere with children's growth and development.

▶ **Adverse Reactions**

Burning; itching; irritation; erythema; dryness; folliculitis; hypertrichosis; pruritus; acneiform eruptions; hypopigmentation; perioral dermatitis; allergic contact dermatitis; numbness of fingers; stinging and cracking or tightening of skin; maceration of the skin; secondary infection; skin atrophy; striae; miliaria; telangiectasia. These may occur more frequently with the use of occlusive dressings.

There also have been reports of development of pustular psoriasis from chronic plaque psoriasis following reduction or discontinuation of potent topical corticosteroids.

Sensitivity to a particular dressing material or adhesive may occur occasionally.

▶ **Administration and Dosage**

Usual dosage: Apply sparingly to affected areas 2 to 4 times daily.

General considerations: Topical corticosteroids have a repository effect; with continuous use, 1 or 2 applications/day may be as effective as 3 or more. Many clinicians advise applying twice daily until clinical response is achieved and then only as frequently as needed to control the condition.

Short-term or intermittent therapy using high-potency prescription agents (eg, every other day, 3 to 4 consecutive days per week, or once per week) may be more effective and cause fewer adverse effects than continuous regimens using lower-potency products.

Only use low-potency agents in children, on large areas, and on body sites especially prone to steroid damage (eg, the face, scrotum, axillae, flexures, and skin folds). Reserve higher-potency agents for areas and conditions resistant to treatment with milder agents.

TOPICAL CORTICOSTEROID PRODUCTS	
Trade name	Doseform
Cortizone•5	**Ointment**: 0.5% hydrocortisone. Excipients.
Cortizone•10	**Ointment**: 1% hydrocortisone. Benzyl alcohol, SD alcohol 40.
Hydrocortisone	**Ointment**: 1% hydrocortisone. Mineral oil, white petrolatum.
Cortaid Maximum Strength	**Ointment**: 1% hydrocortisone (as acetate). Parabens, mineral oil, white petrolatum.
Hydrocortisone Acetate	**Ointment**: 1% hydrocortisone (as acetate). Aloe, white petrolatum.
Cortizone•5	**Cream**: 0.5% hydrocortisone. Parabens, glycerin, mineral oil, white petrolatum, aloe.
Corticaine	**Cream**: 0.5% hydrocortisone. Methylparaben, mineral oil, white petrolatum, menthol, stearyl alcohol, EDTA.
Cortaid Sensitive Skin Formula with Aloe	**Cream**: 0.5% hydrocortisone (as acetate). Aloe, parabens.
Hydrocortisone	**Cream**: 1% hydrocortisone. Aloe, cetearyl alcohol, glycerin, methylparaben.
Cortaid Intensive Therapy	**Cream**: 1% hydrocortisone. Parabens, cetyl alcohol, stearyl alcohol.
Cortizone•10	**Cream**: 1% hydrocortisone. Parabens, glycerin, mineral oil, white petrolatum, cetearyl alcohol, aloe.
Cortaid Maximum Strength	**Cream**: 1% hydrocortisone. Benzyl alcohol, cetearyl alcohol, glycerin, methylparaben, aloe.

TOPICAL CORTICOSTEROID PRODUCTS

Trade name	Doseform
Maximum Strength HydroZone Plus	**Cream**: 1% hydrocortisone. Benzyl alcohol, glycerin, stearyl alcohol.
LanaCort Maximum Strength	**Cream**: 1% hydrocortisone (as acetate). Glycerin, mineral oil, cetyl alcohol, lanolin, EDTA, parabens, menthol, aloe.
HydroZone Plus, Hydrocortisone	**Lotion**: 1% hydrocortisone. Cetyl alcohol.
CortaGel Maximum Strength	**Gel**: 1% hydrocortisone. Ethanol, aloe, EDTA.
CortiCool	**Gel**: 1% hydrocortisone, 45% alcohol, benzethonium chloride
Cortaid Intensive Therapy	**Spray**: 1% hydrocortisone. EDTA, glycerin, 45% SD alcohol 40.

Products listed are representative of currently available and widely distributed brands. Similar products, including regional and private label brands, may also exist.

PATIENT INFORMATION

Topical Corticosteroids

- For external use only. Cleanse affected area of skin prior to application (unless directed otherwise).
- Apply ointments, creams, or gels sparingly in a light film. Rub in gently. Washing or soaking the area before application may increase drug penetration.
- To use a lotion, solution, or gel on your scalp, part your hair, apply a small amount of the medicine on the affected area, and rub it in gently. Protect the area from washing, clothing, rubbing, etc., until the medicine dries. You may wash your hair as usual, but not immediately after applying the medicine.
- Use only as directed. Do not put bandages, dressings, cosmetics, or other skin products over the treated area unless directed by a physician.
- Notify a physician if the condition being treated worsens or if burning, swelling, or redness develop.
- Avoid prolonged use around the eyes, in the genital and rectal areas, and on the face, armpits, and skin creases unless directed by a physician. Avoid contact with the eyes.
- If you forget a dose, apply it as soon as you remember and continue on your regular schedule. If it is almost time for the next application, wait and continue on your regular schedule. Do not apply double doses.
- *For parents of pediatric patients*: Consult a physician. If corticosteroid treatment is recommended, do not use tight-fitting diapers or plastic pants on a child treated in the diaper area; these garments may work like occlusive dressings and cause more of the drug to be absorbed into your child's body. Do not use topical steroids to treat diaper rash.

ANTI-INFECTIVES, TOPICAL

▶ **Actions**

OTC topical anti-infectives may be bactericidal or bacteriostatic. Most inhibit protein synthesis. Bacitracin inhibits cell-wall synthesis. Bacitracin is most effective against gram-positive organisms, polymyxin is more effective against gram-negative organisms, and neomycin has both gram-positive and gram-negative antimicrobial activity.

▶ **Indications**

These antibiotic preparations are used for mixed-infection treatment or prophylaxis in minor cuts, wounds, burns, and skin abrasions, as an aid to healing, and for the treatment of superficial skin infections caused by susceptible organisms amenable to local treatment.

▶ **Contraindications**

Hypersensitivity to any component of the product; ophthalmic use.

▶ **Warnings**

For external use only: Do not use in or near the eyes, nose, mouth, or any mucous membrane.

Systemic therapy: Deeper cutaneous infections may require systemic antibiotic therapy in addition to local treatment. Use caution when applying over large areas of the body or for deep puncture wounds, animal bites, or serious burns.

Neomycin toxicity: Because of the potential nephrotoxicity and ototoxicity of neomycin, use with care in treating extensive burns, trophic ulceration, or other extensive conditions where absorption is possible. Do not apply more than once daily in burn cases where more than 20% of BSA is affected, especially if the patient has impaired renal function or is receiving another aminoglycoside antibiotic concurrently via a parenteral route.

Neomycin hypersensitivity: Chronic application of neomycin sulfate to inflamed skin of individuals with allergic contact dermatitis and chronic dermatoses (eg, chronic otitis externa, stasis dermatitis) increases the possibility of sensitization. Low-grade reddening with swelling, dry scaling, and itching or a failure to heal usually are manifestations of this hypersensitivity. During long-term use of neomycin-containing products, perform periodic examinations and discontinue use if symptoms appear. Symptoms regress upon withdrawal of medication, but avoid neomycin-containing products thereafter. Patients sensitive to neomycin generally can be treated with topical prescription gentamicin.

Superinfection: Prolonged use of topical antibiotics may result in overgrowth of non-susceptible organisms, particularly fungi. Such overgrowth may lead to a secondary infection. Discontinue the drug and take appropriate measures if superinfection occurs.

Children: Safety and effectiveness have not been established.

▶ **Adverse Reactions**

Bacitracin ointment: Allergic contact dermatitis has occurred.

Neomycin: Ototoxicity and nephrotoxicity have occurred (see Warnings) but are highly unlikely with short-term topical use.

MISCELLANEOUS ANTI-INFECTIVE PRODUCTS	
Trade name	**Doseform**
Baciguent	**Ointment**: 500 units bacitracin/g. Mineral oil, white petrolatum.
Neosporin	**Ointment**: 5000 units polymyxin B sulfate, 3.5 mg neomycin, 400 units bacitracin/g. White petrolatum, cottonseed oil, olive oil.
Betadine First Aid Antibiotics + Moisturizer, Polysporin	**Ointment**: 10,000 units polymyxin B sulfate, 500 units bacitracin/g. White petrolatum.

MISCELLANEOUS ANTI-INFECTIVE PRODUCTS	
Trade name	Doseform
Lanabiotic Maximum Strength First Aid & Pain Relief	**Ointment**: 10,000 units polymyxin B sulfate, 5 mg neomycin, 500 units bacitracin, 40 mg lidocaine/g. Aloe, lanolin, mineral oil, petrolatum.
Betadine Plus First Aid Antibiotics + Pain Reliever	**Ointment**: 10,000 units polymyxin B sulfate, 500 units bacitracin, 10 mg pramoxine HCl/g
Maximum Strength Neosporin + Pain Relief, Spectrocin Plus	**Ointment**: 10,000 units polymyxin B sulfate, 3.5 mg neomycin, 500 units bacitracin, 10 mg pramoxine/g. White petrolatum.
Maximum Strength Neosporin + Pain Relief	**Cream**:10,000 units polymyxin B sulfate, 3.5 mg neomycin, 10 mg pramoxine/g. Methylparaben, mineral oil, white petrolatum.

Products listed are representative of currently available and widely distributed brands. Similar products, including regional and private label brands, may also exist.

PATIENT INFORMATION

Miscellaneous Anti-Infectives, Topical

- For external use only. Cleanse affected area of skin prior to application (unless directed otherwise).
- Do not use in or near the eyes.
- Apply a small amount of drug in a thin layer on the affected area 1 to 2 times daily.
- Deeper skin infections may require oral or injectable antibiotic therapy in addition to topical treatment.
- If rash or irritation develops or worsens where the antibiotic is applied, contact a physician.

LOCAL ANESTHETICS, TOPICAL

▶ Actions

Local anesthetics inhibit conduction of nerve impulses from sensory nerves. They are poorly absorbed through intact epidermis.

▶ Indications

Topical anesthesia in many different local skin disorders involving itching and pain, including pain caused by sunburn.

▶ Contraindications

Hypersensitivity to any component of these products; ophthalmic use.

▶ Warnings

Pregnancy: Category B (lidocaine); *Category C* (benzocaine).

Lactation: Lidocaine is excreted in breast milk. Exercise caution when administering any of these drugs to a nursing woman.

Children: Do not use benzocaine in infants younger than 1 year of age. Reduce dosages in children commensurate with age, body weight, and physical condition.

▶ Drug Interactions

Use with caution in patients receiving class I antiarrhythmic drugs because the toxic effects are additive and potentially synergistic.

▶ **Adverse Reactions**

In general, adverse reactions are dose-related and may result from high plasma levels because of excessive dosage, rapid absorption, hypersensitivity, idiosyncrasy, or diminished tolerance. Patients may have hypersensitivity reactions (urticaria, edema, contact dermatitis) or local reactions (burning, stinging, tenderness).

▶ **Administration and Dosage**

Apply to affected area as needed. Ointments and creams may be applied to gauze or a bandage prior to applying on the skin. Duration of local anesthetic effect is relatively brief (20 to 30 minutes). More than three to four applications/day generally is discouraged.

BENZOCAINE

BENZOCAINE PRODUCTS	
Trade name	Doseform
Benzocaine	Cream: 5%

Products listed are representative of currently available and widely distributed brands. Similar products, including regional and private label brands, may also exist.

DIBUCAINE

DIBUCAINE PRODUCTS	
Trade name	Doseform
Dibucaine	Ointment: 1%. Lanolin, white petrolatum.

Products listed are representative of currently available and widely distributed brands. Similar products, including regional and private label brands, may also exist.

LIDOCAINE

LIDOCAINE PRODUCTS	
Trade name	Doseform
L.M.X. 4	Cream: 4% lidocaine. 1.5% benzyl alcohol.
Solarcaine Aloe Extra Burn Relief	Gel: 0.5%. Aloe, glycerin, isopropyl alcohol, menthol, EDTA.
	Spray: 0.5%. Aloe, parabens, EDTA.

Products listed are representative of currently available and widely distributed brands. Similar products, including regional and private label brands, may also exist.

PRAMOXINE HCL

PRAMOXINE HCL PRODUCTS	
Trade name	Doseform
Prax	Lotion: 1%. Cetyl alcohol, glycerin, coconut oil, lanolin, mineral oil, petrolatum.
Pramegel	Gel: 1%. 0.5% menthol, alcohol SD 40.
Itch-X	Gel: 1% pramoxine, 10% benzyl alcohol. Aloe, SD alcohol 40, parabens.
	Spray: 1% pramoxine, 10% benzyl alcohol. Aloe, SD alcohol 40.

Products listed are representative of currently available and widely distributed brands. Similar products, including regional and private label brands, may also exist.

LOCAL ANESTHETIC COMBINATIONS, TOPICAL

TOPICAL LOCAL ANESTHETIC COMBINATION PRODUCTS	
Trade name	Doseform
Foille Medicated First Aid	**Ointment**: 5% benzocaine, 0.1% chloroxylenol. Benzyl alcohol, EDTA in corn oil base.
	Spray: 5% benzocaine, 0.6% chloroxylenol. Benzyl alcohol in corn oil base.
Unguentine Maximum Strength	**Cream**: 5% benzocaine, 2% resorcinol. Aloe, cetyl alcohol, lanolin, methylparaben, mineral oil.
Lanacane	**Cream**: 6% benzocaine, 0.1% benzethonium chloride. Aloe, parabens, castor oil, glycerin, isopropyl alcohol.
Bactine Original First Aid	**Liquid**: 2.5% lidocaine, 0.13% benzalkonium chloride. EDTA.
Bactine Pain Relieving Cleansing Spray	**Spray**: 2.5% lidocaine, 0.13% benzalkonium chloride. EDTA.
Lanacane Maximum Strength	**Spray**: 20% benzocaine, 0.1% benzethonium chloride, 36% ethanol. Aloe.
Dermoplast	**Spray**: 20% benzocaine, 0.2% benzethonium chloride. Methylparaben, aloe, lanolin.
Bactine Pain Relieving Cleansing Wipes	**Wipes**: 1% pramoxine, 0.13% benzalkonium chloride. EDTA.

Products listed are representative of currently available and widely distributed brands. Similar products, including regional and private label brands, may also exist.

PATIENT INFORMATION

Local Anesthetics, Topical

- For external use only. Cleanse affected area of skin prior to application (unless directed otherwise).
- Do not use in the eyes.
- Ointments are more greasy; creams may be preferred in some cases.
- Not intended for prolonged use.
- Some of these products contain tartrazine or sulfites, which can cause allergic-type reactions in susceptible individuals.
- Use the lowest concentration and frequency of application needed for symptom relief to avoid excessive absorption into the blood and serious adverse effects.

VITAMINS A, D, AND E, TOPICAL

▶ Indications

Temporary relief of discomfort caused by sunburn and other minor dermal conditions.

▶ Administration and Dosage

Apply locally to affected skin with gentle massage as needed.

TOPICAL VITAMINS A, D, AND E PRODUCTS	
Trade name	Doseform
Vitamin A and Vitamin D	**Ointment**: Vitamin A, D. Lanolin, white petrolatum.
Lazer Creme	**Cream**: 100,000 IU vitamin A, 3500 IU vitamin E/oz. Parabens.

TOPICAL VITAMINS A, D, AND E PRODUCTS	
Trade name	Doseform
Lobana Derm-ADE	**Cream**: Vitamins A, D, and E. Lanolin, stearyl alcohol, cetyl alcohol, vegetable oil, parabens.
Vitamin E-Cream	**Cream**: 100 IU vitamin E. Cetearyl alcohol, mineral oil, wheat germ oil, parabens, petrolatum.
Alph-E	**Cream**: 6000 IU vitamin E, 600 IU vitamin A, 60 IU vitamin D. Wheat germ oil, emollient base.

Products listed are representative of currently available and widely distributed brands. Similar products, including regional and private label brands, may also exist.

PATIENT INFORMATION

Vitamins A, D, and E, Topical

- For external use only. Cleanse affected area of skin prior to application (unless directed otherwise).
- Do not use in the eyes.
- If the condition worsens or does not improve within three to five days, consult a physician.

CALLUSES
(Tylomas)

DEFINITION

A callus is a thickening of the epidermal layer (hyperkeratosis) that results from chronic, repeated trauma, friction, or pressure. It is usually broad-based and of relatively even thickness.

ETIOLOGY

Calluses are caused by repeated pressure or friction to an area, usually where there is a bony prominence and excessive pronation of the foot. Poor footwear and faulty foot mechanics (usually due to deformity) are common etiologies.

INCIDENCE

Calluses typically occur on the hands or feet and are more common in women.

PATHOPHYSIOLOGY

Vasodilation, then hyperkeratosis and increased epidermal cell turnover, are normal physiological responses to chronic, excessive pressure or friction to the skin. The hyperkeratosis results in increased pressure that results in further hyperkeratosis, thereby setting up a vicious cycle. Unlike corns, calluses do not have a central core.

SIGNS/SYMPTOMS

Calluses are raised areas of tissue that are usually off-white or brownish in color and have the normal pattern of skin ridges on the surface. They range in size from a few millimeters to a few centimeters in diameter. When the horny skin is trimmed away, it reveals only heaped up keratin with preserved skin markings; no black dots are visible.

Diffuse calluses are typically asymptomatic. **Thick calluses** can cause a painful, burning sensation. Calluses can cause serious morbidity in patients with diabetes mellitus or in patients with compromised circulation to the extremities. In these patients, ulceration or infection may occur as a complication.

DIAGNOSTIC PARAMETERS/PHYSICAL ASSESSMENT

Clinical Observation: Base diagnosis on clinical presentation through observation of signs and symptoms described above.

Interview: To help the patient determine if physician referral or self-treatment is warranted, it may be beneficial to ask about the following:

- Location and size of callus.
- Physical appearance of callus.
- Degree of pain or irritation caused by the callus.
- Past attempts to remove calluses and degree of success achieved.

- Ability to perform work functions while treating the callus (treatment needs to stay in contact with callus).
- Other medical conditions (eg, diabetes, compromised circulation).
- Include lifestyle questions about occupation, hobbies, etc. that may be precipitating or confounding callus formation.

TREATMENT

Approaches to therapy: A callus is a physical manifestation of increased mechanical stress; it is not a disease in itself. Therefore, it is important that treatment provides symptomatic relief, determining the cause of the irritation and then removing this cause. Treatment depends on the location and severity of the callus and on the physical condition of the patient. Remove the callus with caution because the callus provides protection to the underlying tissue. Elimination or reduction of the cause of the increased pressure to the affected site is essential. Freezing calluses with liquid nitrogen is sometimes an option for more severe cases.

Nondrug therapy: Relief from calluses is usually provided by debridement. Diffuse calluses can be easily controlled by gentle, regular trimming using a pumice stone or emery board after soaking the tissue in warm water for approximately 15 minutes. Excessive pressure can be relieved with orthotic devices such as pads, rings, *Moleskin*, arch inserts, and foam rubber protective bandages. Low-heeled, soft, well fitting shoes are critical.

Pharmacotherapy: Topical salicylic acid is the only OTC keratolytic agent considered safe and effective by the FDA for the treatment of calluses. Any topical wart medicine with salicylic acid can be used to treat calluses. Two parts propylene glycol to 1 part water under plastic occlusion can be effective.

TOPICAL SALICYLIC ACID

▶ **Actions**

Pharmacology: Salicylic acid is the only OTC product considered safe and effective by the FDA for use as a keratolytic for corns, calluses, and warts. Salicylic acid produces desquamation of the horny layer of skin, while not adversely affecting the structure of the viable epidermis, by dissolving intercellular cement substance. The keratolytic action causes the cornified epithelium to swell, soften, macerate, and then desquamate.

Salicylic acid is keratolytic at concentrations of approximately 2% to 6%. These concentrations generally are used for treatment of dandruff, seborrhea, and psoriasis. Concentrations of 5% to 17% in collodion are safe and effective for the removal of common and plantar warts; up to 40% salicylic acid in plasters is used to remove warts, corns, and calluses.

Salicylic acid preparations, alone or in combination, have also been used to treat dandruff, seborrheic dermatitis, acne, tinea infections, and psoriasis.

Pharmacokinetics: In a study of the percutaneous absorption of salicylic acid in 4 patients with extensive active psoriasis, peak serum salicylate levels never exceeded 5 mg/dL even though more than 60% of the applied salicylic acid was absorbed.

Systemic toxic reactions are usually associated with much higher serum levels (30 to 40 mg/dL). Peak serum levels occurred within 5 hours of the topical application under occlusion.

The major urinary metabolites identified after topical administration differ from those after oral salicylate administration; those derived from percutaneous absorption contain more salicylate glucuronides (42%) and less salicyluric (52%) and salicylic acid (6%).

▶ Indications

A topical aid in the removal of excessive keratin in hyperkeratotic skin disorders, including common and plantar warts, psoriasis, calluses, and corns.

The use of a 40% salicylic acid disk covered with an adhesive strip has been used to aid in the removal of inaccessible splinters in children.

▶ Contraindications

Sensitivity to salicylic acid; prolonged use, especially in infants, diabetics, and patients with impaired circulation; use on moles, birthmarks, or warts with hair growing from them; genital or facial warts; or warts on mucous membranes, irritated skin, or any area that is infected or reddened.

▶ Warnings

Salicylate toxicity: Prolonged use over large areas, especially in young children and those patients with significant renal or hepatic impairment, could result in salicylism. Limit the area to be treated and be aware of signs of salicylate toxicity (eg, nausea, vomiting, dizziness, loss of hearing, tinnitus, lethargy, hyperpnea, diarrhea, psychic disturbances). In the event of salicylic acid toxicity, discontinue use.

Refer to the Aspirin section in the Aches and Pains monograph in the CNS Conditions chapter for additional information on the systemic effects of salicylates.

For external use only: Avoid contact with eyes, eyelids, mucous membranes, and normal skin surrounding warts. If contact with eyes, eyelids, or mucous membranes occurs, immediately flush with tap water for 15 minutes. Avoid inhaling vapors.

Special risk patients: Do not use if diabetes or poor blood circulation exists.

Pregnancy: Category C.

▶ Drug Interactions

Interactions have been reported with topical and oral salicylates. Refer to the Aspirin section in the Aches and Pains monograph in the CNS Conditions chapter for a complete listing of drug interactions.

▶ Adverse Reactions

Local irritation may occur from contact with normal skin surrounding the affected area. If irritation occurs, temporarily discontinue use and take care to apply only to the callus site when treatment is resumed.

▶ Administration and Dosage

For specific instructions for use of these products, refer to individual product labeling.

Apply to affected area. May soak in warm water for 5 minutes prior to use to hydrate skin and enhance the effect. Remove any loose tissue with brush, washcloth, or emery board, and dry thoroughly.

In general, for treatment of calluses, improvement should occur in 1 to 2 weeks; maximum resolution may be expected after 4 to 6 weeks, although application for up to 12 weeks may be necessary. If skin irritation develops or there is no improvement after several weeks, contact a physician.

Storage/Stability: Some products are flammable; keep away from fire or flame. Keep bottle tightly capped and store at room temperature, away from heat.

TOPICAL SALICYLIC ACID PRODUCTS	
Trade name	Doseform
Dr. Scholl's Callus Removers	**Disk**: 40% in a rubber-based vehicle
Dr. Scholl's Cushlin Gel Callus Removers	**Disk**: 40% in a rubber-based vehicle
Dr. Scholl's Extra-Thick Callus Removers	**Disk**: 40% in a rubber-based vehicle
Dr. Scholl's OneStep Callus Removers	**Disk**: 40% in a rubber-based vehicle
Dr. Scholl's Corn/Callus Remover	**Liquid**: 12.6% in flexible collodion base with 18% alcohol, 55% ether, acetone, hydrogenated vegetable oil
Maximum Strength Freezone Corn and Callus Remover	**Liquid**: 17.6%, 33% alcohol, 65.5% ether, castor oil
Maximum Strength Freezone One Step Callus Remover	**Medicated pads**: 40% in a plaster vehicle
Mosco	**Liquid**: 17.6% in a flexible collodion base with 33% alcohol and 65.5% ether
Mediplast	**Plaster**: 40%
Sal-Acid	**Plaster**: 40% in a collodion-like vehicle

Products listed are representative of currently available and widely distributed brands. Similar products, including regional and private label brands, may also exist.

PATIENT INFORMATION
Salicylic Acid

- Follow label directions and package insert instructions.
- For external use only. Avoid contact with eyes, eyelids, face, genitals, mucous membranes, and normal skin surrounding lesion. For liquid products, normal skin may be protected by surrounding the affected area with petrolatum jelly.
- Medication may cause reddening or scaling of skin.
- Contact with clothing, fabrics, plastics, wood, metal, or other materials may cause damage; avoid contact.
- Do not use if you are a diabetic or have poor circulation.
- Do not use on irritated skin or any area that is reddened or infected.
- Wash hands after using this product.
- Keep out of reach of children.
- With liquid products, keep the lid tightly closed and store at room temperature, away from heat, fire, or flame. Do not inhale vapors.

CONTACT DERMATITIS

DEFINITION

Dermatitis simply means inflammation of the skin, without indicating a cause. Contact dermatitis is inflammation resulting from "contact" or exposure of the skin to a substance, and symptoms may be acute, subacute, or chronic.

ETIOLOGY

Allergic contact dermatitis: Allergic contact dermatitis is a skin eruption caused by a delayed hypersensitivity (allergic) reaction to a known or unknown substance. Poison ivy and poison oak dermatitis is the prototype for this type of reaction, but any allergen to which the skin is sensitized (eg, antibiotics, local anesthetics, antiseptics) can be the cause.

Irritant contact dermatitis: Irritant contact dermatitis is a skin eruption caused by exposure to a chemical that is too harsh for the skin. As opposed to allergic dermatitis, which is less common and involves a person's immunologic reaction to a chemical, irritant dermatitis can be induced in almost any person if the concentration of the offending chemical is great enough. Strongly acidic or alkaline drugs can cause obvious symptoms soon after exposure. Mild irritants in soaps or cosmetics, for example, may not produce symptoms immediately.

Photoallergic/Phototoxic contact dermatitis: Occasionally, the addition of sunlight to an offending agent (either systemic or topical) may cause a contact dermatitis. In these cases, the conditions are termed phototoxic dermatitis and photoallergic contact dermatitis.

INCIDENCE

Contact dermatitis is widespread, with irritant dermatitis more prevalent than allergic dermatitis. The incidence varies in different population groups because exposure to different allergens or irritants varies according to lifestyle or environmental conditions. For example, women are more likely than men to manifest allergies to nickel because of their higher usage of jewelry. The incidence of rhus dermatitis (poison ivy or poison oak) is higher in North America than in Europe because of the greater potential for exposure to the plant in North America. Similarly, the incidence of irritant dermatitis is determined by the group being studied; for example, the incidence of irritant dermatitis to cement is much higher in construction workers than in white-collar workers.

PATHOPHYSIOLOGY

In *allergic contact dermatitis*, sensitization to a chemical is the result of a complex interaction of an allergen and the skin, causing altered (sensitized) lymphocytes that react to it. This reaction may develop up to 8 to 10 days after exposure to the allergen. However, once skin is sensitized to a chemical, the reaction occurs more quickly (often within a day or so) upon re-exposure. The ability to become sensitized to a chemical seems to be a genetic trait, with some people having more "allergic" skin than others.

Some factors that can increase a person's likelihood to become sensitized are: Constant exposure to the chemical, application of the chemical to already inflamed skin, and occlusion of the chemical against the skin.

In *irritant contact dermatitis*, an offending chemical or substance causes direct damage to the skin cells, which triggers the release of a variety of chemical mediators of the inflammatory response. Unlike allergic dermatitis, no previous exposure or sensitization to the substance is needed. Strong irritants may produce acute, severe ulcerating damage (eg, "chemical burn"), whereas weak irritants may produce just minor erythema, itching, sensitivity to foreign objects secondary to inflammation, or scaling.

The key distinction between allergic and irritant contact dermatitis is the immunologic mechanism of allergic dermatitis. However, both conditions lead to the common pathway of the inflammatory response.

In the case of *phototoxic contact dermatitis*, a chemical is either on the skin or circulating in the blood stream (in the superficial capillary plexus of the skin) and sufficient sunlight causes a toxic reaction, generally manifested as an exaggerated sunburn. A common example is the tetracycline + sunlight phototoxic reaction. This type of reaction is easily avoided by lowering the amount of incident sunlight energy that a person receives while using the offending agent, generally by not being in the sun or by using a sunblock. (A sunscreen will not be useful in these cases, as the causative sunlight wavelength generally will not be locked out.)

In cases of photoallergic contact dermatitis, the patient is allergic to a chemical moiety, which is induced by the reaction of a drug/chemical (either topical or systemic) plus sunlight energy. Because this represents an allergic reaction rather than a toxic reaction, the incidence of these reactions is smaller, and the amount of either sunlight or offending agent required to cause the reaction is smaller than is seen in a phototoxic reaction. In addition, the time of onset of the 2 reactions are different, with a phototoxic reaction occurring within hours of sunlight exposure, whereas a photoallergic reaction requires several days to occur. Once again, avoidance of sunlight (of the peculiar wavelength that causes the new chemical moiety to be made) is crucial to the course of treatment. Here, though, strict avoidance of the particular wavelength is necessary, because such a small amount of sun is necessary to trigger the reaction.

There is no single specific wavelength that causes the problems associated with photoallergic and phototoxic contact dermatitis. Each chemical has an excitability wavelength that is determined by the chemical itself. This "action spectrum" is determined by each chemical's ability to absorb certain wavelengths, but in general, the wavelengths fall within the UVA range.

SIGNS/SYMPTOMS

Symptoms of acute allergic and irritant contact dermatitis are redness, itching, mild-to-moderate pain, and swelling, and may progress in severe cases to oozing vesicles or bullae. Erythema, scaling, and vesicles may be seen with subacute dermatitis. Chronic contact dermatitis reveals the repeated damage and repair cycle by the skin with hyperkeratosis, lichenification, and fissures.

The distribution of the eruption often gives a clue as to the chemical cause. For example, an eruption on an earlobe may indicate an allergy to the metal in an earring; an eruption on the hands and forearms may indicate irritation from soaps, lotions, or cleaning solutions.

DIAGNOSTIC PARAMETERS/PHYSICAL ASSESSMENT

Clinical Observation: Acute contact dermatitis from a strong irritant will be evidenced by pain, swelling, and ulceration (eg, "chemical burn"). However, most cases of contact dermatitis are due to repeated exposure to an allergen or a mild irritant. Generally the patient will complain of an itchy red rash. The causative chemical may or may not be readily obvious.

Interview: To help determine if the process is allergic or irritant, the patient's history is important. If the eruption developed only recently and is seen only in 1 patient, then it may represent an allergic reaction. For example, a recent trip to the country or a weekend of cleaning out a garden helps to establish poison ivy as a possible cause. If several people who perform the same job at the patient's workplace have recently developed the eruption, then an irritant reaction is the likely cause. Only patch testing can absolutely confirm an allergic dermatitis.

It may be beneficial to ask about the following:

- Description, location, and duration of symptoms.
- A recent new exposure to a chemical or other allergen or a recent new activity in the workplace or at home.
- Chronic exposure to a chemical and the type of work or pleasure activity associated with this exposure.
- The number of people with the same type of rash in the person's immediate circle of friends or coworkers.

TREATMENT

Approaches to therapy: Depending upon the severity, location, and the extent of eruption, health care providers may recommend a non-drug approach, appropriate pharmacotherapy, or referral to a physician for medical evaluation and treatment.

Nondrug therapy: The patient should avoid further exposure to the suspected or known irritant or allergen. The patient should also avoid using any personal care products (eg, soaps, cleansers, lotions) on the lesions. Frequent cool water soaks may help oozing and swelling. Mild skin scaling and itchiness may respond to a bland moisturizer.

Pharmacotherapy: Soaks or wet dressings containing an astringent (eg, aluminum sulfate) might be used for oozing, weeping eruptions, although their efficacy may not be any greater than water alone. Baths containing colloidal oatmeal can relieve itching from extensive pruritic lesions. Topical corticosteroids may be applied 2 to 4 times daily if the dermatitis is confined to a relatively small area; creams and lotions might be preferable for vesicular lesions, whereas the occlusive and moisture-retaining effects of an ointment might be more beneficial for chronic scaling lesions. Take care to use a preparation that does not contain an ingredient to which the patient may be allergic; several cream preparations contain parabens. Oral antihistamines may help control pruritus. Do not use topical antihistamines because they are often allergenic.

WET DRESSINGS AND SOAKS

▶ **Actions**

These dressings, soaks, and baths ease pruritus. Astringents (eg, aluminum acetate) have a drying effect and should be used only if there are weeping lesions. Cool baths containing colloidal oatmeal may be more convenient when lesions are widespread.

▶ **Indications**

To reduce oozing and provide relief from itching from vesicular lesions.

WET DRESSING AND SOAK PRODUCTS	
Trade name	**Doseform**
Aveeno Oilated	**Bath**: 43% natural colloidal oatmeal, mineral oil
Aveeno Regular	**Bath**: 100% natural colloidal oatmeal
Nutra•Soothe	**Bath**: Colloidal oatmeal, oat oil
ActBath	**Effervescent Tablets**: 20% colloidal oatmeal
Dermasil	**Lotion**: Glycerin, dimethicone, sunflower seed oil, petrolatum, borage seed oil, vitamin E acetate, vitamin A palmitate, vitamin D_3, corn oil, EDTA, methylparaben
Alpha Keri Therapeutic Bath, Ultra Derm Bath	**Oil**: Mineral oil, lanolin oil, octoxynol-3
Aveeno Shower & Bath	**Oil**: 5% colloidal oatmeal, mineral oil, glyceryl stearate, PEG 100 stearate, laureth-4, benzyl alcohol, silica benzaldehyde
Cameo	**Oil**: Mineral oil, PEG-8 dioleate, lanolin oil
Lubriderm Bath	**Oil**: Mineral oil, PPG-15, stearyl ether oleth-2, nonoxynol-5
Nutraderm Bath	**Oil**: Mineral oil, lanolin oil, PEG-4 dilaurate, benzophenone-3, butylparaben
RoBathol Bath	**Oil**: Cottonseed oil, alkyl aryl polyether alcohol
Sardo Bath & Shower	**Oil**: Mineral oil, tocopherol
Therapeutic Bath	**Oil**: Mineral oil, lanolin oil

Products listed are representative of currently available and widely distributed brands. Similar products, including regional and private label brands, may also exist.

■ ■ ■

PATIENT INFORMATION
Wet Dressing and Soak Products
- For external use only.
- Avoid overuse and contact with eyes.
- If skin irritation develops or becomes excessive, discontinue use and consult your doctor.

ALUMINUM ACETATE SOLUTION

▶ Indications
Aluminum acetate solution provides an astringent wet dressing for relief of inflammatory conditions of the skin.

▶ Warnings
Discontinue use if intolerance, irritation, or extension of the inflammatory condition being treated occurs. If symptoms persist longer than 7 days, discontinue use and consult a physician.

Do not use plastic or other impervious material to prevent evaporation.

For external use only. Avoid contact with the eyes.

▶ Drug Interactions
Collagenase: The enzyme activity of topical collagenase may be inhibited by aluminum acetate solution because of the metal ion and low pH. Cleanse the site of the solution with repeated washings of normal saline before applying the enzyme ointment.

▶ Administration and Dosage
One packet or tablet in a pint of water produces a modified 1:40 Burow's solution. Apply for 15 to 30 minutes for 4 to 6 times daily. Wetting gauze with the solution is a suggested method for application to smaller, defined areas (eg, hand, arm, face, foot).

ALUMINUM ACETATE SOLUTION PRODUCTS	
Trade name	Doseform
Domeboro Astringent Solution, Pedi-Boro Soak Paks	**Powder, tablets**: Aluminum sulfate and calcium acetate.

Products listed are representative of currently available and widely distributed brands. Similar products, including regional and private label brands, may also exist.

PATIENT INFORMATION
Aluminum Acetate Solution
- For external use only. Do not use in eyes or allow to come in contact with the eye(s) or eyelid(s).
- Do not use if you are allergic to any ingredient of the products.
- Do not use on irritated or broken skin without consulting a physician or pharmacist.
- If the condition persists or worsens, or if irritation develops, discontinue use and consult a physician.
- Apply to affected skin with gentle massage as instructed by a physician.

MISCELLANEOUS EMOLLIENTS

► Actions

These preparations lubricate and moisturize the skin, counteracting dryness and itching. Some of the listed ingredients in products that act as emollients are butyl stearate, cetyl alcohol, glycerin, glyceryl monostearate, isopropyl myristate, isopropyl palmitate, lanolin, lanolin alcohol, mineral oil, petrolatum, propylene glycol stearate, squalene, stearic acid, and stearyl alcohol.

In certain products, some of the aquaphilic chemicals used to attract water to the skin are urea and alpha-hydroxy acids. These chemicals, while useful, often will sting when applied to dry skin.

MISCELLANEOUS EMOLLIENT PRODUCTS	
Trade name	Doseform
Aquaphor	**Ointment:** Petrolatum, mineral oil, ceresin, lanolin alcohol, panthenol, glycerin, bisabolol
Balmex Daily Protective Clear	**Ointment:** White petrolatum, cyclomethicone, dimethicone, polyethylene, silica, mineral oil, tocopheryl acetate
AmLactin	**Cream:** 12% ammonium lactate. Light mineral oil, glyceryl stearate, PEG-100 stearate, propylene glycol, glycerin, magnesium aluminum silicate, laureth-4, polyoxyl 40 stearate, cetyl alcohol, parabens, methylcellulose
AmLactin AP	**Cream:** 12% ammonium lactate, 1% pramoxine hydrochloride
Cutemol	**Cream:** Liquid petrolatum, lanolin alcohols extract, mineral wax, beeswax, acetylated lanolin, isopropyl myristate, sorbitan sesquioleate, sodium tetraborate, imidurea, allantoin, parabens
DML Forte	**Cream:** Petrolatum, propylene glycol dioctanoate, glyceryl stearate, PEG-100 stearate, glycerin, stearic acid, DEA-cetyl phosphate, DEX-panthenol, PVP/Eicosene copolymer, simethicone, benzyl alcohol, cetyl alcohol, silica, EDTA, acrylates/C10-30 alkyl acrylate crosspolymer, triethanolamine, magnesium aluminum silicate
Eucerin Original	**Cream:** Mineral oil, petrolatum, mineral oil, ceresin, lanolin alcohol, methylchloroisothiazolinone, methylisothiazolinone
Geri-Hydrolac 12%	**Cream:** Ammonium lactate (equivalent to 12% lactic acid), light mineral oil, petrolatum, propylene glycol, glycerin, cetyl alcohol, parabens
Hydrisinol	**Cream:** Mineral oil, petrolatum, hydrogenated vegetable oil, lanolin, beeswax, paraffin wax, sulfonated castor oil, parabens
Hydrocerin	**Cream:** Petrolatum, mineral oil, mineral wax, ceresin lanolin alcohol, parabens
Lanolor	**Cream:** Glyceryl stearates, propylene glycol, cetyl esters wax, isopropyl palmitate, cetyl alcohol, lanolin oil, sodium lauryl sulfate, methylparaben, simethicone, polyoxyl 40 stearate, sorbic acid
Minerin	**Cream:** Petrolatum, mineral oil, mineral wax, alcohol, methylchloroisothiazolinone, methylisothiazolinone

MISCELLANEOUS EMOLLIENT PRODUCTS

Trade name	Doseform
Neutrogena Norwegian Formula Hand Cream	**Cream:** Glycerin, sodium cetearyl sulfate, sodium sulfate, parabens
Nutraderm	**Cream:** Mineral oil, sorbitan stearate, stearyl alcohol, sorbitol, citric acid, cetyl esters wax, sodium lauryl sulfate, dimethicone, parabens, diazolidinyl urea
Pen•Kera	**Cream:** Cetyl palmitate, glycerin, mineral oil, polysorbate 60, sorbitan stearate, polyamino sugar condensate, urea, wheat germ glycerides, carbomer 940, triethanolamine, DMDM hydantoin, iodopropynyl butylcarbanate, diazolidinyl urea, dehydroacetic acid
Polysorb Hydrate	**Cream:** Cetyl esters wax, mineral oil, perfume oil bouquet, sorbitan sesquioleale, white petrolatum, white wax
Purpose Dry Skin	**Cream:** Mineral oil, white petrolatum, sweet almond oil, propylene glycol, glyceryl stearate, xanthan gum, steareth-2, steareth-20, sodium lactate, cetyl esters wax, lactic acid
Allercreme Skin	**Lotion:** Mineral oil, sorbitol, triethanolamine, parabens
AmLactin	**Lotion:** 12% ammonium lactate. Light mineral oil, glyceryl stearate, PEG-100 stearate, propylene glycol, glycerin, magnesium aluminum silicate, laureth-4, polyoxyl 40 stearate, cetyl alcohol, parabens, methylcellulose
Aquanil	**Lotion:** Glycerin, benzyl alcohol, sodium laureth sulfate, cetyl alcohol, stearyl alcohol, xanthan gum
Aveeno	**Lotion:** 1% colloidal oatmeal, glycerin, phenylcarbinol, petrolatum, dimethicone, benzyl alcohol
Corn Huskers	**Lotion:** Glycerin, SD alcohol 40, sodium calcium alginate, oleyl sarcosine, methylparaben, guar gum, triethanolamine, calcium sulfate, calcium chloride, fumaric acid, boric acid
Curel Original	**Lotion:** Glycerin, distearyldimonium chloride, petrolatum, isopropyl palmitate, cetyl alcohol, dimethicone, sodium chloride, parabens
Curel Soothing Hands	**Lotion:** Glycerin, petrolatum, distearyldimonium chloride, isopropyl palmitate, cetyl alcohol, aluminum starch octenylsuccinate, dimethicone, *Anthemis nobilis* flower extract, tocopheryl acetate, ascorbyl palmitate, panthenol, parabens, propylene glycol
Curel Ultra Healing	**Lotion:** Glycerin, petrolatum, cetearyl alcohol, behentrimonium chloride, cetyl-PG hydroxyethyl pamitamide, isopropyl palmitate, avena sativa (oat) meal extract, *Eucalyptus globus* leaf extract, *Citrus aurantium dulcis* (orange) oil, cyclomethicone, dimethicone, cholesteryl isostearate, BIS-PEG-15 dimethicone/IPDI copolymer, DMDM hydantoin
Derma Viva	**Lotion:** Mineral oil, glyceryl stearate, laureth-4, lanolin oil, PEG-100 stearate, PEG-40 stearate, PEG-4 dilaurate, trolamine, DSS, parabens

MISCELLANEOUS EMOLLIENT PRODUCTS

Trade name	Doseform
DML	Lotion: Petrolatum, glycerin, methyl glucose sesquistearate, dimethicone, PEG-20 methyl glucose sesquistearate, benzyl alcohol, cyclomethicone, glyceryl stearate, stearic acid, cetyl alcohol, sodium carbomer 941, xanthan gum, magnesium aluminum silicate
Emollia	Lotion: Mineral oil, cetyl alcohol, propylene glycol, white wax, sodium lauryl sulfate, oleic acid, parabens
Epilyt	Lotion: Propylene glycol, glycerin, oleic acid, quaternium-26, lactic acid, BHT
Esotérica Dry Skin Treatment	Lotion: Propylene glycol, dicaprylate/dicapric, mineral oil, glyceryl stearate, cetyl esters wax, hydrolyzed animal protein, dimethicone, TEA-carbomer-941, parabens
Eucerin Daily Replenishing	Lotion: Dimethicone, sunflower seed oil, petrolatum, glycerin, glyceryl stearate SE, octyldodecanol, panthenol, caprylic/capric triglyceride, tocopherol acetate, stearic acid, cholesterol, cetearyl alcohol, lanolin alcohol, carbomer, EDTA, sodium hydroxide, phenoxyethanol, parabens, BHT
Eucerin Plus Intensive Repair	Lotion: Mineral oil, PEG-7 hydrogenated castor oil, isohexadecane, sodium lactate, urea, glycerin, isopropyl palmitate, panthenol, microcrystalline wax, magnesium sulfate, lanolin alcohol, bisabolol, methylchloroisothiazolinone, methylisothiazolinone
Geri-Soft	Lotion: Mineral oil, propylene glycol, cetearyl alcohol, sorbitol, petrolatum, dimethicone, lanolin, castor oil, stearic acid, parabens, stearyl alcohol, EDTA, lemon oil
Geri SS	Lotion: Mineral oil, propylene glycol, cetearyl alcohol, petrolatum, glycerin, dimethicone, colloidal oatmeal, hydrogenated castor oil, parabens, stearyl alcohol, EDTA, lemon oil, tocopheryl acetate
Hydrisinol	Lotion: Propylene glycol stearate SE, hydrogenated vegetable oil, stearic acid, sulfonated castor oil, mineral oil, lanolin, lanolin alcohol, sesame oil, sunflower oil, aloe, triethanolamine, sorbitan stearate, hydroxyethyl cellulose, parabens
Hydrocerin	Lotion: EDTA, lanolin, parabens, mineral oil, PEG-40 sorbitan, peroleate, propylene glycol, sorbitol, water
Jergen's Ash Relief Moisturizer	Lotion: Glycerin, cetearyl alcohol, petrolatum, mineral oil, ceteareth-20, cyclomethicone, dimethicone, theobroma cacao (cocoa) seed butter, butyrospermum parkii (shea butter), tridecyl salicylate, tocopheryl acetate, stearic acid, glyceryl dilaurate, aluminum starch octenylsuccinate, acrylates/C10-30 alkyl acrylate crosspolymer, parabens, DMDM hydantoin, sodium hydroxide
Jergen's Ultra Healing Intense Moisture Therapy	Lotion: Glycerin, distearyldimonium chloride, petrolatum, isopropyl palmitate, cetyl alcohol, dimethicone, parabens, sodium chloride

MISCELLANEOUS EMOLLIENT PRODUCTS

Trade name	Doseform
Keri	**Lotion**: Mineral oil, glycerin, PEG-40 stearate, glyceryl stearate, PEG-100 stearate, PEG-4 dilaurate, laureth-4, aloe, sunflower seed oil, tocopheryl acetate, carbomer, parabens, DMDM hydantoin, iodopropynyl butylcarbamate, sodium hydroxide, EDTA
Lac-Hydrin Five	**Lotion**: 5% ammonium lactate, glycerin, petrolatum, squalane, steareth-2, POE-21-stearyl ether, propylene glycol dioctanoate, cetyl alcohol, dimethicone, cetyl palmitate, magnesium aluminum silicate, diazolidinyl urea, methylchloroisothiazolinone, methylisothiazolone
LactiCare	**Lotion**: Mineral oil, 5% lactic acid, isopropyl palmitate, sodium PCA, stearyl alcohol, ceteareth-20, sodium hydroxide, glyceryl stearate, PEG-100 stearate, myristyl lactate, cetyl alcohol, carbomer, DMDM hydantoin, parabens
Lobana Body	**Lotion**: Mineral oil, triethanolamine stearate, stearic acid, cetyl alcohol, lanolin, potassium stearate, aloe, propylene glycol, parabens
Lubriderm Advanced Therapy	**Lotion**: Cetyl alcohol, glycerin, mineral oil, cyclomethicone, propylene glycol discaprylate/dicaprate, PEG-40 stearate, isopropyl isostearate, emulsifying wax, lecithin, carbomer 940, diazolidinyl urea, titanium dioxide, sodium benzoate, tri (PPG-3 myristyl ether) citrate, EDTA, retinyl palmitate, tocopheryl acetate, sodium pyruvate, iodopropynyl butylcarbamate, sodium hydroxide, xanthan gum
Lubriderm Seriously Sensitive	**Lotion**: Butylene glycol, mineral oil, petrolatum, glycerin, cetyl alcohol, propylene glycol dicaprylate/dicaprate, PEG-40 stearate, C11-13 isoparaffin, glyceryl stearate, tri (PPG-3 myristyl ether) citrate, emulsifying wax, dimethicone, DMDM hydantoin, parabens, carbomer 940, titanium dioxide, EDTA, sodium hydroxide, xanthan gum
Lubriderm Skin Firming	**Lotion**: Isostearic acid, stearic acid, steareth-21, sodium lactate, PPG 12/SMDI copolymer, lactic acid, steareth-2, magnesium aluminum silicate, cetyl alcohol, imidurea, potassium sorbate, xanthan gum
Lubriderm Skin Renewal Firming	**Lotion**: Gluconolactone, propylene glycol, cetearyl glucoside/cetearyl alcohol, cyclomethicone, stearic acid, propylene glycol dicaprylate-dicaprate, C12-15 alkyl benzoate, isohexyl caprate, isocetyl stearate, triethanolamine, dimethicone, glycerin, petrolatum, glyceryl stearate, PEG-100 stearate, cetyl alcohol, emulsifying wax, steareth-2, diazolidinyl urea, EDTA, tocopheryl acetate, glycine, xanthan gum, hydroxyethyl cellulose, iodopropynyl butylcarbamate
Lubriderm Skin Therapy	**Lotion**: Mineral oil, petrolatum, sorbitol, stearic acid, lanolin, lanolin alcohol, cetyl alcohol, glyceryl stearate/PEG-100 stearate, triethanolamine, dimethicone, propylene glycol, microcrystalline wax, tri (PPG-3 myristyl ether) citrate, EDTA, parabens, xanthan gum, methyldibromo glutaronitrile

MISCELLANEOUS EMOLLIENT PRODUCTS

Trade name	Doseform
Lubriskin	**Lotion**: Mineral oil, petrolatum, lanolin, lanolin alcohol, cetearyl alcohol, castor oil, triethanolamine, stearyl alcohol, propylene glycol, parabens, EDTA
Minerin	**Lotion**: Mineral oil, isopropyl myristate, PEG-40 sorbitan peroleate, lanolin acid, glycerin ester, sorbitol, propylene glycol, cetyl palmitate, magnesium sulfate, aluminum stearate, lanolin alcohol, methylchloroisothiazolinone, methylisothiazolinone, BHT
Moisturel	**Lotion**: 3% dimethicone, benzyl alcohol, carbomer, cetyl alcohol, glycerin, laureth-23, magnesium aluminum silicate, petrolatum, potassium sorbate, sodium hydroxide, steareth-2
Neutrogena Body	**Lotion**: Glyceryl stearate, PEG-100 stearate, imidazolidinyl urea, carbomer-954, parabens, sodium lauryl sulfate, triethanolamine
Nutraderm	**Lotion**: Mineral oil, sorbitan stearate, stearyl alcohol, sodium lauryl sulfate, carbomer 940, diazolidinyl urea, parabens, triethanolamine
Shepard's	**Lotion**: Glycerin, sesame oil, vegetable oil, SD alcohol 40-B, propylene glycol, ethoxydiglycol, triethanolamine, glyceryl stearate, cetyl alcohol, simethicone, monoglyceride citrate, parabens
Sofenol 5	**Lotion**: Glycerin, petrolatum, cetearyl alcohol, soluble collagen, dimethicone, PEG-40-stearate, allantoin, sunflower seed oil, kaolin, sorbic acid, carbomer 940, sodium hydroxide
Therapeutic Bath	**Lotion**: Mineral oil, glyceryl stearate, PEG-100 stearate, propylene glycol, PEG-40 stearate, laureth-4, PEG-4 dilaurate, lanolin oil, parabens, quaternium-15, carbomer 934, trolamine, dioctyl sodium sulfosuccinate
Wibi	**Lotion**: Glycerin, SD alcohol 40, PEG-4, PEG-6-32 stearate, PEG-6-32, carbomer-940, PEG-75, parabens, triethanolamine, menthol
Neutrogena Body	**Oil**: Sesame oil, PEG-40 sorbitan peroleate

Products listed are representative of currently available and widely distributed brands. Similar products, including regional and private label brands, may also exist.

PATIENT INFORMATION

Emollients

- For external use only. Do not use in eyes or allow to come in contact with the eye(s) or eyelid(s).
- Do not use if you are allergic to any ingredient of the products.
- Do not use on irritated or broken skin without consulting a physician or pharmacist.
- If the condition persists or worsens or if irritation develops, discontinue use and consult a physician.
- Apply to affected skin with gentle massage as instructed by a physician.

CORTICOSTEROIDS, TOPICAL

▶ **Actions**

The primary therapeutic effect of topical corticosteroids is their anti-inflammatory activity, which is nonspecific (ie, they act against most causes of inflammation, including mechanical, chemical, microbiological, and immunological).

By suppressing DNA synthesis, topical corticosteroids decrease the rate of epidermal cell formation. This property is useful in treating proliferative disorders such as psoriasis, but also can be demonstrated in normal skin.

The amount of corticosteroid absorbed from the skin depends on the intrinsic properties of the drug itself, the vehicle used, the duration of exposure, and the surface area and condition of the skin to which it is applied. In general, absorption is enhanced by increased skin temperature, hydration, application to inflamed or denuded skin, intertriginous areas (eg, eyelids, groin, axilla), or skin surfaces with a thin stratum corneum layer (eg, face, scrotum). Palms, soles, and crusted skin surfaces are less permeable. Occlusive dressings greatly enhance skin penetration, and therefore increase drug absorption.

Infants and children have a higher total body surface-to-body weight ratio that decreases with age. Therefore, proportionately more of any topical medication will be absorbed systemically in this population, which puts infants and children at a greater risk for systemic effects.

Vehicles: Ointments are more greasy and occlusive and are preferred for dry, scaly lesions. Therefore, use creams on oozing lesions or in intertriginous areas where the occlusive effects of ointments may cause maceration and folliculitis. Creams often are preferred by patients for aesthetic reasons, although their water content makes them more drying than ointments. Gels, aerosols, lotions, and solutions are useful on hairy areas. Urea enhances the penetration of hydrocortisone and selected steroids by hydrating the skin. As a general rule, ointments and gels are slightly more potent than creams or lotions. However, optimized vehicles that have been formulated for some products have demonstrated equal potency in cream, gel, and ointment forms. Steroid impregnated tapes are useful for occlusive therapy in small areas.

Occlusive dressings: Occlusive dressings, such as a plastic wrap, increase skin penetration approximately 10-fold by increasing the moisture content of the stratum corneum. Occlusion can be beneficial in resistant cases, but it also may lead to sweat retention and increased bacterial and fungal infections. Additionally, increased absorption of corticosteroids may produce systemic side effects. Therefore, do not use occlusive dressings for longer than 12 hours/day or when using very potent topical corticosteroids or unless directed to do so by a physician.

Relative potency: The relative potency of a product depends on several factors, including the characteristics and concentrations of the drug and the vehicle used.

▶ **Indications**

Relief of inflammatory and pruritic manifestations of a variety of corticosteroid-responsive dermatoses (eg, contact dermatoses, contact dermatitis, rash, pruritus, minor skin inflammation).

Topical corticosteroids are indicated for alternative/adjunctive treatment of psoriasis. More specifically, nonprescription hydrocortisone preparations are indicated for temporary relief of itching or inflammation caused by psoriasis.

▶ **Contraindications**

Hypersensitivity to any component of the product; treatment of rosacea, perioral dermatitis, or acne; use on the face, groin, or axilla (very high or high-potency agents); ophthalmic use (prolonged ocular exposure may cause steroid-induced glaucoma and cataracts).

▶ **Warnings**

Systemic effects: Systemic absorption of chronically applied topical corticosteroids, particularly the high-potency prescription products, has produced reversible hypothalamic-pituitary-adrenal (HPA) axis suppression, Cushing syndrome, hyperglycemia, and glycosuria. Conditions that augment systemic absorption include the application of more potent steroids, use over large surface areas, prolonged use, and the use of occlusive dressings.

As a general rule, little effect on the HPA axis will occur with use of an OTC or prescription topical corticosteroid in amounts of less than 50 g weekly for an adult and 15 g weekly for a small child, without occlusion. To cover the adult body 1 time requires 12 to 26 g.

Local irritation: If local irritation develops, discontinue use and wash affected area with mild soap and water. Medications containing alcohol may produce dry skin or burning sensations/irritation in open lesions. Allergic contact dermatitis usually is diagnosed by observing the failure to heal rather than noting clinical exacerbation, as with most topical products that do not contain corticosteroids.

    Skin atrophy – Skin atrophy is common and may be clinically significant after 3 to 4 weeks of regular use of potent prescription preparations. Atrophy occurs most readily at sites where percutaneous absorption is high.

Patients should exercise caution when using around the eye or in the genital area. The use of high-potency prescription formulations on the face and in intertriginous areas should be avoided because of resulting striae.

Psoriasis: Do not use nonprescription or prescription topical corticosteroids as the sole form of therapy in patients with widespread plaque.

In rare instances, treatment (or withdrawal of treatment) of psoriasis with corticosteroids is thought to have provoked the pustular form of the disease.

Atrophic changes: Certain areas of the body, such as the face, groin, and axillae, are more prone to atrophic changes than other areas of the body following chronic treatment with topical corticosteroids. Frequent observation of the patient is important if these areas are to be treated.

Infections: In the presence of an infection, institute appropriate therapy. If a favorable response does not occur promptly, discontinue the corticosteroid until the infection has been controlled. Treating skin infections with topical corticosteroids can worsen the infection.

For external use only: Avoid ingestion, contact with the eyes, or the inhalation of steroid-containing aerosols.

Vehicles: Many topical corticosteroids are in specially formulated bases designed to maximize their release and potency. Mixing these formulations with other bases or vehicles may affect the potency of the drug far beyond what would normally be expected from the dilution. Exercise caution before mixing; if necessary, contact the manufacturer to determine if there may be an incompatibility.

Occlusive therapy: Discontinue the use of occlusive dressings if infection develops, and institute appropriate therapy.

Pregnancy: Category C. Corticosteroids are teratogenic in animals when administered systemically at relatively low doses. The more potent corticosteroids are teratogenic after dermal application in animals. There are no adequate and well-controlled studies in pregnant women. Therefore, use during pregnancy only if the potential benefits outweigh the potential hazards to the fetus. In pregnant patients, do not use in large amounts or for prolonged periods of time.

Lactation: It is not known whether topical corticosteroid application could result in sufficient systemic absorption to produce detectable quantities in breast milk. Systemic corticosteroids are secreted into breast milk in quantities not likely to have a deleterious effect on the infant. Nevertheless, exercise caution when administering topical corticosteroids to a nursing mother.

Children: Children may be more susceptible to topical corticosteroid-induced HPA axis suppression and Cushing syndrome than adults because of their larger skin surface area-to-body weight ratio.

Hypothalamic-pituitary axis suppression, Cushing syndrome, and intracranial hypertension have occurred in children receiving topical corticosteroids. Manifestations of adrenal suppression include linear growth retardation, delayed weight gain, low plasma cortisol levels, and absence of response to adrenocorticotropic hormone (ACTH) stimulation.

Limit administration to the least amount compatible with effective therapy. Chronic corticosteroid therapy may interfere with children's growth and development.

▶ Adverse Reactions

Burning; itching; irritation; erythema; dryness; folliculitis; hypertrichosis; pruritus; acneiform eruptions; hypopigmentation; perioral dermatitis; allergic contact dermatitis; numbness of fingers; stinging and cracking or tightening of skin; maceration of the skin; secondary infection; skin atrophy; striae; miliaria; telangiectasia. These may occur more frequently with the use of occlusive dressings.

There also have been reports of development of pustular psoriasis from chronic plaque psoriasis following reduction or discontinuation of potent topical corticosteroids.

Sensitivity to a particular dressing material or adhesive may occur occasionally.

▶ Administration and Dosage

Usual dosage: Apply sparingly to affected areas 2 to 4 times daily.

General considerations: Topical corticosteroids have a repository effect; with continuous use, 1 or 2 applications/day may be as effective as 3 or more. Many clinicians advise applying twice daily until clinical response is achieved and then only as frequently as needed to control the condition.

Short-term or intermittent therapy using high-potency prescription agents (eg, every other day, 3 to 4 consecutive days per week, or once per week) may be more effective and cause fewer adverse effects than continuous regimens using lower-potency products.

Only use low-potency agents in children, on large areas, and on body sites especially prone to steroid damage (eg, the face, scrotum, axillae, flexures, and skin folds). Reserve higher-potency agents for areas and conditions resistant to treatment with milder agents.

TOPICAL CORTICOSTEROID PRODUCTS

Trade name	Doseform
Cortizone•5	**Ointment**: 0.5% hydrocortisone. Excipients.
Cortizone•10	**Ointment**: 1% hydrocortisone. Benzyl alcohol, SD alcohol 40.
Hydrocortisone	**Ointment**: 1% hydrocortisone. Mineral oil, white petrolatum.
Cortaid Maximum Strength	**Ointment**: 1% hydrocortisone (as acetate). Parabens, mineral oil, white petrolatum.
Hydrocortisone Acetate	**Ointment**: 1% hydrocortisone (as acetate). Aloe, white petrolatum.
Cortizone•5	**Cream**: 0.5% hydrocortisone. Parabens, glycerin, mineral oil, white petrolatum, aloe.
Corticaine	**Cream**: 0.5% hydrocortisone. Methylparaben, mineral oil, white petrolatum, menthol, stearyl alcohol, EDTA.
Cortaid Sensitive Skin Formula with Aloe	**Cream**: 0.5% hydrocortisone (as acetate). Aloe, parabens.
Hydrocortisone	**Cream**: 1% hydrocortisone. Aloe, cetearyl alcohol, glycerin, methylparaben.
Cortaid Intensive Therapy	**Cream**: 1% hydrocortisone. Parabens, cetyl alcohol, stearyl alcohol.
Cortizone•10	**Cream**: 1% hydrocortisone. Parabens, glycerin, mineral oil, white petrolatum, cetearyl alcohol, aloe.
Cortaid Maximum Strength	**Cream**: 1% hydrocortisone. Benzyl alcohol, cetearyl alcohol, glycerin, methylparaben, aloe.
Maximum Strength HydroZone Plus	**Cream**: 1% hydrocortisone. Benzyl alcohol, glycerin, stearyl alcohol.
LanaCort Maximum Strength	**Cream**: 1% hydrocortisone (as acetate). Glycerin, mineral oil, cetyl alcohol, lanolin, EDTA, parabens, menthol, aloe.
HydroZone Plus, Hydrocortisone	**Lotion**: 1% hydrocortisone. Cetyl alcohol.
CortaGel Maximum Strength	**Gel**: 1% hydrocortisone. Ethanol, aloe, EDTA.
CortiCool	**Gel**: 1% hydrocortisone, 45% alcohol, benzethonium chloride
Cortaid Intensive Therapy	**Spray**: 1% hydrocortisone. EDTA, glycerin, 45% SD alcohol 40.

Products listed are representative of currently available and widely distributed brands. Similar products, including regional and private label brands, may also exist.

PATIENT INFORMATION
Topical Corticosteroids
- For external use only. Cleanse affected area of skin prior to application (unless directed otherwise).
- Apply ointments, creams, or gels sparingly in a light film. Rub in gently. Washing or soaking the area before application may increase drug penetration.
- To use a lotion, solution, or gel on your scalp, part your hair, apply a small amount of the medicine on the affected area, and rub it in gently. Protect the area from washing, clothing, rubbing, etc., until the medicine dries. You may wash your hair as usual, but not immediately after applying the medicine.
- Use only as directed. Do not put bandages, dressings, cosmetics, or other skin products over the treated area unless directed by a physician.
- Notify a physician if the condition being treated worsens or if burning, swelling, or redness develop.
- Avoid prolonged use around the eyes, in the genital and rectal areas, and on the face, armpits, and skin creases unless directed by a physician. Avoid contact with the eyes.
- If you forget a dose, apply it as soon as you remember and continue on your regular schedule. If it is almost time for the next application, wait and continue on your regular schedule. Do not apply double doses.
- *For parents of pediatric patients*: Consult a physician. If corticosteroid treatment is recommended, do not use tight-fitting diapers or plastic pants on a child treated in the diaper area; these garments may work like occlusive dressings and cause more of the drug to be absorbed into your child's body. Do not use topical steroids to treat diaper rash.

ANTIHISTAMINES, ORAL
▶ Actions
Antihistamines competitively antagonize histamine at the H_1-receptor site but do not bind with histamine to inactivate it. Antihistamines do not block histamine release, antibody production, or antigen-antibody interactions. They have antipruritic effects.

▶ Indications
For the relief of mild, uncomplicated allergic skin manifestations of urticaria and angioedema. For the symptomatic relief of allergic and non-allergic pruritic symptoms. These agents have other labeled indications as well.

▶ Contraindications
Hypersensitivity to antihistamines; newborn or premature infants; nursing mothers; narrow-angle glaucoma; stenosing peptic ulcer; symptomatic prostatic hypertrophy; bladder neck obstruction; pyloroduodenal obstruction; lower respiratory tract symptoms (including asthma); MAOI use.

▶ Warnings
Sleep apnea: If possible, avoid sedatives, CNS depressants, and drugs with CNS depressant activity in patients with a history of sleep apnea.

Hypersensitivity reactions: Hypersensitivity reactions may occur, and any of the usual manifestations of drug allergy may develop.

Pregnancy: Category B.

Lactation: Because of the higher risk of adverse effects for infants generally and for newborns and premature infants in particular, antihistamine therapy is contraindicated in nursing mothers.

Children: Antihistamines may diminish mental alertness; conversely, they may occasionally produce excitation, particularly in the young child. Use in children younger than 2 years of age only as directed by a physician.

Elderly: Antihistamines are more likely to cause dizziness, excessive sedation, syncope, toxic confusional states, and hypotension in patients 60 years of age and older. They may also cause paradoxical stimulation, particularly in pediatric and geriatric patients. Dosage reduction or drug discontinuation may be required.

▶ Drug Interactions

Concomitant use of alcohol or other CNS depressants with antihistamines may result in an additive CNS-depressant effect. MAOIs may prolong and intensify the anticholinergic effects of antihistamines.

▶ Adverse Reactions

Adverse reactions of severe magnitude are relatively rare but may include the following: Peripheral, angioneurotic, and laryngeal edema; dermatitis; asthma; lupus erythematosus-like syndrome; urticaria; drug rash; anaphylactic shock; photosensitivity; postural hypotension; palpitations; bradycardia; tachycardia; reflex tachycardia; extrasystoles; faintness; hypertension; hypotension; cardiac arrest; ECG changes; drowsiness, sedation; dizziness; faintness; disturbed coordination; epigastric distress; urinary frequency; dysuria; urinary retention; early menses; induced lactation; gynecomastia; inhibition of ejaculation; hemolytic anemia; hypoplastic anemia; aplastic anemia; thrombocytopenia; leukopenia; agranulocytosis; pancytopenia; thickening of bronchial secretions; tingling, heaviness, and weakness of the hands; thrombocytopenic purpura; excessive perspiration; chills.

DIPHENHYDRAMINE HCL

▶ Administration and Dosage

Tablets, caplets, capsules, and softgels:

Adults and children (12 years of age and older) – 25 to 50 mg every 4 to 6 hours as needed. Do not exceed 300 mg in 24 hours.

Children (6 to 12 years of age) – 12.5 to 25 mg every 4 to 6 hours as needed. Do not exceed 150 mg in 24 hours.

Children (younger than 6 years of age) – Use only as directed by a physician.

Liquid and elixir:

Adults and children (12 years of age and older) – 25 to 50 mg (10 to 20 mL) every 4 to 6 hours as needed. Do not exceed 300 mg (120 mL) in 24 hours.

Children (6 to 12 years of age) – 12.5 to 25 mg (5 to 10 mL) every 4 to 6 hours as need. Do not exceed 150 mg (60 mL) in 24 hours.

Children (younger than 6 years of age) – Use only as directed by a physician.

DIPHENHYDRAMINE HCL PRODUCTS	
Trade name	Doseform
Benadryl Allergy Ultratabs, Diphenhist Captabs[1]	**Tablets**: 25 mg
Children's Benadryl Allergy	**Tablets, chewable**: 12.5 mg. Aspartame, 4.2 mg phenylalanine. Grape flavor.
Maximum Strength AllerMax	**Caplets**: 50 mg. Lactose.
Benadryl Allergy Kapseals	**Capsules**: 25 mg. Lactose.
Benadryl Dye-Free Allergy Liqui-Gels	**Softgels**: 25 mg. Sorbitol, glycerin.
AllerMax Allergy & Cough Formula[2], Children's Benadryl Allergy[3], Children's Benadryl Dye-Free Allergy[4], Genahist[4], Scot-Tussin[5], Siladryl Allergy[6]	**Liquid**: 12.5 mg/5 mL
Banophen	**Elixir**: 12.5 mg/5 mL

Products listed are representative of currently available and widely distributed brands. Similar products, including regional and private label brands, may also exist.

[1] Contains lactose.
[2] Contains 0.5% alcohol, saccharin, sugar, and sorbitol.
[3] Contains sugar and glycerin. Alcohol free.
[4] Contains saccharin, sorbitol, and glycerin. Alcohol and sugar free.
[5] Contains parabens, glycerin, and menthol. Alcohol and sugar free.
[6] Contains parabens, saccharin, and sorbitol.

BROMPHENIRAMINE MALEATE

▶ Administration and Dosage

Adults: 10 mg (range 5 to 20 mg) twice daily. Duration of action is 3 to 12 hours. Do not exceed 40 mg.

Children (younger than 12 years): 0.5 mg/kg/day or 15 mg/kg/day, divided into 3 or 4 doses.

BROMPHENIRAMINE MALEATE PRODUCTS	
Trade name	Doseform
Dimetapp Allergy	**Liqui-gels**: 4 mg

Products listed are representative of currently available and widely distributed brands. Similar products, including regional and private label brands, may also exist.

CHLORPHENIRAMINE MALEATE

▶ Administration and Dosage

Immediate-release tablets:

Adults and children (12 years of age and older) – 4 mg every 4 to 6 hours as needed. Do not exceed 24 mg in 24 hours.

Children (6 to 12 years of age) – 2 mg every 4 to 6 hours as needed. Do not exceed 12 mg in 24 hours.

Children (younger than 6 years of age) – Use only as directed by a physician.

Sustained-release tablets:

Adults and children (12 years of age and older) – 8 to 12 mg at bedtime or every 8 to 12 hours as needed during the day. Do not exceed 24 mg in 24 hours.

Children (younger than 12 years of age) – Use only as directed by a physician.

Liquid:

Adults and children (12 years of age and older) – 4 mg (10 mL) every 4 to 6 hours. Do not exceed 24 mg (60 mL) in 24 hours.

Children (6 to 12 years of age) – 2 mg (5 mL) every 4 to 6 hours. Do not exceed 12 mg (30 mL) in 24 hours.

CHLORPHENIRAMINE MALEATE PRODUCTS	
Trade name	**Doseform**
Chlorpheniramine Maleate	**Tablets**: 4 mg
Teldrin HBP	**Tablets**: 4 mg
Chlor-Trimeton Allergy 4 Hour	**Tablets, immediate-release**: 4 mg. Lactose, sugar, talc.
Chlor-Trimeton Allergy-D 4 Hour	**Tablets, immediate-release**: 4 mg chlorpheniramine maleate, 60 mg pseudoephedrine sulfate. Lactose.
Chlor-Trimeton Allergy 12 Hour	**Tablets, sustained-release**: 12 mg. Lactose, sugar, talc.
Diabetic Tussin (sf)	**Liquid**: 2 mg/5 mL. Saccharin, methylparaben. Alcohol and dye free.
Tricodene (sf)	**Liquid**: 2 mg chlorpheniramine maleate, 10 mg dextromethorphan hydrobromide/5 mL. Saccharin, glycerin, sorbitol. Alcohol free.

Products listed are representative of currently available and widely distributed brands. Similar products, including regional and private label brands, may also exist.
sf = Sugar free.

VITAMINS A, D, AND E, TOPICAL

▶ **Indications**

For temporary relief of discomfort due to minor burns, sunburn, windburn, abrasions, chapped or chafed skin, diaper rash, and other minor non-infected skin irritations.

▶ **Warnings**

For external use only: Avoid contact with the eyes.

Worsened condition: If the conditions worsen or do not improve within 7 days, consult a physician.

▶ **Administration and Dosage**

Apply locally to affected skin with gentle massage.

TOPICAL VITAMINS A, D, AND E PRODUCTS	
Trade name	**Doseform**
Lazer Creme	**Cream**: Vitamins A (3333.3 units/g) and E (116.67 units/g)
Lobana Derm-Ade	**Cream**: Vitamins A, D, and E, moisturizers, emollients, silicone
A and D	**Ointment**: Fish liver oil, cholecalciferol, lanolin, petrolatum, mineral oil

Products listed are representative of currently available and widely distributed brands. Similar products, including regional and private label brands, may also exist.

PATIENT INFORMATION

Vitamins A, D, and E, Topical

- Do not use in eyes or allow to come in contact with eye(s) or eyelid(s).
- Do not use if you are allergic to any ingredient in the product.
- Do not use on irritated or broken skin without consulting your doctor or pharmacist.
- If the condition for which these preparations is used persists or worsens, or if irritation develops, consult your doctor.
- Do not apply over deep or puncture wounds, infections, or lacerations.
- Stinging, burning, itching, or irritation may develop with the use of these products.

VITAMIN E

▶ Indications

Temporary relief of minor skin disorders, such as diaper rash, burns, sunburn, and chapped or dry skin.

▶ Administration and Dosage

For external use only: Avoid contact with the eyes. Apply a thin layer over affected area.

VITAMIN E PRODUCTS	
Trade name	Doseform
Vitamin E	**Cream, lotion, oil**
Vitec	**Cream:** dl-alpha tocopheryl acetate in a vanishing cream base, cetearyl alcohol, sorbitol, propylene glycol, simethicone, glyceryl monostearate, PEG monostearate
Vite E Creme	**Cream:** 50 mg dl-alpha tocopheryl acetate per g

Products listed are representative of currently available and widely distributed brands. Similar products, including regional and private label brands, may also exist.

PATIENT INFORMATION

Vitamin E, Topical

- Do not use in eyes or allow to come in contact with eye(s) or eyelid(s).
- Do not use if you are allergic to any ingredient in the product.
- Do not use on irritated or broken skin without consulting your doctor or pharmacist.
- If the condition for which these preparations is used persists or worsens, or if irritation develops, consult your doctor.
- Do not apply over deep or puncture wounds, infections, or lacerations.
- Stinging, burning, itching, or irritation may develop with the use of these products.

DANDRUFF

DEFINITION

Dandruff is defined as a dry or greasy, noninflammatory condition of the scalp resulting in excessive production of small flakes of dead skin. It is a disease of hyperproliferation that is common and carries no health risks. Dandruff is a precursor to, or a mild form of, seborrheic dermatitis.

ETIOLOGY

The exact etiology of dandruff is unknown; some potential causes include nutritional deficiencies or infection by the fungus *Pityrosporum ovale*. Exacerbating factors for dandruff include emotional stress, poor diet, poor hygiene, changes in weather, allergies, or chemicals or cosmetics applied to the scalp.

INCIDENCE

Dandruff is most prevalent during adolescence and adulthood, with the onset usually occurring in early adulthood. The incidence peaks in adults in their 20s, with approximately 50% of this age group affected. By 30 years of age, approximately 40% of adults are affected. The condition is uncommon in infancy and early childhood.

PATHOPHYSIOLOGY

Dandruff is the result of accelerated epidermal growth. Although increased production and prolonged retention of sebum on the skin may act as an irritant or may alter the epidermal function, there are no data to confirm this; in fact, there is little likelihood that this plays a role in this condition. There is evidence to suggest that the fungus *P. ovale* may be involved, along with multifactorial host conditions (eg, poor hygiene, allergies).

SIGNS/SYMPTOMS

The onset of dandruff is gradual, presenting as dry or greasy, noninflammatory scaling of the scalp that may be diffuse or localized. Itching may be present, but dandruff usually is only a cosmetic problem.

DIAGNOSTIC PARAMETERS/PHYSICAL ASSESSMENT

Clinical Observation: Dandruff is diagnosed by history and observation of the signs and symptoms described above. Patients with dandruff have a noninflammatory, diffuse scaling on the scalp only. There usually is no significant increase in sebum production. Severe itching may indicate signs of inflammatory changes. Examine the patient (including nails and skin) to rule out seborrheic dermatitis or psoriasis. When there is erythema with greasy scaling on the central face or along the eyelid margins, the diagnosis may be more consistent with seborrheic dermatitis.

Interview: To help the patient determine whether physician referral or self-treatment is warranted, it may be beneficial to ask about the following:
• Duration of scalp flaking or other symptoms
• Other skin conditions (specifically on the head or face) and their symptoms
• History of dandruff (including past treatment and treatment results)

TREATMENT

Approaches to therapy: The goal of dandruff therapy is to decrease epidermal hyperproliferation, which will alleviate the unsightly flaking. There is no known cure; treatment is aimed at controlling symptoms.

Symptoms that fail to respond to standard treatment warrant physician referral.

Nondrug therapy: Dandruff symptoms may resolve by improving hygiene and diet and minimizing the use of irritating hair chemicals or cosmetics. Stress reduction is also potentially helpful.

Pharmacotherapy: A variety of OTC topical agents are available for the management of dandruff, including ketoconazole, salicylic acid, selenium sulfide, sulfur, tar derivatives, and zinc pyrithione. For severe cases of dandruff, stronger prescription agents (eg, chloroxine, 10% coal tar) are available.

Topical Agents for Dandruff	
Drug	Action(s)
Benzalkonium chloride, isopropyl alcohol, phenol, menthol	Mild antiseptic
Benzyl alcohol	Weak antimicrobial
Ketoconazole	Antifungal
Menthol	Antipruritic
Salicylic acid, sulfur	Antiseborrheic and keratolytic/keratoplastic
Tar preparations, zinc pyrithione, selenium	Antipruritic, antibacterial, and antiseborrheic

KETOCONAZOLE

▶ **Actions**

Ketoconazole is a broad-spectrum antifungal agent. In vitro studies suggest it impairs the synthesis of ergosterol, a vital component of fungal cell membranes. The therapeutic effect in seborrheic dermatitis and dandruff may be caused by *P. ovale* (*Malassezia ovale*) reduction.

Ketoconazole inhibits the growth of the following common dermatophytes and yeasts by altering the permeability of the cell membrane. Dermatophytes: *Trichophyton rubrum, Trichophyton mentagrophytes, Trichophyton tonsurans, Microsporum canis, Microsporum audouinii, Microsporum gypseum,* and *Epidermophyton floccosum.* Yeasts: *Candida albicans, Candida tropicalis, P. ovale* (*M. ovale*), and *Pityrosporum orbiculare* (*Malassezia furfur*, the organism responsible for tinea versicolor). Development of resistance to the drug has not been reported.

▶ **Indications**

Controls the flaking, scaling, and itching associated with dandruff.

▶ **Contraindications**

Hypersensitivity to any component of the product; broken skin or inflamed scalp.

▶ **Warnings**

For external use only: Avoid contact with the eyes, eyelids, and mucous membranes. If contact occurs, rinse thoroughly with water.

Sensitivity: Discontinue use if sensitivity reactions or chemical irritation develops.

Pregnancy: Category C. There are no adequate and well-controlled studies in pregnant women. Use during pregnancy only if the potential benefits outweigh the possible risks to the fetus.

Lactation: Safety for use in the nursing mother has not been established. Exercise caution when applying on a nursing woman.

Children: Safety and efficacy in children have not been established.

▶ **Adverse Reactions**

Increase in normal hair loss; irritation (less than 1%); abnormal hair texture; scalp pustules; mild dryness of skin; itching; oiliness/dryness of hair and scalp.

▶ **Overdosage**

In the event of ingestion, advise patients to seek professional assistance or contact a poison control center immediately. Supportive measures, including gastric lavage with sodium bicarbonate, may be necessary. Refer to General Management of Acute Overdosage in Appendix B.

▶ **Administration and Dosage**

Wet hair thoroughly. Apply shampoo, lather liberally, rinse thoroughly, and repeat. Use every three to four days for up to eight weeks if needed, or as directed by a physician. Then use only as needed to control dandruff.

Children younger than 12 years of age: Consult a physician.

KETOCONAZOLE PRODUCTS	
Trade name	**Doseform**
Nizoral A-D	**Shampoo:** 1%. EDTA.

Products listed are representative of currently available and widely distributed brands. Similar products, including regional and private label brands, may also exist.

PATIENT INFORMATION

Ketoconazole

- For external use only. Avoid contact with the eyes, eyelids, and mucous membranes. If contact occurs, rinse thoroughly with water.
- Do not use on broken skin or inflamed scalp.
- Rinse thoroughly after each application. Discontinue use and consult a physician if irritation or rash occurs.
- Discontinue use if condition worsens or does not improve in two to four weeks.
- Removal of curl from permed hair may occur.

SELENIUM SULFIDE

▶ **Actions**

Selenium sulfide appears to have a cytostatic effect on cells of the epidermis and follicular epithelium, thus reducing corneocyte production.

▶ **Indications**

Controls itching, flaking, scaling, irritation, and redness associated with dandruff and seborrheic dermatitis.

▶ **Contraindications**

Hypersensitivity to any component of the product; broken skin or inflamed scalp.

▶ **Warnings**

For external use only: Avoid contact with the eyes, eyelids, and mucous membranes. If contact occurs, rinse thoroughly with water.

Sensitivity: Discontinue use if sensitivity reactions or chemical irritation develops.

Pregnancy: Category C. There are no adequate and well-controlled studies in pregnant women. Use during pregnancy only if the potential benefits outweigh the possible risks to the fetus.

Lactation: Safety for use in the nursing mother has not been established. Exercise caution when applying on a nursing woman.

Children: Safety and efficacy in infants have not been established.

▶ **Adverse Reactions**

Scalp irritation; increased hair loss; hair discoloration; oiliness/dryness of the scalp.

▶ **Administration and Dosage**

Massage 5 to 10 mL into wet scalp. Allow to remain on scalp two to three minutes. Rinse thoroughly; repeat application process and rinse thoroughly. Wash hands after treatment. Usually two applications each week for two weeks will control the condition, but the treatment may be used as frequently as once daily. After this, it may be used at less frequent intervals. Do not apply more frequently than required to maintain control. While 1% selenium sulfide lotions and shampoos are available OTC, 2.5% concentrations may be obtained with a prescription.

SELENIUM SULFIDE PRODUCTS	
Trade name	Doseform
Head & Shoulders Intensive Treatment	**Shampoo**: 1%. Cetyl alcohol, stearyl alcohol.
Selsun Blue Medicated Treatment	**Shampoo**: 1%. Menthol.

Products listed are representative of currently available and widely distributed brands. Similar products, including regional and private label brands, may also exist.

PATIENT INFORMATION
Selenium Sulfide
- For external use only. Avoid contact with the eyes, eyelids, and mucous membranes. If contact occurs, rinse thoroughly with water.
- Do not use on broken skin or inflamed scalp.
- Consult a physician before use if you have a condition that covers a large portion of the body.
- Rinse thoroughly after each application. Discontinue use and consult a physician if irritation occurs.
- Discontinue use if condition worsens or does not improve after regular use as directed.
- If using on bleached, tinted, gray, or permed hair, rinse hair for at least five minutes in cool running water.
- May damage jewelry; remove jewelry before using.

TAR DERIVATIVES

▶ **Actions**

Tar derivatives help correct keratinization abnormalities by decreasing epidermal proliferation and dermal infiltration. They also have antipruritic and mild antibacterial actions.

▶ **Indications**

For treatment of scalp psoriasis, eczema, seborrheic dermatitis, dandruff, cradle cap, and other oily, itchy conditions of the body and scalp. These agents may decrease scaling associated with tinea capitis and, therefore, may be used as adjunctive therapy.

▶ **Contraindications**

Hypersensitivity to any component of the product; acute inflammation; open or infected scalp lesions.

▶ **Warnings**

For external use only: Avoid contact with the eyes, eyelids, and mucous membranes. If contact occurs, rinse thoroughly with water.

Sensitivity: Discontinue use and contact a pharmacist or physician if sensitivity reactions (eg, redness, swelling, itching, burning) or chemical irritation occurs.

Pregnancy: Category C. There are no adequate and well-controlled studies in pregnant women. Use during pregnancy only if the potential benefits outweigh the possible risks to the fetus.

Lactation: Safety for use in the nursing mother has not been established. Exercise caution when applying on a nursing woman.

Children: Use on children younger than two years of age only as directed by a physician.

Photosensitivity: Use caution in exposing skin to sunlight after application. It may increase tendency to sunburn for up to 24 hours after application.

▶ **Adverse Reactions**

Minor dermatologic side effects include rash or burning sensation. Photosensitivity or skin discoloration may occur.

▶ **Administration and Dosage**

Refer to the specific product labeling for dosing information. Rub shampoo liberally into scalp. Leave on for several minutes. Rinse thoroughly. Repeat and rinse. Depending on the product, use at least twice per week up to once daily or as directed by a physician. For severe scalp problems, use daily according to product instructions.

TAR DERIVATIVE PRODUCTS	
Trade name	Doseform
DHS Tar	**Shampoo**: 0.5% coal tar
Doak Tar	**Shampoo**: 0.5% coal tar. EDTA, isopropyl alcohol.
Polytar	**Shampoo**: 0.5% coal tar. EDTA, lanolin.
Sebutone	**Shampoo**: 0.5% coal tar. EDTA, lanolin oil, salicylic acid, sulfur.
Tera-Gel	**Shampoo**: 0.5% coal tar. EDTA, parabens.
Ionil T, Zetar	**Shampoo**: 1% coal tar
PC-Tar	**Shampoo**: 1% coal tar. EDTA.
Creamy Tar	**Shampoo**: 2% coal tar. 5.6% ethyl alcohol.
Ionil T Plus	**Shampoo**: 2% coal tar
Neutrogena T/Gel	**Shampoo**: 2% coal tar extract
	Conditioner: 2% coal tar extract in a conditioner base
X•Seb T Pearl, X•Seb T Plus	**Shampoo**: 2% coal tar. EDTA, lanolin, salicylic acid.
Original Therapeutic Strength Denorex	**Shampoo**: 2.5% coal tar. 10.4% alcohol, menthol.
MG217 Extra Strength with Conditioners	**Shampoo**: 3% coal tar
Pentrax 5%	**Shampoo**: 5% coal tar
Original Therapeutic Strength Denorex 2 in 1	**Shampoo/Conditioner**: 2.5% coal tar. 10.4% alcohol, avocado oil, lanolin, menthol.
Tarsum	**Shampoo/Gel**: 2% coal tar. Salicylic acid.

Products listed are representative of currently available and widely distributed brands. Similar products, including regional and private label brands, may also exist.

PATIENT INFORMATION

Tar Derivatives

- For external use only. Avoid contact with the eyes, eyelids, or mucous membranes. If contact occurs, rinse thoroughly with water.
- Rinse thoroughly after each application. Discontinue use and consult a physician if excessive dryness or irritation occurs.
- Consult a physician before use if you have a condition that covers a large portion of the body.
- Discontinue use if condition worsens or does not improve after regular use as directed.
- Tar derivatives increase sensitivity to the sun and may increase tendency to sunburn for up to 24 hours after use. Avoid prolonged exposure to the sun or other forms of ultraviolet light (eg, tanning beds). Use sunscreens and wear protective clothing until tolerance is determined.
- Do not use for prolonged periods (longer than six months) or with psoriasis therapy (eg, phototherapy, prescription drugs) unless instructed by a physician.
- Products containing tar may temporarily discolor blond, gray, bleached, or tinted hair, or cause slight staining of clothing. Clothing stains normally are removed by standard laundry methods.
- Some coal tar products are extremely flammable. Keep away from fire and flame.

PYRITHIONE ZINC

▶ **Actions**

Pyrithione zinc, a cytostatic agent, reduces cell turnover rate. Its action is thought to be caused by a nonspecific toxicity for epidermal cells. The compound strongly binds to hair and external skin layers.

▶ **Indications**

Helps relieve the itching, flaking, and scaling associated with dandruff and seborrheic dermatitis.

▶ **Contraindications**

Hypersensitivity to any component of the product.

▶ **Warnings**

For external use only: Avoid contact with the eyes, eyelids, and mucous membranes. If contact occurs, rinse thoroughly with water.

Sensitivity: Discontinue use if sensitivity reactions or chemical irritation develops.

Pregnancy: Category C. There are no adequate and well-controlled studies in pregnant women. Use during pregnancy only if the potential benefits outweigh the possible risks to the fetus.

Lactation: Safety for use in the nursing mother has not been established. Exercise caution when applying on a nursing woman.

Children: Do not use on children younger than two years of age unless instructed by a physician (*Zincon* only).

▶ **Adverse Reactions**

Skin irritation has occurred rarely.

► **Administration and Dosage**

Apply shampoo; lather, rinse, and repeat. Use at least twice weekly for best results.

Children younger than 2 years of age: Do not use *Zincon* unless instructed by a physician.

PYRITHIONE ZINC PRODUCTS	
Trade name	Doseform
Head & Shoulders, Head & Shoulders Dry Scalp, Pantene Pro-V Anti-Dandruff, Zincon	**Shampoo**: 1%
Fructis Fortifying Anti-Dandruff	**Shampoo**: 1%. Cetyl alcohol, parabens, vitamin B_3, vitamin B_6.
DHS Zinc	**Shampoo**: 2%
Sebulon	**Shampoo**: 2%. Benzyl alcohol.
Everyday Strength Denorex	**Shampoo**: 2%. Menthol.
ZNP	**Bar**: 2%

Products listed are representative of currently available and widely distributed brands. Similar products, including regional and private label brands, may also exist.

PATIENT INFORMATION
Pyrithione Zinc

- For external use only. Avoid contact with eyes, eyelids, and mucous membranes. If contact occurs, rinse thoroughly with water.
- Rinse thoroughly after each application. Discontinue use and consult a physician if irritation, rash, or burning occurs.
- Discontinue use if condition worsens or does not improve after regular use as directed.

ANTISEBORRHEIC COMBINATIONS

► **Indications**

The following ingredients are adjunctive in the management of tinea capitis.

Salicylic acid and **sulfur** are used for antiseborrheic and keratolytic/keratoplastic actions.

Tar preparations are used for their antipruritic, mild antibacterial, or antiseborrheic actions.

Menthol is used as an antipruritic.

Benzalkonium chloride, isopropyl alcohol, phenol, and **menthol** are used as mild antiseptics.

► **Warnings**

For external use only: Avoid contact with the eyes, eyelids, or mucous membranes. If contact occurs, rinse thoroughly with water.

If undue skin irritation, burning, stinging, or itching develops or worsens, discontinue use and consult physician. Preparations containing tar may temporarily discolor blond, bleached, or tinted hair. Slight staining of clothing also may occur.

Children: Do not use on children younger than two years of age unless instructed by a physician.

► **Administration and Dosage**

Follow instructions on the label of the individual products very closely.

ANTISEBORRHEIC COMBINATION PRODUCTS	
Trade name	Doseform
Ionil, Ionil Plus, P & S	Shampoo: 2% salicylic acid
Neutrogena T/Sal	Shampoo: 2% salicylic acid, 2% solubilized coal tar extract
Sebex	Shampoo: 2% salicylic acid, 2% sulfur
Sebulex, Sebulex with Conditioners	Shampoo: 2% salicylic acid, 2% sulfur. EDTA.
Maximum Strength Meted	Shampoo: 3% salicylic acid, 5% sulfur
Sulfoam	Shampoo: 2% sulfur. Parabens.
Sebucare	Lotion: 1.8% salicylic acid. 61% alcohol, dihydrobietyl alcohol.
Scalpicin	Liquid: 3% salicylic acid. Menthol, SD alcohol 40.
P & S	Liquid: Glycerin, mineral oil, phenol

Products listed are representative of currently available and widely distributed brands. Similar products, including regional and private label brands, may also exist.

PATIENT INFORMATION
Antiseborrheic Combinations

- For external use only. Avoid contact with the eyes, eyelids, or mucous membranes. If contact occurs, rinse thoroughly with water.
- Consult a physician before use if you have a condition that covers a large portion of the body.
- Rinse thoroughly after each application. Discontinue use and consult a physician if irritation occurs.
- Discontinue use if condition worsens or does not improve after regular use as directed.
- Do not use on children younger than two years of age.
- Tar derivatives increase sensitivity the sun and may increase tendency to sunburn for up to 24 hours after use. Avoid prolonged exposure to the sun or other forms of ultraviolet light (eg, tanning beds). Use sunscreens and wear protective clothing until tolerance is determined.
- Do not use for prolonged periods (longer than 6 months) or with psoriasis therapy (eg, phototherapy, prescription drugs) unless instructed by a physician.
- Products containing tar may temporarily discolor blond, gray, bleached, or tinted hair, or cause slight staining of clothing. Clothing stains normally are removed by standard laundry methods.

DIAPER RASH

DEFINITION
Diaper rash is defined as an acute, inflammatory reaction of the skin in the diaper area as a result of constant exposure to an adverse local environment.

ETIOLOGY
Diaper rash is caused by a combination of factors, including occlusion, friction, and wetness. The most significant contributing factors include prolonged contact with and irritation from urine and feces, maceration from wet diapers, and impervious diaper coverings. In a high percentage of cases, a secondary infection with *Candida albicans* is involved. Additional contributing factors may include increased local heat and humidity, infrequent diaper changes, inadequate cleaning of the diaper area, and irritants such as intestinal enzymes and soaps.

INCIDENCE
Diaper rash is the most common of all cutaneous pediatric disorders, affecting at least 50% of infants. It is unusual for diaper rash to occur in the first month of life and is most common between 9 and 12 months of age; it can continue for as long as the child is in diapers, but usually occurs in children younger than 2 years of age.

PATHOPHYSIOLOGY
Diaper rash initially presents as a nonallergic, irritant dermatitis. It most commonly occurs on the lower abdomen, inner thighs, and buttocks. Once established, there may be colonization by bacteria and yeast. The frequency of occurrence and severity of rash decrease with the use of disposable diapers and as the frequency of diaper changes increases. It is thought that urinary wetness increases the permeability of the skin to irritants and the pH of the diaper area, which intensifies the activities of fecal proteases and lipases, which are the major irritants responsible for this disorder.

SIGNS/SYMPTOMS
Infants with diaper rash may be irritable and may experience itching and discomfort. The rash is usually well demarcated and erythematous, with exudative patches, but may have a variety of appearances depending on the most significant cause. It often appears where friction is the most pronounced and typically will spare the inguinal creases if caused by friction or irritant dermatitis. Mild diaper rash appears as erythematous, lichenified scaling plaques. More intense involvement is characterized by erythematous papules, vesicles or erosions, oozing, and ulceration. If colonized by *Candida*, a deep red plaque of the inner thighs and genitals occurs with sharp margination, scaling, and pustulovesicular satellite lesions.

DIAGNOSTIC PARAMETERS/PHYSICAL ASSESSMENT

Clinical Observation: Diaper rash is diagnosed by evaluating patient history, clinical presentation, and often by KOH examination of the rash. Evaluate the child to rule out atopic dermatitis or other conditions with a similar appearance. If a long-lasting diaper rash (longer than 3 days) is accompanied by intense erythema and satellite pustules, consider a candidal infection.

Interview: When evaluating an infant with diaper rash, it is important to get an accurate history of skin care and diaper-changing habits. Health care professionals should ask the parent about the following:

- The child's associated signs and symptoms (eg, burning, itching, irritability, diarrhea).
- Duration and location of symptoms.
- Diaper-changing routine.
- Types of diaper and hygiene products used on the baby (eg, strong soaps).
- Current and previous treatments for diaper rash.

TREATMENT

Approaches to therapy: The ideal approach to managing diaper rash is prevention. There are a variety of non-drug techniques and pharmacotherapies that can be used to alleviate the occurrence of diaper rash.

Nondrug therapy: Prevention of diaper rash can be facilitated through frequent diaper changes, cleaning the diaper area thoroughly with warm water after each diaper change and removing traces of feces, keeping the area dry (especially folds and creases), avoiding the use of excessive soaps (eg, soaps containing a deodorant) and commercial diaper wipes, and maintaining a comfortable room temperature. To decrease the alkalinity of cloth diapers because of soap and detergent residue, rinse in diluted acetic acid (1 oz vinegar in 1 gallon water).

Pharmacotherapy: A variety of topical products are available for the management of diaper rash. Many of these products combine a variety of ingredients including antimicrobial agents, corticosteroids, drying agents, occlusive agents, local anesthetic agents, protectants, and lubricants. Because these products are applied topically for a short period of time, it is unlikely that patients will experience systemic side effects or drug interactions. If a secondary bacterial or candidal infection develops, the child may require treatment with a topical antibacterial or antifungal agent. Prior to initiating anti-infective treatment, the patient should be evaluated by a physician. If diaper rash is resistant or nonresponsive to OTC medications, physician referral is warranted. In these cases, prescription antibiotics may be required.

TOPICAL DIAPER RASH PREPARATIONS

▶ **Actions**

Antimicrobial Agents (triclosan, eucalyptol): Minimize bacterial proliferation.

Barrier Agent (zinc oxide): Minimizes urine and fecal contact with the skin.

Local Anesthetic Agent (camphor): Relieves pain, itching, and irritation.

Moisture-Absorbing Agents (calcium carbonate, kaolin): Absorb fluid.

Protectants and Lubricants (petrolatum): Minimize chafing and irritation.

Antifungal Agents (undecylenate): Inhibits fungal cell growth.

▶ Indications

For the management of diaper rash. Some of these ingredients may have other indications.

▶ Warnings

Some practitioners do not recommend the use of products containing cornstarch, which may be metabolized by microorganisms, thus facilitating infection. Evidence to support this hypothesis, however, is unconfirmed.

Powder-based products may be inhaled by the child if used excessively.

▶ Administration and Dosage

Apply to affected area as needed.

DIAPER RASH PRODUCTS	
Trade name	**Doseform**
Diaparene Baby	**Cream:** Mineral oil, petrolatum, aloe, EDTA, diazolidinyl urea, parabens
Diaper Rash	**Ointment:** Zinc oxide, cod liver oil, lanolin, methylparaben, petrolatum, talc
A and D Medicated	**Ointment:** White petrolatum, zinc oxide, benzyl alcohol, cod liver oil, light mineral oil, propylparaben, vitamins A and D
A and D Original	**Ointment:** 53% petrolatum, 15.5% lanolin, cod liver oil, light mineral oil
Balmex	**Ointment:** 11.3% zinc oxide, Balsam Peru, benzoic acid, bismuth subnitrate, borax, mineral oil, silicone
Bottom Better	**Ointment:** 49% petrolatum, 15.5% lanolin, lanolin alcohols, EDTA, parabens
Caldesene	**Ointment:** 40% zinc oxide, BHT, cod liver oil, levomenthol, methylparaben, lanolin, talc, petrolatum
Desitin	**Ointment:** 40% zinc oxide, BHA, cod liver oil, lanolin, methylparaben, petrolatum, talc
Desitin Creamy	**Ointment:** 10% zinc oxide, cyclomethicone, dimethicone, parabens, mineral oil, sodium borate, sorbitan sesquiolate, white petrolatum
Diaper Guard	**Ointment:** 1% dimethicone, 66% white petrolatum, benzalkonium chloride, cocoa butter, colloidal oatmeal, colloidal silicon dioxide, talc, parabens, vitamins A, D_3, and E, zinc oxide
Diaparene Diaper Rash	**Ointment:** Zinc oxide, petrolatum, parabens, imidazolidinyl urea
Flanders Buttocks Ointment	**Ointment:** Zinc oxide, castor oil, Balsam Peru
Johnson's Diaper Rash	**Ointment:** Zinc oxide, mineral oil, glycerin, white petrolatum, lanolin
Dyprotex	**Pads:** 40% micronized zinc oxide, 37.6% petrolatum, 2.5% dimethicone, cod liver oil, aloe
Balmex Baby	**Powder:** Zinc oxide, balsam peru, corn starch, calcium carbonate
Caldesene Baby	**Powder:** 81% talc, 15% zinc oxide
Caldesene Protecting	**Powder:** 81% cornstarch, 15% zinc oxide

DIAPER RASH PRODUCTS

Trade name	Doseform
Desitin Cornstarch with Zinc Oxide	**Powder**: 10% zinc oxide, cornstarch, tribasic calcium phosphate
Diaparene Cornstarch Baby	**Powder**: Cornstarch, aloe
Gold Bond Cornstarch Plus Medicated Baby	**Powder**: Cornstarch, zinc oxide, kaolin
Gold Bond Medicated Baby	**Powder**: Talc, zinc oxide
Mexsana Medicated	**Powder**: Kaolin, eucalyptus oil, camphor, cornstarch, lemon oil, zinc oxide
Protectol	**Powder**: 15% undecylenate, starch, bismuth subgallate, magnesium carbonate, tricalcium phosphate
Triple Action Gold Bond Medicated Baby	**Powder**: 89% talc, 10% zinc oxide
ZBT Baby	**Powder**: Talc, mineral oil

Products listed are representative of currently available and widely distributed brands. Similar products, including regional and private label brands, may also exist.

PATIENT INFORMATION
Diaper Rash Products

- For external use only.
- Avoid contact with the eyes. Rinse with water if this occurs.
- Use powders cautiously. Inhalation may cause chemical pneumonia in the child.
- Do not treat if the skin is broken, because it is more likely to be infected by bacteria or fungi. Consult a physician.
- If condition worsens or if there is no noticeable improvement after 3 days, consult a physician.

■ ■ ■
Dry Skin
(Xerosis)

DEFINITION

Dry skin is defined as skin that looks and feels rough, scaly, and flaky because of decreased water content. It also is known as xerosis, asteatosis, and xeroderma.

ETIOLOGY

Dry skin occurs because of decreased moisture content within the skin. Water is the primary hydration chemical of the skin. The relative amount of water present in the skin is determined by three factors: the rate of water transported to the stratum corneum from the dermis; the rate of water loss from the surface; and the water-binding ability of the epidermis. This means that water loss will increase with decreased ambient humidity; it also will increase with a decreased or defective epidermal stratum corneum (ie, decreased epidermal lipid layer).

INCIDENCE

A genetic tendency appears to be operative in the development of dry skin. True incidence figures for xerosis are unknown; however, it is more common in cold, dry weather. Wind or dry heat also aggravates the condition. Aging of the skin, either in the elderly or in skin that has become atrophic through weathering, often results in dryness because the skin has become thinner. Dry skin tends to occur more often over the shin areas and the extensor surface of the forearms.

Dry skin may be a marker for systemic conditions such as hypothyroidism, lymphoma, sarcoidosis, ichthyosis, and atrophic eczema, as well as a drug-induced phenomenon with lithium, hypervitaminosis-A, and nicotinamide.

PATHOPHYSIOLOGY

With a decreased amount of water in the stratum corneum, the skin is less pliable and more prone to cracking and fissuring when bent. Any condition that either decreases the water flow to the epidermis or increases the water loss to the environment will lead to dry skin. Dry skin is more susceptible to injury from external trauma.

SIGNS/SYMPTOMS

Flaking, scaling skin with accentuation of the skin lines often is observed with dry skin. If the skin becomes irritated, then redness and fissuring with cracked plate-like scaling may ensue. Itching often is present, especially if irritation occurs.

DIAGNOSTIC PARAMETERS/PHYSICAL ASSESSMENT

Clinical Observation: The patient usually is aware of the nature of the problem, although with the elderly the dryness often is not appreciated by the patient (especially when the condition occurs on the back).

Interview: To determine the proper treatment for the patient's dry skin, it may be beneficial to ask about the following:

- Appearance of the skin
- Duration of condition
- Areas of involvement
- Occurrence at certain times of the year (eg, cold, dry weather or during windy conditions with dry heat)
- Treatments attempted and success of such treatments
- Other symptoms involving the skin

TREATMENT

Approaches to therapy: The basic element of treatment is to add moisture or water to the skin. This may be accomplished in two ways: by sealing in or trapping water that is already present and brought to the epidermis by using emollients, or by attracting water to the epidermis by using aquaphilic moisturizers.

If the problem is of recent onset, and especially if the problem is generalized and associated with significant pruritus, redness, and discomfort, the patient should be referred to a physician (preferably a dermatologist) for a generalized evaluation to search for a systemic disorder such as thyroid dysfunction, lymphoma, kidney disease, or sarcoidosis.

Nondrug therapy: Prevention of dry skin is very important. Avoidance of situations that tend to cause or increase dry skin should be encouraged. For example, in a cold, dry environment, humidifying the room air with a cool mist humidifier may be helpful. In addition, those practices that tend to strip oil from the skin, including frequent use of soaps and detergents, frequent use of solvents and overbathing, and use of hot water should be avoided or minimized.

Pharmacotherapy: Some products that may be used to prevent dry skin or relieve symptoms associated with the condition are described below.

EMOLLIENTS

▶ **Actions**

Some of the listed ingredients to look for that act as emollients are cetyl alcohol, glycerin, isopropyl myristate, isopropyl palmitate, lanolin, petrolatum, and stearyl alcohol. Some of the aquaphilic chemicals found in emollients and moisturizers and used to attract water to the skin are dexpanthenol, urea, and topical vitamins A, D, and E.

DEXPANTHENOL

▶ Indications

Relieves itching and aids healing of skin in mild eczemas and dermatoses, such as itching skin, minor wounds, stings, bites, poison ivy, poison oak (dry stage), and minor skin irritations. Also used to treat diaper rash, chafing, and mild skin irritations in infants and children.

▶ Administration and Dosage

For external use only. Avoid contact with the eyes.

Apply a thin layer to affected areas once or twice daily or as instructed by a physician.

DEXPANTHENOL PRODUCTS	
Trade name	Doseform
Panthoderm	**Cream**: 2% in a water-miscible base. Cetyl alcohol, glycerin, menthol, camphor, parabens.

Products listed are representative of currently available and widely distributed brands. Similar products, including regional and private label brands, may also exist.

PATIENT INFORMATION

Dexpanthenol

- For external use only. Do not use in eyes or allow to come in contact with the eye(s) or eyelid(s).
- Do not use if you are allergic to any ingredient of the products.
- Do not use on irritated or broken skin without consulting a physician or pharmacist.
- Stinging, burning, itching, or irritation may develop with the use of these products.
- If the condition persists or worsens or if irritation develops, discontinue use and consult a physician.
- Do not apply over deep or puncture wounds, infections, or lacerations.

UREA (CARBAMIDE)

▶ Indications

Promotes hydration and removes excess keratin in dry skin and hyperkeratotic conditions.

▶ Administration and Dosage

For external use only. Avoid contact with the eyes.

Apply a thin layer 1 to 4 times daily to affected area or as directed by a physician. Rub in completely.

UREA PRODUCTS

Trade name	Doseform
Lanaphilic	**Ointment**: 10%. White petrolatum, stearyl alcohol, isopropyl palmitate, lanolin oil, sorbitol, propylene glycol, sodium lauryl sulfate, lactic acid.
	Ointment: 20%. White petrolatum, stearyl alcohol, isopropyl palmitate, lanolin oil, sorbitol, propylene glycol, sodium lauryl sulfate, lactic acid.
Aqua Care	**Cream**: 10%. Petrolatum, glycerin, lanolin oil, mineral oil, lanolin alcohol, benzyl alcohol.
Nutraplus	**Cream**: 10%. Mineral oil, parabens.
Carmol 20	**Cream**: 20%. Nonlipid vanishing cream base.
Gormel	**Cream**: 20%. Mineral oil, cetyl alcohol, parabens.
Ureacin-20	**Cream**: 20%. Glycerin, mineral oil, parabens, EDTA.
Aqua Care	**Lotion**: 10%. Mineral oil, petrolatum, parabens, cetyl alcohol, lactic acid.
Carmol 10	**Lotion**: 10%. Cetyl alcohol.
Gormel Ten	**Lotion**: 10%. Mineral oil, cetyl alcohol, parabens.
Nutraplus	**Lotion**: 10%. Lanolin alcohol, petrolatum, parabens.
Ureacin-10	**Lotion**: 10%. EDTA, parabens, cetyl alcohol.
Ultra Mide 25	**Lotion**: 25%. Mineral oil, glycerin, lanolin, cetyl alcohol.

Products listed are representative of currently available and widely distributed brands. Similar products, including regional and private label brands, may also exist.

PATIENT INFORMATION

Urea

- For external use only. Do not use in eyes or allow to come in contact with the eye(s) or eyelid(s).
- Do not use if you are allergic to any ingredient of the products.
- Do not use on irritated or broken skin without consulting a physician or pharmacist.
- Stinging, burning, itching, or irritation may develop with the use of these products.
- If the condition persists or worsens or if irritation develops, discontinue use and consult a physician.
- Do not apply over deep or puncture wounds, infections, or lacerations.

VITAMINS A, D, AND E, TOPICAL

► **Indications**

For temporary relief of discomfort caused by minor burns, sunburn, windburn, abrasions, chapped or chafed skin, and other minor noninfected skin irritations, including diaper rash and irritations associated with ileostomy and colostomy skin drainage.

▶ **Warnings**

For external use only. Avoid contact with the eyes.

If the condition worsens or does not improve within 7 days, consult a physician.

▶ **Administration and Dosage**

Apply a thin layer to affected skin with gentle massage as directed by a physician.

TOPICAL VITAMINS A, D, AND E PREPARATIONS	
Trade name	Doseform
Vitamin A and Vitamin D	**Ointment**: Vitamins A and D. Lanolin, white petrolatum, mineral oil.
Lobana Derm-ADE	**Cream**: Vitamins A, D, and E. Lanolin, stearyl alcohol, cetyl alcohol, vegetable oil, parabens, glycerin.
Alph-E	**Cream**: 6,000 international units vitamin E, 600 international units vitamin A, 60 international units vitamin D. Wheat germ oil, emollient base.
Lazer Creme	**Cream**: 100,000 international units vitamin A, 3,500 international units vitamin E/oz. Parabens.

Products listed are representative of currently available and widely distributed brands. Similar products, including regional and private label brands, may also exist.

PATIENT INFORMATION
Vitamins A, D, and E, Topical

- For external use only. Do not use in eyes or allow to come in contact with the eye(s) or eyelid(s).
- Do not use if you are allergic to any ingredient of the products.
- Do not use on irritated or broken skin without consulting a physician or pharmacist.
- Stinging, burning, itching, or irritation may develop with the use of these products.
- If the condition persists or worsens or if irritation develops, discontinue use and consult a physician.
- Do not apply over deep or puncture wounds, infections, or lacerations.

VITAMIN E

▶ **Indications**

For the temporary relief of minor skin disorders such as diaper rash, burns, sunburn, and chapped or dry skin.

▶ **Administration and Dosage**

For external use only. Avoid contact with the eyes.

Apply a thin layer to affected skin with gentle message as directed by a physician.

VITAMIN E PRODUCTS	
Trade name	Doseform
Vitamin E[1]	**Cream, lotion, oil**
Vitec	**Cream**: dl-alpha tocopheryl acetate in vanishing cream base, cetearyl alcohol, sorbitol, propylene glycol, simethicone, glyceryl monostearate, PEG monostearate

VITAMIN E PRODUCTS	
Trade name	Doseform
Vite E Creme	**Cream**: 50 mg dl-alpha tocopheryl acetate/g
Vitamin E-Cream	**Cream**: 100 international units/g. Petrolatum, cetearyl alcohol, mineral oil, wheat germ oil, parabens.
Alph-E-Oil	**Oil**: 28,000 units/oz pure dl-alpha tocopheryl

Products listed are representative of currently available and widely distributed brands. Similar products, including regional and private label brands, may also exist.

[1] May or may not contain aloe.

PATIENT INFORMATION

Vitamin E

- For external use only. Do not use in eyes or allow to come in contact with the eye(s) or eyelid(s).
- Do not use if you are allergic to any ingredient of the products.
- Do not use on irritated or broken skin without consulting a physician or pharmacist.
- Stinging, burning, itching, or irritation may develop with the use of these products.
- If the condition persists or worsens or if irritation develops, discontinue use and consult a physician.
- Do not apply over deep or puncture wounds, infections, or lacerations.

MISCELLANEOUS EMOLLIENTS

► Actions

These preparations lubricate and moisturize the skin, counteracting dryness and itching. Some of the listed ingredients in products that act as emollients are butyl stearate, cetyl alcohol, glycerin, glyceryl monostearate, isopropyl myristate, isopropyl palmitate, lanolin, lanolin alcohol, mineral oil, petrolatum, propylene glycol stearate, squalene, stearic acid, and stearyl alcohol.

In certain products, some of the aquaphilic chemicals used to attract water to the skin are urea and alpha-hydroxy acids. These chemicals, while useful, often will sting when applied to dry skin.

MISCELLANEOUS EMOLLIENT PRODUCTS	
Trade name	Doseform
Aquaphor	**Ointment**: Petrolatum, mineral oil, ceresin, lanolin alcohol, panthenol, glycerin, bisabolol
Balmex Daily Protective Clear	**Ointment**: White petrolatum, cyclomethicone, dimethicone, polyethylene, silica, mineral oil, tocopheryl acetate
AmLactin	**Cream**: 12% ammonium lactate. Light mineral oil, glyceryl stearate, PEG-100 stearate, propylene glycol, glycerin, magnesium aluminum silicate, laureth-4, polyoxyl 40 stearate, cetyl alcohol, parabens, methylcellulose
AmLactin AP	**Cream**: 12% ammonium lactate, 1% pramoxine hydrochloride

MISCELLANEOUS EMOLLIENT PRODUCTS

Trade name	Doseform
Cutemol	**Cream:** Liquid petrolatum, lanolin alcohols extract, mineral wax, beeswax, acetylated lanolin, isopropyl myristate, sorbitan sesquioleate, sodium tetraborate, imidurea, allantoin, parabens
DML Forte	**Cream:** Petrolatum, propylene glycol dioctanoate, glyceryl stearate, PEG-100 stearate, glycerin, stearic acid, DEA-cetyl phosphate, DEX-panthenol, PVP/Eicosene copolymer, simethicone, benzyl alcohol, cetyl alcohol, silica, EDTA, acrylates/C10-30 alkyl acrylate crosspolymer, triethanolamine, magnesium aluminum silicate
Eucerin Original	**Cream:** Mineral oil, petrolatum, mineral oil, ceresin, lanolin alcohol, methylchloroisothiazolinone, methylisothiazolinone
Geri-Hydrolac 12%	**Cream:** Ammonium lactate (equivalent to 12% lactic acid), light mineral oil, petrolatum, propylene glycol, glycerin, cetyl alcohol, parabens
Hydrisinol	**Cream:** Mineral oil, petrolatum, hydrogenated vegetable oil, lanolin, beeswax, paraffin wax, sulfonated castor oil, parabens
Hydrocerin	**Cream:** Petrolatum, mineral oil, mineral wax, ceresin lanolin alcohol, parabens
Lanolor	**Cream:** Glyceryl stearates, propylene glycol, cetyl esters wax, isopropyl palmitate, cetyl alcohol, lanolin oil, sodium lauryl sulfate, methylparaben, simethicone, polyoxyl 40 stearate, sorbic acid
Minerin	**Cream:** Petrolatum, mineral oil, mineral wax, alcohol, methylchloroisothiazolinone, methylisothiazolinone
Neutrogena Norwegian Formula Hand Cream	**Cream:** Glycerin, sodium cetearyl sulfate, sodium sulfate, parabens
Nutraderm	**Cream:** Mineral oil, sorbitan stearate, stearyl alcohol, sorbitol, citric acid, cetyl esters wax, sodium lauryl sulfate, dimethicone, parabens, diazolidinyl urea
Pen•Kera	**Cream:** Cetyl palmitate, glycerin, mineral oil, polysorbate 60, sorbitan stearate, polyamino sugar condensate, urea, wheat germ glycerides, carbomer 940, triethanolamine, DMDM hydantoin, iodopropynyl butylcarbanate, diazolidinyl urea, dehydroacetic acid
Polysorb Hydrate	**Cream:** Cetyl esters wax, mineral oil, perfume oil bouquet, sorbitan sesquioleate, white petrolatum, white wax
Purpose Dry Skin	**Cream:** Mineral oil, white petrolatum, sweet almond oil, propylene glycol, glyceryl stearate, xanthan gum, steareth-2, steareth-20, sodium lactate, cetyl esters wax, lactic acid
Allercreme Skin	**Lotion:** Mineral oil, sorbitol, triethanolamine, parabens
AmLactin	**Lotion:** 12% ammonium lactate. Light mineral oil, glyceryl stearate, PEG-100 stearate, propylene glycol, glycerin, magnesium aluminum silicate, laureth-4, polyoxyl 40 stearate, cetyl alcohol, parabens, methylcellulose

MISCELLANEOUS EMOLLIENT PRODUCTS

Trade name	Doseform
Aquanil	**Lotion:** Glycerin, benzyl alcohol, sodium laureth sulfate, cetyl alcohol, stearyl alcohol, xanthan gum
Aveeno	**Lotion:** 1% colloidal oatmeal, glycerin, phenylcarbinol, petrolatum, dimethicone, benzyl alcohol
Corn Huskers	**Lotion:** Glycerin, SD alcohol 40, sodium calcium alginate, oleyl sarcosine, methylparaben, guar gum, triethanolamine, calcium sulfate, calcium chloride, fumaric acid, boric acid
Curel Original	**Lotion:** Glycerin, distearyldimonium chloride, petrolatum, isopropyl palmitate, cetyl alcohol, dimethicone, sodium chloride, parabens
Curel Soothing Hands	**Lotion:** Glycerin, petrolatum, distearyldimonium chloride, isopropyl palmitate, cetyl alcohol, aluminum starch octenylsuccinate, dimethicone, *Anthemis nobilis* flower extract, tocopheryl acetate, ascorbyl palmitate, panthenol, parabens, propylene glycol
Curel Ultra Healing	**Lotion:** Glycerin, petrolatum, cetearyl alcohol, behentrimonium chloride, cetyl-PG hydroxyethyl pamitamide, isopropyl palmitate, avena sativa (oat) meal extract, *Eucalyptus globus* leaf extract, *Citrus aurantium dulcis* (orange) oil, cyclomethicone, dimethicone, cholesteryl isostearate, BIS-PEG-15 dimethicone/IPDI copolymer, DMDM hydantoin
Derma Viva	**Lotion:** Mineral oil, glyceryl stearate, laureth-4, lanolin oil, PEG-100 stearate, PEG-40 stearate, PEG-4 dilaurate, trolamine, DSS, parabens
DML	**Lotion:** Petrolatum, glycerin, methyl glucose sesquistearate, dimethicone, PEG-20 methyl glucose sesquistearate, benzyl alcohol, cyclomethicone, glyceryl stearate, stearic acid, cetyl alcohol, sodium carbomer 941, xanthan gum, magnesium aluminum silicate
Emollia	**Lotion:** Mineral oil, cetyl alcohol, propylene glycol, white wax, sodium lauryl sulfate, oleic acid, parabens
Epilyt	**Lotion:** Propylene glycol, glycerin, oleic acid, quaternium-26, lactic acid, BHT
Esotérica Dry Skin Treatment	**Lotion:** Propylene glycol, dicaprylate/dicapric, mineral oil, glyceryl stearate, cetyl esters wax, hydrolyzed animal protein, dimethicone, TEA-carbomer-941, parabens
Eucerin Daily Replenishing	**Lotion:** Dimethicone, sunflower seed oil, petrolatum, glycerin, glyceryl stearate SE, octyldodecanol, panthenol, caprylic/capric triglyceride, tocopherol acetate, stearic acid, cholesterol, cetearyl alcohol, lanolin alcohol, carbomer, EDTA, sodium hydroxide, phenoxyethanol, parabens, BHT
Eucerin Plus Intensive Repair	**Lotion:** Mineral oil, PEG-7 hydrogenated castor oil, isohexadecane, sodium lactate, urea, glycerin, isopropyl palmitate, panthenol, microcrystalline wax, magnesium sulfate, lanolin alcohol, bisabolol, methylchloroisothiazolinone, methylisothiazolinone

MISCELLANEOUS EMOLLIENT PRODUCTS

Trade name	Doseform
Geri-Soft	**Lotion:** Mineral oil, propylene glycol, cetearyl alcohol, sorbitol, petrolatum, dimethicone, lanolin, castor oil, stearic acid, parabens, stearyl alcohol, EDTA, lemon oil
Geri SS	**Lotion:** Mineral oil, propylene glycol, cetearyl alcohol, petrolatum, glycerin, dimethicone, colloidal oatmeal, hydrogenated castor oil, parabens, stearyl alcohol, EDTA, lemon oil, tocopheryl acetate
Hydrisinol	**Lotion:** Propylene glycol stearate SE, hydrogenated vegetable oil, stearic acid, sulfonated castor oil, mineral oil, lanolin, lanolin alcohol, sesame oil, sunflower oil, aloe, triethanolamine, sorbitan stearate, hydroxyethyl cellulose, parabens
Hydrocerin	**Lotion:** EDTA, lanolin, parabens, mineral oil, PEG-40 sorbitan, peroleate, propylene glycol, sorbitol, water
Jergen's Ash Relief Moisturizer	**Lotion:** Glycerin, cetearyl alcohol, petrolatum, mineral oil, ceteareth-20, cyclomethicone, dimethicone, theobroma cacao (cocoa) seed butter, butyrospermum parkii (shea butter), tridecyl salicylate, tocopheryl acetate, stearic acid, glyceryl dilaurate, aluminum starch octenylsuccinate, acrylates/C10-30 alkyl acrylate crosspolymer, parabens, DMDM hydantoin, sodium hydroxide
Jergen's Ultra Healing Intense Moisture Therapy	**Lotion:** Glycerin, distearyldimonium chloride, petrolatum, isopropyl palmitate, cetyl alcohol, dimethicone, parabens, sodium chloride
Keri	**Lotion:** Mineral oil, glycerin, PEG-40 stearate, glyceryl stearate, PEG-100 stearate, PEG-4 dilaurate, laureth-4, aloe, sunflower seed oil, tocopheryl acetate, carbomer, parabens, DMDM hydantoin, iodopropynyl butylcarbamate, sodium hydroxide, EDTA
Lac-Hydrin Five	**Lotion:** 5% ammonium lactate, glycerin, petrolatum, squalane, stearth-2, POE-21-stearyl ether, propylene glycol dioctanoate, cetyl alcohol, dimethicone, cetyl palmitate, magnesium aluminum silicate, diazolidinyl urea, methylchloroisothiazolinone, methylisothiazolone
LactiCare	**Lotion:** Mineral oil, 5% lactic acid, isopropyl palmitate, sodium PCA, stearyl alcohol, ceteareth-20, sodium hydroxide, glyceryl stearate, PEG-100 stearate, myristyl lactate, cetyl alcohol, carbomer, DMDM hydantoin, parabens
Lobana Body	**Lotion:** Mineral oil, triethanolamine stearate, stearic acid, cetyl alcohol, lanolin, potassium stearate, aloe, propylene glycol, parabens
Lubriderm Advanced Therapy	**Lotion:** Cetyl alcohol, glycerin, mineral oil, cyclomethicone, propylene glycol discaprylate/dicaprate, PEG-40 stearate, isopropyl isostearate, emulsifying wax, lecithin, carbomer 940, diazolidinyl urea, titanium dioxide, sodium benzoate, tri (PPG-3 myristyl ether) citrate, EDTA, retinyl palmitate, tocopheryl acetate, sodium pyruvate, iodopropynyl butylcarbamate, sodium hydroxide, xanthan gum

MISCELLANEOUS EMOLLIENT PRODUCTS

Trade name	Doseform
Lubriderm Seriously Sensitive	**Lotion:** Butylene glycol, mineral oil, petrolatum, glycerin, cetyl alcohol, propylene glycol dicaprylate/dicaprate, PEG-40 stearate, C11-13 isoparaffin, glyceryl stearate, tri (PPG-3 myristyl ether) citrate, emulsifying wax, dimethicone, DMDM hydantoin, parabens, carbomer 940, titanium dioxide, EDTA, sodium hydroxide, xanthan gum
Lubriderm Skin Firming	**Lotion:** Isostearic acid, stearic acid, steareth-21, sodium lactate, PPG 12/SMDI copolymer, lactic acid, steareth-2, magnesium aluminum silicate, cetyl alcohol, imidurea, potassium sorbate, xanthan gum
Lubriderm Skin Renewal Firming	**Lotion:** Gluconolactone, propylene glycol, cetearyl glucoside/cetearyl alcohol, cyclomethicone, stearic acid, propylene glycol dicaprylate-dicaprate, C12-15 alkyl benzoate, isohexyl caprate, isocetyl stearate, triethanolamine, dimethicone, glycerin, petrolatum, glyceryl stearate, PEG-100 stearate, cetyl alcohol, emulsifying wax, steareth-2, diazolidinyl urea, EDTA, tocopheryl acetate, glycine, xanthan gum, hydroxyethyl cellulose, iodopropynyl butylcarbamate
Lubriderm Skin Therapy	**Lotion:** Mineral oil, petrolatum, sorbitol, stearic acid, lanolin, lanolin alcohol, cetyl alcohol, glyceryl stearate/PEG-100 stearate, triethanolamine, dimethicone, propylene glycol, microcrystalline wax, tri (PPG-3 myristyl ether) citrate, EDTA, parabens, xanthan gum, methyldibromo glutaronitrile
Lubriskin	**Lotion:** Mineral oil, petrolatum, lanolin, lanolin alcohol, cetearyl alcohol, castor oil, triethanolamine, stearyl alcohol, propylene glycol, parabens, EDTA
Minerin	**Lotion:** Mineral oil, isopropyl myristate, PEG-40 sorbitan peroleate, lanolin acid, glycerin ester, sorbitol, propylene glycol, cetyl palmitate, magnesium sulfate, aluminum stearate, lanolin alcohol, methylchloroisothiazolinone, methylisothiazolinone, BHT
Moisturel	**Lotion:** 3% dimethicone, benzyl alcohol, carbomer, cetyl alcohol, glycerin, laureth-23, magnesium aluminum silicate, petrolatum, potassium sorbate, sodium hydroxide, steareth-2
Neutrogena Body	**Lotion:** Glyceryl stearate, PEG-100 stearate, imidazolidinyl urea, carbomer-954, parabens, sodium lauryl sulfate, triethanolamine
Nutraderm	**Lotion:** Mineral oil, sorbitan stearate, stearyl alcohol, sodium lauryl sulfate, carbomer 940, diazolidinyl urea, parabens, triethanolamine
Shepard's	**Lotion:** Glycerin, sesame oil, vegetable oil, SD alcohol 40-B, propylene glycol, ethoxydiglycol, triethanolamine, glyceryl stearate, cetyl alcohol, simethicone, monoglyceride citrate, parabens
Sofenol 5	**Lotion:** Glycerin, petrolatum, cetearyl alcohol, soluble collagen, dimethicone, PEG-40-stearate, allantoin, sunflower seed oil, kaolin, sorbic acid, carbomer 940, sodium hydroxide

MISCELLANEOUS EMOLLIENT PRODUCTS	
Trade name	Doseform
Therapeutic Bath	Lotion: Mineral oil, glyceryl stearate, PEG-100 stearate, propylene glycol, PEG-40 stearate, laureth-4, PEG-4 dilaurate, lanolin oil, parabens, quaternium-15, carbomer 934, trolamine, dioctyl sodium sulfosuccinate
Wibi	Lotion: Glycerin, SD alcohol 40, PEG-4, PEG-6-32 stearate, PEG-6-32, carbomer-940, PEG-75, parabens, triethanolamine, menthol
Neutrogena Body	Oil: Sesame oil, PEG-40 sorbitan peroleate

Products listed are representative of currently available and widely distributed brands. Similar products, including regional and private label brands, may also exist.

PATIENT INFORMATION
Emollients

- For external use only. Do not use in eyes or allow to come in contact with the eye(s) or eyelid(s).
- Do not use if you are allergic to any ingredient of the products.
- Do not use on irritated or broken skin without consulting a physician or pharmacist.
- If the condition persists or worsens or if irritation develops, discontinue use and consult a physician.
- Apply to affected skin with gentle massage as instructed by a physician.

SOAP-FREE CLEANSERS

▶ **Actions**

These products are recommended for patients with sensitive, dry, or irritated skin who may react adversely to common soap products. Therapeutic cleansers include "soap-free" cleansers, which may be adjusted to a neutral pH and are less irritating to sensitive skin, and "modified" soap products, which may contain emollient components or may be adjusted to a neutral or slightly acidic pH.

Cleansers (including synthetic nonsoap cleansers), have a wide range of pH values. Soaps with a high alkaline pH (eg, *Irish Spring, Coast, Lava*) tend to be more irritating to the skin. Those with a lower or neutral pH (eg, *Purpose, Dial, Lever 2000, Neutrogena*) are more easily tolerated. Synthetic detergents (eg, *Cetaphil, Aveeno, Keri*) tend to be mildest.

SOAP-FREE CLEANSERS	
Trade name	Doseform
Cetaphil	Cream: Polyglycerylmethacrylate, propylene glycol, petrolatum, diccaprylyl ether, PEG-5 glyceryl stearate, glycerin, dimethicone, dimethiconol, cetyl alcohol, sweet almond oil, acrylates/C10-30 alkyl acrylate crosspolymer, tocopheryl acetate, phenoxyethanol, benzyl alcohol, EDTA, sodium hydroxide, lactic acid
Aquanil Cleanser	Lotion: Glycerin, cetyl, stearyl, and benzyl alcohols. Lipid free.
Aveeno Daily Moisturizing	Lotion: 1.25% dimethicone, 1% colloidal oatmeal, glycerin, distearyldimonium chloride, petrolatum, isopropyl palmitate, cetyl alcohol, benzyl alcohol, sodium chloride

SOAP-FREE CLEANSERS	
Trade name	Doseform
Cetaphil	**Lotion:** Glycerin, hydrogenated polyisobutane, cetearyl alcohol, cetearth-20, macadamia nut oil, dimethicone, tocopheryl acetate, stearoxytrimethylsilane, stearyl alcohol, panthenol, farnesol, benzyl alcohol, phenoxyethanol, acrylates/C10-30 alkyl acrylate crosspolymer, sodium hydroxide, citric acid
Eucerin Gentle Hydrating Cleanser	**Lotion:** Sodium laureth sulfate, cocamidopropyl betaine, disodium cocamphodiacetate, glycol distearate, PEG-7 glyceryl cocoate, PEG 5 lanolate, cocamide MEA, laureth-10, citric acid, PEG-120 methyl glucose dioleate, lanolin alcohol, imidazolidinyl urea
SFC	**Lotion:** PEG-75, stearyl alcohol, sodium cocoyl isethionate, parabens
Lobana Body Shampoo	**Liquid:** Chloroxylenol in a mild sudsing base with conditioners and emollients
Moisturel	**Liquid:** Cocamidopropyl betaine, diazolidinyl urea, methylchloroisothiazolinone, methylisothiazolinone, methyl gluceth-20, sodium laureth sulfate, laureth-6 carboxylic acid, disodium laureth sulfosuccinate
pHisoDerm, Normal to Dry Skin	**Liquid:** Sodium laureth sulfate, mineral oil, disodium ricinoleamido MEA-sulfosuccinate, cocamidopropylamine oxide, acrylates/C10-30 alkyl acrylate crosspolymer, aloe, *Chamomilia recutita* extract, tocopheryl acetate, diazolidinyl urea, propylene glycol, parabens, triethanolamine, EDTA
pHisoDerm, Normal to Oily Skin	**Liquid:** Sodium laureth sulfate, disodium ricinoleamido MEA-sulfosuccinate, cocamidopropylamine oxide, mineral oil, acrylates/C10-30 alkyl acrylate crosspolymer, aloe, *Chamomilia recutita* extract, tocopheryl acetate, diazolidinyl urea, propylene glycol, parabens, triethanolamine, EDTA
pHisoDerm for Sensitive Skin	**Liquid:** Potassium C12-13 phosphate, lauryl glucoside, sodium laureth sulfate, mineral oil, aloe vera, tocopheryl acetate, acrylates/C10-30 alkyl acrylate crosspolymer, EDTA, propylene glycol, diazolidinyl urea, parabens, citric acid
Purpose Gentle Cleansing Wash	**Liquid:** PEG-80 sorbitan laurate, sodium laureth sulfate, cocamidopropyl betaine, PEG-150 distearate, sodium lauroampho PG-acetate phosphate, quaternium-15, EDTA
Spectro-Jel	**Liquid:** Methyl cellulose, carboxypolymethylene, cetyl alcohol, sorbitan mono-oleate, fumed silica, triethanolamine stearate, glycol polysiloxane, propylene glycol, glycerine, 5% isopropyl alcohol
Sulfoil	**Liquid:** Sulfonated castor oil. Neutral pH.
Lobana Liquid Lather	**Body wash:** Sodium laureth sulfate, sodium lauryl sarcosinate, sodium myristyl sarcosinate, lauramide DEA, linoleamide DEA, octyl hydroxystearate, polyquarternium 7, tetrasodium EDTA, quaternium 15, sodium chloride, citric acid

SOAP-FREE CLEANSERS	
Trade name	**Doseform**
Spectro-Jel	**Gel**: Methyl cellulose, carboxypolymethylene, cetyl alcohol, sorbitan mono-oleate, fumed silica, triethanolamine stearate, glycol polysiloxane, propylene glycol, glycerine, 5% isopropyl alcohol
Lowila Cake	**Bar**: Dextrin, sodium lauryl sulfoacetate, boric acid, urea, sorbitol, mineral oil, PEG-14M, lactic acid, dioctyl sodium sulfosuccinate, cellulose gum
MODIFIED BAR SOAPS	
pHisoDerm Cleansing Bar	**Bar**: Sodium tallowate, sodium cocoate, petrolatum, glycerin, lanolin, titanium dioxide, pentasodium pentetate, tetrasodium etidronate. May also contain sodium palm kernelate.
Oilatum Soap	**Bar**: Sodium palmate, sodium palm kernelate, peanut oil, octyl hydroxystearate, lecithin, glycerin, sodium chloride, titanium dioxide, sodium hydroxide, tetrasodium EDTA, tetrasodium etidronate, o-tolyl biguanide, trisodium HEDTA, glyceryl oleate, corn oil, t-butyl hydroquinone, propylene glycol, citric acid
Cetaphil Antibacterial Gentle Cleansing	**Bar**: Triclosan, sodium cocoyl bethionate, stearic acid, sodium tallowate, sodium dodecylbenzene sulfonate, sodium cocoate, PEG-20, sodium chloride, sodium isothionate, petrolatum, sodium isostearyl lactylate, sucrose laurate, titanium dioxide, pentasodium pentetate, tetrasodium etidronate. May contain sodium palm kernelate.
Cetaphil Gentle Cleansing	**Bar**: Sodium cocoyl isethionate, stearic acid, sodium tallowate, sodium stearate, sodium dodecylbenzene sulfonate, sodium cocoate, PEG-20, sodium chloride, sodium petrolatum, sodium isostearoyl lactylate, sucrose laurate, titanium dioxide, pentasodium pentetate, tetrasodium etidronate. May contain sodium palm kernelate.
Purpose Gentle Cleansing	**Bar**: Sodium tallowate, sodium cocoate, glycerin, sodium chloride, BHT, trisodium HEDTA
Vanicream Cleansing	**Bar**: Sodium cocoyl isethionate, stearic acid, sodium stearate, coconut acids, sodium lauroyl sarcosinate, paraffin wax, sodium cocoate, sodium isethionate, white petrolatum, cetearyl alcohol & ceteareth-20, titanium dioxide, sorbitol, propylene glycol, simethicone, glyceryl monostearate, polyethylene glycol monostearate, sorbic acid, BHT

Products listed are representative of currently available and widely distributed brands. Similar products, including regional and private label brands, may also exist.

PATIENT INFORMATION
Soap-Free Cleansers/Modified Bar Soaps
- For external use only. Do not use in eyes or allow to come in contact with the eye(s) or eyelid(s).
- Do not use if you are allergic to any ingredient of the products.
- Do not use on irritated or broken skin without consulting a physician or pharmacist.
- If the condition persists or worsens, or if irritation develops, discontinue use and consult a physician.
- Apply to affected skin with gentle massage as instructed by your physician.

WET DRESSINGS AND SOAKS

► **Actions**

These dressings, soaks, and baths ease pruritus. Astringents (eg, aluminum acetate) have a drying effect and should be used only if there are weeping lesions. Cool baths containing colloidal oatmeal may be more convenient when lesions are widespread.

► **Indications**

To reduce oozing and provide relief from itching from vesicular lesions.

WET DRESSING AND SOAK PRODUCTS	
Trade name	Doseform
Cameo	**Oil**: Mineral oil, PEG-8 dioleate, lanolin oil, isopropyl myristate
RoBathol	**Oil**: Cottonseed oil, alkyl aryl polyether alcohol
Aveeno Shower & Bath	**Oil**: 5% colloidal oatmeal, mineral oil, laureth-4, quaternium-18, hectorite, benzyl alcohol, benzaldehyde, silica

Products listed are representative of currently available and widely distributed brands. Similar products, including regional and private label brands, may also exist.

PATIENT INFORMATION
Wet Dressing and Soak Products
- For external use only. Do not use in eyes or allow to come in contact with the eye(s) or eyelid(s).
- Do not use if you are allergic to any ingredient of the products.
- Do not use on irritated or broken skin without consulting a physician or pharmacist.
- If the condition persists or worsens, or if irritation develops, discontinue use and consult a physician.
- Apply to affected skin with gentle massage as instructed by a physician.

ALUMINUM ACETATE SOLUTION

▶ **Indications**

Aluminum acetate solution provides an astringent wet dressing for relief of inflammatory conditions of the skin.

▶ **Warnings**

Discontinue use if intolerance, irritation, or extension of the inflammatory condition being treated occurs. If symptoms persist longer than 7 days, discontinue use and consult a physician.

Do not use plastic or other impervious material to prevent evaporation.

For external use only. Avoid contact with the eyes.

▶ **Drug Interactions**

Collagenase: The enzyme activity of topical collagenase may be inhibited by aluminum acetate solution because of the metal ion and low pH. Cleanse the site of the solution with repeated washings of normal saline before applying the enzyme ointment.

▶ **Administration and Dosage**

One packet or tablet in a pint of water produces a modified 1:40 Burow's solution. Apply for 15 to 30 minutes for 4 to 6 times daily. Wetting gauze with the solution is a suggested method for application to smaller, defined areas (eg, hand, arm, face, foot).

ALUMINUM ACETATE SOLUTION PRODUCTS	
Trade name	Doseform
Domeboro Astringent Solution, Pedi-Boro Soak Paks	**Powder, tablets**: Aluminum sulfate and calcium acetate.

Products listed are representative of currently available and widely distributed brands. Similar products, including regional and private label brands, may also exist.

PATIENT INFORMATION

Aluminum Acetate Solution

- For external use only. Do not use in eyes or allow to come in contact with the eye(s) or eyelid(s).
- Do not use if you are allergic to any ingredient of the products.
- Do not use on irritated or broken skin without consulting a physician or pharmacist.
- If the condition persists or worsens, or if irritation develops, discontinue use and consult a physician.
- Apply to affected skin with gentle massage as instructed by a physician.

FOLLICULITIS, FURUNCLES (BOILS), CARBUNCLES

DEFINITION

Folliculitis is defined as an inflammation of the hair follicle caused by infection, chemical irritation, or physical injury. The inflammation can be superficial in the hair follicle (referred to as folliculitis) or deep (referred to as furuncle, carbuncle, or sycosis). In most cases, folliculitis, furuncles, and carbuncles occur on hair-bearing areas that are exposed to friction, perspiration, and maceration, especially the scalp, back of the neck, face, axillae, buttocks, and perineum.

ETIOLOGY

Superficial and deep folliculitides may be caused by a variety of factors. Superficial folliculitis can be caused by bacteria (*Staphylococcus, Proprionobacterium acnes*), fungi (dermatophytes, candida), drugs (eg, steroids, lithium, estrogens), or mechanical forces (eg, shaving, hair acting as foreign bodies, occlusion of follicles by clothing, hats).

Deep folliculitis is typically caused by bacteria and rarely by dermatophytes. Furuncles and carbuncles are usually caused by *S. aureus*. Other organisms, either aerobic (*Escherichia coli, Pseudomonas aeruginosa, Streptococcus faecalis*) or anaerobic (*Bacteroides* sp, *Lactobacillus, Peptococcus* sp, *Peptostreptococcus* sp), may also cause furuncles and carbuncles. In general, the microbiology of abscesses (furuncles and carbuncles) reflects the microflora of the anatomic part of the body involved. Sycosis refers to follicular inflammation of the entire depth of the follicle and may be caused by infection with *S. aureus* or dermatophyte fungi.

INCIDENCE

Incidence rates vary depending on whether folliculitis is superficial or deep. Superficial folliculitis in general is quite common, particularly in adults.

PATHOPHYSIOLOGY

In superficial folliculitis, the inflammation is confined to the upper part of the hair follicle. The pathophysiology of this folliculitis involves the attraction of inflammatory white blood cells (WBCs) to the hair follicle. The cause of the attraction depends on the etiology of the folliculitis (eg, bacteria, fungi, chemical, foreign body). With *Staphylococcus* folliculitis, the bacteria accumulate within the follicle, which then stimulates the inflammatory cascade. The bacteria can gain entrance because of injury, abrasion, or nearby surgical wounds or in the setting of occluded moist skin.

The deeper folliculitides, such as furuncles and carbuncles, may begin as a superficial folliculitis that progresses to the formation of an abscess. An abscess is a walled-off collection of pus (WBCs, bacteria, and necrotic tissue). It is a cavity formed by finger-like loculations of granulation tissue and pus that extends outward along planes of least resistance. They can occur at any site but appear particularly in areas prone to friction or minor trauma, such as the waist, buttocks, groin, thighs, and axillae. Occlusion of these areas by clothing, especially in a patient with hyperhidrosis, encourages bacterial colonization.

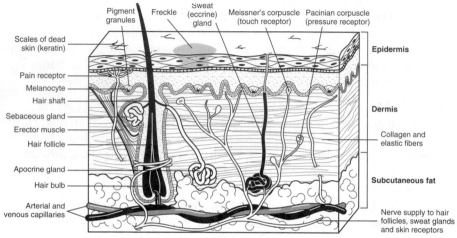

Figure 1. Layers of Skin with Hair Follicle

SIGNS/SYMPTOMS

With superficial folliculitis, one pustule or a group of pustules may appear on any body surface, usually without fever or other systemic symptoms. These follicular pustules or red papules may be tender or sometimes itchy. They typically heal without scarring.

Deep folliculitis is characterized by a swollen, tender, deep red mass that may eventually develop toward the surface, becoming a somewhat larger pustule than that seen in superficial folliculitis. These deeper lesions are painful and may heal with scarring. They usually remain firm and painful for several days before becoming fluctuant. Fever is usually not present, and there are no systemic symptoms.

Carbuncles are aggregates of infected follicles. The infection originates deep in the dermis and subcutaneous tissue, forming a broad, red, swollen, deep, painful mass that drains through multiple openings. Malaise, chills, and fever may occur before or during the active phase. Areas with thick dermis (posterior neck, back, lateral thighs) are the preferred sites.

DIAGNOSTIC PARAMETERS/PHYSICAL ASSESSMENT

Clinical Observation: The diagnosis of folliculitis is based first on clinical examination. The exam can show the presence of inflammation within hair follicles and whether it is superficial or deep but often does not reveal the underlying cause for the folliculitis, particularly superficial folliculitis. A physician may perform a culture, Gram's stain or KOH exam of 1 or more pustules to help determine the etiology as bacterial, fungal, or sterile folliculitis.

Interview: To assist patients in the diagnosis and proper treatment of folliculitis, which would result in physician referral, it may be beneficial to ask about the following:

- Location of the condition.
- Duration of the condition.
- Extent of the condition (ie, area of involvement, superficial vs deep).
- Recurrence or previous experience of this condition.
- Presence of pain or itchiness.
- Description of the pustule.
- Description of systemic symptoms such as fever, chills, or malaise.

TREATMENT

Approaches to therapy: If folliculitis is suspected, physician referral is appropriate, because antibiotic therapy may be required.

Nondrug therapy: Use of antibacterial soap is beneficial but will not treat the condition. Proper cleansing may help avoid the recurrence of this condition.

Pharmacotherapy: There is no effective OTC treatment for folliculitis. If the condition is suspected, physician referral is appropriate, because accurate diagnosis and use of prescription antibiotic therapy may be necessary.

HAIR LOSS
(Alopecia)

Introduction

Hair loss disorders can be classified into 2 groups: Scarring (cicatricial) alopecia or nonscarring (noncicatricial) alopecia. Scarring alopecia can be due to congenital and developmental defects, infectious diseases, chemical or thermal injuries, and various dermatological disorders. Nonscarring alopecia often results from alterations in the hair growth cycle, structural abnormalities of the hair, and inflammatory cutaneous diseases. Androgenetic alopecia, anagen effluvium, telogen effluvium, and alopecia areata are examples of nonscarring alopecia. This monograph will focus on androgenetic alopecia, the most common form of hair loss in humans.

DEFINITION

Androgenetic alopecia (AGA), also commonly referred to as male pattern baldness, is the most common cause of progressive hair loss in men and women. It is an androgen-mediated, autosomal dominant disorder that begins any time after puberty. The pattern of hair loss varies by individual and gender. Men typically experience a bitemporal receding hairline with additional loss at the vertex (crown). The pattern of hair loss in women involves more thinning at the crown with sparing of the anterior hairline.

ETIOLOGY

Genetics: Genetic predisposition to AGA is poorly understood but appears to have a substantial role in the development of this disorder. Although this condition can be hereditary, it may not be genetically homogenous. In general, AGA is believed to be due to an autosomal dominant gene. However, a polygenic inheritance has not been excluded. Some genetic abnormalities have been associated with the presence or absence of androgenetic alopecia. Interestingly, patients with testicular feminization syndrome (a condition involving end-organ insensitivity to androgens) do not experience any degree of AGA.

Androgens: For years it was known that men who had undergone prepubertal castration did not develop male-pattern baldness. Today, there is indisputable evidence that the potent androgen, dihydrotestosterone (DHT), is involved in the pathophysiology of AGA. Compared with the non-balding regions, the balding regions of the scalp of men with AGA contain miniaturized hair follicles and increased amounts of DHT. DHT is responsible for shortening the anagen phase (growth phase) in the normal hair cycle, thereby leading to the production of finer and thinner hypopigmented hair (miniaturized hair).

INCIDENCE

Androgenetic alopecia is the most common type of human hair loss. It affects nearly 50% of men by age 50 and 50% of women age 60 or older. An estimated 40 million American men and 20 million American women are affected by AGA. However, there is racial variation in the incidence of this condition. White males are 4 times as likely to be affected as black males. Asians and American Indians are relatively unaffected by AGA.

PATHOPHYSIOLOGY

Hair growth is a result of follicular activity with alternating periods of growth (anagen) and rest (telogen), separated by a transitional (catagen) phase (see Figure 1). During the anagen phase, follicles increase in length, the dermal papillae grow in size, and keratinized hair is continuously produced. On average, 90% or more of scalp hair is in the anagen phase at any given time. The duration of the anagen phase ranges from 2 to 8 years, with an average duration of 1000 days. At the end of the anagen phase, hair growth stops, and the catagen phase begins. During the catagen phase, cell proliferation stops, hair follicles shorten, and a bulbous enlargement forms at the base of the hair. At any one time, approximately 1% of scalp hair is in the catagen phase, which lasts several weeks. Terminal scalp hair, which contains mature hair with unpigmented club-shaped roots, enters the resting or telogen phase for an average period of 3 months, after which the terminal hair is shed and a new anagen phase begins.

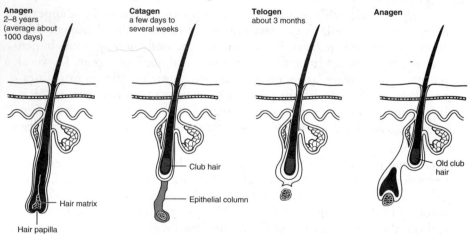

Anagen
2–8 years
(average about
1000 days)

Catagen
a few days to
several weeks

Telogen
about 3 months

Anagen

Club hair

Epithelial column

Hair matrix

Hair papilla

Old club hair

Figure 1. Phases of the Normal Hair Cycle

Approximately 50 to 100 hairs are shed daily from the scalp. When a hair is shed, it is replaced by a new terminal hair from the same follicle. However, in patients with AGA, new hairs are finer in texture and thinner than those shed (see Figure 2). Dihydrotestosterone (DHT) appears to be the specific androgen responsible for AGA. Hair follicle cytoplasm contains an intracellular enzyme, type II 5-α-reductase, which converts testosterone to DHT. The hair follicles of men with male pattern baldness have demonstrated an enhanced 5-α-reductase activity. Testosterone and DHT can reach the hair follicles through systemic circulation. They are also produced locally in the follicle from other weak circulating androgens such as dehydroepiandrosterone and androstenedione. In comparison to testosterone, DHT has a greater binding affinity to androgen receptors, and the resulting complex inhibits adenyl cyclase in the hair bulb, leading to decreased protein synthesis. This in turn shortens the anagen phase, resulting in the production of finer and thinner hair with reduced pigmentation. In women, dehydroepiandrosterone (DHEA) is the major precursor of DHT. DHT and DHEA appear to be responsible for the miniaturization of hair follicles in women with AGA.

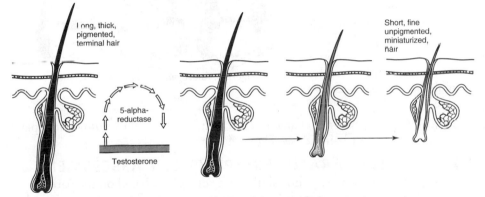

Figure 2. Miniaturization of the Hair Follicle

SIGNS/SYMPTOMS

In the majority of men with AGA, hair loss begins in the frontal region of the head and appears as a receding hairline. This is followed by further hair loss at the crown (vertex) of the head. The area of baldness on the vertex gradually increases over time and joins the receding frontal hairline. Eventually, only a ring of hair around the occipital portion and the marginal parietal area of the scalp remains. The Hamilton-Norwood Scale, which shows gradations of hair loss, is the most common classification for male pattern baldness (see Figure 3).

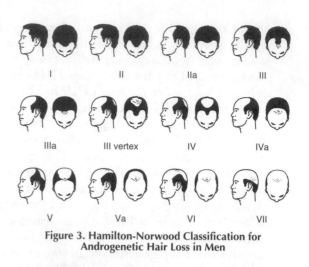

Figure 3. Hamilton-Norwood Classification for Androgenetic Hair Loss in Men

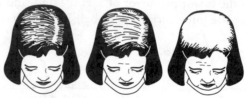

Figure 4. Androgenetic Hair Loss in Women

In women, the pattern is characterized by diffuse central thinning with sparing of the anterior hairline (see Figure 4).

DIAGNOSTIC PARAMETERS/PHYSICAL ASSESSMENT

Clinical Observation: The clinical diagnosis of AGA is based on the patients' clinical presentation, history, hair examination, scalp biopsy, and screening laboratory tests for androgen excess. Rule out other causes of hair loss such as thyroid and other endocrine disorders, poor nutritional status, iron deficiency, drugs, severe infection, systemic disease, and malignancy. Hair samples (hair pluck) are often collected to assess the hair growth cycle and diameter. A common finding in AGA is an increase in the amount of telogen hair from 20% to 35% of the entire scalp hair as compared with less than 20% in normal individuals. A scalp biopsy can be done to confirm the results of the hair pluck test. Seborrheic folliculitis and local dermatitis are commonly seen in patients with AGA. Laboratory assessment for androgen excess has been useful in females with AGA. Plasma testosterone (normal: 20 to 80 ng/dL), DHEA (normal: less than 350 mcg/dL), and androstenedione concentrations are often included in routine screening tests. To exclude other treatable causes of hair thinning, the following tests may be used: Thyroid-stimulating hormone (thyroxine); serum iron, serum ferritin, or total iron binding capacity; and complete blood count. Various drugs may also be associated with the occurrence of alopecia, as listed in the following table:

Drugs Associated with Alopecia		
Amiodarone	Cimetidine	Minoxidil[1]
Angiotensin-converting enzyme inhibitors	Colchicine	Oral contraceptives[1,2]
Anticoagulants	Fluoxetine	Retinoids
Antineoplastic agents	Gold	Sulfasalazine
Antithyroid agents	Interferons	Tricyclic antidepressants
Beta blockers	Lipid lowering agents	Valproic acid
Bromocriptine	Lithium	

[1] Alopecia occurred upon withdrawal of the drug.
[2] Observations made with earlier oral contraceptives with greater androgenic activity and higher estrogen content than those used today.

Interview: To ensure the proper diagnosis and treatment of androgenetic alopecia, it may be beneficial to ask about the following:

- Age of onset of hair thinning or hairline recession.
- Pattern and distribution of hair thinning.
- Health history, including thyroid and other endocrine disorders, autoimmune disorders, malignancy.
- Diet, including adequate intake of protein and iron.
- Family history of thinning hair or balding in parents, siblings, aunts, uncles, or grandparents on both sides of the family.
- Use of medications, including vitamins and chemotherapy.
- Use of anabolic steroids.
- Hair care procedures or hair product use that may contribute to hair breakage.
- Menstrual and pregnancy history, oral contraceptive use (for women only).

TREATMENT

Approaches to therapy: The goal of treatment in AGA is to reduce hair loss and increase scalp coverage. It may be beneficial to advise patients experiencing hair loss to consult a physician for proper diagnosis, discussion of treatment options, and evaluation of the likelihood of response to available treatments.

Nondrug therapy: Non-pharmacological approaches used by individuals with alopecia to conceal hair loss and improve appearance include the following: Wigs, toupees, hair weaves, hair fusion, hair dyeing, permanent waving, sprays, mousses, and scalp camouflage (crayons, creams, sprays). Surgical procedures, including hair transplantation, scalp reduction, transposition flaps, and soft tissue expansion may also be considered.

Pharmacotherapy: Currently there are 2 drugs approved for the treatment of androgenetic alopecia: Topical minoxidil and oral finasteride. Topical minoxidil, a biologic response modifier, is available OTC, but finasteride is available by prescription only. Other agents used topically in the management of alopecia include tretinoin, corticosteroids, and various sensitizing agents. The 2% topical minoxidil solution was first approved in August 1988 as a prescription-only agent for use in males and females with vertex balding secondary to AGA; this formulation later became available as a nonprescription product. In December 1997, a 5% topical minoxidil solution was granted FDA approval; this product is indicated for use only by men with vertex balding. Topical minoxidil is the only OTC product approved for the treatment of AGA.

MINOXIDIL

▶ **Actions**

The mechanism by which minoxidil promotes hair growth is not completely understood. Minoxidil appears to directly stimulate the hair follicles and prolong the anagen phase. It also increases the mean hair shaft diameter and reduces hair loss. Minoxidil opens potassium channels and allows further proliferation and differentiation of epidermal cells in the hair shaft.

▶ **Indications**

The 2% topical minoxidil solution is indicated for the treatment of AGA in men and women. However, the 5% solution is only recommended for use in men; avoid use in women, because it stimulates the growth of facial hair.

▶ **Contraindications**

History of hypersensitivity to minoxidil or to any of the components of the product (ethanol and propylene glycol); use of 5% solution in women.

▶ **Warnings**

Systemic exposure: Prior to initiating treatment with topical minoxidil, it is important to ensure that patients have an otherwise healthy, normal scalp. Local abrasions, dermatitis, or severe sunburn can increase drug absorption and the risk of systemic adverse effects. Topical minoxidil is poorly absorbed from the intact scalp. Therefore, treatment with minoxidil is not associated with a high incidence of systemic side effects. Do not use with other topical agents that are known to enhance cutaneous absorption. Patients with underlying heart disease, including coronary artery disease and congestive heart failure, may be at higher risk for the potential systemic effects of topical minoxidil. Alert these patients to the possibility of angina, fluid retention, tachycardia, and edema, and monitor for increased heart rate, weight gain, or other systemic side effects.

Pregnancy: Category C. Adequate and well-controlled trials have not been conducted in pregnant women receiving topical or oral minoxidil. Oral administration of minoxidil has been associated with increased fetal resorption in rabbits when given at 5 times the maximum recommended dose.

Lactation: There have been reports of minoxidil excretion into the breast milk of women treated with the oral formulation. Because of the potential for adverse effects in nursing infants, do not use topical minoxidil in nursing mothers.

Children: Safety and efficacy have not been established in children younger than 18 years of age.

▶ **Drug Interactions**

Currently, there are no known drug interactions associated with the use of topical minoxidil. However, there is a theoretical possibility for this medication to potentiate orthostatic hypotension in patients taking guanethidine concurrently. Do not use with other topical agents (eg, corticosteroids, retinoids, petrolatum) or agents that are known to enhance absorption.

▶ **Adverse Reactions**

Approximately 25% of patients using topical minoxidil experience some degree of dryness, itching, or erythema of the scalp. These adverse effects are primarily attributed to the vehicle, which contains 60% alcohol in addition to water and propylene glycol. If patients experience these symptoms, advise them to refrain from using this product for several days. Treatment can be resumed once the symptoms have resolved.

The typical systemic effects of oral minoxidil (weight gain, edema, tachycardia, angina) are not commonly seen in patients receiving the topical formulation. This is due to the poor absorption (1.4% bioavailability) of minoxidil from the intact scalp and the low systemic exposure to the drug.

▶ **Administration and Dosage**

Apply a 1 mL total dose of the solution to the affected areas of the scalp twice daily, once in the morning and once at night. Do not exceed a total daily dose of 2 mL. Dry the hair and scalp prior to application. If exposed fingertips are used during application of the product, wash hands immediately afterward. Note that twice-daily application for a minimum of 4 months may be required before individual response to the medication can be evaluated. Onset and degree of hair regrowth may vary among patients. If hair regrowth is noted, continued treatment is *required* indefinitely to *maintain* the newly grown hair.

MINOXIDIL PRODUCTS	
Trade name	**Doseform**
Rogaine for Men, Rogaine for Women	**Topical solution:** 2%. 60% alcohol, propylene glycol, purified water
Rogaine Extra Strength for Men	**Topical solution:** 5%. 30% alcohol, 50% propylene glycol, purified water.

Products listed are representative of currently available and widely distributed brands. Similar products, including regional and private label brands, may also exist.

PATIENT INFORMATION
Minoxidil

- Consult with pharmacist or physician regarding reasonable expectations from therapy. Do not expect immediate or unrealistic results. Some patients may continue to experience hair loss while on topical minoxidil, while others may see a decrease in hair thinning or a noticeable increase in hair growth. Because of the location, extent, or duration of hair loss, some patients may not be appropriate candidates for treatment with topical minoxidil.
- Apply 1 mL of minoxidil solution to a clean, dry scalp twice a day (once in the morning and once at night). No additional benefits are associated with more frequent application of the product. Overuse can lead to an increased incidence of dry, itchy scalp from the alcohol contained in the vehicle.
- Keep scalp dry for 4 hours or longer after application of topical minoxidil. In cases where the scalp becomes wet, reapply the solution.
- Avoid contact of the solution with eyes and mucous membranes. The alcohol in the vehicle can cause burning and stinging. Wash hands immediately after handling the solution with exposed fingertips.
- Continue usual hair care routine while using topical minoxidil. Use hair-styling products, colors, or perms only after the scalp has dried completely following application of the solution. These products do not impair the efficacy of topical minoxidil.
- Do not make up for missed doses by doubling the amount of the solution. When a dose is missed, restart twice-daily application on the next day.
- Use topical minoxidil regularly for a minimum of 4 months before individual response to the medication can be evaluated. If hair growth is experienced, continue to use the medication. Discontinuation of therapy leads to loss of newly grown hair within 3 to 6 weeks.
- Do not use topical minoxidil in the presence of scalp abrasions, infections, open sores, severe sunburn, or scalp psoriasis. These conditions can increase the medication's absorption from the scalp, thereby increasing the risk of side effects.
- Do not use topical minoxidil in combination with other topical products unless clearly directed to do so by a physician.
- If there is no response to treatment after a reasonable time (4 months or longer), consult your health care provider as to whether to discontinue use.

HEAD LICE
(Pediculosis Capitis)

DEFINITION

Pediculosis capitis is a parasitic infestation of the scalp by the head louse, which feeds on scalp and neck blood and deposits its eggs (nits) on the hair. Pediculosis capitis (head lice) is not to be confused with Pediculus humanis corpris (body lice or "cooties") or Phthirus pubis (pubic lice or "crabs"). Infestations of head lice are treated uniquely and are generally very manageable if treated properly.

ETIOLOGY

Pediculosis capitis is caused by the lice subspecies *Pediculus humanus* var. *capitis*. These are wingless, clawed, dorsoventrally flattened insects approximately 3 to 4 mm long (about the size of a small sesame seed) that are obligate ectoparasites of humans. They have 6 legs with claws that grasp the hair shaft. Head lice live mainly on the scalp and nape of the neck of their human host, where they pierce skin with powerful jaws and feed off blood for 30 to 45 minutes every 3 to 4 hours. They change from a whitish-gray to brownish-red color when filled with blood. They deposit their eggs on the hair.

INCIDENCE

The head louse has a worldwide distribution and is still common in many communities. Lice are more common in whites than in blacks and in children than in adults. Infestation is also more prevalent in urban areas than in rural areas because crowded conditions are more conducive to transmission. Head lice may be transmitted by sharing hats, caps, headbands, scarves, barrettes, brushes, combs, or other hair accessories. Lice may be epidemic among elementary school children, becoming most apparent at the beginning of each school year. Other modes of transmission include contaminated clothing, bed liners, pillows, cushions, head rests, furniture backs, infested mattresses and carpets, earphones, and headphones. Poverty, ignorance, and poor hygiene also encourage the spread of lice. However, the occurrence of infestation is not restricted to a particular socioeconomic class, and the presence of head lice does not necessarily allude to poor hygiene or sanitation by the host.

Although head lice are transmissible, the likelihood of an overall epidemic spread is minimal. The basic reproduction rate (a measure that defines the number of secondary infections arising from an index case) is far lower for head lice than for infections due to cold or flu viruses.

PATHOPHYSIOLOGY

The claws on the legs of *P. capitis* are adapted for clinging to hair. Lice and their eggs are not able to burrow into the scalp. The louse is transmitted to the scalp hair by head-to-head contact or shared hair accessories. They may also remain on bedding, scarves, clothing, bed linens, pillows, cushions, head rests, mattresses, carpets, headphones, or upholstered furniture for a short period. Because they are not able to jump or fly, lice are not likely to abandon their preferred habitat. The female louse lives approximately 40 days, mates, and can lay up to 300 eggs over a 20- to 30-day period. These eggs cannot be removed by ordinary washing because they are cemented to hair shafts by a material secreted from the female. To provide a suitable temperature for incubations, the eggs are attached to hair close to the surface of the scalp. A louse hatches from its egg after approximately 8 days of development and begins to feed and grow until it reaches the adult stage 2 to 3 weeks after hatching. Once the louse has emerged, the empty egg case (nit shell) becomes more visible. Mature lice derive nutrients approximately 5 times each day by piercing the skin with their jaws, injecting saliva, which contains an enzyme (hyaluronidase) that thins blood, and sucking blood. They cannot survive for longer than 1 day without access to human blood.

In general, fewer than a dozen active head lice live on the scalp at any time, but there may be hundreds of viable and hatched eggs. With adequate magnification and bright light, the developing louse can be seen within the egg.

SIGNS/SYMPTOMS

Scalp pruritus (itching), which is often intense, is the characteristic manifestation of head lice infection. In addition, infested adults and children may experience loss of sleep, a shortened attention span, and depression. Louse saliva contains foreign proteins and ultimately sensitizes the host to the bites, increasing the itching, irritation, and chance of a secondary infection. Secondary bacterial infection with excoriations and crust, often associated with occipital or cervical lymphadenopathy (lymph node swelling of the neck or back of the head), may occur as a result of scratching.

Head lice are mainly an annoyance in North America. However, body lice (and possibly head lice) create public health concerns overseas because they may transmit some human pathogens.

On close inspection of the scalp, the empty egg cases are easily identified as oval, grayish-white capsules approximately 1 mm in length, firmly cemented to the hairs. They may be viewed as dandruff initially. They occur in greatest density on the parietal and occipital areas of the scalp where the hair is the thickest, and can range from a few to thousands. The adult *P. capitis* louse is frequently not observed because less than 10 lice are present in over half of the cases. Pruritic papular lesions may sometimes be seen at the sites of louse bites.

DIAGNOSTIC PARAMETERS/PHYSICAL ASSESSMENT

Clinical Observation: The diagnosis of head lice is based on clinical findings confirmed under strong light or natural daylight by detection of eggs, egg cases, or lice. Live eggs can be accentuated by Wood's light examination, which causes them to fluoresce white. A magnifying glass will also aid identification. When searching for eggs or head lice, one should wear gloves and begin the search at the nape of the neck or behind the ears where hair is thickest. If a secondary bacterial infection is suspected, obtain bacterial cultures.

Interview: To ensure the proper treatment of head lice and prevent further infestation, it may be beneficial to ask about the following:

- Verify that an accurate diagnosis of lice infestation has been made
- When the nits or lice were initially detected
- Whether family members, schoolmates, or other contacts are known to have lice
- All contacts with the infected individual (eg, family members, schoolmates), because all should be examined and treated
- Past use of or sensitivity to permethrin, pyrethrin, pyrethroids, or pediculicides
- Any treatments attempted and description of treatment (eg, *otc* therapy, home remedy)

TREATMENT

Approaches to therapy: The *goals* of treatment are: 1) To kill the mature lice, nymphs (immature louse), and eggs; 2) to control symptoms; and 3) to prevent or treat secondary infections. Consider treatment only when active lice or viable eggs are visible. Without confirmation, itching of the scalp or the sensation of something crawling on the head does not warrant treatment, nor does evidence of an old infestation (presence of hatched eggs). Once a diagnosis has been confirmed; however, contacts should be treated.

Treatment requires the use of topical pediculicides. Treatment may need to be repeated in 1 week (the time required for eggs to hatch) because eggs are sometimes less likely to be killed than adult lice. Empty egg cases may persist for some time until they are gradually worn away by repeated washing or are treated with a formic acid cream rinse that facilitates their removal. Removal after effective treatment is not necessary but may be psychologically important to the patient. Fomites (objects such as clothing or linens suspected of causing transmission) should be discarded or washed with hot water.

Some people overreact to a minor problem, becoming overzealous in their idea of cleanliness. In some cases, people may believe that an infestation exists, even though several specialists have been unable to confirm the infestation. This belief can be dangerous for the person and those around if they use flammable or toxic substances to remove the infestation, whether it is perceived or real. Do *not* use kerosene to treat head lice infestations. Brown soap, vinegar rinses, and tar soaps are not effective.

Nondrug therapy: The most effective treatment is physically removing the lice and eggs, but this method is also the most time consuming. In a well-lit room, use magnification to locate the insects and remove them with a good louse or nit comb. Hair should be clean and free from tangles. Combing effectiveness may be influenced by hair texture, combing technique, and thoroughness of treatment (time and care expended). Curly hair will be more difficult to work with than straight hair. Selecting a small section of hair, comb down the hair shaft (toward the scalp) to detach the eggs, and clean the louse comb frequently. Eggs that have grown away from the scalp (more than

1 inch) have usually hatched. Viable eggs are found at the base of the hair shaft. Repeat the process (which may take several hours a day for several days) until eggs and active lice are gone.

Food oils (eg, vegetable oil, olive oil) or hair gels have been used to smother the lice, or to improve ease of combing. However, food oils may be difficult to remove from the hair and have been reported to make eggs more difficult to see.

Other methods include heat (eg, use of standard hair dryers; however, care must be taken not to burn the hair or scalp) or shaving the infested hair (including eyelashes or other facial hair). Shaving the infested area is not encouraged, but if shaving is the method selected, take care to avoid injury to the eyes.

Bed linens, towels, night clothes, and stuffed animals should be washed and dried on the hottest setting. Wash brushes, combs, hats, caps, and other hair accessories in hot water (higher than 130°F) each day until the infestation is resolved. Infested objects that cannot be heated in a clothes dryer because of possible shrinkage may be wrapped in a plastic bag and subjected to freezing temperatures (either in a freezer or outdoors) for several days.

Pharmacotherapy: Nonprescription agents used to treat head lice include permethrin 1% cream rinse (eg, *Nix*), the usual treatment of choice. This preparation is applied to the scalp and rinsed off after 10 minutes. Pyrethrins are also available and are the least toxic of the insecticides for humans. They induce nervous system paralysis in insects.

For severe infestations that do not respond to topical nonprescription drug therapy, refer patients to a physician. Prescripton topical agents for the treatment of head lice include lindane and malathion. Lindane has been widely used, but the development of resistance and its toxicity now limit its use. Malathion is an efficient pediculicide with good ovicidal activity and has a residual protective effect against reinfection for up to 6 weeks. It should remain on the scalp for 12 hours before being washed off. Trimethoprim-sulfamethoxazole, available by prescription, can also be used. The antibiotic is ingested by the louse from the patient's blood and affects its symbiotic bacteria, without which the louse cannot survive. It can be given as 80 mg trimethoprim plus 400 mg sulfamethoxazole twice daily for 3 days and repeated 7 to 10 days later.

For secondary bacterial infections, give appropriate systemic antibiotics. Decontamination of other inanimate objects is also an important lice control measure. Contaminated combs, brushes, barettes, and hair clips should be soaked in a pediculocidal shampoo (eg, *RID*) for at least 1 hour. Lice control spray (eg, *RID*) should be used to decontaminate items that cannot be machine washed and dried or soaked (eg, mattresses, chair backs, headrests, headphones, carpets, sofas, pillows). It is always prudent to vacuum frequently when a head lice infestation exists.

PERMETHRIN

▶ Actions

Permethrin is a synthetic pyrethroid that is active against lice, ticks, mites, and fleas. It acts quickly on the parasites' nerve cell membranes to disrupt the sodium channel current, resulting in delayed repolarization, paralysis of the pests, and death.

In vitro data indicate permethrin has pediculicidal and ovicidal activity against *Pediculus humanus* var. *capitis*. The high cure rate (97% to 99%) in patients with head lice demonstrated at 14 days after a single application is attributable to a combination of its pediculicidal and ovicidal activities and its residual persistence on the hair, which may also prevent reinfestation.

Permethrin is rapidly metabolized by ester hydrolysis to inactive metabolites that are excreted in the urine. The amount of permethrin absorbed after a single application of 5% prescription cream has not been determined, but preliminary data suggest it is less than 2% of the amount applied. Residual persistence is detectable on the hair for 10 days or longer following a single application.

▶ Indications

For the single-application treatment of infestation with *Pediculus humanus* var. *capitis* (the head louse) and its eggs. Treatment for recurrences is required in less than 1% of patients because the ovicidal activity may be supplemented by the drug's residual persistence in the hair. If live lice are observed 7 days or longer following the initial application, give a second application.

▶ Contraindications

Hypersensitivity to any synthetic pyrethroid or pyrethrin, chrysanthemums, ragweed, or any component of the product. If hypersensitivity (eg, rash, itching, hives, difficulty breathing) develops, discontinue use.

▶ Warnings

For external use only.

Pruritus, erythema, and edema: Pruritus, erythema, and edema often accompany head lice infestation. Treatment with permethrin may temporarily worsen these conditions, but this is no cause for alarm.

Pregnancy: Category B. There are no adequate and well-controlled studies in pregnant women. Use during pregnancy only if clearly needed.

Lactation: It is not known whether this drug is excreted in breast milk. Because of the evidence for tumorigenic potential of permethrin in animal studies, consider discontinuing nursing temporarily or withholding the drug while the mother is nursing.

Children: Safety and efficacy for use in children younger than 2 months or younger than 2 years (liquid) of age have not been established.

▶ Adverse Reactions

The most frequent adverse reaction is pruritus (itching). Usually a consequence of head lice infestation itself, itching may be temporarily aggravated following treatment.

Mild temporary itching (5.9%); mild transient burning, stinging, tingling, numbness, discomfort (3.4%); mild transient erythema, edema, or rash (2.1%).

▶ **Overdosage**

If ingested, perform gastric lavage, employ general supportive measures, and call a poison control center.

▶ **Administration and Dosage**

Use after the hair has been washed with shampoo, rinsed with water, and towel dried. Apply a sufficient volume to saturate the hair and scalp. Leave on the hair for 10 minutes before rinsing off with water.

A single treatment typically eliminates head lice infestation. If live lice are observed 7 days or longer after the initial application, apply again. Combing of nits is not required for therapeutic efficacy but may be done for cosmetic reasons.

PERMETHRIN PRODUCTS	
Trade name	Doseform
Nix	**Liquid (cream rinse)**: 1% permethrin. Cetyl alcohol, 20% isopropyl alcohol, parabens.
Nix Family Pack (2 treatments)	**Liquid (cream rinse)**: 1% permethrin. Cetyl alcohol, 20% isopropyl alcohol, parabens.

Products listed are representative of currently available and widely distributed brands. Similar products, including regional and private label brands, may also exist.

PATIENT INFORMATION
Permethrin

- Follow instructions provided with each product. Instructions for use vary from product to product.
- For external use only. Avoid contact with the mucous membranes (eg, nose, mouth), acutely inflamed skin, or raw, oozing skin.
- Itching, redness, or swelling of the scalp may occur; notify physician if irritation persists.
- Avoid contact with eyes; flush with water immediately if eye contact occurs.
- Washing and drying pillowcases, sheets, night clothes, towels, stuffed animals, etc. may help eliminate lice and eggs and should be done during an infestation to prevent reinfestation or further infestation of other family members. Combs, brushes, hats, and other hair accessories should be washed in hot water each day until the infestation is eliminated.
- Patient instructions and information are available with the product. Do not exceed the prescribed dosage.

PERMETHRIN SPRAYS

▶ **Indications**

To kill lice and their eggs on garments, bedding, and furniture. Also kills ticks and fleas.

▶ **Warnings**

Decontamination of inanimate objects: Not for use on humans or animals. Keep out of reach of children. If lice infestations should occur on humans, consult a physician or pharmacist for a product safe for human use.

Harmful if swallowed or absorbed through skin. Avoid breathing vapors or spray mist. Avoid contact with skin and eyes. If contact occurs, immediately flush eyes or skin with plenty of water. Consult a physician if irritation persists. If swallowed, do not induce vomiting. Contact a physician immediately.

Food proximity: Do not apply near or directly on food. Cover or remove all food and food processing equipment during application. Do not apply while food is being prepared. After spraying, wash all areas where exposed food will be handled (eg, benches, shelves, tables). All food oriented surfaces or utensils should be covered during treatment or thoroughly washed before use. Remove pets and birds, and cover fish aquariums before spraying.

Extremely flammable: Do not use or store near fire, sparks, or heated surfaces. Do not smoke in use area. Turn off pilot lights in gas appliances and unplug or turn off electical equipment until spraying is complete.

▶ **Administration and Dosage**

Shake well before each use. Remove protective cap. Aim spray opening away from person. Push button to spray. Spray only on garments or objects that cannot be laundered or dry cleaned (eg, mattresses, chair backs, headrests, headphones, carpets, sofas, pillows).

PERMETHRIN SPRAYS	
Trade name	Doseform
A•200[1]	**Spray:** 0.5%
RID[1]	**Spray:** 0.5%
Pronto[1]	**Spray:** 0.4%

Products listed are representative of currently available and widely distributed brands. Similar products, including regional and private label brands, may also exist.

[1] Not for use on humans or animals; for decontamination of inanimate objects.

PATIENT INFORMATION

Permethrin Sprays

- Follow instructions provided with each product. Instructions for use vary from product to product.
- For decontamination of inanimate objects only. Do not use on humans or animals.
- Avoid contact with skin and eyes; flush with water immediately if contact occurs.
- Irritation may occur upon skin contact; notify physician if irritation persists.
- Avoid breathing vapors or spray mist.
- Keep out of reach of children. If swallowed, do not induce vomiting. Consult a physician immediately.
- Use in a well-ventilated area.
- Keep away from food and food processing equipment during application.
- *Extremely flammable:* Store in a cool area away from heat or open flame. Exposure to temperatures above 130°F may cause bursting.
- Washing and drying pillowcases, sheets, night clothes, towels, stuffed animals, etc. may help eliminate lice and eggs and should be done during an infestation to prevent reinfestation or further infestation of other family members. Combs, brushes, hats, and other hair accessories should be washed in hot water each day until the infestation is eliminated.
- Patient instructions and information are available with the product.

MISCELLANEOUS PEDICULICIDES-PYRETHRINS

▶ **Indications**

Treatment of infestations of head lice, body lice, pubic (crab) lice, and their eggs.

▶ **Contraindications**

Hypersensitivity to ingredients; ragweed-sensitization (pyrethrins and permethrins).

▶ **Warnings**

For external use only. Harmful if swallowed or inhaled. May be irritating to the eyes, eyelids, and mucous membranes. In case of contact with eyes, flush with water. Discontinue use and notify physician if irritation or infection occurs.

Infestation of eyelashes or eyebrows: Do not use in these areas. Consult physician.

Reinfestation: To prevent reinfestation, sterilize or treat all clothing and bedding concurrently.

▶ **Administration and Dosage**

Administration and dosage varies. Refer to individual package inserts for information.

MISCELLANEOUS PEDICULICIDES-PYRETHINS	
Trade name	**Doseform[1]**
Tisit	**Liquid**: 0.3% pyrethrins, 2% piperonyl butoxide
	Shampoo: 0.3% pyrethrins, 3% piperonyl butoxide
A•200	**Shampoo**: 0.33% pyrethrins, 4% piperonyl butoxide
Clear	**Shampoo**: 0.33% pyrethrins, 4% piperonyl butoxide. Benzyl alcohol.
Tisit	**Shampoo**: 0.3% pyrethrins, 3% piperonyl butoxide
A•200 Maximum Strength, Pyrinyl Lice, Pyrinyl Plus, RID Maximum Strength	**Shampoo**: 0.33% pyrethrins, 4% piperonyl butoxide. Isopropyl alcohol, castor oil.
R&C	**Shampoo/Conditioner**: 0.33% pyrethrins, 3% piperonyl butoxide
Pronto	**Shampoo/Conditioner**: 0.33% pyrethrins, 4% piperonyl butoxide
Pronto with Creme Rinse Kit	**Shampoo/Conditioner**: 0.33% pyrethrins, 4% piperonyl butoxide
Tisit Blue	**Gel**: 0.3% pyrethrins, 3% piperonyl butoxide
InnoGel Plus	**Gel**: 0.3% pyrethrins, 3% piperonyl butoxide
A•200	**Gel**: 0.33% pyrethrins, 4% piperonyl butoxide
Tisit [2]	**Kit**: 0.3% pyrethrins, 4% piperonyl butoxide (shampoo); 0.4% pyrethrins, 2% piperonyl butoxide (spray)
A•200 [2]	**Kit**: 0.33% pyrethrins, 4% piperonyl butoxide (shampoo); 0.5% permethrin (spray)
Pronto [2]	**Kit**: 0.33% pyrethrins, 4% piperonyl butoxide (shampoo); 0.4% permethrin (spray)
Clear	**Kit**: 0.33% pyrethrins, 4% piperonyl butoxide. Benzyl alcohol (shampoo); hydrolase, isomerase, ligase, lyase, oxidoreductase, transferase, detergents (gel).

MISCELLANEOUS PEDICULICIDES-PYRETHINS	
Trade name	Doseform[1]
RID [2]	**Kit**: 0.33% pyrethrins, 4% piperonyl butoxide (shampoo); 0.5% permethrin (spray)

Products listed are representative of currently available and widely distributed brands. Similar products, including regional and private label brands, may also exist.

[1] Piperonyl butoxide is not an insecticide but it increases the pediculicidal activity of pyrethrins by a factor of 2 to 10 because it impairs the insect's ability to metabolize and detoxify pyrethrins. Effective concentrations of piperonyl butoxide range from 2% to 4%.

[2] The spray component of each kit not for use on humans or animals; for decontamination of inanimate objects only.

PATIENT INFORMATION

Miscellaneous Pediculicides-Pyrethrins

- Follow instructions provided with each product. Instructions for use vary from product to product.
- For external use only. Avoid contact with eyes, eyelids, mucous membranes (eg, nose, mouth), acutely inflamed skin, or raw, oozing skin.
- Avoid contact with eyes: Flush with water immediately if eye contact occurs.
- During use, close eyes tightly and do not open them until product is rinsed out. In addition, cover eyes with washcloth, towel, or other covering during use.
- Keep out of reach of children. If swallowed, contact a poison control center immediately.
- Itching, redness, or swelling of the scalp may occur; notify physician if irritation persists.
- Washing and drying pillowcases, sheets, night clothes, scarves, pillows, cushions, towels, stuffed animals, etc. may help eliminate lice and eggs, and should be done during an infestation to prevent reinfestation or further infestation of other family members. Combs, brushes, hats, and other hair accessories should be washed in hot water each day until the infestation is eliminated.
- Patient instructions and information are available with the product. Do not exceed the prescribed dosage.

IMPETIGO

DEFINITION

Impetigo, also known as impetigo contagiosa or bullous impetigo, is a common bacterial skin disease caused by either group A β-hemolytic streptococci or *Staphylococcus aureus*.

ETIOLOGY

Impetigo contagiosa is generally caused by group A β-hemolytic streptococci bacteria; bullous impetigo is generally caused by *Staphylococcus aureus*. Depending upon the depth of the infection, an impetigo contagiosum lesion that extends into the dermis and causes a shallow ulceration is termed ecthyma.

Usually, an impetigo contagiosa infection begins as a pure streptococcal infection, which may later become secondarily infected with *S. aureus*.

INCIDENCE

Impetigo is a common skin infection that occurs more frequently in children and young adults although it may appear at any age. Impetigo prevalence is higher in countries with a tropical climate; it occurs most frequently in late summer and early fall.

PATHOPHYSIOLOGY

Pathogenic streptococci are not considered to be normal flora of the skin. Hence, it is usually believed that local factors, such as abrasion or puncturing of the skin by insect bites or scratching from a dermatitis, play a role in the development of impetigo with streptococci germs.

Bullous impetigo is probably induced by an epidermolysin produced by *S. aureus*. This is the same epidermolysin that causes scalded skin syndrome.

SIGNS/SYMPTOMS

Impetigo contagiosa usually begins as a small papule that becomes a vesicle-pustule and quickly ruptures to become a honey-colored crust on a red base. Over a period of days, more crusted lesions develop. If left untreated, the lesions often show central clearing. Generally, the legs, arms, face, and trunk (in that order) are infected. Itching is a common symptom. Patients should avoid scratching, if possible, as this may spread the infection.

Bullous impetigo begins as a small vesicle that quickly develops into a bulla. These bullae persist longer than the vesicles of impetigo contagiosa, and when these rupture, a red-based, thin, honey-colored, crusted lesion is produced. These lesions occur most commonly on the face.

Usually, systemic symptoms are not observed although regional lymphadenopathy is commonly seen, especially with impetigo contagiosa when diagnosis and treatment are delayed or neglected. Cellulitis is a potential complication of impetigo.

DIAGNOSTIC PARAMETERS/PHYSICAL ASSESSMENT

Clinical Observation: Honey-colored, crusted lesions on an erythematous base on the exposed areas of the legs, arms, and face, especially in children, are indicative of impetigo. The relative rapid onset of disease, often associated with regional lymphadenopathy but without systemic symptoms, should be sought. Recent damage to the skin, as with insect bites or abrasion, or a recent bout of frequent nose-blowing, will help determine the underlying cause.

Interview: To ensure the proper diagnosis of impetigo contagiosa, it may be beneficial to ask about the following:

• Duration of symptoms/condition.
• Description of condition (especially if on areas of the body not readily apparent, [eg, trunk]).
• Exposure to other individuals with a similar condition (eg, wrestlers will often contract this condition from other wrestlers because of the nature of the sport and subsequent contact).
• Recent abrasion or insect bite before symptoms occurred.

TREATMENT

Approaches to therapy: Because there is no effective OTC treatment, it is important to determine the possibility of impetigo, at which point physician referral is necessary and appropriate.

Nondrug therapy: There is no effective OTC treatment of impetigo. The traditional therapy of soaks, washing with hexachlorophene soap, and topical antibiotics (eg, bacitracin, neomycin, polymyxin) are of little value unless lesions are detected very early, are superficial, and involve only a small area of skin surface.

Pharmacotherapy: Systemic antibiotics (eg, penicillins, tetracyclines, cephalosporins) are the treatment of choice in impetigo contagiosa. Lesions heal promptly with the selection and use of an appropriate systemic antibiotic. It is important to remember to treat the nose with a staph/streptococcal bactericidal agent to cut down on the resident flora of these bacteria.

INSECT BITES AND STINGS

DEFINITION

Insect bites and stings cause local or systemic reactions (mild to fatal) in susceptible individuals. The reaction to bites and stings is the result of toxins or allergens injected by the arthropod. Most reactions are mild. Insect bites and stings produce approximately 50 deaths per year in the US.

ETIOLOGY

The irritation that occurs from insect bites and stings is caused by a variety of substances. Mosquitoes and flies inject irritating salivary secretions. Hymenoptera (ie, bees, wasps, hornets, yellow jackets, fire ants) inject venom containing proteins, amines, and enzymes that cause histamine release in susceptible individuals. The sting from fire ants also contains alkaloids that are irritating. Spiders may inject venoms that are hemolytic, enzymatic, or that may affect the nervous system.

INCIDENCE

Biting arthropods: The most common biting arthropods are nonvenomous and include mosquitoes, ticks, chiggers (redbugs), mites, fleas, lice, and sand, horse, or deer flies. Bites from these arthropods frequently cause local reactions but rarely cause anaphylaxis.

Spiders: In the US, the spiders that cause the most serious reactions in humans are the black widow and the brown recluse.

Hymenoptera: The harvester ant and the fire ant cause most ant sting reactions in humans. Stings from other hymenoptera (eg, bees, wasps, hornets, yellow jackets) cause local reactions in most patients, but can cause anaphylaxis in approximately 4% of the US population. The incidence of anaphylaxis correlates with exposure; the average age of affected individuals is 20 years with an increased frequency in men. Severe reactions and fatalities are more common in adults; fatalities are rare in children. More than 80% of the deaths secondary to anaphylaxis occur within 1 hour of the sting. Approximately 50% of deaths caused by bites or stings from venomous animals are the result of bees or wasps; 14% are caused by poisonous spiders. More deaths occur in the US from bee stings than snakebites.

PATHOPHYSIOLOGY

Insect bites and stings cause local allergic reactions resulting in the release of histamine. The *normal reaction* to an insect bite or sting is sharp, localized pain followed by a small reddened area that resolves within 24 hours. While insect bites may or may not be painful, insect stings are almost always painful. When there is an unusual amount of swelling, itching, and pain at the sting site, the patient is considered to have a severe local reaction. A *toxic reaction* occurs following an episode of simultaneous multiple stings and is the result of histamine-like substances in the venom; it is not truly an allergic reaction. A toxic reaction manifests with GI symptoms, headache, vertigo, syncope, convulsions, and fever. An *immediate systemic reaction* can be mild to severe. Mild reactions are the most common; symptoms occur beyond the sting site and usually include itching, flushing, and urticaria. A *severe systemic reaction* (ie, anaphylaxis) usually occurs 15 to 60 minutes after the sting and has airway involvement (eg, dyspnea, wheezing, chest tightness, hoarseness) and hypotension (eg, disorientation, loss of consciousness, incontinence, nausea, vomiting, abdominal pain). Anaphylaxis is an acute, life-threatening, generalized reaction that results from the release of mediators from mast cells, basophils, and other inflammatory cells. Patients using beta blockers may experience severe and protracted anaphylaxis, and treatment of hypotension may be resistant to therapy. Their reactions may diminish temporarily and then intensify after several hours. Patients who have a history of severe systemic reactions to any insect bite or sting are strongly encouraged to purchase and retain ready access to an *EpiPen Auto Injector* or its equivalent. Such a device contains a dose of epinephrine in a 1:1000 concentration in a 2 mL disposable, prefilled auto injector. Prompt use of an *EpiPen* can save a life. A *delayed systemic reaction* occurs 2 hours to 3 weeks after the sting and manifests as serum sickness (eg, fever, arthralgia, lymphadenopathy, urticaria, angioedema, purpura), neurologic reactions (eg, peripheral neuritis, hemiplegia, encephalopathy), allergic vasculitis, and coagulation defects. The most serious reactions to biting insects are caused by acquired hypersensitivity; the most serious reaction to stinging insects is anaphylaxis.

SIGNS/SYMPTOMS

Biting arthropods: The immediate reaction to a mosquito bite is itching. A delayed reaction, which may occur several hours later, can cause severe, intense burning and itching. Flea bites typically cause itching. Fly bites can cause a painful sting when the fly pierces through the skin and injects its irritating salivary secretions. While the bite from a tick is usually not painful, the tick can serve as a vector for other diseases such as Lyme disease and Rocky Mountain spotted fever. Chiggers attach to skin and suck blood. The bite from chigger larvae releases antigenic salivary and digestive chemicals, including an enzyme that causes cellular degeneration, red papules, and intense itching. Chigger larvae do not burrow into skin, but reside within the papule.

Hymenoptera: The normal reaction to the sting from hymenoptera includes itching, local burning, erythema, and pain that usually subsides within several hours. Severe local reactions cause itching, pain, and an unusual amount of localized swelling. An immediate systemic reaction will manifest as anaphylaxis. With a delayed systemic reaction, there will be urticaria with lymphadenopathy and polyarthritis. The sting from harvester or fire ants causes intense burning and pain.

Spiders: Reaction to spider bites depend on the type of spider. Ninety percent of the time the bite from the brown recluse spider causes little or no pain; sometimes there can be severe local pain and localized swelling 4 to 8 hours after the bite. Within 24 hours, the bite is a painful, purple papule surrounded by a blanched ischemic zone. This lesion progresses to a necrotic, ulcerating wound for as long as a week after the bite. A disfiguring ulcer may result, requiring weeks to heal and possible surgical grafting. Systemic reactions to the brown recluse spider include nausea, vomiting, malaise, chills, sweats, thrombocytopenia, kidney failure, and, rarely, death. The black widow spider causes an initial short, sharp, pinprick-like pain at the bite site followed by systemic reactions including chills, nausea, vomiting, abdominal pain, leg pain, sweating, restlessness, anxiety, headache, dizziness, respiratory distress, increased salivation, and, rarely, death. The syndrome following the bite of the black widow spider may be confused with any medical or surgical condition with acute abdominal symptoms. The symptoms of a black widow spider bite increase in severity for several hours, perhaps a day, and then very slowly become less severe, gradually passing off in 2 or 3 days, except in fatal cases. Residual symptoms such as general weakness, tingling, nervousness, and transient muscle spasm may persist for weeks or months after recovery from the acute stage.

DIAGNOSTIC PARAMETERS/PHYSICAL ASSESSMENT

Biting arthropods: Arthropod bites vary from small papules to large ulcers with swelling and acute pain. Dermatitis may also occur. The most serious bites are complicated by sensitivity reactions. Mosquito bites initiate as wheals that may develop into a swollen papular lesions several hours later. Flea bites are usually grouped, urticarial papules.

Hymenoptera: Unlike arthropod bites, insect stings are almost always associated with pain that tends to be more severe on the extremities than on the trunk or head. The affected area is red with a central punctum (point of projection) surrounded by a white zone and flare zone. There is usually intense local edema around the sting area. Honeybees will leave a stinger. The sting from fire ants begins as a wheal and flare lesion that develops into a sterile pustule at the sting site.

Spiders: The local reaction to the black widow spider bite is unremarkable. The bite from the brown recluse spider looks like a bull's-eye.

Interview: To help patients determine the most appropriate form of treatment, it may be beneficial to ask about the following:

- The type of insect (if known)
- The setting in which the patient was bitten or stung (to help determine the type of insect, if unknown)
- Previous reactions to insect bites or stings
- Previous response to treatments
- Current symptoms, including itching and swelling, difficulty breathing, dizziness, nausea, and abdominal pain
- Description and extent of bite or sting
- Any treatment already administered and how it helped
- Presence/absence of a stinger
- Any known adverse reactions to topical ointments

TREATMENT

Approaches to therapy: Because most treatments for insect bites and stings are of limited value, it is important to use preventative measures such as avoidance, physical barriers (eg, clothing, hats, screens), chemical protection (eg, insect repellents), or administration of venom immunotherapy, which is available by prescription only. When bitten by an insect, flick the insect off the skin and apply ice to the area as soon as possible to relieve pain, retard absorption, and decrease the chemical activity of the venom. Ticks are best removed by grasping close to the skin with tweezers and pulling steadily upward until completely extracted; never squeeze, crush, or puncture the tick. If stung by a bee, remove the stinger by scraping, not by pulling or squeezing.

Nondrug therapy: The best interventions for insect bites and stings are preventative measures.

Biting arthropods – To minimize mosquito bites, perform the following activities: Eliminate water-containing recepticles near the home; treat mosquito breeding sites with insecticides; stay indoors during the late afternoon, early evening, and night; avoid bright-colored clothing; and cover skin with clothing. To minimize bites from ticks, visually inspect the entire body thoroughly after being in wooded areas. Insect repellents are a convenient way to prevent mosquito, flea, tick, and fly bites; none are available that are effective against stinging insects. Insect repellents, available in a variety of forms (ie, creams, lotions, sprays), are applied directly to clothing and skin. They deter insects by producing an offensive vapor barrier but do not kill the insect. Their efficacy is reduced by sweating or washing, and increased temperatures, or high winds. *Avon's Skin-So-Soft* has been used as a natural repellent that works by forming a slippery physical barrier. While it might offer some efficacy in detering mosquitoes, it acts for a limited duration of time (15 minutes to 1.5 hours). Citronella oil, available in lotions, sprays, candles, and incense sticks, is another natural product used to deter mosquitoes that is also of limited efficacy and duration.

The most studied and most commonly used insect repellent is DEET (N,N-diethyl-m-toluanide). It is effective against a variety of insects including mosquitoes, biting fleas, gnats, black flies, and ticks. For adults, a 10% to 30% DEET product is recommended for normal daily activities while a 40% to 50% product is recommended for camping and hiking. Use in children should be restricted to products containing less than 10% DEET; it should not be used in children younger than 2 years old. When using DEET in children, apply the product to clothing, thereby minimizing application to the skin. Local reactions (eg, dermatitis, irritation) can occur with the use of DEET; serious reactions (eg, seizures, allergic reactions, encephalopathy) have also been reported, mostly in children.

DEET-CONTAINING INSECT REPELLENTS	
Products	**% DEET**
Gel	
Cutter Skinsations	7%. Aloe vera, vitamin E.
Repel	7%
Lotion	
Cutter Skinsations	7%. Aloe vera, vitamin E.
Off Skintastic MagiColor[1]	7.5%
Off Skintastic with Sunscreen, Repel, Repel Camp for Kids	10%
Repel and Sun Block, Repel Sun & Bug Stuff, Repel Sportmen Formula	20%
Cutter Outdoorsman	30%
Spray, aerosol	
Cutter Skinsations	7%. Aloe vera, vitamin E.
Cutter All Family	10%
Repel Family Formula[2]	18%
Cutter Backwoods	23%
Off Deepwoods	25%
Repel Sportmen Formula[2]	29%
Cutter Outdoorsman, Off Deepwoods for Sportsmen	30%
Repel Classic Formula	40%
Spray, pump	
Off Skintastic for Kids	5%
Cutter All Family, Off Skintastic with Aloe Vera	7%. Aloe vera.
Cutter Skinsations	7%. Aloe vera, vitamin E.
Repel Sportmen Formula	18%
Cutter Backwoods, Repel Family Formula	23%
Cutter Outdoorsman	30%
Off Deepwoods for Sportsmen, Repel 100	100%
Stick	
Cutter Outdoorsman	30%
Towelettes	
Cutter All Family	7%

* Products listed are representative of currently available and widely distributed brands. Similar products, including regional and private brands, may also exist.
[1] In purple color.
[2] Also available in pocket size.

Permethrin is another available agent that acts as an insecticide and a repellent. It is most effective against lice, ticks, fleas, mites, mosquitoes, and black flies. It is the best available agent for repelling ticks. Permethrin is recommended for use on clothing or camping gear and tents. When using any insect repellent, it is important to remember that these products are pesticides. As such, follow these guidelines:

• Apply only as directed
• Use only on intact skin
• Do not use near eyes or mouth and cautiously near ears
• Avoid breathing aerosol products
• Only apply to exposed skin or clothing
• Do not apply to children's hands

- Once inside, wash treated areas with soap and water
- Wash clothes before rewearing
- If an adverse reaction is suspected, wash immediately and seek medical attention.

Hymenoptera – To minimize exposure to bees and wasps, avoid disturbing hives or activity near flowers or blooming trees; wear long sleeves and protective clothing; avoid wearing leather, bright-colored clothing, or flowery prints; avoid wearing flowers and scented cosmetics; do not walk barefoot outdoors; and keep garbage can lids tightly closed.

Spiders – Spider bites can be minimized by checking stored items before use. Local treatment of the bite is of no value; nothing is gained by applying a tourniquet or attempting to remove venom by incision and suction. If possible, hospitalize the patient for black widow or brown recluse spider bites.

Pharmacotherapy: Biting anthropods (eg, ticks, chiggers, fleas, lice) can be suffocated with a topical application of a lacquer-containing liquid such as *Chiggerid* or clear nail polish. Other agents used to treat insect bites and stings are designed to manage symptoms. Agents available for relieving the itching associated with insect bites include topical antipruritics, topical steroids, and systemic antipruritics. If the patient presents with a systemic reaction, a physician referral is warranted. Emergency kits for those who are hypersensitive to the stings from hymenoptera are available by prescription. If the systemic reaction is severe, prompt medical attention should be sought to handle potential acute respiratory and cardiovascular emergencies.

TOPICAL ANTIHISTAMINE-CONTAINING PRODUCTS

▶ **Actions**

Diphenhydramine (0.5% to 2%) is the antihistamine contained in most topical products to manage symptoms of insect bites and stings. Topical antihistamine containing products often contain multiple additional ingredients. Some have local anesthetic activity and are used to relieve itching. Some transdermal absorption may occur, but not in sufficient quantities to produce significant systemic side effects. They may cause local irritation and sensitization, especially with prolonged use. The actions of selected adjunctive agents are listed in the following table:

Adjunctive Topical Agents for Managing Symptoms of Insect Bites and Stings	
Drug	Use
Benzalkonium chloride, eucalyptol	Bacteriostatic agents
Benzocaine (5% to 20%)	Local anesthetic
Benzyl alcohol (5% to 20%), camphor (0.1% to 3%), menthol (0.1% to 1%), phenol (0.25% to 1%)	Antipruritic effects
Calamine, zinc oxide	Astringents
Chlorobutanol	Antipruritic and antiseptic effects
Isopropyl alcohol	Antiseptic
Pramoxine (0.5% to 1%)	Local anesthetic

▶ **Indications**

Temporary relief of itching due to minor skin disorders including poison ivy, sumac, or oak; sunburn; and insect bites and stings.

▶ **Warnings**

Do not apply to blistered, raw, or oozing areas of the skin, or around the eyes or other mucous membranes (eg, nose, mouth).

▶ **Administration and Dosage**

Apply a thin layer as needed and according to package directions to control symptoms.

TOPICAL ANTIHISTAMINE-CONTAINING PRODUCTS[1]	
Trade name	Doseform
Band-Aid Fast Relief Anti-Itch	**Spray:** 2% diphenhydramine HCl, 0.1% zinc acetate, 12% benzyl alcohol
Benadryl Extra Strength Itch Relief	**Stick:** 2% diphenhydramine HCl, 0.1% zinc acetate. 73.5% alcohol.
	Spray: 2% diphenhydramine HCl, 0.1% zinc acetate. 73.5% alcohol.
Benadryl Extra Strength Itch Stopping	**Cream:** 2% diphenhydramine HCl, 0.1% zinc acetate
	Gel: 2% diphenhydramine HCl
	Spray, pump: 2% diphenhydramine HCl, 0.1% zinc acetate. 73.6% alcohol.
Benadryl Itch Stopping	**Cream:** 1% diphenhydramine HCl, 0.1% zinc acetate
	Gel: 1% diphenhydramine HCl
	Spray, pump: 1% diphenhydramine HCl, 1% zinc oxide. 73.6% alcohol.
CalaGel	**Gel:** 1.8% diphenhydramine HCl, 0.21% zinc acetate
Calamycin Multi-Purpose Medicated	**Lotion:** 2% diphenhydramine, calamine, 5% zinc oxide, 5% benzocaine
Derma-Pax	**Lotion:** 0.5% diphenhydramine HCl
Dermamycin	**Cream:** 2% diphenhydramine HCl
	Spray: 2% diphenhydramine HCl, 1% menthol
Dermarest Clear Anti-Itch with Aloe	**Gel:** 2% diphenhydramine HCl, 2% resorcinol
Dermarest Plus	**Gel:** 2% diphenhydramine HCl, 1% menthol
	Spray: 2% diphenhydramine HCl, 1% menthol
Di-Delamine	**Gel:** 1% diphenhydramine HCl, 0.5% tripelennamine HCl
HC Derma-Pax	**Spray:** 0.5% diphenhydramine HCl, 0.5% hydrocortisone
Soothaderm	**Lotion:** 2.07% pyrilamine maleate, 2.08% benzocaine, 41.35% zinc oxide

Products listed are representative of currently available and widely distributed brands. Similar products, including regional and private label brands, may also exist.

[1] For topical products containing no antihistamine, see the Local Anesthetics-Topical monographs in the Dermatological Conditions chapter.

PATIENT INFORMATION
Topical Antihistamine-Containing Products
- For external use only. Avoid contact with the eyes, nose, or mouth.
- Do not apply to blistered, raw, or oozing areas of the skin.
- If condition persists, recurs after a few days, or if irritation develops, discontinue use.
- Avoid prolonged use (longer than 7 days) or use on extensive skin areas. If symptoms persist for longer than 7 days, contact your doctor.

CAMPHORATED COMPOUNDS

▶ **Warnings**

Apply to dry skin only; may have caustic effects if applied to moist areas.

▶ **Administration and Dosage**

Clean the affected area before applying. Apply with cotton 1 to 3 times daily.

CAMPHORATED COMPOUNDS	
Trade name	Doseform
Campho-phenique Pain Relieving Antiseptic	**Liquid**: 10.8% camphor, 4.7% phenol. Eucalyptus oil, light mineral oil.
	Gel: 10.8% camphor, 4.7% phenol. Eucalyptus oil, glycerin, light mineral oil.

Products listed are representative of currently available and widely distributed brands. Similar products, including regional and private label brands, may also exist.

PATIENT INFORMATION
Camphorated Compounds
- Doses and frequency of use depend on the condition, the area to be treated, individual tolerance, and doseform. Individual products should be reviewed for their use and dosage guidelines. Consult your doctor or pharmacist for product-specific information.
- For external use only. Avoid contact with eyes. If contact occurs, immediately flush with water.
- Do not apply over large areas of the body or in large quantities.
- Consult your doctor before use if you have deep or puncture wounds, animal bites, or serious burns.
- Do not use for longer than 1 week, unless directed by your doctor.
- Stop use and consult your doctor if conditions worsen or if symptoms persist for more than 7 days or clear up and occur again within a few days.
- Discontinue use and consult your doctor if redness, irritation, swelling, or pain increases.
- Clean the affected area and apply liquid with cotton 1 to 3 times daily.
- Do not bandage.
- In case of accidental ingestion, contact your doctor or the Poison Control Center immediately.

CORTICOSTEROIDS, TOPICAL

► **Actions**

The primary therapeutic effect of topical corticosteroids is due to their nonspecific anti-inflammatory activity (ie, they act against most causes of inflammation including mechanical, chemical, microbiological, and immunological). Topical corticosteroids diffuse across cell membranes to interact with cytoplasmic receptors located in the dermal and intradermal cells. The intracellular effects are similar to those of systemic corticosteroids.

► **Indications**

Temporary relief of redness and itching associated with minor skin irritations, inflammation, and rashes caused by eczema, insect bites or stings, poison ivy, poison oak, poison sumac, soaps, detergents, cosmetics, and jewelry. These agents have other labeled indications as well. Do not use these products chronically without consulting a physician.

► **Contraindications**

Hypersensitivity to any component of the formulation; monotherapy in primary bacterial infections such as impetigo, paronychia, erysipelas, cellulitis, angular cheilitis, treatment of rosacea, perioral dermatitis or acne; ophthalmic use or use near the eyes.

► **Warnings**

Local irritation: If local irritation develops, discontinue use and institute appropriate therapy.

For external use only: Avoid ingestion or contact with eyes.

Pregnancy: Category C. Animal studies have shown adverse effects, but there are no adequate studies in humans. Benefits from topical use in pregnant women may be acceptable.

Lactation: It is not known whether topical corticosteroids could result in sufficient systemic absorption to produce detectable quantities in breast milk. Exercise caution when administering topical corticosteroids to a nursing mother.

Children: Children may be more susceptible to topical corticosteroid-induced hypothalamic-pituitary-adrenal (HPA) axis suppression and Cushing syndrome than adults. Consult a physician regarding pediatric use, and limit administration to the least amount compatible with effective therapy.

► **Drug Interactions**

Because these products are low potency and are applied topically for a limited time, systemic absorption is likely to be minimal and drug interactions are unlikely to occur.

► **Adverse Reactions**

Local reactions are rare with short-term use, but may include burning, itching, erythema, dryness, folliculitis, hypertrichosis, acneiform eruptions, hypopigmentation, perioral dermatitis, allergic contact dermatitis, stinging and cracking or tightening of skin, maceration of the skin, and secondary infection. Skin atrophy, striae, miliaria, and telangiectasia would be more likely with chronic use. While systemic absorption has produced reversible HPA axis suppression and other systemic effects, they are unlikely to occur with the application of low-potency agents for a short period of time. Following prolonged application around the eyes, cataracts and glaucoma may develop.

▶ **Administration and Dosage**

Apply sparingly to affected areas 2 to 4 times daily. Use 1% concentration of hydro-cortisone, if well tolerated, for optimal effect. To avoid greasiness, select a cream over an ointment.

TOPICAL CORTICOSTEROID PRODUCTS	
Trade name	**Doseform**
Corticaine, Cortizone•5, Cortizone•5 with Aloe	**Cream:** 0.5% hydrocortisone
Cortaid Intensive Therapy, Cortaid Maximum Strength, Cortizone•10, Dermtex HC, Hytone, Lanacort, Maximum Strength KeriCort-10	**Cream:** 1% hydrocortisone
Hytone	**Cream:** 2.5% hydrocortisone
CortaGel Extra Strength, CortiCool	**Gel:** 1% hydrocortisone
Cortizone•5	**Ointment:** 0.5% hydrocortisone
Cortaid Maximum Strength	**Ointment:** 1% hydrocortisone
	Stick: 1% hydrocortisone.
	Pump Spray: 1% hydrocortisone
Cortizone•10	**Spray:** 1% hydrocortisone
Dermtex HC	**Spray:** 1% hydrocortisone. 1% menthol.

Products listed are representative of currently available and widely distributed brands. Similar products, including regional and private label brands, may also exist.

PATIENT INFORMATION

Topical Corticosteroids

- For external use only.
- Apply ointments, creams, gels, and sprays sparingly in a light film; rub in gently. To avoid greasiness, select a cream over an ointment. Washing or soaking the area before application may increase drug penetration. After application, do not wash or rub the area and keep away from clothing until the lotion dries.
- To use a lotion, solution, or gel on the scalp, part hair, apply a small amount of the medicine on the affected area, and rub it in gently. Wash hair as usual, but not right after applying the medicine.
- Use only as directed. Do not put bandages, dressing, cosmetics, or other skin products over the treated area unless directed by a physician.
- Notify a physician if the condition worsens, or if burning, swelling, or redness develops.
- Avoid prolonged use around the eyes, in the genital and rectal areas, and on the face, armpits, and in skin creases unless directed by a physician. Avoid contact with the eyes.
- If you forget an application, apply it as soon as you remember, and continue on your regular schedule. If it is almost time for the next application, wait and continue on your regular schedule. Do not apply double doses.
- *For parents of pediatric patients:* Consult a physician. If corticosteroid treatment is recommended, do not use tight-fitting diapers or plastic pants on a child treated in the diaper area; these garments may work like occlusive dressings and cause more of the drug to be absorbed into your child's body. Do not use topical steroids to treat diaper rash.

DIPHENHYDRAMINE, ORAL

▶ Actions

Diphenhydramine is an antihistamine that antagonizes histamine at the H_1-receptor site but does not bind with histamine to inactivate it. Antihistamines do not block histamine release, antibody production, or antigen-antibody interactions. The antipruritic (anti-itching) effect is the primary value of diphenhydramine for managing the symptoms of insect bites and stings. Diphenhydramine also has anticholinergic properties (eg, dry eyes, dry mouth, constipation).

▶ Indications

For the symptomatic relief of allergic and nonallergic pruritic symptoms. This agent has other labeled indications as well.

▶ Contraindications

Hypersensitivity to antihistamines; newborn or premature infants; nursing mothers; narrow-angle glaucoma; stenosing peptic ulcer; symptomatic prostatic hypertrophy; bladder obstruction; pyloroduodenal obstruction; lower respiratory tract symptoms (including asthma); use of monoamine oxidase inhibitors.

▶ Warnings

Pregnancy: Category B.

Lactation: Safety for use in the nursing mother has not been established.

Children: Use on children younger than 2 years of age only as directed by a physician.

▶ Drug Interactions

Concomitant use of alcohol or other CNS depressants with antihistamines may have an additive effect. MAOIs may prolong and intensify the anticholinergic effects of antihistamines.

▶ Adverse Reactions

Adverse reactions can be seen in the CNS (eg, drowsiness, restlessness, slowed reaction time, impaired coordination, blurred vision), GI (eg, dry mouth, anorexia), GU (eg, urinary retention), cardiovascular (eg, hypotension, palpitations, tachycardia), and respiratory (eg, thickening of bronchial secretions, chest tightness, wheezing) systems.

▶ Administration and Dosage

Adults: 25 to 50 mg every 6 to 8 hours as needed.

Children (more than 10 kg): 12.5 to 25 mg 3 or 4 times daily as needed.

DIPHENHYDRAMINE HCL PRODUCTS	
Trade name	Doseform
Banophen, Benadryl Allergy Kapseals, Benadryl Dye-Free Allergy Liqui-Gels	**Capsules, soft gels**: 25 mg
Banophen, Diphenydramine HCl, Genahist	**Capsules**: 25 mg
Diphenhist, Diphenhydramine HCl	**Capsules**: 50 mg
Benadryl Allergy	**Tablets, chewable**: 12.5 mg
Banophen, Benadryl Allergy Ultratabs, Diphenhist Captabs	**Tablets**: 25 mg
AllerMax Maximum Strength	**Tablets**: 50 mg
Benadryl Dye-Free Allergy[1], Diphen AF[2]	**Liquid**: 6.25 mg/5 mL

DIPHENHYDRAMINE HCL PRODUCTS	
Trade name	Doseform
AllerMax Allergy & Cough, Banophen, Genahist[3], Scot-Tussin Allergy Relief Formula[2]	**Liquid**: 12.5 mg/5 mL
Diphenhist	**Solution**: 12.5 mg/5 mL
Siladryl	**Elixir**: 12.5 mg/5 mL

Products listed are representative of currently available and widely distributed brands. Similar products, including regional and private label brands, may also exist.

[1] In bubble gum flavor.
[2] In cherry flavor.
[3] In cherry-strawberry flavor.

PATIENT INFORMATION

Diphenhydramine, Oral

- Keep out of reach of children.
- May cause drowsiness; observe caution while driving or performing other tasks requiring coordination, alertness, or physical dexterity.
- Avoid alcohol and other CNS depressants.
- Inform physician of a history of glaucoma, peptic ulcer, urinary retention, or pregnancy before starting this medication.
- May cause nervousness, dry mouth, or insomnia.

PRICKLY HEAT
(Miliaria; Heat Rash)

DEFINITION

Prickly heat, or miliaria rubra, is a sweating disorder that results in an acute, inflammatory, pruritic rash. There are 3 other forms of miliaria that do not result in the characteristic rash of prickly heat.

ETIOLOGY

Prickly heat is caused by occluded eccrine (sweat) glands; the cause of the obstruction is still unknown.

INCIDENCE

Prickly heat may be seen in patients of any age but is most commonly seen in infants and children; 40% of infants may be affected. It is usually seen in warm, humid weather or in patients who are overdressed in cold weather. It can also be seen in patients who are wearing nonporous clothing or in patients who are febrile.

PATHOPHYSIOLOGY

Prickly heat occurs when perspiration cannot reach the skin surface because of duct obstruction and inflammation. Sweat gets trapped in the epidermis or dermis, causing irritation and edema of the stratum corneum. In infants, it is believed that prickly heat is caused by immaturity of the eccrine (sweat) structures, which results in sweat retention.

SIGNS/SYMPTOMS

Prickly heat presents as a rash that creates a tingling, burning, prickling sensation (more so than an itch). Other forms of miliaria are typically asymptomatic.

DIAGNOSTIC PARAMETERS/PHYSICAL ASSESSMENT

Clinical Observation: Miliaria is classified into 4 subtypes: Crystallina, rubra, pustulosa, and profunda. The diagnosis depends on clinical presentation. Miliaria crystallina is usually associated with neonates, after a severe sunburn, or with a febrile illness. It presents as minute (1 to 2 mm), superficial, noninflammatory, vesicular lesions that rupture easily when rubbed. The lesions tend to occur on the head, trunk, or back, and can be few to many in number. Miliaria rubra (common prickly heat) occurs when the sweat duct is occluded deeper, thereby causing inflamed, nonfollicular, erythematous, pruritic papules. Prickly heat lesions may be localized or generalized and typically occur on the neck, scalp, or upper trunk. Miliaria pustulosa occurs when miliaria rubra becomes pustular; the lesions are usually superficial. Miliaria profunda occurs when sweat is retained in the dermis causing noninflammatory, nonpruritic, flesh-colored papules that are firm to touch. Lesions tend to occur on the trunk or the extremities.

Interview: To ensure the proper diagnosis and treatment of prickly heat, it may be beneficial to ask about the following:

• Duration and type of symptoms.
• Concurrent medical conditions.
• Recent use of occlusive dressings or tight-fitting clothes.

TREATMENT

Approaches to therapy: Treatment for prickly heat is symptomatic and prophylactic. The involved skin should be kept cool and dry, and the patient should avoid conditions that cause sweating.

Nondrug therapy: The symptoms of prickly heat can be relieved by providing the patient with a cool, dry environment (eg, air conditioning), eliminating any occlusive fabrics or dressings, reducing fever, avoiding conditions that cause sweating, and taking cool baths.

Pharmacotherapy: A variety of topical products are available for the management of prickly heat. Because these products are applied topically for a short period of time, it is unlikely that patients will experience systemic side effects or drug interactions.

LOCAL ANESTHETICS, TOPICAL

▶ **Actions**

Local anesthetics inhibit conduction of nerve impulses from sensory nerves. They are poorly absorbed through intact epidermis.

▶ **Indications**

Topical anesthesia in many different local skin disorders involving itching and pain, including pain caused by sunburn.

▶ **Contraindications**

Hypersensitivity to any component of these products; ophthalmic use.

▶ **Warnings**

Pregnancy: Category B (lidocaine); *Category C* (benzocaine).

Lactation: Lidocaine is excreted in breast milk. Exercise caution when administering any of these drugs to a nursing woman.

Children: Do not use benzocaine in infants younger than 1 year of age. Reduce dosages in children commensurate with age, body weight, and physical condition.

▶ **Drug Interactions**

Use with caution in patients receiving class I antiarrhythmic drugs because the toxic effects are additive and potentially synergistic.

▶ **Adverse Reactions**

In general, adverse reactions are dose-related and may result from high plasma levels because of excessive dosage, rapid absorption, hypersensitivity, idiosyncrasy, or diminished tolerance. Patients may have hypersensitivity reactions (urticaria, edema, contact dermatitis) or local reactions (burning, stinging, tenderness).

▶ Administration and Dosage

Apply to affected area as needed. Ointments and creams may be applied to gauze or a bandage prior to applying on the skin. Duration of local anesthetic effect is relatively brief (20 to 30 minutes). More than three to four applications/day generally is discouraged.

BENZOCAINE

BENZOCAINE PRODUCTS	
Trade name	Doseform
Benzocaine	**Cream**: 5%

Products listed are representative of currently available and widely distributed brands. Similar products, including regional and private label brands, may also exist.

DIBUCAINE

DIBUCAINE PRODUCTS	
Trade name	Doseform
Dibucaine	**Ointment**: 1%. Lanolin, white petrolatum.

Products listed are representative of currently available and widely distributed brands. Similar products, including regional and private label brands, may also exist.

LIDOCAINE

LIDOCAINE PRODUCTS	
Trade name	Doseform
L.M.X. 4	**Cream**: 4% lidocaine. 1.5% benzyl alcohol.
Solarcaine Aloe Extra Burn Relief	**Gel**: 0.5%. Aloe, glycerin, isopropyl alcohol, menthol, EDTA.
	Spray: 0.5%. Aloe, parabens, EDTA.

Products listed are representative of currently available and widely distributed brands. Similar products, including regional and private label brands, may also exist.

PRAMOXINE HCL

PRAMOXINE HCL PRODUCTS	
Trade name	Doseform
Prax	**Lotion**: 1%. Cetyl alcohol, glycerin, coconut oil, lanolin, mineral oil, petrolatum.
Pramegel	**Gel**: 1%. 0.5% menthol, alcohol SD 40.
Itch-X	**Gel**: 1% pramoxine, 10% benzyl alcohol. Aloe, SD alcohol 40, parabens.
	Spray: 1% pramoxine, 10% benzyl alcohol. Aloe, SD alcohol 40.

Products listed are representative of currently available and widely distributed brands. Similar products, including regional and private label brands, may also exist.

LOCAL ANESTHETIC COMBINATIONS, TOPICAL

TOPICAL LOCAL ANESTHETIC COMBINATION PRODUCTS	
Trade name	Doseform
Foille Medicated First Aid	**Ointment**: 5% benzocaine, 0.1% chloroxylenol. Benzyl alcohol, EDTA in corn oil base.
	Spray: 5% benzocaine, 0.6% chloroxylenol. Benzyl alcohol in corn oil base.

TOPICAL LOCAL ANESTHETIC COMBINATION PRODUCTS	
Trade name	Doseform
Unguentine Maximum Strength	**Cream**: 5% benzocaine, 2% resorcinol. Aloe, cetyl alcohol, lanolin, methylparaben, mineral oil.
Lanacane	**Cream**: 6% benzocaine, 0.1% benzethonium chloride. Aloe, parabens, castor oil, glycerin, isopropyl alcohol.
Bactine Original First Aid	**Liquid**: 2.5% lidocaine, 0.13% benzalkonium chloride. EDTA.
Bactine Pain Relieving Cleansing Spray	**Spray**: 2.5% lidocaine, 0.13% benzalkonium chloride. EDTA.
Lanacane Maximum Strength	**Spray**: 20% benzocaine, 0.1% benzethonium chloride, 36% ethanol. Aloe.
Dermoplast	**Spray**: 20% benzocaine, 0.2% benzethonium chloride. Methylparaben, aloe, lanolin.
Bactine Pain Relieving Cleansing Wipes	**Wipes**: 1% pramoxine, 0.13% benzalkonium chloride. EDTA.

Products listed are representative of currently available and widely distributed brands. Similar products, including regional and private label brands, may also exist.

PATIENT INFORMATION

Local Anesthetics, Topical

- For external use only. Cleanse affected area of skin prior to application (unless directed otherwise).
- Do not use in the eyes.
- Ointments are more greasy; creams may be preferred in some cases.
- Not intended for prolonged use.
- Some of these products contain tartrazine or sulfites, which can cause allergic-type reactions in susceptible individuals.
- Use the lowest concentration and frequency of application needed for symptom relief to avoid excessive absorption into the blood and serious adverse effects.

CORTICOSTEROIDS, TOPICAL

▶ **Actions**

The primary therapeutic effect of topical corticosteroids is their anti-inflammatory activity, which is nonspecific (ie, they act against most causes of inflammation, including mechanical, chemical, microbiological, and immunological).

By suppressing DNA synthesis, topical corticosteroids decrease the rate of epidermal cell formation. This property is useful in treating proliferative disorders such as psoriasis, but also can be demonstrated in normal skin.

The amount of corticosteroid absorbed from the skin depends on the intrinsic properties of the drug itself, the vehicle used, the duration of exposure, and the surface area and condition of the skin to which it is applied. In general, absorption is enhanced by increased skin temperature, hydration, application to inflamed or denuded skin, intertriginous areas (eg, eyelids, groin, axilla), or skin surfaces with a thin stratum corneum layer (eg, face, scrotum). Palms, soles, and crusted skin surfaces are less permeable. Occlusive dressings greatly enhance skin penetration, and therefore increase drug absorption.

Infants and children have a higher total body surface-to-body weight ratio that decreases with age. Therefore, proportionately more of any topical medication will be absorbed systemically in this population, which puts infants and children at a greater risk for systemic effects.

Vehicles: Ointments are more greasy and occlusive and are preferred for dry, scaly lesions. Therefore, use creams on oozing lesions or in intertriginous areas where the occlusive effects of ointments may cause maceration and folliculitis. Creams often are preferred by patients for aesthetic reasons, although their water content makes them more drying than ointments. Gels, aerosols, lotions, and solutions are useful on hairy areas. Urea enhances the penetration of hydrocortisone and selected steroids by hydrating the skin. As a general rule, ointments and gels are slightly more potent than creams or lotions. However, optimized vehicles that have been formulated for some products have demonstrated equal potency in cream, gel, and ointment forms. Steroid impregnated tapes are useful for occlusive therapy in small areas.

Occlusive dressings: Occlusive dressings, such as a plastic wrap, increase skin penetration approximately 10-fold by increasing the moisture content of the stratum corneum. Occlusion can be beneficial in resistant cases, but it also may lead to sweat retention and increased bacterial and fungal infections. Additionally, increased absorption of corticosteroids may produce systemic side effects. Therefore, do not use occlusive dressings for longer than 12 hours/day or when using very potent topical corticosteroids or unless directed to do so by a physician.

Relative potency: The relative potency of a product depends on several factors, including the characteristics and concentrations of the drug and the vehicle used.

▶ **Indications**

Relief of inflammatory and pruritic manifestations of a variety of corticosteroid-responsive dermatoses (eg, contact dermatoses, contact dermatitis, rash, pruritus, minor skin inflammation).

Topical corticosteroids are indicated for alternative/adjunctive treatment of psoriasis. More specifically, nonprescription hydrocortisone preparations are indicated for temporary relief of itching or inflammation caused by psoriasis.

▶ **Contraindications**

Hypersensitivity to any component of the product; treatment of rosacea, perioral dermatitis, or acne; use on the face, groin, or axilla (very high or high-potency agents); ophthalmic use (prolonged ocular exposure may cause steroid-induced glaucoma and cataracts).

▶ **Warnings**

Systemic effects: Systemic absorption of chronically applied topical corticosteroids, particularly the high-potency prescription products, has produced reversible hypothalamic-pituitary-adrenal (HPA) axis suppression, Cushing syndrome, hyperglycemia, and glycosuria. Conditions that augment systemic absorption include the application of more potent steroids, use over large surface areas, prolonged use, and the use of occlusive dressings.

As a general rule, little effect on the HPA axis will occur with use of an OTC or prescription topical corticosteroid in amounts of less than 50 g weekly for an adult and 15 g weekly for a small child, without occlusion. To cover the adult body 1 time requires 12 to 26 g.

Local irritation: If local irritation develops, discontinue use and wash affected area with mild soap and water. Medications containing alcohol may produce dry skin or burning sensations/irritation in open lesions. Allergic contact dermatitis usually is diagnosed by observing the failure to heal rather than noting clinical exacerbation, as with most topical products that do not contain corticosteroids.

> *Skin atrophy* – Skin atrophy is common and may be clinically significant after 3 to 4 weeks of regular use of potent prescription preparations. Atrophy occurs most readily at sites where percutaneous absorption is high.

Patients should exercise caution when using around the eye or in the genital area. The use of high-potency prescription formulations on the face and in intertriginous areas should be avoided because of resulting striae.

Psoriasis: Do not use nonprescription or prescription topical corticosteroids as the sole form of therapy in patients with widespread plaque.

In rare instances, treatment (or withdrawal of treatment) of psoriasis with corticosteroids is thought to have provoked the pustular form of the disease.

Atrophic changes: Certain areas of the body, such as the face, groin, and axillae, are more prone to atrophic changes than other areas of the body following chronic treatment with topical corticosteroids. Frequent observation of the patient is important if these areas are to be treated.

Infections: In the presence of an infection, institute appropriate therapy. If a favorable response does not occur promptly, discontinue the corticosteroid until the infection has been controlled. Treating skin infections with topical corticosteroids can worsen the infection.

For external use only: Avoid ingestion, contact with the eyes, or the inhalation of steroid-containing aerosols.

Vehicles: Many topical corticosteroids are in specially formulated bases designed to maximize their release and potency. Mixing these formulations with other bases or vehicles may affect the potency of the drug far beyond what would normally be expected from the dilution. Exercise caution before mixing; if necessary, contact the manufacturer to determine if there may be an incompatibility.

Occlusive therapy: Discontinue the use of occlusive dressings if infection develops, and institute appropriate therapy.

Pregnancy: Category C. Corticosteroids are teratogenic in animals when administered systemically at relatively low doses. The more potent corticosteroids are teratogenic after dermal application in animals. There are no adequate and well-controlled studies in pregnant women. Therefore, use during pregnancy only if the potential benefits outweigh the potential hazards to the fetus. In pregnant patients, do not use in large amounts or for prolonged periods of time.

Lactation: It is not known whether topical corticosteroid application could result in sufficient systemic absorption to produce detectable quantities in breast milk. Systemic corticosteroids are secreted into breast milk in quantities not likely to have a deleterious effect on the infant. Nevertheless, exercise caution when administering topical corticosteroids to a nursing mother.

Children: Children may be more susceptible to topical corticosteroid-induced HPA axis suppression and Cushing syndrome than adults because of their larger skin surface area-to-body weight ratio.

Hypothalamic-pituitary axis suppression, Cushing syndrome, and intracranial hypertension have occurred in children receiving topical corticosteroids. Manifestations of adrenal suppression include linear growth retardation, delayed weight gain, low plasma cortisol levels, and absence of response to adrenocorticotropic hormone (ACTH) stimulation.

Limit administration to the least amount compatible with effective therapy. Chronic corticosteroid therapy may interfere with children's growth and development.

► **Adverse Reactions**

Burning; itching; irritation; erythema; dryness; folliculitis; hypertrichosis; pruritus; acneiform eruptions; hypopigmentation; perioral dermatitis; allergic contact dermatitis; numbness of fingers; stinging and cracking or tightening of skin; maceration of the skin; secondary infection; skin atrophy; striae; miliaria; telangiectasia. These may occur more frequently with the use of occlusive dressings.

There also have been reports of development of pustular psoriasis from chronic plaque psoriasis following reduction or discontinuation of potent topical corticosteroids.

Sensitivity to a particular dressing material or adhesive may occur occasionally.

► **Administration and Dosage**

Usual dosage: Apply sparingly to affected areas 2 to 4 times daily.

General considerations: Topical corticosteroids have a repository effect; with continuous use, 1 or 2 applications/day may be as effective as 3 or more. Many clinicians advise applying twice daily until clinical response is achieved and then only as frequently as needed to control the condition.

Short-term or intermittent therapy using high-potency prescription agents (eg, every other day, 3 to 4 consecutive days per week, or once per week) may be more effective and cause fewer adverse effects than continuous regimens using lower-potency products.

Only use low-potency agents in children, on large areas, and on body sites especially prone to steroid damage (eg, the face, scrotum, axillae, flexures, and skin folds). Reserve higher-potency agents for areas and conditions resistant to treatment with milder agents.

TOPICAL CORTICOSTEROID PRODUCTS	
Trade name	**Doseform**
Cortizone•5	**Ointment**: 0.5% hydrocortisone. Excipients.
Cortizone•10	**Ointment**: 1% hydrocortisone. Benzyl alcohol, SD alcohol 40.
Hydrocortisone	**Ointment**: 1% hydrocortisone. Mineral oil, white petrolatum.
Cortaid Maximum Strength	**Ointment**: 1% hydrocortisone (as acetate). Parabens, mineral oil, white petrolatum.
Hydrocortisone Acetate	**Ointment**: 1% hydrocortisone (as acetate). Aloe, white petrolatum.
Cortizone•5	**Cream**: 0.5% hydrocortisone. Parabens, glycerin, mineral oil, white petrolatum, aloe.
Corticaine	**Cream**: 0.5% hydrocortisone. Methylparaben, mineral oil, white petrolatum, menthol, stearyl alcohol, EDTA.
Cortaid Sensitive Skin Formula with Aloe	**Cream**: 0.5% hydrocortisone (as acetate). Aloe, parabens.
Hydrocortisone	**Cream**: 1% hydrocortisone. Aloe, cetearyl alcohol, glycerin, methylparaben.

TOPICAL CORTICOSTEROID PRODUCTS	
Trade name	Doseform
Cortaid Intensive Therapy	**Cream**: 1% hydrocortisone. Parabens, cetyl alcohol, stearyl alcohol.
Cortizone•10	**Cream**: 1% hydrocortisone. Parabens, glycerin, mineral oil, white petrolatum, cetearyl alcohol, aloe.
Cortaid Maximum Strength	**Cream**: 1% hydrocortisone. Benzyl alcohol, cetearyl alcohol, glycerin, methylparaben, aloe.
Maximum Strength HydroZone Plus	**Cream**: 1% hydrocortisone. Benzyl alcohol, glycerin, stearyl alcohol.
LanaCort Maximum Strength	**Cream**: 1% hydrocortisone (as acetate). Glycerin, mineral oil, cetyl alcohol, lanolin, EDTA, parabens, menthol, aloe.
HydroZone Plus, Hydrocortisone	**Lotion**: 1% hydrocortisone. Cetyl alcohol.
CortaGel Maximum Strength	**Gel**: 1% hydrocortisone. Ethanol, aloe, EDTA.
CortiCool	**Gel**: 1% hydrocortisone, 45% alcohol, benzethonium chloride
Cortaid Intensive Therapy	**Spray**: 1% hydrocortisone. EDTA, glycerin, 45% SD alcohol 40.

Products listed are representative of currently available and widely distributed brands. Similar products, including regional and private label brands, may also exist.

PATIENT INFORMATION
Topical Corticosteroids

- For external use only. Cleanse affected area of skin prior to application (unless directed otherwise).
- Apply ointments, creams, or gels sparingly in a light film. Rub in gently. Washing or soaking the area before application may increase drug penetration.
- To use a lotion, solution, or gel on your scalp, part your hair, apply a small amount of the medicine on the affected area, and rub it in gently. Protect the area from washing, clothing, rubbing, etc., until the medicine dries. You may wash your hair as usual, but not immediately after applying the medicine.
- Use only as directed. Do not put bandages, dressings, cosmetics, or other skin products over the treated area unless directed by a physician.
- Notify a physician if the condition being treated worsens or if burning, swelling, or redness develop.
- Avoid prolonged use around the eyes, in the genital and rectal areas, and on the face, armpits, and skin creases unless directed by a physician. Avoid contact with the eyes.
- If you forget a dose, apply it as soon as you remember and continue on your regular schedule. If it is almost time for the next application, wait and continue on your regular schedule. Do not apply double doses.
- *For parents of pediatric patients*: Consult a physician. If corticosteroid treatment is recommended, do not use tight-fitting diapers or plastic pants on a child treated in the diaper area; these garments may work like occlusive dressings and cause more of the drug to be absorbed into your child's body. Do not use topical steroids to treat diaper rash.

PSORIASIS

DEFINITION

Psoriasis is a relatively common, potentially genetic, chronic, inflammatory, and proliferative skin disease. It is characterized by sharply demarcated, red or silvery scaly plaques of various sizes, particularly on the extensor prominences (eg, knees, elbows) and scalp. The back, buttocks, nails, eyebrows, axilla, and anogenital areas also may be affected. Psoriasis cases generally may be divided into four groups: classic psoriasis (psoriasis vulgaris), which includes plaque, guttate, and inverse psoriasis; localized pustular psoriasis; generalized pustular psoriasis; and erythrodermic psoriasis. Each type of psoriasis is classified by characteristic lesions, location on the body, and type of scale (if any).

ETIOLOGY

The cause of psoriasis is unknown. A genetic tendency exists for this condition, which is associated with certain human leukocyte antigen (HLA) types. Immunologic abnormalities also play a role.

INCIDENCE

Psoriasis affects 1.5% to 2% of the population in Western countries. The age of onset peaks at 16 to 22 years and again at 57 to 60 years. Women and patients with a family history of psoriasis tend to have an earlier age of onset. The incidence of psoriasis in adult men is equal to the incidence in women.

PATHOPHYSIOLOGY

The principal abnormality characteristic of psoriasis is an alteration of keratinocyte cell kinetics, in which the cell cycle decreases from approximately 311 to approximately 36 hours, resulting in a tremendous increase in the production of epidermal cells; therefore, psoriasis is essentially a proliferative skin disorder. The etiologic basis for this overproduction is unknown. However, changes in the level of cyclic nucleotides, arachidonic acid metabolism, production of cytokines, and expression of adhesion molecules are seen in this condition. Whether these changes are primary or secondary remains to be determined.

SIGNS/SYMPTOMS

The onset of signs and symptoms usually is gradual.

Psoriasis is a papulosquamous skin disorder that consists of scaling papules and plaques. The amount of scaling can be significant, with patients leaving a "trail of scale" wherever they go. Pruritus is relatively common, especially in scalp and anogenital psoriasis. Constitutional symptoms can develop in generalized pustular psoriasis and include arthritis, fever, and chills. Typically, psoriasis involves the scalp, knees, elbows, and lower back, but extracutaneous disease can affect the nails, fingers, spine, and hip. Symptoms tend to intensify and remit at unpredictable intervals.

DIAGNOSTIC PARAMETERS/PHYSICAL ASSESSMENT

Clinical Observation: Psoriasis is diagnosed by clinical presentation. Classic psoriasis (psoriasis vulgaris) is characterized by well-demarcated, red plaques with silvery-white scale. These plaques can be localized, as in chronic plaque psoriasis, or widespread, as in guttate psoriasis. Additionally, generalized psoriasis can be present as erythroderma.

Interview: To assist in the diagnosis of psoriasis, inquire about the following:

- Family history of psoriasis (approximately 50% of patients with psoriasis have a relative with the disease)
- Nature of the lesions (eg, are they red, sharply demarcated, scaling, or episodic? How many lesions exist? Was their onset acute?)
- Presence of the Koebner phenomenon (development of psoriasis in previously traumatized skin)
- Exacerbations by stress, certain drugs (eg, antimalarials), or infections
- Duration of the condition
- Previous treatments and whether they were successful or not
- Areas of the body where the condition exists
- Presence of itching

TREATMENT

Approaches to therapy: The severity of psoriasis will determine appropriate therapy. Nondrug treatment options are limited. In severe or widespread cases, or cases that are refractory to OTC treatment, physician referral is appropriate.

Nondrug therapy: Advise psoriasis patients to avoid factors that may exacerbate the condition, such as certain drugs (eg, antimalarial agents), stress, and local trauma to the skin or nails. Emollients are useful in decreasing pruritus and the amount of scaling. Natural sunlight, in moderation, has been shown to improve psoriasis, particularly guttate psoriasis.

Pharmacotherapy: The type of therapy used depends on several factors: the patient's age, type of psoriasis, site and extent of involvement, previous treatment(s), and the presence of any associated medical disorders. Topical therapy is useful for treating less severe cases, but tachyphylaxis (decreased effectiveness of therapeutic agents with prolonged use) is relatively common. Nonprescription topical therapy options for mildly to moderately severe cases include corticosteroids and tar. Prescription products include anthralin, calcipotriene, and retinoids. Treatment options for widespread disease include phototherapy (UVB/PUVA) or prescription drugs such as systemic retinoids, methotrexate, cyclosporine, hydroxyurea, acitretin, alefacept, efalizumab, and occasionally, systemic steroids.

EMOLLIENTS

▶ **Actions**

Some of the listed ingredients to look for that act as emollients are cetyl alcohol, glycerin, isopropyl myristate, isopropyl palmitate, lanolin, petrolatum, and stearyl alcohol. Some of the aquaphilic chemicals found in emollients and moisturizers and used to attract water to the skin are dexpanthenol, urea, and topical vitamins A, D, and E.

DEXPANTHENOL

▶ **Indications**

Relieves itching and aids healing of skin in mild eczemas and dermatoses, such as itching skin, minor wounds, stings, bites, poison ivy, poison oak (dry stage), and minor skin irritations. Also used to treat diaper rash, chafing, and mild skin irritations in infants and children.

▶ **Administration and Dosage**

For external use only. Avoid contact with eyes.

Apply a thin layer to affected areas once or twice daily or as instructed by a physician.

DEXPANTHENOL PRODUCTS	
Trade name	Doseform
Panthoderm	**Cream**: 2% in a water-miscible base. Cetyl alcohol, glycerin, menthol, camphor, parabens.

Products listed are representative of currently available and widely distributed brands. Similar products, including regional and private label brands, may also exist.

PATIENT INFORMATION

Dexpanthenol

- For external use only. Do not use in eyes or allow to come in contact with the eye(s) or eyelid(s).
- Do not use if you are allergic to any ingredient of the products.
- Do not use on irritated or broken skin without consulting a physician or pharmacist.
- Stinging, burning, itching, or irritation may develop with the use of these products.
- If the condition persists or worsens or if irritation develops, discontinue use and consult a physician.
- Do not apply over deep or puncture wounds, infections, or lacerations.

UREA (CARBAMIDE)

▶ **Indications**

Promotes hydration and removes excess keratin in dry skin and hyperkeratotic conditions, including psoriasis.

▶ **Administration and Dosage**

For external use only. Avoid contact with the eyes.

Apply a thin layer 1 to 4 times daily to affected area or as instructed by a physician. Rub in completely.

UREA PRODUCTS	
Trade name	**Doseform**
Lanaphilic	**Ointment**: 10%. White petrolatum, stearyl alcohol, isopropyl palmitate, lanolin oil, sorbitol, propylene glycol, sodium lauryl sulfate, lactic acid.
	Ointment: 20%. White petrolatum, stearyl alcohol, isopropyl palmitate, lanolin oil, sorbitol, propylene glycol, sodium lauryl sulfate, lactic acid.
Aqua Care	**Cream**: 10%. Petrolatum, glycerin, lanolin oil, mineral oil, lanolin alcohol, benzyl alcohol.
Nutraplus	**Cream**: 10%. Mineral oil, parabens.
Carmol 20	**Cream**: 20%. Nonlipid vanishing cream base.
Gormel	**Cream**: 20%. Mineral oil, cetyl alcohol, parabens.
Ureacin-20	**Cream**: 20%. Glycerin, mineral oil, parabens, EDTA.
Aqua Care	**Lotion**: 10%. Mineral oil, petrolatum, parabens, cetyl alcohol, lactic acid.
Carmol 10	**Lotion**: 10%. Cetyl alcohol.
Gormel Ten	**Lotion**: 10%. Mineral oil, cetyl alcohol, parabens.
Nutraplus	**Lotion**: 10%. Lanolin alcohol, petrolatum, parabens.
Ureacin-10	**Lotion**: 10%. EDTA, parabens, cetyl alcohol.
Ultra Mide 25	**Lotion**: 25%. Mineral oil, glycerin, lanolin, cetyl alcohol.

Products listed are representative of currently available and widely distributed brands. Similar products, including regional and private label brands, may also exist.

PATIENT INFORMATION
Urea

- For external use only. Do not use in eyes or allow to come in contact with the eye(s) or eyelid(s).
- Do not use if you are allergic to any ingredient of the products.
- Do not use on irritated or broken skin without consulting a physician or pharmacist.
- Stinging, burning, itching, or irritation may develop with the use of these products.
- If the condition persists or worsens or if irritation develops, discontinue use and consult a physician.
- Do not apply over deep or puncture wounds, infections, or lacerations.

VITAMINS A, D, AND E, TOPICAL
► **Indications**

For temporary relief of discomfort caused by minor burns, sunburn, windburn, abrasions, chapped or chafed skin, and other minor noninfected skin irritations, including diaper rash and irritations associated with ileostomy and colostomy skin drainage. May be a useful adjunctive agent in the treatment of psoriasis.

▶ **Warnings**

For external use only. Avoid contact with the eyes.

If the condition worsens or does not improve within 7 days, consult a physician.

▶ **Administration and Dosage**

Apply a thin layer to affected skin with gentle massage as instructed by a physician.

TOPICAL VITAMINS A, D, AND E PREPARATIONS	
Trade name	Doseform
Vitamin A and Vitamin D	**Ointment**: Vitamins A and D. Lanolin, white petrolatum, mineral oil.
Lobana Derm-ADE	**Cream**: Vitamins A, D, and E. Lanolin, stearyl alcohol, cetyl alcohol, vegetable oil, parabens, glycerin.
Alph-E	**Cream**: 6,000 international units vitamin E, 600 international units vitamin A, 60 international units vitamin D. Wheat germ oil, emollient base.
Lazer Creme	**Cream**: 100,000 international units vitamin A, 3,500 international units vitamin E/oz. Parabens.

Products listed are representative of currently available and widely distributed brands. Similar products, including regional and private label brands, may also exist.

PATIENT INFORMATION

Vitamins A, D, and E, Topical

- For external use only. Do not use in eyes or allow to come in contact with the eye(s) or eyelid(s).
- Do not use if you are allergic to any ingredient of the products.
- Do not use on irritated or broken skin without consulting a physician or pharmacist.
- Stinging, burning, itching, or irritation may develop with the use of these products.
- If the condition persists or worsens or if irritation develops, discontinue use and consult a physician.
- Do not apply over deep or puncture wounds, infections, or lacerations.

VITAMIN E

▶ **Indications**

For the temporary relief of minor skin disorders such as diaper rash, burns, sunburn, and chapped or dry skin. Vitamin E is of limited adjunctive use in the management of psoriasis.

▶ **Administration and Dosage**

For external use only. Avoid contact with the eyes.

Apply a thin layer to affected skin with gentle message as instructed by a physician.

VITAMIN E PRODUCTS	
Trade name	Doseform
Vitamin E[1]	**Cream, lotion, oil**
Vite E Creme	**Cream**: 50 mg dl-alpha tocopheryl acetate/g

VITAMIN E PRODUCTS	
Trade name	Doseform
Vitamin E-Cream	**Cream**: 100 international units/g. Petrolatum, cetearyl alcohol, mineral oil, wheat germ oil, parabens.
Vitec	**Lotion**: dl-alpha tocopheryl acetate, cetearyl alcohol, sorbitol, propylene glycol, simethicone, glyceryl monostearate, sorbic acid
Alph-E-Oil	**Oil**: 28,000 units/oz.

Products listed are representative of currently available and widely distributed brands. Similar products, including regional and private label brands, may also exist.

[1] May or may not contain aloe.

PATIENT INFORMATION
Vitamin E

- For external use only. Do not use in eyes or allow to come in contact with the eye(s) or eyelid(s).
- Do not use if you are allergic to any ingredient of the products.
- Do not use on irritated or broken skin without consulting a physician or pharmacist.
- Stinging, burning, itching, or irritation may develop with the use of these products.
- If the condition persists or worsens or if irritation develops, discontinue use and consult a physician.
- Do not apply over deep or puncture wounds, infections, or lacerations.

MISCELLANEOUS EMOLLIENTS

▶ Actions

These preparations lubricate and moisturize the skin, counteracting dryness and itching. Some of the listed ingredients in products that act as emollients are butyl stearate, cetyl alcohol, glycerin, glyceryl monostearate, isopropyl myristate, isopropyl palmitate, lanolin, lanolin alcohol, mineral oil, petrolatum, propylene glycol stearate, squalene, stearic acid, and stearyl alcohol.

In certain products, some of the aquaphilic chemicals used to attract water to the skin are urea and alpha-hydroxy acids. These chemicals, while useful, often will sting when applied to dry skin.

MISCELLANEOUS EMOLLIENT PRODUCTS	
Trade name	Doseform
Aquaphor	**Ointment**: Petrolatum, mineral oil, ceresin, lanolin alcohol, panthenol, glycerin, bisabolol
Balmex Daily Protective Clear	**Ointment**: White petrolatum, cyclomethicone, dimethicone, polyethylene, silica, mineral oil, tocopheryl acetate
AmLactin	**Cream**: 12% ammonium lactate. Light mineral oil, glyceryl stearate, PEG-100 stearate, propylene glycol, glycerin, magnesium aluminum silicate, laureth-4, polyoxyl 40 stearate, cetyl alcohol, parabens, methylcellulose
AmLactin AP	**Cream**: 12% ammonium lactate, 1% pramoxine hydrochloride

MISCELLANEOUS EMOLLIENT PRODUCTS

Trade name	Doseform
Cutemol	**Cream**: Liquid petrolatum, lanolin alcohols extract, mineral wax, beeswax, acetylated lanolin, isopropyl myristate, sorbitan sesquioleate, sodium tetraborate, imidurea, allantoin, parabens
DML Forte	**Cream**: Petrolatum, propylene glycol dioctanoate, glyceryl stearate, PEG-100 stearate, glycerin, stearic acid, DEA-cetyl phosphate, DEX-panthenol, PVP/Eicosene copolymer, simethicone, benzyl alcohol, cetyl alcohol, silica, EDTA, acrylates/C10-30 alkyl acrylate crosspolymer, triethanolamine, magnesium aluminum silicate
Eucerin Original	**Cream**: Mineral oil, petrolatum, mineral oil, ceresin, lanolin alcohol, methylchloroisothiazolinone, methylisothiazolinone
Geri-Hydrolac 12%	**Cream**: Ammonium lactate (equivalent to 12% lactic acid), light mineral oil, petrolatum, propylene glycol, glycerin, cetyl alcohol, parabens
Hydrisinol	**Cream**: Mineral oil, petrolatum, hydrogenated vegetable oil, lanolin, beeswax, paraffin wax, sulfonated castor oil, parabens
Hydrocerin	**Cream**: Petrolatum, mineral oil, mineral wax, ceresin lanolin alcohol, parabens
Lanolor	**Cream**: Glyceryl stearates, propylene glycol, cetyl esters wax, isopropyl palmitate, cetyl alcohol, lanolin oil, sodium lauryl sulfate, methylparaben, simethicone, polyoxyl 40 stearate, sorbic acid
Minerin	**Cream**: Petrolatum, mineral oil, mineral wax, alcohol, methylchloroisothiazolinone, methylisothiazolinone
Neutrogena Norwegian Formula Hand Cream	**Cream**: Glycerin, sodium cetearyl sulfate, sodium sulfate, parabens
Nutraderm	**Cream**: Mineral oil, sorbitan stearate, stearyl alcohol, sorbitol, citric acid, cetyl esters wax, sodium lauryl sulfate, dimethicone, parabens, diazolidinyl urea
Pen•Kera	**Cream**: Cetyl palmitate, glycerin, mineral oil, polysorbate 60, sorbitan stearate, polyamino sugar condensate, urea, wheat germ glycerides, carbomer 940, triethanolamine, DMDM hydantoin, iodopropynyl butylcarbanate, diazolidinyl urea, dehydroacetic acid
Polysorb Hydrate	**Cream**: Cetyl esters wax, mineral oil, perfume oil bouquet, sorbitan sesquioleale, white petrolatum, white wax
Purpose Dry Skin	**Cream**: Mineral oil, white petrolatum, sweet almond oil, propylene glycol, glyceryl stearate, xanthan gum, steareth-2, steareth-20, sodium lactate, cetyl esters wax, lactic acid
Allercreme Skin	**Lotion**: Mineral oil, sorbitol, triethanolamine, parabens
AmLactin	**Lotion**: 12% ammonium lactate. Light mineral oil, glyceryl stearate, PEG-100 stearate, propylene glycol, glycerin, magnesium aluminum silicate, laureth-4, polyoxyl 40 stearate, cetyl alcohol, parabens, methylcellulose

MISCELLANEOUS EMOLLIENT PRODUCTS

Trade name	Doseform
Aquanil	**Lotion:** Glycerin, benzyl alcohol, sodium laureth sulfate, cetyl alcohol, stearyl alcohol, xanthan gum
Aveeno	**Lotion:** 1% colloidal oatmeal, glycerin, phenylcarbinol, petrolatum, dimethicone, benzyl alcohol
Corn Huskers	**Lotion:** Glycerin, SD alcohol 40, sodium calcium alginate, oleyl sarcosine, methylparaben, guar gum, triethanolamine, calcium sulfate, calcium chloride, fumaric acid, boric acid
Curel Original	**Lotion:** Glycerin, distearyldimonium chloride, petrolatum, isopropyl palmitate, cetyl alcohol, dimethicone, sodium chloride, parabens
Curel Soothing Hands	**Lotion:** Glycerin, petrolatum, distearyldimonium chloride, isopropyl palmitate, cetyl alcohol, aluminum starch octenylsuccinate, dimethicone, *Anthemis nobilis* flower extract, tocopheryl acetate, ascorbyl palmitate, panthenol, parabens, propylene glycol
Curel Ultra Healing	**Lotion:** Glycerin, petrolatum, cetearyl alcohol, behentrimonium chloride, cetyl-PG hydroxyethyl pamitamide, isopropyl palmitate, avena sativa (oat) meal extract, *Eucalyptus globus* leaf extract, *Citrus aurantium dulcis* (orange) oil, cyclomethicone, dimethicone, cholesteryl isostearate, BIS-PEG-15 dimethicone/IPDI copolymer, DMDM hydantoin
Derma Viva	**Lotion:** Mineral oil, glyceryl stearate, laureth-4, lanolin oil, PEG-100 stearate, PEG-40 stearate, PEG-4 dilaurate, trolamine, DSS, parabens
DML	**Lotion:** Petrolatum, glycerin, methyl glucose sesquistearate, dimethicone, PEG-20 methyl glucose sesquistearate, benzyl alcohol, cyclomethicone, glyceryl stearate, stearic acid, cetyl alcohol, sodium carbomer 941, xanthan gum, magnesium aluminum silicate
Emollia	**Lotion:** Mineral oil, cetyl alcohol, propylene glycol, white wax, sodium lauryl sulfate, oleic acid, parabens
Epilyt	**Lotion:** Propylene glycol, glycerin, oleic acid, quaternium-26, lactic acid, BHT
Esotérica Dry Skin Treatment	**Lotion:** Propylene glycol, dicaprylate/dicapric, mineral oil, glyceryl stearate, cetyl esters wax, hydrolyzed animal protein, dimethicone, TEA-carbomer-941, parabens
Eucerin Daily Replenishing	**Lotion:** Dimethicone, sunflower seed oil, petrolatum, glycerin, glyceryl stearate SE, octyldodecanol, panthenol, caprylic/capric triglyceride, tocopherol acetate, stearic acid, cholesterol, cetearyl alcohol, lanolin alcohol, carbomer, EDTA, sodium hydroxide, phenoxyethanol, parabens, BHT
Eucerin Plus Intensive Repair	**Lotion:** Mineral oil, PEG-7 hydrogenated castor oil, isohexadecane, sodium lactate, urea, glycerin, isopropyl palmitate, panthenol, microcrystalline wax, magnesium sulfate, lanolin alcohol, bisabolol, methylchloroisothiazolinone, methylisothiazolinone

MISCELLANEOUS EMOLLIENT PRODUCTS

Trade name	Doseform
Geri-Soft	**Lotion:** Mineral oil, propylene glycol, cetearyl alcohol, sorbitol, petrolatum, dimethicone, lanolin, castor oil, stearic acid, parabens, stearyl alcohol, EDTA, lemon oil
Geri SS	**Lotion:** Mineral oil, propylene glycol, cetearyl alcohol, petrolatum, glycerin, dimethicone, colloidal oatmeal, hydrogenated castor oil, parabens, stearyl alcohol, EDTA, lemon oil, tocopheryl acetate
Hydrisinol	**Lotion:** Propylene glycol stearate SE, hydrogenated vegetable oil, stearic acid, sulfonated castor oil, mineral oil, lanolin, lanolin alcohol, sesame oil, sunflower oil, aloe, triethanolamine, sorbitan stearate, hydroxyethyl cellulose, parabens
Hydrocerin	**Lotion:** EDTA, lanolin, parabens, mineral oil, PEG-40 sorbitan, peroleate, propylene glycol, sorbitol, water
Jergen's Ash Relief Moisturizer	**Lotion:** Glycerin, cetearyl alcohol, petrolatum, mineral oil, ceteareth-20, cyclomethicone, dimethicone, theobroma cacao (cocoa) seed butter, butyrospermum parkii (shea butter), tridecyl salicylate, tocopheryl acetate, stearic acid, glyceryl dilaurate, aluminum starch octenylsuccinate, acrylates/C10-30 alkyl acrylate crosspolymer, parabens, DMDM hydantoin, sodium hydroxide
Jergen's Ultra Healing Intense Moisture Therapy	**Lotion:** Glycerin, distearyldimonium chloride, petrolatum, isopropyl palmitate, cetyl alcohol, dimethicone, parabens, sodium chloride
Keri	**Lotion:** Mineral oil, glycerin, PEG-40 stearate, glyceryl stearate, PEG-100 stearate, PEG-4 dilaurate, laureth-4, aloe, sunflower seed oil, tocopheryl acetate, carbomer, parabens, DMDM hydantoin, iodopropynyl butylcarbamate, sodium hydroxide, EDTA
Lac-Hydrin Five	**Lotion:** 5% ammonium lactate, glycerin, petrolatum, squalane, steareth-2, POE-21-stearyl ether, propylene glycol dioctanoate, cetyl alcohol, dimethicone, cetyl palmitate, magnesium aluminum silicate, diazolidinyl urea, methylchloroisothiazolinone, methylisothiazolone
LactiCare	**Lotion:** Mineral oil, 5% lactic acid, isopropyl palmitate, sodium PCA, stearyl alcohol, ceteareth-20, sodium hydroxide, glyceryl stearate, PEG-100 stearate, myristyl lactate, cetyl alcohol, carbomer, DMDM hydantoin, parabens
Lobana Body	**Lotion:** Mineral oil, triethanolamine stearate, stearic acid, cetyl alcohol, lanolin, potassium stearate, aloe, propylene glycol, parabens
Lubriderm Advanced Therapy	**Lotion:** Cetyl alcohol, glycerin, mineral oil, cyclomethicone, propylene glycol discaprylate/dicaprate, PEG-40 stearate, isopropyl isostearate, emulsifying wax, lecithin, carbomer 940, diazolidinyl urea, titanium dioxide, sodium benzoate, tri (PPG-3 myristyl ether) citrate, EDTA, retinyl palmitate, tocopheryl acetate, sodium pyruvate, iodopropynyl butylcarbamate, sodium hydroxide, xanthan gum

MISCELLANEOUS EMOLLIENT PRODUCTS

Trade name	Doseform
Lubriderm Seriously Sensitive	**Lotion**: Butylene glycol, mineral oil, petrolatum, glycerin, cetyl alcohol, propylene glycol dicaprylate/dicaprate, PEG-40 stearate, C11-13 isoparaffin, glyceryl stearate, tri (PPG-3 myristyl ether) citrate, emulsifying wax, dimethicone, DMDM hydantoin, parabens, carbomer 940, titanium dioxide, EDTA, sodium hydroxide, xanthan gum
Lubriderm Skin Firming	**Lotion**: Isostearic acid, stearic acid, steareth-21, sodium lactate, PPG 12/SMDI copolymer, lactic acid, steareth-2, magnesium aluminum silicate, cetyl alcohol, imidurea, potassium sorbate, xanthan gum
Lubriderm Skin Renewal Firming	**Lotion**: Gluconolactone, propylene glycol, cetearyl glucoside/cetearyl alcohol, cyclomethicone, stearic acid, propylene glycol dicaprylate-dicaprate, C12-15 alkyl benzoate, isohexyl caprate, isocetyl stearate, triethanolamine, dimethicone, glycerin, petrolatum, glyceryl stearate, PEG-100 stearate, cetyl alcohol, emulsifying wax, steareth-2, diazolidinyl urea, EDTA, tocopheryl acetate, glycine, xanthan gum, hydroxyethyl cellulose, iodopropynyl butylcarbamate
Lubriderm Skin Therapy	**Lotion**: Mineral oil, petrolatum, sorbitol, stearic acid, lanolin, lanolin alcohol, cetyl alcohol, glyceryl stearate/PEG-100 stearate, triethanolamine, dimethicone, propylene glycol, microcrystalline wax, tri (PPG-3 myristyl ether) citrate, EDTA, parabens, xanthan gum, methyldibromo glutaronitrile
Lubriskin	**Lotion**: Mineral oil, petrolatum, lanolin, lanolin alcohol, cetearyl alcohol, castor oil, triethanolamine, stearyl alcohol, propylene glycol, parabens, EDTA
Minerin	**Lotion**: Mineral oil, isopropyl myristate, PEG-40 sorbitan peroleate, lanolin acid, glycerin ester, sorbitol, propylene glycol, cetyl palmitate, magnesium sulfate, aluminum stearate, lanolin alcohol, methylchloroisothiazolinone, methylisothiazolinone, BHT
Moisturel	**Lotion**: 3% dimethicone, benzyl alcohol, carbomer, cetyl alcohol, glycerin, laureth-23, magnesium aluminum silicate, petrolatum, potassium sorbate, sodium hydroxide, steareth-2
Neutrogena Body	**Lotion**: Glyceryl stearate, PEG-100 stearate, imidazolidinyl urea, carbomer-954, parabens, sodium lauryl sulfate, triethanolamine
Nutraderm	**Lotion**: Mineral oil, sorbitan stearate, stearyl alcohol, sodium lauryl sulfate, carbomer 940, diazolidinyl urea, parabens, triethanolamine
Shepard's	**Lotion**: Glycerin, sesame oil, vegetable oil, SD alcohol 40-B, propylene glycol, ethoxydiglycol, triethanolamine, glyceryl stearate, cetyl alcohol, simethicone, monoglyceride citrate, parabens
Sofenol 5	**Lotion**: Glycerin, petrolatum, cetearyl alcohol, soluble collagen, dimethicone, PEG-40-stearate, allantoin, sunflower seed oil, kaolin, sorbic acid, carbomer 940, sodium hydroxide

MISCELLANEOUS EMOLLIENT PRODUCTS	
Trade name	Doseform
Therapeutic Bath	**Lotion**: Mineral oil, glyceryl stearate, PEG-100 stearate, propylene glycol, PEG-40 stearate, laureth-4, PEG-4 dilaurate, lanolin oil, parabens, quaternium-15, carbomer 934, trolamine, dioctyl sodium sulfosuccinate
Wibi	**Lotion**: Glycerin, SD alcohol 40, PEG-4, PEG-6-32 stearate, PEG-6-32, carbomer-940, PEG-75, parabens, triethanolamine, menthol
Neutrogena Body	**Oil**: Sesame oil, PEG-40 sorbitan peroleate

Products listed are representative of currently available and widely distributed brands. Similar products, including regional and private label brands, may also exist.

PATIENT INFORMATION

Emollients

- For external use only. Do not use in eyes or allow to come in contact with the eye(s) or eyelid(s).
- Do not use if you are allergic to any ingredient of the products.
- Do not use on irritated or broken skin without consulting a physician or pharmacist.
- If the condition persists or worsens or if irritation develops, discontinue use and consult a physician.
- Apply to affected skin with gentle massage as instructed by a physician.

CORTICOSTEROIDS, TOPICAL

▶ Actions

The primary therapeutic effect of topical corticosteroids is their anti-inflammatory activity, which is nonspecific (ie, they act against most causes of inflammation, including mechanical, chemical, microbiological, and immunological).

By suppressing DNA synthesis, topical corticosteroids decrease the rate of epidermal cell formation. This property is useful in treating proliferative disorders such as psoriasis, but also can be demonstrated in normal skin.

The amount of corticosteroid absorbed from the skin depends on the intrinsic properties of the drug itself, the vehicle used, the duration of exposure, and the surface area and condition of the skin to which it is applied. In general, absorption is enhanced by increased skin temperature, hydration, application to inflamed or denuded skin, intertriginous areas (eg, eyelids, groin, axilla), or skin surfaces with a thin stratum corneum layer (eg, face, scrotum). Palms, soles, and crusted skin surfaces are less permeable. Occlusive dressings greatly enhance skin penetration, and therefore increase drug absorption.

Infants and children have a higher total body surface-to-body weight ratio that decreases with age. Therefore, proportionately more of any topical medication will be absorbed systemically in this population, which puts infants and children at a greater risk for systemic effects.

Vehicles: Ointments are more greasy and occlusive and are preferred for dry, scaly lesions. Therefore, use creams on oozing lesions or in intertriginous areas where the occlusive effects of ointments may cause maceration and folliculitis. Creams often are preferred by patients for aesthetic reasons, although their water content makes them more drying than ointments. Gels, aerosols, lotions, and solutions are useful on hairy areas. Urea enhances the penetration of hydrocortisone and selected steroids by hydrating the skin. As a general rule, ointments and gels are slightly more potent than creams or lotions. However, optimized vehicles that have been formulated for some products have demonstrated equal potency in cream, gel, and ointment forms. Steroid impregnated tapes are useful for occlusive therapy in small areas.

Occlusive dressings: Occlusive dressings, such as a plastic wrap, increase skin penetration approximately 10-fold by increasing the moisture content of the stratum corneum. Occlusion can be beneficial in resistant cases, but it also may lead to sweat retention and increased bacterial and fungal infections. Additionally, increased absorption of corticosteroids may produce systemic side effects. Therefore, do not use occlusive dressings for longer than 12 hours/day or when using very potent topical corticosteroids or unless directed to do so by a physician.

Relative potency: The relative potency of a product depends on several factors, including the characteristics and concentrations of the drug and the vehicle used.

► **Indications**

Relief of inflammatory and pruritic manifestations of a variety of corticosteroid-responsive dermatoses (eg, contact dermatoses, contact dermatitis, rash, pruritus, minor skin inflammation).

Topical corticosteroids are indicated for alternative/adjunctive treatment of psoriasis. More specifically, nonprescription hydrocortisone preparations are indicated for temporary relief of itching or inflammation caused by psoriasis.

► **Contraindications**

Hypersensitivity to any component of the product; treatment of rosacea, perioral dermatitis, or acne; use on the face, groin, or axilla (very high or high-potency agents); ophthalmic use (prolonged ocular exposure may cause steroid-induced glaucoma and cataracts).

► **Warnings**

Systemic effects: Systemic absorption of chronically applied topical corticosteroids, particularly the high-potency prescription products, has produced reversible hypothalamic-pituitary-adrenal (HPA) axis suppression, Cushing syndrome, hyperglycemia, and glycosuria. Conditions that augment systemic absorption include the application of more potent steroids, use over large surface areas, prolonged use, and the use of occlusive dressings.

As a general rule, little effect on the HPA axis will occur with use of an OTC or prescription topical corticosteroid in amounts of less than 50 g weekly for an adult and 15 g weekly for a small child, without occlusion. To cover the adult body 1 time requires 12 to 26 g.

Local irritation: If local irritation develops, discontinue use and wash affected area with mild soap and water. Medications containing alcohol may produce dry skin or burning sensations/irritation in open lesions. Allergic contact dermatitis usually is diagnosed by observing the failure to heal rather than noting clinical exacerbation, as with most topical products that do not contain corticosteroids.

Skin atrophy – Skin atrophy is common and may be clinically significant after 3 to 4 weeks of regular use of potent prescription preparations. Atrophy occurs most readily at sites where percutaneous absorption is high.

Patients should exercise caution when using around the eye or in the genital area. The use of high-potency prescription formulations on the face and in intertriginous areas should be avoided because of resulting striae.

Psoriasis: Do not use nonprescription or prescription topical corticosteroids as the sole form of therapy in patients with widespread plaque.

In rare instances, treatment (or withdrawal of treatment) of psoriasis with corticosteroids is thought to have provoked the pustular form of the disease.

Atrophic changes: Certain areas of the body, such as the face, groin, and axillae, are more prone to atrophic changes than other areas of the body following chronic treatment with topical corticosteroids. Frequent observation of the patient is important if these areas are to be treated.

Infections: In the presence of an infection, institute appropriate therapy. If a favorable response does not occur promptly, discontinue the corticosteroid until the infection has been controlled. Treating skin infections with topical corticosteroids can worsen the infection.

For external use only: Avoid ingestion, contact with the eyes, or the inhalation of steroid-containing aerosols.

Vehicles: Many topical corticosteroids are in specially formulated bases designed to maximize their release and potency. Mixing these formulations with other bases or vehicles may affect the potency of the drug far beyond what would normally be expected from the dilution. Exercise caution before mixing; if necessary, contact the manufacturer to determine if there may be an incompatibility.

Occlusive therapy: Discontinue the use of occlusive dressings if infection develops, and institute appropriate therapy.

Pregnancy: Category C. Corticosteroids are teratogenic in animals when administered systemically at relatively low doses. The more potent corticosteroids are teratogenic after dermal application in animals. There are no adequate and well-controlled studies in pregnant women. Therefore, use during pregnancy only if the potential benefits outweigh the potential hazards to the fetus. In pregnant patients, do not use in large amounts or for prolonged periods of time.

Lactation: It is not known whether topical corticosteroid application could result in sufficient systemic absorption to produce detectable quantities in breast milk. Systemic corticosteroids are secreted into breast milk in quantities not likely to have a deleterious effect on the infant. Nevertheless, exercise caution when administering topical corticosteroids to a nursing mother.

Children: Children may be more susceptible to topical corticosteroid-induced HPA axis suppression and Cushing syndrome than adults because of their larger skin surface area-to-body weight ratio.

Hypothalamic-pituitary axis suppression, Cushing syndrome, and intracranial hypertension have occurred in children receiving topical corticosteroids. Manifestations of adrenal suppression include linear growth retardation, delayed weight gain, low plasma cortisol levels, and absence of response to adrenocorticotropic hormone (ACTH) stimulation.

Limit administration to the least amount compatible with effective therapy. Chronic corticosteroid therapy may interfere with children's growth and development.

▶ Adverse Reactions

Burning; itching; irritation; erythema; dryness; folliculitis; hypertrichosis; pruritus; acneiform eruptions; hypopigmentation; perioral dermatitis; allergic contact dermatitis; numbness of fingers; stinging and cracking or tightening of skin; maceration of the skin; secondary infection; skin atrophy; striae; miliaria; telangiectasia. These may occur more frequently with the use of occlusive dressings.

There also have been reports of development of pustular psoriasis from chronic plaque psoriasis following reduction or discontinuation of potent topical corticosteroids.

Sensitivity to a particular dressing material or adhesive may occur occasionally.

▶ Administration and Dosage

Usual dosage: Apply sparingly to affected areas 2 to 4 times daily.

General considerations: Topical corticosteroids have a repository effect; with continuous use, 1 or 2 applications/day may be as effective as 3 or more. Many clinicians advise applying twice daily until clinical response is achieved and then only as frequently as needed to control the condition.

Short-term or intermittent therapy using high-potency prescription agents (eg, every other day, 3 to 4 consecutive days per week, or once per week) may be more effective and cause fewer adverse effects than continuous regimens using lower-potency products.

Only use low-potency agents in children, on large areas, and on body sites especially prone to steroid damage (eg, the face, scrotum, axillae, flexures, and skin folds). Reserve higher-potency agents for areas and conditions resistant to treatment with milder agents.

TOPICAL CORTICOSTEROID PRODUCTS	
Trade name	**Doseform**
Cortizone•5	**Ointment**: 0.5% hydrocortisone. Excipients.
Cortizone•10	**Ointment**: 1% hydrocortisone. Benzyl alcohol, SD alcohol 40.
Hydrocortisone	**Ointment**: 1% hydrocortisone. Mineral oil, white petrolatum.
Cortaid Maximum Strength	**Ointment**: 1% hydrocortisone (as acetate). Parabens, mineral oil, white petrolatum.
Hydrocortisone Acetate	**Ointment**: 1% hydrocortisone (as acetate). Aloe, white petrolatum.
Cortizone•5	**Cream**: 0.5% hydrocortisone. Parabens, glycerin, mineral oil, white petrolatum, aloe.
Corticaine	**Cream**: 0.5% hydrocortisone. Methylparaben, mineral oil, white petrolatum, menthol, stearyl alcohol, EDTA.
Cortaid Sensitive Skin Formula with Aloe	**Cream**: 0.5% hydrocortisone (as acetate). Aloe, parabens.
Hydrocortisone	**Cream**: 1% hydrocortisone. Aloe, cetearyl alcohol, glycerin, methylparaben.
Cortaid Intensive Therapy	**Cream**: 1% hydrocortisone. Parabens, cetyl alcohol, stearyl alcohol.
Cortizone•10	**Cream**: 1% hydrocortisone. Parabens, glycerin, mineral oil, white petrolatum, cetearyl alcohol, aloe.
Cortaid Maximum Strength	**Cream**: 1% hydrocortisone. Benzyl alcohol, cetearyl alcohol, glycerin, methylparaben, aloe.

TOPICAL CORTICOSTEROID PRODUCTS	
Trade name	**Doseform**
Maximum Strength HydroZone Plus	**Cream**: 1% hydrocortisone. Benzyl alcohol, glycerin, stearyl alcohol.
LanaCort Maximum Strength	**Cream**: 1% hydrocortisone (as acetate). Glycerin, mineral oil, cetyl alcohol, lanolin, EDTA, parabens, menthol, aloe.
HydroZone Plus, Hydrocortisone	**Lotion**: 1% hydrocortisone. Cetyl alcohol.
CortaGel Maximum Strength	**Gel**: 1% hydrocortisone. Ethanol, aloe, EDTA.
CortiCool	**Gel**: 1% hydrocortisone, 45% alcohol, benzethonium chloride
Cortaid Intensive Therapy	**Spray**: 1% hydrocortisone. EDTA, glycerin, 45% SD alcohol 40.

Products listed are representative of currently available and widely distributed brands. Similar products, including regional and private label brands, may also exist.

PATIENT INFORMATION
Topical Corticosteroids

- For external use only. Cleanse affected area of skin prior to application (unless directed otherwise).
- Apply ointments, creams, or gels sparingly in a light film. Rub in gently. Washing or soaking the area before application may increase drug penetration.
- To use a lotion, solution, or gel on your scalp, part your hair, apply a small amount of the medicine on the affected area, and rub it in gently. Protect the area from washing, clothing, rubbing, etc., until the medicine dries. You may wash your hair as usual, but not immediately after applying the medicine.
- Use only as directed. Do not put bandages, dressings, cosmetics, or other skin products over the treated area unless directed by a physician.
- Notify a physician if the condition being treated worsens or if burning, swelling, or redness develop.
- Avoid prolonged use around the eyes, in the genital and rectal areas, and on the face, armpits, and skin creases unless directed by a physician. Avoid contact with the eyes.
- If you forget a dose, apply it as soon as you remember and continue on your regular schedule. If it is almost time for the next application, wait and continue on your regular schedule. Do not apply double doses.
- *For parents of pediatric patients*: Consult a physician. If corticosteroid treatment is recommended, do not use tight-fitting diapers or plastic pants on a child treated in the diaper area; these garments may work like occlusive dressings and cause more of the drug to be absorbed into your child's body. Do not use topical steroids to treat diaper rash.

TAR-CONTAINING PREPARATIONS

▶ **Actions**

Coal tar: Coal tar and its derivatives are used for their antipruritic, antieczematous, and keratolytic actions to treat psoriasis and other chronic skin disorders.

▶ **Indications**

For the relief and control of itching, irritation, and skin flaking associated with psoriasis and seborrheic dermatitis.

▶ **Contraindications**

Do not use on patients who are sensitive to any component of the product.

▶ **Warnings**

For external use only: Avoid contact with the eyes.

Photosensitivity: Avoid exposure to sunlight for up to 24 hours after using these products. Patients who have a disease characterized by photosensitivity (eg, lupus erythematosus, sunlight allergy) should not use these products.

Application considerations: Do not apply to acutely inflamed or broken skin or to the genital or rectal areas. If the condition covers a large area of the body, consult a physician before using these products.

Discoloration/Staining: Light-colored, bleached, or tinted hair may become temporarily discolored. Slight staining of clothes also may occur; standard laundry procedures will remove most stains.

Do not use with other forms of psoriasis therapy (eg, ultraviolet radiation, drug therapy) unless directed to do so.

Children: Do not use in children younger than 2 years of age.

TAR-CONTAINING PREPARATIONS	
Trade name	**Doseform**
Medotar	**Ointment**: 1% coal tar, 0.5% polysorbate 80, octoxynol-5, zinc oxide, white petrolatum
Taraphilic	**Ointment**: 1% coal tar distillate, 0.5% polysorbate 20, stearyl alcohol, white petrolatum, sorbitol, propylene glycol, sodium lauryl sulfate, parabens
MG217 Medicated	**Ointment**: 2% coal tar (as 10% coal tar solution), petrolatum, cetyl alcohol
Fototar	**Cream**: 2% coal tar in an emollient moisturizing base
MG217 Medicated	**Lotion**: 1% coal tar (as 5% coal tar solution) in a light greaseless moisturizing base with jojoba
Oxipor VHC	**Lotion**: 5% coal tar (25% coal tar solution), 79% alcohol
Estar	**Gel**: Coal tar extract equivalent to 5% coal tar, benzyl alcohol, carbomer 940, glycereth-7 coconate, laureth-4, polysorbate 80, 15.6% SD alcohol 40, simethicone, sorbitol
PsoriGel	**Gel**: 7.5% coal tar solution, 28.3% alcohol
Packer's Pine Tar	**Soap**: Soap base. Pine tar, pine oil, iron oxide, PEG-75
Polytar	**Soap**: 0.5% coal tar (juniper tar, pine tar, coal tar solution, solubilized crude coal tar, octoxynol-9, povidone, sodium borohydride, sodium cocoate, sodium tallowate, trisodium HEDTA)

Products listed are representative of currently available and widely distributed brands. Similar products, including regional and private label brands, may also exist.

■ ■ ■

PATIENT INFORMATION
Tar-Containing Preparations

- If condition covers a large area of the body, worsens, or does not improve or if irritation develops after regular use as directed, consult a physician. Do not use for prolonged periods or with other psoriasis therapies, such as ultraviolet light or prescription drugs, unless directed by a physician.
- May stain clothing or temporarily discolor white, blond, gray, bleached, or tinted hair.
- Skin may tingle during treatment.
- These products may cause sensitivity to sunlight. Avoid prolonged exposure to direct sunlight. Using topical tar plus ultraviolet light may increase one's tendency to sunburn for 24 to 72 hours.
- Do not apply to genital or rectal areas.

■ ■ ■
ROSACEA
(Acne Rosacea)

DEFINITION

Rosacea, which is sometimes inappropriately referred to as "adult acne," is a vascular condition characterized by papules and papulopustules that occur in the central region of the face on a background of prominent erythema and telangiectases, lesions formed by a terminal artery or dilated capillary (see Figure 1). The disease develops through several stages, beginning with episodes of blushing, to permanent erythema on the cheeks and nose, followed by development of papules and pustules, then eventually telangiectases. If the conditions is severe and persistent, it can progress to diffuse hyperplasia of connective tissue with enlarged sebaceous glands causing disfigurement of the nose (rhynophyma).

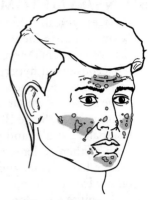

Figure 1. Acne Rosacea

ETIOLOGY

The cause of rosacea is unknown. Possible causes include genetic predisposition, GI diseases, chronic gall bladder disease, hypertension, and *Demodex folliculorum* mites, but a cause-and-effect relationship has not been fully established. It is known that a genetic predisposition exists, particularly for those of Celtic or northern European background. Additionally, there are known triggering factors, such as sunlight and heat. Other exacerbating factors include ingestion of hot liquids, spicy foods, alcohol, caffeine, or anything that causes one to flush or blush.

INCIDENCE

Reliable incidence figures are not available; however, rosacea is a relatively common disease, especially in fair-skinned people. It is estimated that 13 million Americans are affected; this number is increasing as baby boomers reach mid-life. There is no gender predisposition, although the sebaceous gland hyperplasia leading to rhynophyma (ie, red, swollen bumpy nose) occurs mostly in men. Rosacea is common in the 3rd and 4th decades and peaks between 40 to 50 years of age.

PATHOPHYSIOLOGY

Rosacea is sometimes considered a seborrheic disease. However, it is not primarily a disease of sebaceous follicles, in contrast to acne vulgaris. Comedones are absent, and the pustules of rosacea appear to be follicular abscesses, not keratotic plugged pustules as in acne. The condition exacerbates and remits, is progressive, and cosmetic manifestations may become permanent if not properly managed.

SIGNS/SYMPTOMS

Rosacea typically affects the nose, cheeks, chin, forehead, and glabella (a smooth prominence on the frontal bone above the root of the nose). It consists of erythema, erythematous papules and pustules, telangiectases, and sebaceous gland hyperplasia. Some classify rosacea as having 3 stages. Prior to Stage I disease, rosacea manifests as episodic erythema. This can progress to Stage I disease, which consists of persistent, moderate erythema with scattered telangiectases. Stage II consists of persistent erythema, numerous telangiectases, and papules and pustules. Finally, Stage III is characterized by persistent deep erythema, dense telangiectases, papules, pustules and nodules, variable plaque-like edema, and sometimes eventual tissue or sebaceous gland hyperplasia. Eye involvement (usually inflamed eyelids with crusting or matting) is also quite common in rosacea, affecting more than 50% of rosacea patients.

DIAGNOSTIC PARAMETERS/PHYSICAL ASSESSMENT

Clinical Observation: The hallmark signs of rosacea are papules and papulopustules, vivid red erythema, and telangiectases. Comedones (ie, blackheads and whiteheads) are notably absent. In later stages, tissue or sebaceous hyperplasia develops, particularly in men. Eye inflammation (blepharitis, conjunctivitis, iritis, or keratitis) is common. The most frequent eye symptom is inflamed eyelid margins with scales and crusts (similar to seborrheic dermatitis).

If the episodes of rosacea are frequent, persistent, or severe, and if eye signs or symptoms exist, physician referral is necessary.

Interview: To ensure the proper diagnosis and treatment of rosacea, it may be beneficial to ask about the following:

- Patient's age.
- Duration and type of symptoms and whether symptoms have progressively worsened.
- Presence of eye irritation or inflammation.
- Medical history (ask specifically about GI disease, hypertension).
- Family history of rosacea.
- Current medication profile.
- Recent exposure to triggering factors (eg, heat, sunlight, wind, alcohol, caffeine, hot or spicy foods/beverages, use of topical steroids).

TREATMENT

Approaches to therapy: Rosacea can be very difficult to treat. There is no cure. The goal of treatment is to manage symptoms and slow progression of the disease. Treatment schedules for managing symptoms are determined by the severity of the disease. The approach to therapy is 2-fold: Avoidance of exacerbating factors and pharmacotherapy.

Nondrug therapy: An important treatment strategy is avoidance of exacerbating factors. Rosacea patients have sensitive skin. Therefore, all sources of local irritation, such as soaps, alcohol cleansers, astringents, abrasives, and peeling agents must be avoided. Only mild soaps or cleansers are advised. Protection against sunlight is also very important. A broad-spectrum UVA/UVB non-irritating sunscreen with SPF of 15 or larger should be used at least daily. Other items to avoid include caffeine, chocolate, hot liquids, spicy foods, alcohol, and emotional stress. For nonprescription therapy for eye symptoms, see the Blepharitis monograph in the Ophthalmic Conditions chapter.

Pharmacotherapy: Pharmacotherapy is the mainstay treatment for rosacea. This treatment is divided into topical and systemic medications. Do not treat acne rosacea with nonprescription drugs. When acne rosacea is suspected, refer the patient to an appropriate physician, preferably a dermatologist. Prescription topical therapy includes topical antibiotics, metronidazole, imidazoles, and topical tretinoin. Systemic therapy includes prescription drugs such as oral antibiotics (eg, tetracycline, doxycycline) and oral metronidazole.

SEBORRHEIC DERMATITIS

DEFINITION
Seborrheic dermatitis is a chronic inflammatory, erythematous, and scaling condition involving areas rich in sebaceous glands, including the scalp, face, and upper trunk.

ETIOLOGY
The causes of seborrheic dermatitis are unknown although theories regarding the fungal spore *Pityrosporum ovale* or *Malassezia furfur* as the infectious etiology have been suggested. Stress, weather changes, or genetic factors may affect the incidence and severity of seborrheic dermatitis. Symptoms are usually worse during the winter months.

INCIDENCE
The incidence of seborrheic dermatitis has been estimated to be between 3% to 5%. There is no sex or race predilection. The age of occurrence is generally post-puberty although it is also seen in children as young as 2 weeks of age, and, in this case, generally clears by 12 months of age. An abnormally high incidence of the disease is seen in people with CNS disorders, such as stress, strokes, parkinsonism, and brain tumors. It may also be seen, in severe form, in HIV-positive patients.

PATHOPHYSIOLOGY
Because the etiology is often uncertain, the pathophysiology is also unclear. The body's inflammatory response to the high numbers of *M. furfur* is, in some way, related to the cause. Also, increased sebum production is generally seen in disorders that have a high incidence of seborrheic dermatitis (eg, acne, parkinsonism, and other neurologic disorders) and may therefore contribute to the pathophysiology of seborrheic dermatitis.

SIGNS/SYMPTOMS
The hallmark of the disorder is scaling and erythematous patches in typical "seborrheic" areas (eg, scalp, eyebrows, eyelids, behind the ears, in the ear canal, nasolabial folds, bridge of the nose, mid-chest and intertriginous areas such as the groin, umbilical, and inframammary areas). The patches may or may not be pruritic.

The onset of symptoms is usually gradual. The most common form of seborrheic dermatitis is dandruff (dry or greasy diffuse scaling of the scalp with variable degrees of itching). Newborns may experience a thick, yellow crusting of the scalp; this form of seborrheic dermatitis is called "cradle cap."

DIAGNOSTIC PARAMETERS/PHYSICAL ASSESSMENT
Clinical Observation: The typical presentation is generally characteristic (see Signs/Symptoms); however, it may be confused with psoriasis (when the scalp

is involved) or with *Candida albicans* infections (when the inframammary, axillary, or mouth angles are involved).

Interview: To help the patient determine if physician referral or self-treatment is warranted, it is important to consider the age of the patient and the extent of the disease. If the patient is an infant or if the disorder is extensive or very thick, highly inflamed, associated with intense erythema and itching, cosmetically objectionable, or otherwise symptomatic, physician referral should be made.

Topics to ask about include the following:
- History of seborrheic dermatitis. Previous treatment and success.
- Recent significant lifestyle changes.
- Duration of symptoms.
- Symptoms and their severity.
- Areas of the body affected.

TREATMENT

Approaches to therapy: Therapy is dependent upon the location, extent, and severity of the disorder. For scalp seborrheic dermatitis, including dandruff, control can often be achieved with shampoos containing either zinc pyrithione, tar, selenium sulfide, or salicylic acid. Occasionally, the scaling is so thick that the patient must soak the scale overnight with occluded mineral oil before shampooing in the morning. Seborrheic dermatitis of the scalp, body, and face can be generally be controlled with good skin hygeine and judicious use of topical hydrocortisone products.

For infants with "cradle cap," use a mild baby shampoo daily, and rub a hydrocortisone cream into the scalp twice daily. Salicylic acid, 10% in mineral oil, may be effective if lesions are thick. If a yeast (fungus) is suspected as an etiological factor, topical imidazole antifungals may be useful.

Nondrug therapy: No non-drug therapy is currently available for seborrheic dermatitis. Avoidance of exacerbating factors can help control seborrheic dermatitis.

Pharmacotherapy: Several different brands of tar shampoos are available, ranging from less than 1% to 5% concentrations. The shampoos are also available in a wide range of scents, from fairly unpleasant to acceptable. Similarly, many different shampoos containing zinc pyrithione are available in different strengths, with some vehicles being harsher on the hair than others. The OTC hydrocortisone creams/ointments are available in 0.5% and 1% strengths. Use the creams in areas that require a cosmetically acceptable vehicle or in intertriginous areas as they are less greasy than an ointment. Use the ointments if the skin appears to be overly dry.

SELENIUM SULFIDE

▶ **Actions**

Selenium sulfide appears to have a cytostatic effect on cells of the epidermis and follicular epithelium, thus reducing corneocyte production and subsequent scaling.

▶ Indications

Treatment of seborrheic dermatitis of the scalp (including dandruff), tinea versi-color, scalp psoriasis, eczema, "cradle cap," and other oily, itchy, scaling conditions of the body and scalp.

▶ Contraindications

Allergy to any component of the product or acute inflammation; open, oozing, or infected lesions.

▶ Warnings

Hypersensitivity: If sensitivity reactions occur, or symptoms worsen, discontinue use.

For external use only: Avoid contact with the eyes, eyelids, and mucous membranes. If contact occurs, rinse thoroughly with water.

Acute inflammation/exudation: Do not use when these conditions are present; absorption may be increased.

If condition worsens or does not improve after regular use, or if excessive dryness or any undesirable effect occurs, discontinue use and contact your physician.

Children: Safety and efficacy in infants have not been established. Use only upon the advice of a physician.

▶ Adverse Reactions

Skin irritation; greater than normal hair loss; hair discoloration (avoid or minimize by thorough rinsing after treatment); oiliness or dryness of hair and scalp. Minor dermatologic side effects may also include rash or burning sensation. Photosensitivity may occur. May discolor skin.

▶ Overdosage

Accidental oral ingestion:

    Symptoms – Selenium sulfide shampoos have relatively low toxicity if ingested. Nausea, vomiting, and diarrhea usually occur after oral ingestion. There may also be a burning sensation in the mouth and a garlic-like taste/smell to the breath. The detergents found in selenium sulfide shampoos may act as emetics, thereby preventing significant GI absorption of selenium.

    Treatment – Includes usual supportive measures. In cases of accidental ingestion, encourage individuals to call local or regional Poison Control Centers.

▶ Administration and Dosage

Massage 5 to 10 mL of the medicated shampoo into wet scalp. Allow to remain on the scalp for 2 to 3 minutes. Rinse thoroughly. Repeat application and rinse thoroughly. Wash hands well after treatment.

Usually, 2 applications each week for 2 weeks will afford symptom control. After this, it may be used at less frequent intervals - weekly, every 2 weeks, or every 3 or 4 weeks in some cases. Do not apply more frequently than required to maintain control.

SELENIUM SULFIDE PRODUCTS	
Trade name	**Doseform**
Head & Shoulders Intensive Treatment Dandruff Shampoo, Selsun Blue	**Lotion/Shampoo:** 1%

Products listed are representative of currently available and widely distributed brands. Similar products, including regional and private label brands, may also exist.

PATIENT INFORMATION
Selenium Sulfide

- It is important to advise the patient that the condition is chronic, and that the goal of therapy is to control the symptoms of the condition rather than cure it. Consequently, continued shampooing will be necessary.
- For external use only. Avoid contact with the eyes, eyelids, and mucous membranes.
- Do not use on acutely inflamed, oozing, or infected skin.
- If irritation occurs, or symptoms worsen, discontinue use.
- Thoroughly rinse after each application.
- If using on the scalp before or after bleaching, tinting, or permanent waving, rinse hair for five minutes or longer after application with cool running water.
- May damage jewelry; remove before using.

TAR DERIVATIVES

▶ Actions

Tar derivatives help correct keratinization abnormalities by decreasing epidermal proliferation and dermal infiltration. They also have antipruritic and mild antibacterial actions.

▶ Indications

For treatment of scalp psoriasis, eczema, seborrheic dermatitis, dandruff, cradle cap, and other oily, itchy conditions of the body and scalp. These agents may decrease scaling associated with tinea capitis and, therefore, may be used as adjunctive therapy.

▶ Contraindications

Hypersensitivity to any component of the product; acute inflammation; open or infected scalp lesions.

▶ Warnings

For external use only: Avoid contact with the eyes, eyelids, and mucous membranes. If contact occurs, rinse thoroughly with water.

Sensitivity: Discontinue use and contact a pharmacist or physician if sensitivity reactions (eg, redness, swelling, itching, burning) or chemical irritation occurs.

Pregnancy: Category C. There are no adequate and well-controlled studies in pregnant women. Use during pregnancy only if the potential benefits outweigh the possible risks to the fetus.

Lactation: Safety for use in the nursing mother has not been established. Exercise caution when applying on a nursing woman.

Children: Use on children younger than two years of age only as directed by a physician.

Photosensitivity: Use caution in exposing skin to sunlight after application. It may increase tendency to sunburn for up to 24 hours after application.

▶ Adverse Reactions

Minor dermatologic side effects include rash or burning sensation. Photosensitivity or skin discoloration may occur.

▶ **Administration and Dosage**

Refer to the specific product labeling for dosing information. Rub shampoo liberally into scalp. Leave on for several minutes. Rinse thoroughly. Repeat and rinse. Depending on the product, use at least twice per week up to once daily or as directed by a physician. For severe scalp problems, use daily according to product instructions.

TAR DERIVATIVE PRODUCTS	
Trade name	**Doseform**
DHS Tar	**Shampoo**: 0.5% coal tar
Doak Tar	**Shampoo**: 0.5% coal tar. EDTA, isopropyl alcohol.
Polytar	**Shampoo**: 0.5% coal tar. EDTA, lanolin.
Sebutone	**Shampoo**: 0.5% coal tar. EDTA, lanolin oil, salicylic acid, sulfur.
Tera-Gel	**Shampoo**: 0.5% coal tar. EDTA, parabens.
Ionil T, Zetar	**Shampoo**: 1% coal tar
PC-Tar	**Shampoo**: 1% coal tar. EDTA.
Creamy Tar	**Shampoo**: 2% coal tar. 5.6% ethyl alcohol.
Ionil T Plus	**Shampoo**: 2% coal tar
Neutrogena T/Gel	**Shampoo**: 2% coal tar extract
	Conditioner: 2% coal tar extract in a conditioner base
X•Seb T Pearl, X•Seb T Plus	**Shampoo**: 2% coal tar. EDTA, lanolin, salicylic acid.
Original Therapeutic Strength Denorex	**Shampoo**: 2.5% coal tar. 10.4% alcohol, menthol.
MG217 Extra Strength with Conditioners	**Shampoo**: 3% coal tar
Pentrax 5%	**Shampoo**: 5% coal tar
Original Therapeutic Strength Denorex 2 in 1	**Shampoo/Conditioner**: 2.5% coal tar. 10.4% alcohol, avocado oil, lanolin, menthol.
Tarsum	**Shampoo/Gel**: 2% coal tar. Salicylic acid.

Products listed are representative of currently available and widely distributed brands. Similar products, including regional and private label brands, may also exist.

PATIENT INFORMATION

Tar Derivatives

- For external use only. Avoid contact with the eyes, eyelids, or mucous membranes. If contact occurs, rinse thoroughly with water.
- Rinse thoroughly after each application. Discontinue use and consult a physician if excessive dryness or irritation occurs.
- Consult a physician before use if you have a condition that covers a large portion of the body.
- Discontinue use if condition worsens or does not improve after regular use as directed.
- Tar derivatives increase sensitivity to the sun and may increase tendency to sunburn for up to 24 hours after use. Avoid prolonged exposure to the sun or other forms of ultraviolet light (eg, tanning beds). Use sunscreens and wear protective clothing until tolerance is determined.
- Do not use for prolonged periods (longer than six months) or with psoriasis therapy (eg, phototherapy, prescription drugs) unless instructed by a physician.
- Products containing tar may temporarily discolor blond, gray, bleached, or tinted hair, or cause slight staining of clothing. Clothing stains normally are removed by standard laundry methods.
- Some coal tar products are extremely flammable. Keep away from fire and flame.

TAR-CONTAINING PREPARATIONS

▶ Indications

Coal tar: Coal tar (or derivatives) is used for its antipruritic, anti-eczematous and keratoplastic actions. Used in psoriasis and other chronic skin disorders.

Precipitated sulfur: Precipitated sulfur is a keratolytic, antifungal and antiparasitic agent. See the Acne monograph in the Dermatological Condtions chapter.

Salicylic acid: Salicylic acid is a keratolytic agent.

Zinc oxide: Zinc oxide is an astringent, antiseptic and protective agent.

▶ Contraindications

Do not use on patients sensitive to any component.

▶ Warnings

For external use only: Avoid contact with the eyes.

Children: Do not use in children younger than 2 years of age.

▶ Administration and Dosage

Refer to individual package labeling.

TAR-CONTAINING PREPARATIONS	
Trade name	Doseform
Medotar	Ointment: 1% coal tar, 0.5% polysorbate 80, octoxynol–5, zinc oxide, white petrolatum
Taraphilic	Ointment: 1% coal tar, 0.5% polysorbate 20, stearyl alcohol, white petrolatum, sorbitol, propylene glycol, sodium lauryl sulfate, parabens
MG217 Medicated	Ointment: 2% coal tar solution, 1.1% colloidal sulfur, 1.5% salicylic acid

TAR-CONTAINING PREPARATIONS

Trade name	Doseform
Fototar	**Cream**: 2% coal tar in an emollient moisturizing base
Tegrin for Psoriasis	**Cream**: 5% coal tar solution, acetylated lanolin alcohol, 4.7% alcohol, carbomer 934P, glyceryl tribehenate, mineral oil, potassium hydroxide, lanolin alcohol, petrolatum, titanium dioxide, stearyl alcohol
Doak Tar	**Lotion**: 5% Doak tar distillate (equiv. to 2% coal tar)
MG217 for Psoriasis	**Lotion**: 5% coal tar solution in a light greaseless moisturizing base with jojoba
Doak Tar Distillate	**Liquid**: 40% coal tar distillate
Oxipor VHC	**Lotion**: 25% coal tar solution, 79% alcohol
Coal Tar or Carbonis Detergens	**Solution**: 20% coal tar
Estar	**Gel**: Coal tar extract equivalent to 5% coal tar, benzyl alcohol, carbomer 940, glycereth-7 coconate, laureth-4, polysorbate 80, 15.6% SD alcohol 40, simethicone, sorbitol
P & S Plus	**Gel**: 8% coal tar solution (1.6% crude coal tar, 6.4% ethyl alcohol), 2% salicylic acid
PsoriGel	**Gel**: 7.5% coal tar solution, 33% alcohol
Packer's Pine Tar	**Soap**: Soap base, Pine tar, pine oil, iron oxide, PEG-75
Polytar	**Soap**: 1% polytar (juniper tar, pine tar, coal tar solution, solubilized crude coal tar, octoxynol-9, povidone, sodium borohydride, sodium cocoate, sodium tallowate, trisodium HEDTA)
Tegrin Medicated for Psoriasis	**Soap**: 5% coal tar solution, chromium hydroxide green, glycerin, titanium dioxide
Neutrogena T/Derm	**Oil**: 5% solubilized coal tar extract in an oil base

Products listed are representative of currently available and widely distributed brands. Similar products, including regional and private label brands, may also exist.

PATIENT INFORMATION

Tar-Containing Preparations

- If condition covers a large area of the body, worsens, or does not improve, or if irritation develops after regular use as directed, consult your doctor. Do not use for prolonged periods or with other psoriasis therapy, such as ultraviolet light or prescription drugs, unless directed by a physician.
- May stain clothing or temporarily discolor white, blond, gray, bleached, or tinted hair.
- Skin may tingle during treatment.
- *Sensitivity to sunlight:* Avoid prolonged exposure to direct sunlight. Topical tar plus ultraviolet light may increase tendency to sunburn for 24 to 72 hours.
- Do not apply to genital or rectal area.

PYRITHIONE ZINC

▶ Actions

Pyrithione zinc, a cytostatic agent, reduces cell turnover rate, and skin scaling and sloughing. Its action is thought to be caused by a nonspecific toxicity for epidermal cells. The compound strongly binds to hair and external skin layers.

▶ Indications

Pyrithione zinc helps control seborrheic dermatitis of the scalp (dandruff) and body, and assists in controlling dry scalp and its symptoms.

▶ Warnings

For external use only: Avoid contact with the eyes, eyelids, and mucous membranes. If contact occurs, rinse thoroughly with water.

▶ Administration and Dosage

Apply shampoo; lather, rinse, and repeat. Use once or twice weekly.

PYRITHIONE ZINC PRODUCTS	
Trade name	Doseform
Head & Shoulders, Head & Shoulder Dry Scalp, Zincon	Shampoo: 1%
Denorex Advanced Formula, DHS Zinc, Sebulon	Shampoo: 2%
ZNP Bar	Soap: 2%

Products listed are representative of currently available and widely distributed brands. Similar products, including regional and private label brands, may also exist.

PATIENT INFORMATION

Pyrithione Zinc

- For external use only.
- Avoid contact with eyes. If contact occurs, rinse thoroughly with water.
- If condition worsens or does not improve with regular use as directed, discontinue use and contact your doctor.
- May temporarily discolor bleached, tinted, gray, or permed hair; rinse for five minutes.

POVIDONE-IODINE

▶ Actions

Povidone-iodine shampoo is a broad-spectrum antimicrobial agent that liberates free iodine.

▶ Indications

Povidone-iodine shampoo provides temporary relief of scaling and itching due to seborrheic dermatitis of the scalp (dandruff).

▶ Warnings

For external use only: Avoid contact with the eyes, eyelids, and mucous membranes. If contact occurs, rinse thoroughly with water.

Irritation: Discontinue if signs of irritation or inflammation develop or symptoms worsen. These could be symptoms of an allergic/hypersensitivity reaction.

► **Administration and Dosage**

Apply 2 tsp (10 mL) to hair and scalp; use warm water to lather. Rinse. Repeat application. Massage gently into scalp. Allow to remain on scalp for 5 minutes or longer. Work up lather to a golden color using warm water. Rinse scalp thoroughly. Repeat twice weekly until improvement is noted. Thereafter, shampoo weekly.

POVIDONE-IODINE SHAMPOOS	
Trade name	Doseform
Betadine	Shampoo: 7.5%

Products listed are representative of currently available and widely distributed brands. Similar products, including regional and private label brands, may also exist.

PATIENT INFORMATION

Povidone-Iodine Shampoos

- Doses and frequency of use depend on the condition, treated area, individual tolerance, and dosage form. Review individual products for their use and dosage guidelines. Consult a pharmacist or physician for product-specific information.

CORTICOSTEROIDS, TOPICAL

► **Actions**

The primary therapeutic effects of topical corticosteroids are because of their anti-inflammatory activity, which is nonspecific (ie, they act against most causes of inflammation including mechanical, chemical, microbiological, and immunological).

Topical corticosteroids diffuse across cell membranes to interact with cytoplasmic receptors located in the dermal and intradermal cells. The intracellular effects are similar to those that occur with systemic corticosteroids.

At the cellular level, corticosteroids appear to depress formation, release, and activity of the endogenous mediators of inflammation, such as prostaglandins, kinins, histamine, liposomal enzymes, and the complement system.

When corticosteroids are applied to inflamed skin, they inhibit the migration of macrophages and leukocytes into the area. The clinical result is a decrease in edema, erythema, and pruritus.

By suppressing DNA synthesis, topical corticosteroids also have an antimitotic effect on epidermal cells. This property is useful in proliferative, scaling disorders such as psoriasis.

The amount of corticosteroid absorbed from the skin depends on the intrinsic properties of the drug itself, the vehicle used, exposure duration, and the surface area and condition of the skin to which it is applied. In general, absorption will be enhanced by increased skin temperature, hydration, application to inflamed or denuded skin, intertriginous area (eg, eyelids, groin, axilla), or skin surfaces with a thin stratum corneum layer (eg, face, scrotum). Palms, soles, and crusted surfaces are less permeable. Occlusive dressings greatly enhance skin penetration and, therefore, increase drug absorption.

Vehicles: Ointments are more occlusive and "greasy" and are preferred for dry scaly lesions. Use creams on oozing lesions or in intertriginous areas where the occlusive effects of ointments may cause maceration and folliculitis. Creams are often preferred by patients for aesthetic reasons even though their water content makes them more drying than ointments. Gels, aerosols, lotions, and solutions are useful on hairy areas. Urea enhances the penetration of hydrocortisone by hydrating the skin. Steroid impregnated tapes are useful for occlusive therapy on small areas.

▶ **Indications**

Temporary relief of inflammation, redness, or itching associated with minor skin irritations, inflammation and rashes due to eczema, insect bites, poison ivy, poison oak, poison sumac, soaps, detergents, cosmetics, jewelry, seborrheic dermatitis, psoriasis, and external genital and anal itching.

▶ **Contraindications**

Hypersensitivity to any component. When applied to the eyelids or skin near the eyes, the drug may enter the eyes and increase the risk of steroid-induced glaucoma or cataracts with chronic use.

▶ **Warnings**

Systemic effects: Systemic absorption of topical corticosteroids has produced reversible hypothalamic-pituitary-adrenal (HPA) axis suppression, Cushing syndrome, hyperglycemia, and glycosuria. Conditions that augment systemic absorption include the application of the more potent steroids, use over large surface areas, prolonged use, and the addition of occlusive dressings.

If HPA axis suppression is noted, attempt to withdraw the drug, reduce the frequency of application, substitute a less potent steroid, or use a sequential approach with the occlusive technique.

Recovery of HPA axis function and thermal homeostasis is generally prompt and complete upon discontinuation of the drug. Infrequently, signs and symptoms of steroid withdrawal may occur, requiring supplemental systemic corticosteroids.

As a general rule, little effect on the HPA axis will occur with use of a potent, prescription-only topical corticosteroid in amounts of less than 50 g weekly for an adult and 15 g weekly for a small child, without occlusion. To cover the adult body 1 time requires 12 to 26 g.

Local irritation: If local irritation develops, discontinue use and institute appropriate therapy. Medications containing alcohol may produce dry skin or burning sensations/irritation in open lesions. Allergic contact dermatitis is usually diagnosed by observing failure to heal rather than noting clinical exacerbation as with most topical products not containing corticosteroids. Corroborate such an observation with diagnostic patch testing.

> *Skin atrophy* – Skin atrophy is common and may be clinically significant in 3 to 4 weeks with potent prescription-only preparations. Atrophy occurs most readily at sites where percutaneous absorption is high.

Take care when using periorbitally or in the genital area. Avoid chronic use of high-potency, prescription-only topical corticosteroids on the face and in intertriginous areas because of the risk of striae.

Atrophic changes: Certain areas of the body, such as the face, groin, and axillae, are more prone to atrophic changes than other areas of the body following or during chronic treatment with corticosteroids. Frequent observation of the patient is important if these areas are to be treated.

Infections: In the presence of a dermal infection, institute therapy with an appropriate antifungal or antibacterial agent. If a favorable response does not occur promptly, discontinue the corticosteroid until the infection has been controlled. Treating skin infections with topical corticosteroids can extensively worsen the infection.

For external use only: Avoid inhalation of aerosols, ingestion or contact with eyes, eyelids, and mucous membranes.

Pregnancy: Category C. Corticosteroids are teratogenic in animals when administered systemically (eg, orally, by injection) at relatively low dosages. The more potent corticosteroids are teratogenic after dermal application in animals. There are no adequate and well controlled studies in pregnant women. Therefore, use during pregnancy only if the potential benefits outweigh the potential hazards to the fetus. In pregnant patients, do not use extensively; do not use in large amounts or for prolonged periods of time.

Lactation: It is unknown whether topical corticosteroids result in sufficient systemic absorption to produce detectable quantities in breast milk. Systemic corticosteroids are secreted into breast milk in quantities not likely to have a deleterious effect on the infant. Nevertheless, exercise caution when administering topical corticosteroids to a nursing mother.

Children: Children may be more susceptible to topical corticosteroid-induced HPA axis suppression and Cushing syndrome than adults because of a larger skin surface area to body weight ratio.

Limit administration to the least amount compatible with effective therapy at an acceptable level of risk. Chronic corticosteroid therapy may interfere with the growth and development of children.

▶ **Adverse Reactions**

Local: Burning; itching; irritation; erythema; dryness; folliculitis; hypertrichosis; pruritus; acneiform eruptions; hypopigmentation; perioral dermatitis; allergic contact dermatitis; numbness of fingers; stinging and cracking/tightening of skin; maceration of the skin; secondary infection; skin atrophy; striae; miliaria; telangiectasia. These may occur more frequently with occlusive dressings.

Sensitivity to a particular dressing material or adhesive may occur occasionally.

Systemic: Systemic absorption of chronically administered topical corticosteroids has produced reversible HPA axis suppression, manifestations of Cushing syndrome, hyperglycemia, and glycosuria (see Precautions). This is more likely to occur with occlusive dressings, when large areas are treated, and with more potent steroids. Patients with liver failure or children (see Warnings) may be at higher risk. Lightheadedness and hives have been reported rarely.

Following prolonged application around the eyes, cataracts and glaucoma may develop. In diffusely atrophied skin, blood vessels may become visible on the skin surface; telangiectasia and purpura may occur at the trauma site.

The risk of adverse reactions may be minimized by changing to a less potent agent, reducing the dosage or using intermittent therapy.

▶ **Overdosage**

Topical corticosteroids can be absorbed in sufficient amounts to produce systemic effects (see Precautions).

▶ Administration and Dosage

Usual dosage: Apply sparingly to affected areas 2 to 4 times daily.

General considerations: Topical corticosteroids have a repository effect; with continuous use, 1 or 2 applications/day may be as effective as 3 or more. Many clinicians advise applying twice daily until clinical response is achieved and then only as frequently as needed to control the condition.

Short-term or intermittent therapy (eg, every other day, 3 to 4 consecutive days per week, or once per week) using high-potency, prescription-only agents may be more effective and cause fewer adverse effects than continuous regimens using lower-potency products.

Do not discontinue treatment abruptly. After long-term use or after using a potent prescription-only agent, switch to a less potent agent or alternate use of topical corticosteroids and emollient products in order to prevent a rebound effect.

Use low-potency agents in children, on large areas, and on body sites especially prone to steroid damage, such as the face, scrotum, axilla, flexures, and skin folds. Reserve higher-potency agents for areas and conditions resistant to treatment with milder agents; they may be alternated with milder agents.

Treatment with very high-potency topical prescription-only corticosteroids should not exceed 2 consecutive weeks and the total dosage should not exceed 50 g/week because of the potential for these drugs to suppress the HPA axis.

TOPICAL CORTICOSTEROID PRODUCTS	
Trade name	**Doseform**
Cortizone•5	**Ointment**: 0.5% hydrocortisone
Cortizone•10	**Ointment**: 1% hydrocortisone. Parabens.
Bactine Hydrocortisone, Cortizone•5, Dermtex HC with Aloe	**Cream**: 0.5% hydrocortisone. Parabens.
Corticaine	**Cream**: 0.5% hydrocortisone
Cortaid Intensive Therapy, Cortizone•10, DriCort, Maximum Strength KeriCort-10, Procort	**Cream**: 1% hydrocortisone
Maximum Strength Scalpicin	**Liquid**: 1% hydrocortisone
Extra Strength CortaGel, CortiCool	**Gel**: 1% hydrocortisone
Maximum Strength Cortaid	**Pump Spray**: 1% hydrocortisone
Procort	**Spray**: 1% hydrocortisone
Maximum Strength Cortaid Fastick	**Stick, roll-on**: 1% hydrocortisone. Methylparaben.
Cortaid with Aloe	**Ointment**: 0.5% hydrocortisone acetate
Corticaine, Cortaid with Aloe	**Cream**: 0.5% hydrocortisone acetate. Parabens.
Maximum Strength Cortaid	**Ointment**: 1% hydrocortisone acetate
Maximum Strength Lanacort 10 Creme, Maximum Strength Cortaid	**Cream**: 1% hydrocortisone acetate
Anusol HC-1	**Ointment**: Hydrocortisone acetate equivalent to 1% hydrocortisone
Dermtex HC	**Cream**: Hydrocortisone acetate equivalent to 1% hydrocortisone

Products listed are representative of currently available and widely distributed brands. Similar products, including regional and private label brands, may also exist.

■ ■ ■

PATIENT INFORMATION
Topical Corticosteroids

- For external use only.
- Apply ointments, creams, or gels sparingly in a light film; rub in gently. Washing or soaking the area before application may increase drug penetration.
- Use caution with continued (daily) use of hydrocortisone cream, especially when used around the eye areas. Use these products sporadically.
- To use a lotion, solution, or gel on your scalp, part your hair, apply a small amount of the medicine on the affected area, and rub it in gently. Protect the area from washing, clothing, or rubbing until the lotion dries. You may wash your hair as usual but not immediately after applying the medicine.
- Use only as directed. Do not put bandages, dressings, cosmetics, or other skin products over the treated area unless authorized by your physician.
- Notify your physician if the condition worsens, or if burning, swelling, itching, or redness develops.
- Avoid prolonged use around the eyes, in the genital and rectal areas, on the face, in the armpits, and in skin creases unless directed by your physician. Avoid contact with the eyes, eyelids, and mucous membranes.
- If you forget a dose, apply it as soon as you remember and continue on your regular schedule. If it is almost time for the next application, wait and continue on your regular schedule. Do not apply double doses.
- *For parents of pediatric patients:* Do not use tight-fitting diapers or plastic pants on a child treated in the diaper area; these garments may work like occlusive dressings and cause excessive amounts of the drug to be absorbed into your child's body.

ANTISEBORRHEIC COMBINATIONS

▶ Indications

The following ingredients are adjunctive in the management of tinea capitis.

Salicylic acid and **sulfur** are used for antiseborrheic and keratolytic/keratoplastic actions.

Tar preparations are used for their antipruritic, mild antibacterial, or antiseborrheic actions.

Menthol is used as an antipruritic.

Benzalkonium chloride, isopropyl alcohol, phenol, and **menthol** are used as mild antiseptics.

▶ Warnings

For external use only: Avoid contact with the eyes, eyelids, or mucous membranes. If contact occurs, rinse thoroughly with water.

If undue skin irritation, burning, stinging, or itching develops or worsens, discontinue use and consult physician. Preparations containing tar may temporarily discolor blond, bleached, or tinted hair. Slight staining of clothing also may occur.

Children: Do not use on children younger than two years of age unless instructed by a physician.

▶ Administration and Dosage

Follow instructions on the label of the individual products very closely.

ANTISEBBORHEIC COMBINATION PRODUCTS	
Trade name	Doseform
Ionil, Ionil Plus, P & S	**Shampoo**: 2% salicylic acid
Neutrogena T/Sal	**Shampoo**: 2% salicylic acid, 2% solubilized coal tar extract
Sebex	**Shampoo**: 2% salicylic acid, 2% sulfur
Sebulex, Sebulex with Conditioners	**Shampoo**: 2% salicylic acid, 2% sulfur. EDTA.
Maximum Strength Meted	**Shampoo**: 3% salicylic acid, 5% sulfur
Sulfoam	**Shampoo**: 2% sulfur. Parabens.
Sebucare	**Lotion**: 1.8% salicylic acid. 61% alcohol, dihydrobietyl alcohol.
Scalpicin	**Liquid**: 3% salicylic acid. Menthol, SD alcohol 40.
P & S	**Liquid**: Glycerin, mineral oil, phenol

Products listed are representative of currently available and widely distributed brands. Similar products, including regional and private label brands, may also exist.

PATIENT INFORMATION

Antiseborrheic Combinations

- For external use only. Avoid contact with the eyes, eyelids, or mucous membranes. If contact occurs, rinse thoroughly with water.
- Consult a physician before use if you have a condition that covers a large portion of the body.
- Rinse thoroughly after each application. Discontinue use and consult a physician if irritation occurs.
- Discontinue use if condition worsens or does not improve after regular use as directed.
- Do not use on children younger than two years of age.
- Tar derivatives increase sensitivity the sun and may increase tendency to sunburn for up to 24 hours after use. Avoid prolonged exposure to the sun or other forms of ultraviolet light (eg, tanning beds). Use sunscreens and wear protective clothing until tolerance is determined.
- Do not use for prolonged periods (longer than 6 months) or with psoriasis therapy (eg, phototherapy, prescription drugs) unless instructed by a physician.
- Products containing tar may temporarily discolor blond, gray, bleached, or tinted hair, or cause slight staining of clothing. Clothing stains normally are removed by standard laundry methods.

SUNBURN
(Prevention and Treatment)

DEFINITION

Sunburn is an inflammatory reaction of the skin resulting from overexposure to the sun's ultraviolet (UV) light or artificial UV light, particularly UVB.

ETIOLOGY

Sunburn most commonly occurs after prolonged exposure to the sun, but it may also occur after exposure to sunlamps or occupational light sources.

PATHOPHYSIOLOGY

Ultraviolet radiation is divided into different bands based on wavelength. UVA (320 to 400 nm) can cause immediate pigment darkening of preformed melanin but is 1000 times less efficient at producing hyperemia than UVB. UVB (290 to 320 nm) is the most efficient at producing redness and erythema. UVC (200 to 290 nm) is stopped at the outer stratosphere. Photosensitivity occurs when a photon-absorbing chemical in the skin absorbs the energy from UVB, is promoted to an excited state, and then transfers and dissipates that energy. UVB stimulates melanocytes to make melanosomes that react to the UV light by producing melanin. Tolerance to sunlight is based on the amount of melanin in the skin and the person's ability to produce melanin after exposure to the sun. The erythema produced by a sunburn may be a prostaglandin-mediated vasodilatory effect. Peeling is the result of increased epidermal turnover that usually occurs 7 days or longer after a sunburn.

There are 4 major effects seen after skin is exposed to UV radiation. The first is erythema, which occurs 2 to 12 hours after exposure. The severity of erythema is related to skin type, duration of exposure, and amount of protection. The second is short-term tan that occurs early and is caused by increased dispersion and oxidation of melanin; it usually fades after 1 to 2 days. The third is common tan, which is a delayed hyperpigmentation that takes several days to occur; it will fade unless there is regular UV exposure. The fourth is delayed epidermal hyperplasia, which is skin thickening.

SIGNS/SYMPTOMS

The physical signs and symptoms of sunburn appear within 1 to 24 hours and usually begin to subside in 72 hours. The symptoms range from mild erythema to pain, swelling, tenderness, and blister formation. Fever, chills, weakness, and shock can occur if a severe sunburn occurs on a large portion of the body surface. Chronic symptoms of photo-damaged skin include wrinkling, blotchiness, and carcinoma (eg, basal cell carcinoma, squamous cell carcinoma, melanoma). Harmful effects on the eyes can include cataract formation and retinal damage.

DIAGNOSTIC PARAMETERS/PHYSICAL ASSESSMENT

The patient history is usually adequate to assess the clinical picture of a sunburn. It is important to rule out any predisposing factors such as medication, use of photosensitizing agents (eg, dapsone, fluoroquinolones, methoxsalen, nitrofurantoin, phenothiazines, sulfonamides, sulfonylureas, tetracyclines, tricyclic antidepressants), or systemic illness (eg, lupus erythematosus, porphyria, and herpes simplex).

FDA- and AAD-Recognized Skin Categories		
Skin Type	Sun History	Example
I	Always burns easily, never tans, extremely sun-sensitive skin	Red-headed, freckles, Northern Europeans
II	Always burns easily, tans minimally, very sun-sensitive skin	Fair-skinned, fair-haired, blue-eyed Caucasians
III	Sometimes burns, tans gradually to light brown, sun-sensitive skin	Average skin
IV	Burns minimally, always tans to moderate brown, minimally sun-sensitive	Mediterranean-type Caucasians
V	Rarely burns, tans well, sun-insensitive skin	Middle Eastern, some Hispanics, some African-Americans
VI	Never burns, deeply pigmented, sun-insensitive skin	African-Americans
The American Academy of Dermatology suggests that, regardless of skin type, a sunscreen with an SPF of 15 or larger should be used year-round.		

Clinical Observation: History and evaluation of the patient prior to prolonged sun exposure should include expected length of exposure, characteristics of the skin such as light vs dark, age, past experience with sun exposure, where exposure will take place (eg, local pool, beach, in high altitudes, etc.), and any history of sensitivity reactions to suntan or sunblock products.

Interview: If the patient has sunburned, it may be beneficial to ask about the following:

• Degree of pain or discomfort.
• Observation of the skin to detect signs of severe burn, including marked erythema and blisters, which may require physician referral.
• History of sunburn.

TREATMENT

Approaches to therapy: Prevention of sunburn is important and can be best accomplished by avoidance or photoprotection with the use of sunscreens or clothing. Direct sunburn treatment at symptom relief.

Nondrug therapy: To minimize the occurrence of sunburn, clothes should be of tightly woven, light-colored material, covering as much of the body as possible; wide-brimmed hats are also advisable. Outdoor activities should be completed before 10 am or after 3 pm to minimize the most direct and harmful exposure to UVB radiation. If sunburn occurs, pain can be relieved through the use of cool compresses. Emollients may be used to help soothe and relieve dryness. (For more information about emollients, refer to the Dry Skin monograph in the Dermatological Conditions chapter.)

Pharmacotherapy: Prevention of sunburn can be accomplished through the use of sunscreens. Sunscreens are available in 2 forms: 1) Chemical agents that absorb energy in the UVA/UVB range, and 2) physical agents that reduce the absorption of light by the skin. Chemical sunscreens absorb most UVB light but only some UVA light. While they offer the advantage of being invisible after application, they can cause adverse reactions, including a burning or stinging sensation. Chemical sunscreens are rated by their sun protection factor (SPF), a rating that is defined as the amount of time needed to produce minimal erythema from UVB light in individuals wearing sunscreen vs those not wearing sunscreen. As an example, using a product with SPF 15 would permit 15 times as much sun exposure before erythema (redness) would occur. An SPF of 15 blocks 92% of UVB radiation, while an SPF of 30 blocks 96% to 97% of UVB radiation. Scientific evidence shows a point of diminishing returns at SPF levels larger than 30; any benefits that might be derived from using sunscreens with SPFs larger than 30 are negligible. An SPF of 15 or larger for most individuals is recommended by the Skin Cancer Foundation.

Physical sunscreens reflect the UV radiation away from the skin, blocking UVA and UVB radiation. Their effectiveness is less dependent on proper application techniques, but compared with chemical sunscreens, they are usually messy to apply and are often unacceptable cosmetically. The appropriate choice of a sunscreen for a patient is dependent on skin type (ie, those more prone to burning should use a product with a higher SPF) and need for water resistance.

In May 1999, the FDA issued a final monograph on sunscreen products for OTC use. This document establishes conditions under which OTC sunscreen products are generally recognized as safe and effective, and are not misbranded. All sunscreen product ingredients included in the final monograph must have a USP monograph; there are currently 17 such ingredients (see Sunscreen Ingredients table). The final monograph sets standards for SPF values, water resistance testing, and the content and format of labeling, allowing consumers to be better informed. Key points of the final monograph are as follows:

- Labels displaying SPF values of larger than 30 will no longer be allowed. The new maximum SPF that may be displayed on labeling is "30+" or "30-plus."
- Tanning products without a sunscreen must have a prominent warning to the consumer stating that the product does not protect against sunburn.
- The claim "waterproof" is no longer allowed. The new terminology is "water/sweat resistant" (defined as providing protection for 40 minutes of exposure to moisture) or "very water/sweat resistant" (defined as providing protection for 80 minutes of exposure to moisture).
- SPF values are determined after water resistance testing has been conducted.
- The terminology for the amount of protection offered has been standardized to "minimum" for SPF values of 2 to 12, "moderate" for SPF values of 12 to 30, and "high" for SPF values of 30 or higher. The term "sunblock" is no longer allowed.

All products intended for use as sunscreens have the same labeling requirements. These changes must be in place by December 2002.

Sunscreen Ingredients	
Ingredient	UV spectrum (nm)
Benzophenones	**UVA and UVB**
Oxybenzone	270-350
Dioxybenzone	260-380[1]
Sulisobenzone	260-375
PABA and PABA esters	**UVB**
p-aminobenzoic acid	260-313
Padimate O (octyl dimethyl PABA)	290-315
Cinnamates	**UVB[2]**
Cinoxate	270-328
Octocrylene	250-360
Octyl methoxycinnamate	290-320
Salicylates	**UVB[3]**
Homosalate	295-315
Octyl salicylate	260-320
Trolamine salicylate	260-320
Miscellaneous	**UVB**
Menthyl anthranilate	260-380[4]
Avobenzone (butyl-methoxy-dibenzoylmethane; Parsol 1789)	320-400[5]
Phenylbenzimidazole sulfonic acid	290-340
Titanium dioxide	290-700
Red petrolatum	290-365
Zinc oxide	290-700

Chemical is a vertical label spanning the first set of rows (Benzophenones through Phenylbenzimidazole sulfonic acid). *Physical* is a vertical label spanning Titanium dioxide, Red petrolatum, and Zinc oxide.

[1] Values available when used in combination with other screens.
[2] Some UVA spectrum.
[3] Primarily UVB, but has ≈ 1/3 the absorbency of PABA.
[4] Values are for concentrations higher than normally found in nonprescription drugs.
[5] Exclusively UVA absorption.

Treatment options for a sunburn involve the use of oral analgesic agents and
topical local anesthetic agents to help relieve pain and discomfort. Emollients and moisturizers may help soothe dryness. (For further information on
oral analgesics and emollients/moisturizers, refer to the Aches and Pains
monograph in the CNS Conditions chapter and the Dry Skin monograph in
the Dermatological Conditions chapter, respectively.) Topical steroids have
not been shown to be effective at reducing inflammation associated with sunburn. However, with a severe sunburn, oral steroids may be necessary; contact a physician promptly in these situations.

SUNSCREENS

▶ Actions

Sunscreens provide either a chemical or a physical barrier to sunlight. Chemical sunscreens act by absorbing damaging ultraviolet radiation in the UVB range and, in
some cases, a portion or all of the UVA range. After application, they diffuse into the

stratum corneum and adsorb or conjugate with various proteins. Product efficacy is determined by the depth of penetration, binding affinity for the proteins, duration of protection, and other miscellaneous factors.

Chemical agents: Benzophenones, PABA and PABA esters, cinnamates, salicylates, menthyl anthranilate, avobenzone, and phenylbenzimidazole sulfonic acid.

Physical agents: Titanium dioxide, red petrolatum, zinc oxide.

▶ Indications

For the prevention of sunburn caused by overexposure to the sun or in people with predisposing conditions.

▶ Warnings

Children: Do not use sunscreens on infants younger than 6 months years of age. Do not use products with SPFs 3 and lower on children younger than 2 years of age.

▶ Drug Interactions

Because this product is applied topically to intact skin for a short period of time, drug interactions are unlikely to occur.

▶ Adverse Reactions

Contact dermatitis may develop with PABA or its esters, benzophenones, and cinnamates. Physical sunscreens are occlusive; miliaria (heat rash) or folliculitis (inflammation of the hair follicles) may occur.

▶ Administration and Dosage

Apply liberally to all exposed areas (approximately 30 mL [2 tablespoons]) 30 minutes or longer prior to sun exposure to allow for penetration and binding to the skin. Reapply liberally after swimming or excessive sweating.

Sunscreen products include a sun protection factor (SPF) rating. This factor indicates the amount of increased resistance to sunburn the product provides relative to unprotected skin. Effective May 2001, the maximum allowable SPF on labeling is 30+ or 30-plus.

"Water resistant" or "water/sweat resistant" formulas maintain sunburn protection for 40 minutes of sweating or activity in the water. "Very water resistant" or "very water/sweat resistant" formulas maintain sunburn protection for 80 minutes of sweating or activity in the water.

SUNSCREEN PRODUCTS	
Trade name	**Doseform**
Banana Boat Baby (SPF 50), Banana Boat Maximum (SPF 50), Banana Boat Sport Block (SPF 50)	**Lotion:** Octocrylene, octyl methoxycinnamate, oxybenzone, octyl salicylate
Hawaiian Tropic Baby Faces (SPF 50)	**Lotion:** Titanium dioxide, octyl methoxycinnamate, octyl salicylate
Sol Bar Sunscreen (SPF 50)	**Lotion:** Oxybenzone, octyl methoxycinnamate, octocrylene
Coppertone Sport (SPF 48)	**Lotion:** Octyl methoxycinnamate, oxybenzone, octyl salicylate, homosalate. Jojoba oil, parabens, EDTA, aloe, tocopherol.
Hawaiian Tropic (SPF 45+)	**Lotion:** Titanium dioxide, octyl methoxycinnamate, octyl salicylate
BioSun Maximum (SPF 45)	**Lotion:** Octyl methoxycinnamate, oxybenzone, octyl salicylate, octocrylene

SUNSCREEN PRODUCTS

Trade name	Doseform
BullFrog for Babies (SPF 45)	**Lotion:** Octocrylene, octyl methoxycinnamate, benzophenone-3, titanium dioxide, menthyl anthranilate, octyl salicylate. EDTA, sunflower oil, diazolidinyl urea.
BullFrog SuperBlock (SPF 45)	**Lotion:** 10% octocrylene, 7.5% octyl methoxycinnamate, 6% oxybenzone, 5% menthyl anthranilate, 5% octyl salicylate, 4.5% titanium dioxide. EDTA, sunflower oil, diazolidinyl urea.
Coppertone All Day (SPF 45)	**Lotion:** Ethylhexyl p-methoxycinnamate, 2-ethylhexyl salicylate, oxybenzone, homosalate. Polyglyceryl-3 distearate, barium sulfate, benzyl alcohol, aloe extract, jojoba oil, parabens, EDTA, imidazolidinyl urea, tocopherol.
Coppertone Oil Free (SPF 45)	**Lotion:** Ethylhexyl p-methoxycinnamate, 2-ethylhexyl salicylate, oxybenzone, homosalate. Parabens, EDTA, diazolidinyl urea.
Coppertone Shade (SPF 45)	**Lotion:** Ethylhexyl p-methoxycinnamate, 2-ethylhexyl salicylate, oxybenzone, homosalate. Polyglyceryl-3 distearate, barium sulfate, benzyl alcohol, aloe extract, jojoba oil, parabens, EDTA, imidazolidinyl urea, phenethyl alcohol, tocopherol.
Coppertone Water Babies (SPF 45)	**Lotion:** Octyl methoxycinnamate, octyl salicylate, oxybenzone, homosalate. Parabens, EDTA, diazolidinyl urea.
Neutrogena (SPF 45)	**Lotion:** 15% homosalate, 7.5% octyl methoxycinnamate, 6% benzophenone-3, 5% octyl salicylate, 2% avobenzone. Cetyl alcohol, EDTA, parabens, tocopherol.
Coppertone Kids (SPF 40)	**Lotion:** Octyl methoxycinnamate, oxybenzone, octyl salicylate, homosalate. Polyglyceryl-3, benzyl alcohol, aloe extract, jojoba oil, parabens, EDTA, tocopherol. (Also available in Colorblock formula in purple and blue.)
	Foam: Octyl methoxycinnamate, oxybenzone, octyl salicylate, octocrylene. Polyglyceryl-3, barium sulfate, benzyl alcohol, aloe extract, jojoba oil, parabens, EDTA, tocopherol.
BullFrog Body (SPF 36)	**Gel:** 10% octocrylene, 7.5% octyl methoxycinnamate, 3% oxybenzone. Aloe vera gel, isostearyl alcohol, tocopheryl acetate.
BullFrog for Kids (SPF 36)	**Gel:** Benzophenone-3, octocrylene, octyl methoxycinnamate. Aloe, isostearyl alcohol, tocopheryl acetate.
BullFrog Quik (SPF 36)	**Gel:** 10% octocrylene, 7.5% octyl methoxycinnamate, 6% oxybenzone, 5% octyl salicylate. Aloe vera extract, SD alcohol 40, tocopheryl acetate.
	Stick: 7.5% octyl methoxycinnamate, 7% octocrylene, 6% oxybenzone, 5% octyl salicylate. Aloe extract, isostearyl alcohol, tocopheryl acetate.
BullFrog Sport (SPF 36)	**Solution:** 10% octocrylene, 7.5% octyl methoxycinnamate, 6% oxybenzone, 5% octyl salicylate. SD alcohol 40, aloe vera extract, tocopheryl acetate.

SUNSCREEN PRODUCTS

Trade name	Doseform
Elta Block (SPF 32)	**Lotion:** Octyl methoxycinnamate, octyl salicylate, zinc oxide, titanium dioxide. Petrolatum, mineral oil, glyceryl monostearate-450, parabens, diazolidinyl urea.
Banana Boat Kids (SPF 30+), Banana Boat Ultra (SPF 30+)	**Lotion:** Octyl methoxycinnamate, oxybenzone, octyl salicylate
Hawaiian Tropic (SPF 30+)	**Lotion:** Octyl methoxycinnamate, octyl salicylate, titanium dioxide
Bain De Soleil Extended Protection (SPF 30), Bain De Soleil Gentle Block (SPF 30), Bain De Soleil Kids (SPF 30)	**Lotion:** 7.5% octyl methoxycinnamate, 5% octocrylene, 2% oxybenzone, 2% titanium dioxide. Stearyl alcohol, tocopheryl acetate.
BullFrog Body (SPF 30), BullFrog Magic Block (SPF 30), BullFrog Sport (SPF 30)	**Lotion:** 10% octocrylene, 7.5% octyl methoxycinnamate, 6% oxybenzone, 5% octyl salicylate. Aloe vera gel, diazolidinyl urea, EDTA, parabens, tocopheryl acetate.
Coppertone All Day (SPF 30)	**Lotion:** Ethylhexyl p-methoxycinnamate, oxybenzone, 2-ethylhexyl salicylate, homosalate. Glyceryl stearate SE, hydrogenated vegetable oil, benzyl alcohol, parabens, imidazolidinyl urea, aloe extract, jojoba oil, EDTA, tocopherol.
Coppertone Bug & Sun (SPF 30)	**Lotion:** 9.5% N,n-diethyl-m-toluamide, octocrylene, ethylhexyl p-methoxycinnamate, oxybenzone
Coppertone to Go (SPF 30), Coppertone Sport (SPF 30)	**Solution:** Octyl methoxycinnamate, octyl salicylate, homosalate, oxybenzone. SD alcohol 40.
Coppertone Kids (SPF 30)	**Lotion:** Ethylhexyl p-methoxycinnamate, oxybenzone, 2-ethylhexyl salicylate, homosalate. Polyglyceryl-3, barium sulfate, benzyl alcohol, aloe extract, jojoba oil, parabens, EDTA, imidazolidinyl urea, tocopherol. (Also available in Colorblock formula in purple and blue.)
	Stick: Ethylhexyl p-methoxycinnamate, oxybenzone, 2-ethylhexyl salicylate, homosalate. Talc, propylparaben.
Coppertone Kids Spray 'n Splash (SPF 30)	**Lotion:** Ethylhexyl p-methoxycinnamate, oxybenzone, 2-ethylhexyl salicylate, homosalate. Parabens, EDTA, diazolidinyl urea.
Coppertone Shade (SPF 30)	**Gel:** Ethylhexyl p-methoxycinnamate, oxybenzone, homosalate. SD alcohol 40.
	Solution: Octyl methoxycinnamate, octyl salicylate, homosalate, oxybenzone, avobenzone. SD alcohol 40.
	Stick: Ethylhexyl p-methoxycinnamate, oxybenzone, 2-ethylhexyl salicylate, homosalate
Coppertone Oil Free (SPF 30)	**Lotion:** Homosalate, ethylhexyl p-methoxycinnamate, oxybenzone, 2-ethylhexyl salicylate. Glycerol stearate, cetyl alcohol, methylparaben, EDTA, diazolidinyl urea.
Coppertone Sport (SPF 30)	**Lotion:** Octyl methoxycinnamate, oxybenzone, homosalate, octyl salicylate. Diazolidinyl urea, jojoba oil, parabens, EDTA, aloe extract, tocopherol.
	Stick: Octyl methoxycinnamate, oxybenzone, homosalate, octyl salicylate. Talc, propylparaben.

SUNSCREEN PRODUCTS

Trade name	Doseform
Coppertone Water Babies (SPF 30)	**Lotion**: Octyl methoxycinnamate, oxybenzone, octyl salicylate, homosalate. Glyceryl stearate SE, hydrogenated vegetable oil, benzyl alcohol, parabens, tocopherol, imidazolidinyl urea, EDTA.
	Solution: Octyl methoxycinnamate, oxybenzone, octyl salicylate, homosalate. Diazolidinyl urea, parabens, EDTA.
DuraScreen (SPF 30)	**Lotion**: Octyl methoxycinnamate, octyl salicylate, benzophenone-3, phenylbenzidmidazole sulfonic acid, titanium dioxide. Cetearyl alcohol, diazolidinyl urea, parabens.
Fisher-Price Sunscreen for Kids (SPF 30)	**Lotion**: 7.5% octyl methoxycinnamate, 5% octyl salicylate, 3% avobenzone, 3% oxybenzone. Cetyl alcohol, benzyl alcohol, EDTA.
Kiss My Face Sun Block (SPF 30)	**Lotion**: Titanium dioxide, octyl methoxycinnamate. Aloe vera gel, polyglycerol 4 isostearate, hexyl laurate, oat protein complex, soybean oil, diazolidinyl urea, parabens, glycerine, oat beta glucan, coconut oil.
	Solution: Octyl methoxycinnamate, octyl salicylate, benzophenone-3. Palm oil, propylparaben.
Neutrogena Oil-Free (SPF 30)	**Lotion**: 15% homosalate, 7.5% octyl methoxycinnamate, 6% benzophenone-3, 5% octyl salicylate. Isocethyl alcohol, tocopheryl acetate, parabens, diazolidinyl urea, EDTA.
Neutrogena (SPF 30)	**Lotion**: 7.5% octyl methoxycinnamate, 6.5% homosalate, 5% octyl salicylate, 3% benzophenone-3, 2% avobenzone. Cetyl alcohol, tocopheryl acetate, oat extract, EDTA, parabens.
Neutrogena Transparent (SPF 30)	**Gel**: 7.5% octyl methoxycinnamate, 5% homosalate, 5% octyl salicylate, 3% benzophenone-3. SD alcohol 40, tocopheryl acetate.
PreSun Ultra (SPF 30)	**Cream**: 7.5% octyl methoxycinnamate, 5% octyl salicylate, 3% avobenzone, 3% oxybenzone. Cetyl alcohol, benzyl alcohol, EDTA.
	Gel: 7.5% octyl methoxycinnamate, 6% oxybenzone, 5% octyl salicylate, 3% avobenzone. SD alcohol 40.
Shade UVA Guard (SPF 30)	**Lotion**: Ethylhexyl p-methoxycinnamate, oxybenzone, 2-ethylhexyl salicylate, homosalate, avobenzone. Polyglyceryl-3 distearate, barium sulfate, benzyl alcohol, parabens, aloe extract, jojoba oil, tocopherol, phenethyl alcohol, EDTA.
Sol Bar PF (SPF 30)	**Liquid**: Octocrylene. Oxybenzone, octyl methoxycinnamate, SD alcohol 40.
TI•Screen (SPF 30)	**Lotion**: 7.5% octocrylene, 7.5% octyl methoxycinnamate, 6% benzophenone-3, 5% octyl salicylate, 2% avobenzone. Cetyl alcohol, tocopherol acetate, 99% triethanolamine, phenethyl alcohol, parabens, EDTA.
Fisher-Price Sensitive Skin Sunblock for Kids (SPF 28), PreSun Sensitive (SPF 28)	**Cream**: 16% titanium dioxide. C12-15 alcohols benzoate, benzyl alcohol, diazolidinyl urea, magnesium sulfate, polyglyceryl-4.

SUNSCREEN PRODUCTS

Trade name	Doseform
Fisher-Price Spray Mist Sunscreen for Kids (SPF 27), PreSun Ultra (SPF 27)	**Solution:** 7.5% octyl methoxycinnamate, 6% oxybenzone, 5% octyl salicylate, 3% avobenzone. SD alcohol 40.
Banana Boat Action Sport (SPF 25)	**Gel:** Octyl methoxycinnamate, octyl salicylate, homosalate, oxybenzone
BioSun Faces (SPF 25)	**Lotion:** Octyl methoxycinnamate, oxybenzone, octyl salicylate
Neutrogena Sunblock Stick (SPF 25)	**Stick:** Benzophenone-3, octyl methoxycinnamate, octyl salicylate. Castor oil, cetearyl alcohol, sodium cetearyl sulfate, sodium sulfate, propylparaben.
RV Paque (SPF 24)	**Lotion:** Red petrolatum, zinc oxide, cinoxate
Banana Boat Faces Plus (SPF 23)	**Lotion:** Octyl methoxycinnamate, oxybenzone, octyl salicylate. Aloe vera extract.
TI•Screen (SPF 23)	**Solution:** 7.5% octyl methoxycinnamate, 4% octocrylene, 3.5% menthyl anthranilate, 3% benzophenone-3. SD alcohol 40, tocopheryl acetate.
Neutrogena Oil-Free (SPF 20)	**Solution:** 12% homosalate, 7.5% octyl methoxycinnamate, 5% octyl salicylate, 4.5% menthyl anthranilate
TI•Screen Sports (SPF 20)	**Gel:** 7.5% octyl methoxycinnamte, 6% benzophenone-3, 5% octyl salicylate, avobenzone 2%. SD alcohol 40B.
BullFrog Quik (SPF 18)	**Gel:** Benzophenone-3, octyl methoxycinnamate, octyl salicylate. Aloe extract oil, SD alcohol 40, tocopheryl acetate.
Kiss My Face Non-Chemical Sun Block (SPF 18)	**Lotion:** Titanium dioxide. Aloe vera gel, polyglycerol-4 isostearate, hexyl laurate, oat protein complex, soybean oil, diazolidinyl urea, parabens, glycerine, oat beta glucan, coconut oil.
Neutrogena Sensitive Skin (SPF 17)	**Lotion:** Titanium dioxide. Parabens, diazolidinyl urea, polyglyceryl-4 isostearate.
TI•Baby Natural (SPF 16), TI•Screen Natural (SPF 16)	**Lotion:** Titanium dioxide
Hawaiian Tropic (SPF 15+)	**Lotion:** Octyl methoxycinnamate, octyl salicylate, titanium dioxide
Abuval Sport (SPF 15)	**Lotion:** Octyl methoxycinnamate, oxybenzone, octyl salicylate. SD alcohol 40.
Bain de Soleil All Day Extended Protection (SPF 15), Bain de Soleil Mademoiselle (SPF 15)	**Lotion:** 7.5% octyl methoxycinnamate, 4% octocrylen, 2% titanium dioxide, 1% oxybenzone. Stearyl alcohol, tocopheryl acetate.
Bain de Soleil Orange Gelée (SPF 15)	**Lotion:** 5% octyl methoxycinnamate, 4% octocrylen, 3% octyl salicylate, 2% oxybenzone. Aloe, parabens, glycerides, lanolin, mineral oils, palm oil, petrolatums, tocopheryl acetate.
Banana Boat Sport (SPF 15)	**Lotion:** Octyl methoxycinnamate, oxybenzone, octyl salicylate
Coppertone All Day (SPF 15)	**Lotion:** Ethylhexyl p-methoxycinnamate, oxybenzone. Glyceryl stearate SE, hydrogenated vegetable oil, benzyl alcohol, parabens, imidazolidinyl urea, tocopherol, aloe extract, jojoba oil, EDTA.
Coppertone Bug & Sun (SPF 15)	**Lotion:** 9.5% N,n-diethyl-m-toluamide, ethylhexyl p-methoxycinnamate, oxybenzone, 2-ethylhexyl salicylate, homosalate

SUNSCREEN PRODUCTS

Trade name	Doseform
Coppertone to Go (SPF 15), Coppertone Sport (SPF 15)	**Solution**: Octyl methoxycinnamate, octyl salicylate, homosalate, oxybenzone. SD alcohol 40.
Coppertone Oil Free (SPF 15)	**Lotion**: Ethylhexyl p-methoxycinnamate, oxybenzone. Aloe extract, tocopheryl acetate, diazolidinyl urea, parabens, EDTA.
Coppertone Sport (SPF 15)	**Lotion**: Octyl methoxycinnamate, oxybenzone, octyl salicylate. Diazolidinyl urea, parabens, aloe, jojoba oil, EDTA, tocopherol.
Coppertone Sunblock (SPF 15)	**Lotion**: Octyl methoxycinnamate, oxybenzone. Glyceryl stearate SE, hydrogenated palm kernel oil, benzyl alcohol, parabens, aloe, jojoba oil, tocopherol, imidazolidinyl urea, EDTA.
DuraScreen (SPF 15)	**Lotion**: Octyl methoxycinnamate, octyl salicylate, benzophenone-3, titanium dioxide. Cetyl alcohol, chamomile oil, stearyl alcohol, parabens, imidazolidinyl urea.
Hawaiian Tropic Super Waterproof (SPF 15)	**Lotion**: Octyl methoxycinnamate, octyl salicylate, titanium dioxide
Neutrogena Moisturizer (SPF 15)	**Lotion**: 7.5% octyl methoxycinnamate, 5% octyl salicylate, 3% benzophenone-3. Glycerin, glyceryl stearate, diazolidinyl urea, parabens.
Neutrogena (SPF 15)	**Lotion**: 7.5% octyl methoxycinnamate, 3% benzalkonium chloride. Cetyl alcohol, oat extract, tocopheryl acetate, EDTA, parabens, diazolidinyl urea.
PreSun Ultra (SPF 15)	**Cream**: 6% oxybenzone, 5% octyl methoxycinnamate, 5% octyl salicylate, 3% avobenzone. Cetyl alcohol, benzyl alcohol, EDTA.
	Gel: 6% oxybenzone, 5% octyl methoxycinnamate, 5% octyl salicylate, 3% avobenzone. SD alcohol 40.
Ray Block Sunscreen (SPF 15)	**Lotion**: 5% octyl dimethyl PABA, 3% benzophenone-3. SD alcohol.
TI•Screen (SPF 15)	**Lotion**: 7.5% octyl methoxycinnamate, 5% benzophenone-3. Glyceryl monostearate, hybrid safflower oil, stearyl alcohol, cetyl alcohol, parabens.
Bain De Soleil Mademoiselle (SPF 8)	**Lotion**: 7.5% octyl methoxycinnamate, 4% octocrylene, 2% titanium dioxide. Stearyl alcohol, tocopheryl acetate.
Bain De Soleil Orange Gelée (SPF 8)	**Lotion**: 4% octyl methoxycinnamate, 3% octocrylene, 3% octyl salicylate, 1% oxybenzone. Aloe, parabens, hydroxylated milk glycerides, lanolin, mineral oils, palm oil, petrolatums, tocopheryl acetate.
Bain De Soleil Tanning Mist (SPF 8)	**Solution**: 5% octyl methoxycinnamate, 3%, octocrylene, 1% oxybenzone. SD alcohol 3-C, aloe, parabens, lanolin, palm kernel oil, tocopheryl acetate.
Coppertone All Day (SPF 8)	**Lotion**: Ethylhexyl p-methoxycinnamate, oxybenzone. Glyceryl stearate SE, benzyl alcohol, parabens, aloe extract, tocopheryl acetate, jojoba oil, EDTA.
Coppertone Oil Free (SPF 8)	**Lotion**: Ethylhexyl p-methoxycinnamate, oxybenzone. Tocopheryl acetate, aloe extract, diazolidinyl urea, parabens, EDTA.

SUNSCREEN PRODUCTS

Trade name	Doseform
Coppertone Sport (SPF 8)	**Lotion**: Octyl methoxycinnamate, oxybenzone. Diazolidinyl urea, parabens, aloe, jojoba oil, tocopherol, EDTA.
Panama Jack Sunscreen (SPF 8)	**Lotion**: Ethylhexyl p-methoxycinnamate, 2-ethylhexyl salicylate
Hawaiian Tropic Golden Tanning (SPF 6)	**Lotion**: Octyl methoxycinnamate, octyl salicylate
Bain De Soleil Mega Tan (SPF 4)	**Lotion**: 3.5% octyl methoxycinnamate, 1% octocrylene. Aloe, cetyl alcohol, eucalyptus oil, lanolin, mineral oil, palm oil.
Bain De Soleil Orange Gelée (SPF 4)	**Lotion**: 2.5% octyl methoxycinnamate, 0.5% octyl salicylate. Parabens, mineral oils, petrolatums.
Bain De Soleil Tanning Mist (SPF 4)	**Solution**: 3% octyl methoxycinnamate, 2% octocrylene. SD alcohol 3-C, aloe, parabens, lanolin, palm kernel oil, tocopheryl acetate.
Bain De Soleil Tropical Deluxe (SPF 4)	**Lotion**: 3% octyl methoxycinnamate, 0.5% octyl salicylate. Aloe, cetyl alcohol, eucalyptus oil, lanolin, mineral oils, palm oil.
Banana Boat Dark Tanning (SPF 4)	**Lotion**: Padimate O
	Oil: Padimate O, octyl methoxycinnamate. Aloe, tocopheryl acetate.
Coppertone Gold (SPF 4)	**Oil**: Homosalate, oxybenzone. Mineral oil, aloe extract, tocopheryl acetate, propylparaben.
Coppertone Sunscreen (SPF 4)	**Lotion**: Octyl methoxycinnamate, oxybenzone. Glyceryl stearate SE, benzyl alcohol, parabens, aloe, jojoba oil, tocopherol, EDTA.
Hawaiian Tropic Dark Tanning (SPF 4)	**Lotion**: Ethylhexyl p-methoxycinnamate, 2-ethylhexyl salicylate, menthyl anthranilate
Panama Jack Dark Tanning (SPF 4)	**Lotion**: Octyl methoxycinnamate
	Oil: Octyl dimethyl PABA. Mineral oil, peanut oil, aloe extract, olive oil, sweet almond oil, propylparaben.
Banana Boat Dark Tanning (SPF 2)	**Oil**: Padimate O, octyl methoxycinnamate
Coppertone Gold (SPF 2)	**Oil**: Homosalate. Mineral oil, aloe, tocopherol.
Coppertone Gold Tan Magnifier (SPF 2)	**Oil**: Triethanolamine salicylate. Glycerin, lanolin oil, macadamia nut oil, olive oil, sweet almond oil, aloe extract, jojoba oil, tocopheryl acetate, coconut oil, diazolidinyl urea, parabens.
Lip Balms	
Hawaiian Tropic 45 Plus (SPF 45+)	**Lip balm**: Octocrylene, octyl methoxycinnamate, octyl salicylate, homosalate
Blistex Ultra Protection (SPF 30)	**Lip balm**: 7.4% octyl methoxycinnamate, 5.2% oxybenzone, 5% octyl salicylate, 4.8% menthyl anthranilate, 4.5% homosalate, 3% dimethicone. Parabens, tocopheryl linoleate.
ChapStick Ultra (SPF 30)	**Lip balm**: 30% white petrolatum, 7.5% octyl methoxycinnamate, 7% octocrylene, 5% octyl salicylate, 5% oxybenzone. Aloe extract, cetyl alcohol, parabens, modified lanolin, oleyl alcohol, tocopherol.
Coppertone Little Licks (SPF 30)	**Lip balm**: Ethylhexyl p-methoxycinnamate, oxybenzone, 2-ethylhexyl salicylate. Talc, propylparaben, aloe extract, tocopheryl acetate.

SUNSCREEN PRODUCTS

Trade name	Doseform
Blistex DCT (SPF 20)	**Lip balm**: 7.3% octyl methoxycinnamate, 4.5% oxybenzone, petrolatum. Tocopherol, aloe extract, lanolin.
ChapStick Flava-Craze (SPF 15)	**Lip balm**: 38.7% white petrolatum, 7.5% octyl methoxycinnamate, 3.5% oxybenzone. Cetyl alcohol, parabens, lanolin, light mineral oil.
Coppertone Aloe and Vitamin E (SPF 15)	**Lip balm**: Ethylhexyl p-methoxycinnamate, oxybenzone. Hydrogenated vegetable oil, petrolatum, propylparaben, aloe, extract, tocopheryl acetate.
Coppertone Natural Fruit (SPF 15)	**Lip balm**: Ethylhexyl p-methoxycinnamate, oxybenzone. Hydrogenated vegetable oil, petrolatum, propylparaben.
TI•Screen (SPF 15)	**Lip balm**: 7.5% octyl methoxycinnamate, 5% oxybenzone. Petrolatum.
Blistex Regular (SPF 10)	**Lip balm**: 6.6% padimate O, 2.5% oxybenzone, 2% dimethicone. Lanolin, parabens, mineral oil, petrolatum.

Products listed are representative of currently available and widely distributed brands. Similar products, including regional and private label brands, may also exist.

PATIENT INFORMATION
Sunscreens
- Follow directions on product container concerning frequency of application; reapply after swimming or sweating. Reapplication does not extend the protection period.
- For external use only. Avoid contact with the eyes. Do not swallow.
- If irritation or rash occurs, discontinue use and wash remaining product off the skin.
- PABA may permanently stain clothing yellow.
- Wear protective eye coverings or sunglasses; UV light can cause corneal damage.
- Do not use on infants younger than 6 months of age. For children younger than 2 years of age, do not use sunscreens with SPFs 3 or lower.
- Keep out of reach of children. In case of accidental ingestion, seek professional assistance or contact a poision control center immediately.

LOCAL ANESTHETICS, TOPICAL
► **Actions**

Local anesthetics inhibit conduction of nerve impulses from sensory nerves. They are poorly absorbed through intact epidermis.

► **Indications**

For topical anesthesia in many different local skin disorders including pain caused by sunburn.

► **Contraindications**

Hypersensitivity to any component of these products; ophthalmic use.

► **Warnings**

Pregnancy: Category B (lidocaine); *Category C* (benzocaine).

Lactation: Lidocaine, and probably prilocaine, are excreted in breast milk. Exercise caution when administering any of these drugs to a nursing woman.

Children: Do not use benzocaine on infants younger than 1 year of age. Reduce dosages in children commensurate with age, body weight, and physical condition.

► **Drug Interactions**

Use with caution in patients receiving Class I antiarrhythmic drugs because the toxic effects are additive and potentially synergistic.

► **Adverse Reactions**

Adverse reactions are, in general, dose-related and may result from high plasma levels caused by excessive dosage or rapid absorption, hypersensitivity, idiosyncrasy, or diminished tolerance. Patients may have hypersensitivity reactions (urticaria, edema, contact dermatitis) or local reactions (burning, stinging, tenderness).

► **Administration and Dosage**

Apply to affected area as needed. Ointments and creams may be applied to gauze or to a bandage prior to applying to the skin.

BENZOCAINE

BENZOCAINE PRODUCTS	
Trade name	Doseform
Dermoplast	**Solution**: 20%. 0.5% menthol, methylparaben, aloe vera oil, acetylated lanolin alcohol.
Foille Plus	**Solution**: 20%. 0.15% benzethonium chloride, benzyl alcohol, SD alcohol 40.
Lanacane	**Solution**: 20%. 0.1% benzethonium chloride, 36% ethanol, aloe extract.
Solarcaine	**Solution**: 20%. 0.13% triclosan, SD alcohol 40, tocopheryl acetate.
Americaine	**Suspension**: 20%
Lanacane	**Cream**: 6%. 0.1% benzethonium chloride, aloe, parabens, sulfated castor oil, glycerin, glyceryl stearate SE, isopropyl alcohol.
Foille Medicated First Aid	**Ointment**: 5%. 0.1% chloroxylenol, benzyl alcohol, calcium. EDTA, corn oil.
Benzocaine	**Cream**: 5%
Foille Medicated First Aid	**Suspension**: 5%. 0.6% chloroxylenol, benzyl alcohol, corn oil.

Products listed are representative of currently available and widely distributed brands. Similar products, including regional and private label brands, may also exist.

DIBUCAINE

DIBUCAINE PRODUCTS	
Trade name	Doseform
Dibucaine	**Ointment**: 1%. Lanolin, white petrolatum, acetone sodium bisulfite.
Nupercainal	**Ointment**: 1%. Acetone sodium bisulfite, lanolin, light mineral oil, white petrolatum.

Products listed are representative of currently available and widely distributed brands. Similar products, including regional and private label brands, may also exist.

LIDOCAINE

LIDOCAINE PRODUCTS	
Trade name	**Doseform**
Xylocaine	**Ointment**: 2.5%
Solarcaine Aloe Extra Burn Relief	**Suspension**: 0.5%. Aloe vera, tocopherol, urea, parabens, EDTA.
	Gel: 0.5%. Aloe vera gel, glycerin, 0.06% isopropyl alcohol, diazolidinyl urea, menthol, EDTA.

Products listed are representative of currently available and widely distributed brands. Similar products, including regional and private label brands, may also exist.

BUTAMBEN PICRATE

BUTAMBEN PICRATE PRODUCTS	
Trade name	**Doseform**
Butesin Picrate	**Ointment**: 1%. Anhydrous lanolin, parabens, mineral oil.

Products listed are representative of currently available and widely distributed brands. Similar products, including regional and private label brands, may also exist.

PRAMOXINE HCL

PRAMOXINE HCL PRODUCTS	
Trade name	**Doseform**
Tronothane HCl	**Cream**: 1%. Cetyl alcohol, glycerin, sodium lauryl sulfate, parabens.
Prax	**Lotion**: 1%. Mineral oil, lanolin, cetyl alcohol, glycerin, 0.1% potassium sorbate, 0.1% sorbic acid.
Itch-X	**Solution**: 1%. Benzyl alcohol, aloe vera gel, SD alcohol 40.
	Gel: 1%. Benzyl alcohol, aloe vera gel, diazolidinyl urea, parabens, SD alcohol 40.

Products listed are representative of currently available and widely distributed brands. Similar products, including regional and private label brands, may also exist.

LOCAL ANESTHETIC COMBINATIONS, TOPICAL

TOPICAL LOCAL ANESTHETIC PRODUCTS	
Trade name	**Doseform**
Bactine First Aid	**Liquid**: 0.13% benzalkonium chloride, 2.5% lidocaine HCl
Dermacoat	**Solution**: 4.5% benzocaine, p-chloro-m-xylenol, menthol, isopropyl alcohol.
Solarcaine	**Lotion**: Benzocaine, triclosan. Mineral oil, stearyl alcohol, cetyl alcohol, benzyl alcohol, aloe extract, tocopheryl acetate, menthol, camphor, parabens, EDTA.
	Solution: 20% benzocaine, 0.13% triclosan. SD alcohol 40, tocopheryl acetate.

Products listed are representative of currently available and widely distributed brands. Similar products, including regional and private label brands, may also exist.

PATIENT INFORMATION
Local Anesthetics, Topical

- For external use only. Do not use in the eyes.
- Ointments are more greasy; creams may be preferred in some cases.
- Not intended for prolonged use.
- Some of these products contain tartrazine or sulfites, which can cause allergic-type reactions in susceptible individuals.
- Use the lowest dose needed for relief of symptoms to avoid excessive absorption into the blood and serious adverse effects.
- May not be appropriate for use on children younger than 2 years of age; refer to the product label.
- Keep out of reach of children. In case of accidental ingestion, seek professional assistance or contact a poision control center immediately.

VITAMINS A, D, AND E, TOPICAL

▶ Indications

For temporary relief of discomfort caused by sunburn and other minor dermal conditions.

▶ Administration and Dosage

Apply locally to affected skin with gentle massage.

TOPICAL VITAMINS A, D, AND E PREPARATIONS	
Trade name	**Doseform**
A and D	**Ointment**: 1% dimethicone, 10% zinc oxide. Aloe extract, benzyl alcohol, cod liver oil containing vitamins A and D, glyceryl oleate, light mineral oil.
Lazer Creme	**Cream**: Vitamin A (3333.3 units/g) and E (116.67 units/g), parabens, diazolidinyl urea
Lobana Derm-Ade	**Cream**: Vitamins A (1500 units/g) , D, and E, silicone, lanolin oil, glycerin, stearyl alcohol, cetyl alcohol, parabens

Products listed are representative of currently available and widely distributed brands. Similar products, including regional and private label brands, may also exist.

PATIENT INFORMATION
Vitamins A, D, and E, Topical

- For external use only; avoid contact with the eyes.
- If the condition worsens or does not improve within 7 days, consult a physician.

VITAMIN E

VITAMIN E PRODUCTS	
Trade name	**Doseform**
Vitamin E	**Oil**: 100% concentrate
Vitec	**Lotion**: dl-alpha tocopheryl acetate, cetearyl alcohol, sorbitol, propylene glycol, simethicone, glyceryl monostearate

Products listed are representative of currently available and widely distributed brands. Similar products, including regional and private label brands, may also exist.

PATIENT INFORMATION
Vitamin E
- Do not use in the eyes or allow to come in contact with the eye(s) or eyelid(s).
- Do not use if you are allergic to any ingredient of the products.
- Do not use on irritated or broken skin without consulting a pharmacist or physician.
- If the condition for which these preparations is used persists or worsens, or if irritation develops, discontinue use and consult a physician.
- Do not apply over deep or puncture wounds, infections, or lacerations.
- Stinging, burning, itching, or irritation may develop with the use of these products.

TOPICAL ANTIHISTAMINE-CONTAINING PRODUCTS

▶ Actions
Topical antihistamines are used for their anesthetic effects and to relieve itching.

▶ Indications
Temporary relief of itching due to minor skin disorders, including poison ivy, sumac, or oak; sunburn; and insect bites and stings.

▶ Warnings
Do not apply to blistered, raw, or oozing areas of the skin or around the eyes or other mucous membranes (eg, nose, mouth).

▶ Administration and Dosage
Apply as needed and according to package directions to control symptoms.

TOPICAL ANTIHISTAMINE-CONTAINING PRODUCTS	
Trade name	**Doseform**
Benadryl Extra Strength Itch Relief	**Stick**: 2% diphenhydramine HCl, 0.1% zinc acetate. Alcohol, glycerin.
Benadryl Extra Strength Itch Stopping	**Cream**: 2% diphenhydramine HCl, 0.1% zinc acetate. Cetyl alcohol, diazolidinyl urea, parabens.
	Gel: 2% diphenhydramine HCl. SD alcohol 38B, diazolidinyl urea, glycerin, parabens.
	Solution: 2% diphenhydramine HCl, 0.1% zinc acetate. Alcohol, glycerin.
Benadryl Original Strength Itch Stopping	**Cream**: 1% diphenhydramine HCl, 0.1% zinc acetate. Cetyl alcohol, diazolidinyl urea, parabens.
	Gel: 1% diphenhydramine HCl. SD alcohol 38B, diazolidinyl urea, glycerin, parabens.
	Solution: 1% diphenhydramine HCl, 0.1% zinc acetate. Alcohol, glycerin.
Caladryl	**Lotion**: 8% calamine, 1% pramoxine HCl. SD alcohol 38B, diazolidinyl urea, parabens.
Caladryl Clear	**Lotion**: 1% pramoxine HCl, 0.1% zinc acetate. SD alcohol 38B, diazolidinyl urea, glycerin, parabens.
Caladryl for Kids	**Cream**: 8% calamine, 1% pramoxine HCl. Cetyl alcohol, diazolidinyl urea, parabens.
Cala-gen	**Lotion**: 8% calamine, 1% pramoxine HCl. SD alcohol 38B, diazolidinyl urea, parabens.

TOPICAL ANTIHISTAMINE-CONTAINING PRODUCTS

Trade name	Doseform
CalaGel	**Gel**: 1.8% diphenhydramine HCl, 0.21% zinc acetate, 0.15% benzethonium chloride. EDTA, sodium metabisulfite, menthol.
Calamycin	**Lotion**: 5% zinc oxide, 5% benzocaine, 2% diphenhydramine HCl. Calamine, isopropyl alcohol.
Calamycin Cool & Clear	**Solution**: 1% pramoxine HCl, 0.1% zinc acetate. Aloe vera gel, SDA alcohol.
Dermamycin	**Cream**: 2% diphenhydramine HCl. Cetyl alcohol, methylparaben.
	Solution: 2% diphenhydramine HCl, 1% menthol. Methylparaben, SDA alcohol.
Dermarest	**Gel**: 2% diphenhydramine HCl, 2% resorcinol. Aloe vera gel, menthol, methylparaben.
Di-Delamine	**Gel**: 1% diphenhydramine HCl, 0.5% tripelennamine HCl, 0.12% benzalkonium chloride. Menthol.
Soothaderm	**Lotion**: 4.14% zinc oxide, 0.21% benzocaine, 0.21% pyrilamine maleate. Silicone oil, simethicone, parabens, propylene glycol, camphor, menthol, wysteria oil, apple blossom oil, isopropyl alcohol.

Products listed are representative of currently available and widely distributed brands. Similar products, including regional and private label brands, may also exist.

PATIENT INFORMATION

Topical Antihistamine-Containing Products

- For external use only. Avoid contact with the eyes.
- If condition persists, recurs after a few days, or if irritation develops, discontinue use.
- Avoid prolonged use (longer than 7 days) or use on extensive skin areas.
- Do not apply to blistered, raw, or oozing areas of the skin or around the eyes or other mucous membranes (eg, nose, mouth).
- May not be appropriate for use on children younger than 2 years of age; refer to the product label.
- Keep out of reach of children. In case of accidental ingestion, seek professional assistance or contact a poision control center immediately.

TINEA CAPITIS
(Ringworm of the Scalp)

DEFINITION

Tinea capitis is a superficial dermatophyte fungal infection of the scalp with invasion of hair shafts. The acute infection is characterized by follicular inflammation with painful, boggy nodules that sometimes drain pus and, on rare occasions, can cause a scarring alopecia (hair loss). The subacute and chronic infection is characterized by the presence of scaling patches and plaques.

ETIOLOGY

Dermatophytes are fungi composed of three groups of organisms: *Microsporum*, *Trichophyton*, and *Epidermophyton*. Only *Microsporum* and *Trichophyton* species invade hair and cause tinea capitis.

Microsporum species produce small- and large-spored hair infection, meaning the organism grows on the outside as well as within the hair shaft. The most common *Microsporum* species that causes tinea capitis is *M. canis* (Europe and the US); *M. audouinii* (West Africa) is less common.

Trichophyton species can cause a large-spored external infection and an internal infection of the hair follicle. The most common species include *T. tonsurans* (in the US); *T. violaceum* and *T. schoenleinii* are less common.

INCIDENCE

True incidence rates for tinea capitis are unknown, but estimates range from 5% to 20% of population at risk. This population primarily consists of children four to 14 years of age. Tinea capitis is caused by *T. tonsurans* in 90% of cases in the US. Blacks and Hispanics are more commonly infected by *T. tonsurans*, whereas whites are infected more commonly by *Microsporum* species.

PATHOPHYSIOLOGY

The fungi spores that cause tinea capitis can come from animal-to-human contact (zoophilic), human-to-human contact (anthropophilic), or soil-to-human contact (geophilic—a rare cause of tinea capitis). The contact may occur from use of a contaminated inanimate object (eg, a comb, cap, hat, scarf, barrette, headband, earphones, pillow). Spores are trapped by scalp hairs with subsequent infection beginning in the perifollicular stratum corneum. Following incubation, fungal filaments known as hyphae (a branching cell characteristic of filamentous fungi growth) generally spread into and around the hair shaft and descend into the follicle (see Figure 1). The hyphae then can penetrate the midportion of the hair and descend within the internal portion of the hair. There, they proliferate and divide into arthrospores, which can remain within the hair shaft (endothrix) or penetrate the cortex of the hair onto its surface (ectothrix).

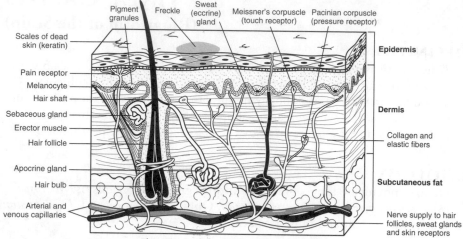

Figure 1. Layers of Skin with Hair Follicle

SIGNS/SYMPTOMS

Clinically, patients may have only a few symptoms with localized lesions or they may experience extensive, inflamed lesions. Tinea capitis can be divided into four types of infection:

"Gray patch" ringworm: Round patches of hair loss with brittle hair. The hair shaft breaks off close to the scalp surface. Scaling also may be present (*M. audouinii, M. canis*).

"Black dot" ringworm: More diffuse, poorly circumscribed areas of hair loss. The hair shaft breaks off at the level of the scalp. The hair left behind in the infected follicle appears as a black dot on clinical exam. The appearance can be variable with diffuse scaling; minimal hair loss is a possibility. The degree of inflammation also is variable (*T. tonsurans, T. violaceum*).

"Kerion": Boggy, elevated, purulent, inflamed nodules and plaques that are painful and drain pus. Hairs fall out or can be pulled out easily but do not break off. Healing often occurs with scarring alopecia (hair loss). Kerions develop in approximately 10% of cases.

"Favus": Severe, chronic ringworm, with yellowish adherent crusts on the scalp (scutula). The borders of the infected lesions represent areas of advancing disease and are often polycyclic in shape. The center of the infected area becomes atrophic, scarred, and nearly devoid of hair. Favus also may involve glabrous (nonhair-bearing) skin and nails (*T. schoenleinii*).

Associated systemic findings may include regional lymphadenopathy, particularly posterior occipital and cervical nodes in tinea capitis of long duration.

DIAGNOSTIC PARAMETERS/PHYSICAL ASSESSMENT

Clinical Observation: Refer any child who presents with scaling or areas of hair loss to a physician for evaluation of tinea capitis. Because the scalp symptoms are similar to alopecia areata, psoriasis, seborrheic dermatitis, or a bacterial infection, the diagnosis of tinea should be confirmed. Examination of scalp with a Wood lamp may show bright green fluorescence of hair shafts if the infection is caused by *M. audouinii*, *M. canis*, or *T. schoenleinii* (*T. tonsurans*, the most common cause of tinea capitis in the US, does not fluoresce). Microscopic examination of broken hairs scraped from the scalp and stained with 10% potassium hydrochloride may show hyphae. Fungal culture of hairs in the involved area requires a few weeks to grow and would confirm the diagnosis of tinea capitis.

Interview: Tinea capitis usually is transmitted by human-to-human contact, and localized epidemics are common in classrooms or group environments. If a patient is suspected of having tinea capitis, it may be useful to determine:

- Recent diagnosis of tinea capitis in a classmate, playmate, or family member
- Contact by the patient with a new cat or dog
- Recent borrowing/wearing of a potentially contaminated cap, hat, barrette, headband, scarf, or comb

TREATMENT

Approaches to therapy: Treatment for tinea capitis depends on the clinical presentation of either inflammatory or noninflammatory disease. Therapy will include systemic (oral) and topical medicines. It is important to remember that tinea capitis can resolve spontaneously within one year, although few people would want to live with an untreated or undertreated condition.

Nondrug therapy: It is useful to restrict the patient's contact with other individuals who might become infected. Near the end of the course of systemic antifungal therapy, cutting the distal infected hair may be useful to curb reinfection and can help decrease the amount of scaling in the scalp; however, this will not clear the disease and foster healing. Nonprescription antidandruff shampoos can help decrease the amount of scaling in the scalp but will *not* clear the infection; prescription therapy is required.

Pharmacotherapy: Nonprescription drugs cannot cure tinea capitis; their role in the treatment of tinea capitis is limited and adjunctive only. Treat tinea capitis with a systemic antifungal such as griseofulvin. The usual dose is 1 g/day of the microcrystalline variety or 0.5 g/day of the ultramicrosized drug. For children, the dose of griseofulvin is 10 to 12 mg/kg/day. Continue therapy until a clinical and laboratory cure is obtained, usually after four to eight weeks of drug therapy. Alternative systemic antifungal drugs include fluconazole and itraconazole.

For inflammatory tinea capitis and kerions, oral corticosteroids may be helpful in reducing the inflammation and risk of scarring. The usual dose is 1 mg/kg/day prednisolone combined with appropriate systemic antifungal therapy. Family members and close contacts should be examined and treated if necessary.

Adjunctive therapies for managing tinea capitis are listed below.

SELENIUM SULFIDE

► **Actions**

Selenium sulfide appears to have a cytostatic effect on cells of the epidermis and follicular epithelium, thus reducing corneocyte production.

► **Indications**

Treatment of dandruff, seborrheic dermatitis of the scalp, and tinea versicolor; adjunctive therapy for managing tinea capitis.

► **Contraindications**

Hypersensitivity to any component of the product; broken skin or inflamed scalp.

► **Warnings**

For external use only: Avoid contact with the eyes, eyelids, and mucous membranes. If contact occurs, rinse thoroughly with water.

Sensitivity: Discontinue use and contact a pharmacist or physician if sensitivity reactions (eg, redness, swelling, itching, burning) occur.

Pregnancy: Category C. There are no adequate and well-controlled studies in pregnant women. Use during pregnancy only if the potential benefits outweigh the possible risks to the fetus.

Lactation: Safety for use in the nursing mother has not been established. Exercise caution when applying on a nursing woman.

Children: Safety and efficacy in infants have not been established.

► **Adverse Reactions**

Scalp irritation; increased hair loss; hair discoloration; oiliness/dryness of hair and scalp.

► **Administration and Dosage**

Massage 5 to 10 mL into wet scalp. Allow to remain on scalp two to three minutes. Rinse thoroughly; repeat application process and rinse thoroughly. Wash hands after treatment. Usually, two applications each week for two weeks will afford control of the condition, but the treatment may be used as frequently as once daily. After this, it may be used at less frequent intervals (weekly, every two weeks, or even every three or four weeks in some cases). Do not apply more frequently than required to maintain control. While 1% selenium sulfide lotion and shampoos are available OTC, 2.5% concentrations may be obtained with a prescription.

SELENIUM SULFIDE PRODUCTS	
Trade name	Doseform
Head & Shoulders Intensive Treatment	**Shampoo**: 1%. Cetyl alcohol, stearyl alcohol.
Selsun Blue Medicated Treatment	**Shampoo**: 1%. Menthol.

Products listed are representative of currently available and widely distributed brands. Similar products, including regional and private label brands, may also exist.

PATIENT INFORMATION
Selenium Sulfide
- For external use only. Avoid contact with the eyes, eyelids, and mucous membranes. If contact occurs, rinse thoroughly with water.
- Do not use on broken skin or inflamed scalp.
- Consult a physician before use if you have a condition that covers a large portion of the body.
- Rinse thoroughly after each application. Discontinue use and consult a physician if irritation occurs.
- Discontinue use if condition worsens or does not improve after regular use as directed.
- If using on bleached, tinted, gray, or permed hair, rinse hair for at least five minutes in cool running water.
- May damage jewelry; remove before using.

TAR DERIVATIVES

▶ Actions
Tar derivatives help correct keratinization abnormalities by decreasing epidermal proliferation and dermal infiltration. They also have antipruritic and mild antibacterial actions.

▶ Indications
For treatment of scalp psoriasis, eczema, seborrheic dermatitis, dandruff, cradle cap, and other oily, itchy conditions of the body and scalp. These agents may decrease scaling associated with tinea capitis and, therefore, may be used as adjunctive therapy.

▶ Contraindications
Hypersensitivity to any component of the product; acute inflammation; open or infected scalp lesions.

▶ Warnings
For external use only: Avoid contact with the eyes, eyelids, and mucous membranes. If contact occurs, rinse thoroughly with water.

Sensitivity: Discontinue use and contact a pharmacist or physician if sensitivity reactions (eg, redness, swelling, itching, burning) or chemical irritation occurs.

Pregnancy: Category C. There are no adequate and well-controlled studies in pregnant women. Use during pregnancy only if the potential benefits outweigh the possible risks to the fetus.

Lactation: Safety for use in the nursing mother has not been established. Exercise caution when applying on a nursing woman.

Children: Use on children younger than two years of age only as directed by a physician.

Photosensitivity: Use caution in exposing skin to sunlight after application. It may increase tendency to sunburn for up to 24 hours after application.

▶ Adverse Reactions
Minor dermatologic side effects include rash or burning sensation. Photosensitivity or skin discoloration may occur.

▶ Administration and Dosage

Refer to the specific product labeling for dosing information. Rub shampoo liberally into scalp. Leave on for several minutes. Rinse thoroughly. Repeat and rinse. Depending on the product, use at least twice per week up to once daily or as directed by a physician. For severe scalp problems, use daily according to product instructions.

TAR DERIVATIVE PRODUCTS	
Trade name	**Doseform**
DHS Tar	**Shampoo**: 0.5% coal tar
Doak Tar	**Shampoo**: 0.5% coal tar. EDTA, isopropyl alcohol.
Polytar	**Shampoo**: 0.5% coal tar. EDTA, lanolin.
Sebutone	**Shampoo**: 0.5% coal tar. EDTA, lanolin oil, salicylic acid, sulfur.
Tera-Gel	**Shampoo**: 0.5% coal tar. EDTA, parabens.
Ionil T, Zetar	**Shampoo**: 1% coal tar
PC-Tar	**Shampoo**: 1% coal tar. EDTA.
Creamy Tar	**Shampoo**: 2% coal tar. 5.6% ethyl alcohol.
Ionil T Plus	**Shampoo**: 2% coal tar
Neutrogena T/Gel	**Shampoo**: 2% coal tar extract
	Conditioner: 2% coal tar extract in a conditioner base
X•Seb T Pearl, X•Seb T Plus	**Shampoo**: 2% coal tar. EDTA, lanolin, salicylic acid.
Original Therapeutic Strength Denorex	**Shampoo**: 2.5% coal tar. 10.4% alcohol, menthol.
MG217 Extra Strength with Conditioners	**Shampoo**: 3% coal tar
Pentrax 5%	**Shampoo**: 5% coal tar
Original Therapeutic Strength Denorex 2 in 1	**Shampoo/Conditioner**: 2.5% coal tar. 10.4% alcohol, avocado oil, lanolin, menthol.
Tarsum	**Shampoo/Gel**: 2% coal tar. Salicylic acid.

Products listed are representative of currently available and widely distributed brands. Similar products, including regional and private label brands, may also exist.

PATIENT INFORMATION

Tar Derivatives

- For external use only. Avoid contact with the eyes, eyelids, or mucous membranes. If contact occurs, rinse thoroughly with water.
- Rinse thoroughly after each application. Discontinue use and consult a physician if excessive dryness or irritation occurs.
- Consult a physician before use if you have a condition that covers a large portion of the body.
- Discontinue use if condition worsens or does not improve after regular use as directed.
- Tar derivatives increase sensitivity to the sun and may increase tendency to sunburn for up to 24 hours after use. Avoid prolonged exposure to the sun or other forms of ultraviolet light (eg, tanning beds). Use sunscreens and wear protective clothing until tolerance is determined.
- Do not use for prolonged periods (longer than six months) or with psoriasis therapy (eg, phototherapy, prescription drugs) unless instructed by a physician.
- Products containing tar may temporarily discolor blond, gray, bleached, or tinted hair, or cause slight staining of clothing. Clothing stains normally are removed by standard laundry methods.
- Some coal tar products are extremely flammable. Keep away from fire and flame.

ANTISEBORRHEIC COMBINATIONS

▶ **Indications**

The following ingredients are adjunctive in the management of tinea capitis.

Salicylic acid and **sulfur** are used for antiseborrheic and keratolytic/keratoplastic actions.

Tar preparations are used for their antipruritic, mild antibacterial, or antiseborrheic actions.

Menthol is used as an antipruritic.

Benzalkonium chloride, **isopropyl alcohol**, **phenol**, and **menthol** are used as mild antiseptics.

▶ **Warnings**

For external use only: Avoid contact with the eyes, eyelids, or mucous membranes. If contact occurs, rinse thoroughly with water.

If undue skin irritation, burning, stinging, or itching develops or worsens, discontinue use and consult physician. Preparations containing tar may temporarily discolor blond, bleached, or tinted hair. Slight staining of clothing also may occur.

Children: Do not use on children younger than two years of age unless instructed by a physician.

▶ **Administration and Dosage**

Follow instructions on the label of the individual products very closely.

ANTISEBORRHEIC COMBINATION PRODUCTS	
Trade name	Doseform
Ionil, Ionil Plus, P & S	**Shampoo:** 2% salicylic acid
Neutrogena T/Sal	**Shampoo:** 2% salicylic acid, 2% solubilized coal tar extract
Sebex	**Shampoo:** 2% salicylic acid, 2% sulfur
Sebulex, Sebulex with Conditioners	**Shampoo:** 2% salicylic acid, 2% sulfur. EDTA.
Maximum Strength Meted	**Shampoo:** 3% salicylic acid, 5% sulfur
Sulfoam	**Shampoo:** 2% sulfur. Parabens.
Sebucare	**Lotion:** 1.8% salicylic acid. 61% alcohol, dihydrobietyl alcohol.
Scalpicin	**Liquid:** 3% salicylic acid. Menthol, SD alcohol 40.
P & S	**Liquid:** Glycerin, mineral oil, phenol

Products listed are representative of currently available and widely distributed brands. Similar products, including regional and private label brands, may also exist.

PATIENT INFORMATION
Antiseborrheic Combinations

- For external use only. Avoid contact with the eyes, eyelids, or mucous membranes. If contact occurs, rinse thoroughly with water.
- Consult a physician before use if you have a condition that covers a large portion of the body.
- Rinse thoroughly after each application. Discontinue use and consult a physician if irritation occurs.
- Discontinue use if condition worsens or does not improve after regular use as directed.
- Do not use on children younger than two years of age.
- Tar derivatives increase sensitivity the sun and may increase tendency to sunburn for up to 24 hours after use. Avoid prolonged exposure to the sun or other forms of ultraviolet light (eg, tanning beds). Use sunscreens and wear protective clothing until tolerance is determined.
- Do not use for prolonged periods (longer than 6 months) or with psoriasis therapy (eg, phototherapy, prescription drugs) unless instructed by a physician.
- Products containing tar may temporarily discolor blond, gray, bleached, or tinted hair, or cause slight staining of clothing. Clothing stains normally are removed by standard laundry methods.

TINEA CORPORIS
(Ringworm of the Body; Tinea Circinata)

DEFINITION

Tinea corporis is a superficial dermatophyte fungal infection of the skin on the trunk and limbs excluding the scalp, face, feet, hands, and groin. Clinical manifestations result from invasion and proliferation of fungi in the stratum corneum.

ETIOLOGY

Dermatophytes are fungi and are composed of 3 groups of organisms: *Microsporum*, *Trichophyton*, and *Epidermophyton*. All known dermatophytes can produce tinea corporis. The 3 most common causative organisms are *T. rubrum*, *M. canis*, and *T. mentagrophytes*; however, endemic species in certain geographic areas can influence which organism is the most common. Tinea corporis is most often caused by a *Trichophyton* species in the US.

Variants of tinea corporis include the following:

- *Bullous tinea corporis* - Blister-like lesions usually due to *T. rubrum*.
- *Kerion of glabrous (non-hair-bearing) skin* - Inflamed, pustular lesions.
- *Majocchi's granuloma* - Deeper, perifollicular, granulomatous inflammation.

INCIDENCE

True incidence rates for tinea corporis are unknown. The infection can occur in individuals of any age. Children have an increased incidence of tinea corporis caused by zoophilic organisms (animal-to-human transmission), particularly *M. canis* (from cats and dogs). Adults, on the other hand, develop tinea corporis from anthropophilic organisms (human-to-human transmission) and zoophilic organisms.

PATHOPHYSIOLOGY

The organism responsible for tinea corporis may be transmitted by direct contact with other infected individuals or inanimate fomites (carriers), such as those found on clothing and furniture (anthropophilic) or by direct contact with infected animals (zoophilic). A reservoir of infection elsewhere on the body, such as on the feet, scalp, or groin area, may also be the source of tinea corporis.

The organism infects the skin by first invading the stratum corneum, especially under warm, moist, occlusive conditions. After a 1- to 3-week incubation period, outward spread occurs. The active advancing border can continue to spread, leaving a relative clearing in the center of the lesion. Most organisms causing tinea corporis are located in the stratum corneum of the skin, but hair follicle involvement can occur and tends to be more inflammatory.

SIGNS/SYMPTOMS

- Symptoms of tinea corporis are usually limited to skin lesions commonly found on the buttocks and around the waist. Most lesions of tinea corporis are asymptomatic but itching may be present, particularly in areas where sweat is retained, such as in skin folds and areas where clothing (eg, elastic bands) fit tightly.
- Zoophilic (animal-transmitted) infections appear as circular, bright red, sharply marginated, scaling plaques. Often only a single plaque is present but occasionally more may be seen. Each plaque is usually smaller than 5 cm (approximately 2 inches) in diameter. Plaques are often solid, although annular forms can be seen.
- Anthropophilic infections appear as the classic annular, scaling, red plaque with central clearing. Incomplete forms may be present such that only fragments of the circles are seen as arciform plaques. The amount of scale present and extent of area affected are highly variable.

DIAGNOSTIC PARAMETERS/PHYSICAL ASSESSMENT

Clinical Observation: Because the clinical presentation may appear similar to psoriasis or eczema, examine specimens with 10% potassium hydroxide (KOH) for branching hyphae in the stratum corneum. With a negative KOH examination, a fungal culture is imperative. Four weeks of incubation are required before the culture results are known.

Interview: Because tinea corporis can be spread by contact with pets or with infected humans, it may be beneficial to ask about the following:

- Description, location, and duration of signs and symptoms of the condition.
- History of tinea corporis (either in adolescence or adulthood).
- Other family members who have symptoms or who have been examined for tinea infections.
- Description of any past self-treatment, including success of treatment, and recurrence of the condition.
- Pets with skin conditions.
- Exposure to contaminated surfaces (eg, public shower facilities).
- Whether friends or classmates have had recent tinea infections.

TREATMENT

Approaches to therapy: For isolated lesions of tinea corporis, topical agents, including various *otc* products, are the most effective. For widespread or inflammatory lesions, systemic prescription agents are required.

Nondrug therapy: Instruct patients to wear loose clothing and avoid occlusive fabrics or elastic that retain heat and moisture. Wash contaminated clothing and bedding, and avoid sources of reinfection, such as health clubs and contaminated showers. Treat pet dogs or cats, if necessary, by a veterinarian.

Pharmacotherapy: Nonprescription topical drugs used for the treatment of localized superficial dermatophyte infections include miconazole nitrate 1%, clotrimazole 2%, terbinafine 1%, tolnaftate 1%, and undecylenic acid. These agents are effective against most dermatophytes. Prescription topical medicines for tinea corporis include econazole, ketoconazole, and ciclopirox olamine. Systemic oral agents include griseofulvin, ketoconazole, itraconazole, fluconazole, and terbinafine.

MICONAZOLE NITRATE

► **Actions**

Miconazole alters cellular membrane permeability and interferes with mitochondrial and peroxisomal enzymes, resulting in intracellular necrosis and fungal death. It inhibits growth of the common dermatophytes, *Trichophyton rubrum, T. mentagrophytes, Epidermophyton floccosum, Candida albicans*, and the active organism in tinea versicolor, *Malassezia furfur*.

► **Indications**

Tinea pedis (athlete's foot), tinea cruris (jock itch), and tinea corporis (ringworm) caused by *T. rubrum, T. mentagrophytes*, and *E. floccosum*.

► **Contraindications**

Hypersensitivity to miconazole or any component of the product.

► **Warnings**

For external use only: Avoid contact with the eyes, eyelids, and mucous membranes.

Sensitivity: If a reaction occurs suggesting sensitivity or chemical irritation (eg, itching, burning, irritation, redness, swelling), discontinue use and contact a pharmacist or physician.

Children: Do not use on children younger than 2 years of age unless directed by a physician.

► **Adverse Reactions**

Infrequent reports of irritation, burning, maceration (softening of the skin due to excessive moisture), and allergic contact dermatitis.

► **Administration and Dosage**

Cream and solution: Apply a thin layer of medication to affected areas twice daily, morning and evening (once daily in patients with tinea versicolor). Solution is preferred in intertriginous areas (areas of skin folds); if cream is used, apply sparingly to avoid maceration effects.

Powder: Spray or sprinkle liberally over affected area morning and evening. Early relief of symptoms occurs in most patients; clinical improvement may be seen within 2 to 3 days after beginning treatment. However, candida, tinea cruris, and tinea corporis should be treated daily for 2 weeks or longer, and tinea pedis for 1 month or longer, to reduce chance of recurrence. If no clinical improvement is observed after 1 month, reevaluate the diagnosis. Patients with tinea versicolor usually exhibit clinical and mycological clearing in 2 weeks.

MICONAZOLE NITRATE PRODUCTS	
Trade name	**Doseform**
Micatin, Podiatrx-AF	**Cream**: 2%
Micatin, Lotrimin AF, Zeasorb-AF	**Powder**: 2%
Lotrimin AF, Micatin	**Spray Powder**: 2%
	Solution: 2%
Fungoid Tincture	**Solution**: 2%

Products listed are representative of currently available and widely distributed brands. Similar products, including regional and private label brands, may also exist.

PATIENT INFORMATION

Miconazole Nitrate

- For external use only. Avoid contact with eyes, eyelids, and mucous membranes.
- Apply after cleansing affected area unless directed otherwise.
- Do not apply to blistered, oozing, or raw skin.
- If condition persists or worsens, or if irritation (burning, itching, stinging, redness) occurs, discontinue use and notify a pharmacist or physician.
- Use for full treatment time, even if symptoms improve. Strict compliance is crucial to a good therapeutic outcome. Notify a pharmacist or physician if there is no improvement after treating for 2 consecutive weeks (*Candida* infections, tinea cruris, and tinea corporis) or 4 consecutive weeks (tinea pedis).

CLOTRIMAZOLE

▶ **Actions**

Antifungal agent that impairs the synthesis of ergosterol, a component of the fungus cell membrane, ultimately causing the destruction of the fungus cell membrane, rendering the fungus nonviable.

Clotrimazole, a broad-spectrum antifungal agent, inhibits growth of pathogenic dermatophytes, yeasts, and *Malassezia furfur*. Exhibits fungistatic and fungicidal activity in vitro against isolates of *Trichophyton rubrum*, *T. mentagrophytes*, *Epidermophyton floccosum*, *Microsporum canis*, and *Candida* sp, including *C. albicans*. No single-step or multiple-step resistance to clotrimazole has developed during successive passages of *C. albicans* and *T. mentagrophytes*.

▶ **Indications**

Topical treatment of tinea pedis (athlete's foot), tinea cruris (jock itch), and tinea corporis (ringworm) due to *T. rubrum*, *T. mentagrophytes*, *E. floccosum*, and *M. canis*.

▶ **Contraindications**

Hypersensitivity to clotrimazole or any product component.

▶ **Warnings**

For external use only: Avoid contact with the eyes, eyelids, and mucous membranes.

If irritation, burning, itching, redness, or other signs of sensitivity develop, discontinue use, contact a pharmacist or physician, and institute appropriate first aid therapy.

Pregnancy: Category B. In clinical trials, vaginal use in pregnant women in their second and third trimesters has not been associated with ill effects. Consult an obstetrician or gynecologist prior to use in pregnancy.

There are no adequate and well-controlled studies in pregnant women during the first trimester of pregnancy. Use only if clearly indicated during the first trimester.

Lactation: Topical preparations are known to be excreted in breast milk. Use with caution.

▶ **Adverse Reactions**

Adverse reactions are usually limited to the local application sites. Erythema, stinging sensation, pruritis, and general irritation of the skin may occur. Local allergic reactions have been seen on the skin from the components of the topical spray products.

▶ **Administration and Dosage**

Gently massage into affected and surrounding skin areas twice daily, morning and evening. Clinical improvement, with relief of pruritus, usually occurs within the first week of treatment. If patient shows no clinical improvement after 4 weeks, reevaluate the diagnosis.

CLOTRIMAZOLE PRODUCTS	
Tradename	Doseform
Lotrimin AF, Mycelex OTC	Cream: 1%
	Solution: 1%

Products listed are representative of currently available and widely distributed brands. Similar products, including regional and private label brands, may also exist.

PATIENT INFORMATION
Clotrimazole

- For external use only. Avoid contact with the eyes, eyelids, and mucous membranes.
- Apply after cleansing affected area unless directed otherwise.
- Do not apply to blistered, oozing, or raw skin.
- If condition persists or worsens, or if irritation occurs, discontinue use, and notify a pharmacist or physician.
- Use the medication for the full 4-week treatment time even though the symptoms may have improved. Notify a pharmacist or physician if no improvement is observed after 4 weeks of treatment.
- Inform a pharmacist or physician if the area of application shows signs of increased irritation (eg, redness, itching, burning, blistering, swelling, oozing) indicative of possible sensitization.
- Do not use in children younger than 2 years of age unless directed by a physician.

TOLNAFTATE

▶ **Actions**

Effective in the treatment of superficial fungus infections (eg, ringworm, athlete's foot, jock itch) of the skin.

▶ **Indications**

Treatment of tinea pedis (athlete's foot), tinea cruris (jock itch), or tinea corporis (ringworm) due to infection with *Trichophyton rubrum*, *T. mentagrophytes*, *T. tonsurans*, *Microsporum canis*, *M. audouini*, and *Epidermophyton floccosum* and for tinea versicolor due to *Malassezia furfur*.

In onychomycosis (fungal infection of nails), in chronic scalp infections in which fungi are numerous and widely distributed in skin and hair follicles, where kerion has formed, and in fungal infections of palms and soles, use tolnaftate concurrently with other antifungal agents for adjunctive local benefit in these lesions.

Powder and powder aerosol: May also be used prophylactically against athlete's foot.

▶ **Contraindications**

Hypersensitivity to miconazole or any component of the product.

▶ **Warnings**

Sensitization or irritation: Discontinue treatment if sensitization or irritation occur.

Nail/Scalp infections: Not recommended as sole therapy for these infections. May be used as adjunctive therapy to systemic treatment.

If symptoms do not improve after 10 consecutive days of use as recommended by the labeling, discontinue use unless otherwise directed.

For external use only: Keep out of eyes, and avoid contact with eyelids and mucous membranes.

Reevaluate patient: If no improvement occurs after 4 consecutive weeks of daily therapy, reevaluate the patient.

If irritation, burning, itching, redness, or other signs of sensitivity develop, discontinue use, contact a pharmacist or physician, and institute appropriate first aid therapy.

▶ **Adverse Reactions**

A few cases of sensitization (eg, redness, stinging, itching, burning) have been confirmed; mild irritation has occurred.

▶ **Administration and Dosage**

Only small quantities are required. Apply thin layers of the drug twice a day for 2 to 3 weeks, although 4 to 6 weeks may be required if the skin has thickened. Continue twice-daily treatment to maintain remission.

The choice of vehicle is important for these products. Ointments, creams, and liquids are used as primary therapy. In general, powders are used as adjunctive therapy, but they may be acceptable as primary therapy in very mild conditions.

TOLNAFTATE PRODUCTS	
Trade name	**Doseform**
NP•27, Tinactin, Ting	**Cream**: 1%
NP•27, Tinactin	**Solution**: 1%
Quinsana Plus, Tinactin	**Powder**: 1%
Tinactin	**Spray Liquid**: 1%
Aftate for Athlete's Foot, Tinactin	**Spray Powder**: 1%

Products listed are representative of currently available and widely distributed brands. Similar products, including regional and private label brands, may also exist.

PATIENT INFORMATION
Tolnaftate

- For external use only. Avoid contact with the eyes, eyelids, or mucous membranes.
- Cleanse affected area with soap and water and dry thoroughly before applying product.
- For athlete's foot, wear well-fitting, ventilated shoes; change shoes and socks at least once a day. A dusting of powder into socks and shoes may be beneficial.

TERBINAFINE

▶ **Actions**

Terbinafine exerts its antifungal effect by inhibiting squalene epoxidase, a key enzyme in sterol biosynthesis in fungi. This action results in a deficiency in ergosterol and a corresponding accumulation of squalene within the fungal cell and causes fungal cell death.

Terbinafine is active against most strains of the following organisms both in vitro and in clinical infections: *Epidermophyton floccosum*; *Trichophyton mentagrophytes*; *T. rubrum*.

▶ Indications

Topical treatment of the following dermatologic infections: Interdigital tinea pedis (athlete's foot), tinea cruris (jock itch), or tinea corporis (ringworm of the body) due to *E. floccosum*, *T. mentagrophytes*, or *T. rubrum*.

▶ Contraindications

Hypersensitivity to terbinafine or any component of the product.

▶ Warnings

For external use only: Not for oral, ophthalmic, or intravaginal use.

Irritation/Sensitivity: If irritation or sensitivity develops, discontinue treatment and institute appropriate therapy.

Pregnancy: Category B. There are no adequate and well-controlled studies in pregnant women.

Lactation: Decide whether to discontinue nursing or the drug, taking into account the importance of the drug to the mother. Nursing mothers should not apply to the breast.

Children: Safety and efficacy in children younger than 12 years of age have not been established.

▶ Adverse Reactions

In clinical trials, 0.2% of patients discontinued therapy because of adverse events and 2.3% reported adverse reactions. These reactions included the following: irritation (1%); burning (0.8%); itching, dryness (0.2%).

▶ Overdosage

Acute overdosage with topical application is unlikely because of the limited absorption and would not be expected to lead to serious adverse effects.

▶ Administration and Dosage

Cream: Apply to cover the affected and immediately surrounding areas once daily until clinical signs and symptoms are significantly improved. In many patients, this occurs by day 7 of therapy. Duration of therapy should be for a minimum of 1 week and should not exceed 2 weeks.

Many patients treated with durations of therapy of 1 to 2 weeks continue to improve during the 2 to 4 weeks after drug therapy has been completed. As a consequence, patients should not be considered therapeutic failures until they have been observed for a period of 2 to 4 weeks post-therapy.

If successful outcome is not achieved during the posttreatment observation period, review the diagnosis.

Spray: First, wash the infected area with soap and water and dry completely. Do not cover the treated skin with any bandages. Wash your hands with soap and water after touching the infected skin so that you do not spread the infection on yourself or to others.

For ringworm, spray the infected skin and surrounding area once a day (morning or night) for 1 week or as directed by a doctor.

Many people experience symptom relief after the completion of 1 week of treatment. Spray as directed. Skin may continue to show some signs of infection described above until the outer layer of the treated skin naturally replaces itself. Skin replacement takes longer on some parts of the body than others. If no improvement is seen within 2 weeks, consult a physician.

TERBINAFINE PRODUCTS	
Trade name	Doseform
Lamisil AT	**Cream**: 1%. Benzyl, cetyl, and stearyl alcohols.
	Solution: 1%. Ethanol.
	Spray: 1%. Ethanol.

Products listed are representative of currently available and widely distributed brands. Similar products, including regional and private label brands, may also exist.

PATIENT INFORMATION
Terbinafine
- For external use only. Use as directed; avoid contact with eyes, nose, mouth, or other mucous membranes.
- Apply after cleansing and drying the affected area. Wash hands after applying the medication to the affected areas.
- Use the medication for the recommended treatment time. Strict adherence to the dosage schedule is essential for optimal clinical response.
- Inform a pharmacist or physician if the area of application shows signs of increased irritation or possible sensitization (redness, itching, burning, blistering, swelling, or oozing).
- Avoid the use of occlusive dressings unless otherwise directed.
- Do not use on children younger than 12 years of age unless directed by a physician.

BUTENAFINE

▶ **Actions**

Antifungal agent that impairs the synthesis of ergosterol, a component of the fungus cell membrane, ultimately causing the destruction of the fungus cell membrane, rendering the fungus nonviable.

Butenafine is active against most strains of the following microorganisms both in vitro and in clinical infections: *Malassezia furfur, Epidermophyton floccosum, Trichophyton mentagrophytes, T. rubrum,* and *T. tonsurans.*

▶ **Indications**

Topical treatment of the following dermatologic infections: interdigital tinea pedis (athlete's foot), tinea cruris (jock itch), or tinea corporis (ringworm of the body) due to *E. floccosum, T. mentagrophytes, T. rubrum,* or *T. tonsurans.*

▶ **Contraindications**

Hypersensitivity to butenafine or any component of the product.

▶ **Warnings**

For external use only: For topical use only. Do not use in mouth, eyes, or vagina.

Irritation/Sensitivity: If irritation or sensitivity develops, discontinue treatment and institute appropriate therapy. Patients known to be sensitive to allylamine antifungals should use butenafine with caution; it is possible that these drugs may be cross-reactive.

Pregnancy: Category B. There are no adequate and well-controlled studies in pregnant women. Use during pregnancy only if clearly needed.

Lactation: It is not known if butenafine is excreted in breast milk. Exercise caution when administering to a breastfeeding woman. Breastfeeding mothers should avoid application of butenafine cream to the breast.

Children: Do not use on children younger than 12 years of age unless directed by a physician.

▶ **Adverse Reactions**

Burning/stinging, itching, and worsening of the condition (approximately 1%); contact dermatitis; erythema, irritation, and itching (less than 2%). No patient treated with butenafine discontinued treatment due to an adverse event.

In provocative testing in over 200 subjects, there was no evidence of allergic contact sensitization for either cream or vehicle base.

▶ **Administration and Dosage**

First, wash the infected area with soap and water and dry completely. Apply sufficient butenafine to cover the affected area and immediate surrounding skin. Wash hands with soap and water after use to avoid spreading infection.

Apply butenafine once daily for 2 weeks. If a patient shows no clinical improvement after the treatment period, consult a physician.

BUTENAFINE PRODUCTS	
Trade name	Doseform
Lotrimin Ultra	Cream: 1%. Benzyl and cetyl alcohol, white petrolatum.

Products listed are representative of currently available and widely distributed brands. Similar products, including regional and private label brands, may also exist.

PATIENT INFORMATION

Butenafine

- For external use only. Use as directed; avoid contact with eyes, nose, mouth, or other mucous membranes.
- Apply after cleansing and drying the affected area. Wash hands after applying the medication to the affected area(s).
- Use the medication for the recommended treatment time. Strict adherence to the dosage schedule is essential for optimal clinical response.
- Inform a pharmacist or physician if the area of application shows signs of increased irritation or possible sensitization (redness, itching, burning, blistering, swelling, or oozing).
- Avoid the use of occlusive dressings unless otherwise directed.
- Do not use on children younger than 12 years of age unless directed by a physician.

UNDECYLENIC ACID AND DERIVATIVES

▶ Indications

Antifungal and antibacterial agents for treatment of tinea corporis (ringworm), tinea pedis (athlete's foot), exclusive of the nails and hairy areas. Also recommended for the relief and prevention of diaper rash, itching, burning and chafing, prickly heat, tinea cruris (jock itch), excessive perspiration and irritation in the groin area, and bromhidrosis (foul-smelling perspiration).

▶ Contraindications

Allergy or sensitivity to the preparation or its components.

▶ Warnings

Patients with impaired circulation, including diabetic patients, should consult a physician before using.

For external use only: Avoid inhaling and contact with the eyes or other mucous membranes.

Children: Do not use in children younger than 2 years of age except on advice of physician.

▶ Administration and Dosage

Cleanse and dry area well; rub, massage, or spray on. Apply as directed. For dosage guidelines, refer to the specific package labeling.

▶ Product Selection

The choice of vehicle is important for these products. Ointments and creams are used as primary therapy. In general, powders are used as adjunctive therapy, but they may be acceptable as primary therapy in very mild conditions.

UNDECYLENIC ACID AND DERIVATIVES PRODUCTS	
Trade name	Doseform
Gordochom	**Solution**: 25% undecylenic acid and chloroxynol in an oily base
Elon Dual Defense Anti-Fungal Formula	**Solution**: 25% undecylenic acid. Ethyl alcohol, lime oil, tea tree oil.
Blis-To-Sol	**Powder**: 12% zinc undecylenate and bentonite, talc, thymo, zinc oxide
Pedi-Pro	**Powder**: 1% bonzalkonium chloride, zinc undecylenate, corn starch, kaolin, aluminum chlorhydroxide, phenoxyisopropanol. Menthol.
Breeze Mist	**Powder**: Aluminum chlorohydrate, cyclomethine, undecylenic acid. Menthol.

Products listed are representative of currently available and widely distributed brands. Similar products, including regional and private label brands, may also exist.

PATIENT INFORMATION
Undecylenic Acid and Derivatives

- For external use only. Avoid contact with the eyes, nose, mouth, or other mucous membranes.
- Cleanse and dry the area to be treated before application.
- Apply with caution to blistered, raw skin, or oozing skin, or skin over a deep puncture wound.
- Patients with decreased circulation, including diabetic patients, should consult their physician before using undecylenic acid.
- Allergic reactions may occur. If the condition worsens or if irritation, burning, redness, swelling, or stinging persists, discontinue use, and notify pharmacist or physician.
- Use these medications for the full treatment time, even if the symptoms improve.
- Notify a pharmacist or physician if there is no improvement after 4 weeks.
- Do not use in children younger than 2 years of age unless directed by a physician.

TINEA CRURIS
(Jock Itch)

DEFINITION

Tinea cruris is a dermatophyte, or mold-type, fungal infection of the inguinal area, which includes the upper inner thighs, pubic area, perineal and perianal areas, and buttocks.

ETIOLOGY

The causative organisms include the dermatophytes *Trichophyton rubrum*, *T. mentagrophytes*, *Epidermophyton floccosum*, and occasionally lesser-seen dermatophytes. Occasionally, *Candida albicans* can resemble tinea cruris, but this organism is a yeast, not a mold. Tight-fitting clothing, such as swimsuits, and moisture, such as sweating, predisposes the development of the infection. A concurrence of tinea of the hands and feet is also frequently seen.

INCIDENCE

The disease is generally observed after puberty, mostly in males. It is diagnosed more frequently in the tropics and in climates with warm, moist weather.

PATHOPHYSIOLOGY

Pathophysiology of tinea cruris is not well defined. Tight-fitting undergarments or clothing and moisture predisposes the patient to the condition, and the presence of tinea pedis and tinea manuum may serve as a source for infection.

SIGNS/SYMPTOMS

The upper, inner thigh is most often involved, with symmetrical scaling, erythematous arcuate, or polycyclic patches seen spreading posteriorly to involve the perianal or buttocks area and anteriorly to involve the pubic area. The scrotum is generally spared. Itching may or may not be seen, although significant pruritus is common. The eruption is generally chronic and spreading in nature.

DIAGNOSTIC PARAMETERS/PHYSICAL ASSESSMENT

Clinical Observation: Dry, erythematous, scaling, arcuate (arch-shaped) patches in the inguinal area indicate a tinea infection. If the area is moist with small pustules and includes the scrotum, a yeast infection must be considered.

Once the diagnosis is made, treatment is often successful with 1 of many OTC products available. In addition, keeping the area dry with absorbent powder or talc and avoiding tight-fitting clothes or wet swimsuits will help prevent recurrences.

Interview: To ensure the diagnosis and proper treatment of tinea cruris, it may be beneficial to ask about the following:

- Duration of symptoms.
- Description of symptoms (eg, pain, redness, itching).
- Location of condition, especially scrotal involvement, or a similar condition on hands or feet.
- Use of tight-fitting undergarments or clothing or prolonged exposure to wet swimsuits.
- Previous occurrence of condition.
- Description of any attempted treatments and success of such treatments.

TREATMENT

Approaches to therapy: Recurrent disease is common. Treat concurrent fungal infection of the feet and hands.

When the issue of "transmission to others" is raised, note that another person may come in contact with the infecting fungal organisms, but that innate resistance to the fungi is the most important factor in determining whether transfer of infection occurs.

Nondrug therapy: Control aggravating factors. Preventive measures include avoidance of tight-fitting undergarments or clothing and of prolonged exposure to wet swimsuits or high-humidity situations. In addition, stress the use of absorbent powders in the affected areas.

Pharmacotherapy: The available topical creams include the imidazole and undecylenate classes. These are represented by clotrimazole (eg, *Lotrimin A/F*), miconazole (eg, *Micatin*), undecylenic acid/zinc undecylenate (eg, *Cruex*), tolnaftate (eg, *Ting*), and terbinafine (*Lamisil AT*).

MICONAZOLE NITRATE

▶ **Actions**

Miconazole alters cellular membrane permeability and interferes with mitochondrial and peroxisomal enzymes, resulting in intracellular necrosis. It inhibits growth of the common dermatophytes, *Trichophyton rubrum*, *T. mentagrophytes*, *Epidermophyton floccosum*, *Candida albicans*, and the active organism in tinea versicolor, *Malassezia furfur*.

▶ **Indications**

Tinea pedis (athlete's foot), tinea cruris, and tinea corporis (ringworm) caused by *T. rubrum*, *T. mentagrophytes*, and *E. floccosum*.

Relieves itching, cracking, burning, scaling, and discomfort that can accompany these conditions.

▶ **Contraindications**

Hypersensitivity to miconazole or any components of the product.

▶ **Warnings**

If there is no improvement of jock itch within 2 weeks, discontinue use, and consult a pharmacist or physician.

For external use only: Avoid contact with the eyes.

Sensitivity: If a reaction occurs suggesting sensitivity or chemical irritation, discontinue use.

Children: Do not use in children younger than 2 years of age unless directed by a physician.

► **Adverse Reactions**

Isolated reports of irritation, burning, maceration, and allergic contact dermatitis.

► **Administration and Dosage**

Early relief of symptoms (2 to 3 days) occurs in most patients; clinical improvement may be seen fairly soon after treatment. However, treat tinea cruris for at least 2 weeks to reduce chance of recurrence. If no clinical improvement occurs after 2 weeks, reevaluate diagnosis. Patients with tinea versicolor usually exhibit clinical and mycological clearing in 2 weeks.

Cream and lotion: Cover affected areas twice daily, morning and evening. Lotion is preferred in intertriginous areas; if cream is used, apply sparingly to avoid maceration effects.

Powder: Spray or sprinkle liberally over affected area, morning and evening.

Spray: Clean the affected area and dry thoroughly. Shake can well before using. Hold can about 6 inches from the area to be treated. Apply a thin layer over affected area twice daily (morning and night) or as directed. Supervise children in the use of this product. Use daily for 2 weeks. If conditions persist longer, consult a physician. This product is not effective on the scalp or nails.

MICONAZOLE NITRATE PRODUCTS	
Trade name	Doseform
Micatin, Neosporin AF Jock Itch	Cream: 2%
Lotrimin AF, Micatin, Ting	Spray powder: 2%
Micatin	Spray: 2%
Zeasorb-AF	Powder: 2%

Products listed are representative of currently available and widely distributed brands. Similar products, including regional and private label brands, may also exist.

PATIENT INFORMATION

Miconazole Nitrate

- For external use only. Avoid contact with the eyes, eyelids, and mucous membranes.
- Apply after cleansing affected area unless directed otherwise.
- If condition persists or worsens or if irritation (burning, itching, stinging, redness) occurs, discontinue use, and notify a pharmacist or physician.
- Use for full treatment time, even if symptoms improve. Notify a pharmacist or physician if there is no improvement after 2 weeks.
- Do not use in children younger than 2 years of age unless directed by a physician.

CLOTRIMAZOLE

▶ **Actions**

Clotrimazole, a broad-spectrum antifungal agent, inhibits growth of pathogenic dermatophytes, yeasts, and *Malassezia furfur*. It exhibits fungistatic and fungicidal activity in vitro against isolates of *Trichophyton rubrum*, *T. mentagrophytes*, *Epidermophyton floccosum*, *Microsporum canis*, and *Candida* sp, including *C. albicans*. No single-step or multiple-step resistance to clotrimazole has developed during successive passages of *C. albicans* and *T. mentagrophytes*.

▶ **Indications**

Topical treatment of tinea pedis (athlete's foot), tinea cruris, and tinea corporis (ringworm) due to *T. rubrum*, *T. mentagrophytes*, *E. floccosum*, and *M. canis*.

▶ **Contraindications**

Hypersensitivity to clotrimazole or any product component.

▶ **Warnings**

For external use only: Avoid contact with the eyes.

Sensitivity: If irritation or sensitivity develops, discontinue use, and notify a pharmacist or physician.

Pregnancy: Category B. In clinical trials, use of vaginally applied clotrimazole in pregnant women in their second and third trimesters has not been associated with ill effects.

There are, however, no adequate and well-controlled studies in pregnant women during the first trimester of pregnancy. Use only if clearly indicated during the first trimester.

Lactation: It is not known whether this drug is excreted in breast milk. Exercise caution when applying on a nursing mother.

Children: Do not use in children younger than 2 years of age unless directed by a physician.

▶ **Adverse Reactions**

Erythema; stinging; blistering; peeling; edema; pruritus; urticaria; burning; general skin irritation.

▶ **Administration and Dosage**

Gently massage into affected and surrounding skin areas twice daily, morning and evening. Clinical improvement, with relief of pruritus, usually occurs within the first week of treatment. If patient shows no clinical improvement after 4 weeks, reevaluate the diagnosis.

CLOTRIMAZOLE PRODUCTS	
Trade name	**Doseform**
Lotrimin AF, Mycelex OTC	**Cream:** 1%
	Solution: 1%

Products listed are representative of currently available and widely distributed brands. Similar products, including regional and private label brands, may also exist.

PATIENT INFORMATION

Clotrimazole

- For external use only. Avoid contact with the eyes.
- Apply after cleansing affected area unless directed otherwise.
- If condition persists or worsens or if irritation (burning, itching, stinging, redness) occurs, discontinue use, and notify a pharmacist or physician.
- Use the medication for the full treatment time even though the symptoms may have improved.
- Notify a pharmacist or physician if there is no improvement after 4 weeks of treatment.
- Inform a pharmacist or physician if the area of application shows signs of increased irritation (eg, redness, itching, burning, blistering, swelling, oozing) indicative of possible sensitization.
- Do not use in children younger than 2 years of age unless directed by a physician.

TOLNAFTATE

▶ Actions

Effective in the treatment of superficial fungal infections (eg, ringworm, athlete's foot, jock itch) of the skin.

▶ Indications

Treatment of tinea pedis (athlete's foot), cruris (jock itch), or corporis (ringworm) due to infection with *Trichophyton rubrum*, *T. mentagrophytes*, *T. tonsurans*, *Microsporum canis*, *M. audouini*, and *Epidermophyton floccosum*, and for tinea versicolor due to *Malassezia furfur*.

Effectively soothes and relieves the painful symptoms of jock itch, including itching, chafing, and burning.

▶ Contraindications

Hypersensitivity to tolnaftate or any component of the product.

▶ Warnings

If symptoms do not improve after 10 to 14 days of use as recommended by the labeling, discontinue use unless otherwise directed.

For external use only. Keep out of eyes.

Reevaluate patient if no improvement occurs after 4 weeks.

Sensitization or irritation: Discontinue treatment.

Nail/Scalp infections: Not recommended for these infections except as adjunctive therapy to systemic treatment.

Children: Do not use in children younger than 2 years of age unless directed by a physician.

▶ Adverse Reactions

A few cases of sensitization have been confirmed; mild irritation has occurred.

▶ Administration and Dosage

Only small quantities are required. Treatment twice a day for 2 or 3 weeks is usually adequate, although 4 to 6 weeks may be required if the skin has thickened. Continue treatment to maintain remission.

Spray powder: Wash the affected area and dry thoroughly. Shake can well. Spray a thin layer of the product over the affected area twice daily (morning and evening) or as directed. Supervise children in the use of this product. Use daily for 2 weeks. If condition persists longer, consult a physician.

► **Product Selection**

The choice of vehicle is important for these products. Creams and liquids are used as primary therapy. In general, powders are used as adjunctive therapy, but they may be acceptable as primary therapy in very mild conditions.

TOLNAFTATE PRODUCTS	
Trade name	**Doseform**
Tinactin	**Cream**: 1%. Cetearyl alcohol, mineral oil.
Ting	**Cream**: 1%. White petrolatum.
Quinsana Plus	**Powder**: 1%. Talc.
Tinactin	**Powder**: 1%
Tinactin	**Solution**: 1%. SD alcohol 40.
Absorbine Jr	**Liquid**: 1%. Iodine, menthol, wormwood oil.
Absorbine Jr	**Gel**: SD alcohol 40. Menthol, tea tree oil.
Tinactin, Ting	**Spray**: SD alcohol 40.
Tinactin	**Spray Powder**: 1%. SD alcohol 40, talc.
Tinactin	**Wipes**: 1% SD alcohol 40.

Products listed are representative of currently available and widely distributed brands. Similar products, including regional and private label brands, may also exist.

PATIENT INFORMATION

Tolnaftate

- For external use only. Avoid contact with the eyes.
- Cleanse and dry the area to be treated before application.
- Apply after cleansing affected area unless directed otherwise.
- If condition persists or worsens, or if irritation occurs, discontinue use and notify a pharmacist or physician.
- Do not use in children younger than 2 years of age unless directed by a physician.

TERBINAFINE

► **Actions**

Terbinafine exerts its antifungal effect by inhibiting squalene epoxidase, a key enzyme in sterol biosynthesis in fungi. This action results in a deficiency in ergosterol and a corresponding accumulation of squalene within the fungal cell, causing fungal cell death.

Terbinafine is active against most strains of the following organisms both in vitro and in clinical infections: *Epidermophyton floccosum*; *Trichophyton mentagrophytes*; *T. rubrum*; *T. tonsurans.*

► **Indications**

Topical treatment of the following dermatologic infections: interdigital tinea pedis (athlete's foot), tinea cruris (jock itch), or tinea corporis (ringworm of the body) due to *E. floccosum*, or *T. mentagrophytes, T. rubrum, T. tonsuras.*

▶ **Contraindications**

Hypersensitivity to terbinafine or any component of the product.

▶ **Warnings**

For external use only: For topical use only. Do not use in mouth, eyes, or vagina.

Irritation/Sensitivity: If irritation or sensitivity develops, discontinue treatment and institute appropriate therapy.

Pregnancy: Category B. There are no adequate and well-controlled studies in pregnant women. Use during pregnancy only if clearly needed.

Lactation: Decide whether to discontinue breastfeeding or the drug, taking into account the importance of the drug to the mother. Breastfeeding mothers should not apply to the breast.

Children: Safety and efficacy in children younger than 12 years of age have not been established.

▶ **Adverse Reactions**

In clinical trials, 0.2% of patients discontinued therapy because of adverse events, and 2.3% reported adverse reactions. These reactions included the following: irritation (1%); burning (0.8%); itching, dryness (0.2%).

▶ **Overdosage**

Acute overdosage with topical application is unlikely because of the limited absorption and would not be expected to lead to serious adverse effects.

▶ **Administration and Dosage**

Cream: Apply to cover the affected and immediately surrounding areas once daily until clinical signs and symptoms are significantly improved. In many patients, this occurs by day 7 of therapy. Duration of therapy should be for a minimum of 1 week and should not exceed 2 weeks.

Many patients treated with durations of therapy of 1 to 2 weeks continue to improve during the 2 to 4 weeks after drug therapy has been completed. As a consequence, patients should not be considered therapeutic failures until they have been observed for a period of 2 to 4 weeks after therapy.

If a successful outcome is not achieved during the posttreatment observation period, review the diagnosis.

Spray: First, wash the infected area with soap and water and dry completely. Do not cover the treated skin with any bandages. Wash your hands with soap and water after touching the infected skin so that you do not spread the infection on yourself or to others.

For jock itch, spray the infected skin and surrounding area once a day (morning or night) for 1 week or as directed by a physician.

Many people experience relief of their symptoms after the completion of 1 week of treatment. Spray as directed. Skin may continue to show some signs of infection until the outer layer of the treated skin naturally replaces itself. Skin replacement takes longer on some parts of the body than others. If no improvement is seen within 2 weeks, consult a physician.

TERBINAFINE PRODUCTS	
Trade name	Doseform
Lamisil AT	Cream: 1%. Benzyl, cetyl, and stearyl alcohols.
	Solution: 1%. Ethanol.
	Spray: 1%. Ethanol.

Products listed are representative of currently available and widely distributed brands. Similar products, including regional and private label brands, may also exist.

PATIENT INFORMATION
Terbinafine

- For external use only. Use as directed. Avoid contact with the eyes, nose, mouth or other mucous membranes.
- Cleanse and dry the area to be treated before application. Wash hands after applying the medication onto affected areas.
- Use the medication for the recommended treatment time. Strict adherence to the dosage schedule is essential for optimal clinical response.
- Inform a pharmacist or physician if the area of application shows signs of increased irritation or possible sensitization (redness, itching, burning, blistering, swelling, or oozing).
- Avoid the use of occlusive dressings unless otherwise directed.
- Do not use in children younger than 12 years of age unless directed by a physician.

BUTENAFINE

► Actions

Antifungal agent that impairs the synthesis of ergosterol, a component of the fungus cell membrane, ultimately causing the destruction of the fungus cell membrane, rendering the fungus nonviable.

Butenafine is active against most strains of the following microorganisms both in vitro and in clinical infections: *Malassezia furfur*, *Epidermophyton floccosum*, *Trichophyton mentagrophytes*, *T. rubrum*, and *T. tonsurans*.

► Indications

Topical treatment of the following dermatologic infections: Interdigital tinea pedis (athlete's foot), tinea cruris (jock itch), or tinea corporis (ringworm of the body) due to *E. floccosum*, *T. mentagrophytes*, *T. rubrum*, or *T. tonsurans*.

► Contraindications

Hypersensitivity to butenafine or any component of the product.

► Warnings

For external use only: Not for oral, ophthalmic, or intravaginal use.

Irritation/Sensitivity: If irritation or sensitivity develops, discontinue treatment and institute appropriate therapy. Patients known to be sensitive to allylamine antifungals should use butenafine with caution; it is possible that these drugs may be cross-reactive.

Pregnancy: Category B. There are no adequate and well-controlled studies in pregnant women. Use during pregnancy only if clearly needed.

Lactation: It is not known if butenafine is excreted in breast milk. Exercise caution when administering to a breastfeeding woman. Breastfeeding mothers should avoid application of butenafine cream to the breast.

Children: Do not use on children younger than 12 years of age unless directed by a physician.

▶ **Adverse Reactions**

Burning/stinging, itching, and worsening of the condition (approximately 1%); contact dermatitis; erythema, irritation, and itching (less than 2%). No patient treated with butenafine discontinued treatment due to an adverse event.

In provocative testing in over 200 subjects, there was no evidence of allergic contact sensitization for either cream or vehicle base.

▶ **Administration and Dosage**

First wash the infected area with soap and water and dry completely. Apply sufficient butenafine to cover the affected area and immediately surrounding skin. Wash hands with soap and water after use to avoid spreading infection. Apply butenafine once daily for 2 weeks. If a patient shows no clinical improvement after the treatment period, consult a physician.

BUTENAFINE PRODUCTS	
Trade name	Doseform
Lotrimin Ultra	**Cream:** 1%. Benzyl and cetyl alcohol, white petrolatum.

Products listed are representative of currently available and widely distributed brands. Similar products, including regional and private label brands, may also exist.

PATIENT INFORMATION

Butenafine

- For external use only. Use as directed; avoid contact with eyes, nose, mouth, or other mucous membranes. Wash hands after applying the medication to the affected area(s).
- Cleanse and dry the area to be treated before application.
- Use the medication for the recommended treatment time. Strict adherence to the dosage schedule is essential for optimal clinical response.
- Inform a pharmacist or physician if the area of application shows signs of increased irritation or possible sensitization (redness, itching, burning, blistering, swelling, or oozing).
- Avoid the use of occlusive dressings unless otherwise directed.
- Do not use on children younger than 12 years of age unless directed by a physician.

UNDECYLENIC ACID AND DERIVATIVES

▶ **Indications**

Antifungal and antibacterial agents for treatment of tinea pedis (athlete's foot), exclusive of the nails and hairy areas. Also recommended for the relief and prevention of diaper rash, itching, burning and chafing, prickly heat, tinea cruris (jock itch), excessive perspiration and irritation in the groin area, and bromhidrosis (foul-smelling perspiration).

▶ Contraindications

Allergy or sensitivity to the preparation or its components.

▶ Warnings

Patients with impaired circulation, including diabetic patients, should consult a physician before using.

For external use only: Avoid inhaling and contact with the eyes or other mucous membranes.

Children: Do not use in children younger than 2 years of age except on advice of physician.

▶ Administration and Dosage

Cleanse and dry area well; rub, massage, or spray on. Apply as directed. For dosage guidelines, refer to specific package labeling.

▶ Product Selection

The choice of vehicle is important for these products. Ointments and creams are used as primary therapy. In general, powders are used as adjunctive therapy, but they may be acceptable as primary therapy in very mild conditions.

UNDECYLENIC ACID AND DERIVATIVES PRODUCTS	
Trade name	Doseform
Gordochom	**Solution**: 25% undecylenic acid and chloroxynol in an oily base
Elon Dual Defense Anti-Fungal Formula	**Solution**: 25% undecylenic acid. Ethyl alcohol, lime oil, tea tree oil.
Blis-To-Sol	**Powder**: 12% zinc undecylenate, bentonie, talc, thymo, zinc oxide
Pedi-Pro	**Powder**: 1% bonzalkonium chloride, zinc undecylenate, corn starch, kaolin, aluminum chlorhydroxide, phenoxyisopropanol. Menthol.
Breeze Mist	**Powder**: Aluminum chlorohydrate, cyclomethione, undecylenic acid. Menthol.

Products listed are representative of currently available and widely distributed brands. Similar products, including regional and private label brands, may also exist.

PATIENT INFORMATION

Undecylenic Acid and Derivatives

- For external use only. Avoid contact with the eyes, nose, mouth, or other mucous membranes.
- Cleanse and dry the area to be treated before application.
- Apply with caution to blistered, raw, oozing skin, or skin over a deep puncture wound.
- Patients with decreased circulation, including diabetic patients, should consult their physician before using undecylenic acid.
- Allergic reactions may occur. If the condition worsens or if irritation, burning, redness, swelling, or stinging persists, discontinue use, and notify pharmacist or physician.
- Use these medications for the full treatment time, even if the symptoms improve.
- Notify a pharmacist or physician if there is no improvement after 4 weeks.
- Do not use in children younger than 2 years of age unless directed by a physician.

TINEA VERSICOLOR
(Pityriasis Versicolor)

DEFINITION

Tinea versicolor is a mild, chronically recurring fungal infection of the stratum corneum caused by *Pityrosporum* species and characterized by discrete, scaly, discolored, or depigmented areas predominantly on the upper trunk.

ETIOLOGY

Tinea versicolor is caused by the fungus *Malassezia furfur*, but historically, the synonyms *P. ovale*, *P. orbiculare*, and *M. ovalis*, have been used interchangeably. *M. furfur* is considered part of the normal flora of the skin and is common in sebum-rich areas of the skin. *M. furfur* is a dimorphic, lipophilic organism that converts from the saprophytic yeast to the parasitic mycelial form associated with clinical disease.

INCIDENCE

True incidence rates for tinea versicolor are unknown. It occurs primarily in adults between 20 and 45 years of age and is usually established by the early twenties, particularly in the summer or in warm climates. In seasonal climates, tinea versicolor usually resolves on its own in autumn.

PATHOPHYSIOLOGY

Tinea versicolor represents an opportunistic infection in the skin. The organism is considered normal flora, but under certain conditions (ie, warm, humid environment, inherited predisposition, endogenous or exogenous Cushing disease, immunosuppression, or malnourished state), *M. furfur* converts to the mycelial form.

The hypopigmentation that occurs may be caused by the formation of dicarboxylic acids that competitively inhibit tyrosinase. These dicarboxylic acids form from enzymatic oxidation of fatty acids in skin surface lipids by *M. furfur*.

SIGNS/SYMPTOMS

The most common presentation consists of scaly, hypopigmented or hyperpigmented, round or oval macules on the chest or back and less commonly on the abdomen, proximal extremities, or face. The scale is fine and dustlike and may only be noticed by lightly scraping the involved area. The color of the lesions varies from white (especially in dark-skinned individuals) to reddish-brown or fawn-colored (in fair-skinned people). The eruption is usually noticed after sun exposure because lesions often fail to tan. Pruritus is mild or absent.

DIAGNOSTIC PARAMETERS/PHYSICAL ASSESSMENT

Clinical Observation: The diagnosis of tinea versicolor can usually be made based on clinical appearance. Lesions that are imperceptible may become apparent by use of Wood light, which fluoresces the lesions to a yellow or brown color. Direct microscopic exam of scale prepared with potassium hydroxide (KOH) can be used to confirm the diagnosis. One sees short, stubby hyphae and round spores (sometimes referred to as "spaghetti and meatballs").

Interview: To aid in the proper diagnosis and treatment of tinea versicolor, it may be beneficial to ask about the following:

• Location and extent of infection
• Description of symptoms, including duration
• Patient's exposure to a warm, humid environment
• Allergies to topical medications
• Family history of tinea versicolor or preexisting medical conditions that may predispose the patient to tinea versicolor (eg, Cushing disease, immunosuppression, malnutrition)
• Attempted treatment and its efficacy

TREATMENT

Approaches to therapy: Treatment for tinea versicolor is typically requested because patients have an uneven tan. It is important to stress that tinea versicolor is not contagious; it is simply an overgrowth of an organism that is always present in the skin.

Pharmacotherapy: Several topical OTC products are useful in treating tinea versicolor. Nonprescription topical agents that have been used include: 1% ketoconazole; 2% miconazole; 1% clotrimazole; 1% tolnaftate; 25% sodium thiosulfate; sulfur/salicylic acid soaps or shampoos (eg, *Sebulex*); 1% selenium sulfide; or keratolytic agents such as 50% propylene glycol. Soaps with zinc pyrithione (for a list of products, see the Dandruff monograph in the Dermatological Conditions chapter) may help prevent recurrence.

For more severe or persistent cases of tinea versicolor, physician referral is warranted. The most widely used prescription agent is 2.5% selenium sulfide lotion. Various prescription-strength topical antifungals can be used, but because a large surface area is to be treated, lotion formulations, such as oxiconazole, are preferred. Systemic drugs are not usually necessary to treat tinea versicolor but are sometimes used because of their convenient dosing (eg, itraconazole 200 mg/day for 5 days or a single-dose of fluconazole 400 mg). Systemic azole antifungals of varying doses and topical agents have been used to prevent recurrence. However, topical prophylactic treatment is often associated with low patient compliance. Because disease recurrence is impossible to predict, it is preferable to treat the condition when it occurs rather than prophylactically.

SELENIUM SULFIDE

▶ **Actions**

Selenium sulfide appears to have a cytostatic effect on cells of the epidermis and follicular epithelium, thus reducing corneocyte production and subsequent scaling.

▶ Indications

Although not an FDA-approved indication, selenium sulfide is used for the treatment of tinea versicolor. This agent has other labeled indications as well.

▶ Contraindications

Allergy to any component of the product.

▶ Warnings

Irritation: Selenium sulfide may irritate the skin, especially in the genital area and in skin folds. Rinse these areas thoroughly after application.

Acute inflammation/exudation: Do not use when present; absorption may be increased.

For external use only: Avoid contact with eyes. If contact occurs, rinse thoroughly with tap water.

Hypersensitivity: If hypersensitivity reactions occur, discontinue use.

Pregnancy: Category C.

Children: Safety and efficacy in infants have not been established.

▶ Drug Interactions

Because this product is applied topically to intact skin for a short period of time, drug interactions are unlikely to occur.

▶ Adverse Reactions

Skin irritation; greater than normal hair loss; hair discoloration; oiliness or dryness of the scalp.

▶ Overdosage

Symptoms: Selenium sulfide shampoos generally have low toxicity if ingested. Nausea, vomiting, and diarrhea usually occur after oral ingestion. There may also be a burning sensation in the mouth and a garlic-like taste or smell to the breath. The detergents found in selenium sulfide shampoos may act as emetics, thereby preventing significant GI absorption of selenium.

Treatment: Treatment includes usual supportive measures.

▶ Administration and Dosage

Apply 5 to 10 mL of the medicated shampoo onto affected areas after showering, and allow it to remain for 5 to 10 minutes before rinsing thoroughly. Wash hands after treatment. Alternatively, applications can be left overnight and washed off the following morning. Treatment is usually continued for the next 7 to 14 days or longer depending on symptom severity. Do not apply more frequently than required to maintain control. While 1% selenium sulfide lotions and shampoos are available OTC, 2.5% concentrations may be obtained with a prescription.

SELENIUM SULFIDE PRODUCTS	
Trade name	**Doseform**
Selsun Blue	**Lotion:** 1%
Head & Shoulders Intensive Treatment	**Shampoo:** 1%
Selsun Blue	**Shampoo:** 1%

Products listed are representative of currently available and widely distributed brands. Similar products, including regional and private label brands, may also exist.

PATIENT INFORMATION
Selenium Sulfide

- For external use only. Avoid contact with the eyes, mouth, and vagina. In case of contact, flush thoroughly. Do not use on acutely inflamed skin.
- Work up a lather and apply shampoo to all affected areas. It is preferable to treat the entire trunk, including the neck, arms, and legs, down to the knees, even when small areas are affected.
- If irritation occurs, discontinue use. Thoroughly rinse after application.
- May damage jewelry; remove before using.
- For tinea versicolor on the scalp, rinse hair for five minutes or longer in cool tap water if using these products before or after bleaching, tinting, or permanently waving hair.
- Use only as directed. Do not put bandages, dressings, cosmetics, or other skin products over the treated area unless directed by a physician.
- If you forget an application, apply it as soon as you remember and continue on your regular schedule. If it is almost time for the next application, wait and continue on your regular schedule. Do not apply double applications.
- Depigmented spots may remain after tinea versicolor is treated.
- If you are pregnant, consult your obstetrician/gynecologist prior to using.

MICONAZOLE

▶ Actions

Miconazole alters cellular membrane permeability and interferes with mitochondrial and peroxisomal enzymes, resulting in intracellular necrosis. It inhibits growth of the common dermatophytes, *Trichophyton rubrum*, *T. mentagrophytes*, *Epidermophyton floccosum*, *Candida albicans*, and the active organism in tinea versicolor, *Malassezia furfur*.

▶ Indications

Although not an FDA-approved indication, miconazole is used for the treatment of tinea versicolor. This agent has other labeled indications as well.

▶ Contraindications

Allergy or sensitivity to the preparation or its components.

▶ Warnings

Sensitivity: If a reaction occurs suggesting sensitivity or chemical irritation, discontinue use.

For topical use only: Do not use in mouth, eyes, or vagina.

Pregnancy: Consult an obstetrician/gynecologist prior to use in pregnancy.

Lactation: Topical preparations are excreted in breast milk.

▶ Drug Interactions

There are no known drug/drug or drug/food interactions with topical miconazole.

▶ Adverse Reactions

Isolated reports of irritation, burning, maceration, and allergic contact dermatitis.

▶ **Administration and Dosage**

Follow dosing guidelines for individual products. Twice-daily application of most topical creams, sprays, solutions, or powders is recommended. Creams, sprays, solutions, and powders are applied generously to all involved areas. Continue treatment for 2 weeks or longer following resolution of symptoms.

MICONAZOLE NITRATE PRODUCTS	
Trade name	Doseform
Micatin	Cream: 2%
Desenex, Lotrimin AF, Micatin, Zeasorb-AF	Powder: 2%
Cruex, Desenex, Lotrimin AF, Micatin, Ting	Spray Powder: 2%
Desenex, Lotrimin AF, Micatin	Spray: 2%

Products listed are representative of currently available and widely distributed brands. Similar products, including regional and private label brands, may also exist.

PATIENT INFORMATION

Miconazole

- For external use only. Avoid contact with the eyes, mouth, and vagina. In case of contact, flush thoroughly.
- If condition persists or worsens or if irritation (eg, burning, itching, stinging, redness) occurs, discontinue use and notify physician.
- Use for full treatment time, even if symptoms improve. Notify physician if there is no improvement after treatment period has passed.
- It is preferable to treat the entire trunk, including the neck, arms, and legs, down to the knees, even when small areas are affected.
- Apply creams, solutions, and powders sparingly in a light film; rub in gently.
- Use only as directed. Do not put bandages, dressings, cosmetics, or other skin products over the treated area unless directed by a physician.
- If you forget an application, apply it as soon as you remember and continue on your regular schedule. If it is almost time for the next application, wait and continue on your regular schedule. Do not apply double applications.
- Depigmented spots may remain after tinea versicolor is treated.
- If you are pregnant, consult your obstetrician/gynecologist prior to using the topical antifungal agents.

CLOTRIMAZOLE

▶ **Actions**

Clotrimazole, a broad-spectrum antifungal agent, inhibits growth of pathogenic dermatophytes, yeasts, and *Malassezia furfur*. It exhibits fungistatic and fungicidal activity in vitro against isolates of *Trichophyton rubrum*, *T. mentagrophytes*, *Epidermophyton floccosum*, *Microsporum canis*, and *Candida* sp, including *C. albicans*. No single- or multiple-step resistance to clotrimazole has developed during successive passages of *C. albicans* and *T. mentagrophytes*.

▶ **Indications**

Although not an FDA-approved indication, clotrimazole is used for the treatment of tinea versicolor. This agent has other labeled indications as well.

▶ **Contraindications**

Allergy or sensitivity to the preparation or its components.

▶ **Warnings**

For topical use only: Do not use in mouth, eyes, or vagina.

Pregnancy: Category B. In clinical trials, vaginal use in pregnant women in their second and third trimesters has not been associated with ill effects.

However, there are no adequate and well-controlled studies in pregnant women during the first trimester of pregnancy. Use only if clearly needed during the first trimester.

Lactation: It is unknown whether this drug is excreted in breast milk. Exercise caution with use in nursing mothers.

▶ **Drug Interactions**

There are no known drug/drug or drug/food interactions with topical clotrimazole.

▶ **Adverse Reactions**

Erythema; stinging; blistering; peeling; edema; pruritus; urticaria; burning; general skin irritation.

▶ **Administration and Dosage**

Gently massage into affected and surrounding skin areas twice daily, morning and evening. Clinical improvement, with relief of pruritus, usually occurs within the first week of treatment. If patient shows no clinical improvement after 4 weeks, reevaluate the diagnosis.

CLOTRIMAZOLE PRODUCTS	
Trade name	Doseform
Desenex, Lotrimin AF	**Cream**: 1%
Lotrimin AF	**Lotion**: 1%
Lotrimin AF	**Solution**: 1%

Products listed are representative of currently available and widely distributed brands. Similar products, including regional and private label brands, may also exist.

■ ■ ■

PATIENT INFORMATION

Clotrimazole

- For external use only. Avoid contact with the eyes, mouth, and vagina. In case of contact, flush thoroughly.
- Apply after cleansing affected area (unless directed otherwise).
- It is preferable to treat the entire trunk, including the neck, arms, and legs, down to the knees, even when small areas are affected.
- Apply creams and solutions sparingly in a light film; rub in gently.
- Use only as directed. Do not put bandages, dressings, cosmetics, or other skin products over the treated area, unless directed by a physician.
- If you forget an application, apply it as soon as you remember and continue on your regular schedule. If it is almost time for the next application, wait and continue on your regular schedule. Do not apply double applications.
- If the condition persists or worsens or if irritation occurs, discontinue use and notify physician.
- Use the medication for the full treatment time even though symptoms may have improved. Notify physician if no improvement is seen after 4 weeks of treatment.
- Inform a physician if the area of application shows signs of increased irritation (eg, redness, itching, burning, blistering, swelling, oozing) indicative of possible sensitization.
- Depigmented spots may remain after tinea versicolor is treated.
- If you are pregnant, consult your obstetrician/gynecologist prior to using the topical antifungal agents.

TOLNAFTATE

▶ Actions

Effective in the treatment of superficial fungal infections of the skin.

▶ Indications

Although not an FDA-approved indication, tolnaftate is used for the treatment of tinea versicolor. This agent has other labeled indications as well.

▶ Warnings

Sensitization or irritation: Discontinue treatment if sensitization or irritation occur.

Nail/Scalp infections: Not recommended for these infections except as adjunctive therapy to systemic treatment.

Duration of treatment: If symptoms do not improve after 2 to 4 weeks of use as recommended by labeling, discontinue use unless otherwise directed, and refer patient to a physician for evaluation.

For topical use only: Do not use in mouth, eyes, or vagina.

Pregnancy: Consult an obstetrician/gynecologist prior to use in pregnancy.

Lactation: Topical preparations are known to be excreted in breast milk. Exercise caution when administering to a nursing mother.

▶ Drug Interactions

There are no known drug/drug or drug/food interactions with topical tolnaftate.

▶ Adverse Reactions

Adverse reactions are usually limited to the local application sites. Erythema, blistering of skin, stinging sensation, pruritus, and general irritation of the skin may occur. Local allergic reactions have been seen on the skin from the components of the topical spray products.

▶ Administration and Dosage

Only small quantities are required. Treatment twice a day for 2 or 3 weeks is usually adequate although 4 to 6 weeks may be required if the skin has thickened. Continue treatment to maintain remission.

▶ Product Selection

The choice of vehicle is important for these products. Creams, liquids, and solutions are used as primary therapy. In general, powders are used as adjunctive therapy, but they may be acceptable as primary therapy in very mild conditions.

TOLNAFTATE PRODUCTS

Trade name	Doseform
Tinactin, Ting	**Cream**: 1%
Quinsana Plus, Tinactin	**Powder**: 1%
Tinactin	**Solution**: 1%
Absorbine Jr	**Liquid**: 1%
Absorbine Jr	**Gel**: 1%
Tinactin	**Spray Powder**: 1%
Tinactin, Ting	**Spray**: 1%

Products listed are representative of currently available and widely distributed brands. Similar products, including regional and private label brands, may also exist.

PATIENT INFORMATION

Tolnaftate

- For external use only. Avoid contact with the eyes, mouth, and vagina. In case of contact, flush thoroughly.
- Cleanse skin with soap and water and dry thoroughly before applying product.
- Apply cream, solution, or powder to all affected areas. It is preferable to treat the entire trunk, including the neck, arms, and legs, down to the knees, even when small areas are affected.
- Apply cream, solution, or powder sparingly in a light film; rub in gently.
- Use only as directed. Do not put bandages, dressings, cosmetics, or other skin products over the treated area unless directed by a physician.
- If you forget an application, apply it as soon as you remember and continue on your regular schedule. If it is almost time for the next application, wait and continue on your regular schedule. Do not apply double applications.
- Depigmented spots may remain after tinea versicolor is treated.
- If you are pregnant, consult your obstetrician/gynecologist prior to using the topical antifungal agents.

KETOCONAZOLE

▶ **Actions**

Ketoconazole impairs ergosterol synthesis, which is a vital component of fungal cell membranes.

▶ **Indications**

Although not an FDA-approved indication, ketoconazole is used for the treatment of tinea versicolor. This agent has other labeled indications as well.

▶ **Contraindications**

Allergy or sensitivity to the drug or any of its components; use on broken skin or inflamed scalp.

▶ **Warnings**

For external use only: Avoid contact with the eyes, eyelids, and mucous membranes.

Sensitivity: If sensitivity or chemical irritation occurs, discontinue use.

Pregnancy: Category C.

Lactation: Safety for use in the nursing mother has not been established; exercise caution.

Children: Safety and efficacy in children younger than 12 years of age have not been established.

▶ **Drug Interactions**

Because this product is applied topically to intact skin for a short period of time, drug interactions are unlikely.

▶ **Adverse Reactions**

Skin irritation; greater than normal hair loss; abnormal hair texture; scalp pustules; mild dryness of skin; itching; oiliness/dryness of hair and scalp.

▶ **Overdosage**

In the event of ingestion, advise patients to seek professional assistance or contact a poison control center immediately. Supportive measures, including gastric lavage with sodium bicarbonate, may be necessary. Refer to General Management of Acute Overdosage in Appendix B.

▶ **Administration and Dosage**

Wet hair thoroughly; apply shampoo; generously lather; rinse thoroughly; repeat. Use every 3 to 4 days for up to 8 weeks if needed, or as directed by a physician. Then use only as needed to control dandruff.

Children younger than 12 years of age: Consult a physician.

KETOCONAZOLE PRODUCTS	
Trade name	**Doseform**
Nizoral A-D	**Shampoo:** 1%

Products listed are representative of currently available and widely distributed brands. Similar products, including regional and private label brands, may also exist.

PATIENT INFORMATION
Ketoconazole

- For external use only. Avoid contact with the eyes, eyelids, and mucous member-anes. In case of contact, rinse eyes thoroughly with water.
- Do not use on broken skin or inflamed scalp.
- Discontinue use if irritation occurs. Rinse thoroughly after each application.
- Discontinue use if rash appears or condition worsens or does not improve in 2 to 4 weeks; these may be signs of serious condition, consult physician.
- Removal of curl from permanently waved hair may occur.
- If pregnant or nursing, consult physician prior to use.
- Do not use if allergic to any component of the product.

DEFINITION

Common warts (also known as verrucae) are defined as benign, epidermal growths caused by the human papilloma virus (HPV).

INCIDENCE

Warts occur in 7% to 10% of the population. They can occur in any age group but are most common in children between 12 and 16 years of age; they rarely are seen in the elderly. Warts are seen more commonly in patients with an immune deficiency disorder or in those receiving immunosuppressive therapy; lesions can be disseminated widely in the immunocompromised patient. Previously infected patients are at a three times greater risk for reinfection.

PATHOPHYSIOLOGY

Warts are spread by direct contact with the virus or through autoinoculation. HPV enters through the skin surface, often through a site of recent trauma. Once the virus enters the skin surface, it uses the host-cell resources to replicate. A defective cell-mediated immunity predisposes an individual to developing warts. The number of virus particles produced is related to the type and age of the wart (eg, new lesions and plantar warts have a higher virus load than old lesions or common warts). The more numerous the virus particles, the more infectious the lesion. The incubation period of HPV is between one to 12 months, with an average period of two to three months.

SIGNS/SYMPTOMS

Wart tissue is not inherently painful; patients with common warts are usually asymptomatic. Exposed warts are cosmetically objectionable. Physical symptoms typically occur only when the wart becomes awkward because of its size or appearance. Plantar warts may become painful, particularly when walking or running.

DIAGNOSTIC PARAMETERS/PHYSICAL ASSESSMENT

There are three common clinical features of warts. They disrupt the normal skin lines; they frequently have thrombosed capillaries visible on the surface (seen as black pinpoint dots); and they most commonly occur at trauma sites. Paring or shaving of a wart results in punctate bleeding points from the capillaries that feed the wart. Three of the most frequently occurring classes of warts are common, plantar, and flat warts. The diagnosis is based on clinical presentation.

Common warts: Common warts can occur anywhere on the body but are often seen on the hands, knees, and areas surrounding the fingernails. They are sharply demarcated, rough-surfaced, round or irregular, firm papules that grow to 2 to 10 mm in diameter over several weeks to months. Common warts may be light gray, yellow, brown, or grayish-black in color.

Plantar: Plantar warts occur on the plantar surface of the foot, usually on the pressure points of the heel and metatarsal heads (see Plantar Warts in the Podiatric Conditions chapter). They appear as hyperkeratotic lesions that may be flat or raised.

Flat warts: Flat warts mainly affect children and generally occur on the hands, forearms, face, and neck. They appear as small (1 to 3 mm), soft, flesh- or tan-colored, flat-topped lesions.

Clinical Observation: Examine the wart if possible (do not touch warts), and try to verify the patient's diagnosis by its physical characteristics.

Interview: To determine treatment intervention processes, it may be beneficial to ask about the following:

• Additional symptoms (eg, pain, drainage) besides the presence of the wart
• History of warts
• Prior successful treatment
• Sensitivity to sulfites
• Medication profile (eg, chronic aspirin therapy)
• Presence of predisposing (immunocompromising) diseases or drug therapies (eg, chronic corticosteroid use)

TREATMENT

Approaches to therapy: When evaluating treatment options for warts, it is important to remember that they are benign, cutaneous growths that often disappear spontaneously (20% to 30% within six months, 50% within one year, and 66% within two years). Take into consideration the patient's age, underlying health status, and the number and location of warts. It should present no harm to the patient and should cause no scarring and minimal side effects. There is no need to remove every wart that may be present. Preventing the spread of warts also is important; wash hands frequently, avoid picking at the lesions, and cover new warts (which tend to be more infectious) with an occlusive dressing, particularly when showering.

Nondrug therapy: A variety of techniques have been used to treat warts, including benign neglect (where warts are allowed to spontaneously resolve), hypnotherapy, tape occlusion (applied for 6½ days with a ½-day of rest for 2 weeks), and intermittent flattening of the lesion using a pumice stone or callus file (especially for plantar warts).

The most common nondrug therapies for warts include physical measures, such as cryotherapy, laser treatments, and surgical excision.

Pharmacotherapy:

Salicylic acid – Salicylic acid is a safe and effective topical treatment of warts, and there are several topical products available. Prior to the application of medication, it often is helpful to soak the wart in warm water for several minutes and then file the surface with a nail file or pumice stone.

Cimetidine – Cimetidine (eg, *Tagamet, Tagamet HB*) has been studied in the treatment of warts in doses of 25 to 40 mg/kg/day, usually for three to four months. Results have been variable, but the higher doses may be more effective. It should not be first-line therapy but may offer an alternative. Cimetidine does have a significant adverse reaction and drug interaction profile.

Cryotherapy – Cryotherapy is another method of treatment for warts. This method freezes and kills the affected cells. As a result of freezing, a blister may form under the wart. The frozen skin falls off after 10 to 14 days. In the meantime, new skin is already growing under the blister.

TOPICAL SALICYLIC ACID

▶ **Actions**

Pharmacology: Salicylic acid is the only OTC product considered safe and effective by the Food and Drug Administration for use as a keratolytic for corns, calluses, and warts. Salicylic acid produces desquamation of the horny layer of skin, while not affecting the structure of the viable epidermis, by dissolving intercellular cement substance. The keratolytic action causes the cornified epithelium to swell, soften, macerate, and then desquamate.

Salicylic acid is keratolytic at concentrations of approximately 2% to 6%. These concentrations generally are used for treatment of dandruff, seborrhea, and psoriasis. Concentrations of 5% to 17% in collodion are safe and effective for the removal of common and plantar warts; concentrations up to 40% in plasters are used to remove warts, corns, and calluses.

Salicylic acid preparations, alone or in combination, also have been used to treat dandruff, seborrheic dermatitis, acne, tinea infections, and psoriasis.

Pharmacokinetics: In a study of the percutaneous absorption of salicylic acid in 4 patients with extensive active psoriasis, peak serum salicylate levels never exceeded 5 mg/dL, even though more than 60% of the applied salicylic acid was absorbed. Systemic toxic reactions usually are associated with much higher serum levels (30 to 40 mg/dL). Peak serum levels occurred within 5 hours of a topical application under an occlusive dressing.

The major urinary metabolites identified after topical administration differ from those after oral salicylate administration; those derived from percutaneous absorption contain more salicylate glucuronides (42%), and less salicyluric (52%) and salicylic acid (6%).

▶ **Indications**

A topical aid in the removal of excessive keratin in hyperkeratotic skin disorders, including common and plantar warts, psoriasis, calluses, and corns.

▶ **Contraindications**

Sensitivity to salicylic acid; prolonged use, especially in children younger than 2 years of age, diabetic patients, and patients with impaired circulation; use on moles, birthmarks, or warts with hair growing from them, genital warts or warts on the face or mucous membranes; use on irritated skin, or any area that is infected or reddened.

▶ **Warnings**

Salicylate toxicity: Prolonged use over large areas, especially in young children and those patients with significant renal or hepatic impairment, could result in salicylism. Limit the area to be treated, and be aware of signs of salicylate toxicity (eg, nausea, vomiting, dizziness, loss of hearing, tinnitus, lethargy, hyperpnea, diarrhea, psychic disturbances). In the event of salicylic acid toxicity, discontinue use.

Refer to the Aspirin section in the Aches and Pains monograph in the CNS Conditions chapter for additional information on the systemic effects of salicylates.

For external use only: Avoid contact with eyes, eyelids, mucous membranes, and normal skin surrounding warts. If contact with eyes or mucous membranes occurs, immediately flush with tap water for 15 minutes. Avoid inhaling vapors.

Special risk patients: Do not use in diabetic patients or patients with poor circulation.

Pregnancy: Category C.

▶ **Drug Interactions**

Interactions have been reported with topical and oral salicylates. Refer to the Aspirin section in the Aches and Pains monograph for a complete listing.

▶ **Adverse Reactions**

Local irritation may occur from contact with normal skin surrounding the affected area. If irritation occurs, temporarily discontinue use and take care to apply only to the wart site when treatment is resumed.

▶ **Administration and Dosage**

For specific instructions for use of these products, refer to individual product labeling.

Before application, wash the affected area or soak it in warm water for 5 minutes prior to use to hydrate skin and enhance the keratolytic effect. Remove any loose tissue with brush, washcloth, or emery board. Dry thoroughly. Apply to affected area.

In general, for treatment of warts, improvement should occur in 1 to 2 weeks; maximum resolution may be expected after 4 to 6 weeks of use, although application for up to 12 weeks may be necessary. If skin irritation develops or there is no improvement after several weeks, contact a physician.

Storage/Stability: Some products are flammable; keep away from fire or flame. Keep bottle tightly capped and store at room temperature away from heat.

TOPICAL SALICYLIC ACID PRODUCTS	
Trade name	Doseform
Gordofilm	**Liquid**: 16.7% in a flexible collodion base
Compound W	**Liquid**: 17% with collodion, 21.2% alcohol, 63.6% ether, camphor, castor oil, menthol
Dr. Scholl's Clear Away	**Liquid**: 17% in a flexible collodion with 17% alcohol, 52% ether, acetone
DuoFilm	**Liquid**: 17% in flexible collodion with 15.8% alcohol, castor oil, and 42.6% ether
Occlusal-HP	**Liquid**: 17% in polyacrylic vehicle base containing ethyl acetate, isopropyl alcohol
Off-Ezy Wart Remover Kit	**Liquid**: 17% in collodion-like vehicle with 21% alcohol, 65% ether, and acetone
Salactic Film	**Liquid**: 17% in flexible collodion vehicle, 2.7% isopropyl alcohol
Tinamed Wart Remover	**Liquid**: 17% with 16.5% alcohol ethyl lactate, flexible collodion.
Wart-Off Maximum Strength	**Liquid**: 17% in flexible collodion with 26.3% alcohol, propylene glycol dipelargonate, and t-butyl alcohol
freezone Maximum Strength	**Liquid**: 17.6% with 33% alcohol, 65.5% ether.
Mosco Callus & Corn Remover	**Liquid**: 17.6% in a flexible collodion base with 33% alcohol and 65.5% ether

TOPICAL SALICYLIC ACID PRODUCTS	
Trade name	**Doseform**
Compound W	**Gel**: 17% with 67.5% alcohol, camphor, castor oil, collodion, colloidal silicon dioxide
Dr. Scholl's Clear Away	**Gel**: 17% with alcohol, ether, aloe extract, flexible collodion.
DuoPlant	**Gel**: 17% in flexible collodion with 57.6% alcohol, 16.42% ether
Sal-Plant	**Gel**: 17% in flexible collodion vehicle, 2.5% isopropyl alcohol
Trans-Ver-Sal PlantarPatch	**Transdermal patch**: 15% in natural karaya gum base with PEG-300, propylene glycol, quaternium-15
Trans-Ver-Sal PediaPatch	**Transdermal patch**: 15% in natural karaya gum base with PEG-300, propylene glycol, quaternium-15
Trans-Ver-Sal AdultPatch	**Transdermal patch**: 15% in natural karaya gum base with PEG-300, propylene glycol, quaternium-15
DuoFilm	**Transdermal patch**: 40% in a rubber-based vehicle
DuoFilm Patch for Kids	**Transdermal patch**: 40% in a rubber-based vehicle
Compound W One Step Wart Remover	**Medicated pads**: 40% in a plaster vehicle. Lanolin, rubber.
Compound W One Step Wart Remover for Kids	**Medicated pads**: 40% in a plaster vehicle. Lanolin, rubber.
Curad Mediplast	**Medicated pads**: 40%. Natural rubber, lanolin.
Dr. Scholl's Clear Away One Step for Kids	**Medicated pads**: 40% in a rubber-based vehicle
Sal-Acid	**Medicated plaster**: 40% in a plaster vehicle
Dr. Scholl's Clear Away	**Medicated discs**: 40% in a rubber-based vehicle
Dr. Scholl's Clear Away One Step	**Medicated strips**: 40% in a rubber-based vehicle

Products listed are representative of currently available and widely distributed brands. Similar products, including regional and private label brands, may also exist.

PATIENT INFORMATION
Salicylic Acid

- For external use only. Avoid contact with eyes, eyelids, face, genitals, mucous membranes, and normal skin surrounding lesion.
- Medication may cause reddening or scaling of skin when used on open skin lesions.
- Contact with clothing, fabrics, plastics, wood, metal, or other materials may cause damage; avoid contact.
- Do not use if you have diabetes or poor peripheral circulation.
- Do not use on irritated skin or any area that is reddened or infected.
- Contact a physician if the wart becomes very red (or redness spreads around the wart or red streaks appear), irritated or sore, or if it begins draining fluid. Also report any numbness or tingling around the site or if more warts begin to appear.
- Wash hands after using this product.
- Keep out of the reach of children.

FREEZING PRODUCTS

▶ **Actions**

Freezing kills both the virus and the infected site. When the applicator is pressed on the wart, freezing begins within a few seconds and the skin turns white. As a result of freezing, a blister may form under the wart within a few days. The frozen skin with the treated wart falls off after about 10 to 14 days. In the meantime, new healthy skin forms under the blister.

▶ **Indications**

For removing common and plantar warts.

▶ **Contraindications**

Hypersensitivity to the products; children younger than 4 years of age; diabetic patients, and patients with poor blood circulation; use on areas with thin skin, such as the face, armpits, breasts, buttocks, or genitals; use on moles, birthmarks, or warts with hair growing from them, genital warts, or warts on the face or mucous membranes; use on irritated skin, or on any area that is infected, reddened or showing any signs of inflammation, such as itching or swelling.

▶ **Warnings**

For external use only: Avoid contact with eyes, eyelids, mucous membranes, and normal skin surrounding warts. If contact with eyes or mucous membranes occurs, immediately flush with tap water for 15 minutes. Use only in well-ventilated areas. The treated area may be sensitive for a few days. Avoid inhaling vapors.

Pregnancy: Category X. Do not use if you are pregnant.

Lactation: Do not use if you are breastfeeding.

▶ **Adverse Reactions**

A stinging, itching, aching feeling may occur during and after freezing that quickly decreases after the area thaws for common warts. For plantar warts, the feeling may last 24 hours after the area thaws. If the aching or stinging feeling continues beyond 3 hours for common warts and 24 hours for plantar warts, see a physician.

Blistering; changes in skin coloring from white to red; possible changes in skin pigmentation.

► **Administration and Dosage**

For specific instructions for use of these products, refer to individual product labeling.

Before application, plantar warts may be soaked in warm water for 5 minutes, dried thoroughly, and the area filed with an emery board.

Only 1 treatment is necessary in most cases for each common wart. Common warts usually are gone 2 weeks after treatment. Plantar warts may require more than 1 treatment. If a wart or part of it is still there 2 weeks after treatment, you may then safely treat it again. Do not treat each wart for more than 4 times total. If 4 treatments have not removed the wart, ask a doctor and do not treat additional warts. Do not apply with any other method of wart removal because it is uncertain how the combination may affect your skin. Combination usage may result in serious burns and permanent scarring of the skin.

If there is more than 1 wart on a finger or toe, only treat 1 wart at a time. Do not begin treatment of another wart until 2 weeks after the final treatment of the previous wart.

Storage/stability: Highly flammable; keep away from fire or flame. Store at room temperature away from heat.

FREEZING PRODUCTS	
Trade name	**Doseform**
Dr. Scholl's Freeze Away, Wartner	**Aerosol spray**: Dimethyl ether and propane

Products listed are representative of currently available and widely distributed brands. Similar products, including regional and private label brands, may also exist.

PATIENT INFORMATION

Freezing Products

- Use these products only if you are sure the skin condition is a common or plantar wart.
- For external use only. Avoid contact with the eyes, eyelids, genitals, mucous membranes, and normal skin surrounding the lesion. Contact with the eyes may cause blindness. Do not rub or touch the eyes with your hands if applied to the hands. If the product gets into the eyes, flush with water for 15 minutes and get medical help immediately.
- Do not use if you have diabetes or poor blood circulation.
- Do not use on irritated skin or any area that is reddened or infected.
- Do not swallow or inhale. Contents are toxic and may cause serious internal damage.
- Do not use if you are pregnant or breastfeeding.
- Wash your hands after using this product.
- Keep out of the reach of children.
- Store at room temperature and away from heat.

SUPERFICIAL WOUND CARE
(Cuts & Abrasions)

DEFINITION

An *abrasion* is an acute, superficial wound that involves the scraping away of a portion of the epidermis. In some instances, it may not involve loss of any skin layers and consists primarily of reddened, unbroken skin. A *puncture* wound involves penetration of the epidermis, dermis, and potentially deeper tissue. A *laceration* refers to a linear cut involving the same potential layers as a puncture.

ETIOLOGY

A rubbing or friction injury to the epidermal portion of the skin results in an abrasion, which can extend to the uppermost layer of the dermis. Punctures and lacerations result from a foreign body or instrument that has pierced or cut the skin, respectively.

INCIDENCE

Approximately 25 million people are afflicted with various acute and chronic wounds in need of intervention each year. Nearly 10 million wounds are treated in the emergency department annually. Annual worldwide expenditure on wound care is estimated to be approximately $7 billion.

PATHOPHYSIOLOGY

Within minutes of injury, surface wounds begin the repair process. Wound healing consists of 3 overlapping stages:

- inflammatory
- proliferative
- remodeling

Inflammatory phase, which lasts approximately 3 to 4 days, is the body's immediate response to injury. During this phase, hemostasis and subsequent inflammation prepare the wound for tissue development. Intense vasoconstriction, platelet aggregation, and activation of the clotting cascade prevent blood loss during the first few minutes after injury. Once hemostasis is reached, polymorphonuclear neutrophil (PMN) leukocytes absorb or engulf most of the bacteria or debris in the wound, marking the beginning of the acute inflammatory stage. Macrophages function as phagocytes, releasing growth factors to stimulate epithelial mitogenesis and endothelial angiogenesis. The final portion of the inflammatory phase involves the migration of new epithelial cells over the denuded area of the wound, providing a one-cell-thick layer of new skin for the wound.

The **proliferative** phase, beginning approximately 3 days after the injury and lasting approximately 3 weeks, involves the formation of a granulation tissue layer. Granulation tissue is comprised of new connective tissue (fibroblast and collagen), capillaries, and inflammatory cells. Epithelial cells, which have moved to the top layer of the skin, begin to fill in the wound. Wound contraction, which involves the mobilization and pulling together of the wound, is completed by the smooth muscle cells.

The last (and longest) repair phase is **remodeling**, which occurs when the wound is completely closed by connective tissue and resurfaced by epithelial cells. This phase usually begins at approximately week 3 and may continue for up to 2 years. In remodeling, collagen synthesis and breakdown replaces the existing weak collagen with high-tensile strength collagen, resulting in a scar. Such scars typically have approximately 75% of the strength of the original skin.

SIGNS/SYMPTOMS

Symptoms may include pain, burning, and itching in and around the wound bed. Signs may include bleeding, erythema, edema, drainage, and induration in the affected area. Any change in the color and texture of the wound bed, as indicated by increased edema, erythema, and odorous or purulent drainage, may signify an infection of the wound. Fever, flu-like symptoms, and leukocytosis are frequently associated with systemic infections.

DIAGNOSTIC PARAMETERS/PHYSICAL ASSESSMENT

Clinical Observation: Baseline and ongoing evaluation of the following wound characteristics are critical in determining whether the current wound management is effective or a prompt referral for physician evaluation is indicated.

- Wound color:
    red - healthy and healing
    yellow - infected
    black - necrotic
- Wound size and depth
- Condition of wound margins and surrounding skin
- Presence of foreign materials or necrotic tissue
- Amount and type of exudate (purulent, odorous)
- Peripheral tissue edema or induration
- Anatomical location of wound

Interview: It is important to assess a patient's medical and physical status to identify any systemic factors that can affect the overall wound-healing process.

- Patient's overall nutritional status
- Patient's age and weight
- Coexisting diabetes mellitus or other acute or chronic medical condition
- Immunodeficiency
- Current medications

TREATMENT

Approaches to therapy: After performing an initial assessment of the wound, counsel the patient to do the following:

- Elevate the wound above the level of the heart to assist in pain relief and venous return. This should control any throbbing pain and slow bleeding and swelling.

- Clean any dirt from the wound with normal saline (if available) or mild soap and water. Mild soap and water are usually sufficient to clean minor wounds. Normal saline has quickly emerged as the "gold standard" for wound cleansing. Selection of and closure with an appropriate dressing are the final and critical steps in wound management. Most superficial wounds can be covered with a *Band-Aid* or other adhesive bandage.
- Use only properly diluted antiseptic solutions.
- Use an occlusive dressing that will completely cover the wound and will keep the wound site from drying out.
- Changing the dressing can remove layers of new skin, thereby delaying healing. Replace the occlusive dressing only if it no longer adheres to the skin, or if the wound is exposed to dirt.
- Pain can be relieved with OTC NSAIDs, acetaminophen, or salicylates.
- An unpleasant odor may indicate that the wound is infected. A tetanus shot may be needed. Consult a physician.

For optimal healing of more severe wounds, select a dressing with the following needs in mind:

- Control of excess exudate by absorption
- Maintenance of a moist wound environment
- Oxygen permeability
- Ease in removal without disrupting delicate new tissue
- Appropriate size and contour for the affected body part
- Comfort and convenience
- Cost-effectiveness

For minor wounds, consider the various features of the bandages in recommendations for patients:

- *Contour* - Consider high-stretch flexible fabric that conforms to the skin despite flexing or friction.
- *Size* - Select an appropriate size and shape to adequately protect the wound bed.
- *Allergenicity* - Consider hypo-allergenic adhesive closure in sensitive patients.
- *Medicated bandages* - Some products contain a benzalkonium chloride pad that claims to "kill germs and prevent infection." In selecting these products, it is important to evaluate whether application of the antiseptic agent is even necessary if a wound has been adequately cleansed. In addition, consider the cost-effectiveness and the actual clinical efficacy of these products.

Pharmacotherapy: To help prevent superficial skin infection in minor cuts and scrapes, topical nonprescription antibiotics and antiseptic preparations can be useful but may not be necessary. Puncture wounds or other more serious or deeper tissue infections may require prescription-strength antibiotics (either topical or systemic) and should be assessed by a physician.

ANTISEPTIC PREPARATIONS
▶ **Indications**
The goal of wound cleansing or antisepsis is to remove necrotic tissue, excess wound exudate, dressing residue, and metabolic waste from the wound surface with as little chemical and mechanical trauma as possible. In general, normal saline is considered to

be the "gold standard" for wound cleansing. Antiseptic agents may not be necessary in most superficial, clean wounds and should not be used on healthy granulating tissue because of their toxicity.

Active Ingredient	Actions	Indications
Benzalkonium chloride	Cationic surfactant with antimicrobial effects on gram-positive and gram-negative bacteria but not on spores. The antimicrobial activity may involve the disruption of cell membranes and denaturation of lipoprotein of microbes.	First-aid antiseptic
Camphorated compounds	Antibacterial agent.	First-aid antiseptic
Chlorhexidine gluconate	Antimicrobial effects against gram-positive and gram-negative bacteria, such as *Pseudomonas aeruginosa*.	Skin wound cleanser
Hydrogen peroxide	Antimicrobial oxidizing agent. When hydrogen peroxide comes in contact with blood and tissue fluids, oxygen is enzymatically released, which has a physical cleansing effect on a wound. The duration of action is only as long as the period of active oxygen release (fizzing).	First-aid antiseptic and wound cleanser
Iodine	Broad antimicrobial spectrum against bacteria, fungi, virus, spores, protozoa, and yeast.	First-aid antiseptic pre-op skin preparation. 2% iodine and 2.5% sodium iodide are used as antiseptics for superficial wounds. Do not use strong iodine solution (*Lugol's*) as an antiseptic.
Isopropyl alcohol	Stronger bactericidal activity and lower surface tension than ethanol.	First-aid antiseptic
Phenolic compounds	Bacteriostatic at low concentration and bactericidal and fungicidal at higher concentrations.	First-aid antiseptic
Povidone-iodine	Less potent bactericidal activity than iodine.	First-aid antiseptic and skin cleanser
Sodium hypochlorite	Germicidal agent effective against vegetative bacteria, viruses, and, to some degree, against spores and fungi.	Skin antiseptic
Triclosan	Bacteriostatic agent with activity against gram-positive and gram-negative bacteria.	Skin disinfectant

► Contraindications

In general, hypersensitivity to the active antiseptic ingredient listed.

► Warnings

In general, antiseptic agents are to be applied to intact skin surrounding the wound because direct application of antiseptics to the wound bed can cause tissue irritation.

BENZALKONIUM CHLORIDE

► Actions

Benzalkonium chloride (BAC), a cationic surface-active agent, is also a rapidly acting anti-infective agent with a moderately long duration of action. It is active against bacteria and some viruses, fungi, and protozoa at proper concentrations. Bacterial spores are resistant. Solutions are bacteriostatic or bactericidal according to their concentration. The exact mechanism of bactericidal action is unknown but may be due to enzyme inactivation. Solutions also have deodorant, wetting, detergent, keratolytic, and emulsifying activities.

▶ Indications

Aqueous solutions in appropriate dilutions: Antisepsis of skin, mucous membranes, and wounds; treatment of wounds.

Tinctures and sprays: Treatment of minor skin wounds and abrasions.

▶ Contraindications

Do not use in occlusive dressings, casts, and anal or vaginal packs because irritation or chemical burns may result.

▶ Warnings

Diluents: Use sterile water for injection as a diluent for aqueous solutions intended for deep wounds. Otherwise, use freshly distilled water. Tap water containing metallic ions and organic matter may reduce antibacterial potency. Do not use resin deionized water because it may contain pathogenic bacteria.

Storage: Organic, inorganic, and synthetic materials and surfaces may adsorb sufficient quantities to significantly reduce the antibacterial potency in solutions, resulting in serious contamination of solutions with viable pathogenic bacteria. Do not use corks to stopper bottles containing BAC solution. Do not store cotton, wool, rayon, or other materials in solutions. Use sterile gauze sponges and fiber pledgets to apply solutions to the skin, and store in separate containers; immerse in BAC solutions immediately prior to application.

Soaps: BAC solutions are inactivated by soaps and anionic detergents; therefore, rinse thoroughly if these agents are employed prior to BAC use.

Sterilization: Do not rely on antiseptic solutions to achieve complete sterilization; they do not destroy bacterial spores and certain viruses, including the etiologic agent of infectious hepatitis, and may not destroy *Mycobacterium tuberculosis* and other bacteria. In addition, when applied to the skin, BAC may form a film under which bacteria remain viable.

Flammable solvents: The tinted tincture and spray contain flammable organic solvents; do not use near an open flame or cautery.

Eyes/Mucous membranes: If solutions stronger than 1:3000 enter the eyes, irrigate immediately and repeatedly with water; obtain medical attention promptly. Do not use concentrations over 1:5000 on mucous membranes, except the vaginal mucosa (see recommended dilutions). Keep the tinted tincture and spray, which contain irritating organic solvents, away from the eyes or other mucous membranes.

Inflamed/Irritated tissues: Solutions used must be more dilute than those used on normal tissues (see recommended dilutions).

▶ Adverse Reactions

Solutions in normal concentrations have low systemic and local toxicity and are generally well tolerated, although a rare individual may exhibit hypersensitivity.

▶ Overdosage

(Systemic—via accidental ingestion/poisoning):

Symptoms – Marked local GI tract irritation (eg, nausea, vomiting) may occur after ingestion. Signs of systemic toxicity include restlessness, apprehension, weakness, confusion, dyspnea, cyanosis, collapse, convulsions, and coma. Death occurs as a result of respiratory muscle paralysis.

Treatment – Immediately administer several glasses of mild soap solution, milk, or egg whites beaten in water. This may be followed by gastric lavage with a mild soap solution. Avoid alcohol as it promotes absorption. Contact a Poison Control Center immediately.

To support respiration, clear airway and administer oxygen; employ artificial respiration if necessary. If convulsions occur, a short-acting parenteral barbiturate may be given with caution.

▶ Administration and Dosage

Thoroughly rinse anionic detergents and soaps from the skin or other areas prior to use of solutions because they reduce the antibacterial activity of BAC.

Incompatibilities: The following are incompatible with BAC solutions: iodine, silver nitrate, fluorescein, nitrates, peroxide, lanolin, potassium permanganate, aluminum, kaolin, pine oil, zinc sulfate, zinc oxide, yellow oxide of mercury.

Recommended dilutions for specific applications of BAC solutions:

Deeply infected wounds – 1:3000 to 1:20,000 aqueous solution.

Denuded skin and mucous membranes – 1:5000 to 1:10,000 aqueous solution.

Minor wounds/lacerations – 1:750 tincture or spray.

Oozing and open infections – 1:2000 to 1:5000 aqueous solution.

Wet dressings – Less than 1:5000 aqueous solution.

Clean the affected area and apply a thin layer 1 to 3 times daily. Cover with sterile bandage if desired. Do not use for longer than 1 week.

BENZALKONIUM CHLORIDE PRODUCTS	
Trade name	**Doseform**
Benza	**Solution:** 0.13%
Zephiran	**Solution, aqueous:** 1:750
Bactine	**Liquid:** 0.13% with 2.5% lidocaine. EDTA.
Benza	**Tincture:** 0.13%, 10% alcohol
Bactine	**Spray:** 0.13% with 2.5% lidocaine. EDTA.
Gold Bond First Aid Antiseptic	**Spray:** 0.13% with 1% menthol
Medi-Quik	**Spray:** 0.135% with 2% lidocaine
Band-Aid	**Foam:** 0.13%
Bactine	**Wipes:** 0.13% with 1% pramoxine HCl. EDTA.
Gold Bond First Aid Antiseptic	**Wipes:** 0.13% with 1% menthol

Products listed are representative of currently available and widely distributed brands. Similar products, including regional and private label brands, may also exist.

PATIENT INFORMATION
Benzalkonium Chloride

- Doses and frequency of use depend on the condition, the area to be treated, individual tolerance, and doseform. Individual products should be reviewed for their use and dosage guidelines. Consult your doctor or pharmacist for product-specific information.
- For external use only. Avoid contact with eyes. If contact occurs, immediately flush with water.
- Do not apply over large areas of the body or in large quantities.
- Do not apply over raw surfaces or blistered areas.
- Consult your doctor before use if you have deep or puncture wounds, animal bites, or serious burns.
- Do not use for longer than 1 week, unless directed by your doctor.
- Stop use and consult your doctor if conditions worsen or if symptoms persist for more than 7 days or clear up and occur again within a few days.
- Discontinue use and consult your doctor if redness, irritation, swelling, or pain increases.
- Benzalkonium chloride's effects are deactivated by soap.
- Clean the affected area and apply a thin layer 1 to 3 times daily. Cover with sterile bandage if desired.

CAMPHORATED COMPOUNDS

▶ Warnings
Apply to dry skin only; may have caustic effects if applied to moist areas.

▶ Administration and Dosage
Clean the affected area before applying. Apply with cotton 1 to 3 times daily.

CAMPHORATED COMPOUNDS	
Trade name	Doseform
Campho-phenique Pain Relieving Antiseptic	**Liquid**: 10.8% camphor, 4.7% phenol. Eucalyptus oil, light mineral oil.
	Gel: 10.8% camphor, 4.7% phenol. Eucalyptus oil, glycerin, light mineral oil.

Products listed are representative of currently available and widely distributed brands. Similar products, including regional and private label brands, may also exist.

PATIENT INFORMATION
Camphorated Compounds

- Doses and frequency of use depend on the condition, the area to be treated, individual tolerance, and doseform. Individual products should be reviewed for their use and dosage guidelines. Consult your doctor or pharmacist for product-specific information.
- For external use only. Avoid contact with eyes. If contact occurs, immediately flush with water.
- Do not apply over large areas of the body or in large quantities.
- Consult your doctor before use if you have deep or puncture wounds, animal bites, or serious burns.
- Do not use for longer than 1 week, unless directed by your doctor.
- Stop use and consult your doctor if conditions worsen or if symptoms persist for more than 7 days or clear up and occur again within a few days.
- Discontinue use and consult your doctor if redness, irritation, swelling, or pain increases.
- Clean the affected area and apply liquid with cotton 1 to 3 times daily.
- Do not bandage.
- In case of accidental ingestion, contact your doctor or the Poison Control Center immediately.

CHLORHEXIDINE GLUCONATE

▶ **Actions**

Provides an antimicrobial effect against a wide range of microorganisms, including gram-positive and gram-negative bacteria such as *Pseudomonas aeruginosa*.

▶ **Indications**

Skin wound cleanser.

▶ **Contraindications**

Hypersensitivity to chlorhexidine gluconate or any component of the product.

▶ **Warnings**

There have been several case reports of anaphylaxis following disinfection with 0.05% to 1% chlorhexidine. Symptoms included generalized urticaria, bronchospasm, cough, dyspnea, wheezing, and malaise. Symptoms resolved following therapy with various agents including oxygen, aminophylline, epinephrine, corticosteroids, or antihistamines. Refer to Management of Acute Hypersensitivity Reactions.

For external use only: Keep out of eyes, ears, and mouth; if this accidentally occurs, rinse out promptly and thoroughly with water. Do not use as a preoperative skin preparation of the face or head (except *Hibiclens* liquid).

Excessive heat: Avoid exposing the drug to excessive heat (higher than 40°C [104°F]).

Routine use: Do not use routinely on wounds involving more than superficial layers of skin or for repeated general skin cleansing of large body areas, except in those patients whose underlying condition makes it necessary to reduce the bacterial population of the skin.

Deafness: May cause deafness when instilled in the middle ear. Take particular care in the presence of a perforated eardrum to prevent exposure of inner ear tissues.

Lactation: In one case report, a mother sprayed chlorhexidine gluconate on her breasts to prevent mastitis. Her 2-day-old infant developed bradycardia episodes after breastfeeding; symptoms resolved when the topical chlorhexidine was discontinued by the mother.

▶ **Adverse Reactions**

Irritation; dermatitis; photosensitivity (rare); deafness (see Warnings). Sensitization and generalized allergic reactions have occurred, especially in the genital areas. If adverse reactions occur, discontinue use immediately. If severe, contact a physician.

▶ **Administration and Dosage**

Skin wound and general skin cleanser: Rinse affected area thoroughly with water. Apply a sufficient amount to cover skin or wound area and wash gently. Rinse again thoroughly.

CHLORHEXIDINE GLUCONATE PRODUCTS	
Trade name	Doseform
Dyna-Hex 2	**Liquid:** 2%. 4% isopropyl alcohol.
Operand	**Liquid:** 4%
Betasept, Dyna-Hex, Hibiclens	**Liquid:** 4%. 4% isopropyl alcohol.
Hibistat Germicidal Hand Rinse	**Rinse:** 0.5%. 70% isopropyl alcohol.
Hibistat	**Wipes:** 0.5%. 70% isopropyl alcohol.

Products listed are representative of currently available and widely distributed brands. Similar products, including regional and private label brands, may also exist.

PATIENT INFORMATION
Chlorhexidine Gluconate

- Doses and frequency of use depend on the condition, the area to be treated, individual tolerance, and doseform. Individual products should be reviewed for their use and dosage guidelines. Consult your doctor or pharmacist for product-specific information.
- For external use only. Avoid contact with eyes, ears, and mouth, or mucous membranes. If contact occurs, immediately flush with water.
- Consult your doctor before use if you have deep or puncture wounds, animal bites, or serious burns.
- Discontinue use and consult your doctor if redness, irritation, swelling, or pain increases.
- In case of accidental ingestion, contact your doctor or the Poison Control Center immediately.

HYDROGEN PEROXIDE

▶ **Warnings**

Do not use in abscesses, and do not apply bandages before the compound dries.

▶ **Adverse Reactions**

Generally safe, nonirritating, and noncorrosive.

▶ **Administration and Dosage**

Use on intact skin is of minimal value because the release of nascent oxygen is too slow. Do not use in abscesses. Do not apply bandages before the compound dries.

HYDROGEN PEROXIDE PRODUCTS	
Trade name	**Doseform**
Hydrogen Peroxide	**Solution**: 3%

Products listed are representative of currently available and widely distributed brands. Similar products, including regional and private label brands, may also exist.

PATIENT INFORMATION

Hydrogen Peroxide

- Doses and frequency of use depend on the condition, the area to be treated, individual tolerance, and doseform. Individual products should be reviewed for their use and dosage guidelines. Consult your doctor or pharmacist for product-specific information.
- For external use only. Avoid contact with eyes. If contact occurs, immediately flush with water.
- Do not apply over large areas of the body or in large quantities.
- Consult your doctor before use if you have deep or puncture wounds, animal bites, or serious burns.
- Do not use for longer than 1 week, unless directed by your doctor.
- Stop use and consult your doctor if conditions worsen or if symptoms persist for more than 7 days or clear up and occur again within a few days.
- Discontinue use and consult your doctor if redness, irritation, swelling, fever, or pain develop.
- In case of accidental ingestion, contact your doctor or the Poison Control Center immediately.
- Clean the affected area and apply a thin layer 1 to 3 times daily. Cover with sterile bandage if desired.

IODINE

▶ **Indications**

Iodine preparations are used externally for their broad microbicidal spectrum against bacteria, fungi, viruses, spores, protozoa, and yeasts. Iodine may be used to disinfect intact skin preoperatively. Potassium iodide is added to increase the solubility of the iodine. Sodium iodide is present to stabilize the tincture and make it miscible with water in all proportions.

▶ **Contraindications**

Hypersensitivity to iodine.

▶ **Warnings**

For external use only: Avoid contact with the eyes and mucous membranes.

Highly toxic: Highly toxic if ingested. Sodium thiosulfate is the most effective chemical antidote.

Staining: Iodine preparations stain skin and clothing.

Occlusive dressings: Do not use with occlusive dressings or bandages.

▶ **Adverse Reactions**

Iodine tincture may be irritating to the tissue.

▶ **Administration and Dosage**

Do not use with occlusive dressing or bandages.

IODINE PRODUCTS	
Trade name	Doseform
Mild Iodine Tincture	**Solution:** 2% iodine and 2.4% sodium iodide in 47% alcohol, purified water
Strong Iodine Tincture	**Solution:** 7% iodine and 5% potassium iodide in 85% alcohol

Products listed are representative of currently available and widely distributed brands. Similar products, including regional and private label brands, may also exist.

PATIENT INFORMATION
Iodine

- Doses and frequency of use depend on the condition, the area to be treated, individual tolerance, and doseform. Individual products should be reviewed for their use and dosage guidelines. Consult your doctor or pharmacist for product-specific information.
- For external use only. Avoid contact with eyes or mucous membranes. If contact occurs, immediately flush with water.
- Do not apply over large areas of the body or in large quantities.
- Consult your doctor before use if you have deep or puncture wounds, animal bites, or serious burns.
- Do not use for longer than 1 week, unless directed by your doctor.
- Stop use and consult your doctor if conditions worsen or if symptoms persist for more than 7 days or clear up and occur again within a few days.
- Discontinue use and consult your doctor if redness, irritation, swelling, or pain develop.
- In case of accidental ingestion, contact your doctor or the Poison Control Center immediately.
- Highly toxic if ingested.
- May stain skin and clothing or fabrics.
- Use only in well-ventilated areas. Fumes may be harmful.
- Clean the affected area and apply a thin layer 1 to 3 times daily. Do not use with tight-fitting dressings.

ISOPROPYL ALCOHOL

▶ Warnings

Flammable; keep away from fire or flame.

▶ Adverse Reactions

Greater potential for drying the skin than alcohol.

▶ Administration and Dosage

May apply on intact skin 1 to 3 times daily.

ISOPROPYL ALCOHOL PRODUCTS	
Trade name	Doseform
Isopropyl Alcohol	**Liquid:** 70% (typically)

Products listed are representative of currently available and widely distributed brands. Similar products, including regional and private label brands, may also exist.

PATIENT INFORMATION
Isopropyl Alcohol

- Doses and frequency of use depend on the condition, the area to be treated, individual tolerance, and doseform. Individual products should be reviewed for their use and dosage guidelines. Consult your doctor or pharmacist for product-specific information.
- For external use only. Avoid contact with eyes or mucous membranes. If contact occurs, immediately flush with water.
- Do not apply over large areas of the body or in large quantities.
- Consult your doctor before use if you have deep or puncture wounds, animal bites, or serious burns.
- Do not use for longer than 1 week, unless directed by your doctor.
- Stop use and consult your doctor if conditions worsen or if symptoms persist for more than 7 days or clear up and occur again within a few days.
- Discontinue use and consult your doctor if redness, irritation, swelling, or pain develop.
- In case of accidental ingestion, contact your doctor or the Poison Control Center immediately.
- Use only in well-ventilated areas. Fumes may be harmful.
- Clean the affected area and apply a thin layer 1 to 3 times daily. Cover with sterile bandage if desired.

PHENOLIC COMPOUNDS

▶ Warnings

May only be used on the skin as a keratolytic or chemical peel because, in aqueous solutions of more than 1%, it is a primary irritant.

▶ Adverse Reactions

In aqueous solutions of more than 1%, it is a primary irritant and should not be used on the skin except as a keratolytic or peeling agent.

▶ Administration and Dosage

Clean the affected area. Apply with cotton 1 to 3 times daily.

PHENOLIC COMPOUNDS	
Trade name	**Doseform**
Castellani Paint Modified	**Liquid**: 1.5% phenol. 13% SD alcohol 40B

Products listed are representative of currently available and widely distributed brands. Similar products, including regional and private label brands, may also exist.

■ ■ ■

PATIENT INFORMATION
Phenolic Compounds

- Doses and frequency of use depend on the condition, the area to be treated, individual tolerance, and doseform. Individual products should be reviewed for their use and dosage guidelines. Consult your doctor or pharmacist for product-specific information.
- For external use only. Avoid contact with eyes. If contact occurs, immediately flush with water.
- Do not apply over large areas of the body or in large quantities.
- Consult your doctor before use if you have deep or puncture wounds, animal bites, or serious burns.
- Do not use for longer than 1 week, unless directed by your doctor.
- Stop use and consult your doctor if conditions worsen or if symptoms persist for more than 7 days or clear up and occur again within a few days.
- Discontinue use and consult your doctor if redness, irritation, swelling, or pain develop.
- In case of accidental ingestion, contact your doctor or the Poison Control Center immediately.
- Cleanse affected area as directed. Check individual package labels for directions.
- May stain skin and clothing or fabrics.
- Clean the affected area and apply a thin layer 1 to 3 times daily. Do not bandage.

POVIDONE-IODINE

► Actions
Water soluble complex of iodine with povidone. Povidone-iodine contains 9% to 12% available iodine. It retains the bactericidal activity of iodine but is less potent, and therefore causes less irritation to skin and mucous membranes.

► Warnings
Hypothyroidism: A 6-week-old infant developed low serum total thyroxine concentration and high thyroid stimulating hormone concentration following maternal use of topical povidone-iodine during pregnancy and lactation. In 1 study, the use of povidone-iodine solution on very-low birthweight infants resulted in neonatal hypothyroidism. In contrast, women who used povidone-iodine douche daily for 14 days did not develop overt hypothyroidism; however, there was a significant increase in serum total iodine concentration and urine iodine excretion. Use with caution during pregnancy and lactation and in infants.

Open wounds: Avoid solutions containing a detergent if treating open wounds with povidone-iodine. The value of povidone-iodine on open wounds has not been established.

► Adverse Reactions
Hypothyroidism may develop when used to treat large wounds in patients with abnormal renal function. May cause a hypersensitivity reaction.

► Administration and Dosage
Unlike iodine tincture, treated areas may be bandaged.

POVIDONE-IODINE PRODUCTS	
Trade name	Doseform
Betadine, Efodine	Ointment: 10%
Povidone-Iodine, Operand	Solution: 10%
Betadine, Minidyne	Solution: 10%. Dibasic sodium phosphate, glycerin.
Betadine	Solution, swab aid: 10%. Dibasic sodium phosphate, glycerin.
Betadine	Solution, swabsticks: 10%. Dibasic sodium phosphate, glycerin.
Betadine	Solution, prepstick: 10%
Betadine	Solution, prepstick plus: 10%. Alcohol.
Operand	Gel: 10%
Betadine	Aerosol: 5%. Dibasic sodium phosphate, glycerin.
Operand	Douche: 10%
Betadine	Skin cleanser: 7.5%
Operand	Whirlpool concentrate: 10%
Operand	Periwash kit: 10%
Operand	Scrub: 7.5%

Products listed are representative of currently available and widely distributed brands. Similar products, including regional and private label brands, may also exist.

PATIENT INFORMATION
Povidone-Iodine

- Doses and frequency of use depend on the condition, the area to be treated, individual tolerance, and doseform. Individual products should be reviewed for their use and dosage guidelines. Consult your doctor or pharmacist for product-specific information.
- For external use only. Avoid contact with eyes or mucous membranes. If contact occurs, immediately flush with water.
- Do not apply over large areas of the body or in large quantities.
- Consult your doctor before use if you have deep or puncture wounds, animal bites, or serious burns.
- Do not use for longer than 1 week, unless directed by your doctor.
- Stop use and consult your doctor if conditions worsen or if symptoms persist for more than 7 days or clear up and occur again within a few days.
- Discontinue use and consult your doctor if redness, irritation, swelling, or pain increases.
- In case of accidental ingestion, contact your doctor or the Poison Control Center immediately.
- Clean the affected area and apply a thin layer 1 to 3 times daily. Cover with sterile bandage if desired.

SODIUM HYPOCHLORITE

▶ **Actions**

Sodium hypochlorite has germicidal, deodorizing, and bleaching properties. It is effective against vegetative bacteria and viruses and, to some degree, against spores and fungi.

► **Indications**

Applied topically to the skin as an antiseptic.

► **Warnings**

Avoid eye contact with this solution. Use with caution as chemical burns may be produced.

Chemical burns: Chemical burns may be produced; avoid eye contact with this solution.

► **Administration and Dosage**

Administer as lavage solution for wounds.

SODIUM HYPOCHLORITE PRODUCTS	
Trade name	Doseform
Dakin's Half Strength	**Solution:** 0.25%
Dakin's Full Strength	**Solution:** 0.5%

Products listed are representative of currently available and widely distributed brands. Similar products, including regional and private label brands, may also exist.

PATIENT INFORMATION

Sodium Hypochlorite

- Doses and frequency of use depend on the condition, the area to be treated, individual tolerance, and doseform. Individual products should be reviewed for their use and dosage guidelines. Consult your doctor or pharmacist for product-specific information.
- For external use only. Avoid contact with eyes or mucous membranes. Chemical burns may be produced. If contact occurs, immediately flush with water.
- Do not apply over large areas of the body or in large quantities.
- Consult your doctor before use if you have deep or puncture wounds, animal bites, or serious burns.
- Do not use for longer than 1 week, unless directed by your doctor.
- Stop use and consult your doctor if conditions worsen or if symptoms persist for more than 7 days or clear up and occur again within a few days.
- Discontinue use and consult your doctor if redness, irritation, swelling, or pain increases.
- In case of accidental ingestion, contact your doctor or the Poison Control Center immediately.

TRICLOSAN

► **Actions**

Triclosan, a bis-phenol disinfectant, is a bacteriostatic agent with activity against a wide range of gram-positive and gram-negative bacteria.

► **Indications**

Skin cleanser. May use as hand/body wash, shampoo, or bed or towel bath.

► **Contraindications**

Use on burned or denuded skin or mucous membranes; routine prophylactic total body bathing.

Not a surgical scrub; do not use in preparation for surgery.

▶ **Warnings**

Septi-Soft is not a surgical scrub and should not be used in preparation for surgery. Avoid contact with the eyes.

For external use only: Avoid contact with the eyes.

▶ **Administration and Dosage**

Dispense a small amount (5 mL) on hands, rub thoroughly for 30 seconds, rinse thoroughly, and dry.

TRICLOSAN PRODUCTS	
Trade name	Doseform
Septi-Soft	Solution: 0.25%. Glycerin, emollients.

Products listed are representative of currently available and widely distributed brands. Similar products, including regional and private label brands, may also exist.

PATIENT INFORMATION
Triclosan

- Doses and frequency of use depend on the condition, the area to be treated, individual tolerance, and doseform. Individual products should be reviewed for their use and dosage guidelines. Consult your doctor or pharmacist for product-specific information.
- For external use only. Avoid contact with eyes or mucous membranes. If contact occurs, immediately flush with water.
- Do not apply over large areas of the body or in large quantities.
- Consult your doctor before use if you have deep or puncture wounds, animal bites, or serious burns.
- Do not use for longer than 1 week, unless directed by your doctor.
- Stop use and consult your doctor if conditions worsen or if symptoms persist for more than 7 days or clear up and occur again within a few days.
- Discontinue use and consult your doctor if redness, irritation, swelling, or pain increases.
- In case of accidental ingestion, contact your doctor or the Poison Control Center immediately.
- Dispense a small amount (5 mL) on hands, rub thoroughly for 30 seconds, rinse thoroughly, and dry.

FIRST-AID ANTIBIOTICS

▶ **Indications**

Infection in minor cuts, burns, wounds, and scrapes may be alleviated by topical OTC antibiotics (eg, tetracycline, bacitracin/neomycin/polymyxin B sulfate combination). The pharmacist should assess the wound and possible infection before recommending any topical product. Consider referral to a physician in the following situations:

- Uncertainty over cause of infection.
- Top layer of skin is missing from a large area.
- Wound continues to drain a large amount of exudate. Draining and pain are aided by lancing.
- Infection is widespread.
- Deep lesions cover a wide area of skin.

- Underlying illness (eg, diabetes, systemic infection, immune deficiency), which may predispose patients to serious abrasions.
- Unsuccessful initial attempt at treatment or worsened condition.

Active Ingredient	Actions	Indications
Bacitracin	Polypeptide bactericidal antibiotic that inhibits cell wall synthesis in several gram-positive organisms.	Help prevent infection in minor cuts, burns, wounds, and scrapes.
Neomycin	Aminoglycoside antibiotic that exerts its bacterial activity by inhibiting protein synthesis in gram-negative organisms and some species of *Staphylococcus*.	Help prevent infection in minor cuts, burns, wounds, and scrapes.
Polymyxin B Sulfate	Polypeptide antibiotic effective against several gram-negative organisms by altering cell wall permeability.	Help prevent infection in minor cuts, burns, wounds, and scrapes.

► **Contraindications**

Hypersensitivity to any of the listed ingredients. Do not use in eyes or in external ear canal if the eardrum is perforated.

► **Warnings**

For topical use only. Deeper cutaneous infections may require systemic antibiotic therapy in addition to local treatment. Because of the potential nephrotoxicity and ototoxicity of neomycin, use with care in treating extensive burns, trophic ulceration, or other extensive conditions where absorption is possible. Do not apply more than once daily in burn cases where more than 20% of body surface is affected, especially if the patient has impaired renal function or is receiving other aminoglycoside antibiotics concurrently. Chronic application of neomycin to inflamed skin of individuals with allergic contact dermatitis increases the possibility of sensitization.

Neomycin: Low-grade reddening with swelling, dry scaling, and itching, or a failure to heal are usually manifestations of this hypersensitivity. During long-term use of neomycin-containing products, perform periodic examinations and discontinue use if symptoms appear. These symptoms regress upon withdrawal of medication, but avoid neomycin-containing products thereafter.

Cross-sensitization: Sensitization is frequent, and patients may experience cross-reaction to gentamicin.

► **Drug Interactions**

None significant.

► **Adverse Reactions**

Bacitracin: Allergic contact dermatitis has been reported. Case reports of anaphylaxis.

Neomycin: Ototoxicity and nephrotoxicity have been reported with its use.

Polymyxin B sulfate: Rare sensitizer.

BACITRACIN

► **Administration and Dosage**

Clean the affected area and apply a thin layer 1 to 3 times daily. Cover with sterile bandage if desired. Do not use for longer than 1 week.

BACITRACIN PRODUCTS	
Trade name	Doseform
Bacitracin Zinc	**Ointment**: 500 units/g. White petrolatum.
Q-Tips Treat & Go	**Swabs**: 500 units/g. White petrolatum, mineral oil.

Products listed are representative of currently available and widely distributed brands. Similar products, including regional and private label brands, may also exist.

NEOMYCIN

▶ Administration and Dosage

Clean the affected area and apply a thin layer 1 to 3 times daily. Cover with sterile bandage if desired. Do not use for longer than 1 week.

NEOMYCIN PRODUCTS	
Trade name	Doseform
Neomycin	**Ointment**: 3.5 mg neomycin (as sulfate)/g

Products listed are representative of currently available and widely distributed brands. Similar products, including regional and private label brands, may also exist.

POLYMYXIN B SULFATE AND NEOMYCIN

▶ Administration and Dosage

Clean the affected area and apply a thin layer 1 to 3 times daily. Cover with sterile bandage if desired. Do not use for longer than 1 week.

POLYMYXIN B SULFATE/NEOMYCIN PRODUCTS	
Trade name	Doseform
Neosporin Plus Pain Relief	**Cream**: 10,000 units polymyxin B sulfate, 3.5 mg neomycin, 10 mg pramoxine/g. Methylparaben, mineral oil, white petrolatum.

Products listed are representative of currently available and widely distributed brands. Similar products, including regional and private label brands, may also exist.

POLYMYXIN B SULFATE AND BACITRACIN

▶ Administration and Dosage

Clean the affected area and apply a thin layer 1 to 3 times daily. Cover with sterile bandage if desired. Do not use for longer than 1 week.

POLYMYXIN B SULFATE/BACITRACIN PRODUCTS	
Trade name	Doseform
Betadine First Aid Antibiotics + Moisturizer	**Ointment**: 10,000 units polymyxin B sulfate, 500 units bacitracin/g
Polysporin	**Ointment**: 10,000 units polymyxin B sulfate, 500 units bacitracin/g. White petrolatum.
Betadine Plus First Aid Antibiotics + Pain Reliever	**Ointment**: 10,000 units polymyxin B sulfate, 500 units bacitracin, 1% pramoxine HCl/g

Products listed are representative of currently available and widely distributed brands. Similar products, including regional and private label brands, may also exist.

POLYMYXIN B SULFATE, NEOMYCIN, AND BACITRACIN

▶ Administration and Dosage

Clean the affected area and apply a thin layer 1 to 3 times daily. Cover with sterile bandage if desired. Do not use for longer than 1 week.

POLYMYXIN B SULFATE/NEOMYCIN/BACITRACIN PRODUCTS	
Trade name	Doseform
Triple Antibiotic	**Ointment:** 5000 units polymyxin B sulfate, 3.5 mg neomycin, 400 units bacitracin/g. White petrolatum.
Neosporin, Neosporin To Go	**Ointment:** 5000 units polymyxin B sulfate, 3.5 mg neomycin, 400 units bacitracin/g. White petrolatum, oils.
Maximum Strength Neosporin Plus	**Ointment:** 10,000 units polymyxin B sulfate, 3.5 mg neomycin, 500 units bacitracin, 40 mg lidocaine/g. White petrolatum.
Tri-Biozene, Neosporin Plus Pain Relief	**Ointment:** 10,000 units polymyxin B sulfate, 3.5 mg neomycin, 500 units bacitracin, 10 mg pramoxine HCl/g. White petrolatum.
Lanabiotic Ointment	**Ointment:** 10,000 units polymyxin B sulfate, 3.5 mg neomycin, 500 units bacitracin, 40 mg lidocaine/g. White petrolatum, mineral oil.
Bactine Pain Relieving Protective Antibiotic	**Ointment:** 10,000 units polymyxin B sulfate, 3.5 mg neomycin, 500 units bacitracin, 1% pramoxine hydrochloride/g. White petrolatum.

Products listed are representative of currently available and widely distributed brands. Similar products, including regional and private label brands, may also exist.

PATIENT INFORMATION

First-Aid Antibiotics

- Doses and frequency of use depend on the condition, the area to be treated, individual tolerance, and doseform. Individual products should be reviewed for their use and dosage guidelines. Consult your doctor or pharmacist for product-specific information.
- For external use only. Avoid contact with eyes or mucous membranes. If contact occurs, immediately flush with water.
- Do not apply over large areas of the body or in large quantities.
- Do not apply over raw surfaces or blistered areas.
- Consult your doctor before use if you have deep or puncture wounds, animal bites, or serious burns.
- Do not use for longer than 1 week, unless directed by your doctor.
- Stop use and consult your doctor if conditions worsen or if symptoms persist for more than 7 days or clear up and occur again within a few days.
- Discontinue use and consult your doctor if redness, irritation, swelling, or pain increases.
- In case of accidental ingestion, contact your doctor or the Poison Control Center immediately.
- Clean the affected area and apply a thin layer 1 to 3 times daily. Cover with sterile bandage if desired.

GI/GU
CONDITIONS

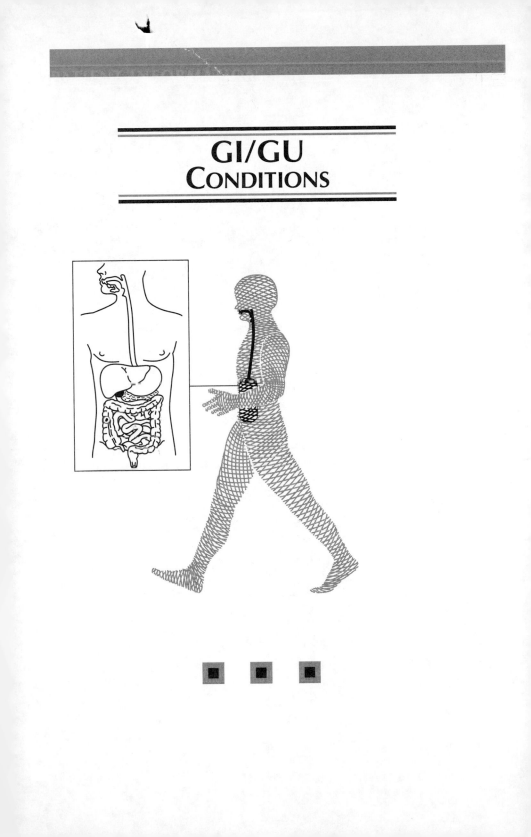

NONPRESCRIPTION DRUG THERAPY
TABLE OF CONTENTS

■ ■ ■

GI/GU CONDITIONS

INTRODUCTION

The gastrointestinal (GI) system consists of the GI tract (mouth, pharynx, esophagus, stomach, intestines, and rectum) and the secretory organs (liver, salivary glands, pancreas, and gall bladder). The GI tract facilitates the absorption of nutrients, water, and electrolytes. It also eliminates waste and kills microbes. Because numerous drugs are administered orally, the GI tract plays a very important role in drug absorption.

The stomach mixes, stores, and controls the emptying of food into the small intestine. It secretes acid (from the parietal cells) and proteolytic enzymes (pepsin) which aid in digestion. The acid also kills microbes ingested with food. Epithelial cells line the surface of the stomach and the duodenum. The mucus and bicarbonate secreted by these epithelial cells form the mucosal barrier which protects the stomach lining from the highly acidic environment. A breakdown in the mucosal barrier, due to drugs (eg, NSAIDs) or *H. pylori*, may lead to GI ulceration. Food is mixed with luminal contents and propelled through the GI tract by peristalsis. Peristalsis is the rhythmic contraction of smooth muscles along the GI tract. Disorders that affect the nervous system (eg, diabetes), drugs that slow GI motility (eg, opioids), low dietary fiber, and GI surgery retard GI motility. Infections and certain drugs (eg, antibiotics) may cause diarrhea.

Most absorption and digestion takes place in the small intestine. The small intestine is divided into 3 segments. The duodenum and jejunum are the first 2 segments, which is where most absorption occurs. The ileum is the longest segment and leads into the large intestine or colon.

In the colon, undigested materials are concentrated by the absorption of salt and water and acted upon by bacteria. The final product (feces) passes into the rectum and is excreted by defecation.

Numerous conditions directly affect the GI tract. Viral and bacterial infections, peptic ulcer disease (PUD), Zollinger-Ellison syndrome, stress ulcers, gastro-esophageal reflux disorder (GERD), ulcerative colitis, enzyme deficiencies (eg, lactase deficiency), and GI cancers are some of the more common conditions that affect the GI tract. Systemic illnesses such as diabetes and hypothyroidism also affect GI function. Ingestion of toxic substances (alcohol and tobacco) may increase the likelihood of developing ulcers. The effects of drugs on the GI tract should not be ignored. Chronic use of nonsteroidal anti-inflammatory drugs (NSAIDs) and systemic steroids also predispose patients to developing ulcers. NSAIDs can cause also acute GI injury. Other GI side effects of medications include diarrhea (eg, antibiotics, laxatives) and constipation (eg, verapamil, opioids). Apart from alcohol and tobacco, lifestyle factors such as diet, physical activity, and fluid intake also affect GI function. The elderly have a higher likelihood of having systemic illnesses and serious GI conditions. Practitioners should have a high level of suspicion when the elderly have frequent or severe GI complaints.

Diagnosis of GI conditions outside of a doctor's office is quite challenging. Because many GI conditions present with nonspecific symptoms, radiology or endoscopy is often needed to rule out serious pathology. However, obtaining a detailed medical, family, and social history could alert the practitioner to patients that need to be referred to a physician. In general, the elderly, patients with severe pain, systemic illnesses (eg, diabetes, hypothyroidism), significant weight loss, blood loss, fevers, and symptoms refractive to OTC therapy should be referred to a physician for further evaluation. Indeed, persistent GI complaints may be the first manifestation of serious pathology. Patients with symptoms that persist for longer than 2 weeks should also be referred to a physician. Inappropriate self-medication or duration of self-medication may mask symptoms of serious disease and prevent patients from seeking appropriate medical therapy.

Before recommending OTC therapy, practitioners should identify lifestyle factors that may cause or contribute to the observed symptoms. Current drug therapy should also be taken into consideration. In some instances, lifestyle modification or a change in drug therapy is all that may be needed. In recommending an OTC product, practitioners should consider the contraindications, side effects, drug interactions, cost, and the efficacy of each OTC agent. Patients should be adequately counseled on the appropriate use of these agents. They should also be made aware that some of these agents have not been adequately studied for some conditions for which they are commonly used. In addition, encourage patients to return for follow-up and to see a physician if symptoms persist or worsen.

Finally, GI complaints are common. Pharmacists can alleviate pain and suffering by appropriately referring patients and managing those conditions that may be amenable to self-treatment. Recognizing that the observed symptoms may be an adverse drug reaction could avoid a costly work-up, while correctly identifying conditions that are not suitable for OTC therapy could prevent serious complications. Patients do not always ask questions. The pharmacist should be proactive in counseling patients who purchase OTC products.

BOWEL PREPS

DEFINITION

Bowel preps are used to evacuate bowel contents prior to diagnostic procedures (eg, barium studies, flexible sigmoidoscopy, colonoscopy) and colonoscopic procedures.

Barium administration via nasogastric tube into the jejunum or by enema into the rectum facilitates radiologic study of small bowel diseases and certain colonic diseases. Barium is a useful diagnostic tool for the identification of diverticulosis, motility disturbances, displacement of colon by extrinsic lesions, loss of haustral markings in chronic ulcerative colitis, and intestinal fistulas.

The technique of flexible fiberoptic sigmoidoscopy makes it possible to examine the lower 40 to 60 cm of the colon. This range is important because approximately half of all colorectal neoplasms lie in the distal 50 cm of the bowel. A rectal carcinoma that can be missed on routine barium enema studies can be easily visualized and biopsied through the sigmoidoscope. In addition, sigmoidoscopy can easily detect early tissue changes associated with ulcerative colitis. Colonoscopy offers the same diagnostic advantages as sigmoidoscopy, but with colonoscopy, the entire length of the colon from cecum to anus can be examined. During sigmoidoscopy or colonoscopy, minor surgical procedures (eg, biopsy, polypectomy) may be done.

SIGNS/SYMPTOMS

The major clinical manifestations of bowel disease are motility disturbances or changes in bowel habit, abdominal pain and distention, and gastrointestinal (GI) or rectal bleeding. Decreased or increased bowel motility, or alternating between these two states, can occur with bowel disease. Abdominal pain can be poorly localized, intermittent, colicky, or visceral in nature, depending on the etiology of the disease.

GI bleeding caused by bowel disease may be detected as occult bleeding or, rarely, brisk hemorrhage. In general, bleeding from the stomach or small intestine results in black, tarry stools, whereas colonic and rectal bleeding usually presents as bright red blood or clots. The appearance of blood alone is insufficient for an accurate diagnosis. Any persistent change in bowel habit, abdominal pain, or rectal bleeding should be referred to a physician immediately.

TREATMENT

Approaches to therapy: The purpose of bowel prep use is to thoroughly cleanse the colon to remove debris and allow good GI tissue visualization and possible biopsy. Patients should strictly adhere to the bowel preparation regimen to avoid unsatisfactory visualization and the need to repeat the radiographic or endoscopic procedure.

Bowel preparation for sigmoidoscopy usually begins the day before the procedure, whereas preparation for colonoscopy and barium enema studies may require a few days. Bowel preparation often is individualized based on the patient's condition. Modified or minimum bowel cleansing is used in patients with inflammatory bowel disease, diarrhea of unknown cause, or GI bleeding to avoid adversely affecting the evaluation. The physician may have asked the patient to follow individualized instructions or to follow the written instructions of a particular bowel prep kit. The pharmacist should ask about the instructions given to the patient. The pharmacist also should ask when the GI procedure is scheduled to ensure that the patient has sufficient time to completely follow the bowel prep regimen.

Nondrug therapy: Dietary restrictions and high fluid intake are necessary for one to several days before the GI procedure. Specific dietary instructions may have been provided by the physician, or via written instructions in bowel prep products. Only clear liquids (eg, clear soups and gelatin) are allowed during the 18 to 24 hours before the procedure, and nothing is to be eaten at breakfast on the day of the procedure. Water, clear juices (eg, apple, white grape), carbonated and noncarbonated flavored drinks, and plain coffee or tea are considered clear liquids. Avoid grape juice, orange juice, or other pulp-containing juices. To ensure a high fluid intake, clear liquids are scheduled at specific times before the procedure.

Depending on the patient's condition and the procedure to be done, patients may need to stop iron supplements or drugs that decrease GI motility, such as anticholinergics or codeine. If biopsy or polypectomy is anticipated, the patient may need to stop antiplatelet drugs (eg, aspirin, nonsteroidal anti-inflammatory drugs [NSAIDs]) and anticoagulants. If the patient is taking any of these medications and has not been given instructions for them, the pharmacist should discuss these medications with the physician to determine if actions are required.

Pharmacotherapy: Oral and rectal laxatives may be used as bowel preps; both are generally included before colonoscopy or barium studies, but only one might be included before sigmoidoscopy. Oral electrolyte solutions for bowel cleansing also are available by prescription. Enemas often are given 1 to 2 hours before the procedure, and may be self-administered at home or administered by a physician. Some bowel prep kits include enemas for self-administration. Enemas may consist of tap water, saline, concentrated electrolyte solutions, or stimulant laxatives. Some patients may be instructed to use more than one enema.

LAXATIVES
▶ **Actions**

For a complete discussion of laxatives, refer to the Constipation monograph.

Osmotic laxatives usually contain magnesium citrate or sodium phosphate, and produce a hyperosmotic effect in the GI tract; the increased intraluminal pressure promotes evacuation. Also, magnesium stimulates the release of cholecystokinin, a hormone that increases bowel motility and fluid secretion. The onset of action is 0.5 to 3 hours when given orally; enemas containing sodium phosphate act quickly, usually within 2 to 15 minutes.

Stimulant laxatives, such as bisacodyl and senna, have a direct irritant effect on the colonic mucosa to promote evacuation. Onset of action ranges from 6 to 10 hours after oral administration. Bowel evacuation occurs within 0.25 to 1 hour after rectal suppositories, and within 20 minutes after enema preparations.

▶ Indications

For use as part of a bowel cleansing regimen to remove intestinal debris and prepare the colon for radiologic and endoscopic procedures. These agents have other labeled indications as well (see the Constipation monograph in the GI Conditions chapter).

▶ Contraindications

Hypersensitivity to any ingredient; nausea, vomiting, or other symptoms of appendicitis; fecal impaction; intestinal obstruction; undiagnosed abdominal pain.

Fleet Phospho-soda: Congenital megacolon; bowel obstruction; ascites; congestive heart failure (CHF); kidney disease; children younger than 5 years of age.

▶ Warnings

Bisacodyl tablets are enteric coated and should not be chewed or crushed.

Rectal bleeding or failure to have a bowel movement may indicate a serious medical problem, and the patient should inform the physician immediately.

Special risk patients: These products should not be used when abdominal pain, nausea, or vomiting is present. Sodium-containing laxatives should not be used in patients with megacolon, bowel obstruction, imperforate anus, or CHF. Caution is required in patients with borderline edema, CHF, hypertension, or in those on a sodium restricted diet. Use *Fleet Phospho-soda* with caution in patients with impaired renal function, heart disease, acute myocardial infarction, unstable angina, preexisting electrolyte disturbances, increased risk for electrolyte disturbances (eg, dehydration, GI obstruction, gastric retention, bowel perforation, colitis, inability to take adequate oral fluid, taking diuretics or other medications that affect electrolytes), debilitated patients, and who are taking medications known to prolong the QT interval. Do not give any other sodium phosphate preparations concomitantly with *Fleet Phospho-soda*.

Renal function impairment: Cautiously use products containing phosphate, sodium, potassium, or magnesium in patients with renal dysfunction to avoid hyperphosphatemia, hypernatremia, hypermagnesemia, acidosis, or hypocalcemia.

Pregnancy: Use only on the advice of a health care professional.

Lactation: Use only on the advice of a health care professional.

Children: Use in children younger than 6 years of age only on the advice of a health care professional.

▶ Drug Interactions

Avoid administration of milk, antacids, H_2 antagonists, or proton pump inhibitors 1 to 2 hours before bisacodyl tablets; coadministration may cause the enteric coating to dissolve, resulting in gastric lining irritation or dyspepsia.

▶ **Adverse Reactions**

Adverse reactions may include abdominal cramping, diarrhea, nausea, vomiting, perianal irritation, or fainting; and bloating, flatulence, or rectal burning may occur with enemas.

▶ **Administration and Dosage**

Follow directions in the package labeling and those provided by your health care practitioner exactly to ensure optimum results and to avoid repeat examination.

Most laxatives require dose adjustments for children 6 to 12 years of age and are not recommended for children younger than 6 years of age.

BISACODYL

▶ **Administration and Dosage**

Tablets: Bisacodyl tablets should be taken whole, not chewed or crushed, and not within 1 to 2 hours of antacids, milk, H_2 antagonists, or proton pump inhibitors.

Adults and children 12 years of age and older – 10 to 15 mg (usually 10) in a single dose once daily. Up to 30 mg has been used for preparation of lower GI tract for diagnostic or surgical procedures.

Children 6 to younger than 12 years of age – 5 mg once daily.

Suppositories and enemas: Suppositories and enemas act quickly. Encourage patients to retain suppositories for 15 to 20 minutes. Most suppositories exert a laxative effect within 15 to 60 minutes in adults. The onset of action may be much faster in children. Enemas may exert their laxative effect in less than 5 to 15 minutes. Refer to Appendix D, Administration Techniques, for administration guidelines.

Suppositories:

Adults – 10 mg once daily to induce bowel movement.

Children 6 to younger than 12 years of age – 5 mg once daily.

Enemas:

Adults and children 12 years of age and older – One bottle (as a single daily dose).

Children younger than 12 years of age – Do not use. Consult a physician.

BISACODYL PRODUCTS	
Trade name	**Doseform**
Veracolate	**Tablets, enteric coated**: 5 mg
Gentlax	**Tablets, enteric coated**: 5 mg. Sugar, sucrose.
Alophen, Stimulant Laxative	**Tablets, enteric coated**: 5 mg. Lactose, sugar.
Dulcolax	**Tablets, enteric coated**: 5 mg. Lactose, methylparaben, propylparaben, sucrose.
Correct-Tabs	**Tablets, delayed release**: 5 mg. Sugar.
Doxidan	**Tablets, delayed release**: 5 mg. Lactose, sugar, methylparaben, propylparaben, sucrose.
Bisacodyl Uniserts, Dulcolax	**Suppositories**: 10 mg
Fleet Bisacodyl	**Disposable enema**: 10 mg/30 mL

Products listed are representative of currently available and widely distributed brands. Similar products, including regional and private label brands, may also exist.

SALINE LAXATIVES

▶ Administration and Dosage

With all laxatives, it is wise to initiate dosing at the lower end of the dosage range. Increase subsequent doses if necessary. Dosing recommendations for individual products vary, but usual dosage ranges are as follows:

Magnesium citrate liquid:

> *Adults and children 12 years of age and older* – ½ to 1 full bottle (148 to 296 mL).

> *Children 6 to younger than 12 years of age* – ⅓ to ½ bottle (99 to 148 mL).

> *Children younger than 6 years of age* – Consult a physician.

Magnesium hydroxide liquid:

> *Adults and children 12 years of age and older* – 15 to 30 mL (concentrate) or 30 to 60 mL (regular), at bedtime or upon rising, followed by a full glass of liquid.

> *Children 6 to younger than 12 years of age* – 7.5 to 15 mL (concentrate) or 15 to 30 mL (regular), followed by a full glass of liquid. Do not use dosage cup.

> *Children 2 to 5 years of age* – 2.5 to 7.5 mL (concentrate) or 5 to 15 mL (regular), followed by a full glass of liquid. Do not use dosage cup.

> *Children younger than 2 years of age* – Consult a physician.

Magnesium hydroxide/mineral oil liquid:

> *Adults and children 12 years of age and older* – 30 to 60 mL at bedtime or upon rising, followed by a full glass of liquid.

> *Children 6 to 11 years of age* – 5 to 15 mL at bedtime or upon rising, followed by a full glass of liquid. Do not use dosage cup.

> *Children younger than 6 years of age* – Consult a physician.

Magnesium hydroxide chewable tablets:

> *Adults and children 12 years of age and older* – Chew 6 to 8 tablets, preferably before bedtime, followed by a full glass of water.

> *Children 6 to younger than 12 years of age* – Chew 3 to 4 tablets, preferably before bedtime, followed by a full glass of water.

> *Children 2 to 5 years of age* – Chew 1 to 2 tablets, preferably before bedtime, followed by a full glass of water.

> *Children younger than 2 years of age* – Consult a physician.

Monobasic sodium phosphate monohydrate/dibasic sodium phosphate heptahydrate solution:

> *Adults and children 12 years of age and older* – 20 to 45 mL.

> *Children 10 to 11 years of age* – 10 to 20 mL.

> *Children 5 to 9 years of age* – 5 to 10 mL.

> *Children younger than 5 years of age* – Do not use.

SALINE LAXATIVE PRODUCTS	
Trade name	Doseform
Phillips' Antacid/Laxative	**Tablets, chewable**: 311 mg magnesium hydroxide. Sucrose. Mint flavor.
Phillips' M-O Lubricant Laxative	**Liquid**: 300 mg magnesium hydroxide, 1.25 mL mineral oil/5 mL. Original and mint flavors.
Phillips' Milk of Magnesia	**Liquid**: 400 mg magnesium hydroxide/5 mL. Sorbitol, sugar (cherry formula). Original, mint, and cherry flavors.
Phillips' Milk of Magnesia Concentrated Laxative/Antacid	**Liquid**: 800 mg magnesium hydroxide/5 mL. Sorbitol, sugar. Strawberry creme flavor.
Fleet Phospho-soda	**Solution**: 2.4 g monobasic sodium phosphate monohydrate, 0.9 g dibasic sodium phosphate heptahydrate/5 mL. Unflavored and ginger-lemon flavors.
Magnesium Citrate	**Solution**: 1.745 g magnesium citrate/30 mL. Lemon flavor. Sugar free.

Products listed are representative of currently available and widely distributed brands. Similar products, including regional and private label brands, may also exist.

PATIENT INFORMATION

Laxatives (used as bowel preps)

- Carefully follow directions provided in package labeling or by your health care practitioner to ensure optimum results and avoid repeat examinations.
- Shake saline laxative solutions well before taking.
- Do not use in the presence of abdominal pain, nausea, or vomiting. Inform a physician of these symptoms.

MISCELLANEOUS BOWEL EVACUANTS

▶ Warnings

Children: Because bowel prep kit products are designed for adults, they are not recommended for children younger than 12 years of age. If used in children, dose adjustments may be required.

▶ Administration and Dosage

Follow directions in the package labeling and those provided by your health care practitioner exactly to ensure optimum results and to avoid repeat examination.

MISCELLANEOUS BOWEL EVACUANTS	
Trade name	Description
Tridrate Bowel Evacuant Kit	**Kit**: 300 mL *Tridate* solution: Magnesium citrate. 3 *Tridate* tablets: 5 mg bisacodyl. 1 *Tridate* suppository: 10 mg bisacodyl.
Evac-Q-Kwik	**Kit**: 300 mL *Evac-Q-Mag* solution: Magnesium citrate. Sugar free. Lemon flavor. 3 *Evac-Q-Tab* tablets: 5 mg bisacodyl. Lactose, sugar. 1 *Evaq-Q-Kwik* suppository: 10 mg bisacodyl.

MISCELLANEOUS BOWEL EVACUANTS	
Trade name	**Description**
X-Prep Bowel Evacuant Kit-1	**Kit**: 74 mL *X-Prep* liquid: Standardized senna concentrate, 130 mg sennosides. Parabens, sucrose. 2 *Senokot-S* tablets: 50 mg docusate sodium, standardized senna concentrate, 8.6 mg sennosides. Lactose. 1 *Rectolax* suppository: 10 mg bisacodyl.
X-Prep Bowel Evacuant Kit-2	**Kit**: 74 mL *X-Prep* liquid: Standardized senna concentrate, 130 mg sennosides. Parabens, sucrose. 1 packet (30 g) *Citralax* granules: 8 g magnesium citrate, 5.3 g magnesium sulfate (equal to 1.6 g magnesium/packet). Sucrose. 1 *Rectolax* suppository: 10 mg bisacodyl.
Fleet Prep Kit 1	**Kit**: 45 mL *Fleet Phospho-soda* solution: 21.6 g monobasic sodium phosphate, 8.1 g dibasic sodium phosphate. 4 *Fleet* enteric-coated tablets: 5 mg bisacodyl. 1 *Fleet* suppository: 10 mg bisacodyl.
Fleet Prep Kit 2	**Kit**: 45 mL *Fleet Phospho-soda* solution: 21.6 g monobasic sodium phosphate, 8.1 g dibasic sodium phosphate. 4 *Fleet* enteric-coated tablets: 5 mg bisacodyl. 1 *Fleet Bagenema* enema unit: 9 mL liquid castile soap.
Fleet Prep Kit 3	**Kit**: 45 mL *Fleet Phospho-soda* solution: 21.6 g monobasic sodium phosphate, 8.1 g dibasic sodium phosphate. 4 *Fleet* enteric-coated tablets: 5 mg bisacodyl. 1 *Fleet Bisacodyl* enema: 10 mg/30 mL bisacodyl.
Fleet Phospho-soda ACCU PREP	**Kit**: Six 15 mL bottles *Fleet Phospho soda* solution: 9.9 g dibasic sodium phosphate, monobasic sodium phosphate/15 mL. 4 *Fleet Pain-Relief Pre-Moistened Anorectal* pads: 1% pramoxine hydrochloride, 12% glycerin/pad. EDTA, menthol.

Products listed are representative of currently available and widely distributed brands. Similar products, including regional and private label brands, may also exist.

PATIENT INFORMATION

Bowel Preps

- Exact adherence (compliance) to instructions is critical for optimal results so that repeat examination is avoided. Instructions for some products have pictures accompanying the written text. Consult a physician or pharmacist regarding the proper use of oral bowel evacuants, suppositories, and enemas, which can easily be misused.
- Bowel preparations should be purchased well in advance of need so that there will be time to use the product correctly. If time guidelines are not adhered to, a recommendation to reschedule the test would be prudent.
- Abdominal cramping and other possible GI effects may occur. Kit instructions have explicit directions about proper use of the product, but few list adverse effects, so consult a pharmacist or physician. Higher doses, used for complete bowel evacuation, are more likely to cause adverse effects than usual laxative doses. Life-style adjustments may need to be made.

PATIENT INFORMATION (continued)

Bowel Preps (continued)

- Make certain to know exactly what constitutes a "light meal" and a "clear liquid." A light meal can include clear, fat-free soups; small portions of skinless chicken, turkey, or fish (not fried); white bread (no butter or mayonnaise); or plain *Jell-O*. Clear soups are chicken, beef, or vegetable bouillon. Clear fluids are transparent, and examples include apple juice, soft drinks, and plain coffee or tea. Avoid vegetables, fruit, nuts, fats, butter, milk, cheese, beef, pork, lamb, or whole grain cereals. Grape juice, orange juice, or other pulpy juices are not allowed. If in doubt about a certain food, contact a pharmacist or physician or avoid the food entirely.

- Make sure to have an accurate way to measure 8 oz of fluid. Pharmacists may provide an empty 8 oz prescription bottle. Patients can drink more, but not less, than recommended amounts. Drink the full amount of liquid at all required times, as instructed.

- If you have CHF or kidney impairment, make sure the prescribing physician, perhaps not the primary care physician, is aware of the medical condition. For example, magnesium citrate could be a better saline laxative than sodium phosphate in a patient with CHF, but sodium phosphate may be preferable in the renally impaired patient. An alternative product may be offered and the change justified by the pharmacist or physician.

- Keep in mind when bowel movement may occur (6 to 10 hours or overnight after oral tablets; within a few hours after an oral saline laxative; within an hour after a suppository; within 15 minutes after an enema). Know where toilet facilities are and remain close to toilets after the fast-acting preps.

- If the prep includes oral bisacodyl, the tablets are not to be chewed or crushed and should not be taken within 1 to 2 hours of drinking milk or taking antacids, H_2 antagonists, or proton pump inhibitors.

- If the prep includes a suppository, check to see that it is firm, not soft, and, if necessary, hold the wrapped suppository under cold water for 1 to 2 minutes until firm. Remove the wrapper and insert the suppository as far into the rectum as possible. An immediate urge to remove the suppository means that it was not inserted far enough. If possible, written material, including drawings, may be provided on proper insertion of suppositories (refer to Appendix D).

- If self-administering an enema, follow instructions carefully. Bisacodyl enemas require shaking. Remove the protective covering from the enema tip, carefully insert the enema tip without force, and remain close to the toilet. If possible, written material, including drawings, may be provided on proper use of enemas.

- If rectal bleeding occurs or a bowel movement does not occur, inform a physician immediately.

CONSTIPATION

DEFINITION

Constipation is an abnormally slow movement of feces through the large intestine (colon) and is generally associated with dry, hard feces in the descending branch of the colon. This typically results in infrequent or difficult evacuation and often is followed by a sense of incomplete evacuation.

Note: To place the definition of constipation in its proper context, one must also understand that regularity is the easy passage of soft, well-formed stools on a regular basis, regardless of the interval between stools. "Normal" refers to what is normal for the individual, and wide variations may be seen among individuals.

ETIOLOGY

Constipation is a symptom rather than a disease. It is caused by a variety of factors including the following:

Lifestyle factors: Faulty bowel habits and failure to respond promptly to the physiological urge to defecate; inactivity or lack of physical exercise; lack of adequate dietary fiber; inadequate (less than 1,500 mL) daily fluid intake; excessive intake of constipating foods (eg, processed cheese); nervous tension/mental stress; fear of straining after surgery or because of illness.

Drug therapy: Analgesics (natural, semisynthetic, and synthetic opioids); anesthesia (general); antacids in which aluminum and calcium salts are the sole antacid or dominant antacid in a combination formulation; anticholinergics (eg, benztropine, trihexyphenidyl, hyoscyamine, scopolamine, atropine); antidepressants (particularly those with significant anticholinergic activity); antihistamines (eg, diphenhydramine); antihypertensives (varying degrees); antipsychotics (particularly those with significant anticholinergic activity); bismuth salts; diuretics; iron salts; irritant laxatives (when used on a chronic basis).

Medical conditions: Cancer of the gastrointestinal (GI) tract; diabetes mellitus (autonomic neuropathy); diminished neurological stimulation caused by advancing age; diverticular disease; GI adhesions or strictures; hernia; hypothyroidism (untreated); hypercalcemia; irritable bowel syndrome; multiple sclerosis; Parkinson disease; pregnancy; rectal/anal narrowing (stenosis); stroke.

INCIDENCE

The incidence of constipation is difficult to predict because many individuals self-treat constipation with nonprescription drugs. It is estimated that more than 4 million people in the United States experience constipation frequently, with tens of millions more experiencing infrequent, episodic constipation. Constipation requires approximately 2.5 million physician office visits per year. Sales of nonprescription laxatives exceed $1 billion per year.

PATHOPHYSIOLOGY

Approximately 95% of nutrient and drug absorption occurs in the small intestine. The primary function of the large intestine is to facilitate elimination of unabsorbed waste. Various mixing and propulsive movements under neurological control occur in the large intestine. Solid waste is moved systematically toward the descending and sigmoid colon and rectum through involuntary, coordinated physiologic processes. Defecation occurs when the wall of the rectum is distended by feces, the anal sphincter relaxes, intra-abdominal pressure increases, and abdominal muscles tighten.

SIGNS/SYMPTOMS

Constipation usually produces one or more symptoms. Constipation of mild to moderate severity may produce a dull headache, loss of appetite, lack of energy, or a feeling of fatigue. As constipation worsens, the above symptoms may be accompanied by abdominal distention, bloating, lower abdominal discomfort or pain, and lower back pain.

DIAGNOSTIC PARAMETERS/PHYSICAL ASSESSMENT

Clinical Observation: Through interview and clinical observation, health professionals should discern whether the classic symptoms of constipation are present or not, and if so, what is/are the most probable etiological cause(s).

Interview: In addition to recording symptoms, direct core questions to the following:

- Nature and appearance of stool
- Bowel habits
- Occupation/lifestyle
- Level of physical activity
- Bulk content in regular diet
- Presence of constipating food(s) in regular diet
- Daily fluid intake
- Anxiety/stress level
- History of laxative use/abuse
- Current medication profile to determine presence of constipating drugs (prescription and nonprescription) in the drug regimen (regularly consumed or as needed)
- Allergies/hypersensitivities/intolerance to drugs (prescription and nonprescription)
- Recent illness (nature, severity, progression, chronology)
- History of surgery, injuries, hospitalizations
- Current medical condition(s)
- Pregnancy status

Promptly refer any patient whose symptoms include blood in the feces, nausea, vomiting, and acute abdominal pain persisting 7 to 10 days or longer, or patients who are unresponsive or inappropriately responsive to adequate laxative therapy to a physician for a thorough medical evaluation.

TREATMENT

Approaches to therapy: Evaluate patients requesting treatment for constipation using the previous diagnostic parameters, which take into account the multiple etiologies of constipation. Depending on the etiology, acuity, and severity of the constipation, health care providers may recommend: (1) a nondrug approach to managing constipation, (2) a laxative to treat constipation, or (3) immediate referral to a physician for medical evaluation.

Nondrug therapy: Nondrug approaches to managing constipation may be effective in treating mild constipation, but many of the nondrug measures work best to prevent recurrence of mild, moderate, or severe constipation rather than to treat existing constipation, which often requires laxative therapy. Nondrug management processes include alterations in diet, increased fluid intake, exercise, stress management, and avoidance of constipating drugs, if feasible. Constipation caused by organic pathology requires medical evaluation and follow-up.

Pharmacotherapy: The pharmacotherapeutic management of constipation involves the use of various laxatives. Laxatives are not to be viewed as interchangeable. The different laxative types act by different mechanisms, and clinical situations generally exist in which the etiology of constipation, as well as patient-specific factors, lead the health care provider to a few products, or perhaps a single product, best suited to the individual. In addition to treating constipation, laxatives also are used to:

- Manage irritable bowel syndrome (IBS)
- Prevent constipation in immobile patients
- Retrain a laxative-dependent colon
- Evacuate the small intestine and large intestine prior to surgery or proctoscopic or sigmoidoscopic exam
- Ease elimination and straining at times when patients should not strain at defecation (eg, after heart attack, abdominal or anorectal surgery, or childbirth)

LAXATIVES

▶ **Actions**

The various types of laxatives act by different mechanisms. Consider the following when selecting a laxative:

- Etiology and severity of constipation
- The laxative's mechanism, site, and onset of action
- Drug-drug interaction potential
- Side effect profile
- Dosage form most likely to be tolerated/accepted by the patient (eg, chewable tablet or wafer, regular tablet, powder, liquid, syrup, emulsion, granules, suppository, enema)
- Palatability of the laxative
- Pregnancy status
- Complicating organic pathology

The 6 types of laxatives are:
- Bulk
- Stimulant
- Saline
- Surfactant
- Lubricant
- Hyperosmotic

▶ **Warnings**

Because of possible carcinogenic risk, laxative products containing phenolphthalein have been discontinued or reformulated as of 1997. In 1999, the FDA issued a final rule establishing that phenolphthalein generally is not recognized as safe and effective. Products manufactured with this ingredient may not be marketed in the future without an approved NDA. Some reformulated products have retained their original trade names. If patients still have laxative products containing phenolphthalein, advise them to dispose of these products and select an alternative product.

Individual products: Individual laxative products work differently. Encourage patients to start with the smallest recommended dose. Increase subsequent doses if necessary.

BULK LAXATIVES

▶ **Indications**

Bulk laxatives are nonabsorbable agents that expand, take up water, provide bulk, and stimulate the distention reflex and intestinal motility. They are a good initial choice for uncomplicated constipation in adults, elderly patients, and pregnant women. The bulk laxatives are mild, and approximate the normal intestinal physiology better than other laxatives.

▶ **Contraindications**

There are few absolute contraindications to bulk laxative use.

Bulk laxatives are contraindicated in individuals with intestinal ulcerations, intestinal narrowing (stenosis), or severe intestinal adhesions because of the risk of intestinal obstruction.

▶ **Warnings**

Casual use: Casual use of laxatives is strongly discouraged.

Esophageal/intestinal obstruction: Esophageal/intestinal obstruction may occur if the bulk laxatives in powder or granular forms are not mixed and administered properly. Strict attention to and compliance with the manufacturer's mixing and administration recommendations are crucial. If choking, chest pain, salivation, or an impaired swallowing reflex follow the administration of a bulk laxative, patients should seek immediate medical attention.

Diabetic patients: Carefully evaluate the sugar (dextrose) content of the bulk laxatives before recommending bulk laxatives to diabetic patients. Patients with phenylketonuria should avoid the artificial sweetener aspartame. Evaluate sodium content for patients on sodium-restricted diets.

▶ **Drug Interactions**

Although debated, bulk laxatives do not appear to interact adversely with other drugs to a significant extent or to interfere with the absorption of nutrients from dietary products.

▶ **Adverse Reactions**

Bulk laxatives are not absorbed systemically, so the incidence of adverse effects is low and the severity level is minor. Some flatulence (gas) and borborygmus (intestinal rumbling) may occur secondary to bacterial activity. Allergic reactions to bulk laxatives are very rare.

▶ **Administration and Dosage**

With all laxatives, it is wise to initiate dosing at the lower end of the dosage range. Subsequent doses may be increased if necessary.

Because the onset of action of bulk laxatives is slow (12 to 72 hours), it may be necessary to take the bulk laxative for up to 3 days to see an effect. The bulk laxatives generally are employed alone but may be combined with a surfactant laxative (eg, docusate) in some situations. Carefully follow manufacturer recommended mixing and administration procedures.

The effectiveness of bulk laxatives may be enhanced by increasing daily fluid intake.

POLYCARBOPHIL

▶ **Actions**

Calcium polycarbophil is a hydrophilic agent. As a bulk laxative, it retains free water within the intestinal lumen and indirectly opposes dehydrating forces of the bowel, promoting well-formed stools. In diarrhea, when the intestinal mucosa is incapable of absorbing water at normal rates, it absorbs free fecal water, forming a gel and producing formed stools. Thus, in both diarrhea and constipation, it works by restoring a more normal moisture level and providing bulk. The onset of action of polycarbophil is 24 to 72 hours. Its primary sites of action are the small and large intestine.

▶ **Indications**

Treatment of constipation or diarrhea associated with conditions such as irritable bowel syndrome and diverticulosis; acute nonspecific diarrhea.

▶ **Warnings**

Take these products with 240 mL (8 oz) or more of water or other fluid. Taking these products without enough liquid may cause choking.

▶ **Administration and Dosage**

When using these products as laxatives, drink 240 mL (8 oz) water or other liquid with each dose.

Adults: Usual dose is 1 g 1 to 4 times/day or as needed. Do not exceed 4 g in 24 hours.

Children (6 to 12 years of age): Usual dose is 500 mg 1 to 3 times/day or as needed. Do not exceed 2 g/day.

Children (younger than 6 years of age): Consult a physician.

POLYCARBOPHIL PRODUCTS	
Trade name	**Doseform**
Konsyl Fiber	**Tablets**: 500 mg polycarbophil
Fiber-Lax	**Tablets**: 625 mg calcium polycarbophil (equivalent to 500 mg polycarbophil)
Equalactin	**Tablets, chewable**: 625 mg calcium polycarbophil (equivalent to 500 mg polycarbophil). Dextrose. Citrus flavor.
FiberCon	**Caplets**: 625 mg calcium polycarbophil (equivalent to 500 mg polycarbophil)

POLYCARBOPHIL PRODUCTS	
Trade name	**Doseform**
Fiber-Lax	**Captabs**: 625 mg calcium polycarbophil (equivalent to 500 mg polycarbophil)

Products listed are representative of currently available and widely distributed brands. Similar products, including regional and private label brands, may also exist.

PSYLLIUM

► Actions

Psyllium acts primarily in the small and large intestine, producing a laxative effect in 12 to 72 hours.

► Administration and Dosage

Adults: 3 to 12 g in 240 mL (8 oz) liquid 1 to 3 times/day as needed.

Children (6 to 12 years of age): One-half the adult dose in 240 mL (8 oz) liquid 1 to 3 times/day as needed.

Children (younger than 6 years of age): Consult a physician.

PSYLLIUM PRODUCTS	
Trade name	**Doseform**
Fibro-XL	**Capsules**: 675 mg psyllium husk powder
Metamucil	**Wafers**: ≈ 3.4 g psyllium mucilloid, 17 g carbohydrate, 20 mg sodium, 5 g fat, 120 calories/dose. Apple crisp, cinnamon spice flavors.
Serutan	**Granules**: 2.5 g psyllium, < 0.03 g sodium per heaping tsp. Sucrose.
Konsyl	**Powder**: 6 g psyllium, 3 calories, 4.1 mg sodium/tsp
Bulk-K	**Powder**: 4.725 g psyllium hydrophilic mucilloid
Hydrocil Instant	**Powder**: 3.5 g psyllium hydrophilic mucilloid, 10 calories, 3 mg sodium/rounded tsp
Konsyl-D	**Powder**: 3.4 g psyllium hydrophilic mucilloid, 14 calories, 2.3 mg sodium, 24 mg potassium per tsp. Dextrose.
Metamucil	**Powder**: ≈ 3.4 g psyllium hydrophilic mucilloid/dose
Metamucil, Orange Flavor	**Powder**: ≈ 3.4 g psyllium hydrophilic mucilloid, 12 g carbohydrate (sucrose), 5 mg sodium, 45 calories/dose
Metamucil, Sugar Free	**Powder**: ≈ 3.4 g psyllium hydrophilic mucilloid, 0.3 g carbohydrate, < 10 mg sodium, 31 mg potassium/dose
Metamucil, Sugar Free	**Powder**: ≈ 3.4 mg psyllium hydrophilic mucilloid, 1.4 mg carbohydrate, < 10 mg sodium, 31 mg potassium/dose. 25 mg phenylalanine, aspartame. Orange flavor.
Modane Bulk	**Powder**: ≈ 3.4 g psyllium per rounded tsp. Dextrose.
Natural Vegetable	**Powder**: 3.4 g psyllium hydrophilic mucilloid with dextrose, < 10 mg sodium/dose
Reguloid, Orange Flavor	**Powder**: ≈ 3.4 g psyllium mucilloid per rounded tsp. Sucrose, < 0.01 g sodium, 30 calories.

PSYLLIUM PRODUCTS	
Trade name	**Doseform**
Reguloid, Sugar Free	**Powder**: ≈ 3.4 g psyllium hydrophilic mucilloid per rounded tsp. 6 mg phenylalanine per tsp, aspartame, maltodextrin.
Reguloid, Sugar Free	**Powder**: ≈ 3.4 g psyllium hydrophilic mucilloid per rounded tsp. 30 mg phenylalanine per tsp, aspartame. Orange flavor.
Reguloid	**Powder**: ≈ 3.4 g psyllium hydrophilic mucilloid per rounded tsp. Dextrose, < 0.01 g sodium, ≈ 14 calories/7 g.
Syllact	**Powder**: 3.3 g psyllium seed husks per rounded tsp. Dextrose, parabens, saccharin sodium.
V-Lax	**Powder**: 50% psyllium hydrophilic mucilloid, 50% dextrose/dose

Products listed are representative of currently available and widely distributed brands. Similar products, including regional and private label brands, may also exist.

MISCELLANEOUS BULK LAXATIVES

▶ Actions

Methylcellulose acts primarily in the small and large intestine and produces a laxative effect in 12 to 72 hours.

▶ Administration and Dosage

Take with a 240 mL (8 oz) glass of water or other fluid, and encourage additional fluid intake.

Citrucel:

Adults – 1 heaping tbsp (10.2 g) 1 to 3 times/day as needed.

Children (6 to 12 years of age) – One-half the adult dose once daily.

MISCELLANEOUS BULK LAXATIVE PRODUCTS	
Trade name	**Doseform**
FiberChoice, FiberChoice (sf)	**Tablets, chewable**: 2 g fructan
Citrucel	**Caplets**: 500 mg methylcellulose
Fiber Therapy	**Caplets**: 500 mg methylcellulose. Sorbitol, talc.
Citrucel (sf)	**Powder**: 2 g methylcellulose/tbsp. Aspartame, 52 mg phenylalanine. Orange flavor.
Maltsupex	**Powder**: 8 g malt soup extract per level scoop
Fiberall (sf)	**Powder**: Psyllium hydrophilic mucilloid, wheat bran, < 10 mg sodium, < 60 mg potassium/dose. Contains additional nutrients. Aspartame, phenylalanine. Orange flavor.
Benefiber (sf)	**Powder**: 3 g partially hydrolyzed guar gum/tbsp

Products listed are representative of currently available and widely distributed brands. Similar products, including regional and private label brands, may also exist.

sf = Sugar free

PATIENT INFORMATION
Bulk Laxatives

- Patient instructions accompany each product. Read these instructions carefully before use, preferably before leaving the pharmacy, in case of any questions.
- Give direct attention to proper dietary fiber intake, adequate fluid intake, and regular exercise.
- Do not use in the presence of abdominal pain, nausea, or vomiting.
- Take these products with 240 mL (8 oz) or more of water or other fluid. Taking these products without enough liquid may cause choking.
- Laxative use is usually a temporary measure; do not use longer than 1 week without consulting a physician. When regularity returns, discontinue use. Prolonged, frequent, or excessive use may result in dependence or electrolyte imbalance.
- Notify a physician if unrelieved constipation, rectal bleeding, or symptoms of electrolyte imbalance (eg, muscle cramps or pain, weakness, dizziness) occur.

STIMULANT LAXATIVES

▶ **Indications**

Stimulant laxatives produce local irritation in the intestinal tract and increase peristaltic activity. They also may alter the cell permeability of the intestine and increase electrolyte secretion and fluid accumulation in the intestine, further stimulating peristaltic activity.

Generally, do not employ stimulant laxatives as the laxative of first choice, although in some cases they are first-line therapy. Stimulant laxatives may be required in patients taking potent opioids. Do not use stimulant laxatives for longer than 1 week without medical evaluation. Castor oil as a laxative is best reserved for use when thorough evacuation of the intestinal tract is required (eg, prior to abdominal or intestinal diagnostic or surgical procedures).

▶ **Contraindications**

There are few absolute contraindications to laxative use.

Do not use laxatives in general (stimulant laxatives in particular) in the presence of nausea, vomiting, abdominal pain, suspected appendicitis, or when blood in the feces is present or suspected. Do not coadminister bisacodyl as the enteric-coated tablet with certain prescription or nonprescription drugs (see Drug Interactions).

▶ **Warnings**

Casual use: Casual use of laxatives is strongly discouraged.

Overuse/Abuse: Stimulant laxatives frequently are overused and abused. When used chronically, the stimulant laxatives may damage physiologic neurological colon function, thus producing chronic, drug-induced constipation and laxative dependency ("cathartic colon").

Urine discoloration: The stimulant laxative senna may produce a yellowish-brown urine discoloration in an acidic urine and a reddish-violet discoloration in an alkaline urine; counsel patients accordingly.

Onset: Castor oil may produce a laxative effect in 2 to 6 hours. When selecting a laxative, take into account social activities, work schedule, and bedtime.

Bisacodyl tablets: The stimulant laxative bisacodyl, in its tablet form, is enteric-coated to prevent release in the stomach and irritation of the gastric mucosa. Do not break, crush, or chew the tablet. Gastric acid reduction allows the enteric coating to dissolve prematurely in the stomach, producing abdominal pain and cramping.

▶ **Drug Interactions**

Bisacodyl tablets interact with antacids, H_2 antagonists (eg, cimetidine, famotidine, nizatidine, ranitidine), and proton pump inhibitors (eg, lansoprazole, omeprazole).

▶ **Adverse Reactions**

Adverse effects induced by stimulant laxatives are dose-related. All stimulant laxatives may produce abdominal cramping, profuse diarrhea, fluid depletion, electrolyte depletion, and laxative dependency with chronic use. Some nursing mothers using senna-containing preparations have reported a brownish discoloration of breast milk and subsequent diarrhea in the nursing child.

▶ **Administration and Dosage**

With all laxatives, it is wise to initiate dosing at the lower end of the dosage range. Increase subsequent doses if necessary.

SENNA

▶ **Actions**

Senna acts primarily in the large intestine, producing a laxative effect in 6 to 12 hours.

▶ **Administration and Dosage**

Dosing recommendations for individual products vary widely. Read instructions on package labeling carefully.

SENNA PRODUCTS	
Trade name	**Doseform**
Dr. Edwards'	**Tablets:** 8.6 mg sennosides
Senna Plus	**Tablets:** 8.6 mg sennosides. Tartrazine, mineral oil.
SennaCon, Senokot	**Tablets:** 8.6 mg sennosides. Glycerin, lactose, talc.
Regular Strength Ex-Lax	**Tablets:** 15 mg sennosides. Sucrose, talc.
Rite Aid Laxatives	**Tablets:** 15 mg sennosides. EDTA, parabens, sucrose, talc.
Double-Strength SenokotXTRA	**Tablets:** 17 mg sennosides. Glycerin, lactose, talc.
Maximum Strength Ex-Lax	**Tablets:** 25 mg sennosides. Sucrose, talc.
Regular Strength Ex-Lax Chocolated	**Pieces, chewable:** 15 mg sennosides. Hydrogenated palm kernel oil.
Fletcher's Castoria	**Liquid:** 33.3 mg/mL senna concentrate. Sucrose, parabens. Alcohol free. Rootbeer flavor.
Senokot	**Syrup:** 8.8 mg sennosides/tsp. Parabens, sucrose.
Children's Senokot	**Syrup:** 8.8 mg sennosides/tsp. Parabens, sucrose. Chocolate flavor.
Senokot	**Granules:** 15 mg sennosides/tsp. Sucrose.

Products listed are representative of currently available and widely distributed brands. Similar products, including regional and private label brands, may also exist.

CASTOR OIL

▶ Actions

Castor oil acts primarily in the small intestine, producing a laxative effect in 2 to 6 hours.

▶ Administration and Dosage

The taste and texture of castor oil and mineral oil are objectionable to most patients. The emulsion dosage form is somewhat more palatable. Chilling and mixing with fruit juices or carbonated beverages may help mask the unpleasant taste.

Liquid:

Adults (12 years of age and older) – 15 to 60 mL as needed.

Children (2 to 11 years of age) – 5 to 15 mL as needed.

Children (younger than 2 years of age) – Consult a physician.

Emulsion:

Adults (12 years of age and older) – 15 to 60 mL as needed.

Children (2 to 11 years of age) – 5 to 30 mL as needed.

Children (younger than 2 years of age) – Consult a physician.

CASTOR OIL PRODUCTS	
Trade name	Doseform
Purge	**Liquid**: 95% castor oil. Lemon flavor.
Emulsoil	**Emulsion**: 66% castor oil w/w with emulsifying agents. Parabens.

Products listed are representative of currently available and widely distributed brands. Similar products, including regional and private label brands, may also exist.

BISACODYL

▶ Actions

Bisacodyl acts primarily in the large intestine, producing a laxative effect in 15 to 60 minutes (suppositories or enema) or 6 to 12 hours (tablets).

▶ Administration and Dosage

Tablets: Swallow whole; do not crush or chew. Do not take within 1 to 2 hours of antacids, prescription or nonprescription H_2 antagonists, proton pump inhibitors, or milk.

Adults – 10 to 15 mg (usually 10 mg) in a single dose once daily as needed. Up to 30 mg has been used for preparation of lower GI tract for diagnostic or surgical procedures.

Children (6 to 12 years of age) – 5 mg once daily as needed.

Suppositories and enemas: Suppositories and enemas act quickly. Encourage patients to retain suppositories for 15 minutes. Most suppositories exert a laxative effect within 15 to 60 minutes in adults. The onset of action may be much faster in children. Enemas may exert their laxative effect in less than 5 to 15 minutes. Refer to Appendix D, Administration Techniques, for guidelines on administering these doseforms.

Suppositories:

> *Adults* – 10 mg once daily to induce bowel movement as needed.

> *Children (6 to 12 years of age)* – 5 mg once daily as needed.

Enemas:

> *Adults and children (12 years of age and older)* – One prepackaged bottle (as a single daily dose) as needed.

> *Children (younger than 12 years of age)* – Do not use.

BISACODYL PRODUCTS	
Trade name	**Doseform**
Dulcolax	**Tablets:** 5 mg bisacodyl. Sucrose, parabens, lactose, talc.
Correctol, Feen-a-mint, Fleet Stimulant Laxative, Modane Tablets, Time-Capp Stimulant Laxative, Alophen	**Tablets:** 5 mg bisacodyl. Lactose, sugar.
Gentlax	**Tablets:** 5 mg bisacodyl. Confectioner's sugar, sucrose.
Veracolate	**Tablets:** 5 mg bisacodyl
Correct-tabs	**Tablets, delayed-release:** 5 mg bisacodyl. Sugar.
Doxidan	**Tablets, delayed-release:** 5 mg bisacodyl. Lactose, sugar, parabens, sucrose
Dulcolax, Bisacodyl Uniserts, Fleet Bisacodyl, Bisa-lax	**Suppositories:** 10 mg bisacodyl
Fleet Bisacodyl	**Disposable enema:** 10 mg/30 mL bisacodyl

Products listed are representative of currently available and widely distributed brands. Similar products, including regional and private label brands, may also exist.

PATIENT INFORMATION
Stimulant Laxatives

- Patient instructions accompany each product. Read these instructions carefully before use, preferably before leaving the pharmacy, in case of any questions.
- Give direct attention to proper dietary fiber intake, adequate fluids, and regular exercise.
- Do not use in the presence of abdominal pain, nausea, or vomiting.
- Laxative use is usually a temporary measure; do not use longer than 1 week without consulting a physician. When regularity returns, discontinue use. Prolonged, frequent, or excessive use may result in dependence or electrolyte imbalance.
- Notify a physician if unrelieved constipation, rectal bleeding, or symptoms of electrolyte imbalance (eg, muscle cramps or pain, weakness, dizziness) occur.
- Take with a full glass of water or juice.
- Swallow bisacodyl tablets whole; do not take within 1 to 2 hours of antacids, prescription or nonprescription H_2 antagonists, proton pump inhibitors, or milk.
- Pink-red, red-violet, or red-brown discoloration of alkaline urine and yellow-brown discoloration of acidic urine may occur with senna.

SALINE LAXATIVES

▶ Indications

The saline laxatives as oral liquids contain high concentrations of electrolytes (eg, magnesium, sodium, sulfate, phosphate, biphosphate) that produce a hypertonic state in the colon. This osmotic gradient draws water into the colon, increases the internal colon pressure, and stimulates intestinal movement. The oral liquids work throughout the colon; the saline enemas act only on the distal colon. Oral saline laxatives generally produce a laxative effect in 30 minutes to 3 hours.

Do not routinely use saline laxatives in their liquid or enema dosage form to treat uncomplicated constipation. Generally, reserve the oral agents for single-dose or short-term use when acute but thorough evacuation of the colon is required (eg, prior to diagnostic, radiologic, or surgical procedures) or when other agents are contraindicated or poorly tolerated.

▶ Contraindications

There are few absolute contraindications to saline laxative use.

Do not use the saline laxatives chronically. Do not use the saline laxatives in individuals who cannot tolerate fluid loss or shifts in electrolyte levels.

Do not use laxatives in general in the presence of nausea, vomiting, abdominal pain, suspected appendicitis, or when blood in the feces is present or suspected.

▶ Warnings

Casual use: Casual use of laxatives is strongly discouraged.

Special patient populations: Administer saline laxatives containing magnesium with caution in renally impaired patients and the elderly; 15% to 20% of oral magnesium is absorbed systemically and may accumulate to toxic levels with overuse. Many saline laxatives also contain large quantities of sodium and phosphate. Use saline laxatives cautiously in patients with sodium restriction and with the knowledge of their physician. Phosphate levels may increase in patients with significant renal impairment.

▶ Adverse Reactions

Excessive use of saline laxatives may produce hypotension, muscle weakness, electrocardiogram changes, sedation, lethargy, impaired coordination, delayed reaction time, abdominal cramping, excessive diuresis, nausea, vomiting, and dehydration.

▶ Administration and Dosage

With all laxatives, it is wise to initiate dosing at the lower end of the dosage range. Subsequent doses may be increased if necessary. Dosing recommendations for individual products vary, but usual dosage ranges are as follows:

Liquid:

Adults – 15 to 30 mL (concentrate) or 30 to 60 mL (regular), followed by a full glass of liquid as needed.

Children (6 to 12 years of age) – 7.5 to 15 mL (concentrate) or 15 to 30 mL (regular), followed by a full glass of liquid as needed.

Children (2 to 5 years of age) – 2.5 to 7.5 mL (concentrate) or 5 to 15 mL (regular), followed by a full glass of liquid as needed.

Children (younger than 2 years of age) – Consult a physician.

Chewable tablets:

Adults – Chew 6 to 8 tablets, preferably before bedtime, followed by a full glass of water as needed.

Children (6 to 12 years of age) – Chew 3 to 4 tablets, preferably before bedtime, followed by a full glass of water as needed.

Children (2 to 5 years of age) – Chew 1 to 2 tablets, preferably before bedtime, followed by a full glass of water as needed.

Children (younger than 2 years of age) – Consult a physician.

Enema:

Adults – 1 bottle (ready to use enema) as needed.

Children (5 to 11 years of age) – 1 bottle (Children's Strength) or as directed by physician.

Children (2 to 5 years of age) – One-half bottle (Children's Strength) or as directed by physician.

Children (younger than 2 years of age) – Do not use.

SALINE LAXATIVE PRODUCTS	
Trade name	**Doseform**
Phillips' Antacid/Laxative	**Tablets, chewable:** 311 mg magnesium hydroxide. Sugar. Mint flavor.
Concentrated Phillips' Milk of Magnesia	**Liquid:** 800 mg magnesium hydroxide/5 mL. Sugar, sorbitol. Strawberry creme flavor.
Phillips' M-O Lubricant Laxative	**Liquid:** 300 mg magnesium hydroxide, 1.25 mL mineral oil/5 mL. Mint flavor.
Phillips' Milk of Magnesia	**Liquid:** 400 mg magnesium hydroxide/4 mL. Saccharin (mint formula), sugar, sorbitol (cherry formula). Original, mint, and cherry flavors.
Fleet Phospho-Soda	**Solution:** 2.4 g sodium phosphate, 0.9 g sodium biphosphate/5 mL. Sugar free.
Fleet Ready-to-Use Enema	**Disposable enema:** 19 g sodium phosphate, 7 g sodium diphosphate (prepackaged) unit dose

Products listed are representative of currently available and widely distributed brands. Similar products, including regional and private label brands, may also exist.

PATIENT INFORMATION

Saline Laxatives

- Patient instructions accompany each product. Read these instructions carefully before use, preferably before leaving the pharmacy, in case of any questions.
- Give direct attention to proper dietary fiber intake, adequate fluids, and regular exercise.
- Do not use in the presence of abdominal pain, nausea, or vomiting.
- Laxative use is usually a temporary measure; do not use longer than 1 week without consulting a physician. When regularity returns, discontinue use. Prolonged, frequent, or excessive use may result in dependence or electrolyte imbalance.
- Notify a physician if unrelieved constipation, rectal bleeding, or symptoms of electrolyte imbalance (eg, muscle cramps or pain, weakness, dizziness) occur.
- Take with a full glass of water or juice.

SURFACTANT LAXATIVES

▶ **Actions**

Surfactant laxatives work primarily in the small and large intestine, producing a mild laxative effect in 24 to 72 hours.

▶ **Indications**

The surfactant properties of docusate have led to it being called an emollient laxative, a stool softener, and a "wetting" agent. Docusate lowers surface tension and increases the entry of water into the fecal mass, thus softening the stool and facilitating passage.

Docusate is best suited to prevent, rather than treat, constipation. Docusate is useful for preventing constipation in those who should not strain during defecation (eg, patients with acute perianal disease or hemorrhoids; after rectal, abdominal, or eye surgery; after labor and delivery; after heart attack; patients with abdominal hernia or severe hypertension).

▶ **Contraindications**

There are few absolute contraindications to laxative use.

Do not use laxatives in general in the presence of nausea, vomiting, abdominal pain, suspected appendicitis, or when blood in the feces is present or suspected.

▶ **Warnings**

Casual use: Casual use of laxatives is strongly discouraged.

▶ **Drug Interactions**

Generally, do not take surfactant laxatives containing docusate with mineral oil. The surfactant laxative docusate may increase the absorption of mineral oil if administered concurrently.

▶ **Adverse Reactions**

The surfactant laxative docusate is generally nontoxic; rash and abdominal discomfort occur rarely.

▶ **Administration and Dosage**

With all laxatives, it is wise to initiate dosing at the lower end of the dosage range. Subsequent doses may be increased if necessary.

Combine surfactant laxatives with bulk laxatives in some situations. Carefully follow manufacturer recommended mixing and administration procedures.

The effectiveness of surfactant laxatives may be enhanced by increased fluid intake. Docusate may not exert its full pharmacological effect until the patient has completed 3 to 5 days of once-daily dosing.

DOCUSATE SODIUM

▶ **Administration and Dosage**

Adults and children (12 years of age and older): 50 to 500 mg/day (typical daily dosage is 100 to 200 mg) as needed.

Children (6 to 12 years of age): 40 to 120 mg/day as needed.

Children (3 to 6 years of age): 20 to 60 mg/day as needed.

Children (younger than 3 years of age): 10 to 40 mg/day as needed.

DOCUSATE SODIUM PRODUCTS

Trade name	Doseform
Colace	**Capsules**: 50 mg. Sorbitol, glycerin.
Colace, Modane Soft	**Capsules**: 100 mg
Fleet Sof-lax	**Gelcaps**: 100 mg
Diocytn	**Gelcaps**: 100 mg. Glycerin, sorbitol.
Phillips' Liqui-Gels	**Liquigels**: 100 mg. Glycerin, parabens, sorbitol, 5.2 mg sodium.
DSS	**Softgels**: 100 mg
Genasoft	**Softgels**: 100 mg. Glycerin, methylparaben.
DOS, DOK	**Softgels**: 100 mg. Glycerin, sorbitol.
Sulfolax	**Softgels**: 240 mg
DOS, DOK	**Softgels**: 250 mg. Glycerin, parabens, sorbitol.
Colace	**Liquid**: 10 mg/mL
Colace (sf)	**Syrup**: 60 mg/15 mL. Glycerin, saccharin, sorbitol. Alcohol free.

Products listed are representative of currently available and widely distributed brands. Similar products, including regional and private label brands, may also exist.

DOCUSATE CALCIUM

▶ Administration and Dosage

Adults: 240 mg/day as needed.

Children (6 years of age and older): 50 to 150 mg/day as needed.

DOCUSATE CALCIUM PRODUCTS

Trade name	Doseform
Surfak Liquigels	**Capsules**: 50 mg
Sulfolax Calcium, Surfak Liquigels	**Capsules**: 240 mg. Parabens, sorbitol.
DC	**Softgels**: 240 mg. Corn oil, glycerin, sorbitol.

Products listed are representative of currently available and widely distributed brands. Similar products, including regional and private label brands, may also exist.

PATIENT INFORMATION

Surfactant Laxatives

- Patient instructions accompany each product. Read these instructions carefully before use, preferably before leaving the pharmacy, in case of any questions.
- Give direct attention to proper dietary fiber intake, adequate fluids, and regular exercise.
- Do not use in the presence of abdominal pain, nausea, or vomiting.
- Laxative use is usually a temporary measure; do not use longer than 1 week without consulting a physician. In some cases, chronic therapy may be indicated to prevent recurrence of constipation.
- Notify a physician if unrelieved constipation occurs or worsens.
- Take with a full glass of water or juice.

LUBRICANT LAXATIVES

► **Actions**

Lubricant laxatives act primarily in the large intestine, producing a laxative effect in 6 to 8 hours.

► **Indications**

The only lubricant laxative is mineral oil, which lubricates the colon, rectum, and anal canal, allowing easier passage of stools. Mineral oil has limited utility; in most cases, docusate may be used instead.

► **Contraindications**

There are few absolute contraindications for lubricant laxative use.

Avoid using the lubricant laxative mineral oil at bedtime, in the very young, elderly, debilitated patients, and bedridden patients because of the risk of aspirating mineral oil into the lungs, causing lipid pneumonitis, bacterial pneumonia, or pulmonary fibrosis.

► **Warnings**

Casual use: Casual use of laxatives is strongly discouraged.

Mineral oil seepage: Generally, do not take surfactant laxatives containing docusate with mineral oil. The lubricant laxative mineral oil may seep from the rectum and soil clothing and cause anal inflammation and itching. These effects are less likely with the mineral oil emulsion.

► **Drug Interactions**

Fat-soluble vitamins: In general, do not use surfactant laxatives containing docusate with mineral oil. The lubricant laxative mineral oil may decrease absorption of the fat-soluble vitamins (vitamins A, D, E, and K), although the clinical significance of this interaction has not been established.

► **Adverse Reactions**

The lubricant laxative mineral oil is absorbed systemically in small amounts. Chronic, excessive use may produce foreign body reactions in the lymph nodes, spleen, liver, and intestinal mucosa. Chronic use also may impair tissue repair and wound healing in the intestinal tract.

► **Administration and Dosage**

With all laxatives, it is wise to initiate dosing at the lower end of the dosage range. Subsequent doses may be increased if necessary.

The taste and texture of mineral oil is objectionable to most patients. The emulsion dosage form is somewhat more palatable. Chilling and mixing with fruit juices or carbonated beverages may help mask the unpleasant taste.

MINERAL OIL

► **Administration and Dosage**

Although usual directions are to give at bedtime, caution is advised because of the risk of lipid pneumonitis.

Adults: 5 to 45 mL as needed.

Children: 5 to 20 mL as needed.

Enema:

> *Adult* – 1 bottle as needed.
>
> *Children (2 to 12 years of age)* – One-half of a bottle as needed.
>
> *Children (younger than 2 years of age)* – Do not use.

MINERAL OIL PRODUCTS	
Trade name	**Doseform**
Fleet Mineral Oil Oral Lubricant Laxative	**Solution:** Mineral oil
Liqui-Doss (sf)	**Emulsion:** Mineral oil. Alcohol free.
Kondremul Plain	**Emulsion:** 55% mineral oil. Glycerin, mapaline triple oil.
Fleet Ready-to-Use Mineral Oil Enema	**Enema:** 118 mL mineral oil

Products listed are representative of currently available and widely distributed brands. Similar products, including regional and private label brands, may also exist.

sf = Sugar free.

PATIENT INFORMATION

Lubricant Laxatives

- Patient instructions accompany each product. Read these instructions carefully before use, preferably before leaving the pharmacy, in case of any questions.
- Give direct attention to proper dietary fiber intake, adequate fluids, and regular exercise.
- Do not use in the presence of abdominal pain, nausea, or vomiting.
- Laxative use is usually a temporary measure; do not use for longer than 1 week without consulting a physician. When regularity returns, discontinue use. Prolonged, frequent, or excessive use may result in dependence or electrolyte imbalance.
- Notify a physician if unrelieved constipation, rectal bleeding, or symptoms of electrolyte imbalance (eg, muscle cramps or pain, weakness, dizziness) occur.
- Take with a full glass of water or juice.
- Administer mineral oil on an empty stomach.

HYPEROSMOTIC LAXATIVES

▶ Indications

The hyperosmotic agent most widely employed as a laxative is the suppository form of glycerin. An enema doseform also is available. The hyperosmotic agents pull fluid into the colon, provoke peristaltic activity and generally are employed for short-term, episodic use to evacuate the lower bowel. Glycerin suppositories are most widely used in pediatric patients younger than 2 years of age but also may be used by adults.

▶ Contraindications

There are few absolute contraindications to hyperosmotic laxative use.

▶ Warnings

Casual use: Casual use of laxatives is strongly discouraged.

▶ Adverse Reactions

The hyperosmotic glycerin suppository may produce local irritation.

▶ Administration and Dosage

With all laxatives, it is wise to initiate dosing at the lower end of the dosage range. Increase subsequent doses if necessary.

Suppositories and enemas act quickly. Encourage patients to retain suppositories for 15 minutes. Most suppositories exert a laxative effect within 15 to 60 minutes in adults. The onset of action may be much faster in children. Enemas may exert their laxative effect in less than 5 to 15 minutes.

GLYCERIN

▶ Actions

Glycerin acts primarily in the large intestine, producing a laxative effect in 2 to 15 minutes (rectal liquid) or 15 to 60 minutes (rectal suppositories).

▶ Administration and Dosage

Suppositories: Suppositories and enemas act quickly. Encourage patients to retain suppositories for 15 minutes. Most suppositories exert a laxative effect within 15 to 60 minutes in adults. The onset of action may be much faster in children. Enemas may exert their laxative effect in less than 5 to 15 minutes.

Insert 1 suppository high in the rectum and retain 15 minutes; it need not melt to produce laxative action. Refer to Appendix D, Administration Techniques, for guidelines on inserting suppositories.

Rectal liquid: With gentle, steady pressure, insert stem with tip pointing toward navel. Squeeze until nearly all the liquid is expelled, then remove. A small amount of liquid will remain in unit.

GLYCERIN PRODUCTS	
Trade name	**Doseform**
Sani-Supp	**Suppositories**: 82.5% glycerin
Fleet Child Glycerin Suppositories	**Suppositories**: 1 g glycerin
Children's Colace	**Suppositories**: 1.2 g glycerin
Fleet Glycerin Suppositories	**Suppositories**: 2 g glycerin
Colace	**Suppositories**: 2.1 g glycerin
Fleet Glycerin Suppositories Maximum Strength	**Suppositories**: 3 g glycerin
Fleet Glycerin Laxative	**Rectal applicators (liquid)**: 5.6 g glycerin/ 5.5 mL
Fleet Babylax	**Rectal liquid**: 2.3 g glycerin/2.3 mL

Products listed are representative of currently available and widely distributed brands. Similar products, including regional and private label brands, may also exist.

PATIENT INFORMATION

Hyperosmotic Laxatives

- Patient instructions accompany each product. Read these instructions carefully before use, preferably before leaving the pharmacy, in case of any questions.
- Give direct attention to proper dietary fiber intake, adequate fluids, and regular exercise.
- Do not use in the presence of abdominal pain, nausea, or vomiting.
- Laxative use is usually a temporary measure; do not use longer than 1 week without consulting a physician. When regularity returns, discontinue use. Prolonged, frequent, or excessive use may result in dependence or electrolyte imbalance.
- Notify a physician if unrelieved constipation, rectal bleeding, or symptoms of electrolyte imbalance (eg, muscle cramps or pain, weakness, dizziness) occur.

MISCELLANEOUS LAXATIVES

SODIUM BICARBONATE/POTASSIUM BITARTRATE

▶ Administration and Dosage

Suppositories and enemas act quickly. Encourage patients to retain suppositories for 15 minutes. Most suppositories exert a laxative effect within 15 to 60 minutes in adults. Onset of action may be much faster in children. Enemas may exert a laxative effect in less than 5 to 15 minutes.

Moisten suppository with warm water, then insert high in rectum. Refer to Appendix D, Administration Techniques, for guidelines on inserting suppositories.

SODIUM BICARBONATE/POTASSIUM BITARTRATE PRODUCTS	
Trade name	Doseform
Ceo-Two	**Suppositories**: Sodium bicarbonate and potassium bitartrate in a water-soluble polyethylene glycol base.

Products listed are representative of currently available and widely distributed brands. Similar products, including regional and private label brands, may also exist.

PATIENT INFORMATION

Miscellaneous Laxatives

- Patient instructions accompany each product. Read these instructions carefully before use, preferably before leaving the pharmacy, in case of any questions.
- Give direct attention to proper dietary fiber intake, adequate fluids, and regular exercise.
- Do not use if experiencing abdominal pain, nausea, or vomiting.
- Laxative use usually only a temporary measure; do not use for longer than 1 week without consulting a physician. When regularity returns, discontinue use. Prolonged, frequent, or excessive use may result in dependence or electrolyte imbalance.
- Notify a physician if unrelieved constipation, rectal bleeding, or symptoms of electrolyte imbalance (eg, muscle cramps or pain, weakness, dizziness) occur.

COMBINATION LAXATIVES

▶ Administration and Dosage

For specific information on individual ingredients in these combinations, refer to the preceding monographs.

Adults and children (12 years of age and older): Usual starting dose is 2 tablets once daily as needed. Do not exceed 4 tablets twice daily.

Children (6 to 12 years of age): Usual starting dose is 1 tablet once daily as needed. Do not exceed 2 tablets twice daily.

Children (2 to 6 years of age): Usual starting dose is one-half tablet once daily as needed. Do not exceed 1 tablet twice daily.

Children (younger than 2 years of age): Consult a physician.

COMBINATION LAXATIVE PRODUCTS

Trade name	Doseform
Senokot-S, Peri-Colace	**Tablets**: 8.6 mg sennosides, 50 mg docusate sodium. Lactose, talc.
Peri-Colace, Peri-Dos	**Capsules**: 30 mg casanthranol, 100 mg docusate sodium
Genasoft Plus	**Softgels**: 30 mg casanthranol, 100 mg docusate sodium. Glycerin, sorbitol.
Fleet Sof-lax Overnight	**Gelcaps**: 30 mg casanthranol, 100 mg docusate sodium

Products listed are representative of currently available and widely distributed brands. Similar products, including regional and private label brands, may also exist.

PATIENT INFORMATION

Combination Laxatives

- Patient instructions accompany each product. Read these instructions carefully before use, preferably before leaving the pharmacy, in case of any questions.
- Use exactly as prescribed.
- Do not use if experiencing abdominal pain, nausea, or vomiting.
- Laxative use is usually a temporary measure; do not use for longer than 1 week. When regularity returns, discontinue use. Prolonged, frequent, or excessive use may result in dependence or electrolyte imbalance.
- Notify a physician if unrelieved constipation, rectal bleeding, or symptoms of electrolyte imbalance (eg, muscle cramps or pain, weakness, dizziness) occur.
- Pink-red, red-violet, or red-brown discoloration of alkaline urine may occur with senna.
- Take with a full glass of water or juice.

DEFINITION

Diarrhea is defined as an abnormally frequent discharge or abnormal volume increase of semisolid or fluid fecal matter from the bowel. The condition usually is acute but may be chronic and can be mild to severe (or even life-threatening in rare cases). A relatively large amount of water is excreted in diarrhea. Normally, this water is reabsorbed within the intestinal tract.

Acute diarrhea: Acute diarrhea is characterized by abrupt onset of frequent loose stools lasting less than two weeks. It may be accompanied by abdominal pain, malaise, and flatulence. Acute diarrhea most often subsides in 1 to 3 days.

Chronic diarrhea: Chronic diarrhea is characterized by frequent passage of unformed stools that lasts four weeks or longer.

Traveler's diarrhea: Traveler's diarrhea is the presence of frequent loose stools (10 or more daily) in a person who is traveling or has done so recently, usually to a foreign country with different sanitation standards, social conditions, or climate. Nausea, abdominal cramps, and, less frequently, vomiting or fever, may accompany the diarrhea.

Diarrhea also may be classified as acute vs chronic, infectious vs noninfectious, or by the pathophysiological mechanism involved. The pathophysiological mechanisms involved divide diarrhea into four groups or types:

- Osmotic (decreased absorption of fluid)
- Secretory (increased secretion of fluid)
- Exudative
- Motility disorders

Osmotic diarrhea: Osmotic diarrhea occurs when the ingested solute is not absorbed fully, thus drawing fluid into the intestinal lumen. Saline cathartic excess or a lactase deficiency (lactose intolerance) are common causes of osmotic diarrhea.

Secretory diarrhea: Secretory diarrhea typically occurs when the small or large intestine secretes rather than absorbs water and electrolytes. This type of diarrhea most often is caused by viruses and bacteria.

Exudative diarrhea: Exudative diarrhea produces an outpouring of plasma, proteins, mucus, and blood into the stool. This type of diarrhea usually is caused by mucosal inflammation or ulceration caused by inflammatory disorders (eg, ulcerative colitis, Crohn disease) or certain types of cancer.

Motility disorders: Motility disorders caused by conditions such as diabetic neuropathy or irritable bowel syndrome may decrease gastrointestinal (GI) transit time and prevent the reabsorption of ingested material.

ETIOLOGY

Various diseases and conditions (particularly viral or bacterial intestinal infections), drug administration (especially antibiotics), food or water contamination (eg, parasites, bacterial toxins), stress, and changes in diet are the most common causes of diarrhea.

Selected Etiologics Associated with Diarrhea		
Allergy	**Bacterial**	**Dietary**
Foods Drugs	*Salmonella sp.* *Shigella sp.* *Staphylococci sp.* *Streptococci sp.* *Escherichia coli* *Clostridia sp.*	Food intolerance (gluten, lactose) Sorbitol, fructose
Endocrine/Metabolic	**Inflammatory**	**Neurogenic**
Diabetic neuropathy Hyperthyroidism (untreated)	Regional enteritis (Crohn disease) Ulcerative colitis	Irritable bowel syndrome
Parasitic	**Viral**	**Other**
Ascaris *Entamoeba histolytica* *Giardia lamblia* *Trichinella spiralis*	Norwalk virus Rotavirus AIDS	Fecal impaction Neoplasm (GI) Malabsorption disorder (eg, chronic pancreatitis, bile duct obstruction, celiac disease, tropical sprue)

Traveler's diarrhea is caused by bacteria in 80% of cases. Enterotoxigenic *Escherichia coli* is most often the causative organism, although viruses or the change in diet/living habits associated with traveling also are possible causes.

Acute diarrhea usually results from diet, infection, toxicity, or drug administration.

Infectious diarrhea typically is transmitted by fecal-to-oral transmission via contaminated food or water. Improperly cooked meat, particularly ground meat, contaminated by *E. coli* and other bacteria is becoming a seemingly greater problem in the United States. Foods that serve as good culture media for bacteria (eg, tuna salad, chicken salad, cottage cheese) should be avoided if one is not sure whether these foods have been properly refrigerated.

A partial list of drugs capable of inducing diarrhea as a side effect are included below:

Drugs Capable of Inducing Diarrhea as a Side Effect			
Antibiotics*	**Antihypertensives**	**Cardiac Drugs**	**Lipid-Lowering Agents**
Cephalosporins Clindamycin Macrolide antibiotics Penicillins Quinolone antibiotics Sulfonamides Tetracyclines	Guanabenz Guanethidine Methyldopa	ACE inhibitors Beta-blockers Calcium channel blockers Digoxin Diuretics Procainamide Quinidine	Clofibrate Gemfibrozil Statins

Drugs Capable of Inducing Diarrhea as a Side Effect			
Prokinetic Agents	**Psychiatric Agents**	**Miscellaneous**	
Bethanechol	Benzodiazepines	Colchicine	
Metoclopramide	Lithium	Cancer chemo-	
Neostigmine	SSRI antidepressants	therapies	
		Levodopa	
		NSAIDs	
		Theophylline	

* Antibiotic-associated diarrhea may be caused by an overgrowth of antibiotic-resistant bacteria or fungi or from a toxin produced by *Clostridium difficile.*

Chronic diarrhea may be multifactorial and can be difficult to diagnose. Laxative abuse (common), stress, or stomach or colon cancer may cause chronic diarrhea along with a variety of other medical conditions. Chronic diarrhea requires a thorough medical evaluation.

INCIDENCE

Diarrhea occurs frequently as a symptom of a variety of medical conditions and a side effect of certain drugs. Because self-treatment with OTC antidiarrheals is common, the incidence of diarrhea is difficult to determine. Nonetheless, some statistics are available: annually, more than 250,000 hospital admissions and more than 8 million physician visits may be attributed to cases of diarrhea. In the United States, in children younger than 5 years of age, an average of 2 to 2.5 episodes of diarrhea are seen per child per year, and more than 400 children die from complications caused by diarrhea each year in the United States. Worldwide, the estimated diarrhea-associated mortality rate is approximately 4.5 million per year.

PATHOPHYSIOLOGY

Diarrhea usually is preceded by retention of excess water, fluid, or electrolytes in the bowel caused by nonabsorbable solutes (osmotic diarrhea), inflammation or ulceration (exudative diarrhea), an increase in secretion (secretory diarrhea), or abnormal intestinal motility (motility disorder), which stimulate GI contractions or decrease GI transit time.

SIGNS/SYMPTOMS

Signs and symptoms may vary, depending on the patient's age, general health, and the cause, duration, and severity of the diarrhea. The condition may be accompanied by the presence of blood, mucus, pus in the stool, or stool discoloration. Other signs and symptoms may include fever, abdominal pain, vomiting, anorexia, malaise, flatulence, and weight loss. The onset may be acute or chronic. Blood present in the stool may suggest inflammatory, infectious, or neoplastic disease. Pus may indicate inflammation or infection. Fever and bloody diarrhea may suggest bacterial invasion or the presence of toxins. Green stools are associated with infection caused by *Salmonella* or *E. coli.* Watery, nonbloody mucus may indicate small bowel enteritis. Marked vomiting implies viral enteritis. Fecal incontinence and nocturnal diarrhea may be associated with rectal sphincter dysfunction resulting from neurologic problems.

DIAGNOSTIC PARAMETERS/PHYSICAL ASSESSMENT

Clinical Observation: Because of the nature of the condition, observation usually will be performed only by the patient. Patients with temperatures higher than 101°F, nighttime diarrhea, bloody diarrhea, severe abdominal cramps, symptoms of dehydration, or diarrhea not subsiding within 3 to 5 days should be referred to a physician for evaluation.

Interview: To determine whether physician assessment or self-treatment is warranted, it may be beneficial to ask patients about the following:

- Onset/duration of diarrhea
- Frequency of the patient's bowel movements in relation to normal bowel habits
- Physical description of the stool, including consistency, color, odor, and presence/absence of blood or mucus
- Vomiting
- Age
- Hydration status (eg, excessive thirst, decreased urination, lethargy)
- Medication profile (eg, recent or current use of antibiotics or other prescription or nonprescription agents)
- Any recently diagnosed medical conditions (especially diabetes, irritable bowel syndrome, ulcer, or cardiovascular disease)
- Recent consumption of nonchlorinated river, lake, or pond water
- Recent eating habits. Are these a change in usual diet?
- Similar symptoms among family members, friends, or coworkers
- Recent travel history
- Diarrhea accompanied by fever or other symptoms
- Pregnancy status
- Past use of antidiarrheal products (frequency and efficacy)
- Recent or prolonged use of laxatives

TREATMENT

Approaches to therapy: Patients should be evaluated utilizing the above diagnostic parameters. The goals of therapy should be to (1) identify and treat the cause of the diarrhea, (2) prevent fluid/electrolyte loss, and (3) relieve symptoms. Symptomatic relief should not lead to the assumption that the underlying causes of diarrhea are cured; however, sometimes symptomatic relief is the best possible outcome, especially with uncomplicated, self-limiting diarrhea. Depending on various factors (eg, symptoms, duration, frequency), health care providers may recommend one of the following:

- A nondrug approach
- Appropriate pharmacotherapy
- Immediate referral to a physician for medical evaluation

The pediatric population, frail elderly patients, pregnant women, and patients in whom diarrhea has been present for longer than 3 to 5 days should be referred to a physician.

> *Traveler's diarrhea* – Prophylaxis of traveler's diarrhea is controversial; some health care practitioners advise against prophylaxis and recommend treatment only if symptoms appear. When used, prophylaxis includes prescription antibiotics (eg, doxycycline, trimethoprim-sulfamethoxazole,

ciprofloxacin) and nonprescription bismuth subsalicylate. If antibiotics are preferred as prophylactic agents, physician referral is warranted. However, bismuth subsalicylate is available without a prescription and also is effective prophylaxis. Prophylactic medications for traveler's diarrhea should be started on the day of arrival and taken continuously throughout the duration of visit as well as 1 to 2 days after returning to the United States; however, therapy should not exceed 21 days, even if foreign travel is still in progress.

Treatment of traveler's diarrhea may consist of antibiotics, loperamide, bismuth subsalicylate, fluid/electrolyte therapy, or a combination of these medications.

Nondrug therapy: Diarrhea often is a self-limiting condition managed by adequate rehydration with clear liquids for 24 hours and a bland diet on the second day. A regular diet may be resumed within 2 to 3 days.

Pharmacotherapy: If it is determined that treatment of diarrhea is necessary, a number of OTC agents are available for the management of diarrhea. These include bulk-forming agents (eg, polycarbophil), adsorbents, antibacterial/anti-inflammatory agents, loperamide, and oral rehydration solutions. Depending on the patient and severity/duration of the diarrhea, physician referral may be warranted.

ANTIDIARRHEAL AGENTS/ADSORBENTS

▶ Actions

Activated attapulgite, kaolin, and pectin are used for their adsorbent and protectant actions. Bismuth salts have antacid and adsorbent properties.

▶ Indications

Symptomatic treatment of diarrhea by reducing intestinal motility or adsorbing fluid.

▶ Contraindications

Hypersensitivity to the product or any of its ingredients.

▶ Warnings

Diarrhea from other causes: Do not use antiperistaltic agents for diarrhea associated with pseudomembranous enterocolitis or in diarrhea caused by toxigenic bacteria.

Salicylate: Systemic absorption may occur from bismuth subsalicylate; therefore, do not use this product without consulting a physician if the patient has salicylate sensitivity, a bleeding disorder, or bloody or black stool.

Kaolin-Pectin: Not recommended for use in children younger than 12 years of age.

▶ Drug Interactions

Kaolin-Pectin: May delay clindamycin absorption and decrease lincomycin absorption.

▶ Administration and Dosage

Attapulgite:

> *Adults and children (older than 12 years of age)* – 1.5 g (2 tablets or 2 tablespoonsful) after each loose stool, for a maximum of 6 doses (9 g; 12 tablets or 12 tablespoonsful) in 24 hours.

Children (6 to 11 years of age) – 750 mg (1 tablet or 1 tablespoonful) after each loose stool, for a maximum of 6 doses (4.5 g) in 24 hours.

Children (3 to 5 years of age) – 375 mg (½ tablet or ½ tablespoonful) after each loose stool, for a maximum of 6 doses (2.25 g) in 24 hours.

Kaolin-Pectin:

Adults and children (older than 12 years of age) – Dose varies according to product. Usual dosage range is 15 to 120 mL after each loose stool.

ANTIDIARRHEAL COMBINATION PRODUCTS	
Trade name	Doseform
Diarrest	**Tablets**: Activated attapulgite. Sugar free.
Kaopectate Maximum Strength	**Caplets**: 750 mg attapulgite. Parabens, sucrose. May contain talc.
K-Pek	**Suspension**: 750 mg attapulgite/15 mL. Methylparaben, sucrose.
Kaodene Non-Narcotic	**Suspension**: 3.888 g kaolin, 17.3 mg bismuth subsalicylate/30 mL. Sucrose.
Kaolin-Pectin	**Suspension**: 5.83 g kaolin, 130 mg pectin/30 mL

Products listed are representative of currently available and widely distributed brands. Similar products, including regional and private label brands, may also exist.

PATIENT INFORMATION
Antidiarrheal Combinations
- Patient instructions accompany each product. Read instructions carefully before use. If any questions regarding product use arise, contact your pharmacist or physician.
- Notify a physician if diarrhea does not subside after more than 2 days or if high fever, abdominal pain, or abdominal distention occurs.
- Do not use these products in the presence of abdominal pain, nausea, or vomiting.
- It is important to drink sufficient amounts of clear fluids to prevent dehydration that may accompany diarrhea.
- Shake liquid well before using.
- Swallow tablets and caplets whole with a glass of water. Do not chew.

BISMUTH SUBSALICYLATE
▶ Actions
Bismuth subsalicylate appears to have antisecretory and antimicrobial effects in vitro, and may have some anti-inflammatory effects. The salicylate moiety provides the antisecretory effect, while the bismuth moiety may exert direct antimicrobial effects against bacterial and viral enteropathogens.

▶ Indications
For control of diarrhea, including traveler's diarrhea, within 24 hours of onset; indigestion without causing constipation; nausea; relief of abdominal cramps.

▶ Contraindications
Hypersensitivity to the product or any of its ingredients.

▶ Warnings

Impaction: Impaction may occur in infants and debilitated patients; therefore, consult a physician before using this product in these patients. If constipation occurs, discontinue use and consult a physician.

Radiological examinations: Bismuth is radiopaque; therefore, bismuth subsalicylate may interfere with radiologic examinations of the GI tract. Patients should not use this product if a radiological examination is scheduled.

Reye syndrome: Children and teenagers who have recovered or are recovering from chicken pox or flu should not use this product. When using this product, if changes in behavior with nausea and vomiting occur, consult a physician because these symptoms could be an early sign of Reye syndrome.

Salicylate: Systemic absorption may occur; therefore, do not use this product without consulting a physician if the patient has salicylate sensitivity, a bleeding disorder, or bloody or black stool.

Pregnancy: Category C. Safety has not been established. Use only when clearly needed and if the potential benefits to the mother outweigh the possible risks to the fetus.

Lactation: It is not known whether bismuth subsalicylate is excreted in breast milk. Safety for use in the nursing mother has not been established.

▶ Drug Interactions

Aspirin: Because bismuth subsalicylate contains salicylate, overdosage of salicylates may occur if aspirin is administered concurrently. If taken with aspirin and ringing of the ears occurs, discontinue use.

Corticosteroids: May reduce salicylate levels, decreasing the efficacy of bismuth subsalicylate.

Methotrexate: Bismuth subsalicylate may reduce renal elimination of methotrexate, increasing toxicity.

Tetracyclines: Bismuth subsalicylate may reduce the GI absorption and bioavailability of tetracyclines, decreasing their efficacy.

Warfarin: While nonacetylated salicylates appear to be free of antiplatelet effects, a salicylate ion interaction may occur if warfarin is administered concurrently.

▶ Administration and Dosage

Adults and children (12 years of age and older): 524 mg (2 tablets) or 30 mL (2 tablespoonsful).

Children:

> *9 to 11 years of age* – 262 mg (1 tablet) or 15 mL (1 tablespoonful).
>
> *6 to 8 years of age* – 174 mg (⅔ tablet) or 10 mL (2 teaspoonsful).
>
> *3 to 5 years of age* – 87 mg (⅓ tablet) or 5 mL (1 teaspoonful).
>
> *Younger than 3 years of age* – Consult a physician.

Repeat dosage every 30 minutes to 1 hour as needed, up to 8 doses in 24 hours. Use until diarrhea stops but for no more than 2 days. For the maximum strength products, do not exceed 4 doses in a 24-hour period.

Note: The adult prophylactic dose to prevent traveler's diarrhea is 30 mL (2 tablespoonsful) or 2 tablets 4 times daily with meals and at bedtime.

BISMUTH SUBSALICYLATE PRODUCTS

Trade name	Doseform
Bismatrol, Pink Bismuth (sf)	**Tablets, chewable**: 262 mg (102 mg total salicylate). Mannitol, saccharin.
Pepto-Bismol (sf)	**Tablets, chewable**: 262 mg. Mannitol, saccharin. Cherry flavor.
	Caplets: 262 mg. Mannitol.
	Liquid: 262 mg/15 mL. Saccharin. Cherry flavor.
Children's Kaopectate	**Liquid**: 87 mg/5 mL. Sucrose. Cherry flavor.
Diotame, Pink Bismuth (sf)	**Liquid**: 262 mg/15 mL
Kaopectate	**Liquid**: 262 mg/15 mL. Sucrose. Regular and peppermint flavors.
Bismatrol Maximum Strength, Pepto-Bismol Maximum Strength (sf)	**Liquid**: 525 mg/15 mL. Saccharin.
Extra Strength Kaopectate	**Liquid**: 525 mg/15 mL. Sucrose. Peppermint flavor.

Products listed are representative of currently available and widely distributed brands. Similar products, including regional and private label brands, may also exist.

sf = Sugar free.

PATIENT INFORMATION
Bismuth Subsalicylate

- Patient instructions accompany each product. Read instructions carefully before use. If any questions regarding product use arise, contact your pharmacist or physician.
- Notify a physician if diarrhea does not subside after more than 2 days or if high fever, abdominal pain, or abdominal distention occurs.
- Discontinue use if taking with other salicylate-containing products (eg, aspirin) and ringing in the ears occurs.
- Do not use to treat nausea or vomiting in children or teenagers with the flu or chickenpox without consulting a physician.
- Consult a physician before use if you have mucus in the stool or are taking medication for diabetes, gout, arthritis, or anticoagulation.
- It is important to drink sufficient amounts of clear fluids to prevent dehydration that may accompany diarrhea.
- Shake liquid well before using.
- Swallow caplets whole with a glass of water. Do not chew.
- Chewable tablets may be chewed or allowed to dissolve in the mouth. Do not swallow whole.
- May cause temporary and harmless darkening of the tongue or stool.

LOPERAMIDE (MOTILITY INHIBITOR)

► Actions

Loperamide slows intestinal motility and affects water and electrolyte movement through the bowel. It inhibits peristalsis by a direct effect on intestinal wall muscles. It reduces daily fecal volume, increases viscosity and bulk density, and diminishes the loss of fluid and electrolytes. Tolerance to the antidiarrheal effect has not been observed.

▶ **Indications**

For control of symptoms of diarrhea, including traveler's diarrhea.

▶ **Contraindications**

Hypersensitivity to the product or any of its ingredients; patients with bloody diarrhea, a body temperature higher than 101°F, or who must avoid constipation.

▶ **Warnings**

Acute diarrhea: Do not use loperamide in acute diarrhea associated with organisms that penetrate the intestinal mucosa (enteroinvasive *E. coli, Salmonella,* and *Shigella*) or in pseudomembranous colitis associated with broad-spectrum antibiotics.

Acute ulcerative colitis: In some patients with acute ulcerative colitis, agents that inhibit intestinal motility or delay intestinal transit time may induce toxic megacolon. Discontinue therapy promptly if abdominal distention occurs or if other adverse symptoms develop in patients with acute ulcerative colitis.

Fluid/Electrolyte depletion: Fluid/electrolyte depletion may occur in patients who have diarrhea. The use of loperamide does not preclude administration of appropriate fluid and electrolyte therapy.

Pregnancy: Category B. Safety has not been established. Use only when clearly needed and if the potential benefits to the mother outweigh the possible risks to the fetus.

Lactation: It is not known whether loperamide is excreted in breast milk. Safety for use in the nursing mother has not been established.

Children: Not recommended for use in children younger than 2 years of age. Use loperamide with special caution in young children because of the greater variability of response in this age group. Dehydration may further influence the variability of response. A loperamide dosage has not been established for children in the treatment of chronic diarrhea.

▶ **Adverse Reactions**

Adverse experiences are generally minor and self-limiting; they are more commonly observed during the treatment of chronic diarrhea: abdominal pain, distention, or discomfort; constipation; dry mouth; nausea; vomiting; tiredness; drowsiness or dizziness; hypersensitivity reactions (including skin rash).

▶ **Overdosage**

Symptoms: Constipation, CNS depression, and GI irritation may occur.

Treatment: Activated charcoal administered promptly after loperamide ingestion can reduce the amount of drug absorbed into systemic circulation. Monitor patient for signs of CNS depression for 24 hours or longer; if CNS depression is observed, administer naloxone. Children may be more sensitive to CNS effects than adults. It is important to contact a local poison control center or emergency room if overdosage is suspected.

▶ **Administration and Dosage**

Adults and children (12 years of age and older): 4 mg (2 tablets or 4 teaspoonful) after first loose bowel movement, then 2 mg (1 tablet or 2 teaspoonful) after each subsequent loose bowel movement. Do not exceed 8 mg (4 tablets or 8 teaspoonful) in 24 hours and use for no more than 2 days.

Children 9 to 11 years of age (60 to 95 lbs): 2 mg (1 tablet or 2 teaspoonful) after first loose bowel movement, then 1 mg (½ tablet or 1 teaspoonful) after each subsequent loose bowel movement. Do not exceed 6 mg (3 tablets or 6 teaspoonsful) in 24 hours and use for no more than 2 days.

Children 6 to 8 years of age (48 to 59 lbs): 2 mg (1 tablet or 1 teaspoonful) after first loose bowel movement, then 1 mg (½ tablet or 1 teaspoonful) after each subsequent loose bowel movement. Do not exceed 4 mg (2 tablets or 4 teaspoonsful) in 24 hours and use for no more than 2 days.

Children younger than 6 years of age: Consult a physician.

LOPERAMIDE PRODUCTS	
Trade name	Doseform
Imodium Advanced	**Tablets, chewable:** 2 mg loperamide, 125 mg simethicone. Saccharine, sorbitol, sucrose. Mint flavor.
	Caplets: 2 mg loperamide, 125 mg simethicone
Imodium A-D, K-Pek	**Caplets:** 2 mg
Imodium A-D	**Liquid:** 1 mg/5 mL. Glycerin, sorbitol, sucrose.

Products listed are representative of currently available and widely distributed brands. Similar products, including regional and private label brands, may also exist.

PATIENT INFORMATION
Loperamide
- Patient instructions accompany each product. Read instructions carefully before use. If any questions regarding product use arise, contact your pharmacist or physician.
- Notify a physician if diarrhea does not subside after more than 2 days or if high fever, abdominal pain, or abdominal distention occurs.
- Consult a physician before use if you have a fever, mucus in the stool, a history of liver disease, or if you are taking antibiotics.
- It is important to drink sufficient amounts of clear fluids to prevent dehydration that may accompany diarrhea.
- Shake liquid well before using.
- Swallow caplets whole with a glass of water. Do not chew.
- Chewable tablets may be chewed or allowed to dissolve in the mouth. Do not swallow whole.
- May cause drowsiness or dizziness; observe caution while driving or performing other tasks requiring alertness, coordination, or physical dexterity until tolerance is determined.

POLYCARBOPHIL

▶ **Actions**

Calcium polycarbophil is a metabolically inert hydrophilic agent. In diarrhea, when the intestinal mucosa is incapable of absorbing water at normal rates, calcium polycarbophil absorbs free fecal water, forming a gel and producing formed stools. Thus, in diarrhea it works by restoring a more normal moisture level and providing bulk.

▶ **Indications**

Treatment of constipation or diarrhea associated with conditions such as irritable bowel syndrome and diverticulosis; acute nonspecific diarrhea.

► **Contraindications**

Hypersensitivity to the product or any of its ingredients; nausea, vomiting, or other symptoms of appendicitis; fecal impaction; intestinal obstruction; undiagnosed abdominal pain.

► **Warnings**

Impaction or obstruction: Impaction or obstruction may be caused by bulk-forming agents. Use in patients with intestinal ulcerations, stenosis, or disabling adhesions may be hazardous. Patients with these conditions should consult a physician before using a bulk-forming agent.

Rectal bleeding/failure to respond: Rectal bleeding or failure to respond may indicate a serious condition that may require further medical attention.

Pregnancy: Safety has not been established. Use only when clearly needed and if the potential benefits to the mother outweigh the possible risks to the fetus.

Lactation: It is not known whether polycarbophil is excreted in breast milk. Safety for use in the nursing mother has not been established.

Children: Dosage is product specific. Administer with caution.

► **Adverse Reactions**

Diarrhea; nausea; vomiting; perianal irritation; fainting; bloating; flatulence; cramps.

► **Administration and Dosage**

Adults and children (12 years of age and older): 1 g (2 tablets or caplets) 1 to 4 times daily, as needed, not to exceed 4 g (8 tablets or caplets) in 24 hours.

Children:

> *6 to 11 years of age* – 500 mg (1 tablet or caplet) 1 to 4 times daily, as needed, not to exceed 2 g (4 tablets or caplets) in 24 hours.

> *Younger than 6 years of age* – Products vary. Consult product labeling for specific guidelines or consult a physician.

For severe diarrhea, repeat dose every 30 minutes; do not exceed maximum daily dose. A full glass of liquid should be taken with each dose.

POLYCARBOPHIL PRODUCTS	
Trade name	**Doseform**
Konsyl Fiber	**Tablets**: 500 mg polycarbophil
Fiber-Lax	**Tablets**: 625 mg calcium polycarbophil (equivalent to 500 mg polycarbophil)
	Captabs: 625 mg calcium polycarbophil (equivalent to 500 mg polycarbophil)
Equalactin	**Tablets, chewable**: 625 mg calcium polycarbophil (equivalent to 500 mg polycarbophil). Dextrose. Citrus flavor.
FiberCon	**Caplets**: 625 mg calcium polycarbophil (equivalent to 500 mg polycarbophil)

Products listed are representative of currently available and widely distributed brands. Similar products, including regional and private label brands, may also exist.

PATIENT INFORMATION
Polycarbophil

- Patient instructions accompany each product. Read instructions carefully before use. If any questions regarding product use arise, contact your pharmacist or physician.
- Take with a full glass (8 ounces) of water or juice. Taking these products without enough liquid may cause choking. Do not take these products if you have difficulty swallowing.
- Notify a physician immediately if you experience chest pain, vomiting, or difficulty swallowing or breathing after taking this medication.
- Notify a physician if diarrhea does not subside after more than 2 days or if high fever, abdominal pain, or abdominal distention occurs.
- Do not use these products in the presence of abdominal pain, nausea, or vomiting.
- Discontinue use and notify a physician if use for 1 week has no effect or if rectal bleeding occurs.
- Consult a physician before use if you have noticed a sudden change in bowel habits that persists over a period of 2 weeks.
- It is important to drink sufficient amounts of clear fluids to prevent dehydration that may accompany diarrhea.
- Swallow tablets and caplets whole with a glass of water. Do not chew.
- Chewable tablets may be chewed or allowed to dissolve in the mouth. Do not swallow whole.

ORAL ELECTROLYTE MIXTURES

▶ **Actions**

When used properly, mixtures with electrolytes, water, and glucose prevent dehydration or achieve rehydration and maintain strength and feeling of well-being. They contain sodium, chloride, potassium, and bicarbonate to replace depleted electrolytes and restore acid-base balance. Glucose facilitates sodium transport, which aids in sodium and water absorption.

▶ **Indications**

Maintenance of water and electrolytes following corrective parenteral therapy for severe diarrhea; maintenance to replace mild to moderate fluid losses when food and liquid intake are discontinued; restoration of fluids and minerals lost because of diarrhea and vomiting in infants and children.

▶ **Contraindications**

Severe, continuing diarrhea or other critical fluid losses; intractable vomiting; prolonged shock; renal dysfunction (ie, anuria, oliguria). These conditions require parenteral therapy.

▶ **Administration and Dosage**

Individualize dosage. Follow guidelines on product labeling.

ORAL ELECTROLYTE MIXTURE PRODUCTS

Trade name	Doseform
Pedialyte Singles	**Solution**: 10.6 mEq sodium, 4.7 mEq potassium, 8.3 mEq chloride, 4.7 g dextrose, 1.2 g fructose, 24 calories/8 oz. Apple and cherry flavors.
Pedialyte Freezer Pops	**Solution**: 45 mEq sodium, 20 mEq potassium, 35 mEq chloride, 25 g dextrose, 100 calories/L. Blue raspberry, cherry, grape, and orange flavors.
Pedia-Pop	**Solution**: 45 mEq sodium, 20 mEq potassium, 35 mEq chloride, 30 mEq citrate/L
Naturalyte	**Solution**: 45 mEq sodium, 20 mEq potassium, 35 mEq chloride, 30 mEq citrate, 20 g dextrose, 5 g fructose, 100 calories/L. Apple, bubble gum, fruit, and grape flavors.
	Solution: 45 mEq sodium, 20 mEq potassium, 35 mEq chloride, 30 mEq citrate, 25 g dextrose, 100 calories/L. Unflavored.
Pediatric Electrolyte	**Solution**: 45 mEq sodium, 20 mEq potassium, 35 mEq chloride, 30 mEq citrate, 20 g dextrose, 5 g fructose, 100 calories/L. Apple, bubble gum, cherry, fruit, and grape flavors.
	Solution: 45 mEq sodium, 20 mEq potassium, 35 mEq chloride, 30 mEq citrate, 25 g dextrose, 100 calories/L. Unflavored.
CeraLyte 50	**Solution**: 50 mEq sodium, 20 mEq potassium, 30 mEq citrate/L. Natural and lemon flavors.
	Powder for solution: 50 mEq sodium, 20 mEq potassium, 30 mEq citrate/L. Mixed berry, orange, and plum mango flavors.
Enfalyte	**Solution**: 50 mEq sodium, 25 mEq potassium, 45 mEq chloride, 34 mEq citrate, 30 g rice syrup solids, 126 calories/L
Pedialyte	**Solution**: 45 mEq sodium, 20 mEq potassium, 35 mEq chloride, 20 g dextrose, 5 g fructose, 100 calories/L. Fruit, grape, and bubble gum flavors.
	Solution: 45 mEq sodium, 20 mEq potassium, 35 mEq chloride, 25 g dextrose, 100 calories/L. Unflavored.
Rehydralyte	**Solution**: 75 mEq sodium, 20 mEq potassium, 65 mEq chloride, 30 mEq citrate, 25 g dextrose, 100 calories/L
CeraLyte 70	**Powder for solution**: 70 mEq sodium, 20 mEq potassium, 30 mEq citrate/L. Chicken broth, lemon, and natural rice flavors.
CeraLyte 90	**Powder for solution**: 90 mEq sodium, 20 mEq potassium, 30 mEq citrate/L. Chicken broth, lemon, and natural rice flavors.

Products listed are representative of currently available and widely distributed brands. Similar products, including regional and private label brands, may also exist.

■ ■ ■

PATIENT INFORMATION
Oral Electrolyte Mixtures

- Patient instructions accompany each product. Read instructions carefully before use. If any questions regarding product use arise, contact your pharmacist or physician.
- Notify a physician if diarrhea does not subside after more than 2 days or if high fever, abdominal pain, or abdominal distention occurs.
- Do not use these products in the presence of abdominal pain, nausea, or vomiting.

DYSPEPSIA

DEFINITION
Dyspepsia describes a constellation of nonspecific upper abdominal symptoms. Patients refer to dyspepsia by the general term of "upset stomach." These symptoms are similar to complaints experienced by patients with many GI disorders. Dyspepsia may be further divided into organic dyspepsia, which is associated with many diseases, or functional (nonulcer) dyspepsia, which has no identified cause.

ETIOLOGY
Organic dyspepsia: A number of agents and diseases are associated with organic dyspepsia. The following is a list of some conditions that may contribute to organic dyspepsia:

- Food intolerance (eg, caffeine, alcohol, spicy food, soft drinks).
- Medications (eg, aspirin/NSAIDs, antibiotics [eg, penicillins, erythromycin, tetracycline], quinidine, iron).
- GI disorders (eg, peptic ulcer disease, gastroesophageal reflux, irritable bowel syndrome, gastric carcinomas, malabsorption disorders, gastric infections).
- Pancreatobiliary disorders (eg, pancreatitis, pancreatic cancer, cholclithiasis).
- Systemic disorders (diabetes, renal insufficiency, thyroid disease, hyperparathyroidism).

Note: Patients with known or suspected organic dyspepsia should be referred to a physician. It is only discussed here for completeness of the monograph.

Functional dyspepsia: By definition, patients in this group have no identifiable cause for chronic or recurrent dyspepsia. The etiology of this condition has not been clearly defined. Because patients with functional dyspepsia have symptoms that are also experienced by patients with other functional GI disorders, such as irritable bowel syndrome (IBS) and noncardiac chest pain, it may be part of a continuum of these disorders in some cases. Other proposed etiologies for this condition include GI motor abnormalities, visceral hypersensitivity, *Helicobacter pylori* infection and psychological factors. None of the proposed etiologies are proven to cause functional dyspepsia. Moreover, gastric acid hypersecretion is not a cause of functional dyspepsia because these patients have normal acid production.

INCIDENCE
Dyspepsia is highly prevalent in the adult population. The incidence of dyspepsia varies widely depending on the study population and the symptoms included in the definition of dyspepsia. If heartburn and regurgitation are included in the definition, the incidence is between 32% to 54%. If heartburn is excluded, the incidence approaches 26%. Dyspepsia is more prevalent in women and decreases with age. The prevalence of functional dyspepsia is higher than organic dyspepsia.

PATHOPHYSIOLOGY

The pathophysiology of functional dyspepsia has thus far remained elusive because the etiology is poorly understood. It has been proposed that gastric distension after meals or minor irritants (certain foods) produce pain in these patients because they may have an inherent hypersensitivity to pain. Abnormal gastric motility, which is present in 25% to 60% of patients with functional dyspepsia, has also been proposed as a mechanism. However, the presence or absence of gastric hypomotility does not correlate with symptoms. Other proposed mechanisms include *H. pylori*-induced gastritis and the influence of psychosocial parameters. Thus far, the role of *H. pylori* in functional dyspepsia is still controversial. Although patients with functional dyspepsia who seek treatment may have a higher incidence of phobias or anxiety, a causal relationship has not been established. It is possible that these personality traits could influence how a patient responds to the symptoms. The pathophysiology of functional dyspepsia is still unknown.

Note: The pathophysiology of organic dyspepsia is not presented because it is beyond the scope of this monograph. Patients with known or suspected organic dyspepsia should be referred to a physician.

SIGNS/SYMPTOMS

The classical symptoms of dyspepsia are vague complaints of pain or discomfort primarily centered in the upper abdomen. Patients often complain of abdominal bloating or distention, early satiety, belching, flatulence, nausea, anorexia, and heartburn.

DIAGNOSTIC PARAMETERS/PHYSICAL ASSESSMENT

Clinical Observation: Because of the nature of the condition, clinical observation usually is done by the patient. The most common alarm symptoms of organic disease are unintentional weight loss (more than 3 kg), bleeding, and severe or chronic symptoms. Patients who are older than 45 years of age or have a history suggesting the possibility of organic disease should be referred to a physician.

Interview: Because the diagnosis of functional dyspepsia is one of exclusion and the symptoms are non-specific, practitioners need a detailed history before recommending OTC drug therapy. In addition to addressing the nature of the symptoms, questions should address the following:

• History of GI disorders in the patient or family members (IBS, GERD, PUD, cancer).
• Unintentional weight loss.
• GI bleeding (tarry stool).
• Association of symptoms with specific foods or beverages.
• Current medications.
• Concurrent medical problems (eg, diabetes, thyroid disorder).
• Psychiatric history (eg, anxiety, depression).

The presence of any of the above factors could suggest organic disease.

TREATMENT

Approaches to therapy: After carefully evaluating the patient, practitioners should refer all patients with moderate-to-severe symptoms to a physician. Start patients who have mild or minor symptoms on non-drug or drug therapy with the advice to see a physician if symptoms worsen or do not resolve within 2 weeks.

Nondrug therapy: Patients with functional dyspepsia may benefit from reassurance and lifestyle modification. In cases where the cause of symptoms may be due to medications, alcohol, or food intolerance, counsel patients accordingly. A physician referral may be necessary if an organic disorder is suspected.

Pharmacotherapy: Prescription antisecretory agents (histamine H_2 antagonists, proton pump inhibitors) and antacids are frequently used in the management of functional dyspepsia. Available evidence indicates that these agents are only slightly better than placebo. However, patients who have heartburn may experience relief. OTC histamine H_2 antagonists have not been evaluated fully in the management of dyspepsia. A short trial of two weeks or less may be appropriate. If the patient is under the care of a physician, a four-week trial may be appropriate.

HISTAMINE H_2 ANTAGONISTS

▶ **Actions**

Histamine H_2 receptors in gastric parietal cells control acid secretion. Histamine H_2 receptor antagonists decrease acid production by competing reversibly with histamine at the H_2 receptor. These agents also decrease food-, insulin-, and caffeine-induced secretions. They have no anticholinergic properties and no effect on H_1 receptors.

▶ **Indications**

For the relief of symptoms of episodic and uncomplicated heartburn, acid indigestion, and sour stomach.

▶ **Contraindications**

Hypersensitivity to individual agents or other histamine H_2 receptor antagonists.

▶ **Warnings**

Pregnancy: Category B. There are no adequate and well-controlled studies in pregnant women. Use during pregnancy only if the potential benefits outweigh the possible risks to the fetus.

Lactation: Cimetidine and ranitidine are excreted in human breast milk. Avoid cimetidine in nursing mothers. Exercise caution in administering ranitidine to lactating mothers. It is not known whether famotidine is excreted in human breast milk. However, it is excreted in the breast milk of rats. Do not use famotidine in nursing mothers unless the benefits to the mother outweigh the risks to the fetus.

Children: OTC use of H_2 antagonists is not recommended in children younger than 12 years of age. In addition, cimetidine is not recommended in children younger than 16 years of age.

▶ Drug Interactions

Drugs metabolized by cytochrome P450: Significant drug interactions with H_2 antagonists primarily occur with cimetidine. Cimetidine inhibits the metabolism of certain drugs metabolized by the cytochrome P450 system, thereby leading to increased drug levels and toxicity. Through this mechanism, cimetidine inhibits the clearance of drugs such as warfarin, theophylline, phenytoin, propranolol, nifedipine, metronidazole, carbamazepine, sulfonylureas, quinidine, cisapride, alcohol, caffeine, and benzodiazepines.

Carmustine: Cimetidine results in increased bone marrow suppression.

Itraconazole and ketoconazole: H_2 antagonists decrease the absorption of itraconazole and ketoconazole by decreasing gastric acidity.

Metformin: Cimetidine may increase serum plasma levels of metformin by reducing its renal clearance.

Procainamide: Cimetidine and ranitidine may increase serum plasma levels of procainamide by reducing its renal clearance.

Drug-food interactions: Food may increase the bioavailability of famotidine and nizatidine. This interaction is unlikely to be clinically relevant with OTC doses of H_2 antagonists.

▶ Adverse Reactions

H_2 antagonists generally are well tolerated. The most common adverse reactions are headache, fatigue, and diarrhea. Prolonged use of cimetidine may lead to gynecomastia. Reversible confusional states (eg, psychosis, delirium, agitation, depression) have been reported in elderly patients. Gynecomastia and confusion are more likely with the higher prescription doses of cimetidine.

CIMETIDINE

▶ Administration and Dosage

Relief of symptoms: Take 200 mg (one tablet) with a glass of water or other fluid as needed. Do not exceed 400 mg (two tablets) in 24 hours.

Prevention of symptoms: Take 200 mg (one tablet) with a glass of water or other fluid 30 minutes or less before eating food or drinking beverages that cause heartburn, acid indigestion, or sour stomach. Do not exceed 400 mg (two tablets) in 24 hours.

Cimetidine should not be given to children younger than 12 years of age unless directed by a physician.

CIMETIDINE PRODUCTS	
Trade name	**Doseform**
Cimetidine, *Tagamet HB 200*	**Tablets**: 200 mg
Tagamet HB 200	**Suspension**: 200 mg/5 mL

Products listed are representative of currently available and widely distributed brands. Similar products, including regional and private label brands, may also exist.

RANITIDINE

▶ Administration and Dosage

Take tablets with fluid and swallow them whole.

Usual dosage: May be used up to twice daily (up to 2 tablets in 24 hours).

RANITIDINE PRODUCTS	
Trade name	Doseform
Ranitidine (sf)	**Tablets**: 75 mg. Lactose. Sodium free.
Zantac 75 (sf)	**Tablets**: 75 mg. Sodium free.
Zantac 150 (sf)	**Tablets**: 150 mg.

Products listed are representative of currently available and widely distributed brands. Similar products, including regional and private label brands, may also exist.

sf = Sugar free.

FAMOTIDINE

▶ Administration and Dosage

Take the nonchewable tablets and gelcaps with fluid and swallow them whole.

Relief of symptoms: Swallow one tablet or gelcap with a glass of water or chew one chewable tablet.

Prevention of symptoms: Swallow one tablet or gelcap with a glass of water or chew one chewable tablet at any time 15 to 60 minutes before eating food or drinking beverages that cause heartburn.

10 mg: Take 10 mg once or twice daily as needed. Do not exceed 20 mg (two tablets or gelcaps) in 24 hours.

20 mg: Take 20 mg once or twice daily as needed. Do not exceed more than 40 mg (two tablets) in 24 hours.

FAMOTIDINE PRODUCTS	
Trade name	Doseform
Famotidine, *Pepcid AC*	**Tablets**: 10 mg
Maximum Strength Pepcid AC	**Tablets**: 20 mg. Talc.
Pepcid AC Chewable	**Tablets, chewable**: 10 mg. Aspartame, lactose, 1.4 mg phenylalanine.
Pepcid AC Gelcaps	**Gelcaps**: 10 mg

Products listed are representative of currently available and widely distributed brands. Similar products, including regional and private label brands, may also exist.

NIZATIDINE

▶ Administration and Dosage

Take tablets with fluid and swallow them whole.

Usual dosage: Take 75 mg once or twice daily as needed. Do not exceed 150 mg (two tablets) in 24 hours.

NIZATIDINE PRODUCTS	
Trade name	Doseform
Axid AR	**Tablets**: 75 mg

Products listed are representative of currently available and widely distributed brands. Similar products, including regional and private label brands, may also exist.

HISTAMINE H₂ ANTAGONIST COMBINATIONS

▶ Administration and Dosage

Do not swallow tablet whole; chew completely.

Usual dosage: Do not use more than two chewable tablets in 24 hours. Do not give to children younger than 12 years of age unless directed by a physician.

HISTAMINE H$_2$ ANTAGONIST PRODUCTS	
Trade name	Doseform
Pepcid Complete	**Tablets, chewable**: 10 mg famotidine. 800 mg calcium carbonate, 165 mg magnesium hydroxide. Lactose, sugar.

Products listed are representative of currently available and widely distributed brands. Similar products, including regional and private label brands, may also exist.

PATIENT INFORMATION

Histamine H$_2$ Antagonists

- Patient instructions accompany each product. Read these instructions carefully before use, preferably before leaving the pharmacy in case of any questions.
- Do not use the maximum daily doses of these agents for two weeks or more, except under the advice of a physician.
- Histamine H$_2$ antagonists may interact with certain prescription drugs. If you are presently taking a prescription drug, do not take a histamine H$_2$ antagonist without checking with a physician or pharmacist.
- If symptoms worsen or persist for two weeks or more, contact a physician.
- Store at room temperature in a tight container away from light.

ANTACIDS

▶ **Actions**

Antacids increase gastric and duodenal pH by neutralizing acid. They do not affect the production of gastric acid. By raising gastric pH, antacids also inhibit the activity of the pepsin.

▶ **Indications**

Symptomatic relief of conditions associated with hyperacidity such as heartburn, gastroesophageal reflux, acid indigestion, sour stomach, gastritis, and peptic ulcers.

▶ **Contraindications**

There are no specific contraindications to the use of antacids. If possible, avoid magnesium-containing antacids in patients with marked renal failure (see Warnings).

▶ **Warnings**

Congestive heart failure, hypertension, and sodium-restricted diets: Some products have a high sodium content, which may interfere with low-sodium diets and the management of hypertension or congestive heart failure.

Renal insufficiency: These patients are at an increased risk for developing aluminum intoxication, hypermagnesemia, hypercalcemia, and other electrolyte imbalance. If possible, avoid use of magnesium-containing antacids, including magaldrate, in patients where marked renal failure (Ccr 30 mL/min or less) is known or suspected.

Pregnancy: Pregnant women should consult a physician before using antacids.

Lactation: Lactating women should consult a physician before using antacids.

▶ **Drug Interactions**

Antacids, administered concurrently with other drugs, can significantly decrease the absorption of iron salts, quinolones (eg, ciprofloxacin, ofloxacin), ketoconazole, and tetracyclines. Antacids may also decrease the absorption of digoxin, isoniazid, phenytoin, and quinidine. These interactions can be minimized by separating drug administration by 2 hours.

▶ **Adverse Reactions**

Constipation/diarrhea: Magnesium-dominant antacids may cause diarrhea, while aluminum- and calcium-dominant antacids may cause constipation.

Milk alkali syndrome: An acute illness, presents with headaches, nausea, vomiting, weakness, alkalosis, and hypercalcemia that has developed during the use of high-dose calcium carbonate concomitantly with sodium bicarbonate.

Electrolyte imbalance: Hypernatremia, hypermagnesemia, hypercalcemia, and hypophosphatemia may occur with the chronic use of antacids, especially in renal failure.

Alkalosis: Prolonged use of antacids containing sodium bicarbonate may result in systemic alkalosis.

Rebound hyperacidity: Dose-related rebound hyperacidity has been reported with antacids.

MAGNESIUM HYDROXIDE

▶ **Administration and Dosage**

Note: There are numerous antacid formulations. Many combination antacids contain $Mg(OH)_2$ as one of the primary ingredients. Patients should follow the product labeling for appropriate instructions. Doses used for the management of conditions associated with hyperacidity can be used for the management of dyspepsia.

Tablets: 622 mg to 1244 mg up to 4 times daily as needed.

Liquid: 5 to 15 mL up to 4 times daily as needed.

Liquid, concentrated: 2.5 to 7.5 mL up to 4 times daily as needed.

MAGNESIUM HYDROXIDE PRODUCTS	
Trade name	**Doseform**
Phillips' Chewable	**Tablets, chewable**: 311 mg
Milk of Magnesia, Phillips' Milk of Magnesia, Dulcolax Milk of Magnesia (sf)	**Liquid**: 400 mg/5 mL
Concentrated Phillips' Milk of Magnesia	**Liquid, concentrated**: 800 mg/5 mL

Products listed are representative of currently available and widely distributed brands. Similar products, including regional and private label brands, may also exist.

sf = Sugar free.

PATIENT INFORMATION

Magnesium Hydroxide

- If symptoms worsen or persist for longer than 2 weeks, consult a physician.
- Do not exceed the recommended doses for these agents, and do not use maximum daily doses for longer than 2 weeks unless otherwise directed by a physician.
- Magnesium-dominant products may cause diarrhea.
- Shake liquid antacids prior to use.
- Sodium content is generally low but varies. Check package label if you are on a sodium-restricted diet or have heart disease or high blood pressure.

MAGNESIUM OXIDE

▶ **Administration and Dosage**

Note: There are numerous antacid formulations. Patients should follow the product labeling for appropriate instructions. Doses used for the management of conditions associated with hyperacidity can be used for the management of dyspepsia.

Tablets: 400 to 800 mg/day.

Capsules: 140 mg 3 to 4 times daily.

MAGNESIUM OXIDE PRODUCTS	
Trade name	Doseform
Mag-Ox 400	**Tablets**: 400 mg
Maox	**Tablets**: 420 mg
Uro-Mag	**Capsules**: 140 mg

Products listed are representative of currently available and widely distributed brands. Similar products, including regional and private label brands, may also exist.

PATIENT INFORMATION

Magnesium Oxide

- If symptoms worsen or persist for longer than 2 weeks, consult a physician.
- Do not exceed the recommended doses for these agents, and do not use maximum daily doses for longer than 2 weeks unless otherwise directed by a physician.
- Magnesium-dominant products may cause diarrhea.
- Shake liquid antacids prior to use.
- Sodium content is generally low but varies. Check package label if you are on a sodium-restricted diet or have heart disease or high blood pressure.

ALUMINUM HYDROXIDE GEL

▶ **Administration and Dosage**

Note: There are numerous antacid formulations. Many combination antacids contain an aluminum salt as one of the ingredients. Patients should follow the product labeling for appropriate instructions. Doses used for the management of conditions associated with hyperacidity can be used for the management of dyspepsia.

Capsules/Tablets: 500 to 1500 mg 3 to 6 times daily as needed between meals and at bedtime.

Suspension: 5 to 30 mL as needed between meals and at bedtime.

ALUMINUM HYDROXIDE GEL PRODUCTS	
Trade name	Doseform
Amphojel	**Tablets**: 300 mg
Alu-Tab	**Tablets**: 500 mg
Amphojel	**Tablets**: 600 mg
Alu-Cap	**Capsules**: 400 mg
Amphojel	**Suspension**: 320 mg/5 mL
AlternaGEL	**Liquid**: 600 mg/5 mL

Products listed are representative of currently available and widely distributed brands. Similar products, including regional and private label brands, may also exist.

PATIENT INFORMATION
Aluminum Hydroxide Gel

- If symptoms worsen or persist for longer than 2 weeks, consult a physician.
- Do not exceed the recommended doses for these agents, and do not use maximum daily doses for longer than 2 weeks unless directed otherwise by a physician.
- Aluminum-dominant products may cause constipation.
- Shake liquid antacids prior to use.
- Sodium content is generally low but varies. Check package label if you are on a sodium-restricted diet or have heart disease or high blood pressure.

ALUMINUM CARBONATE GEL

▶ Administration and Dosage

Note: There are numerous antacid formulations. Many combination antacids contain an aluminum salt as one of the ingredients. Patients should follow the product labeling for appropriate instructions. Doses used for the management of conditions associated with hyperacidity can be used for the management of dyspepsia.

Capsules/Tablets: 2 every 2 hours, up to 12 times daily as needed.

Suspension: 10 mL every 2 hours, up to 12 times daily as needed.

ALUMINUM CARBONATE GEL PRODUCTS	
Trade name	Doseform
Basaljel	**Tablets:** Equiv. to 608 mg dried aluminum hydroxide gel or 500 mg aluminum hydroxide
	Capsules: Equiv. to 608 mg dried aluminum hydroxide gel or 500 mg aluminum hydroxide
	Suspension: Equiv. to 400 mg aluminum hydroxide/5 mL

Products listed are representative of currently available and widely distributed brands. Similar products, including regional and private label brands, may also exist.

PATIENT INFORMATION
Aluminum Carbonate

- If symptoms worsen or persist for longer than 2 weeks, consult a physician.
- Do not exceed the recommended doses for these agents, and do not use maximum daily doses for longer than 2 weeks unless directed otherwise by a physician.
- Aluminum-dominant products may cause constipation.
- Shake liquid antacids prior to use.
- Sodium content is generally low but varies. Check package label if you are on a sodium-restricted diet or have heart disease or high blood pressure.

CALCIUM CARBONATE

▶ Administration and Dosage

Note: There are numerous antacid formulations. Many combination antacids contain a calcium salt as one of the ingredients. Patients should follow the product labeling for appropriate instructions. Doses used for the management of conditions associated with hyperacidity can be used for the management of dyspepsia.

Tablets/Lozenges: 0.5 to 1.5 g as needed.

CALCIUM CARBONATE PRODUCTS	
Trade name	Doseform
Titralac Extra Strength	**Tablets**: 750 mg. Saccharin.
Amitone	**Tablets, chewable**: 350 mg
Mallamint, Instant Relief Titralac	**Tablets, chewable**: 420 mg
Antacid, Tums	**Tablets, chewable**: 500 mg
Quick Dissolve Maalox	**Tablets, chewable**: 600 mg
Alka-Mints	**Tablets, chewable**: 850 mg
Chooz	**Gum tablets**: 500 mg
Mylanta	**Lozenges**: 600 mg

Products listed are representative of currently available and widely distributed brands. Similar products, including regional and private label brands, may also exist.

PATIENT INFORMATION
Calcium Carbonate

- If symptoms worsen or persist for longer than 2 weeks, consult a physician.
- Do not exceed the recommended doses for these agents, and do not use maximum daily doses for longer than 2 weeks unless directed otherwise by a physician.
- Calcium-dominant products may cause constipation.
- Shake liquid antacids prior to use.
- Sodium content is generally low but varies. Check package label if you are on a sodium-restricted diet or have heart disease or high blood pressure.

MAGALDRATE (ALUMINUM MAGNESIUM HYDROXIDE SULFATE)

▶ Administration and Dosage

Note: There are numerous antacid formulations patients should follow the product labeling for appropriate instructions. Doses used for the management of conditions associated with hyperacidity can be used for the management of dyspepsia.

Suspension/Liquid: 5 to 10 mL between meals and at bedtime as needed.

MAGALDRATE PRODUCTS	
Trade name	Doseform
Iosopan	**Suspension**: 540 mg/5 mL

Products listed are representative of currently available and widely distributed brands. Similar products, including regional and private label brands, may also exist.

PATIENT INFORMATION
Magaldrate

- If symptoms worsen or persist for longer than 2 weeks, consult a physician.
- Do not exceed the recommended doses for these agents, and do not use maximum daily doses for longer than 2 weeks unless directed otherwise by a physician.
- Shake liquid antacids prior to use.

SODIUM BICARBONATE

▶ **Administration and Dosage**

0.3 to 2 g 1 to 4 times daily as needed.

Note: There are numerous antacid formulations. Patients should follow the product labeling for appropriate instructions. Doses used for the management of conditions associated with hyperacidity can be used for the management of dyspepsia.

SODIUM BICARBONATE PRODUCTS	
Trade name	Doseform
Bell/ans	Tablets: 520 mg

Products listed are representative of currently available and widely distributed brands. Similar products, including regional and private label brands, may also exist.

PATIENT INFORMATION

Sodium Bicarbonate

- If symptoms worsen or persist for longer than 2 weeks, consult a physician.
- Do not exceed the recommended doses for these agents, and do not use maximum daily doses for longer than 2 weeks unless directed otherwise by a physician.
- Sodium content is generally low but varies. Check package label if you are on a sodium-restricted diet or have heart disease or high blood pressure.

SODIUM CITRATE

▶ **Administration and Dosage**

30 mL daily as needed.

Note: There are numerous antacid formulations. Patients should follow the product labeling for appropriate instructions. Doses used for the management of conditions associated with hyperacidity can be used for the management of dyspepsia.

SODIUM CITRATE PRODUCTS	
Trade name	Doseform
Citra pH	Solution: 2.7 g/30 mL

Products listed are representative of currently available and widely distributed brands. Similar products, including regional and private label brands, may also exist.

PATIENT INFORMATION

Sodium Citrate

- If symptoms worsen or persist for longer than 2 weeks, consult a physician.
- Do not exceed the recommended doses for these agents, and do not use maximum daily doses for longer than 2 weeks unless directed otherwise by a physician.
- Calcium-dominant products may cause constipation.
- Shake liquid antacids prior to use.
- Sodium content is generally low but varies. Check package label if you are on a sodium-restricted diet or have heart disease or high blood pressure.

ANTACID COMBINATIONS

▶ **Administration and Dosage**

See individual products for administration and dosage guidelines.

ANTACID COMBINATION PRODUCTS

Trade name	Doseform
Capsules and Tablets	
Maalox	**Tablets**: 200 mg aluminum hydroxide, 200 mg magnesium hydroxide. Saccharin, sorbitol.
Mintox, RuLox #1	**Tablets**: 200 mg aluminum hydroxide, 200 mg magnesium hydroxide. Saccharin.
Titralac Plus	**Tablets**: 420 mg calcium carbonate, 21 mg simethicone. Saccharin, 1.1 mg sodium.
Alenic Alka	**Tablets**: 80 mg aluminum hydroxide, 20 mg magnesium trisilicate, sodium bicarbonate, calcium stearate. Sugar, 18.4 mg sodium.
Foamicon	**Tablets**: 80 mg aluminum hydroxide, alginic acid, sodium bicarbonate, 20 mg magnesium trisilicate, calcium stearate. Sugar, sucrose, 18.4 mg sodium.
Genaton	**Tablets**: 80 mg aluminum hydroxide. alginic acid, sodium bicarbonate, 20 mg magnesium trisilicate. Sucrose, sugar, 18.4 mg sodium.
Gaviscon	**Tablets**: 80 mg aluminum hydroxide, alginic acid, sodium bicarbonate, 20 mg magnesium trisilicate, calcium stearate. Sucrose, 18.4 mg sodium.
Double Strength Gaviscon-2	**Tablets**: 160 mg aluminum hydroxide, alginic acid, sodium bicarbonate, 40 mg magnesium trisilicate. Sucrose, 36.8 mg sodium.
Gaviscon Extra Strength Relief Formula, Extra Strength Genaton	**Tablets**: 160 mg aluminum hydroxide, 105 mg magnesium carbonate, alginic acid, sodium bicarbonate, calcium stearate. Sucrose, 29.9 mg sodium.
Extra Strength Alenic Alka	**Tablets**: 160 mg aluminum hydroxide, 105 mg magnesium carbonate. 29.9 mg sodium.
Mylanta	**Tablets**: 200 mg aluminum hydroxide, 200 mg magnesium hydroxide, 20 mg simethicone. Sorbitol, 0.77 mg sodium.
RuLox Plus	**Tablets**: 200 mg aluminum hydroxide, 200 mg magnesium hydroxide, 25 mg simethicone. Sugar, saccharin, dextrose.
Gelusil	**Tablets**: 200 mg aluminum hydroxide, 200 mg magnesium hydroxide, 25 mg simethicone. Sorbitol, sugar.
Mintox Plus	**Tablets**: 200 mg aluminum hydroxide, 200 mg magnesium hydroxide, 25 mg simethicone. Saccharin, sucrose.
Mylanta Double Strength	**Tablets**: 400 mg aluminum hydroxide, 400 mg magnesium hydroxide, 40 mg simethicone. Saccharin, sorbitol.
Tempo	**Tablets**: 133 mg aluminum hydroxide, 81 mg magnesium hydroxide, 414 calcium carbonate, 20 mg simethicone. Corn syrup, sorbitol, 3 mg sodium.
Calcium Rich Rolaids	**Tablets**: 80 mg magnesium hydroxide, 412 mg calcium carbonate. 0.4 mg sodium.
Advanced Formula Di-Gel	**Tablets**: 128 mg magnesium hydroxide, 280 mg calcium carbonate, 20 mg simethicone. Sucrose.
Gas-X with Maalox	**Tablets**: 500 mg calcium carbonate, 125 mg simethicone. Dextrose, talc, mannitol. Wild berry and orange flavors.

ANTACID COMBINATION PRODUCTS

Trade name	Doseform
Capsules and Tablets	
Riopan Plus Double Strength	**Tablets**: 1080 mg magaldrate, 20 mg simethicone. Saccharin, sorbitol, sucrose.
Almacone	**Tablets, chewable**: 200 mg aluminum hydroxide, 200 mg magnesium hydroxide, 20 mg simethicone
Mi-Acid Gelcaps, Mylanta Gelcaps	**Capsules**: 311 mg calcium carbonate, 232 mg magnesium carbonate. Parabens, EDTA.
Liquids	
Alamag	**Suspension**: 225 mg aluminum hydroxide, 200 mg magnesium hydroxide. Sorbitol, sucrose, parabens, < 1.25 mg sodium.
Maalox, Magnox	**Suspension**: 225 mg aluminum hydroxide, 200 mg magnesium hydroxide. Saccharin, sorbitol, parabens.
Alamag Plus	**Suspension**: 225 mg aluminum hydroxide, 200 mg magnesium hydroxide, 25 mg simethicone. Parabens, saccharin, sorbitol.
Antacid	**Suspension**: 225 mg aluminum hydroxide, 200 mg magnesium hydroxide
Mintox, RuLox	**Suspension**: 225 mg aluminum hydroxide, 200 mg magnesium hydroxide. Parabens, saccharin, sorbitol.
Aludrox	**Suspension**: 307 mg aluminum hydroxide, 103 mg magnesium hydroxide, simethicone. Saccharin, sorbitol, parabens.
Extra Strength Maalox	**Suspension**: 500 mg aluminum hydroxide, 450 mg magnesium hydroxide, 40 mg simethicone. Parabens, saccharin, sorbitol.
Maalox Therapeutic Concentrate	**Suspension**: 600 mg aluminum hydroxide, 300 mg magnesium hydroxide. Parabens, sorbitol.
Kudrox Double Strength	**Suspension**: 500 mg aluminum hydroxide, 450 mg magnesium hydroxide, 40 mg simethicone. Parabens, saccharin, sorbitol.
Mygel	**Suspension**: 200 mg aluminum hydroxide, 200 mg magnesium hydroxide, 20 mg simethicone
Alumina, Magnesia, and Simethicone	**Suspension**: 213 mg aluminum hydroxide, 200 mg magnesium hydroxide, 20 mg simethicone. Parabens, sorbitol.
Mygel II	**Suspension**: 400 mg aluminum hydroxide, 400 mg magnesium hydroxide, 40 mg simethicone
Extra Strength RuLox Plus	**Suspension**: 500 mg aluminum hydroxide, 450 mg magnesium hydroxide, 40 mg simethicone. Saccharin, sorbitol, parabens.
Lowsium Plus, Magaldrate Plus	**Suspension**: 540 mg magaldrate, 40 mg simethicone
Riopan Plus	**Suspension**: 540 mg magaldrate, 40 mg simethicone. Saccharin, sorbitol.
Riopan Plus Double Strength	**Suspension**: 1080 mg magaldrate, 40 mg simethicone. Saccharin, sorbitol.
Extra Strength Mintox Plus	**Liquid**: 500 mg aluminum hydroxide, 450 mg magnesium hydroxide, 40 mg simethicone. Parabens, saccharin, sorbitol.

ANTACID COMBINATION PRODUCTS

Trade name	Doseform
Liquids	
Gaviscon Extra Strength Relief Formula	**Liquid**: 254 mg aluminum hydroxide, 237.5 mg magnesium carbonate, simethicone, sodium alginate. Parabens, EDTA, saccharin, sorbitol.
Alenic Alka	**Liquid**: 95 mg aluminum hydroxide, 358 mg magnesium carbonate. EDTA, saccharin, sorbitol, parabens, 1.7 mEq sodium/tbsp.
Gaviscon	**Liquid**: 31.7 mg aluminum hydroxide, 119.3 mg magnesium carbonate, sodium alginate. EDTA, saccharin, sorbitol, parabens, 13 mg sodium.
Genaton	**Liquid**: 31.7 mg aluminum hydroxide, 137.3 mg magnesium carbonate, sodium alginate. EDTA, saccharin, sorbitol, 13 mg sodium.
Marblen	**Liquid**: 520 mg calcium carbonate, 400 mg magnesium carbonate
Titralac Plus	**Liquid**: 500 mg calcium carbonate, 20 mg simethicone. Parabens, saccharin, sorbitol, 0.15 mg sodium.
Almacone	**Liquid**: 200 mg aluminum hydroxide, 200 magnesium hydroxide, 20 mg simethicone
Di-Gel	**Liquid**: 200 mg aluminum hydroxide, 200 magnesium hydroxide, 20 mg simethicone. Saccharin, sorbitol, parabens.
Mi-Acid	**Liquid**: 200 mg aluminum hydroxide, 200 magnesium hydroxide, 20 mg simethicone. Parabens, sorbitol.
Mylanta	**Liquid**: 200 mg aluminum hydroxide, 200 magnesium hydroxide, 20 mg simethicone. Sorbitol, 0.68 mg sodium.
Almacone Double Strength	**Liquid**:400 mg aluminum hydroxide, 400 mg magnesium hydroxide, 40 mg simethicone. Parabens, sorbitol.
Antacid Double Strength	**Liquid**: 400 mg aluminum hydroxide, 400 mg magnesium hydroxide, 40 mg simethicone. Parabens, sorbitol, sucrose, < 1.25 mg sodium.
Mi-Acid II	**Liquid**: 400 mg aluminum hydroxide, 400 mg magnesium hydroxide, 40 mg simethicone. Parabens, sorbitol, sucrose.
Mylanta Double Strength	**Liquid**: 400 mg aluminum hydroxide, 400 mg magnesium hydroxide, 40 mg simethicone. Sorbitol, parabens.
Isopan Plus	**Liquid**: 540 mg magaldrate, 40 mg simethicone
Powder and Effervescent Tablets	
Alka-Seltzer Gold	**Tablets, effervescent**: 958 mg sodium bicarbonate (heat-treated), 832 citric acid 312 mg potassium bicarbonate. 311 mg sodium.
Alka-Seltzer	**Tablets, effervescent**: 1700 mg sodium bicarbonate, 325 mg aspirin, 1000 mg citric acid. 9 mg phenylalanine, 506 mg sodium.
Alka-Seltzer Original	**Tablets, effervescent**: 1916 mg sodium bicarbonate (heat-treated), 325 mg aspirin, 1000 mg citric acid. 567 mg sodium.

ANTACID COMBINATION PRODUCTS

Trade name	Doseform
Powder and Effervescent Tablets	
Extra Strength Alka-Seltzer	**Tablets, effervescent**: 1985 mg sodium bicarbonate (heat-treated), 500 mg aspirin, 1000 mg citric acid. 588 mg sodium.
Citrocarbonate	**Granules, effervescent**: 780 mg sodium bicarbonate, 1820 mg sodium citrate anhydrous. 700.6 mg sodium.
Sparkles	**Granules, effervescent**: 2000 mg sodium bicarbonate, 1500 mg citric acid, simethicone

Products listed are representative of currently available and widely distributed brands. Similar products, including regional and private label brands, may also exist.

PATIENT INFORMATION

Antacid Combinations

- *Chewable tablets:* Thoroughly chew before swallowing and follow with a glass of water.
- *Liquids:* Shake liquid antacids before use.
- *Effervescent tablets:* Allow tablet to completely dissolve in water and allow most of the bubbling to stop before drinking.
- Magnesium-containing products may act as a laxative in large doses and cause diarrhea.
- Aluminum- and calcium-containing products may cause constipation.
- Antacids may interact with certain prescription medications. If you are taking a prescription drug, do not take an antacid without checking with your physician or pharmacist.
- Taking too much of these products can cause the stomach to secrete excess stomach acid.

FLATULENCE

DEFINITION

Flatulence is the expulsion of gas (flatus) via the rectum. Excessive passage of flatus is embarrassing, but it is rarely an indicator of a major digestive disorder.

ETIOLOGY

Although the passage of flatus is normal, the frequency and volume varies widely. It is affected by malabsorption (eg, lactose intolerance) and disorders of gastric motility (eg, irritable bowel syndrome). Dietary composition (eg, lactose, starches, legumes), drugs (eg, antibiotics, bowel preps), and changes in colonic pH also contribute to excessive gas production. In healthy American men and women, the average frequency of flatulence is 10 times per day. Less than 25 times per day is considered normal. The frequency of the passage of flatus is not related to age or sex.

PATHOPHYSIOLOGY

Flatus is formed by the action of colonic bacteria on dietary carbohydrates. Carbohydrates reach the colon when malabsorption or ingestion of nonabsorbable or poorly absorbed carbohydrates occurs. Anaerobic fermentation of carbohydrates results in the production of hydrogen, carbon dioxide, and methane. Nitrogen and oxygen are also present in flatus but are primarily derived from swallowed air. In addition to producing gases, colonic bacteria also consume gases. Excessive production of flatus is an imbalance of gas production and consumption by colonic bacteria.

SIGNS/SYMPTOMS

Patients generally complain of "too much gas." This may be accompanied by abdominal cramps, belching, bloating, discomfort, or audible bowel sounds. Although individuals often assume that these symptoms are caused by excessive gas production, this may not always be true.

DIAGNOSTIC PARAMETERS/PHYSICAL ASSESSMENT

Clinical Observation: It is difficult to objectively confirm the complaint of excessive rectal gas production. Although some individuals may actually pass excessive flatus, a good proportion may have a misconception of what is abnormal. More than 25 passages per day of flatus may be considered abnormal.

Interview: The first step is to determine whether a problem actually exists and to discern the nature of the complaint. Because patients sometimes attribute abdominal bloating and distention or discomfort to too much gas, it is important to determine whether the patient actually passes excessive gas via the rectum. A detailed history should be obtained from each patient. Pertinent questions should address the following:

- Nature of symptoms: Onset, duration, frequency, what relieves symptoms.
- Diet: Consumption of legumes, starch, prunes, lactose-containing products.
- Medications: Narcotics, antibiotics, calcium channel blockers.
- Surgical history: Abdominal surgery.
- Medical history: Peptic ulcer disease (PUD), gastroesophageal reflux disease (GERD), malabsorption, irritable bowel syndrome.
- Systemic diseases: Diabetes, hypothyroidism.

TREATMENT

Approaches to therapy: Individuals with a history suggestive of GI disease (eg, PUD, GERD, irritable bowel syndrome) or systemic disease should be referred to a physician for further evaluation. If appropriate, advise patients to discontinue medications that may be responsible for the observed symptoms. Patients with lactose intolerance should be managed appropriately (see Lactose Intolerance monograph).

Nondrug therapy: Because gas production may be dependent on the consumption of carbohydrates, patients may benefit from dietary modification. Restricting the consumption of beans and other legumes, wheat, and fruit may help alleviate flatulence.

CHARCOAL

▶ **Actions**

Charcoal is an adsorbent, detoxicant, and soothing agent. It reduces the volume of intestinal gas and relieves related discomfort.

▶ **Indications**

For the relief of intestinal gas, diarrhea, and GI distress associated with indigestion and accompanying cramps or odor.

Also used as an antidote in drug overdoses and for the prevention of nonspecific pruritus associated with kidney dialysis treatment.

▶ **Contraindications**

Do not use in children younger than 3 years of age.

▶ **Warnings**

Diarrhea: If diarrhea persists for longer than 2 days or is accompanied by fever, consult physician.

High dosage, prolonged use: High dosage or prolonged use does not cause side effects or harm the patient's nutritional state.

Children: Do not administer to children younger than 3 years of age.

▶ **Drug Interactions**

Charcoal interferes with the absorption of numerous drugs. Activated charcoal can adsorb drugs while they are in the GI tract. A list of drugs that interact with charcoal is not provided because the list is exhaustive and not all drugs have been evaluated. Administer charcoal 2 hours before or 1 hour after other medications.

Drug-food interactions: Milk, ice cream, or sherbet may decrease the adsorptive capacity of activated charcoal.

▶ **Adverse Reactions**

GI: May cause vomiting, constipation, diarrhea, and black stools. Overdosage may lead to bowel obstruction.

Pulmonary: Aspiration of charcoal may lead to airway obstruction.

▶ **Administration and Dosage**

Adults: 500 to 520 mg after meals or at the first sign of discomfort. May repeat as needed up to 4.16 g/day.

CHARCOAL PRODUCTS	
Trade name	Doseform
Charcoal Plus DS	**Tablets:** 250 mg
CharcoCaps	**Capsules:** 260 mg

Products listed are representative of currently available and widely distributed brands. Similar products, including regional and private label brands, may also exist.

PATIENT INFORMATION

Charcoal

- If symptoms persist, consult a physician for further evaluation.
- Charcoal interferes with the absorption of other medications. Administer 2 hours before or 1 hour after other medications.
- Avoid foods that may contribute to the development of symptoms.
- Charcoal will turn stools black.

SIMETHICONE

▶ **Actions**

The defoaming action of simethicone prevents the formation of mucus-surrounded gas pockets in the GI tract and alters the surface tension of gas bubbles. This leads to coalescence and easier elimination of gas by belching or passing of flatus.

▶ **Indications**

Simethicone is used in the management of flatulence and various conditions that may lead to gaseous distention and pain.

▶ **Contraindications**

Hypersensitivity to simethicone.

▶ **Adverse Reactions**

Simethicone does not appear to cause adverse reactions.

▶ **Administration and Dosage**

Capsules: 125 mg after each meal and at bedtime.

Tablets: 40 to 125 mg after each meal and at bedtime. Thoroughly chew tablets.

Drops: Take after meals and at bedtime. Shake well before using. Mix with water or infant formula for ease of administration.

Adults – 40 to 80 mg 4 times daily as needed. Do not exceed 500 mg/day.

Children (2 to 12 years of age) – 40 mg 4 times daily as needed.

Children (younger than 2 years of age) – 20 mg 4 times daily as needed. Do not exceed 240 mg/day.

SIMETHICONE PRODUCTS	
Trade name	Doseform
Maalox Anti-Gas	**Tablets**: 80 mg
Extra Strength Maalox Anti-Gas	**Tablets**: 150 mg
Almacone	**Tablets, chewable**: 20 mg
Gas Relief, Gas-X, Major-Con, Mylanta Gas	**Tablets, chewable**: 80 mg
Extra Strength Gas-X, Maximum Strength Gas Relief, Maximum Strength Mylanta Gas	**Tablets, chewable**: 125 mg
Maximum Strength Mylanta Gas Gelcaps	**Capsules**: 62.5 mg
Maximum Strength Phazyme 125 Softgels, Extra Strength Gas-X Softgels	**Capsules**: 125 mg
Alka-Seltzer Gas Relief	**Capsules**: 125 mg
Fast Acting Mylanta	**Liquid**: 20 mg/5 mL
Fast Acting Mylanta Maximum Strength	**Liquid**: 40 mg/5 mL
Infants' Mylicon Drops, Flatulex, Gas Relief, Mylicon	**Drops**: 40 mg/0.6 mL
Gerber Gas	**Drops**: 40 mg/0.6 mL. Saccharin calcium, 0.15 mg sodium/0.6 mL

Products listed are representative of currently available and widely distributed brands. Similar products, including regional and private label brands, may also exist.

PATIENT INFORMATION
Simethicone
- If symptoms persist, consult a physician for further evaluation.
- Avoid foods that may contribute to the development of symptoms.

CHARCOAL AND SIMETHICONE

▶ **Actions**

Charcoal reduces the volume of gas. Simethicone disperses and prevents the formation of mucus-surrounded gas pockets, and allows for their elimination.

▶ **Indications**

For the relief of gas pain and associated symptoms.

▶ **Administration and Dosage**

One tablet 3 times daily and at bedtime as needed.

CHARCOAL AND SIMETHICONE PRODUCTS	
Trade name	Doseform
Flatulex	**Tablets**: 250 mg activated charcoal, 80 mg simethicone
Maximum Strength Flatulex	**Tablets**: 250 mg activated charcoal, 125 mg simethicone

Products listed are representative of currently available and widely distributed brands. Similar products, including regional and private label brands, may also exist.

PATIENT INFORMATION
Charcoal and Simethicone
- If symptoms persist, consult a physician for further evaluation.
- Charcoal interferes with the absorption of other medications. Administer 2 hours before or 1 hour after other medications.
- Avoid foods that may contribute to the development of symptoms.
- Charcoal will turn stools black.

GASTRITIS

DEFINITION

Gastritis is an inflammation of the gastric mucosa. It is not a single disease, but a manifestation of a heterogeneous group of disorders, which cause mucosal inflammation by various mechanisms. Gastritis is further classified into acute erosive or hemorrhagic, nonerosive (chronic), and distinctive (specific) gastritis. These divisions are based on the pattern of endoscopic or histologic findings. Nonerosive gastritis is further divided into type A and type B gastritis.

ETIOLOGY

Erosive or hemorrhagic gastritis: Erosive or hemorrhagic gastritis is associated with drugs (aspirin, NSAIDs, alcohol, iron), stress ulcers, mechanical trauma (nasogastric tubes, endoscopy), ischemia, and gastroesophageal reflux. The cause may also be idiopathic.

Nonerosive gastritis (type B): Nonerosive gastritis (type B) is most commonly a result of *H. pylori* infection. Crohn's disease, reactive gastropathy, and lymphocytic and atrophic gastritis are also associated with type B gastritis.

Nonerosive gastritis (type A): Nonerosive gastritis (type A) is believed to be autoimmune and is less common than type B.

Distinctive types of gastritis are chiefly caused by non-*H. pylori* infections. These infections can be bacterial (tuberculosis), viral (cytomegalovirus, herpesvirus), fungal (*Candida albicans*, histoplasmosis), or parasitic (*Cryptosporidium*). These types of gastritis are most often seen in immunocompromised patients.

INCIDENCE

Given the many conditions that may cause gastritis, the true incidence is difficult to estimate. The three most common causes of gastritis are aspirin or NSAIDs, alcohol, and *H. pylori* infection. Approximately 50% of patients taking aspirin or NSAIDs develop acute gastric erosions. Although NSAIDs are infamous for causing ulcers, NSAID-induced erosions and hemorrhages develop more frequently. Acute or chronic alcohol ingestion may lead to gastritis. Gastritis may be present in approximately 50% of chronic alcoholics.

H. pylori infection is the most common chronic infection in humans. *H. pylori* is primarily acquired during childhood, and the rate of infection declines to 0.3% to 0.5% per year in adults. Within the same socioeconomic group, at age 60, *H. pylori* is present in approximately 50% of whites and more than 80% of Hispanics or blacks. According to some studies, 80% of *H. pylori*-infected individuals develop gastritis. More recent studies indicate that *H. pylori* is present in approximately 60% of patients with chronic gastritis.

PATHOPHYSIOLOGY

Erosive/Hemorrhagic gastritis:

Aspirin and NSAIDs – Aspirin and NSAIDs induce mucosal damage through direct injury and by inhibition of prostaglandins. Direct injury is primarily responsible for acute mucosal damage. For instance, denudation of surface epithelium can be seen within a few minutes of aspirin ingestion. NSAIDs are weak acids that are unionized at gastric pH levels and therefore lipid soluble. Lipid solubility enables NSAIDs to freely diffuse into mucosal cells. High intracellular levels of NSAIDs are responsible for the local toxic effects. After 1 to 2 weeks of chronic aspirin and NSAID use, prostaglandin inhibition becomes a major factor. These agents inhibit the enzyme cyclooxygenase, which is responsible for the production of prostaglandins. Prostaglandins are a group of fatty acids that protect the mucosa against damage. Therefore, a decrease in prostaglandin production predisposes the mucosa to gastric acid.

Alcohol – Ethanol is lipid soluble and therefore readily penetrates the gastric mucosa where it disrupts intercellular tight junctions formed by gastric epithelial cells. Disruption of these tight junctions compromises the integrity of the gastric mucosal barrier, predisposing the mucosa to damage from stomach acid.

Nonerosive gastritis:

H. pylori – Damages gastric mucosa through direct cytotoxicity and the production of inflammatory mediators. Cytokines and phospholipases produced by *H. pylori* directly interfere with the integrity of gastric epithelium. Ammonia and related compounds, which are byproducts of urease activity, may also contribute to mucosal damage. *H. pylori* stimulates local and systemic immune responses. Stimulation of the immune system leads the production of interleukins, interferons, and immunoglobulins. The net result is inflammation and damage to the gastric mucosa.

SIGNS/SYMPTOMS

Most cases of gastritis are asymptomatic. When present, symptoms include nausea, vomiting, anorexia, epigastric pain, or upper GI bleeding. GI bleeding often brings the condition to medical attention. It manifests as hematemesis, melena, or occult blood in feces. In some cases, patients may present with anemia. Left unnoticed, gastritis may progress to gastric ulcers that may perforate and hemorrhage.

DIAGNOSTIC PARAMETERS/PHYSICAL ASSESSMENT

Clinical Observation: Gastritis is diagnosed objectively by endoscopy.

Interview: To determine which patients to refer for further evaluation, practitioners need a detailed history addressing the following:

- The nature and duration of symptoms.
- GI bleeding (hematemesis, tarry stool, and melena).
- Current medications (prescription and OTC).
- History of peptic ulcer disease.

- Unintentional weight loss.
- Symptoms related to anemia (pallor, fatigue, headache, lightheadedness, and dyspnea).
- Frequency and quantity of alcohol consumption.

The patient response to questioning may prompt practitioners to refer the patient to a physician. In addition, refer chronic alcoholics and individuals with symptoms that have been present for longer than 2 weeks.

TREATMENT

Approaches to therapy: The management of acute erosive gastritis is nonpharmacologic. Discontinuation of the causative agent (NSAIDs, alcohol) leads to resolution within a few days. Antacids may help alleviate symptoms. The use of nonprescription H_2 receptor antagonists has not been evaluated. However, in the absence of contraindications they may be tried. Always refer patients with hemorrhagic gastritis and chronic gastritis to a physician for further evaluation.

Pharmacotherapy: Prescription antisecretory agents (histamine H_2 antagonists) and antacids are used frequently in the management of functional gastritis. Patients who have heartburn may experience relief. A short trial of two weeks or less with OTC therapy may be safe and effective. If the patient is under the care of a physician, a four-week trial may be appropriate.

HISTAMINE H_2 ANTAGONISTS

▶ Actions

Histamine H_2 receptors in gastric parietal cells control acid secretion. Histamine H_2 receptor antagonists decrease acid production by competing reversibly with histamine at the H_2 receptor. These agents also decrease food-, insulin-, and caffeine-induced secretions. They have no anticholinergic properties and no effect on H_1 receptors.

▶ Indications

For the relief of symptoms of episodic and uncomplicated heartburn, acid indigestion, and sour stomach.

▶ Contraindications

Hypersensitivity to individual agents or other histamine H_2 receptor antagonists.

▶ Warnings

Pregnancy: Category B. There are no adequate and well-controlled studies in pregnant women. Use during pregnancy only if the potential benefits outweigh the possible risks to the fetus.

Lactation: Cimetidine and ranitidine are excreted in human breast milk. Avoid cimetidine use in nursing mothers. Exercise caution in administering ranitidine to lactating mothers. It is not known whether famotidine is excreted in human breast milk. However, it is excreted in the breast milk of rats. Do not use famotidine in nursing mothers unless the benefits to the mother outweigh the risks to the fetus.

Children: OTC use of H_2 antagonists is not recommended in children younger than 12 years of age. In addition, cimetidine is not recommended in children younger than 16 years of age.

▶ **Drug Interactions**

Drugs metabolized by cytochrome P450: Significant drug interactions with H_2 antagonists primarily occur with cimetidine. Cimetidine inhibits the metabolism of certain drugs metabolized by the cytochrome P450 system, thereby leading to increased drug levels and toxicity. Through this mechanism, cimetidine inhibits the clearance of drugs such as warfarin, theophylline, phenytoin, propranolol, nifedipine, metronidazole, carbamazepine, phenytoin, sulfonylureas, quinidine, cisapride, alcohol, caffeine, and benzodiazepines.

Carmustine: Cimetidine results in increased bone marrow suppression.

Itraconazole and ketoconazole: H_2 antagonists decrease the absorption of itraconazole and ketoconazole by decreasing gastric acidity.

Metformin: Cimetidine may increase serum plasma levels of metformin by reducing its renal clearance.

Procainamide: Cimetidine and ranitidine may increase serum plasma levels of procainamide by reducing its renal clearance.

Drug-food interactions: Food may increase the bioavailability of famotidine and nizatidine. This interaction is unlikely to be clinically relevant with OTC doses of H_2 antagonists.

▶ **Adverse Reactions**

H_2 antagonists generally are well tolerated. The most common adverse reactions are headache, fatigue, and diarrhea. Prolonged use of cimetidine may lead to gynecomastia. Reversible confusional states (eg, psychosis, delirium, agitation, depression) have been reported in elderly patients. Gynecomastia and confusion are more likely with the higher prescription doses of cimetidine.

CIMETIDINE

▶ **Administration and Dosage**

Relief of symptoms: Take 200 mg (one tablet) with a glass of water or other fluid as needed. Do not exceed 400 mg (two tablets) in 24 hours.

Prevention of symptoms: Take 200 mg (one tablet) with a glass of water or other fluid 30 minutes or less before eating food or drinking beverages that cause heartburn, acid indigestion, or sour stomach. Do not exceed 400 mg (two tablets) in 24 hours.

Cimetidine should not be given to children younger than 12 years of age unless directed by a physician.

CIMETIDINE PRODUCTS	
Trade name	**Doseform**
Cimetidine, *Tagamet HB 200*	**Tablets**: 200 mg
Tagamet HB 200	**Suspension**: 200 mg/5 mL

Products listed are representative of currently available and widely distributed brands. Similar products, including regional and private label brands, may also exist.

RANITIDINE

▶ **Administration and Dosage**

Take tablets with fluid and swallow them whole.

Usual dosage: May be used up to twice daily (up to 2 tablets in 24 hours).

RANITIDINE PRODUCTS	
Trade name	Doseform
Ranitidine (sf)	**Tablets**: 75 mg. Lactose. Sodium free.
Zantac 75 (sf)	**Tablets**: 75 mg. Sodium free.
Zantac 150 (sf)	**Tablets**: 150 mg.

Products listed are representative of currently available and widely distributed brands. Similar products, including regional and private label brands, may also exist.

sf = Sugar free.

FAMOTIDINE

▶ Administration and Dosage

Take the nonchewable tablets and gelcaps with fluid and swallow them whole.

Relief of symptoms: Swallow one tablet or gelcap with a glass of water or chew one chewable tablet.

Prevention of symptoms: Swallow one tablet or gelcap with a glass of water or chew one chewable tablet at any time 15 to 60 minutes before eating food or drinking beverages that cause heartburn.

10 mg: Take 10 mg once or twice daily as needed. Do not exceed 20 mg (two tablets or gelcaps) in 24 hours.

20 mg: Take 20 mg once or twice daily as needed. Do not exceed more than 40 mg (two tablets) in 24 hours.

FAMOTIDINE PRODUCTS	
Trade name	Doseform
Famotidine, Pepcid AC	**Tablets**: 10 mg
Maximum Strength Pepcid AC	**Tablets**: 20 mg. Talc.
Pepcid AC Chewable	**Tablets, chewable**: 10 mg. Aspartame, lactose, 1.4 mg phenylalanine.
Pepcid AC Gelcaps	**Gelcaps**: 10 mg

Products listed are representative of currently available and widely distributed brands. Similar products, including regional and private label brands, may also exist.

NIZATIDINE

▶ Administration and Dosage

Take tablets with fluid and swallow them whole.

Usual dosage: Take 75 mg once or twice daily as needed. Do not exceed 150 mg (two tablets) in 24 hours.

NIZATIDINE PRODUCTS	
Trade name	Doseform
Axid AR	**Tablets**: 75 mg

Products listed are representative of currently available and widely distributed brands. Similar products, including regional and private label brands, may also exist.

HISTAMINE H$_2$ ANTAGONIST COMBINATIONS

▶ Administration and Dosage

Do not swallow tablet whole; chew completely.

Usual dosage: Do not use more than two chewable tablets in 24 hours. Do not give to children younger than 12 years of age unless directed by a physician.

HISTAMINE H₂ ANTAGONIST PRODUCTS	
Trade name	Doseform
Pepcid Complete	**Tablets, chewable**: 10 mg famotidine. 800 mg calcium carbonate, 165 mg magnesium hydroxide. Lactose, sugar.

Products listed are representative of currently available and widely distributed brands. Similar products, including regional and private label brands, may also exist.

PATIENT INFORMATION
Histamine H₂ Antagonists

- Patient instructions accompany each product. Read these instructions carefully before use, preferably before leaving the pharmacy in case of any questions.
- Do not use the maximum daily doses of these agents for two weeks or more, except under the advice of a physician.
- Histamine H₂ antagonists may interact with certain prescription drugs. If you are presently taking a prescription drug, do not take a histamine H₂ antagonist without checking with a physician or pharmacist.
- If symptoms worsen or persist for two weeks or more, contact a physician.
- Store at room temperature in a tight container away from light.

ANTACIDS

▶ Actions
Antacids increase gastric and duodenal pH by neutralizing acid. They do not affect the production of gastric acid. By raising gastric pH, antacids also inhibit the activity of the pepsin.

▶ Indications
Symptomatic relief of conditions associated with hyperacidity such as heartburn, gastroesophageal reflux, acid indigestion, sour stomach, gastritis, and peptic ulcers.

▶ Contraindications
There are no specific contraindications to the use of antacids. If possible, avoid magnesium-containing antacids in patients with marked renal failure (see Warnings).

▶ Warnings
Congestive heart failure, hypertension, and sodium-restricted diets: Some products have a high sodium content, which may interfere with low-sodium diets and the management of hypertension or congestive heart failure.

Renal insufficiency: These patients are at an increased risk for developing aluminum intoxication, hypermagnesemia, hypercalcemia, and other electrolyte imbalances. If possible, avoid use of magnesium-containing antacids, including magaldrate, in patients where marked renal failure (Ccr 30 mL/min or less) is known or suspected.

Pregnancy: Pregnant women should consult a physician before using antacids.

Lactation: Lactating women should consult a physician before using antacids.

▶ Drug Interactions
Antacids administered concurrently with other drugs can significantly decrease the absorption of iron salts, quinolones (eg, ciprofloxacin, ofloxacin), ketoconazole, and

tetracyclines. Antacids may also decrease the absorption of digoxin, isoniazid, phenytoin, and quinidine. These interactions can be minimized by separating drug administration by 2 hours.

▶ **Adverse Reactions**

Constipation/diarrhea: Magnesium-dominant antacids may cause diarrhea, while aluminum- and calcium-dominant antacids may cause constipation.

Milk alkali syndrome: As an acute illness, the syndrome presents with headache, nausea, vomiting, weakness, alkalosis, and hypercalcemia that has developed during the use of high-dose calcium carbonate concomitantly with sodium bicarbonate.

Electrolyte imbalance: Hypernatremia, hypermagnesemia, hypercalcemia, and hypophosphatemia may occur with the chronic use of antacids, especially in renal failure.

Alkalosis: Prolonged use of antacids containing sodium bicarbonate may result in systemic alkalosis.

Rebound hyperacidity: Dose-related rebound hyperacidity has been reported with antacids.

MAGNESIUM HYDROXIDE

▶ **Administration and Dosage**

Note: There are numerous antacid formulations. Many combination antacids contain $Mg(OH)_2$ as one of the primary ingredients. Patients should follow the product labeling for appropriate instructions. Doses used for the management of conditions associated with hyperacidity can be used for the management of gastritis.

Tablets: 622 mg to 1244 mg up to 4 times daily as needed.

Liquid: 5 to 15 mL up to 4 times daily as needed.

Liquid, concentrated: 2.5 to 7.5 mL up to 4 times daily as needed.

MAGNESIUM HYDROXIDE PRODUCTS	
Trade name	Doseform
Phillips' Chewable	**Tablets, chewable**: 311 mg
Milk of Magnesia, Phillips' Milk of Magnesia, Dulcolax Milk of Magnesia (sf)	**Liquid**: 400 mg/5 mL
Concentrated Phillips' Milk of Magnesia	**Liquid**: 800 mg/5 mL

Products listed are representative of currently available and widely distributed brands. Similar products, including regional and private label brands, may also exist.

sf = Sugar free.

PATIENT INFORMATION

Magnesium Hydroxide

- If symptoms worsen or persist for longer than 2 weeks, consult a physician.
- Do not exceed the recommended doses for these agents, and do not use maximum daily doses for longer than 2 weeks unless directed otherwise by a physician.
- Magnesium-dominant products may cause diarrhea.
- Shake liquid antacids prior to use.
- Sodium content is generally low but varies. Check package label if you are on a sodium-restricted diet or have heart disease or high blood pressure.

MAGNESIUM OXIDE

▶ Administration and Dosage

Note: There are numerous antacid formulations. Patients should follow the product labeling for appropriate instructions. Doses used for the management of conditions associated with hyperacidity can be used for the management of gastritis.

Capsules: 140 mg 3 to 4 times daily.

Tablets: 400 to 800 mg/day.

MAGNESIUM OXIDE PRODUCTS	
Trade name	Doseform
Mag-Ox 400	**Tablets**: 400 mg
Maox	**Tablets**: 420 mg
Uro-Mag	**Capsules**: 140 mg

Products listed are representative of currently available and widely distributed brands. Similar products, including regional and private label brands, may also exist.

PATIENT INFORMATION

Magnesium Oxide

- If symptoms worsen or persist for longer than 2 weeks, consult a physician.
- Do not exceed the recommended doses for these agents, and do not use maximum daily doses for longer than 2 weeks unless directed otherwise by a physician.
- Magnesium-dominant products may cause diarrhea.
- Sodium content is generally low but varies. Check package label if you are on a sodium-restricted diet or have heart disease or high blood pressure.

ALUMINUM HYDROXIDE GEL

▶ Administration and Dosage

Note: There are numerous antacid formulations. Many combination antacids contain an aluminum salt as one of the ingredients. Patients should follow the product labeling for appropriate instructions. Doses used for the management of conditions associated with hyperacidity can be used for the management of gastritis.

Tablets/Capsules: 500 to 1500 mg 3 to 6 times daily as needed between meals and at bedtime.

Suspension: 5 to 30 mL as needed between meals and at bedtime.

ALUMINUM HYDROXIDE GEL PRODUCTS	
Trade name	Doseform
Amphojel	**Tablets**: 300 mg
Alu-Tab	**Tablets**: 500 mg
Amphojel	**Tablets**: 600 mg
Alu-Cap	**Capsules**: 400 mg
Dialume	**Capsules**: 500 mg
Amphojel	**Suspension**: 320 mg/5 mL
AlternaGEL	**Liquid**: 600 mg/5 mL

Products listed are representative of currently available and widely distributed brands. Similar products, including regional and private label brands, may also exist.

PATIENT INFORMATION
Aluminum Hydroxide

- If symptoms worsen or persist for longer than 2 weeks, consult a physician.
- Do not exceed the recommended doses for these agents, and do not use maximum daily doses for longer than 2 weeks unless directed otherwise by a physician.
- Aluminum-containing products may cause constipation.
- Liquid antacids should be shaken prior to use.
- Sodium content is generally low but varies. Check package label if you are on a sodium-restricted diet or have heart disease or high blood pressure.

ALUMINUM CARBONATE GEL

▶ Administration and Dosage

Note: There are numerous antacid formulations. Many combination antacids contain an aluminum salt as one of the ingredients. Patients should follow the product labeling for appropriate instructions. Doses used for the management of conditions associated with hyperacidity can be used for the management of gastritis.

Capsules/Tablets: 2 every 2 hours up to 12 times daily as needed.

Suspension: 10 mL every 2 hours up to 12 times daily as needed.

ALUMINUM CARBONATE GEL PRODUCTS	
Trade name	Doseform
Basaljel	**Tablets**: Equiv. to 608 mg dried aluminum hydroxide gel or 500 mg aluminum hydroxide
	Capsules: Equiv. to 608 mg dried aluminum hydroxide gel or 500 mg aluminum hydroxide
	Suspension: Equiv. to 400 mg aluminum hydroxide/5 mL

Products listed are representative of currently available and widely distributed brands. Similar products, including regional and private label brands, may also exist.

PATIENT INFORMATION
Aluminum Carbonate Gel

- If symptoms worsen or persist for longer than 2 weeks, consult a physician.
- Aluminum-containing products may cause constipation.
- Shake liquid antacids prior to use.
- Do not exceed the recommended doses for these agents, and do not use maximum daily doses for longer than 2 weeks unless directed otherwise by a physician.
- Sodium content is generally low but varies. Check package label if you are on a sodium-restricted diet or have heart disease or high blood pressure.

CALCIUM CARBONATE

▶ Administration and Dosage

Note: There are numerous antacid formulations. Patients should follow the product labeling for appropriate instructions. Doses used for the management of conditions associated with hyperacidity can be used for the management of gastritis.

Tablets/Lozenges: 0.5 to 1.5 g as needed.

CALCIUM CARBONATE PRODUCTS	
Trade name	Doseform
Titralac Extra Strength	**Tablets**: 750 mg. Saccharin.
Amitone	**Tablets, chewable**: 350 mg
Mallamint, Instant Relief Titralac	**Tablets, chewable**: 420 mg
Antacid, Tums	**Tablets, chewable**: 500 mg
Quick Dissolve Maalox	**Tablets, chewable**: 600 mg
Alka-Mints	**Tablets, chewable**: 850 mg
Chooz	**Gum tablets**: 500 mg
Mylanta	**Lozenges**: 600 mg

Products listed are representative of currently available and widely distributed brands. Similar products, including regional and private label brands, may also exist.

PATIENT INFORMATION

Calcium Carbonate

- If symptoms worsen or persist for longer than 2 weeks, consult a physician.
- Do not exceed the recommended doses for these agents and do not use maximum daily doses for longer than 2 weeks unless directed otherwise by a physician.
- Calcium-dominant products may cause constipation.
- Sodium content is generally low but varies. Check package label if you are on a sodium-restricted diet or have heart disease or high blood pressure.

MAGALDRATE (ALUMINUM MAGNESIUM HYDROXIDE SULFATE)

▶ Administration and Dosage

Note: There are numerous antacid formulations. Patients should follow the product labeling for appropriate instructions. Doses used for the management of conditions associated with hyperacidity can be used for the management of gastritis.

Suspension/Liquid: 5 to 10 mL between meals and at bedtime as needed.

MAGALDRATE	
Trade name	Doseform
Riopan	**Suspension**: 560 mg/5 mL
Iosopan	**Liquid**: 540 mg/5 mL

Products listed are representative of currently available and widely distributed brands. Similar products, including regional and private label brands, may also exist.

PATIENT INFORMATION

Magaldrate

- If symptoms worsen or persist for longer than 2 weeks, consult a physician.
- Do not exceed the recommended doses for these agents, and do not use maximum daily doses for longer than 2 weeks unless directed otherwise by a physician.
- Shake liquid antacids prior to use.

SODIUM BICARBONATE

▶ **Administration and Dosage**

0.3 to 2 g 1 to 4 times daily as needed.

SODIUM BICARBONATE PRODUCTS	
Trade name	Doseform
Bell/ans	Tablets: 520 mg

Products listed are representative of currently available and widely distributed brands. Similar products, including regional and private label brands, may also exist.

SODIUM CITRATE

▶ **Administration and Dosage**

30 mL daily as needed.

Note: There are numerous antacid formulations. Patients should follow the product labeling for appropriate instructions. Doses used for the management of conditions associated with hyperacidity can be used for the management of gastritis.

SODIUM CITRATE PRODUCTS	
Trade name	Doseform
Citra pH	Solution: 450 mg

Products listed are representative of currently available and widely distributed brands. Similar products, including regional and private label brands, may also exist.

PATIENT INFORMATION

Sodium Citrate

- If symptoms worsen or persist for longer than 2 weeks, consult a physician.
- Do not exceed the recommended doses for these agents, and do not use maximum daily doses for longer than 2 weeks unless directed otherwise by a physician.
- Calcium-dominant products may cause constipation.
- Shake liquid antacids prior to use.
- Sodium content is generally low but varies. Check package label if you are on a sodium-restricted diet or have heart disease or high blood pressure.

ANTACID COMBINATIONS

▶ **Administration and Dosage**

See individual products for administration and dosage guidelines.

ANTACID COMBINATION PRODUCTS	
Trade name	Doseform
Capsules and Tablets	
Maalox	Tablets: 200 mg aluminum hydroxide, 200 mg magnesium hydroxide. Saccharin, sorbitol.
Mintox, RuLox #1	Tablets: 200 mg aluminum hydroxide, 200 mg magnesium hydroxide. Saccharin.
Titralac Plus	Tablets: 420 mg calcium carbonate, 21 mg simethicone. Saccharin, 1.1 mg sodium.
Alenic Alka	Tablets: 80 mg aluminum hydroxide, 20 mg magnesium trisilicate, sodium bicarbonate, calcium stearate. Sugar, 18.4 mg sodium.

ANTACID COMBINATION PRODUCTS

Trade name	Doseform
Capsules and Tablets	
Foamicon	**Tablets**: 80 mg aluminum hydroxide, alginic acid, sodium bicarbonate, 20 mg magnesium trisilicate, calcium stearate. Sugar, sucrose, 18.4 mg sodium.
Genaton	**Tablets**: 80 mg aluminum hydroxide. alginic acid, sodium bicarbonate, 20 mg magnesium trisilicate. Sucrose, sugar, 18.4 mg sodium.
Gaviscon	**Tablets**: 80 mg aluminum hydroxide, alginic acid, sodium bicarbonate, 20 mg magnesium trisilicate, calcium stearate. Sucrose, 18.4 mg sodium.
Double Strength Gaviscon-2	**Tablets**: 160 mg aluminum hydroxide, alginic acid, sodium bicarbonate, 40 mg magnesium trisilicate. Sucrose, 36.8 mg sodium.
Gaviscon Extra Strength Relief Formula, Extra Strength Genaton	**Tablets**: 160 mg aluminum hydroxide, 105 mg magnesium carbonate, alginic acid, sodium bicarbonate, calcium stearate. Sucrose, 29.9 mg sodium.
Extra Strength Alenic Alka	**Tablets**: 160 mg aluminum hydroxide, 105 mg magnesium carbonate. 29.9 mg sodium.
Mylanta	**Tablets**: 200 mg aluminum hydroxide, 200 mg magnesium hydroxide, 20 mg simethicone. Sorbitol, 0.77 mg sodium.
RuLox Plus	**Tablets**: 200 mg aluminum hydroxide, 200 mg magnesium hydroxide, 25 mg simethicone. Sugar, saccharin, dextrose.
Gelusil	**Tablets**: 200 mg aluminum hydroxide, 200 mg magnesium hydroxide, 25 mg simethicone. Sorbitol, sugar.
Mintox Plus	**Tablets**: 200 mg aluminum hydroxide, 200 mg magnesium hydroxide, 25 mg simethicone. Saccharin, sucrose.
Mylanta Double Strength	**Tablets**: 400 mg aluminum hydroxide, 400 mg magnesium hydroxide, 40 mg simethicone. Saccharin, sorbitol.
Tempo	**Tablets**: 133 mg aluminum hydroxide, 81 mg magnesium hydroxide, 414 calcium carbonate, 20 mg simethicone. Corn syrup, sorbitol, 3 mg sodium.
Calcium Rich Rolaids	**Tablets**: 80 mg magnesium hydroxide, 412 mg calcium carbonate. 0.4 mg sodium.
Advanced Formula Di-Gel	**Tablets**: 128 mg magnesium hydroxide, 280 mg calcium carbonate, 20 mg simethicone. Sucrose.
Riopan Plus Double Strength	**Tablets**: 1080 mg magaldrate, 20 mg simethicone. Saccharin, sorbitol, sucrose.
Gas-X with Maalox	**Tablets**: 500 mg calcium carbonate, 125 mg simethicone. Dextrose, mannitol, talc. Wild berry and orange flavors.
Almacone	**Tablets, chewable**: 200 mg aluminum hydroxide, 200 mg magnesium hydroxide, 20 mg simethicone
Mi-Acid Gelcaps, Mylanta Gelcaps	**Capsules**: 311 mg calcium carbonate, 232 mg magnesium carbonate. Parabens, EDTA.
Liquids	
Alamag	**Suspension**: 225 mg aluminum hydroxide, 200 mg magnesium hydroxide. Sorbitol, sucrose, parabens, < 1.25 mg sodium.

ANTACID COMBINATION PRODUCTS	
Trade name	Doseform
Liquids	
Maalox, Magnox	**Suspension**: 225 mg aluminum hydroxide, 200 mg magnesium hydroxide. Saccharin, sorbitol, parabens.
Alamag Plus	**Suspension**: 225 mg aluminum hydroxide, 200 mg magnesium hydroxide, 25 mg simethicone. Parabens, saccharin, sorbitol.
Antacid	**Suspension**: 225 mg aluminum hydroxide, 200 mg magnesium hydroxide
Mintox, RuLox	**Suspension**: 225 mg aluminum hydroxide, 200 mg magnesium hydroxide. Parabens, saccharin, sorbitol.
Aludrox	**Suspension**: 307 mg aluminum hydroxide, 103 mg magnesium hydroxide, simethicone. Saccharin, sorbitol, parabens.
Extra Strength Maalox	**Suspension**: 500 mg aluminum hydroxide, 450 mg magnesium hydroxide, 40 mg simethicone. Parabens, saccharin, sorbitol.
Maalox Therapeutic Concentrate	**Suspension**: 600 mg aluminum hydroxide, 300 mg magnesium hydroxide. Parabens, sorbitol.
Kudrox Double Strength	**Suspension**: 500 mg aluminum hydroxide, 450 mg magnesium hydroxide, 40 mg simethicone. Parabens, saccharin, sorbitol.
Mygel	**Suspension**: 200 mg aluminum hydroxide, 200 mg magnesium hydroxide, 20 mg simethicone
Alumina, Magnesia, and Simethicone	**Suspension**: 213 mg aluminum hydroxide, 200 mg magnesium hydroxide, 20 mg simethicone. Parabens, sorbitol.
Mygel II	**Suspension**: 400 mg aluminum hydroxide, 400 mg magnesium hydroxide, 40 mg simethicone
Extra Strength RuLox Plus	**Suspension**: 500 mg aluminum hydroxide, 450 mg magnesium hydroxide, 40 mg simethicone. Saccharin, sorbitol, parabens.
Lowsium Plus, Magaldrate Plus	**Suspension**: 540 mg magaldrate, 40 mg simethicone
Riopan Plus	**Suspension**: 540 mg magaldrate, 40 mg simethicone. Saccharin, sorbitol.
Riopan Plus Double Strength	**Suspension**: 1080 mg magaldrate, 40 mg simethicone. Saccharin, sorbitol.
Extra Strength Mintox Plus	**Liquid**: 500 mg aluminum hydroxide, 450 mg magnesium hydroxide, 40 mg simethicone. Parabens, saccharin, sorbitol.
Gaviscon Extra Strength Relief Formula	**Liquid**: 254 mg aluminum hydroxide, 237.5 mg magnesium carbonate, simethicone, sodium alginate. Parabens, EDTA, saccharin, sorbitol.
Alenic Alka	**Liquid**: 95 mg aluminum hydroxide, 358 mg magnesium carbonate. EDTA, saccharin, sorbitol, parabens, 1.7 mEq sodium/tbsp.
Gaviscon	**Liquid**: 31.7 mg aluminum hydroxide, 119.3 mg magnesium carbonate, sodium alginate. EDTA, saccharin, sorbitol, parabens, 13 mg sodium.
Genaton	**Liquid**: 31.7 mg aluminum hydroxide, 137.3 mg magnesium carbonate, sodium alginate. EDTA, saccharin, sorbitol, 13 mg sodium.

ANTACID COMBINATION PRODUCTS

Trade name	Doseform
Liquids	
Marblen	**Liquid**: 520 mg calcium carbonate, 400 mg magnesium carbonate
Titralac Plus	**Liquid**: 500 mg calcium carbonate, 20 mg simethicone. Parabens, saccharin, sorbitol, 0.15 mg sodium.
Almacone	**Liquid**: 200 mg aluminum hydroxide, 200 magnesium hydroxide, 20 mg simethicone
Di-Gel	**Liquid**: 200 mg aluminum hydroxide, 200 magnesium hydroxide, 20 mg simethicone. Saccharin, sorbitol, parabens.
Mi-Acid	**Liquid**: 200 mg aluminum hydroxide, 200 magnesium hydroxide, 20 mg simethicone. Parabens, sorbitol.
Mylanta	**Liquid**: 200 mg aluminum hydroxide, 200 magnesium hydroxide, 20 mg simethicone. Sorbitol, 0.68 mg sodium.
Almacone Double Strength	**Liquid**:400 mg aluminum hydroxide, 400 mg magnesium hydroxide, 40 mg simethicone. Parabens, sorbitol.
Antacid Double Strength	**Liquid**: 400 mg aluminum hydroxide, 400 mg magnesium hydroxide, 40 mg simethicone. Parabens, sorbitol, sucrose, < 1.25 mg sodium.
Mi-Acid II	**Liquid**: 400 mg aluminum hydroxide, 400 mg magnesium hydroxide, 40 mg simethicone. Parabens, sorbitol, sucrose.
Mylanta Double Strength	**Liquid**: 400 mg aluminum hydroxide, 400 mg magnesium hydroxide, 40 mg simethicone. Sorbitol, parabens.
Isopan Plus	**Liquid**: 540 mg magaldrate, 40 mg simethicone
Powder and Effervescent Tablets	
Alka-Seltzer Gold	**Tablets, effervescent**: 958 mg sodium bicarbonate (heat-treated), 832 citric acid 312 mg potassium bicarbonate. 311 mg sodium.
Alka-Seltzer	**Tablets, effervescent**: 1700 mg sodium bicarbonate, 325 mg aspirin, 1000 mg citric acid. 9 mg phenylalanine, 506 mg sodium.
Alka-Seltzer Original	**Tablets, effervescent**: 1916 mg sodium bicarbonate (heat-treated), 325 mg aspirin, 1000 mg citric acid. 567 mg sodium.
Extra Strength Alka-Seltzer	**Tablets, effervescent**: 1985 mg sodium bicarbonate (heat-treated), 500 mg aspirin, 1000 mg citric acid. 588 mg sodium.
Citrocarbonate	**Granules, effervescent**: 780 mg sodium bicarbonate, 1820 mg sodium citrate anhydrous. 700.6 mg sodium.
Sparkles	**Granules, effervescent**: 2000 mg sodium bicarbonate, 1500 mg citric acid, simethicone

Products listed are representative of currently available and widely distributed brands. Similar products, including regional and private label brands, may also exist.

PATIENT INFORMATION

Antacid Combinations

- *Chewable tablets:* Thoroughly chew before swallowing and follow with a glass of water.
- *Liquids:* Shake liquid antacids before use.
- *Effervescent tablets:* Allow tablet to completely dissolve in water and allow most of the bubbling to stop before drinking.
- Magnesium-containing products may act as a laxative in large doses and cause diarrhea.
- Aluminum- and calcium-containing products may cause constipation.
- Antacids may interact with certain prescription medications. If you are taking a prescription drug, do not take an antacid without checking with your physician or pharmacist.
- Taking too much of these products can cause the stomach to secrete excess stomach acid.

Heartburn and GERD

DEFINITION

Heartburn, or pyrosis, also referred to as indigestion or sour stomach, is a substernal burning sensation that may radiate upward to the throat and neck region and generally occurs following a meal. Heartburn may be occasional or frequent. *Occasional* heartburn is defined as heartburn that occurs once a week or less. *Frequent* heartburn is defined as heartburn that occurs 2 or more days per week. The burning tends to wax and wane and often worsens with activities that potentiate gastroesophageal reflux (eg, lying down, bending over). Heartburn usually occurs when the gastric pH is less than 4. Heartburn is the most common symptom associated with gastroesophageal reflux disease (GERD) but is a common complaint of healthy people as well. Heartburn associated with GERD is more persistent and severe and results from chronic reflux of stomach contents into the esophagus.

ETIOLOGY

Heartburn is caused by irritation and inflammation of the esophageal mucosa by the retrograde movement of gastric contents into the esophagus. Anatomical factors, lower esophageal sphincter (LES) pressure, esophageal clearing, mucosal resistance, and gastric emptying normally control the damaging effects of gastric acid. Any disruption in this balance of defense mechanisms and aggressive factors that favor gastroesophageal reflux can lead to heartburn.

INCIDENCE

It is estimated that 7% of all adults (approximately 20 million) experience heartburn daily, and approximately 25% of women experience heartburn during pregnancy. Approximately 35% to 50% of healthy adults experience heartburn at least once a month. Approximately 50 million Americans experience frequent heartburn (ie, heartburn symptoms 2 or more days per week). Overall, it is estimated that heartburn symptoms occur over 7 billion times per year in the US. Pathologic changes in the esophageal mucosa may occur in up to 40% of adults with heartburn symptoms. Symptoms, however, do not correlate well with pathologic evidence of esophageal inflammation or erosion, as indicated by studies that identified 65% of esophagitis patients complaining of heartburn but only 6% to 32% of heartburn patients having evidence of esophagitis.

Esophageal complications in patients with reflux esophagitis include esophageal ulcers (5%), peptic stricture (4% to 20%), and Barrett esophagus, a histologic change in esophageal mucosa (10%). Barrett esophagus occurs at a much higher rate (44%) in patients with peptic stricture. The development of Barrett esophagus is associated with a 30% to 80% incidence of stricture formation and a 5% to 10% incidence of esophageal adenocarcinoma.

National surveys estimate 13% of adults take medication more than once a week for indigestion/heartburn, and approximately 50% of those who self-medicate for reflux symptoms may have esophagitis.

PATHOPHYSIOLOGY

Normal defense mechanisms such as anatomic factors, LES pressure, esophageal clearance, mucosal resistance, and gastric emptying protect the esophagus from the erosive effects of occasional reflux. When these compensatory mechanisms are exceeded, symptoms or injury can result. Patient lifestyle factors also play a very important role in the occurrence of heartburn.

Anatomic barriers may be compromised in the presence of a hiatal hernia, which can displace the LES from its usual position; however, not all patients with hiatal hernias experience heartburn. Insufficient LES pressure may occur as a result of any one of three mechanisms: 1) An atonic or hypotonic esophageal sphincter, 2) stress reflux that results when intra-abdominal pressure exceeds that of the LES, or 3) intermittent sphincter relaxations, which are generally associated with eating and swallowing. The esophageal clearance factors referred to as peristalsis, gravity, and salivary flow can be negatively affected by motility disorders, a supine position, and age, respectively, resulting in prolonged contact time between the acid-reflux and the sensitive esophageal mucosa. The duration of this contact time is the principal factor contributing to mucosal irritation and erosion. Disturbances in the secretion of mucus by glands in the esophageal mucosa can also contribute to inflammation of the esophagus by decreasing or altering the mucosal barrier. Delayed gastric emptying as well as an increase in gastric volume may be other factors inducing gastroesophageal reflux.

Patient factors that increase the incidence of reflux include obesity, wearing tight garments, pregnancy, smoking, and bending over or lying down immediately after eating. The quality, quantity, and timing of meals are also important lifestyle factors that can affect the occurrence of reflux. Fatty meals delay the gastric emptying rate, increase gastric volume, and decrease LES pressure, all of which increase both the frequency and the amount of esophageal reflux. Excessive consumption of food and beverages, as well as eating late at night, also increase the occurrence of reflux.

A small amount of reflux into the esophagus is a normal physiologic occurrence. However, chronic, recurrent reflux can lead to GERD and if left untreated may progress to severe complications such as mucosal injury, ulceration, stricture formation, perforation, pharyngeal or oral disturbances, hemorrhage, and possibly premalignant, metaplastic changes in the esophageal epithelium (ie, Barrett esophagus).

SIGNS/SYMPTOMS

A warm or burning sensation in the chest, which usually fluctuates in intensity, may radiate upward to the throat and neck. Heartburn often worsens following activities that potentiate gastroesophageal reflux (eg, lying down, bending over).

Other symptoms accompanying heartburn that are indicative of more severe reflux and possible GERD include regurgitation (usually 1 to 2 hours after eating), hypersalivation, dysphagia (difficulty swallowing), odynophagia (painful swallowing), esophageal bleeding, and chest pain. Coughing, morning hoarseness, hiccups, asthma, bronchospasm, and recurrent pneumonia are more atypical but may also represent complications of severe reflux.

DIAGNOSTIC PARAMETERS/PHYSICAL ASSESSMENT

Clinical Observation: Because of the nature of this condition, the most useful tool for patient assessment is the interview.

Interview: Symptomatology and the presence of risk factors can be identified by a brief clinical history. The following topics should be addressed:

- Description of heartburn: onset, severity, and duration of pain; movement of pain to neck, jaw, or arm; what relieves pain.
- Description of eating habits (what is normally eaten, quantities eaten, and when).
- Medications currently used to treat heartburn: success and length of treatment.
- Hoarseness; difficulty or pain when swallowing food; cough; shortness of breath; recent weight loss without trying; any changes in bowel function or black tarry stool.
- Smoking habits.
- Alcohol consumption pattern.
- Current medication profile (prescription, OTC medications, or herbal products).

It is important to differentiate between patients with classic heartburn and those with more serious symptoms that might warrant physician referral. Physician referral should be considered in the following situations:

- Atypical presentation of symptoms.
- Patient fails to respond to self-treatment after more than 2 weeks of regular treatment with OTC products.
- Symptoms include dysphagia, odynophagia, hemorrhaging, nausea/vomiting, early satiety, or chest pain.
- Patients experience chest pain that feels like a crushing pressure on chest with radiating pain to the neck, arm, and/or back
- Symptoms suggest the possibility of associated disease (eg, peptic ulcer disease).
- Patient presents with recent unexplained weight loss.

Identifying the following risk factors can help determine lifestyle factors that may contribute to reflux and can later serve to guide nondrug therapy.

Dietary Risk Factors

- Foods that decrease LES pressure and stimulate cholecystokinin release (eg, fats, chocolate, alcohol, peppermint, spearmint, onions, garlic).
- Acidic foods that have a direct irritant effect on the esophageal mucosa (eg, hot spices, citric juice, tomatoes, caffeine, vinegars).
- Foods that stimulate gastric acid production (eg, cola, milk, alcohol).
- Eating habits that increase gastric volume (eg, overconsumption of foods and beverages, large meals).
- Lack of foods that augment LES pressure (eg, protein-rich meals).

Nondietary Risk Factors
- Habits that increase spontaneous esophageal sphincter relaxation (eg, smoking).
- Factors that increase intra-abdominal pressure (eg, obesity, tight-fitting clothes, pregnancy, lifting or straining).
- Habits that mechanically facilitate reflux (eg, bending over or lying down within 2 hours of eating).

Pharmacologic Risk Factors
- Agents that have a direct irritant effect on the esophageal mucosa (eg, tetracycline, quinidine, potassium chloride, iron salts, aspirin, NSAIDs). If these agents cannot be avoided, they should be taken with plenty of water or food.
- Agents that reduce LES pressure and promote reflux (eg, nicotine, anticholinergics, alpha blockers, beta agonists, calcium channel blockers, progestins, theophylline, benzodiazepines, dopamine, narcotics, nitrates). Avoid these agents if possible.

Symptomatology must then be used to differentiate between patients with classic reflux symptoms amenable to nondrug or OTC therapy and those with more severe symptoms suggesting complications of chronic reflux that necessitate medical attention.

▶ **Classic symptoms**
- Mild or intermittent heartburn
- Regurgitation (the effortless movement of food from the esophagus into the mouth, not to be confused with vomiting)
- Brackish taste in the mouth
- Bloating

▶ **Complicated, esophageal symptoms**
- Moderate to severe or persistent heartburn
- Hemorrhaging
- Neck or chest pain
- Dysphagia or odynophagia
- Early satiety

▶ **Complicated, extraesophageal symptoms**
- Laryngitis or chronic hoarseness
- Nausea and vomiting
- Wheezing/asthma/bronchospasm
- Unexplained weight loss
- Chronic cough (longer than 3 weeks)
- Recurrent pneumonia

Refer patients with symptoms of complicated esophageal or complicated extroesophageal chronic reflux to a physician for medical evaluation.

TREATMENT
Approaches to therapy: The options for pharmacist-directed management of uncomplicated, classic heartburn include dietary or lifestyle modifications, alginic acid, antacids, OTC histamine H$_2$ antagonists, and omeprazole (a pro-

ton pump inhibitor). Omeprazole is available as *Prilosec OTC* tablets at the prescription strength of 20 mg for the treatment of frequent heartburn. The goals of therapy are:

1.) Alleviate or eliminate symptoms.
2.) Decrease the occurrence of reflux.
3.) Protect and limit or prevent damage to the esophageal mucosa.
4.) Prevent complications or recurrences.

Less disease-specific goals include avoiding side effects and drug interactions, recommending cost-effective therapy, and providing patient satisfaction.

Nondrug therapy: Many patients can control mild infrequent heartburn symptoms with dietary or lifestyle modifications. The risk factors identified during the interview can be utilized at this time to outline a nondrug approach for therapy.

Advise patients to eat frequent, small, protein-rich meals and to avoid foods that worsen reflux, eating late at night, and reclining within 2 hours after eating. Advise smokers and overweight patients to quit smoking and lose weight, respectively. Drug therapy reviews can be performed to identify drugs that might be aggravating symptoms.

In addition to improving patient-specific risk factors, advise patients to elevate the head of the bed 6 to 8 inches or to sleep on a foam wedge. This measure uses gravity to increase esophageal clearance and may reduce the irritating effects of nocturnal reflux.

ANTACIDS

▶ Actions
Antacids neutralize gastric acidity, resulting in an increase in the pH of the stomach contents.

▶ Indications
Hyperacidity: Symptomatic relief of upset stomach associated with hyperacidity (heartburn, gastroesophageal reflux, acid indigestion, and sour stomach); hyperacidity associated with peptic ulcer and gastric hyperacidity.

Unlabeled uses: Antacids with aluminum and magnesium hydroxides or aluminum hydroxide alone effectively prevent significant stress ulcer bleeding. Antacids are also effective in the treatment and maintenance therapy of duodenal ulcer and may be effective in treating gastric ulcer. Antacids can also be recommended for early-stage GERD.

▶ Contraindications
There are no specific contraindications to the use of antacids. If possible, avoid magnesium-containing antacids in patients with marked renal failure (see Warnings).

▶ Warnings
Sodium content: Sodium content of some antacids may be significant. Use a low-sodium preparation in patients with hypertension, congestive heart failure, marked renal failure, or for those on restricted or low-sodium diets. The sodium content of most commercial antacid preparations is found in the product listings.

Acid rebound: Antacids may cause dose-related rebound hyperacidity because they may increase gastric secretion or serum gastrin levels. Early data implicated calcium carbonate as the only agent that caused "acid rebound"; however, it is now clear most antacids may have this effect.

Renal function impairment: Use magnesium-containing products with caution, particularly when more than 50 mEq of magnesium is given daily. Hypermagnesemia and toxicity may occur due to decreased renal clearance of the magnesium ion. Approximately 5% to 20% of oral magnesium salts can be systemically absorbed.

Prolonged use of aluminum-containing antacids in patients with renal failure may result in or worsen dialysis osteomalacia. Elevated tissue aluminum levels contribute to the development of the dialysis encephalopathy and osteomalacia syndromes. Small amounts of aluminum are absorbed from the GI tract and renal excretion of aluminum is impaired in renal failure. Aluminum is not well removed by dialysis because it is bound to albumin and transferrin, which do not cross dialysis membranes. As a result, aluminum is deposited in bone, and dialysis osteomalacia may develop when large amounts of aluminum are ingested orally by patients with impaired renal function.

Pregnancy: Pregnant women should consult a physician before using an antacid.

▶ **Drug Interactions**

Antacid Drug Interactions[1]					
Drug	Aluminum salts	Calcium salts	Magnesium salts	Sodium bicarbonate	Magnesium-aluminum combinations
Allopurinol	↓				
Amphetamines				↑	
Benzodiazepines	↑		↓	↓	↓
Captopril					↓
Chloroquine	↓		↓		↓
Corticosteroids	↓		↓		↓
Dicumarol			↑		
Digoxin	↓		↓		
Ethambutol	↓				
Flecainide				↑	
Fluoroquinolones		↓			↓
Histamine H₂ antagonists	↓		↓		↓
Hydantoins		↓	↓		↓
Iron salts	↓	↓	↓	↓	↓
Isoniazid	↓				
Ketoconazole				↓	↓
Levodopa					↑
Lithium				↓	
Methenamine				↓	
Methotrexate				↓	
Nitrofurantoin			↓		
Penicillamine	↓		↓		↓
Phenothiazines	↓		↓		↓
Quinidine		↑	↓	↑	↑
Salicylates		↓		↓	↓

Antacid Drug Interactions[1]					
Drug	**Aluminum salts**	**Calcium salts**	**Magnesium salts**	**Sodium bicarbonate**	**Magnesium-aluminum combinations**
Sodium polysterene sulfonate					+[2]
Sulfonylureas			↓	↓	↓
Sympathomimetics				↓	
Tetracyclines	↓	↓	↓	↓	↓
Thyroid hormones	↓				
Ticlopidine	↓		↓		↓
Valproic acid					↑

[1] Pharmacologic effect increased (↑) or decreased (↓) by antacids.
[2] Concomitant use may cause metabolic alkalosis in patients with renal function impairment.

Antacids may interact with drugs by:

1.) Increasing the gastric pH or altering disintegration, dissolution, solubility, ionization, and gastric emptying time. Absorption of weakly acidic drugs is decreased, possibly resulting in decreased drug effect (eg, digoxin, phenytoin, chlorpromazine, isoniazid). Weakly basic drug absorption is increased, possibly resulting in toxicity or adverse reactions (eg, pseudoephedrine, levodopa).

2.) Adsorbing or binding drugs to their surface may result in decreased bioavailability (eg, tetracycline). Magnesium trisilicate and magnesium hydroxide have the greatest ability to adsorb drugs; calcium carbonate and aluminum hydroxide have an intermediate ability to adsorb drugs.

3.) Increasing urinary pH may affect the rate of drug elimination. The effect is inhibition of the excretion of basic drugs (eg, quinidine, amphetamines) and enhanced excretion of acidic drugs (eg, salicylates). Sodium bicarbonate has the most pronounced effect on urinary pH.

Staggering the administration times of the interacting drug and the antacid by at least 2 hours will often help avoid undesirable drug interactions.

▶ **Adverse Reactions**

Magnesium-containing antacids: Laxative effect (saline cathartic) may cause diarrhea; hypermagnesemia in renal failure patients (see Warnings).

Aluminum-containing antacids: Constipation (may lead to intestinal obstruction); aluminum-intoxication, osteomalacia, and hypophosphatemia (see Precautions); accumulation of aluminum in serum, bone, and the CNS (aluminum accumulation may be neurotoxic); encephalopathy.

Antacids: Dose-dependent rebound hyperacidity and milk-alkali syndrome (see Warnings).

Milk-alkali syndrome: Milk-alkali syndrome, an acute illness with symptoms of headache, nausea, irritability, and weakness, or a chronic illness with alkalosis, hypercalcemia, and possibly, renal impairment, has occurred following the concurrent use of high-dose calcium carbonate and sodium carbonate.

Hypophosphatemia: Prolonged use of aluminum-containing antacids may result in hypophosphatemia in patients with normal phosphate levels if phosphate intake is not adequate. In its more severe forms, hypophosphatemia can lead to anorexia, malaise, muscle weakness, and osteomalacia.

▶ **Administration and Dosage**

Administration and dosage depends on the condition being treated and the agent being used. See individual products for specific information. Liquid doseforms are usually preferred because of their rapid action and greater activity; however, tablets may be more acceptable and convenient, particularly when patients are away from home or where the liquid would be inconvenient to carry. Other doseforms are available but do not appear to offer any significant advantage.

MAGNESIUM HYDROXIDE

▶ **Indications**

Neutralize gastric acid.

▶ **Drug Interactions**

Magnesium salt antacids reduce the pharmacologic effect of the following drugs if taken together: benzodiazepines, chloroquine, corticosteroids, digoxin, histamine H_2 antagonists, hydantoins, iron salts, nitrofurantoin, penicillamine, phenothiazines, tetracyclines, and ticlopidine. The pharmacologic effects of dicumarol, quinidine, and sulfonylureas are increased.

▶ **Administration and Dosage**

Liquid: 5 to 15 mL up to 4 times daily as needed.

Liquid, concentrated: 2.5 to 7.5 mL up to 4 times daily as needed.

Tablets: 622 to 1244 mg up to 4 times daily as needed.

MAGNESIUM HYDROXIDE PRODUCTS	
Trade name	Doseform
Phillips' Chewable	**Tablets, chewable**: 311 mg. Sucrose.
Phillips' Milk of Magnesia	**Liquid**: 400 mg/5 mL. Original, mint[1], and cherry[2] flavors.
Dulcolax Milk of Magnesia (sf)	**Liquid**: 400 mg/5 mL.
Concentrated Phillips' Milk of Magnesia	**Liquid**: 800 mg/5 mL. Sorbitol, sugar.

Products listed are representative of currently available and widely distributed brands. Similar products, including regional and private label brands, may also exist.

sf = Sugar free.
[1] Saccharin.
[2] Sorbitol, sugar.

■ ■ ■

PATIENT INFORMATION
Magnesium Hydroxide
- Antacids may interact with certain prescription drugs. If you are presently taking a prescription drug, do not take an antacid without checking with a physician or pharmacist.
- Magnesium-containing products may act as a saline cathartic in larger doses and produce a laxative effect that may cause diarrhea.
- Notify physician if relief is not obtained or there are symptoms that suggest bleeding, such as black tarry stools or "coffee-ground" vomit.
- Taking too much of these products can cause the stomach to secrete excess stomach acid. Consult a physician or pharmacist about the appropriate dose. Do not use the maximum daily dose of antacids for more than 2 weeks, except under the supervision of a physician.
- If symptoms worsen or persist for more than 2 weeks, consult a physician.
- *Chewable tablets:* Thoroughly chew before swallowing. Follow with a glass of water.
- *Liquids:* Shake bottle well before use.

MAGNESIUM OXIDE

▶ Indications
Neutralizes gastric acid.

Treatment of magnesium deficiencies or magnesium depletion from malnutrition, restricted diet, alcoholism, or magnesium-depleting drugs.

▶ Drug Interactions
Magnesium salt antacids reduce the pharmacologic effect of the following drugs: benzodiazepines, chloroquine, corticosteroids, digoxin, histamine H_2 antagonists, hydantoins, iron salts, nitrofurantoin, penicillamine, phenothiazines, tetracyclines, and ticlopidine. The pharmacologic effects of dicumarol, quinidine, and sulfonylureas are increased.

▶ Administration and Dosage
Tablets: 400 to 800 mg/day as needed.

Capsules: 140 mg 3 to 4 times daily as needed.

MAGNESIUM OXIDE PRODUCTS	
Trade name	Doseform
Mag-Ox 400 (sf)	**Tablets**: 400 mg
Maox	**Tablets**: 420 mg
Uro-Mag (sf)	**Capsules**: 140 mg

Products listed are representative of currently available and widely distributed brands. Similar products, including regional and private label brands, may also exist.

sf = Sugar free

> ## PATIENT INFORMATION
> ### Magnesium Oxide
> - Antacids may interact with certain prescription drugs. If you are presently taking a prescription drug, do not take an antacid without checking with a physician or pharmacist.
> - Notify physician if relief is not obtained or if there are any symptoms that suggest bleeding, such as black tarry stools or "coffee-ground" vomit.
> - Taking too much of these products can cause the stomach to secrete excess stomach acid. Consult a physician or pharmacist about the appropriate dose. Do not use the maximum daily dosage of antacids for more than 2 weeks, except under the supervision of a physician.
> - If symptoms worsen or persist for more than 2 weeks, consult a physician.
> - Magnesium-containing products may cause diarrhea.

ALUMINUM HYDROXIDE GEL

▶ Indications

Neutralizes gastric acid.

Unlabeled uses: Aluminum hydroxide has been used to reduce phosphate absorption in patients with chronic renal failure.

▶ Drug Interactions

Aluminum salt antacids reduce the pharmacologic effects of the following drugs if taken together: allopurinol, chloroquine, corticosteroids, digoxin, ethambutol, histamine H_2 antagonists, iron salts, isoniazid, penicillamine, phenothiazines, tetracyclines, thyroid hormones, and ticlopidine. The pharmacologic effects of benzodiazepines are increased.

▶ Administration and Dosage

Capsules/Tablets: 500 to 1500 mg 3 to 6 times daily between meals and at bedtime as needed.

Suspension: 5 to 30 mL between meals and at bedtime as needed.

ALUMINUM HYDROXIDE GEL PRODUCTS	
Trade name	Doseform
Aluminum Hydroxide Gel USP	**Liquid**: 320 mg/5 mL. Butylparaben, saccharin, sorbitol, 1.6 mg sodium.
AlternaGEL	**Liquid**: 600 mg/5 mL. Parabens, sorbitol.

Products listed are representative of currently available and widely distributed brands. Similar products, including regional and private label brands, may also exist.

━ ━ ■

PATIENT INFORMATION

Aluminum Hydroxide Gel

- Antacids may interact with certain prescription drugs. If you are presently taking a prescription drug, do not take an antacid without checking with a physician or pharmacist.
- Notify physician if relief is not obtained or if there are any symptoms that suggest bleeding, such as black tarry stools or "coffee-ground" vomit.
- Taking too much of these products can cause the stomach to secrete excess stomach acid. Consult a physician or pharmacist about the appropriate dose. Do not use the maximum daily dosage of antacids for more than 2 weeks, except under the supervision of a physician.
- If symptoms worsen or persist for more than 2 weeks, consult a physician.
- Aluminum-containing products may cause constipation.
- *Liquids:* Shake liquid antacids prior to use.
- *Chewable tablets:* Thoroughly chew before swallowing. Follow with a glass of water.

CALCIUM CARBONATE

▶ Indications

Neutralizes gastric acid.

Treatment of calcium deficiency states (ie, postmenopausal/senile osteoporosis).

Unlabeled uses: Calcium carbonate also may be used to bind phosphate.

▶ Drug Interactions

Calcium salt antacids reduce the pharmacologic effects of the following drugs: fluoroquinolones, hydantoins, iron salts, salicylates, and tetracyclines. The pharmacologic effects of quinidine are increased.

▶ Administration and Dosage

Tablets/Lozenges: 0.5 to 1.5 g as needed.

CALCIUM CARBONATE PRODUCTS	
Trade name	**Doseform**
Titralac	**Tablets**: 420 mg. Saccharin, 1.1 mg sodium.
Children's Mylanta	**Tablets, chewable**: 400 mg. Sugar, sorbitol.
Amitone	**Tablets, chewable**: 420 mg. Sorbitol.
Mallamint	**Tablets, chewable**: 420 mg
Antacid	**Tablets, chewable**: 500 mg. Sucrose, dextrose.
Dicarbosil	**Tablets, chewable**: 500 mg. Sucrose.
Quick Dissolve Regular Strength Maalox	**Tablets, chewable**: 600 mg. Aspartame, dextrose, lemon flavor.
Alka-Mints	**Tablets, chewable**: 850 mg. Sorbitol, sugar, spearmint flavor.
Quick Dissolve Maximum Strength Maalox	**Tablets, chewable**: 1000 mg. Aspartame, dextrose, wintergreen flavor.
Tums Maximum Strength	**Tablets, chewable**: 1000 mg. Sucrose.
Surpass	**Gum tablets**: 300 mg
Surpass Extra Strength	**Gum tablets**: 450 mg

CALCIUM CARBONATE PRODUCTS	
Trade name	Doseform
Chooz (sf)	Gum tablets: 500 mg. Aspartame, sorbitol. Sodium free, mint flavor.

Products listed are representative of currently available and widely distributed brands. Similar products, including regional and private label brands, may also exist.

sf = sugar free

PATIENT INFORMATION
Calcium Carbonate

- Antacids may interact with certain prescription drugs. If you are presently taking a prescription drug, do not take an antacid without checking with a physician or pharmacist.
- Notify physician if relief is not obtained or if there are any symptoms that suggest bleeding, such as black tarry stools or "coffee-ground" vomit.
- Taking too much of these products can cause the stomach to secrete excess stomach acid. Consult a physician or pharmacist about the appropriate dose. Do not use the maximum daily dosage of antacids for more than 2 weeks, except under the supervision of a physician.
- If symptoms worsen or persist for more than 2 weeks, consult a physician.
- Calcium-containing products may cause constipation.
- *Chewable tablets:* Thoroughly chew before swallowing. Follow with a glass of water.

MAGALDRATE (ALUMINUM MAGNESIUM HYDROXIDE SULFATE)

▶ **Indications**

Neutralizes gastric acid.

▶ **Administration and Dosage**

5 to 10 mL between meals and at bedtime as needed.

MAGALDRATE PRODUCTS	
Trade name	Doseform
Losopan	Suspension: 540 mg/5 mL. Saccharin, sorbitol, parabens.
Losopan Plus	Suspension: 540 mg, simethicone 40 mg/5 mL. Saccharin, sorbitol, parabens, 1.5 mg sodium.

Products listed are representative of currently available and widely distributed brands. Similar products, including regional and private label brands, may also exist.

PATIENT INFORMATION

Magaldrate

- Antacids may interact with certain prescription drugs. If you are presently taking a prescription drug, do not take an antacid without checking with a physician or pharmacist.
- Notify physician if relief is not obtained or if there are any symptoms that suggest bleeding, such as black tarry stools or "coffee-ground" vomit.
- Taking too much of these products can cause the stomach to secrete excess stomach acid. Consult a physician or pharmacist about the appropriate dose. Do not use the maximum daily dosage of antacids for more than 2 weeks, except under the supervision of a physician.
- If symptoms worsen or persist for more than 2 weeks, consult a physician.
- *Liquids:* Shake liquid antacids prior to use.

SODIUM BICARBONATE

▶ Indications

Neutralizes gastric acid.

▶ Administration and Dosage

0.3 to 2 g one to four times daily as needed.

SODIUM BICARBONATE PRODUCTS	
Trade name	**Doseform**
Sodium Bicarbonate	**Tablets:** 325 mg

Products listed are representative of currently available and widely distributed brands. Similar products, including regional and private label brands, may also exist.

PATIENT INFORMATION

Sodium Bicarbonate

- Antacids may interact with certain prescription drugs. If you are presently taking a prescription drug, do not take an antacid without checking with a physician or pharmacist.
- Notify physician if relief is not obtained or if there are any symptoms that suggest bleeding, such as black tarry stools or "coffee-ground" vomit.
- Taking too much of these products can cause the stomach to secrete excess stomach acid. Consult a physician or pharmacist about the appropriate dose. Do not use the maximum daily dosage of antacids for more than 2 weeks, except under the supervision of a physician.
- If symptoms worsen or persist for more than 2 weeks, consult a physician.

SODIUM CITRATE

▶ Indications

Neutralizes gastric acid.

▶ Administration and Dosage

30 mL daily as needed.

SODIUM CITRATE PRODUCTS	
Trade name	**Doseform**
Citra pH	**Solution**: 450 mg/5 mL. Sucrose, parabens.

Products listed are representative of currently available and widely distributed brands. Similar products, including regional and private label brands, may also exist.

PATIENT INFORMATION
Sodium Citrate

- Antacids may interact with certain prescription drugs. If you are presently taking a prescription drug, do not take an antacid without checking with a physician or pharmacist.
- Notify physician if relief is not obtained or if there are any symptoms that suggest bleeding, such as black tarry stools or "coffee-ground" vomit.
- Taking too much of these products can cause the stomach to secrete excess stomach acid. Consult a physician or pharmacist about the appropriate dose. Do not use the maximum daily dosage of antacids for more than 2 weeks, except under the supervision of a physician.
- If symptoms worsen or persist for more than 2 weeks, consult a physician.
- *Liquids:* Shake liquid antacids prior to use.

ANTACID COMBINATIONS

▶ Administration and Dosage
See individual products for administration and dosage guidelines.

ANTACID COMBINATION PRODUCTS	
Trade name	**Doseform**
Capsules and Tablets	
Alenic Alka	**Tablets, chewable**: 80 mg aluminum hydroxide, 20 mg magnesium trisilicate, Sugar, butterscotch flavor, 0.8 mEq sodium.
Genaton	**Tablets, chewable**: 80 mg aluminum hydroxide, 20 mg magnesium trisilicate. Alginic acid, sodium bicarbonate, sucrose, sugar, 0.8 mEq sodium.
Gaviscon	**Tablets, chewable**: 80 mg aluminum hydroxide, 20 mg magnesium trisilicate. Sucrose, alginic acid, sodium bicarbonate, ≈ 0.8 mEq sodium.
Gaviscon Extra Strength	**Tablets, chewable**: 160 mg aluminum hydroxide, 105 mg magnesium carbonate. Sorbitol, alginic acid, sodium bicarbonate, ≈ 1.3 mEq sodium.
Extra Strength Alenic Alka	**Tablets, chewable**: 160 mg aluminum hydroxide, 105 mg magnesium carbonate. 1.3 mEq sodium, sucrose, butterscotch flavor.
RuLox #1	**Tablets, chewable**: 200 mg aluminum hydroxide, 200 mg magnesium hydroxide. Saccharin, sorbitol, mint flavor.
Almacone	**Tablets, chewable**: 200 mg aluminum hydroxide, 200 mg magnesium hydroxide, 20 mg simethicone. Sodium free. Sugar.
Gelusil	**Tablets, chewable**: 200 mg aluminum hydroxide, 200 mg magnesium hydroxide, 25 mg simethicone. Sorbitol, sugar.

ANTACID COMBINATION PRODUCTS

Trade name	Doseform
Capsules and Tablets	
Maalox	**Tablets, chewable**: 225 mg aluminum hydroxide, 200 mg magnesium hydroxide. Saccharin, sorbitol, parabens, cherry and lemon flavor.
Advanced Formula Di-Gel	**Tablets, chewable**: 280 mg calcium carbonate, 128 mg magnesium hydroxide, 20 mg simethicone. Sodium free. Sucrose.
Gas Ban	**Tablets**: 300 mg calcium carbonate, 40 mg simethicone. Sorbitol.
Gas-X with Maalox	**Tablets**: 500 mg calcium carbonate, 125 mg simethicone. Dextrose, mannitol, talc. Wild berry and orange flavors.
Titralac Plus	**Tablets, chewable**: 420 mg calcium carbonate, 21 mg simethicone. Saccharin, 1.5 mg sodium.
Calcium Rich Rolaids	**Tablets, chewable**: 550 mg calcium carbonate, 110 mg magnesium hydroxide. Dextrose, sucrose. Original, spearmint, and cherry flavors.
Rolaids Extra Strength	**Tablets, chewable**: 675 mg calcium carbonate, 135 mg magnesium hydroxide. Dextrose, sucrose. Strawberry and tropical punch flavors.
Mylanta Ultra Tabs	**Tablets, chewable**: 700 mg calcium carbonate, 300 mg magnesium hydroxide. Sorbitol, sugar. Cherry and mint flavors.
Mylanta Gelcaps	**Capsules**: 550 mg calcium carbonate, 125 mg magnesium carbonate. Parabens, EDTA.
Liquids	
Alamag	**Suspension**: 225 mg aluminum hydroxide, 200 mg magnesium hydroxide/5 mL. Sorbitol, saccharin, parabens, 0.5 mg sodium.
Alamag Plus	**Suspension**: 225 mg aluminum hydroxide, 200 mg magnesium hydroxide, 25 mg simethicone/5 mL. Parabens, saccharin, sorbitol, 0.5 mg sodium.
Mintox	**Suspension**: 225 mg aluminum hydroxide, 200 mg magnesium hydroxide/5 mL. Mint flavor.
Kudrox Double Strength	**Suspension**: 500 mg aluminum hydroxide, 450 mg magnesium hydroxide, 40 mg simethicone/5 mL. Parabens, saccharin, sorbitol.
Extra Strength RuLox Plus	**Suspension**: 500 mg aluminum hydroxide, 450 magnesium hydroxide, 40 mg simethicone/5 mL. Saccharin, sorbitol, parabens. Sodium free.
Lowsium Plus	**Suspension**: 540 mg magaldrate, 40 mg simethicone/ 5 mL. Parabens, saccharin, sorbitol.
Riopan Plus	**Suspension**: 540 mg magaldrate, 40 mg simethicone/ 5 mL. Saccharin, sorbitol, mint flavor.
Gaviscon	**Liquid**: 95 mg aluminum hydroxide, 358 mg magnesium carbonate/15 mL. EDTA, saccharin, sorbitol, ≈ 1.7 mEq sodium, mint flavor.
Genaton	**Liquid**: 95 mg aluminum hydroxide, 358 mg magnesium carbonate/15 mL. EDTA, saccharin, sorbitol, 30 mg sodium/15 mL, mint flavor.

ANTACID COMBINATION PRODUCTS

Trade name	Doseform
Liquids	
Almacone	**Liquid**: 200 mg aluminum hydroxide, 200 magnesium hydroxide, 20 mg simethicone/5 mL. Sorbitol, parabens.
Mylanta	**Liquid**: 200 mg aluminum hydroxide, 200 magnesium hydroxide, 20 mg simethicone/5 mL. Original[1], cherry[2], mint[2], and lemon[2] flavors.
Gaviscon Extra Strength	**Liquid**: 508 mg aluminum hydroxide, 475 mg magnesium carbonate/10 mL. EDTA, saccharin, sorbitol, ≈ 0.9 mEq sodium, mint flavor.
Almacone Double Strength	**Liquid**: 400 mg aluminum hydroxide, 400 mg magnesium hydroxide, 40 mg simethicone/5 mL. Parabens, sorbitol.
Antacid Double Strength	**Liquid**: 400 mg aluminum hydroxide, 400 mg magnesium hydroxide, 40 mg simethicone/5 mL. Parabens, sorbitol, saccharin, 1.4 mg sodium. Lemon-mint flavor.
Maalox Maximum Strength	**Liquid**: 500 mg aluminum hydroxide, 400 mg magnesium hydroxide, 40 mg simethicone/5 mL. Parabens, saccharin, sorbitol, cherry flavor.
Mylanta Supreme	**Liquid**: 400 mg calcium carbonate, 135 mg magnesium hydroxide/5 mL. Saccharin, sorbitol. Cherry and mint flavors.
Powder and Effervescent Tablets	
Alka-Seltzer Gold	**Tablets, effervescent**: 958 mg sodium bicarbonate (heat-treated), 832 mg citric acid, 312 mg potassium bicarbonate, 299 mg sodium
Alka-Seltzer	**Tablets, effervescent**: 1700 mg sodium bicarbonate (heat-treated), 1000 mg citric acid, 325 mg aspirin. Aspartame, cherry[3] and lemon lime[4] flavors.
Alka-Seltzer Original	**Tablets, effervescent**: 1916 mg sodium bicarbonate (heat-treated), 1000 mg citric acid, 325 mg aspirin, 568 mg sodium
Extra Strength Alka-Seltzer	**Tablets, effervescent**: 1985 mg sodium bicarbonate (heat-treated), 1000 mg citric acid, 500 mg aspirin, 588 mg sodium
Citrocarbonate	**Granules, effervescent**: 780 mg sodium bicarbonate, 1820 mg sodium citrate anhydrous, 700.6 mg sodium

Products listed are representative of currently available and widely distributed brands. Similar products, including regional and private label brands, may also exist.

[1] Parabens, sorbitol.
[2] Parabens, sorbitol, saccharin.
[3] 12 mg phenylalanine, 504 mg sodium.
[4] 9 mg phenylalanine, 504 mg sodium.

PATIENT INFORMATION

Antacid Combinations

- Magnesium-containing products may act as a laxative in large doses and cause diarrhea.
- Aluminum- and calcium-containing products may cause constipation.
- Antacids may interact with certain prescription medications. If you are taking a prescription drug, do not take an antacid without first checking with a physician or pharmacist.
- Taking too much of these products can cause the stomach to secrete excess stomach acid.
- *Chewable tablets:* Chew tablets thoroughly before swallowing and follow with a glass of water.
- *Liquids:* Shake liquid antacids before use.
- *Effervescent tablets:* Allow tablet to completely dissolve in water, and allow most of the bubbling to stop before drinking.

HISTAMINE H_2 ANTAGONISTS

▶ Actions

Histamine H_2 antagonists are reversible competitive blockers of histamine at the H_2 receptors, particularly those in the gastric parietal cells. As inhibitors of gastric acid secretion, they inhibit secretions caused by histamine, muscarinic agonists, and gastrin. They have no anticholinergic activity and no effect on H_1 receptors.

▶ Indications

For the relief of symptoms of episodic and uncomplicated heartburn, acid indigestion, and sour stomach.

▶ Contraindications

Hypersensitivity to individual agents or other H_2 antagonists.

▶ Warnings

Pregnancy: Category B. There are no adequate and well-controlled studies in pregnant women. Use during pregnancy only if the potential benefits outweigh the possible risks to the fetus.

Lactation: Cimetidine and ranitidine are excreted in human breast milk. Avoid cimetidine in nursing mothers. Exercise caution in administering ranitidine to lactating mothers. It is not known whether famotidine is excreted in human breast milk. However, it is excreted in the breast milk of rats. Do not use famotidine in nursing mothers unless the benefits to the mother outweigh the risks to the fetus.

Children: OTC use of H_2 antagonists is not recommended in children younger than 12 years of age. In addition, cimetidine is not recommended in children younger than 16 years of age.

▶ Drug Interactions

Drugs metabolized by cytochrome P450: Significant drug interactions with H_2 antagonists primarily occur with cimetidine. Cimetidine inhibits the metabolism of certain drugs metabolized by the cytochrome P450 system, thereby leading to increased drug levels and toxicity. Through this mechanism, cimetidine inhibits the clearance of drug such as warfarin, theophylline, phenytoin, propranolol, nifedepine, metronidazole, carbamazepine, sulfonylureas, quinidine, alcohol, caffeine, and benzodiazepines.

Carmustine: Cimetidine results in increased bone marrow suppression.

Itraconazole and ketoconazole: H_2 antagonists decrease the absorption of itraconazole and ketoconazole by decreasing gastric acidity.

Metformin: Cimetidine may increase serum plasma levels of metformin by reducing its renal clearance.

Procainamide: Cimetidine and ranitidine may increase serum plasma levels of procainamide by reducing its renal clearance.

Drug-food interactions: Food may increase the bioavailability of famotidine and nizatidine. This interaction is unlikely to be clinically relevant with OTC doses of H_2 antagonists.

▶ **Adverse Reactions**

H_2 antagonists generally are well tolerated. The most common adverse reactions are headache, fatigue, and diarrhea. Prolonged use of cimetidine may lead to gynecomastia. Reversible confusional states (eg, psychosis, delirium, agitation, depression) have been reported in elderly patients. Gynecomastia and confusion are more likely with the higher prescription doses of cimetidine.

▶ **Product Selection**

The following table presents a comparison of OTC histamine H_2 antagonists, which may be helpful for drug selection and use.

Comparison of OTC Histamine H_2 Antagonists								
Agent	Dosage form	Strength (mg)	Duration of action (h)	Half-life (h)	Urinary excretion (%)	Inhibition of CYP450	Inhibition of alcohol dehydrogenase	Daily dosage
Cimetidine	tablet, suspension	200	4 to 6	1.5 to 2.5	50	+++	+	200 mg bid prn (400 mg/day)
Famotidine	tablet, chewable tablet, gelcap	10	6 to 10	2.5 to 4.0	30	–	–	10 mg bid prn (20 mg/day)
Famotidine	tablet	20	6 to 10	2.5 to 4.0	30	–	–	20 mg bid prn (40 mg/day)
Nizatidine	tablet	75	6 to 8	1 to 2	> 90	–	+	75 mg bid prn (150 mg/day)
Ranitidine	tablet	75	6 to 8	2 to 3	30	+	+	75 mg bid prn (150 mg/day)

- none
+ low
+++ high

CIMETIDINE

▶ **Administration and Dosage**

Relief of symptoms: Take 200 mg (one tablet) with a glass of water or other fluid as needed. Do not exceed 400 mg (two tablets) in 24 hours.

Prevention of symptoms: Take 200 mg (one tablet) with a glass of water or other fluid 30 minutes or less before eating food or drinking beverages that cause heartburn, acid indigestion, or sour stomach. Do not exceed 400 mg (two tablets) in 24 hours.

Cimetidine should not be given to children younger than 12 years of age unless directed by a physician.

CIMETIDINE PRODUCTS	
Trade name	Doseform
Cimetidine, *Tagamet HB 200*	**Tablets**: 200 mg
Tagamet HB 200	**Suspension**: 200 mg/5 mL

Products listed are representative of currently available and widely distributed brands. Similar products, including regional and private label brands, may also exist.

RANITIDINE

▶ **Administration and Dosage**

Take tablets with fluid and swallow them whole.

Usual dosage: May be used up to twice daily (up to 2 tablets in 24 hours).

RANITIDINE PRODUCTS	
Trade name	Doseform
Ranitidine (sf)	**Tablets**: 75 mg. Lactose. Sodium free.
Zantac 75 (sf)	**Tablets**: 75 mg. Sodium free.
Zantac 150 (sf)	**Tablets**: 150 mg.

Products listed are representative of currently available and widely distributed brands. Similar products, including regional and private label brands, may also exist.

sf = Sugar free.

FAMOTIDINE

▶ **Administration and Dosage**

Take the nonchewable tablets and gelcaps with fluid and swallow them whole.

Relief of symptoms: Swallow one tablet or gelcap with a glass of water or chew one chewable tablet.

Prevention of symptoms: Swallow one tablet or gelcap with a glass of water or chew one chewable tablet at any time 15 to 60 minutes before eating food or drinking beverages that cause heartburn.

10 mg: Take 10 mg once or twice daily as needed. Do not exceed 20 mg (two tablets or gelcaps) in 24 hours.

20 mg: Take 20 mg once or twice daily as needed. Do not exceed more than 40 mg (two tablets) in 24 hours.

FAMOTIDINE PRODUCTS	
Trade name	Doseform
Famotidine, *Pepcid AC*	**Tablets**: 10 mg
Maximum Strength Pepcid AC	**Tablets**: 20 mg. Talc.
Pepcid AC Chewable	**Tablets, chewable**: 10 mg. Aspartame, lactose, 1.4 mg phenylalanine.
Pepcid AC Gelcaps	**Gelcaps**: 10 mg

Products listed are representative of currently available and widely distributed brands. Similar products, including regional and private label brands, may also exist.

NIZATIDINE

▶ **Administration and Dosage**

Take tablets with fluid and swallow them whole.

Usual dosage: Take 75 mg once or twice daily as needed. Do not exceed 150 mg (two tablets) in 24 hours.

NIZATIDINE PRODUCTS	
Trade name	Doseform
Axid AR	Tablets: 75 mg

Products listed are representative of currently available and widely distributed brands. Similar products, including regional and private label brands, may also exist.

HISTAMINE H₂ ANTAGONIST COMBINATIONS

▶ Administration and Dosage

Do not swallow tablet whole; chew completely.

Usual dosage: Do not use more than two chewable tablets in 24 hours. Do not give to children younger than 12 years of age unless directed by a physician.

HISTAMINE H₂ ANTAGONIST PRODUCTS	
Trade name	Doseform
Pepcid Complete	Tablets, chewable: 10 mg famotidine. 800 mg calcium carbonate, 165 mg magnesium hydroxide. Lactose, sugar.

Products listed are representative of currently available and widely distributed brands. Similar products, including regional and private label brands, may also exist.

PATIENT INFORMATION

Histamine H₂ Antagonists

- Patient instructions accompany each product. Read these instructions carefully before use, preferably before leaving the pharmacy in case of any questions.
- Do not use the maximum daily doses of these agents for two weeks or more, except under the advice of a physician.
- Histamine H₂ antagonists may interact with certain prescription drugs. If you are presently taking a prescription drug, do not take a histamine H₂ antagonist without checking with a physician or pharmacist.
- If symptoms worsen or persist for two weeks or more, contact a physician.
- Store at room temperature in a tight container away from light.

PROTON PUMP INHIBITORS

▶ Actions

Proton pump inhibitors (PPIs) are the most powerful inhibitors of gastric acid secretion. They block the final step of acid production at its source, the acid pumps that produce gastric acid.

OMEPRAZOLE MAGNESIUM

▶ Indications

Indicated for treatment of frequent heartburn (2 or more days a week) in adults 18 years of age and older.

▶ Contraindications

Hypersensitivity to omeprazole; pain or difficulty swallowing food; vomiting with blood; bloody or black stools.

▶ Warnings

Hepatic function impairment: Use with caution in patients with severe liver disease. However, no dosing adjustment is required.

Renal function impairment: Use with caution in patients with severe kidney disease. However, no dosing adjustment is required.

Pregnancy: Category C. Use during pregnancy only if the potential benefit to the mother justifies the unknown potential risk to the fetus. Patients should consult with their doctor before use.

Lactation: Because of the potential for serious adverse reactions in the nursing infant, decide whether to discontinue nursing or to discontinue the drug, taking into account the importance of the drug to the mother.

Children: Safety and effectiveness in children have not been established.

Elderly: Bioavailability of omeprazole may be increased. However, no dosing adjustment is required.

► Drug Interactions

PPIs cause a profound and long-lasting inhibition of gastric acid secretion; therefore it is theoretically possible that omeprazole may interfere with the absorption of drugs where gastric pH is an important determination of bioavailability (eg, ketoconazole, ampicillin, iron salts, digoxin, cyanocobalamin). Patients should consult a doctor or pharmacist if they are taking warfarin, an antifungal or anti-yeast medication, diazepam, or digoxin.

► Adverse Reactions

Infrequently occurring adverse effects include headache, diarrhea, constipation, upset stomach, vomiting, stomach pain, cough, dizziness, and rash.

► Administration and Dosage

Take 1 tablet with a glass of water before eating in the morning (preferably 30 to 60 minutes before eating). Do not crush or chew the tablet; swallow whole. Take every day for 14 days. Do not take more than 1 tablet per day. Do not use for more than 14 days or more often than every 4 months unless directed by a doctor.

May require 1 to 4 days for full effect, although some patients experience complete relief of symptoms within 24 hours.

The 14-day course of therapy may be repeated every 4 months.

OMEPRAZOLE MAGNESIUM	
Trade name	Doseform
Prilosec OTC	**Tablet, delayed-release**: 20.6 mg (equivalent to 20 mg omeprazole). Available as 14, 28, or 42 tablet packages.

Products listed are representative of currently available and widely distributed brands. Similar products, including regional and private label brands, may also exist.

PATIENT INFORMATION
Omeprazole Magnesium

- Take once a day with water in the morning (preferably 30 to 60 minutes before eating) if you suffer from frequent heartburn (heartburn 2 or more days per week). Take every day for 14 days. Do not change the dose or stop taking this medicine unless advised to do so by your doctor.
- Omeprazole must be taken daily to be effective, do not take on an "as needed" basis.
- Do not crush or chew the tablets. This will decrease the effectiveness.
- It may take 1 to 4 days for full effect. Some patients experience complete relief of symptoms within 24 hours. Make sure to take the entire 14 days of therapy.
- Do not take for more than 14 consecutive days or more often than every 4 months unless directed by a doctor.
- Antacids may be used with this medicine.
- Stop use and consult a doctor if heartburn continues or worsens, if you need to take this medicine for more than 14 days, or if you need to take more than 1 course of treatment every 4 months.
- Heartburn over 3 months may be a sign of a more serious condition; consult a doctor.
- Consult a doctor or pharmacist before using this medicine if you have heartburn with light-headedness, sweating, or dizziness; chest pain or shoulder or arm pain with shortness of breath; sweating; pain spreading to arms, neck, or shoulder; light-headedness; frequent chest pain; frequent wheezing, particularly with heartburn; unexplained weight loss; nausea or vomiting; or stomach pain.
- Inform your doctor if you are pregnant, become pregnant, plan on becoming pregnant, or are breastfeeding.

HEMORRHOIDS
(Piles)

DEFINITION

Painful swellings at the anal area caused by a varicose condition of the hemorrhoidal veins.

ETIOLOGY

Hemorrhoids may be precipitated by pregnancy, straining at stool, constipation, prolonged sitting or standing, and anal infection. They may be symptomatic following passage of a large firm stool, urgent defecation (eg, explosive diarrhea), or partial obstruction of the anal canal.

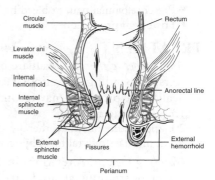

Figure 1. Hemorrhoids

INCIDENCE

Symptomatic hemorrhoids occur in approximately 5% of the population older than 50 years of age and are uncommon in people younger than 30 years of age, except in pregnancy.

PATHOPHYSIOLOGY

Hemorrhoids arise from varices (eg, dilation) of the venous hemorrhoidal plexus and may be internal or external.

SIGNS/SYMPTOMS

Signs and symptoms are usually mild and include anal pain, bleeding, itching, and burning. More severe symptoms may involve incontinence, rectal protrusion of hemorrhoids, increased bleeding, mucus accumulation, fissure, ulceration, infection, prolapse, and thrombosis. Anemia may occur secondary to chronic blood loss.

DIAGNOSTIC PARAMETERS/PHYSICAL ASSESSMENT

Clinical Observation: Clinical presence will usually be reported by the patient or by previous diagnosis by a physician. Confirm hemorrhoids by proctologic examination. Precede treatment with sigmoidoscopy and barium enema to rule out bleeding caused by polyps or other GI pathology (eg, colon cancer, colitis, ulceration).

Interview: To help the patient determine if a physician referral or self-treatment is warranted, ask about the following:

- History of previous physician diagnosis and examination to rule out carcinoma or polyps
- Previous symptoms
- Current symptoms

- Pregnancy status
- Dietary habits
- Bowel habits and presence of constipation
- Current medication history
- Presence of anal pain or bleeding
- History of protrusion

TREATMENT

Approaches to therapy: Evaluate patients using the above diagnostic parameters. Depending on various factors (eg, symptoms, duration, recurrence), health care providers may recommend the following:
1.) A nondrug approach,
2.) appropriate pharmacotherapy, or
3.) immediate referral to a physician for medical evaluation.

Nondrug therapy: Alterations in diet (high-bulk diet), avoidance of prolonged sitting or straining at stool, sitz bath 2 to 3 times daily for 15 to 20 minutes, and anal hygiene may provide relief of hemorrhoidal symptoms. Without treatment, hemorrhoidal symptoms usually resolve within several days but may take several weeks.

Pharmacotherapy: Once it is determined that drug treatment is necessary, there are a number of topical and systemic OTC agents available for symptomatic relief. However, these remedies offer limited and transient therapeutic benefit. The use of stool softeners or bulk laxatives may also be beneficial for patients with constipation or straining at stool, which may precipitate or aggravate hemorrhoids.

PSYLLIUM

▶ **Actions**

Promotes bowel evacuation by taking up fluid, expanding, and providing well-formed intestinal bulk.

▶ **Indications**

For relief of occasional constipation and to induce regularity.

▶ **Contraindications**

Hypersensitivity to any ingredient.

Intestinal obstruction; fecal impaction.

▶ **Warnings**

Do not use this product without consulting a physician if abdominal pain, nausea, undiagnosed rectal bleeding, diagnosed esophageal narrowing, difficulty swallowing, or vomiting is present.

▶ **Adverse Reactions**

Esophageal, gastric, small intestinal, and rectal obstruction; gas.

▶ **Administration and Dosage**

Powder (3 to 3.4 g), granules (2.5 to 4 g) mixed with 8 oz of liquid (eg, cool water, fruit juice, milk) per labeled instructions. Consume wafers with 8 oz of liquid. An additional glass of liquid after each dose will increase effectiveness. May be taken

1 to 3 times daily for 2 to 3 days, depending on the need and response. Chronic constipation may be managed prophylactically with daily psyllium treatment.

PSYLLIUM PRODUCTS	
Trade name	**Doseform**
Metamucil	**Capsules**: 0.52 g psylluim husk, 3 g carbohydrates, 10 calories per dose (6 capsules)
Perdiem	**Granules**: 4.03 g psyllium, 1.8 mg sodium, 36.1 mg potassium, 4 calories per rounded tsp (6 g)
Syllact	**Powder**: 3.3 g psyllium seed husks, ≈ 14 calories per rounded tsp
V-Lax	**Powder**: 3.4 g psyllium hydrophilic mucilloid per dose. Dextrose.
Konsyl-D	**Powder**: 3.4 g psyllium hydrophlic mucilloid, < 5 mg sodium, 14 calories per rounded tsp (6.5 g). Dextrose.
Reguloid, Sugar Free Regular Flavor	**Powder**: ≈ 3.4 g psyllium hydrophilic mucilloid, 6 mg phenylalanine per rounded tsp. Aspartame, maltodextrin.
Reguloid, Sugar Free Orange Flavor	**Powder**: ≈ 3.4 g psyllium hydrophilic mucilloid, 30 mg phenylalanine per rounded tsp. Aspartame, maltodextrin.
Reguloid, Regular Flavor	**Powder**: ≈ 3.4 g psyllium, < 0.01 g sodium, ≈ 14 calories per rounded tsp. Dextrose.
Reguloid, Orange Flavor	**Powder**: ≈ 3.4 g psyllium, < 0.01 g sodium, 30 calories per tbsp. Sucrose.
Metamucil, Sugar Free, Regular Flavor	**Powder**: ≈ 3.4 g psyllium husk, 5 g carbohydrates, 4 mg sodium, 20 calories per rounded tsp (5.4 g). Maltodextrin.
Metamucil, Sugar Free, Orange Flavor	**Powder**: ≈ 3.4 g psyllium husk, 5 g carbohydrates, 5 mg sodium, 25 mg phenylalanine, 20 calories per rounded tsp (5.8 g). Aspartame, maltodextrin.
Metamucil, Regular Flavor	**Powder**: ≈ 3.4 g psyllium husk, 6 g carbohydrates, 3 mg sodium, 25 calories per rounded tsp (7 g). Sucrose.
Metamucil, Orange Flavor	**Powder**: ≈ 3.4 g psyllium husk, 10 g carbohydrates, 5 mg sodium, 40 calories per rounded tbsp (11 g). Sucrose.
Hydrocil Instant	**Powder**: 3.5 g psyllium hydrophilic mucilloid per dose (3.7 g)
Fiberall, Orange Flavor	**Powder**: 3.5 g psylium hydrophillic mucilloid, 5 g carbohydrates, 20 calories per rounded tbsp (10 g). Phenylalanine.
Konsyl, Sugar Free Easy Mix Formula	**Powder**: 6 g psyllium hydrophilic mucilloid, < 5 mg sodium per rounded tsp (6.3 g). Maltodextrin.
Konsyl, Sugar Free	**Powder**: 6 g psyllium hydrophilic mucilloid, 0.5 g carbohydrates, < 5 mg sodium, 3 calories per rounded tsp (6 g)
Metamucil (Apple Crisp or Cinnamon Spice Flavor)	**Wafers**: ≈ 3.4 g psyllium hydrophilic mucilloid, 20 mg sodium, 17 g carbohydrates, 120 calories per wafer

Products listed are representative of currently available and widely distributed brands. Similar products, including regional and private label brands, may also exist.

[1] Contains sucrose.

PATIENT INFORMATION
Psyllium

- Patient instructions accompany each product. Read these instructions carefully before use, preferably before leaving the pharmacy, in case you have any questions. Instructions for proper use must be strictly followed.
- Do not use this product without consulting your physician if abdominal pain, nausea, undiagnosed rectal bleeding, diagnosed esophageal narrowing, difficulty swallowing, or vomiting is present.
- Mix this product with liquid to avoid obstructing the throat or esophagus. An additional glass of water or other liquid will increase effectiveness.
- Consult your physician if anorectal symptoms do not improve within 7 days, or if profuse bleeding, protrusion, seepage, or moderate to severe pain occurs or continues.
- Tell your physician if you are pregnant, become pregnant, plan to become pregnant, or are breastfeeding.

POLYCARBOPHIL

▶ Actions

Calcium polycarbophil is a hydrophilic agent. In diarrhea, when the intestinal mucosa is incapable of absorbing water at normal rates, it absorbs free fecal water, forming a gel, and producing formed stools. Thus, in diarrhea, it works by restoring a more normal moisture level and providing bulk.

▶ Indications

Treatment of constipation associated with conditions such as irritable bowel syndrome and diverticulosis.

▶ Warnings

Impaction or obstruction: Impaction or obstruction may be caused by bulk-forming agents. In patients with intestinal ulcerations, stenosis, or disabling adhesions use may be hazardous. Patients with these conditions should consult a physician before using a bulk-forming agent.

▶ Administration and Dosage

Adults: 1 g 1 to 4 times daily or as needed. Do not exceed 6 g/day.

Children (6 years of age and older): 500 mg 1 to 3 times daily or as needed. Do not exceed 3 g/day.

Children (3 to 6 years of age): 500 mg 1 to 2 times daily or as needed. Do not exceed 1.5 g/day.

For severe diarrhea, repeat dose every 30 minutes; do not exceed maximum daily dose. To treat or prevent constipation, the doses should be separated by several hours.

POLYCARBOPHIL PRODUCTS	
Trade name	Doseform
FiberCon, FiberNorm, Phillips' FiberCaps	**Caplets**: 625 mg calcium polycarbophil (equiv. to 500 mg polycarbophil)
Fiber-Lax, Konsyl	**Tablets**: 625 mg calcium polycarbophil (equiv. to 500 mg polycarbophil)

POLYCARBOPHIL PRODUCTS	
Trade name	Doseform
Equalactin	**Tablets, chewable**: 625 mg calcium polycarbophil (equiv. to 500 mg polycarbophil). Dextrose.

Products listed are representative of currently available and widely distributed brands. Similar products, including regional and private label brands, may also exist.

PATIENT INFORMATION

Polycarbophil

- Patient instructions accompany each product. Read these instructions carefully before use, preferably before leaving the pharmacy in case you have questions.
- Do not use these products in the presence of abdominal pain, nausea, vomiting, undiagnosed rectal bleeding, or difficulty swallowing.
- Drink sufficient amounts of fluids to prevent dehydration that may accompany diarrhea.
- Contact your physician if diarrhea does not subside after a few days, or if abdominal pain, abdominal distention, or fever occurs.
- Tell your physician if you are pregnant, become pregnant, plan to become pregnant, or are breastfeeding.

METHYLCELLULOSE

▶ Administration and Dosage

Citrucel:

> *Adults and children (12 years of age and older)* – 1 heaping tbsp (19 g) in 8 oz cold water 1 to 3 times daily.

> *Children (6 to 12 years of age)* – Half the adult dose in 4 oz cold water 1 to 3 times daily.

Maltsupex:

> *Tablets:*

> *Adults* – 12 to 64 g/day. Initially, 4 tablets 4 times daily (meals and bedtime).

> *Powder:*

> *Adults* – Up to 32 g twice daily for 3 or 4 days, then 16 to 32 g at bedtime.

> *Children (6 to 12 years of age)* – Up to 16 g twice daily for 3 to 4 days.

> *Children (2 to 6 years)* – 8 g twice daily for 3 or 4 days.

> *Infants, (older than 1 month [bottlefed])* – 8 to 16 g daily in formula for 3 or 4 days, then 4 to 8 g daily in formula.

> *Infants (older than 1 month [breastfed])* – 4 g in 2 to 4 oz water or fruit juice twice daily for 3 or 4 days.

> *Liquid:*

> *Adults* – 2 tbsp twice daily for 3 or 4 days, then 1 to 2 tbsp at bedtime.

> *Children (6 to 12 years of age)* – 1 to 2 tbsp once or twice daily for 3 or 4 days.

> *Children (2 to 6 years of age)* – ½ tbsp once or twice daily for 3 or 4 days.

Infants (older than 1 month [bottlefed]) – ½ to 2 tbsp daily in formula for 3 or 4 days, then 1 to 2 tsp daily in formula.

Infants (older than 1 month [breastfed]) – 1 to 2 tsp in 2 to 4 oz water or fruit juice once or twice daily for 3 or 4 days.

METHYLCELLULOSE PRODUCTS	
Trade name	Doseform
Maltsupex	**Tablets, coated**: 750 mg malt soup extract per tbsp
Citrucel	**Caplets**: 0.5 g methlycellulose
Maltsupex	**Liquid**: 16 g malt soup extract per tbsp
Maltsupex	**Powder**: 8 g malt soup extract per scoop
Citrucel, Sugar Free Orange Flavor	**Powder**: 2 g methylcellulose, 6.5 g carbohydrates, 24 calories per tbsp. Aspartame, phenylalanine.
Citrucel Clear-Mix	**Powder**: 2 g methylcellulose, 9 g carbohydrates, 36 calories per tbsp
Citrucel, Orange Flavor	**Powder**: 2 g methylcellulose, 15 g carbohydrates, 60 calories per tbsp
UniFiber	**Powder**: Powdered cellulose

Products listed are representative of currently available and widely distributed brands. Similar products, including regional and private label brands, may also exist.

PATIENT INFORMATION
Methylcellulose

- Patient instructions accompany each product. Read these instructions carefully before use, preferably before leaving the pharmacy, in case you have any questions.
- Take with a full glass of water or juice.
- Do not use in the presence of abdominal pain, nausea, vomiting, or difficulty swallowing.
- Laxative use is only a temporary measure; do not use for longer than 1 week. When regularity returns, discontinue use. Prolonged, frequent, or excessive use may result in dependence or electrolyte imbalance.
- Notify your physician if unrelieved constipation, rectal bleeding, or symptoms of electrolyte imbalance (eg, muscle cramps or pain, weakness, dizziness) occurs.
- Direct attention to proper dietary fiber intake, adequate fluids, and regular exercise.
- Tell your physician if you are pregnant, become pregnant, plan to become pregnant, or are breastfeeding.

DOCUSATE SALTS

▶ Actions

Facilitate stool softening by lowering surface tension and increasing penetration of stool by water.

▶ Indications

Docusate salts are indicated for preventing hardening of stool and constipation in patients who should not strain during defecation (eg, after surgery, post-MI).

▶ **Contraindications**

Hypersensitivity to any ingredient.

Vomiting, nausea, or other symptoms of appendicitis, acute surgical abdomen, fecal impaction, intestinal obstruction, undiagnosed abdominal pain, rectal bleeding, and coadministration of mineral oil.

▶ **Warnings**

Pregnancy: Safety not established. Use only if directed by a physician.

Lactation: Safety not established. Use only if directed by a physician.

▶ **Drug Interactions**

Mineral oil: Docusate may increase absorption of mineral oil from the GI tract, leading to toxicity if use of both agents is chronic.

▶ **Adverse Reactions**

Nausea; diarrhea; rash; perianal irritation; bad taste (liquid formulation).

DOCUSATE SODIUM

▶ **Administration and Dosage**

Adults and children (older than 12 years of age): 50 to 500 mg/day (usually 100 to 200 mg/day)

Children (6 to 12 years of age): 40 to 120 mg/day.

Children (3 to 6 years of age): 20 to 60 mg/day.

Children (younger than 3 years of age): 10 to 40 mg/day.

DOCUSATE SODIUM PRODUCTS	
Trade name	Doseform
Ex-Lax, Gentle Strength	**Caplets**: 65 mg, 10 mg sennosides. Lactose, methylparaben, 5 mg sodium.
Ex-Lax, Stimulant Free	**Caplets**: 100 mg. Methylparaben, 8 mg sodium.
Colace	**Capsules**: 50 mg
Colace[1], DSS, Phillips' Liqui-Gels[1],[2], Regulax SS	**Capsules**: 100 mg
DSS, D.O.S. Softgels[2]	**Capsules**: 250 mg
Colace[1],[3], Diocto[1],[4], Docu	**Syrup**: 20 mg/5 mL
Colace, Diocto[1], Docu	**Liquid**: 50 mg/5 mL

Products listed are representative of currently available and widely distributed brands. Similar products, including regional and private label brands, may also exist.

[1] Contains parabens.
[2] Contains sorbitol.
[3] Contains alcohol, menthol, sucrose.
[4] Contains 60 mg sodium/15 mL.

PATIENT INFORMATION
Docusate Sodium

- Patient instructions accompany each product. Read these instructions carefully before use, preferably before leaving the pharmacy, in case you have any questions.
- Swallow capsules whole; do not chew.
- Take with a full glass of water or other fluid to increase efficacy.
- Mix liquid forms, excluding syrup, with fruit juice or milk to mask unpleasant taste.
- Do not take mineral oil while taking this product.
- Consult your physician if anorectal symptoms do not improve within 7 days, or if profuse bleeding, protrusion, seepage, or moderate to severe pain occurs or continues.
- Tell your physician if you are pregnant, become pregnant, plan to become pregnant, or are breastfeeding.

DOCUSATE CALCIUM

▶ **Administration and Dosage**

Adults: 240 mg.

DOCUSATE CALCIUM PRODUCTS	
Trade name	**Doseform**
DC Softgels[1], *Surfak Liquigels*	**Capsules**: 240 mg

Products listed are representative of currently available and widely distributed brands. Similar products, including regional and private label brands, may also exist.

[1] Contains sorbitol.

PATIENT INFORMATION
Docusate Calcium

- Patient instructions accompany each product. Read these instructions carefully before use, preferably before leaving the pharmacy, in case of questions.
- Swallow capsules whole; do not chew.
- Take with a full glass of water or other fluid to increase the efficacy.
- Do not take mineral oil while taking this product.
- Consult your physician if anorectal symptoms do not improve within 7 days, or if profuse bleeding, protrusion, seepage, or moderate to severe pain occurs or continues.
- Tell your physician if you are pregnant, become pregnant, plan to become pregnant, or are breastfeeding.

ANORECTAL PREPARATIONS (TOPICAL)

▶ **Actions**

Symptomatic relief and perianal hygiene.

Anticholinergics: Inhibit acetylcholine systemically but are not effective in ameliorating local anorectal symptoms.

Antiseptics (benzalkonium chloride, phenylmercuric nitrate): Present as preservatives. Not considered to have therapeutic value.

Astringents (hamamelis water [witch hazel], zinc oxide): Coagulate protein in skin cells, protecting the underlying tissue and decreasing cell volume; reduce mucus and other secretions; relieve anorectal irritation and inflammation.

Counterirritants (camphor): Evoke a feeling of comfort, cooling, tingling, or warmth, distracting the patient from the perception of pain and itching.

Emollients/protectants (bismuth salts, cocoa butter, glycerin, lanolin, mineral oil, petrolatum, shark oil, zinc oxide): Lubricate skin; prevent irritation of the anorectal area and water loss from the stratum corneum by forming a physical barrier on the skin; allow easier evacuation of stool; serve as a base or carrier of pharmacologic ingredients.

Keratolytics (resorcinol): May help to expose underlying tissue to therapeutic agents by causing sloughing of the epidermis.

Local anesthetics (benzocaine, pramoxine): Inhibit conduction of nerve impulses from sensory nerves; relieve pain.

Wound-healing agents (balsam Peru, skin respiratory factor, yeast cell derivatives): Effectiveness has not been demonstrated conclusively, but agents are claimed to promote wound healing and tissue repair.

Vasoconstrictors (ephedrine, phenylephrine): Reduce swelling and congestion of anorectal tissue.

▶ **Indications**

For the symptomatic relief of discomfort associated with hemorrhoids, particularly pain, itching, and burning.

▶ **Contraindications**

Hypersensitivity to any ingredient.

Benzalkonium chloride: Use in anal packs may cause irritation or chemical burns.

Ephedrine, phenylephrine: Concurrent use of monoamine oxidase inhibitors.

▶ **Warnings**

Methemoglobinemia (benzocaine): Do not use benzocaine as a local anesthetic in patients with congenital or idiopathic methemoglobinemia or in children younger than 12 years of age who are receiving methemoglobin-inducing drugs.

Mucous membranes (benzalkonium chloride): Do not use concentrations more than 1:5000 on rectal mucous membranes.

Pregnancy:

> *Benzocaine – Category C.* Safety not established. Do not use during pregnancy unless directed by a physician.

Children: Do not use benzocaine in infants younger than 1 year of age.

▶ **Drug Interactions**

Monoamine oxidase inhibitors: Because of systemic absorption of ephedrine and phenylephrine through mucous membranes, severe hypertensive reactions may occur with concurrent administration of a monoamine oxidase inhibitor (eg, phenelzine).

▶ **Adverse Reactions**

Local anesthetics (benzocaine): Hypersensitivity; methemoglobinemia; burning; stinging; tenderness; sloughing.

HAMAMELIS WATER (WITCH HAZEL)

▶ **Actions**

Hamamelis water, also known as witch hazel, is a mild astringent prepared from twigs of *Hamamelis virginiana*; the distillate is then adjusted with an appropriate amount of alcohol.

▶ **Indications**

Temporary relief of anal or vaginal irritation and itching, hemorrhoids, postepisiotomy discomfort, and hemorrhoidectomy discomfort.

For more information on Witch Hazel, see the Complementary Therapies chapter.

▶ **Warnings**

Worsened condition: If symptoms worsen or do not improve within 7 days, consult a physician.

Bleeding: In case of rectal bleeding, consult a physician promptly.

For external use only: Avoid contact with the eyes.

▶ **Administration and Dosage**

Apply locally up to 6 times daily or after each bowel movement.

HAMAMELIS WATER (WITCH HAZEL) PRODUCTS	
Trade name	Doseform
Witch Hazel	**Liquid**: 86%. 14% alcohol.
Witch Hazel	**Pads**: 50%. 7% alcohol, glycerin, methylparaben, aloe vera gel.
A•E•R	**Pads**: 50%. 12.5% glycerin, methylparaben.

Products listed are representative of currently available and widely distributed brands. Similar products, including regional and private label brands, may also exist.

PATIENT INFORMATION

Hamamelis Water (Witch Hazel)

• For external use only. Avoid contact with the eyes.

• Patient instructions accompany each product. Read these instructions carefully before use, preferably before leaving the pharmacy, in case you have any questions.

• Consult your physician if anorectal symptoms do not improve within 7 days, or if profuse bleeding, protrusion, seepage, or moderate to severe pain occurs or continues.

• Tell your physician if you are pregnant, become pregnant, plan to become pregnant, or are breastfeeding.

LOCAL ANESTHETIC-CONTAINING TOPICAL RECTAL PRODUCTS

▶ **Administration and Dosage**

Apply to affected area using the recommended technique.

Administer the lowest concentration and quantity possible that provides adequate anesthesia (relief of pain, itching, and burning).

LOCAL ANESTHETIC-CONTAINING TOPICAL RECTAL PRODUCTS

Trade name	Doseform
ProctoFoam	**Aerosol Foam**: 1% pramoxine HCl. Cetyl alcohol, parabens.
Tronolane	**Cream**: 1% pramoxine HCl
Americaine	**Ointment**: 20% benzocaine, 0.1% benzalkonium chloride
Medicone	**Ointment**: 20% benzocaine, mineral oil, white petrolatum, methylparaben
Nupercainal	**Ointment**: 1% dibucaine, acetone sodium bisulfite, lanolin, mineral oil, white petrolatum
Anusol	**Ointment**: 1% pramoxine HCl, 12.5% zinc oxide, mineral oil

Products listed are representative of currently available and widely distributed brands. Similar products, including regional and private label brands, may also exist.

PATIENT INFORMATION
Local Anesthetic-Containing Topical Rectal Products

- For external use only.
- Patient instructions accompany each product. Read these instructions carefully before use, preferably before leaving the pharmacy, in case you have any questions.
- Consult your physician if anorectal symptoms do not improve within 7 days, or if profuse bleeding, protrusion, seepage, or moderate to severe pain occurs or continues.
- Maintain normal bowel movements by proper diet, adequate fluid intake, and regular exercise.
- Avoid scratching or rubbing area, washing with strong or scented soaps, or eating spicy foods, peppers, or tomatoes.
- Tell your physician if you are pregnant, become pregnant, plan to become pregnant, or are breastfeeding.

TOPICAL PERIANAL HYGIENE PRODUCTS

▶ Administration and Dosage

Apply to affected area using the recommended technique (see individual product information).

TOPICAL PERIANAL HYGIENE PRODUCTS

Trade name	Doseform
Balneol Soothing Perianal Cleansing	**Lotion**: Mineral oil, lanolin oil, methylparaben
Sensi-Care Perineal/Skin Cleanser	**Solution**: Sodium C_{12-14} olefin sulfonate, disodium cocoamphodiacetate
Tucks	**Pads**: 50% hamamelis water, glycerin, alcohol, urea, parabens
Preparation H Medicated Wipes	**Pads**: 50% hamamelis water, aloe, urea, parabens

Products listed are representative of currently available and widely distributed brands. Similar products, including regional and private label brands, may also exist.

PATIENT INFORMATION
Topical Perianal Hygiene Products

- For external use only.
- Patient instructions accompany each product. Read these instructions carefully before use, preferably before leaving the pharmacy, in case you have any questions.
- Consult your physician if anorectal symptoms do not improve within 7 days, or if profuse bleeding, protrusion, seepage, or moderate to severe pain occurs or continues.
- Maintain normal bowel movements by proper diet, adequate fluid intake, and regular exercise.
- Avoid scratching or rubbing area, washing with strong or scented soaps, or eating spicy foods, peppers, or tomatoes.
- Tell your physician if you are pregnant, become pregnant, plan to become pregnant, or are breastfeeding.

MISCELLANEOUS TOPICAL ANORECTAL COMBINATION PRODUCTS

► Administration and Dosage

Apply to affected area using the recommended technique (see individual product information).

Refer to Appendix D, Administration Techniques, for guidelines on inserting suppositories.

MISCELLANEOUS TOPICAL ANORECTAL COMBINATION PRODUCTS	
Trade name	Doseform
Formulation R	**Cream**: 0.25% phenylephrine HCl, 18% petrolatum, 12% glycerin
Preparation H	**Cream**: 0.25% phenylephrine HCl, 18% petrolatum, 12% glycerin, 3% shark liver oil, cetyl and stearyl alcohols, EDTA, glyceryl oleate and stearate, lanolin, parabens
Hemorid	**Cream**: 1% pramoxine HCl, 0.25% phenylephrine HCl, 30% white petrolatum, 20% mineral oil, aloe vera gel, parabens, cetyl and stearyl alcohols
Preparation H Cooling Gel	**Gel**: 0.25% phenylephrine HCl, 50% witch hazel, aloe gel, EDTA, parabens
Hemorid	**Ointment**: 0.25% phenylephrine HCl, 1% pramoxine HCl, 82.15% white petrolatum, 12.5% mineral oil, aloe vera
Formulation R	**Ointment**: 0.25% phenylephrine HCl, 71.9% petrolatum, 14% mineral oil, lanolin, parabens
Preparation H	**Ointment**: 0.25% phenylephrine HCl, 71.9% petrolatum, 14% mineral oil, 3% shark liver oil, glycerin, lanolin, lanolin alcohol, parabens, tocopherol
Preparation H	**Suppositories**: 0.25% phenylephrine HCl, 3% shark liver oil, 85.5% cocoa butter, parabens
Anusol	**Suppositories**: 51% topical starch, benzyl alcohol

Products listed are representative of currently available and widely distributed brands. Similar products, including regional and private label brands, may also exist.

PATIENT INFORMATION
Miscellaneous Topical Anorectal Combination Products

- Patient instructions accompany each product. Read these instructions carefully before use, preferably before leaving the pharmacy, in case you have any questions.
- For external use only.
- If you are using anorectal preparations containing ephedrine or phenylephrine, notify your physician if insomnia, dizziness, weakness, tremor, or irregular heart beat occurs.
- Consult your physician if anorectal symptoms do not improve within 7 days, or if profuse bleeding, protrusion, seepage, or moderate to severe pain occurs or continues.
- Maintain normal bowel movements by proper diet, adequate fluid intake, and regular exercise.
- Avoid scratching or rubbing area, washing with strong or scented soaps, or eating spicy foods, peppers, or tomatoes.
- Tell your physician if you are pregnant, become pregnant, plan to become pregnant, or are breastfeeding.

LACTOSE INTOLERANCE

DEFINITION

Lactose intolerance is the inability to appropriately digest lactose (a disaccharide) to the monosaccharides glucose and galactose because of a lactase enzyme deficiency. Lactase is produced in the cells that line the small intestine; a lack of the enzyme can result in gas, bloating, abdominal cramping, and diarrhea.

ETIOLOGY

Lactose or "milk" intolerance is thought to be an inherited trait that typically manifests during puberty or late adolescence. Lactose intolerance also is racially linked. This condition can occur secondary to diseases of the GI tract, such as viral and bacterial enteritis and Crohn's disease.

INCIDENCE

Lactose intolerance occurs to varying degrees of severity in approximately 10% to 20% of whites in the US, and in 80% to 90% of patients with African and Asian heritage, as well as American Indians. Approximately 60% of patients with Jewish or Mediterranean ancestry also experience lactose intolerance.

PATHOPHYSIOLOGY

The normal pathophysiology of lactose breakdown occurs in the following manner: Lactose reaches the digestive system and is broken down by lactase into glucose and galactose. The galactose is broken down further by the liver to form glucose. From there it enters the bloodstream and increases blood glucose levels. The deficiency of lactase in the GI mucosa causes ingested lactose (a disaccharide) to remain undigestible and unconverted to 2 monosaccharides (glucose and galactose) in the GI tract. Lactose subsequently causes osmotic diarrhea and gas caused by its fermentation by GI bacteria. This can occur 30 minutes to 2 hours after ingestion of dairy products.

SIGNS/SYMPTOMS

Symptoms include bloating, abdominal cramps, flatus, nausea, borborygmi (ie, GI "rumbling" sounds), and diarrhea soon after consumption of products containing lactose. Lactose intolerance may cause weight loss in children.

DIAGNOSTIC PARAMETERS/PHYSICAL ASSESSMENT

Clinical Observation: Patients with lactose intolerance will report GI disturbances after consuming products high in lactose (eg, milk, ice cream, other dairy products) and will report the absence of symptoms after consuming little or no dairy products. In complicated cases where concomitant GI conditions are present, a specific and noninvasive hydrogen breath test is available to physicians. The breath hydrogen test is thought to be the most accurate and the least time-consuming diagnostic procedure. Its accuracy can be affected by food, medication, and cigarette smoking. This test measures the amount of hydrogen in the breath. It is performed by drinking a lactose-containing liquid, and then analyzing the breath at regular intervals. If the patient is intolerant, the hydrogen levels are increased. A more invasive and less recommended test includes the lactose intolerance test, which consists of the patient fasting before the test and then drinking a lactose-containing liquid. Blood samples are taken over a 2-hour period to measure glucose. Glucose levels do not rise if the patient is intolerant. Other tests are the fecal analysis test, which measures the amount of acid in the stool, and small bowel biopsy, neither of which are recommended unless under extreme and difficult circumstances.

Interview: A quick and simple interview and history of the patient will often reveal the diagnosis. It may be beneficial to ask about the following:

- Description of symptoms.
- What was eaten or what beverage(s) was consumed in the several hour period before the patient experienced symptoms.
- Family members with lactose intolerance (or GI symptoms similar to the patient's).
- Racial/ethnic background of patient. (Patients of ethnic backgrounds in which lactase deficiency is common increase the likelihood of this diagnosis.)
- Existing GI conditions or other diseases. (This may help determine whether the patient has secondary lactase deficiency or, possibly, diarrhea not related to lactose intolerance.)

TREATMENT

Approaches to therapy: Avoiding lactose-containing products is the simplest treatment. However, for individuals who want to consume such products, lactase replacement therapy is readily available *otc* and is considered safe and effective.

Nondrug therapy: A lactose-free or minimized diet is the simplest treatment to prevent symptoms. Often, patients will not notice symptoms when consuming less than 8 oz/day of milk or the lactose equivalent from other dairy products. If patients choose this form of therapy, strongly encourage calcium supplementation. The benefits of yogurt and milk fortified with lactase-producing bacteria (eg, *Lactobacillus acidophilus* and *Bifidobacteria* sp.) currently are being studied. There appears to be an improvement in GI symptoms in lactose-intolerant patients who are taking these products.

Pharmacotherapy: Prescription and OTC medications may contain lactose as a filler. Pharmacists may need to compound medication using different fillers such as calcium carbonate, citric acid, sodium bicarbonate, microcrystalline cellulose, sodium chloride, ginger root powder, or methylcellulose.

Nonprescription products containing lactase enzyme are available. Technically, these products are nutritional supplements and not drugs by definition. However, for the purposes of this monograph, they will be included in this section.

LACTASE ENZYME PRODUCTS

▶ Actions

Enzymatically breaks down the disaccharide lactose into 2 monosaccharides, glucose and galactose, which are readily absorbed and do not produce a hyperosmotic state in the intestinal tract.

▶ Indications

Lactose intolerance.

▶ Warnings

If the patient experiences any unusual symptoms unrelated to his or her condition and for which there is no explanation other than a possible link to the lactase-containing product, the patient should discontinue the product and contact a physician. These lactase-containing products are safe in pregnant, breastfeeding, and pediatric patients.

▶ Adverse Reactions

None reported.

▶ Administration and Dosage

Lactase is available in 3 dosage forms and their respective doses are as follows:

Liquid: 5 to 15 drops/quart of milk, based on the lactose conversion level desired.

Tablets: 1 to 3 tablets with the first bite of dairy food or beverage. (*Lactaid* may be chewed or swallowed.) Do not take more than 6 tablets at a time.

Capsules: 1 to 2 capsules taken with milk or dairy products. If the patient is severely intolerant to lactose, increase the dosage until a satisfactory dose is achieved.

LACTASE ENZYME PRODUCTS	
Trade name	**Doseform**
Lactrase	**Capsules:** 250 mg standardized lactase enzyme
Lactaid Original[1]	**Caplets:** 3000 FCC lactase units
	Drops: 1250 U/drop. Lactase enzyme
Lactaid Extra Strength	**Caplets:** 4500 FCC lactase units
Lactaid Ultra	**Caplets:** 9000 FCC lactase units
Dairy Ease	**Tablets, chewable:** 3000 FCC lactase units
Lactaid Ultra Chewables	**Tablets, chewable:** 9000 FCC lactase units

Products listed are representative of currently available and widely distributed brands. Similar products, including regional and private label brands, may also exist.

[1] *Lactaid* also manufactures a brand of milk that has had the lactose "predigested" at the dairy. The reduction in lactose is 70% or 100% in various forms of milk, ranging from fat-free to low-fat. *Lactaid* milk also is available in a calcium-fortified formulation.

PATIENT INFORMATION
Lactase Enzyme Products
- Place dose of liquid directly into milk, shake gently, and refrigerate for 24 hours.
- Take capsule or tablet with first bite of lactose-containing product.
- Begin with the lowest recommended dose and increase to a dosage that provides relief.
- If dairy intake is minimal, calcium supplementation is most likely warranted.
- If your condition worsens or if you experience any problems, consult your physician.

NAUSEA AND VOMITING

DEFINITION

Nausea is a feeling of discomfort associated with an inclination to vomit. Vomiting is the expulsion of stomach contents through the mouth.

ETIOLOGY

Nausea and vomiting may be associated with GI, cardiovascular, infectious, metabolic, neurologic, or psychological disease processes, and may accompany such conditions as pregnancy, medication administration or withdrawal, motion sickness, or surgical procedures. Factors that may influence the occurrence of nausea include age of the patient, prior experience, clinical setting, psychological conditioning, and response to sight, smell, and taste stimuli.

PATHOPHYSIOLOGY

The neurologic pathways controlling nausea are poorly understood, although an interrelationship between the GI tract and CNS is involved. Impulses from various etiologies stimulate the vomiting center in the brain. The vomiting center triggers a series of responses from the closely located salivary, respiratory, and vasomotor centers, resulting in symptoms of nausea, salivation, perspiration, pallor, and changes in heart and respiratory rates. Stimulation of vagus and phrenic nerves causes lowering of the diaphragm, strong abdominal muscle contractions, opening of the gastric cardia, reduction of esophageal sphincter pressure, and reversal of peristalsis of the stomach and small bowel. These actions result in the symptoms of retching. Retching causes the expulsion of stomach contents through the esophagus and mouth, which is vomiting.

SIGNS/SYMPTOMS

The primary symptom is queasiness that may be accompanied by salivation, increased respiration and heart rate, sweating, and paleness. However, numerous signs and symptoms may be present in association with the underlying cause, some of which include fever, abdominal pain, diarrhea, and headache. Severe vomiting may lead to dehydration and metabolic disturbances, including metabolic alkalosis, hyponatremia, hypokalemia, or hypochloremia. These complications are especially a risk in small children. Thirst and minimal urine volume signal dehydration.

DIAGNOSTIC PARAMETERS/PHYSICAL ASSESSMENT

Clinical Observation: Because of the nature of the condition, the clinical observation will usually occur only by the patient and is a subjective experience. Acute onset of nausea and vomiting is usually due to viral gastroenteritis ("flu") or ingestion of toxins or disagreeable substances, including drugs.

Chronic nausea and vomiting may indicate a serious underlying GI, neurologic, metabolic, or psychological disorder, and these patients should be referred to a physician.

Interview: To determine if physician referral or self-treatment is warranted, ask about the following:

- Frequency, duration, and severity of nausea and vomiting.
- Timing of nausea with respect to meals or activity.
- Concomitant medications or changes in medication.
- Recent radiation therapy or medical procedure.
- Behavioral changes.
- Changes in food ingestion.
- Presence of other signs and symptoms (eg, fever, diarrhea, headache, abdominal pain, discomfort).
- Similar illness in family members.
- Possibility of pregnancy (especially before starting drug administration).

TREATMENT

Approaches to therapy: Evaluate patients using the above diagnostic parameters. The main effort would be to identify and treat the underlying cause. Depending on various factors (eg, symptoms, duration, recurrence), health care providers may recommend either (1) a non-drug approach, (2) approved pharmacotherapy, or (3) immediate referral to a physician for medical evaluation.

Nondrug therapy: Dietary modification may be appropriate when nausea is associated with certain foods or beverages. Nausea related to motion may resolve if one can assume a stable position (eg, looking forward in a moving vehicle). Change of environment may help avoid disturbing odors or other stimuli. Eating small meals is helpful. Frequent snacks of crackers may decrease nausea of pregnancy. Give water and clear liquids to rehydrate the patient who has been vomiting. Electrolyte supplementation may be necessary with prolonged vomiting.

Pharmacotherapy: Treatment is usually directed at the underlying cause. OTC antiemetics/anticholinergics/antihistamines may be useful in the patient with nausea due to motion sickness or dizziness. Taking these drugs 1 to 2 hours before, and during motion exposure (eg, car, air, and sea travel) may prevent nausea from occurring. Antacids may offer relief in nausea associated with indigestion; the reader may refer to the Treatment section in the Heartburn and GERD monograph for more information on these agents. Phosphorated carbohydrate solutions are available to relieve nausea due to intestinal flu or upset stomach, but the FDA has concluded that their efficacy is not established.

BISMUTH SUBSALICYLATE

▶ **Actions**

Bismuth subsalicylate appears to have antisecretory (salicylate moiety) adsorbent and antimicrobial (bismuth moiety) effects in vitro, as well as some anti-inflammatory effects.

▶ Indications

Control of diarrhea (including traveler's diarrhea, within 24 hours of onset), indigestion, nausea, and abdominal cramps.

▶ Warnings

Impaction: Consult a physician before this product is used in an infant or debilitated patient. If constipation occurs, discontinue use and consult physician.

Radiological examinations: Bismuth is radiopaque; therefore, bismuth subsalicylate may interfere with radiologic examinations of the GI tract. Do not use this product if a radiological examination is scheduled.

Salicylate: Systemic absorption may occur; therefore, if the patient has salicylate sensitivity or a bleeding disorder, do not use this product without consulting a physician.

Pregnancy: Do not use during pregnancy without consulting a physician.

▶ Drug Interactions

Aspirin: Because bismuth subsalicylate contains salicylate, overdosage of salicylates may occur if aspirin is administered concurrently. If taken with aspirin and ringing of the ears occurs, discontinue use.

Corticosteroids: May reduce salicylate levels, decreasing the efficacy of bismuth subsalicylate.

Methotrexate: Bismuth subsalicylate may reduce renal elimination of methotrexate, increasing toxicity.

Tetracyclines: Bismuth subsalicylate may reduce the absorption of tetracycline, decreasing their efficacy.

▶ Administration and Dosage

Adults: 2 tablets or 30 mL.

Children:

> *(9 to 12 years of age)* – 1 tablet or 15 mL.

> *(6 to 9 years of age)* – ⅔ tablet or 10 mL.

> *(3 to 6 years of age)* – ⅓ tablet or 5 mL.

> *(younger than 3 years of age)* – Consult physician.

Repeat dosage every 30 minutes to 1 hour, as needed, up to 8 doses in 24 hours.

BISMUTH SUBSALICYLATE PRODUCTS	
Trade name	**Doseform**
Pepto-Bismol	**Tablets:** 262 mg
Bismatrol, Pepto-Bismol, Pink Bismuth	**Tablets, chewable:** 262 mg
Pink Bismuth	**Liquid:** 130 mg/15 mL
Pepto-Bismol, Pink Bismuth	**Liquid:** 262 mg/15 mL
Bismatrol Extra Strength, Pink Bismuth Maximum Strength	**Liquid:** 524 mg/15 mL
Pepto-Bismol Maximum Strength	**Liquid:** 525 mg/15 mL

Products listed are representative of currently available and widely distributed brands. Similar products, including regional and private label brands, may also exist.

PATIENT INFORMATION

Bismuth Subsalicylate
• Shake liquid well before using.
• Chew tablets or allow them to dissolve in the mouth.
• Stool may temporarily appear gray-black.

ANTIEMETIC/ANTIHISTAMINIC/ANTICHOLINERGIC AGENTS

▶ Actions

Cyclizine, meclizine, and dimenhydrinate have antiemetic, anticholinergic, and antihistaminic properties. These agents reduce the sensitivity of the labyrinthine apparatus. The action may be mediated through nerve pathways to the vomiting center and other CNS centers.

▶ Indications

Cyclizine, meclizine, and dimenhydrinate prevent and treat nausea, vomiting, and dizziness of motion sickness. Do not use in pregnancy unless recommended by your doctor.

▶ Contraindications

Dimenhydrinate is contraindicated in neonates.

▶ Warnings

Cyclizine, dimenhydrinate, and meclizine may cause drowsiness or dizziness; use caution while driving or performing tasks requiring alertness, coordination, or physical dexterity.

Other conditions (cyclizine, dimenhydrinate, and meclizine): If the patient has glaucoma, obstructive disease of the GI or GU tract or possible prostatic hypertrophy, consult a physician because appropriate monitoring is needed.

Pregnancy: Use cyclizine, dimenhydrinate, or meclizine only if directed by physician. Meclizine appears to present the lowest risk of teratogenicity and is the drug many physicians generally recommend in treating nausea and vomiting during pregnancy.

Lactation:

> *Cyclizine or meclizine* – Safety not established. Use only if directed by physician.

> *Dimenhydrinate* – Small amounts of dimenhydrinate are excreted in breast milk. Decide whether to temporarily discontinue nursing or the drug, taking into account the importance of the drug to the mother.

Children:

> *Cyclizine or meclizine* – Do not use in children younger than 12 years of age.

> *Dimenhydrinate* – Do not use in children younger than 2 years of age unless directed by physician.

▶ Adverse Reactions

Cyclizine, dimenhydrinate, and meclizine:

> *CNS* – Drowsiness; restlessness; excitation; nervousness; insomnia; euphoria; blurred vision; diplopia; vertigo; tinnitus; auditory and visual hallucinations.

> *Dermatologic* – Urticaria; rash.

GI – Dry mouth; anorexia; nausea; vomiting; diarrhea; constipation; cholestatic jaundice (cyclizine).

GU – Urinary frequency; difficult urination; urinary retention.

Cardiovascular – Decreased blood pressure; palpitations; increased heart rate.

Other – Dry nose and throat; photosensitivity; hemolytic anemia (dimenhydrinate); thickening of bronchial secretions (dimenhydrinate).

CYCLIZINE

▶ Administration and Dosage

Start treatment 1 to 2 hours before exposure to stimulus (eg, car, air, or boat travel) to prevent nausea and vomiting.

Adults: 50 mg every 4 to 6 hours as needed. Do not exceed 200 mg/day.

Children (6 to 12 years of age): 25 mg every 6 to 8 hours as needed. Do not exceed 75 mg/day.

CYCLIZINE PRODUCTS	
Trade name	Doseform
Marezine	**Tablets**: 50 mg

Products listed are representative of currently available and widely distributed brands. Similar products, including regional and private label brands, may also exist.

PATIENT INFORMATION

Cyclizine

- Cyclizine may cause drowsiness or dizziness; use caution while driving or performing tasks requiring alertness, coordination, or physical dexterity.
- Cyclizine may have additive effects with alcohol and CNS depressants (eg, sedatives, tranquilizers). Use with caution or avoid alcohol and CNS depressants.

DIMENHYDRINATE

▶ Administration and Dosage

Start treatment 1 to 2 hours before exposure to stimulus (eg, car, air, or boat travel) to prevent nausea and vomiting.

Adults: 50 to 100 mg every 6 hours as needed. Do not exceed 400 mg in 24 hours.

Children (6 to 12 years of age): 25 to 50 mg every 6 to 8 hours as needed. Do not exceed 150 mg in 24 hours.

Children (2 to 6 years of age): Up to 25 mg every 6 to 8 hours as needed. Do not exceed 75 mg in 24 hours.

DIMENHYDRINATE PRODUCTS	
Trade name	Doseform
Calm X, Dramamine, Motion Sickness Relief	**Tablets**: 50 mg
Dramamine	**Tablets, chewable**: 50 mg
Dramamine	**Liquid**: 15.62 mg/5 mL

Products listed are representative of currently available and widely distributed brands. Similar products, including regional and private label brands, may also exist.

PATIENT INFORMATION

Dimenhydrinate

- *Chewable tablets:* Thoroughly chew before swallowing and follow with a glass of water.
- Dimenhydrinate may cause drowsiness or dizziness; use caution while driving or performing tasks requiring alertness, coordination, or physical dexterity.
- Dimenhydrinate may have additive effects with alcohol and CNS depressants (eg, sedatives, tranquilizers). Use with caution or avoid alcohol and CNS depressants.

MECLIZINE

▶ Administration and Dosage

Start treatment 1 to 2 hours before exposure to stimulus (eg, car, air, or boat travel) to prevent nausea and vomiting.

Adults and children (12 years of age and older): 25 to 50 mg/day as needed. Do not exceed 50 mg/day.

MECLIZINE PRODUCTS	
Trade name	Doseform
Meclizine HCl	**Tablets:** 25 mg
Bonine	**Tablets, chewable:** 25 mg

Products listed are representative of currently available and widely distributed brands. Similar products, including regional and private label brands, may also exist.

PATIENT INFORMATION

Meclizine

- *Chewable tablets:* Thoroughly chew before swallowing and follow with a glass of water.
- Meclizine may cause drowsiness or dizziness; use caution while driving or performing tasks requiring alertness, coordination, or physical dexterity.
- Meclizine may have additive effects with alcohol and CNS depressants (eg, sedatives, tranquilizers). Use with caution or avoid alcohol and CNS depressants.

PHOSPHORATED CARBOHYDRATE SOLUTION

▶ Actions

Phosphorated carbohydrate solution is thought to act on the wall of the GI tract to reduce smooth muscle contraction and delay emptying time.

▶ Indications

For relief of nausea and vomiting.

▶ Warnings

Diabetes: Avoid this product because it contains carbohydrates.

Hereditary fructose intolerance: Do not use this product.

▶ Adverse Reactions

Abdominal pain; diarrhea.

▶ **Administration and Dosage**

Epidemic and other functional vomiting, or nausea and vomiting caused by psychogenic factors:

>   *Adults* – 13 or 30 mL at 15-minute intervals until vomiting ceases. Do not take for longer than 1 hour (5 doses). If first dose is rejected, resume same dosage schedule in 5 minutes.

>   *Infants and children* – 5 or 10 mL at 15-minute intervals until vomiting ceases. Do not take for longer than 1 hour (5 doses).

Morning sickness: 15 to 30 mL on arising; repeat every 3 hours or when nausea threatens.

Motion sickness: 5 mL doses for young children; 15 mL doses for older children and adults.

PHOSPHORATED CARBOHYDRATE SOLUTION PRODUCTS	
Trade name	Doseform
Emetrol, Nausea Relief	**Solution**: 1.87 g dextrose, 1.87 g fructose, 21.5 mg phosphoric acid
Nausetrol	**Solution**: Dextrose, fructose, orthophosphoric acid with controlled hydrogen ion concentration

Products listed are representative of currently available and widely distributed brands. Similar products, including regional and private label brands, may also exist.

PATIENT INFORMATION

Phosphorated Carbohydrate Solution

• Patient instructions accompany each product. Read these instructions before use, preferably before leaving the pharmacy, in case of questions.

• Notify physician if symptoms are not relieved or recur often.

OSTOMY CARE

DEFINITION

Ostomy can be literally defined as "an opening into." It is a surgical opening from the intestines or ureters to the surface of the abdomen for the purpose of discharging feces and urine. The stoma is the actual end of the ureter or the small or large intestines that can be seen protruding from the abdominal wall. There may or may not be an exteriorization of the opening. The opening may be temporary or permanent. The ostomy is further classified according to its location, such as colostomy, ileostomy, or urostomy.

Characteristics of the Ideal Stoma Construction
- Red.
- Round.
- Lumen at apex.
- Adequate protrusion (at least 1 cm).
- Mucocutaneous junction intact/approximated.

A **colostomy** is an opening created anywhere along the large intestine or colon. Stool is diverted out through an abdominal stoma.

A permanent colostomy is classified according to the location along the colon. An ascending colostomy is a relatively rare procedure and is located on the right side of the abdomen. Stools diverted out this stoma are watery with a continuous flow and includes the presence of active digestive enzymes. Along the transverse colon is the transverse colostomy which may have 1 or 2 openings producing liquid and semi-formed stool possibly containing digestive enzymes. It is located in the upper abdomen and can be right- or left-sided. The

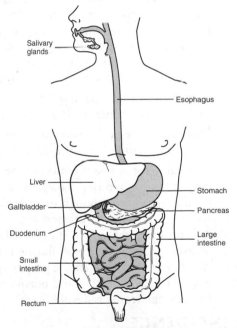

Figure 1. Digestive Tract

sigmoid or descending colostomy is the more common procedure and is usually located on the lower left side of the abdomen. The end of the sigmoid or the descending colon is brought out to form a stoma that produces formed stools without the presence of digestive enzymes.

A temporary colostomy is performed to divert the flow of feces from the distal part of the colon to allow it to rest or heal. This technique allows the closure of the stoma once the condition requiring the surgery has been resolved. Temporary colostomies include the loop and double-barrel colostomy. A loop colostomy involves a loop of the transverse colon or ileum supported by a subcutanous rod. The loop is partially severed and the mucosa is sutured to the skin to create 2 stomas: One that discharges stool and another that discharges mucus. The double-barrel colostomy involves the creation of 2 stomas by bringing out both the proximal and distal end. The proximal end is the functioning stoma that discharges feces. The non-functioning stoma created by the distal end secretes mucus.

Colostomies are performed in patients with cancer, inflammatory disease, congenital malformations, abscesses, fistulas, obstructions, and perforations.

An **ileostomy** is an opening created in the ileum or distal end of the small intestine. The stool consistency is typically loose to liquid, which requires a pouch to be worn at all times. The stoma is located in the right lower abdominal quadrant.

Ileostomies are performed in patients with ulcerative colitis, Crohn disease, familial polyposis, cancer, necrotizing enterocolitis, and vascular infarct involving the large intestine. A permanent ileostomy is constructed when the entire colon, rectum, and anus are removed (total proctocolectomy). When the disease is confined to the colon, a temporary ileostomy (loop ileostomy) with an ilealanal reservoir can be constructed.

A **urostomy** is an opening created in the urinary tract to divert urine proximal from a dysfunctional or diseased portion of the urinary tract.

Urostomies are performed when the bladder is bypassed or removed because of cancer, trauma, or severe dysfunction.

Normally, the stoma is moist and beefy red. However, the color of a GI stoma may vary from red to pink and that of a urinary diversion may be pink. The ideal protrusion is enough to allow stool or urine drainage into the pouch without spillage onto the peristomal skin. The stoma is measured in inches or millimeters and tends to shrink within 6 to 8 weeks after surgery. Weekly measurement are necessary during this period or when the patient experiences weight gain or loss to ensure proper appliance fit. Because the stomal mucosa is very fragile, bleeding and oozing may normally occur upon cleaning. Because the stoma is devoid of pain nerve fibers, it is not painful.

INCIDENCE

It is estimated that approximately 100,000 ostomy surgeries are performed annually in the US.

DIAGNOSTIC PARAMETERS/PHYSICAL ASSESSMENT

Most problems associated with an ostomy can be resolved through clinical observation and interview.

Clinical Observation: Clinical observation is appropriate only when the facility has a treatment room and an Enterostomal Therapy Nurse (ET Nurse) on staff to conduct the physical exam.

Interview: To help the pharmacist determine if self-treatment or an ET nurse or physician referral is warranted, it is beneficial to ask about the following:

- Type and duration of ostomy.
- Type, location, size, and appearance of stoma.
- Type of appliance used for stoma.
- Skin appearance or problems of area surrounding stoma.
- Odor or gas control.
- Changes in output appearance.
- Concurrent prescription and OTC medications, supplements, and herbal products.

Common concerns of people with ostomies are odor, gas, dietary considerations, and sexual activity. Other ostomy-related problems are mechanical breakdown, chemical breakdown, rashes, and allergic reaction. The following table covers possible causes and interventions for ostomy-related problems.

Ostomy-Related Concerns/Problems			
Concerns/Problems	Possible Causes	Appearance	Treatment
Odor	Leaking or inadequately closed pouch. Odor-causing foods (eg, asparagus, broccoli, eggs, fish, garlic).	N/A	Refer to ET nurse to reevaluate pouching system. Ingest foods that prevent odor (eg, buttermilk, cranberry juice, parsley, yogurt).
Gas	Swallowed air, skipping meals, drinking beer/soda, certain foods (eg, cabbage, broccoli, mushrooms, brussel sprouts, peas).	N/A	Simethicone preparations. Foods such as crackers, toast, and yogurt can help prevent gas.
Dietary problems	Gas/odor-causing foods. *Ileostomy*–Food blockage, usually from foods that are not easily digested.	Food blockage–Watery output with abdominal cramping, distension, nausea, or vomiting.	Chew foods thoroughly, avoid foods that are not easily digested (eg, popcorn, skins, peanuts) or caused upset in the past, add new foods one at a time. Drink at least 2 quarts of liquids per day. Food blockage intervention.[1]
Sexual activity	*Physical*–disruption in nerves/vascular supply to sexual organs. *Psychological*–change in body image/self esteem. *Social*–fear of rejection.	N/A	ET nurse consultation or physician referral for assistive devices or medications. Provide reassurance and encouragement.
Mechanical breakdown	Frequent removal of wafer/pouch resulting in stripping of epidermis or inappropriate removal of tape.	Erythematous, raw, moist, and painful.	Refer to ET nurse to reevaluate pouching system and patient's technique. Pouch designed for 4 to 7 days of use. Stoma powder to raw area followed by skin sealant.
Chemical breakdown	Frequent leakage. Irritation due to exposure of skin to stool or urine.	Erythema or raw, moist skin. Tingly to painful irritation.	ET nurse to reevaluate pouching system. Stoma powder to raw area followed by skin sealant.
Fungal rash (*Candida*)	Excessive moisture or adverse reaction to antibiotic therapy.	Papular rash with satellite lesions and itching.	Antifungal powder followed by a skin sealant.
Allergic reaction	Can be caused by any ostomy product.	Erythematous vesicular rash.	Refer to ET nurse to reevaluate pouching system. Corticosteroid cream or spray (not ointment).

[1] *Food blockage intervention:* Drink warm liquids, assume a knee-chest position, and massage peristomal area. Sometimes a warm bath can help to relax and pass the blockage. If symptoms persist, patients should notify their physician.

Effects of Food on Ostomy Function	
Food	Effect
Fish, eggs, asparagus, garlic, beans, turnips, cabbage family vegetables (onions, broccoli, cauliflower, cabbage)	Stool odor
Beans, beer, carbonated beverages, cucumbers, cabbage family vegetables	Gas
Seafood, asparagus	Urine odor
Bananas, rice, bread, cheese, tapioca, pasta, pretzels, applesauce	Thicken stool
Beans, fruits, raw vegetables, spiced foods, greasy foods, prune or grape juice, chocolate	Loosen stools

TREATMENT

Pharmacotherapy: The extensive variety of ostomy products can create confusion in product selection. This decision-making process is simplified by understanding the purpose of each product while considering the principles of ostomy management. Some of these principles include maintenance of peristomal integrity, collection and containment of damage, odor control, ease of application, and cost-effectiveness. The term appliance refers to the combination of the skin barrier and pouch that attaches to the abdomen by the adhesive faceplate and fits over and around the stoma to collect the diverted output. When choosing an appliance or accessory, consider stoma size, type of ostomy, stoma construction, abdomen characteristics, factors affecting the patient's ability to administer self-care (eg, visual acuity, manual dexterity, mental status, general physical condition), patient preference, and cost and availability of product.

Accesories:

Skin sealants – Skin sealants are liquids and are available in the form of wipes, sprays, gels, ointments, and roll-ons. Skin sealants are designed to lay down a synthetic coat on the skin to prevent actual contact of the skin with adhesives. These products also prevent stripping of the top layer of epidermis when the appliance is removed.

Deodorants – These accessories may be taken internally, used to clean appliances, or sprayed into the air. Some of these products may or may not be used on skin or objects that come into contact with the skin. Although aspirin was used at one time as an inexpensive deodorant in pouches, advise patients not to do so because of the risk of stoma ulcerations. Patients have also used charcoal filters and *Tic-Tacs* inside the pouch as deodorizers.

SKIN BARRIERS

▶ Actions

Skin barriers are designed to provide a smooth surface for attaching the pouch and may be used to fill in the gaps between appliance and skin to prevent spillage of urine or stool or to protect the skin peristomally by forming a transparent, waterproof film. Barriers also provide an environment that promotes healing of skin and prevention of future irritation. (Skin barriers come in the form of rigid or flexible faceplates, sheets, creams, sprays, wafers, rings, pastes, and powders, and also may be incorporated into pouches.) They may be sterile or non-sterile and have precut, custom-cut, or cut-to-fit openings.

SKIN BARRIER PRODUCTS	
Trade name	**Description**
Face Plates and Barriers with Flanges, Convexity, etc.	
Assura Convex Skin Barrier Flange with Belt Loops Pre-Cut	Deep convexity attached to long lasting skin barrier; latex-free. Stoma sizes: 13 mm, 19 mm, 22 mm, 25 mm, 29 mm, 32 mm, 38 mm, 44 mm, 47 mm.
Assura Custom Cut Skin Barrier Flange with Belt Loops	Flexible skin barrier for secure, long lasting wear; latex-free. Stoma sizes: 1/2-inch to 1 1/2-inch, 1/2-inch to 2 1/4-inch.
Coloplast Convex Skin Barrier	Stoma sizes from 3/4-inch to 1 1/2-inch with built in convexity.
Coloplast Two-Piece Post-Op Skin Barrier Flange	Custom cut with *Micropore* tape. Stoma sizes: up to 2 3/4-inch, up to 4-inch.
SUR-FIT AutoLock Durahesive Flexible	White collar. Flange sizes: 1 3/8-inch, 1 3/4-inch, 2 1/4-inch, 2 3/4-inch; box of 5.
Soft Guard XL	Wafer with flange: 4-inch by 4-inch.
Torbot Plastic Faceplate	Reusable, convex barrier
Films, pastes, powders, creams	
Bard Protective Barrier	**Film**: Apply before appliance or water; available as 5.5 oz spray and individual wipes.
Barrier	**Cream**: Available in 4 fluid ounze and 8 fluid ounce tubes, packaged 2 dozen per case.
HolliHesive	**Paste**: 2.2 oz, 4.5 oz tubes.
Dansac Soft	**Paste**: Synthetic paste to be used with any synthetic skin barrier or as skin protection.
Nu-Hope Karaya	**Powder**: 3.5 oz, 16 oz bottles.
Rings, wafers, sheets, seals	
ReliaSeal Skin Barrier Adhesive Disc	**Starter openings**: 1/2-inch, 3/4-inch, 1-inch, 1 1/4-inch, 1 1/2-inch
Eakin Cohesive	**Seals**: 2-inch small (box of 20), 4-inch large (box of 10).
HolliSeal Skin Barrier	**Sheets**: 4-inch by 4-inch.
Nu-Hope Skin Barriers	**Sheets**: 4-inch by 4-inch, 5-inch by 5-inch, 6-inch by 6-inch; Rings: 2-inch, 3 1/2-inch, 4-inch (w/precut openings from 1/2-inch to 1 3/4-inch).
Healskin Karaya	**Washers**: Cut-to-fit or precut all-flexible.

Products listed are representative of currently available and widely distributed brands. Similar products, including regional and private label brands, may also exist.

ADHESIVES AND REMOVERS

▶ **Actions**

Adhesives: Adhesives are silicon- or latex-based and are occasionally needed in addition to the pouch adhesive for securing external devices to the skin. It is important to allow the adhesive to completely dry before application to prevent irritation of the skin. If leakage is a frequent problem, it is best to evaluate the appropriateness of the pouching system before deciding to add extra adhesives.

Removers: These solvents are used to remove build-up of adhesives on the skin. Most solvents are oil-based, so it is important to thoroughly wash the skin after each use.

ADHESIVE AND REMOVER PRODUCTS

Trade name	Description
Torbot Cement	Contains zinc oxide to relieve irritation.
Foam Pad Cement	For use only with foam pads and plastic faceplates.
Torbot Regular Solvent Adhesive Remover	Clear, hydrocarbon liquid.
Bard Adhesive and Barrier Film Remover	Individual wipes.
Medical Adhesive	3.2 oz. spray.
Universal Remover for Adhesives and Barriers	6 oz. pump spray.
Nu-Hope Adhesive	1 oz., 3 oz. cement.

Products listed are representative of currently available and widely distributed brands. Similar products, including regional and private label brands, may also exist.

CAPS AND PLUGS

▶ Actions

Stoma caps and plugs are only appropriate for patients with a descending/sigmoid colostomy that is well controlled by irrigation. These accessories are opaque, supplied in different lengths and sizes, and may be 1- or 2-pieces. They may also have other features including contour, adhesives, deodorizing filters, and barrier films. The stoma cap covers the stoma and has an absorptive layer for absorbing mucus but no capacity for collecting stools. The stoma plug is inserted into the stoma and snapped to a 2-piece wafer or fastened to the skin surrounding the stoma to prevent fecal leakage. This accessory may be used for a short duration to provide temporary continence in descending/sigmoid colostomy patients who do not irrigate. A training and adaptation period must be provided by an ET nurse or ostomy specialist for patients using the plug. Patients may experience spontaneous dislodgement of the plug due to massive peristalsis or intolerable cramping.

CAP AND PLUG PRODUCTS

Trade name	Description
Assura One-Piece	**Stoma cap**: Opaque, with filter for odor control; mini security pouch with flexible skin barrier; latex-free. Stoma size: 19 to 64 mm.
Coloplast One-Piece Conseal	**Plug**: Lengths: 1 1/2-inch, 2-inch. Stoma sizes: 3/4-inch to 1 1/4-inch, 3/4-inch to 2-inch.
Coloplast Two-Piece with Filter	**Stoma cap**: Opaque. Stoma sizes up to 1 1/4-inch, up 1 3/4-inch, up to 2-inch.
CenterPointLock Two-Piece Ostomy System	**Stoma cap**: With opaque odor-barrier film, deodorizing filter, flange. Pouch sizes from 1 1/2-inch to 2 3/4-inch.
Guardian Two-Piece Ostomy System	**Stoma cap**: With opaque odor-barrier film, deodorizing filter, flange. Stoma cap openings from 1-inch to 2 1/2-inch.
Stoma Cap	**Cap**: With microporous or standard adhesive, transparent odor-barrier film, deodorizing filter. Stoma cap openings: 2-inch, 3-inch.
Dansac Contour I Mini	**Cap**: Opaque; with thin barrier, absorption pad. Stoma sizes from 3/4-inch to 2-inch.

Products listed are representative of currently available and widely distributed brands. Similar products, including regional and private label brands, may also exist.

BELTS AND BINDERS

► **Actions**

These are available in adjustable sizes from pediatric to extra-large. An elastic ostomy belt provides support on each side of the pouch to hold it against the skin. However, it should be loose enough to leave room for 2 finger-lengths between the skin and the belt. Those patients with stomas along the belt line are better managed with binders, because the belt may ride up and dislodge the pouch or cause the system opening to cut into the stoma. Binders provide support along the circumference of the peristomal region and are beneficial in patients with peristomal hernias and stomal prolapse.

BELT AND BINDER PRODUCTS	
Trade name	Description
Assura Stomy	**Belt**: Elastic, 90% cotton/10% rayon with flexible polypropylene clasps; for use with all *Assura* 1- and 2-piece systems; no need for belt retainer ring; also for use with irrigation systems; fits waist sizes up to 48 inches.
Coloplast Ostomy	**Belt**: Adjustable.
DuoLOCK Curved Tail Closures	**Binder**: 10 per box.
Ostomy Appliance	**Belt**: Adjustable.
Adjustable Ostomy	**Belt**: Sizes: 17-inch to 26-inch (small), 26-inch to 43-inch (medium), 29-inch to 49-inch (large).

Products listed are representative of currently available and widely distributed brands. Similar products, including regional and private label brands, may also exist.

OSTOMY POUCHES

► **Actions**

The ideal pouch collects and contains the drainage, is odorproof, protects the peristomal skin region, is easy to use, and provides 4 to 7 days wear time. It is emptied when it is ⅓ full to prevent leakage and to keep the weight of the contents from pulling the pouch away from the skin.

Fecal pouches are available as closed-end and drainable. **Closed-end pouches** cannot be emptied and are most suitable for individuals with well-regulated descending or sigmoid colostomies. **Drainable pouches** are open at the bottom to allow emptying whenever necessary. Pouch closures are provided for simple sealing of the pouch. Drainable pouches are best for individuals with ileostomy, ascending, or transverse colostomies. **Urinary pouches** have spouts at the bottom for drainage of urine and an antireflux valve to prevent the pooling of urine onto the stoma and peristomal skin. Each box of pouches comes with an adapter so the pouch can be connected to a bedside drainage bag. Pouches are also available in 1- and 2-piece systems. The 1-piece pouch has the barrier and pouch all in one. These pouches generally have a low profile and are easy to apply. The 2-piece systems have a barrier with a flange that adheres to the body and a pouch that "snaps" on. This allows easy access to the stoma for changing of the pouch without removing the barrier. The decision to use a 1- or 2-piece design is dependent on several factors including the type of ostomy the patient has and the patient's general health. For example, patients with diminished eyesight or lacking dexterity and strength may have difficulties in assembling the pieces of a 2-piece system. Pouches can further be classified as **disposable** and **reusable**. The advantage of a reusable pouch is decreased cost over time. Disposable pouches are discarded every 4 to 7 days. The disadvantages of reusable pouches are that they tend to be heavier and more time-consuming to apply, clean, and maintain.

According to the Wound Ostomy Continence Nursing standards of ostomy care, patients with a flat, firm abdomen can use a flexible or nonflexible system. A flexible system usually consists of a paper tape border and a non-flexible system uses a full skin-barrier wafer and is less pliable. A firm abdomen with lateral (toward the stoma) creases or folds requires a flexible system, which enhances adherence by matching the pouch to the patient's contours. In a patient with deep creases, a flabby abdomen, or a retracted, flushed, or concave stoma in relation to the peristomal area, a convex appliance with a stoma belt is required. This system presses into the tissue surrounding the stoma causing it to protrude, which prevents leaks and decreases the risk of skin breakdown.

For additional information regarding ostomy care, the following organizations may be contacted:

- United Ostomy Association, 19772 MacArthur Blvd., Suite 200, Irvine, CA 92612-2405, (800) 826-0826
- Wound, Ostomy and Continence Nurses Society, 1550 S. Coast Highway, Suite 201, Laguna Beach, CA 92651; (888) 224-9626
- Crohn's & Colitis Foundation, 386 Park Avenue South, 17th floor, New York, NY 10016; (800) 343-3637

ONE-PIECE OSTOMY SYSTEMS

ONE-PIECE OSTOMY SYSTEMS	
Trade name	**Description**
Drainable Pouch Products	
Disposable Ileostomy Pouch with Brass Belt Adaptor	**Pouch**: Opaque, transparent, or custom.
Disposable Ileostomy Pouch with Fibre Belt Adaptor	**Pouch**: Opaque or transparent.
Disposable Ileostomy Pouch with Small Fibre Belt Adaptor	**Pouch**: Opaque or transparent.
Disposable Ileostomy Pouch with Hypo-Allergenic Adhesive	**Pouch**: Opaque or transparent.
Disposable Ileostomy Pouch with Adhesive Foam	**Pouch**: Opaque or transparent.
Atlantic Disposable Pouch with Square Stomahesive Wafer	**Pouch**: Opaque white or transparent.
Atlantic Disposable Pouch with Circular Stomahesive Wafer	**Pouch**: Opaque white or transparent.
Atlantic Disposable Pouch with Circular Stomahesive Wafer and Brass Belt Adapter	**Pouch**: Opaque and transparent.
Disposable Pouch with ReliaSeal Wafer and Brass Belt Adapter	**Pouch**: Opaque and transparent.
Disposable Pouch with ReliaSeal Wafer and Fibre Belt Adapater	**Pouch**: Opaque white and transparent.
Post-Op-Ileostomy-Colostomy Drain	**Pouch**: Opaque white and transparent.
Poly Post Op	**Pouch**: Transparent.
Vinyl Pouch	**Pouch**: Opaque.
Premium Pouch with Karaya 5 Seal	**Pouch**: Transparent.
Bard Drainable Adhesive	**Pouch**: Stoma sizes: $9/16$-inch to $1\,3/8$-inch with opening widths $9/16$-inch to $2\,3/8$-inch.

ONE-PIECE OSTOMY SYSTEMS

Trade name	Description
Drainable Pouch Products	
Active Life Convex One-Piece Drainable Pouch with Durahesive Skin Barrier, 12" Transparent	**Pouch**: Nine sizes from 3/4-inch to 2-inch; 1 tail closure per box, 5 per box.
FirstChoice Drainable	**Pouch**: With cut-to-fit skin barrier, backing, tape or adhesive, transparent or opaque odor-barrier film. Stoma sizes custom cut up to 2 1/2 inches.
FirstChoice Drainable	**Pouch**: Opaque, transparent.
FirstChoice	**Pouch**: Transparent.
Karaya Seal Drainable	**Pouch**: With *Karaya 5 Seal Ring*, belt tabs, adhesive, transparent or opaque odor-barrier film. Stoma sizes from 5/8-inch to 2 1/2-inch. Pouch lengths from 9 inches to 16 inches.
Active Life 10"	**Pouch**: Opaque.
Active Life 12"	**Pouch**: Opaque, transparent.
Active Life Convex 12"	**Pouch**: Transparent.
Active Life 12" Drainable Custom	**Pouch**: Transparent.
Max-E Pouch Open-End Drain	**Pouch**: Transparent.
Special Odor Barrier Drain	**Pouch**: Transparent.
Odor Barrier Drain	**Pouch**: Transparent.
Open-End Drain	**Pouch**: Blue.
Premier Drainable Mini-Pouches	**Pouch**: With or without cut-to-fit or precut skin barrier, backing, tape, transparent odor-barrier film, *ComfortWear Panel*. Stoma sizes custom cut up to 2 1/2 inches or precut from 3/4-inch to 2-inch.
Dansac Contour I	**Pouch**: Transparent or opaque; drainable; with tapered, flexible skin barriers and soft backing. Stoma sizes from 5/8-inch to 2 1/2-inch.
11" Standard	**Pouch**: Opaque, transparent.
10" Drainable Small	**Pouch**: Transparent, opaque.
Post-Op	**Pouch**: Transparent.
Colostomy/Ileostomy	**Pouch**: Transparent, opaque.
9" Urostomy	**Pouch**: Opaque, transparent.
Nu-Hope Drainable	**Pouch**: Various features. Stoma sizes from 1/2-inch to 2-inch and custom cut oval.
Urinary Pouch Products	
Atlantic White Rubber Urostomy Pouch with 3 3/4" Flange	**Flange**: Flat or moderate convex.
Assura One-Piece Convex Urostomy Custom Cut	**Pouch**: 375 mL, one-piece, soft absorbent backing, anti-reflux valve, secure outlet closure, simple locking connector for night drainage; latex-free; transparent. Sizes: 13 to 32 mm, 13 to 44 mm.
FirstChoice	**Pouch**: Transparent, cut-to-fit.
Premier	**Pouch**: Transparent.
Premier Flextend	**Pouch**: Transparent.
Lo-Profile	**Pouch**: Transparent.
9" (Brief)	**Pouch**: Transparent.
12" (Short)	**Pouch**: Transparent.
Active Life Convex Urostomy	**Pouch**: Transparent.

ONE-PIECE OSTOMY SYSTEMS

Trade name	Description
Urinary Pouch Products	
Bongort Trim 'n Fit with Anti-Reflux Valve-Cut-To-Fit	**Pouch:** Transparent in small, medium, or large.
SUR-FIT Natura Urostomy, Transparent Small	**Pouch:** Four flange sizes from 1¼-inch to 2¼-inch; 10 pouches and 2 night drainage adapters per box.
Marlen's Ultra	**Pouch:** For ileostomy, colostomy, and urostomy; small and medium sizes. Stoma openings from 12 mm to 50 mm; available in shallow or deep convexity.
Nu-Hope Urinary	**Pouch:** Custom cut oval any size or precut from ½-inch to 2-inch.
E-Z Drain	**Pouch:** Transparent, white, beige.
"All Flexible" Plastic	**Pouch:** Transparent, white, beige.
Closed Pouch Products	
FirstChoice Closed	**Pouch:** Opaque, transparent.
Premium Pouch with Karaya 5 Seal	**Pouch:** Opaque.
Mini Pouch	**Pouch:** Transparent.
Filter Pouch	**Pouch:** Transparent.
Pouch with Karaya 5 Seal Ring	**Pouch:** Transparent.
HolliGard Seal	**Pouch:** Transparent.
Active Life Pre-Cut Closed End	**Pouch:** Opaque, transparent.
Active Life Closed End	**Pouch:** Opaque, transparent.
Bard Closed-End Adhesive	**Pouch:** Stoma sizes: 1⁵⁄₁₆-inch to 1³⁄₁₆-inch.
Assura One-Piece Closed Mini	**Pouch:** Precut 5-inch; odor proof film with integrated charcoal filter for odor control; latex-free. Opaque: 25 mm, 32 mm, 38 mm, 44 mm. Transparent: 25 mm, 32 mm.
Closed Mini-Pouch	**Pouch:** With transparent odor-barrier film, belt tabs. Stoma sizes from 1 inch to 3 inches.
Dansac Combi Colo F	**Pouch:** Opaque; closed; with filter, standard adhesive, and cloth backing. Stoma sizes from 1 inch to 1½ inches. Pouch lengths from 7½ inches to 8½ inches.
Marlen's Ultra	**Pouch:** For ileostomy, colostomy, and urostomy; available in small-medium; stoma opening from ½ inch to 2 inches; available in shallow or deep convexity.
8 ¼" Closed	**Pouch:** Opaque, transparent.
Bongort 1-Piece Ostomy	**Pouch:** Urinary and colostomy pouches with adhesive face plates. Small, medium, large sizes.
Atlantic "O-Dor-Less"	**Pouch:** Disposable or reusable; with precut, convex, flat, or semi-rigid barriers.

Products listed are representative of currently available and widely distributed brands. Similar products, including regional and private label brands, may also exist.

TWO-PIECE OSTOMY SYSTEMS

TWO-PIECE OSTOMY SYSTEMS	
Trade name	Description
Drainable Pouches and Sleeves	
"O-dor-less" Plastic	**Sleeve**: Opaque, transparent.
"O-dor-less" Ileostomy	**Pouch**: Black rubber, opaque white.
Atlantic White Rubber	**Pouch**: Opaque white.
"O-dor-less" Plastic	**Pouch**: Opaque, transparent.
Atlantic Polyethylene Plastic	**Pouch**: Transparent.
Guardian Drainable	**Pouch**: Opaque, transparent.
Guardain Drainable with Replaceble Filter	**Pouch**: Transparent.
SUR-FIT Natura 10" Drainable	**Pouch**: Opaque.
SUR-FIT Natura 12" Drainable	**Pouch**: Opaque, transparent.
SUR-FIT 14" Drainable	**Pouch**: Transparent.
Coloplast Two-Piece Small Drainable, 10"	**Pouch**: Opaque. Stoma sizes: Up to 1¼ inch, up to 1¾-inch, up to 2 inches.
CenterPointLock Two-Piece Ostomy System: Drainable Mini-Pouch	**Pouch**: With opaque odor-barrier film, deodorizing filter, flange. Stoma sizes from 1½ inches to 2¾-inches.
Dansac Contour II	**Pouch**: Transparent or opaque; drainable; with floating flanges and wafers with tapered, flexible skin barriers, soft backing. Stoma sizes from ½ Inch to 2¾ inches.
10" Drainable	**Pouch**: Opaque.
11" Drainable	**Pouch**: Opaque, transparent.
8 ¼" Closed with Filtrodor Filter	**Pouch**: Opaque.
Soft & Secure	**Pouch**: Closed or drainable; for urinary and colostomy use. Small, medium, large sizes. Flange sizes from 1½ inches to 2¾ inches.
Torbot Rubber	**Pouch**: Reusable with convex barrier.
VPI Non-Adhesive Colostomy Systems	**Pouch**: Drainable (8 inches) with belt, closure clip. O-ring seal sizes: 1¼ inch, 1½ inches, 2 inches, 2½ inches.
Urinary Pouch Products	
Atlantic White Rubber	**Pouch**: Small, regular.
SUR-FIT Urostomy	**Pouch**: Transparent.
SUR-FIT Natura Urostomy with Accuseal Tap-Standard	**Pouch**: Opaque, transparent.
Sure-Fit Natura Ostomy with Accuseal Tap-Small	**Pouch**: Opaque.
Assura Two-Piece Urostomy	**Pouch**: Soft, moisture-absorbent backing, antireflux valve, secure outlet closure, simple locking connector for night drainage bag attachment; secure; lock-ring system; latex-free. Standard opaque or transparent: 25 cm, 375 mL capacity. Stoma sizes: ½ inch to 1½ inches, ½ inch to 1¾ inches, ½ inch to 2¼ inches. Small transparent 18 cm, 250 mL capacity. Stoma sizes: ½ inch to 1½ inches to 1¾ inches.
2 piece Ileal Bladder Set-Adult	**Pouch**: Regular, large.
Coloplast Two-Piece Small Urostomy	**Pouch**: Transparent. Stoma sizes up to 1¼ inch, up to 1¾ inch, up to 2 inches, 100 mL.

TWO-PIECE OSTOMY SYSTEMS	
Trade name	**Description**
Urinary Pouch Products	
CenterPointLock Two-Piece Ostomy System: Premier Series Urostomy	**Pouch**: With opaque odor-barrier, *ComfortWear Panel*, flange. Stoma sizes from 1½ inches to 2¾ inches.
Guardian Two-Piece Ostomy System: Urostomy	**Pouch**: With transparent odor-barrier, flange, drain tube adapters. Pouch sizes: 1 inch, 1½ inches, 2 inches.
Closed Pouch Products	
Guardian Closed Mini-Pouch	**Pouch**: Opaque.
Guardian Closed	**Pouch**: Opaque, transparent.
SUR-FIT Natura Closed-End with Filter	**Pouch**: Opaque.
SUR-FIT Natura Closed	**Pouch**: Opaque.
SUR-FIT Mini-Pouches	**Pouch**: Opaque.
Assura Two-Piece Closed Mini	**Pouch**: 5-inch, soft, moisture-absorbent backing, filter for odor control; secure; lock-ring system; latex-free; opaque. Stoma sizes: ½ inch to 1½ inches, ½ inch to 1¾ inches.
CenterPointLock Two-Piece Ostomy System: Closed Mini-Pouch	**Pouch**: With opaque odor-barrier film, deodorizing filter, flange. Stoma sizes from 1½ inches to 2¾ inches.
Guardian Two-Piece Ostomy System: Closed Mini-Pouch	**Pouch**: With opaque odor-barrier film, deodorizing filter, flange. Stoma sizes from 1 inch to 2½ inches.
Dansac Contour II	**Pouch**: Transparent or opaque; closed; with floating flanges and wafers with tapered, flexible skin barriers, soft backing. Stoma sizes from ½ inch to 2¾ inches.

Products listed are representative of currently available and widely distributed brands. Similar products, including regional and private label brands, may also exist.

PATIENT INFORMATION
Ostomy Care

- Drink 6 to 8 glasses of non-caffeinated liquid every day including water, milk, juice, or decaffeinated tea, coffee, or soft drinks.
- Avoid injuring the stoma after changing the appliance by ensuring the skin barrier opening is at least 3 mm (⅛ inch) larger than the stoma diameter. When using new barrier wafers (eg, *Eakin* or *Colly-Seels*), these work best when the barrier opening is the "same" size as the stoma.
- Before starting colostomy irrigation, fill the tube with water to expel air. If the irrigation bag is placed at too high a level, the increased flow of water could cause cramps. Do not irrigate during a bout of diarrhea.
- Use cool to lukewarm water for cleaning your appliance. Hot water has a tendency to seal in odors, particularly in plastics.
- Drinking cranberry juice may help clear the urine and reduce odors.
- For medicines to work quickly, drink plenty of water to help them dissolve faster and to decrease the chance of irritation to the esophagus. Ileostomates should take only liquid medicine. (Those with fast output should take only liquid medicines or soft dissolving pills for quick absorption.) Gelcaps may not dissolve fast enough to be absorbed by those who have little or no colon. Remind your physician of your ostomy when you need a prescription.

PATIENT INFORMATION (continued)

Ostomy Care (continued)

- To thicken output, ileostomates may eat apple sauce, oatmeal, bananas, cheese, creamy peanut butter, boiled rice, tapioca, and boiled milk.
- If carbonated drinks result in gas problems, a shake of salt or sugar will cause fizzing; when the fizzing stops, the beverage will be flat enough to drink.
- Avoid swallowing air, which sometimes occurs from chewing gum, gulping food, or drinking liquids through straw.
- Drinking orange juice may help to prevent odor problems after eating eggs or fish.
- Waiting too long between meals may increase gas production.
- Yogurt helps to control gas formation and buttermilk helps to soothe an irritated bowel; unlike milk, they will not cause diarrhea.
- When ill with a virus and associated diarrhea, eat pretzels; they are easily digested, and the salt helps your electrolyte balance.
- Clean urostomy tubing for night drainage by using 1 part vinegar to 2 parts water.
- Mouthwash, toothpaste, or a sprinkle of cinnamon in the pouch will help to dispel odor upon emptying.
- Diarrhea may be caused by foods and beverages containing caffeine (eg, coffee, tea, chocolate, cola beverages).
- Drinking lots of water each day ensures a good flow of urine. Ostomy patients, especially ileostomates, should increase fluid intake during hot weather.
- Chew solid food thoroughly before swallowing.
- Leaving a little air in the pouch after emptying will allow wastes to flow down easily. Also, small amounts of oil (eg, salad oil, baby oil) may be inserted in the pouch and massaged to coat the inside and make it easier to empty contents (especially for colostomates).
- Because the section of intestine (ileum) that was used to create the urostomy conduit secretes mucus, it is common to see mucus in the urine.
- Salt in the urine will deposit crystals on the stoma and faceplate; rubbing the crystals on the stoma may cause bleeding. Clean the crystals from the appliance by soaking in a solution of one part vinegar and two parts water.
- Micropore tape can be waterproofed by covering it with *Skin Prep* after it is in place.
- Wearing a cotton cover over the appliance will keep you cool. The cover can be made at home or purchased ready-made.
- To avoid splashing, float some toilet paper in the toilet bowel before emptying the pouch.
- Itching under the appliance could be a sign of dehydration. Taking 2 or 3 glasses of water over a short period may relieve the problem and prevent an early appliance change.
- Use ammonia to clean up *Karaya Powder* from the bathroom floor; water makes it gummy or sticky.

PATIENT INFORMATION (continued)

Pouch Change Procedure

1.) Gather supplies: Pouch with attached solid skin barrier wafer; stoma pattern; scissors; skin barrier paste; tissues; small container with warm water; pouch closure clip; plastic bag.

2.) Prepare pouch. Trace stoma pattern onto solid skin barrier wafer surface of pouch and cut out. Remove protective paper backing from adhesive surface of pouch. Set pouch aside.

3.) Remove soiled pouch. Empty pouch. Gently remove pouch from skin by pushing down on skin while peeling adhesive away. A dampened tissue or cloth can assist in breaking the bond of the adhesive to the skin. Discard the soiled pouch in plastic bag. The best and easiest way of doing this is to wrap the used appliance in newspaper, tie it up inside a plastic bag, and then dispose of it with the household rubbish. Alternatively, some local authorities operate a collection service of stoma appliances, and many appliance companies supply sealable plastic bags for disposal.

4.) Cleanse the stoma and the skin. With a dry tissue, wipe stool, mucus, or skin barrier residue from stoma and skin. With moistened tissue or cloth gently cleanse the stoma skin. Dry skin (fan skin or dab with dry cloth).

5.) Apply clean pouch. Apply a bead of skin barrier paste immediately around the stoma. (This may instead be applied directly to the cut edge of skin barrier on pouch in step 2 if preferred.) Apply pouch to wrinkle-free skin (patient may need to stand at this point or use one hand to pull skin taut). Massage skin barrier immediately around the stoma to enhance adherence. Examine adhesive surface to eliminate wrinkles from tape and ensure that skin is smooth under adhesive. Apply pouch closure clip.

PINWORM INFECTION
(Enterobiasis)

DEFINITION
Enterobiasis is a GI infection caused by nematodes of the genus *Enterobius*, especially *E. vermicularis* (pinworm).

ETIOLOGY
E. vermicularis is an intestinal parasite. The adult female migrates to the perianal region and lays approximately 10,000 eggs that become infective within hours. Once transmitted to a host, the eggs hatch, and the larvae reach maturity in approximately 1 month. The lifespan of the adult is approximately 2 months.

INCIDENCE
Globally, enterobiasis affects approximately 300 people per million (0.03%), although some estimate a prevalence of 15% to 20% in the US alone, with the majority of those infected being children.

PATHOPHYSIOLOGY
Enterobiasis results from the transfer of eggs from the perianal area of an infected individual to fomites (eg, bedding, clothing, toys), where the eggs are picked up by a new host, introduced into the mouth, and consequently swallowed. Airborne eggs may be inhaled and then swallowed. The eggs hatch, releasing larvae in the small intestines. After a few weeks, the mature female worm migrates to the perianal area to deposit eggs. The deposited eggs may cause intense irritation and itching. Reinfestation, or autoinfection, is also very common, as well as cross-contamination between family members and institutionalized patients.

SIGNS/SYMPTOMS
Some cases of enterobiasis are symptom-free. However, the most common symptom is perianal pruritus (itching) caused by movements of the migrating female and deposited eggs. Excoriation may be present due to the itching. Severe cases have caused abdominal pain, weight loss, and appendicitis because of intestinal lumen obstruction, although no causal relationship has been demonstrated. In rare cases, migration into the female genital tract can lead to vulvovaginitis and pelvic or peritoneal granulomas. Because of the intense itching and scratching associated with this disease, dermatitis and secondary bacterial superinfections have been reported rarely.

DIAGNOSTIC PARAMETERS/PHYSICAL ASSESSMENT
Clinical Observation: Symptomatology is generally the prelude to physical assessment but is often extremely limited. Occasionally, the female worm (approximately 8 to 13 mm in length) may be found in the perianal region within 1 to 2 hours after the infected patient has gone to bed for the night.

Commonly, a diagnosis is made by detecting the eggs deposited in the peri-anal region by applying clear cellulose acetate tape (eg, *Scotch* tape) to the peri-anal region in the morning and then examining the tape under a microscope.

Interview: When a child experiences anal itching, it may be beneficial to ask about the following:

- Onset/duration of symptoms (worm migration and egg deposition usually occurs at night).
- Family members or contacts with similar symptoms. Pinworm infections are eas-ily transmitted by contamination of clothing or bedding among children in households or child care environments.
- Presence of additional symptoms (other than itching), such as abdominal pain or painful urination. Such symptoms may suggest intestinal or urethral compli-cations, which occur rarely.

TREATMENT

Approaches to therapy: Enterobiasis is generally self-limiting and can be con-trolled through nonpharmacologic means plus medication.

Nondrug therapy: Most infections can be handled successfully with proper per-sonal hygiene. Because this is often difficult with children, and parents feel uncomfortable knowing their children are infected by a parasite, pharmaco-logical management is usually provided.

All undergarments, nightclothes, and bed linens should be laundered daily until the patient is free of worms based on the *Scotch* tape test.

Pharmacotherapy: Pyrantel pamoate is the only OTC agent available for treat-ment of pinworm infections. Although the drug is given as a single dose, check the patient for several consecutive days to ensure that he or she is worm-free by using the *Scotch* tape test. Other household members may also be treated to ensure eradication and to prevent reinfection.

PYRANTEL PAMOATE

▶ **Actions**

Pyrantel pamoate is a depolarizing neuromuscular blocker that causes complete paraly-sis of the worm.

▶ **Indications**

For the treatment of roundworm and pinworm infections.

▶ **Contraindications**

Hypersensitivity to pyrantel; pregnant women (see Warnings); patients with hepatic disease.

▶ **Warnings**

Pregnancy: Very little of the drug is absorbed from the GI tract, and animal studies have not shown harm to the fetus. However, avoid using in pregnant women unless directed by a physician.

Children: Safety and efficacy for use in children younger than 2 years of age have not been established.

▶ **Drug Interactions**

Theophylline serum levels increased in a pediatric patient following pyrantel pamoate administration, but further study is needed because very little of the drug is systemically absorbed.

▶ **Adverse Reactions**

Adverse effects are infrequent, and those that occur are mainly GI-related, including anorexia, nausea, vomiting, abdominal cramps, and diarrhea. Other extremely rare reactions include headache, drowsiness, dizziness, insomnia, rash, and elevated liver enzymes.

▶ **Administration and Dosage**

A single dose of 11 mg/kg (5 mg/lb) is often sufficient. The maximum dose is 1 g. This dose may be repeated in 2 weeks and given without regard to food or time of day.

PYRANTEL PAMOATE PRODUCTS	
Trade name	**Doseform**
Reese's Pinworm	**Capsules**: 180 mg pyrantel pamoate (equiv. to 62.5 mg pyrantel base)
Antiminth	**Oral suspension**: 50 mg pyrantel (as pamoate) per mL
Pin-Rid, Pin-X, Reese's Pinworm, Ascarel, Verm-Rid	**Liquid**: 50 mg pyrantel (as pamoate) per mL

Products listed are representative of currently available and widely distributed brands. Similar products, including regional and private label brands, may also exist.

PATIENT INFORMATION

Pyrantel Pamoate

- Dosage is based on weight.
- May be taken with food, milk, juice, or on an empty stomach anytime during the day.
- Shake liquid formulations well before measuring doses.
- Be certain to take the entire dose.
- Using a laxative to facilitate removal of the parasites is not necessary.
- Strict hygiene is essential as spread to other family members and reinfection are common.
- Change and launder undergarments, bed linens, towels, and nightclothes daily until the patient is free of infection.

CONTRACEPTION

DEFINITION

Contraception: Contraception is the voluntary prevention of the union of an ovum (egg) with sperm or prevention of uterine implantation of a fertilized egg. Conception is defined as the union of ovum with sperm and subsequent uterine implantation.

Normal menstrual cycle/Fertile period: The menstrual cycle consists of 4 phases and, on average, lasts approximately 28 days (see Figure 1 on the following page). The cycle is regulated by the hypothalamus, pituitary gland, ovaries, and the endometrial lining via a biofeedback mechanism.

The **follicular** phase encompasses the proliferative or estrogen-dominant phase. At the beginning of the follicular phase, estrogen levels are low, thus enabling the follicle-stimulating hormone-releasing factor (FSH-RF) to be released from the hypothalamus. This in turn stimulates the anterior pituitary to produce the follicle-stimulating hormone (FSH) and luteinizing hormone (LH). FSH stimulates several follicles in the ovary and LH initiates estrogen secretion by the follicles. The increase in estrogen stimulates the luteinizing hormone-releasing factor (LRF) from the hypothalamus to produce more LH from the anterior pituitary. FSH is inhibited, thus decreasing the number of follicles. Dominant follicles remain and as they mature, produce increased amounts of estrogen, which is responsible for the endometrial growth (proliferative stage).

The **ovulatory** phase takes place when the pituitary releases a surge of LH and the dominant follicle is released. The LH is also responsible for the formation of the corpus luteum. This phase usually occurs on day 14 or 15 of a 28-day cycle.

After ovulation, the **luteal** or **secretory** phase is characterized by the production of estrogen and an increased amount of progesterone by the corpus luteum. Progesterone is responsible for endometrial thickening in preparation for implantation of the fertilized ovum. If implantation does not occur by the 23rd to 25th day, the corpus luteum regresses and circulating estrogen and progesterone diminish. Because the endometrium cannot be maintained with decreased levels of hormones, it sloughs off and the **menstrual** phase begins. If implantation does occur, human chorionic gonadotropin (HCG) is produced by placental trophoblasts within a week of conception and replaces LH in maintaining the secretory capacity of the corpus luteum. The period of viability of the ovum (egg) is approximately 6 to 24 hours, while the period of viability of sperm is 48 to 60 hours. During a given menstrual cycle, a woman's "fertile period" generally consists of 4 days surrounding ovulation (2 days prior to ovulation, the day of ovulation, and the subsequent day).

Pregnancy: Pregnancy or gestation is the condition of the female from conception (ie, union of the sperm and ovum and subsequent uterine implantation) until childbirth. Contraception may be defined as the voluntary control of childbearing by preventing the union of ovum and sperm or retarding uterine implantation of a fertilized egg. Methods of contraception involve drug and nondrug approaches. Over-the-counter methods of contraception include use of male and female condoms, spermicides, periodic abstinence, and withdrawal. Thus, the male and female condom prevent the union of the ovum and sperm by acting as mechanical barriers, preventing the transmission of semen into the vagina.

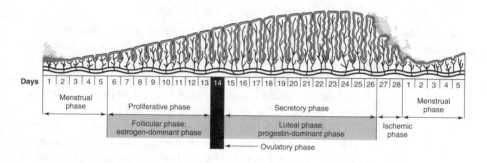

Figure 1. The Menstrual Cycle

INCIDENCE

It has been estimated that more than 60% of women of reproductive age in the US use some method of contraception, including condoms (6 million users), female sterilization (approximately 10 million users), and oral contraceptives (approximately 11 million users). Due to the fear of sexually transmitted diseases, condom use has increased. More than half (56%) of all pregnancies are unintended. Among women who experience unintended pregnancies, 44% have abortions, 43% give birth, and 13% experience miscarriage.

Sexually transmitted diseases: A sexually transmitted disease (STD) is an infection that can be passed on to others through sexual contact. There are 24 recognized STDs. These include HIV/AIDS, gonorrhea, syphilis, chlamydia, genital herpes, genital warts, pelvic inflammatory disease, and hepatitis. In the US, there are 12 million new cases of STDs per year (66% occur in patients under the age of 25). If this rate remains constant, 1 in 4 Americans will at some point contract an STD. Compared with men, women are twice as likely to become infected with an STD as a result of a single act of unprotected sex. Long-term effects of STDs may be serious or fatal, but transmission of STDs may be prevented by total sexual abstinence, remaining in a mutually monogamous relationship with an uninfected individual, or using a barrier contraceptive method, preferably a condom with a spermicide.

DIAGNOSTIC PARAMETERS/PHYSICAL ASSESSMENT

Selection of contraceptive methods: Selection of a method of contraception is extremely personal and individualistic. Religious beliefs, future reproductive plans, and many other factors may influence contraceptive selection. Some additional factors for patients to consider when deciding on a method of contraception include safety, efficacy, simplicity of use, cost, reversibility, acceptability to user and partner, and potential complications from use. The following table documents contraceptive effectiveness among couples who initiate use of a contraceptive method and use it consistently and correctly. Patients should be informed that the success of any method of contraception depends, to a great extent, on the reliability and consistency of the user.

The following table gives ranges of pregnancy rates reported for various means of contraception. *The effectiveness of these means of contraception (except IUD, medroxyprogesterone injection, levonorgestrel implants, vasectomy, and tubal ligation) depends on the degree of adherence to the methods of proper use.*

Pregnancy Rates for Various Means of Contraception (%)[1]		
Method of Contraception	Typical[2]	Lowest[3]
Oral Contraceptives		
Combination (estrogen/progestin)	0.1 to 0.34	0.1
Progestin only	0.5 to 1.5	0.5
Mechanical/Chemical		
Cervical cap[4]		
Multiparous	40	26
Nulliparous	20	9
Male condom without spermicide	12 to 14	3
Male condom with spermicide	4 to 6	1.8
Diaphragm[4]	20	6
Female condom	21	5
IUD	≤ 1 to 2	≤ 1 to 1.5
Levonorgestrel implants	≤ 1	≤ 1
Medroxyprogesterone injection	≤ 1	≤ 1
Spermicide alone	20 to 22	6
Rhythm (all types)	25	1 to 9
Vasectomy/Tubal Ligation	≤ 1	≤ 1
Withdrawal	40 to 50	30
No contraception	85	85

[1] During first year of continuous use.
[2] A typical couple who initiated a method that was either not always used correctly or was not used with every act of sexual intercourse, and who experienced an accidental pregnancy.
[3] The method of birth control was always used correctly with every act of sexual intercourse but the couple still experienced an accidental pregnancy.
[4] Used with spermicide.

Interview: To help determine whether physician referral or self-selection of the method of contraception is preferable, it is beneficial to ask about the following:

• Past experience with contraception
• Current method of contraception

- Current preference for contraceptive method
- Partner's preference for contraceptive method
- Physical, physiologic, or religious considerations limiting contraceptive use
- Role of contraceptive method in preventing STDs

TREATMENT

Approaches to therapy:

Over-the-counter contraceptives – Health care providers may recommend nondrug approaches, appropriate pharmacotherapy, or physician referral for patients attempting to select a method of contraception. The focus of this discussion is on contraceptives available without a prescription. These include male condoms, female condoms, and spermicides. Such agents are the contraceptive methods most often used by the teen population unwilling to seek physician involvement, or by patients who are unable or do not want to take a physician-assisted approach to contraception and in whom sterilization is not an option. As much as possible, patients should be made aware of all contraceptive options, including those that require physician referral.

In many cases, patients have limited accurate knowledge of basic reproductive physiology, sex education, and the implications and consequences of STDs and unwanted pregnancies. Community pharmacists have a unique accessibility to patients that enables them to educate and counsel patients seeking information as well as serve "at risk" populations with regard to contraception. Thus, pharmacists may assist in prevention of the sometimes devastating medical, social, and economic consequences of STDs and unwanted pregnancies.

Nondrug therapy:

High-risk contraception – High-risk methods of contraception include periodic abstinence and withdrawal.

Periodic abstinence – Also referred to as natural family planning or the "rhythm" method, this method of contraception requires avoidance of intercourse during presumed fertile days. Various techniques, such as the calendar method, the basal body temperature method, the cervical mucus method, the symptothermal method, or the use of in-home ovulation detection devices, may be used to identify times of ovulation, when unprotected intercourse is to be avoided. However, patients should be aware that times of ovulation are difficult to predict because of the erratic nature of the menstrual cycle, and 20% to 24% of women practicing periodic abstinence experience pregnancy in the first year of use. Additionally, this method confers no protection against STDs.

Withdrawal – Withdrawal, or coitus interruptus, involves unprotected intercourse until ejaculation is imminent. At that point, the male abruptly withdraws. This method is associated with a high pregnancy rate due to a lack of self-control and the presence of viable sperm in involuntary urethral secretions of the stimulated male. Again, this method provides no protection against transmission of STDs.

Douching – Douching should not be considered a contraceptive method. Insemination may occur as soon as 90 seconds after ejaculation. Furthermore, douching is ineffective in removing sperm from the upper reproductive tract and may actually propel viable sperm into the cervix.

MALE CONDOMS

▶ Actions

Male condoms are sheaths worn over the erect penis at the time of coitus. The male condom acts as a barrier that collects and prevents semen from entering the vagina. Condoms are typically made of latex, polyurethane, or lamb intestinal tissue; however, condoms derived from natural animal tissue do not prevent passage of viral organisms (eg, HIV, hepatitis). Condoms made of intestinal tissue are also typically more expensive. Male condoms are available in various colors, styles, shapes, and thicknesses. They may have reservoir tips, ribs, or studs, or be lubricated (with or without spermicide). Condoms are typically 7.5 inches long and 1.4 inches in diameter at their opening. Condom quality is monitored by the FDA; the federal standard for condom breakage is 4/1000 tested. Breakage may be minimized by proper use.

▶ Guidelines for Use

Patients who select male condoms as a method of contraception should be aware of the following guidelines for proper use:

- Use only fresh condoms (ie, those that have not been previously opened) that have been stored in a cool, dry place (not a wallet or car glove compartment).
- Always use latex condoms unless an allergy or hypersensitivity to latex exists in the male user or partner.
- Do not test condoms for leaks before use; this increases the likelihood of tearing.
- To extend contraceptive protection, condom use by the male and vaginal spermicide use by the female is encouraged.
- Always have a vaginal spermicide product available in case of condom breakage or leakage. Insert the spermicide in the vagina as soon as possible if condom breakage or leakage occurs. In such cases, emergency contraception ("morning after pill") should be considered for use within 72 hours.
- Fingernails or jewelry may tear condoms.
- To prevent both pregnancy and disease transmission, unroll the condom onto the erect penis before the penis comes into any contact with the vagina. If the user begins to put the condom on inside-out, discard that condom and use a fresh one.
- If a reservoir-tipped condom is not being used, leave half an inch between the end of the condom and the tip of the penis by pinching the condom as it is unrolled. This allows space for ejaculate and decreases risk of breakage.
- If one's partner experiences vaginal dryness, provide additional lubrication to reduce friction and decrease the risk of breakage or tearing. Use only water-based lubricants (eg, *H-R Lubricating Jelly, Astroglide, Ortho-Gynol*) because oil-based lubricants (eg, mineral or baby oil, petroleum jelly, or vaginal creams

such as *Vagisil* or *Premarin*) may weaken condoms and increase breakage. Spermicides may also be used as lubricants; these also increase the condom's contraceptive efficacy.

- Withdraw the penis immediately after ejaculation. Hold the rim of the condom during withdrawal to prevent the condom from slipping off.
- Examine the condom for tears and discard.
- If the condom has torn, immediately insert spermicidal foam, cream, or jelly with a high concentration of spermicide into the vagina and consider emergency contraception ("morning after pill") use within 72 hours.

Do not use contraceptive suppositories or vaginal film; the efficacy of these products may be limited. Patients should be aware of lubricants that are safe/unsafe to use with latex condoms. Examples of safe lubricants are contraceptive foams, creams, and jellies, such as *H-R Lubricating Jelly*, *Astroglide*, and *Ortho-Gynol*. Unsafe lubricants include oils (eg, baby, coconut, olive, mineral), petroleum jelly, or vaginal creams (eg, *Monistat*, *Vagisil*, *Premarin*). Pharmacists should recommend use of reputable brands of lubricants and make patients aware of condoms' increased efficacy when used with spermicides.

MALE CONDOMS	
Trade name	Description
Condoms with Spermicidal Lubricants	
Beyond Seven Plus	**Condoms**: 12.5% nonoxynol-9
Trojan Supra Microsheer Polyurethane Ultra-thin	**Condoms**: 8% nonoxynol-9
Class Act Ultra Thin & Sensitive, Trojan-Enz*, Trojan-Enz Large*, Trojan Extra Strength, Trojan Magnum*, Trojan Pleasure Mesh*, Trojan Plus 2 Ultra Fit*, Trojan Ribbed*, Trojan Shared Sensation*, Trojan Ultra Fit*, Trojan Ultra Pleasure*, Trojan Ultra Texture*, Trojan Ultra Thin*, Trojan Very Sensitive*	**Condoms**: 7% nonoxynol-9
Kimono Sensation Plus	**Condoms**: 6.5% nonoxynol-9
Durex Extra Sensitive*, Durex High Sensation*, Durex Natural Feeling*, Durex Pure Protection, Durex Ultimate Feeling*, Durex Ultra Comfort*	**Condoms**: 5% nonoxynol-9
Kling-Tite Naturalamb, LifeStyles, LifeStyles Extra Strength, LifeStyles Ribbed, LifeStyles Ultra Sensitive	**Condoms**: 2.5% nonoxynol-9

MALE CONDOMS	
Trade name	**Description**
Condoms with Nonspermicidal Lubricants	
Beyond Seven, Beyond Seven Ribs & Dots, Class Act Ribbed & Sensitive*, Class Act Smooth Sensation*, Class Act Ultra Thin & Sensitive*, Crown, Durex Avanti Superthin Non-Latex, Durex Colors & Scents*, Durex Enhanced Pleasure, Durex Extra Sensitive*, Durex Extra Strength*, Durex Intense Sensation, Durex High Sensation Ribbed*, Durex Pure Protection*, Durex Ultimate Feeling, Durex Ultra Comfort*, inSpiral, Kama Sutra, Kama Sutra Studded, Kama Sutra Ultrathin, Kimono MicroThin, Kimono MicroThin Ultra-Sensitive, Kimono Sensation, Kling-Tite Naturalamb, LifeStyles Assorted Colors, LifeStyles Large, LifeStyles Luscious Flavors, LifeStyles Ribbed, LifeStyles Snugger Fit, LifeStyles Studded*, LifeStyles Tuxedo Black, LifeStyles Ultra Lubricated, LifeStyles Ultra Sensitive*, LifeStyles Ultra Strength*, LifeStyles Xtra Pleasure*, Pleasure Plus, Sheik Super Thin, Trojan-Enz*, Trojan-Enz Large*, Trojan Extended Pleasure Climax Control¹*, Trojan Extra Strength*, Trojan Magnum*, Trojan Magnum XL*, Trojan Pleasure Mesh*, Trojan Plus Ultra Fit*, Trojan Ribbed*, Trojan Shared Sensation*, Trojan Ultra Pleasure, Trojan Ultra Texture*, Trojan Ultra Thin*, Trojan Very Sensitive*	**Condoms:** Lubricated
Nonlubricated Condoms	
Kling-Tite Naturalamb, LifeStyles Non-Lubricated, LifeStyles Vibra-Ribbed, Trojan Non-Lubricated, Trojan-Enz Non-Lubricated*	**Condoms**

Products listed are representative of currently available and widely distributed brands. Similar products, including regional and private label brands, may also exist.

* Reservoir-tipped.
¹ Contains benzocaine 4%.

FEMALE CONDOMS

▶ Actions

The female condom was developed to provide a means for women to gain greater control of protecting themselves against pregnancy and STDs. The female condom is a polyurethane pouch. It is thinner than the male condom, is prelubricated, and is supplied with additional lubricant. It is resistant to degradation by oil-based lubricants. On the female condom, an inner circular ring fits over the cervix and an outer ring protects external genitalia. Like the male condom, this type of condom is for one-time use. However, it may be inserted up to 8 hours before intercourse. Remove the female condom immediately after intercourse, before the woman stands up. Patients should be aware that the efficacy of the female condom is only marginally acceptable, even when it is used properly. With typical use in the general population, its efficacy is below average (see table). When used properly, the female condom is a good method of prevention of STD transmission, but its below-average reported efficacy for contraception in typical use may also be a cause for skepticism about its value for prevention of STD transmission. Some users note disadvantages of the female condom, such as difficulty inserting, relatively poor acceptance by user and partner, expense, associated vaginal irritation, decreased sensation in some women, and possible "squeaking" if lubrication is inadequate.

▶ Guidelines for Use

Female condoms are worn inside the vaginal canal at the time of coitus. The female condom acts as a barrier that prevents semen from entering the vagina, and is typically made of polyurethane with an inner and outer ring. The inner ring (which has a closed end) is inserted into the vaginal canal behind the pubic bone. A drop of lubricant may be added to aid insertion. Once the condom has been inserted, if the woman can feel the inner ring, or has any pain or discomfort, insert the inner ring higher. The outer ring and about 1 inch of the condom should remain outside the vagina.

FEMALE CONDOMS	
Trade name	Description
Reality	**Kit**: 3 polyurethane condoms, 3 tubes of lubricant, patient instruction leaflet

Products listed are representative of currently available and widely distributed brands. Similar products, including regional and private label brands, may also exist.

PATIENT INFORMATION

Condoms

- Use only fresh condoms (ie, those that have not been previously opened) that have been stored at room temperature.
- Always use latex condoms unless allergies to latex exist (male or partner) or you are in a monogamous relationship with someone you know is not infected with human immunodeficiency virus (HIV). The HIV and hepatitis B virus may pass through condoms made from natural animal tissue.
- Do not test condoms for leaks before use as this increases the likelihood of tearing.
- To extend contraceptive protection, condom use by the male and vaginal spermicide use by the female is encouraged.
- Always have a vaginal spermicidal product available in case of condom breakage or leakage. Insert the spermicide in the vagina as soon as possible if condom breakage or leakage occurs.
- Fingernails or jewelry may tear condoms.
- If pregnancy is medically contraindicated, consult your physician for a contraception program.

SPERMICIDES

▶ Actions

Spermicidal foams, creams, jellies, suppositories, and films contain an active ingredient in an inert vehicle. The active ingredient immobilizes and kills sperm to varying degrees depending on quantity and concentration, while the vehicle provides the additional benefit of creating a mechanical barrier over the cervical opening. Most spermicides contain nonoxynol-9. Another spermicidal agent is octoxynol-9. All vaginal spermicides may be used in combination with male and female condoms. Use with diaphragms and cervical caps is strongly recommended. Patients should be advised to routinely use products with high concentrations of spermicide (8% or more), if tolerated. Possibly due to superior distribution and adherence, contraceptive foams appear to have better efficacy rates than other vaginal spermicides when used without other forms of contraception. While gels and foams are less messy, creams have the best lubricating qualities. Vaginal contraceptive suppositories have low contraceptive efficacy and should not be routinely recommended. Dissolution rates are unpredictable and distribution may be poor. Contraceptive films are paper-thin, 2-inch squares that contain 28% nonoxynol-9. Because experience with contraceptive film is limited, routine recommendations are discouraged.

▶ Guidelines for Use

- Instruct patients to read labeling carefully.
- If using foam, shake container well (approximately 20 times) before use.
- All vaginal spermicides are effective soon after insertion, but insertion more than 60 minutes before intercourse requires reapplication of a full dose to ensure efficacy.
- If using foam, cream, or gel, use supplied applicator to apply required amount near the cervix. Do not assume that 1 full applicator is the appropriate dose; check labeling instructions. Typically, 1 full application is good for only 1 act of intercourse.
- Delay douching until at least 8 hours after intercourse. Douching dilutes or removes spermicide and may propel viable sperm into the uterus.
- Allergic reactions or contact dermatitis occur rarely (1% or less).
- When spermicides are used with a diaphragm or cervical cap, fill the device (concave side) one-third with spermicide and position over the cervix.
- A spermicide-filled diaphragm or cervical cap may be inserted up to 1 hour before intercourse. Leave diaphragm in place for at least 6 hours after intercourse; the cervical cap may be left in place for up to 48 hours. If intercourse occurs again before removal of the diaphragm or cervical cap, apply another full dose of spermicide.
- Vaginal contraceptive suppositories must be inserted at least 10 to 15 minutes before intercourse and require vaginal moisture for dissolution.
- Vaginal contraceptive film is placed on the tip of the finger, inserted intravaginally, and positioned at the cervical opening. The spermicide is activated by vaginal secretions and should be allowed at least 5 minutes to dissolve before intercourse occurs.

SPERMICIDE PRODUCTS	
Trade name	**Doseform**
Koromex, Ortho Options Delfen, VCF	**Foam:** 12.5% nonoxynol-9
Ortho Options Conceptrol	**Gel:** 4% nonoxynol-9
Advantage-S	**Gel:** 3.5% nonoxynol-9
Koromex	**Gel:** 3% nonoxynol-9
K-Y Plus	**Gel:** 2.2% nonoxynol-9
Aqua Lube Plus	**Gel:** 1% nonoxynol-9
Gynol II Extra Strength Contraceptive	**Jelly:** 3% nonoxynol-9
Gynol II Contraceptive	**Jelly:** 2% nonoxynol-9
Ortho Options Ortho-Gynol	**Jelly:** 1% octoxynol-9
VCF Vaginal Contraceptive Film	**Film:** 28% nonoxynol-9
Ortho Options	**Film:** 10% nonoxynol-9
Encare, Semicid	**Vaginal inserts:** 100 mg nonoxynol-9

Products listed are representative of currently available and widely distributed brands. Similar products, including regional and private label brands, may also exist.

PATIENT INFORMATION

Spermicides

- To achieve maximum contraceptive protection, carefully follow the manufacturer's instructions for use.
- *Contraceptive foam:* Shake the aerosol canister thoroughly before use.
- Apply spermicides at least 15 minutes (but no more than 1 hour) before intercourse to ensure effectiveness. If intercourse is delayed more than 1 hour after insertion or is repeated at any time, another applicatorful must be used.
- Insert/Apply products high in the vagina, near the cervix.
- Do not douche within 6 hours after intercourse. Premature douching may dilute the spermicide and propel viable sperm into the uterus.
- Vaginal suppositories (inserts) must dissolve and be dispersed before intercourse. Vaginal contraceptive suppositories are not as effective a mechanical barrier over the cervical opening as spermicidal foams, creams, jellies, and gels.
- Do not insert vaginal contraceptive suppositories into the urinary opening (urethra) or rectum.
- Contact your pharmacist or physician if vaginal, penile, or genital burning, itching, irritation, or painful urination follow use.
- Used alone, these agents are not as effective in preventing pregnancy as oral contraceptives or certain combination methods of contraception (eg, use of a condom plus spermicide).
- If pregnancy is medically contraindicated, consult your physician for a contraception program.
- These products have not been shown to offer significant protection against sexually transmitted diseases. Condoms (male or female) are recommended to prevent transmission of such diseases.

EMERGENCY CONTRACEPTION

DEFINITION

Emergency contraception consists of short-term therapy (2 to 4 dosage units) with one of two products currently available (*Plan B* and *Preven*). Emergency contraception is to be used only to prevent pregnancy following unprotected intercourse or a known or suspected contraceptive failure (eg, condom rupture, tear, or leakage). Directions for use of emergency contraceptives (commonly referred to as the "morning after pill") must be strictly adhered to. Emergency contraception is not the same as, and should not be confused with, the controversial abortion pill, mifepristone (*Mifeprex*).

INCIDENCE

Approximately 3.2 million unintended pregnancies occur annually in the US. This figure represents about one-half of all pregnancies. Among teenagers, over 80% of pregnancies are unintended. In the US, approximately 1400 teenagers become mothers each day. Of the 3.2 million unintended pregnancies per year, approximately 50% are caused by a contraceptive failure and approximately 50% occur because no standard contraceptive method was used during intercourse. Approximately 700,000 potentially fertile couples have intercourse on any given day and use no method of contraception. One in two women 15 to 44 years of age report they have experienced an unintended pregnancy. More than 1 million unplanned pregnancies are terminated by medical abortion each year.

DIAGNOSTIC PARAMETERS/PHYSICAL ASSESSMENT

Selection of emergency contraceptive: Emergency contraceptives are available over-the-counter (OTC) in a few states, but manufacturers of emergency contraceptives plan to petition the FDA for OTC status. Pending nonprescription (OTC) status, many of the nation's more than 40,000 obstetrician-gynecologists, and other medical prescribers, believe they should offer sexually active women of childbearing age advance prescriptions for an emergency contraceptive so that it will be available in the home if and when it is needed.

Interview: In interviewing patients to determine whether an emergency contraceptive is warranted, it is appropriate to ask about the following:

- When did unprotected intercourse occur (day and hour)?
- Have more than 72 hours elapsed since unprotected intercourse occurred?
- Where were you in your menstrual cycle when unprotected intercourse occurred?
- Have you used an emergency contraceptive before? If yes, which one(s)?
- If you have used an emergency contraceptive before, did you experience any side effects?
- Are you, or do you think you are, pregnant now?

- Do you understand that the emergency contraceptive will not work if you are already pregnant? Emergency contraceptives do not induce abortions (miscarriages).

TREATMENT

EMERGENCY CONTRACEPTIVES

► Actions

The two emergency contraceptives currently available (*Plan B* and *Preven*) contain different ingredients but work the same way. *Plan B* contains only a progestin (hormone) known as levonorgestrel. *Preven* contains both a progestin (levonorgestrel) and an estrogen (ethinyl estradiol). *Preven* also is known as the Yupze regimen.

Both emergency contraceptives act by blocking the release of an egg (ovulation) from a woman's ovaries or preventing a fertilized egg from being implanted in the uterus. The emergency contraceptives will not work if a fertilized egg already has been implanted in the uterine wall.

Efficacy: If 100 women experienced unprotected intercourse during the second or third week of their menstrual cycle, when ovulation is most likely, 8 would become pregnant. Emergency contraceptives are not 100% effective. *Preven*, on average, reduces the risk of pregnancy 75%. *Plan B* reduces risk of pregnancy by about 89%.

The sooner an emergency contraceptive is taken after unprotected intercourse, the more effective it will be. *Plan B* prevents 95% of expected pregnancies if taken within 24 hours after unprotected intercourse, thus reducing the expected pregnancy rate from 8% to 0.4%. If *Plan B* treatment is delayed 25 to 48 hours, effectiveness declines to 85%. Effectiveness of both *Plan B* and *Preven* declines sharply 72 hours after unprotected intercourse. Use 72 hours after unprotected intercourse is not approved by the FDA.

Emergency contraceptives are not effective in women who are already pregnant. They do not induce an abortion (miscarriage).

► Contraindications

- Known or suspected pregnancy.
- Hypersensitivity to any component in the product.
- Undiagnosed abnormal genital bleeding.
- Use before menarche.

► Warnings

- Do not use routinely as a contraceptive.
- Not effective in terminating an existing pregnancy.
- Do not use 72 hours after unprotected intercourse.
- Contact your doctor or pharmacist if vomiting occurs within 1 hour of taking either dose of the medication. This is necessary to determine whether an antinausea medication and/or repeat dose of the emergency contraceptive are necessary.

Precautions: Emergency contraceptives do not protect against HIV infection or any other sexually transmitted disease.

Do not use during lactation.

► Drug Interactions

No clinically significant drug-drug interactions have been reported to date.

► **Adverse Reactions**

The most common adverse effects of *Plan B* and *Preven* are nausea and vomiting. The incidence of nausea with *Plan B* is approximately 25% and is substantially higher with *Preven*. Premedication with an antinausea drug (eg, *Bonine*, *Dramamine*) may be appropriate.

Other adverse effects include fatigue, headache, breast tenderness, and diarrhea.

► **Administration and Dosage**

Patients who use emergency contraceptives after unprotected intercourse should be aware of the following guidelines for proper use:

Plan B: Consists of 2 tablets, each containing 0.75 mg of the progestin levonorgestrel. The first tablet is to be followed by the second tablet 12 hours later.

Preven: Available in a kit that contains a pregnancy test and 4 tablets. Each tablet contains 0.05 mg of the estrogen ethinyl estradiol and 0.25 mg of the progestin levonorgestrel. The initial dose of 2 tablets is to be followed by the 2 remaining tablets 12 hours later. If a positive pregnancy result is obtained, the patient should not take any of the 4 pills in the kit.

EMERGENCY CONTRACEPTIVES	
Trade name	Doseform
Plan B	**Tablets:** 0.75 mg levonorgestrel. In blister packages of 2.
Preven Emergency Contraceptive Pills	**Tablets:** 0.25 mg levonorgestrel; 0.05 mg ethinyl estradiol. In blister packages of 4. Includes patient labeling.
Preven Emergency Contraceptive Kit	**Tablets:** 0.25 mg levonorgestrel; 0.05 mg ethinyl estradiol. In blister packages of 4. Includes pregnancy testing kit and detailed patient labeling.

Products listed are representative of currently available and widely distributed brands. Similar products, including regional and private label brands, may also exist.

PATIENT INFORMATION

Emergency Contraceptives

- Follow dosage instructions precisely.
- Take as soon as possible but no later than 72 hours after unprotected intercourse.
- Some people experience nausea and vomiting when taking an emergency contraceptive. If vomiting occurs within 1 hour of taking either of the 2 doses of an emergency contraceptive, contact your doctor or pharmacist. A repeat dose and/or antinausea medication may be necessary.
- Do not use routinely as a contraceptive. Discuss long-term contraceptive protection with your doctor.
- An emergency contraceptive will not terminate an existing pregnancy and should not be used in an attempt to induce an abortion.
- Do not use emergency contraceptives if pregnancy is known or suspected, during lactation, before menarche, or in the presence of undiagnosed and abnormal genital bleeding.
- Modest disruption of the next menstrual cycle may occur, but most women experience their next menses within 3 to 7 days of the expected date.
- If menses doses not occur within 3 weeks of taking an emergency contraceptive, contact your physician.
- Emergency contraceptives do not appear to impair a return to normal ovulation and fertility.
- Emergency contraceptives do not protect against HIV infection or any other sexually transmitted disease.
- Additional information on emergency contraception may be obtained from the *Plan B* Web site (www.go2planb.com), the *Preven* Web site (www.preven.com), or the Office of Population Research Web site (www.not-2-late.com). At the www.getthepill.com Web site, women can complete a questionnaire and, for a $20 fee, a doctor will call in a prescription to the patient's pharmacy. The $20 fee does not cover the cost of the prescription. Educational pamphlets on emergency contraception are available from the American College of Obstetrics and Gynecology by telephone (1-800-762-2264 ext. 830) or online (www.acog.com).

URINARY INCONTINENCE

DEFINITION

Urinary incontinence (UI) is a major health problem that often leads to disability and dependency. UI is defined as the involuntary loss of bladder control causing a problematic leakage of urine. Stress, urge, overflow, and functional UI are the most commonly occurring classifications (for a more detailed discussion on the specific types of UI, see the Pathophysiology section).

ETIOLOGY

Anatomic, physiologic, and nonurogenital abnormalities are etiologic factors in UI. UI is often caused by changes in the body due to disease; aging per se does not cause UI.

INCIDENCE

UI is often misdiagnosed by health care providers and underreported by patients. Many patients and health care providers erroneously dismiss UI as a normal part of aging because the incidence of the disorder increases with age. Patients who suffer with the condition are often too embarrassed to seek help and are unaware of available treatment options.

Data indicate approximately 13 million Americans (in community and institutional settings) suffer from UI; the annual estimated cost is over $15 billion. In the elderly, UI is estimated to afflict 1 out of 10 people 65 years of age and older and 50% or more of all long-term care residents. Caregiver data indicate similar findings: approximately 53% of the homebound elderly reportedly suffer from UI. Random sampling that evaluates persistent UI in the hospitalized elderly reveal 11% of patients are diagnosed with the problem upon admission; discharge data reveal an increase to 23%. Prevalence rates in the community of 15% to 35% have been reported in people older than 60 years of age. In this group, prevalence is two times greater in women than men.

UI can affect younger individuals. Reports from people 15 to 64 years of age indicate women are more likely to suffer from UI. Among men and women in this age group, prevalence rates range from 1.5% to 5% and 10% to 30% in men and women, respectively.

PATHOPHYSIOLOGY

Stress UI is urine leakage caused by increased abdominal pressure in the absence of a bladder contraction. Urethral hypermotility, or loss of support of the urethrovesical junction, is the most common cause. Increased intra-abdominal pressure and displacement of the urethra and bladder neck may result from this hypermotility. Outside the abdominal cavity, displacement of the bladder neck disproportionately increases bladder pressure to the increased urethral pressure.

The ensuing pressure inhibits complete closure of the internal sphincter and urine loss occurs. In females, abnormalities in the pelvic floor muscles or urethral sphincter commonly arise from pregnancy, vaginal childbirth, hysterectomy, and menopause. Prostate disorders, urethral stricture, neurologic problems, or detrusor failure are possible problems in males.

Urge UI (also referred to as overactive bladder) is the inability to delay micturition due to increased bladder contractility. Detrusor hyperreflexia often results from spontaneous bladder contractions in the presence of neurologic disease; the normal flow of messages between the brain, spinal cord, and urinary system may become disrupted. Pelvic organ prolapse in the presence of urethral blockage can result from detrusor instability and hyperreflexia. CNS disorders (eg, Parkinson's disease, multiple sclerosis, stroke), detrusor instability, obstruction, and carcinoma of the lower urinary tract can cause urge UI.

Overflow UI is urine leakage caused by an over distention of the bladder. The bladder may fail to contract because the nerves have become desensitized and unable to detect bladder fullness. The condition may manifest as a frequent dribbling. Several disease processes may cause overflow UI: Under activity of the detrusor muscle (caused by drugs, fecal impaction, diabetic neuropathy, spinal cord injury), urethral obstruction from prostate problems, and uterine prolapse.

Functional UI is leakage of urine that results from the inability to utilize the toilet properly. Causes are usually nonurogenital in origin (eg, decreased mobility, cognitive impairment). Diagnosis of functional incontinence may be difficult because patients often have mixed types of UI.

SIGNS/SYMPTOMS

Symptoms of UI include subjective complaints of involuntary loss of urine/bladder control ranging from mild leakage to uncontrollable wetting, urinary urgency, dysuria, frequency, and perineal irritation.

Each type of incontinence has its own pattern of signs and symptoms. However, individuals with mixed incontinence have a combination of signs and symptoms, which are listed below.

Urge Incontinence (Overactive Bladder)
- Tendency to wet themselves if they cannot get to the toilet immediately
- Get up frequently at night to urinate
- Urinate at least every 2 hours
- Feel they have a weak bladder; consumption of beverages seems to cause urination out of proportion to amount of fluid consumed
- Wet the bed at night

Stress Incontinence
- Leak urine when coughing, sneezing, or laughing
- Use the toilet frequently in order to avoid accidents
- Avoid exercise because of the fear of leaking urine
- Sleep through the night, but experience urinary leakage when arising
- May leak urine when getting up from a seated position

Overflow Incontinence
- Get up frequently at night to urinate
- Urination takes a long time; the stream of urine is weak with no force (ie, dribbling stream)
- Urinate small volumes and do not feel completely empty afterward
- Dribble urine throughout the day
- Feel the urge to urinate but sometimes cannot

DIAGNOSTIC PARAMETERS/PHYSICAL ASSESSMENT

Clinical Observation: Because of the nature of this disorder, observation will usually be apparent only to the patient, patient's family and friends, and caregiver. People in close contact with the patient may inquire about the persistent smell of urine or observance of wetness while in the company of the patient. UI is often a reversible disorder and may be a symptom of another disease process. All patients suspected of UI should be referred to a physician for further evaluation and physical examination.

Interview: Pharmacists may recommend products beneficial in the management of UI. Pending medical evaluation, complete a proper patient assessment and history prior to suggesting products that will aid in management of the condition. The interview should contain, but not be limited to, inquiries concerning the following:

- Onset and duration of urine leakage problems
- Difficulty making it to the toilet without an accident
- Getting up to urinate more than 2 times per night
- Urinating more than 8 times in 24 hours
- Characteristics such as stress, urge, dribbling
- Precipitating events (eg, cough, sneeze, laughter, exercise, surgery, new medications)
- Specific urinary symptoms (pain, hesitancy, urgency, frequency, hematuria, nocturia)
- Weak stream of urine and dribbling with little or no force
- Feel a need to urinate again after going to the toilet
- Experience frequent constipation
- Fluid intake amount and type
- Depression and mental status changes
- Use of protective products
- Concurrent disease states
- Nonprescription and prescription medications
- Previous treatments (if any) and their effect on UI

TREATMENT

Approaches to therapy: Treatment of UI should be designed to meet the patient's needs. After appropriate medical evaluation, the health care provider may recommend several options that consist of behavioral techniques, surgery, prescription medications, and management products.

Nondrug therapy: Behavioral techniques such as pelvic muscle exercises (ie, Kegel exercises), biofeedback, and bladder training can help control incontinence episodes. These techniques can assist the patient in recognizing when the bladder is filling and may help delay voiding until appropriate facilities are reached.

Surgery may be useful in correcting structural abnormalities (eg, abnormally positioned urinary bladder, obstruction).

Patients may benefit from the use of absorbent pads and underclothing to absorb moisture. Use of the products often allows the patient to continue daily activities without disruption or concern for embarrassing situations.

Pharmacotherapy: Medications are often prescribed to treat incontinence and will vary depending on the type and etiology of the problem. Pseudoephedrine (30 to 60 mg 3 times daily) is often used to treat stress UI. Urge and stress incontinence may benefit from imipramine (10 to 25 mg 3 times daily). Oxybutynin (2.5 to 5 mg 3 to 4 times daily) and propantheline (7.5 to 30 mg 3 times daily) are often successful in treating urge incontinence.

DISPOSABLE SHIELDS, GUARDS, AND UNDERGARMENTS

▶ **Actions**

Disposable incontinence products absorb and retain moisture. These products are usually constructed of highly absorbent materials (ie, rayon, cotton, polyester fibers); many products utilize deodorants to control odor or substances that gelatinize liquids and retain the gelled substance in the pad's matrix to prevent leakage.

▶ **Indications**

Disposable shields are worn in addition to regular underwear and are used for light incontinence and absorb 60 to 360 mL of fluid. Most products have gathered sides to prevent leakage.

Disposable guards are worn in addition to regular underwear and are used for light-to-moderate incontinence; the content of absorbent fibers used is more substantial than in disposable shields.

Disposable undergarments and briefs are used for heavy incontinence to total loss of continence control and guard against side leakage for comfortable protection. These products replace regular underwear and absorb 360 to 1100 mL of fluid.

▶ **Warnings**

Skin infections and pressure ulcers: Immobile patients with UI should be checked frequently for signs of macerated skin and skin infections. Consult a health care professional if skin becomes irritated.

Urinary tract infections: Patients with UI (especially in combination with fecal incontinence) may be at increased risk for urinary tract infections. Caution should be taken to thoroughly clean the skin. Advise patients of the signs and symptoms of urinary tract infection.

Flammable: These products do not retard flames. Avoid use near flames and other sources of ignition.

▶ **Adverse Reactions**

Hypersensitivity reactions: Many products utilize deodorants for odor control. Patients with sensitive skin may need to use fragrance-free products.

▶ **Guidelines for USe**

Read and follow instructions for use on the package labeling. Lotions and powders can jeopardize the integrity of taped fasteners; avoid contaminating taped fasteners with lotions and powders. Promptly change soiled products as soon as possible after soiling events or every 2 to 4 hours. Soiled undergarments should be disposed of in appropriate receptacles. Do not flush these products.

Guards and shields: Remove strip covering adhesive. Anchor adhesive strip on the underside of the guard/shield to underwear. Men should wear close-fitting undergarments when using incontinence guards/shields.

Disposable briefs: Disposable briefs with intact sides are worn as regular underwear. The absorbent side of the product is worn against the skin. Disposable briefs with fasteners should be snuggly fastened, but avoid fastening too tightly. Do not discard reusable fasteners.

DISPOSABLE SHIELDS, GUARDS, AND UNDERGARMENTS	
Trade name	**Description**
Depend Disposable Protective Underwear	*Absorbency:* Heavy. S/M fits waist sizes 28 to 40 inches, hip sizes 34 to 46 inches, and weights of 115 to 119 lbs. L fits waist sizes 38 to 50 inches, hip sizes 44 to 54 inches, and weights of 170 to 260 lbs. Breathable, stretch panels for close fit, elastic design, and *Ultra ABSORB-LOC* to quickly absorb liquid.
Depend Easyfit Undergarments with Elastic Leg/Adjustable Straps	*Absorbency:* Regular. Fits hip sizes up to 65 inches. Reusable velcro tabs. *Ultra ABSORB-LOC* to quickly absorb liquid, *StrongBond* fibers in absorbent core.
Depend Fitted Briefs	*Absorbency:* Regular overnight. M fits waist sizes 19 to 34 inches, hip sizes 26 to 41 inches, and weights of 110 to 170 lbs. L fits waist sizes 35 to 49 inches, hip sizes 42 to 54 inches, and weights of > 170 lb. Wetness indicator, 6 *EasyGrip* tabs for close fit, and *Ultra ABSORB-LOC* to quickly absorb liquid.
Depend Guards for Men	*Absorbency:* Light (12 inches).
Depend Undergarments with Elastic Leg/Button Straps	*Absorbency:* Regular; extra. Fits hip sizes up to 65 inches. *Ultra ABSORB-LOC* to quickly absorb liquid.
Poise Pads	*Absorbency:* Light (8 1/2 inches); Regular (8 1/2 inches); Extra (9 1/2 inches); Extra Plus (11 inches). Ultra absorbency with side shields (11 inches); Ultra Plus with side shields (13 inches). *Dry-Touch* layer and granules to quickly absorb liquid and control odors.
Serenity Bladder Control Guards	*Absorbency:* Regular; super; super plus. *Drylater Plus* for drier protection and *Odasorb* system to help control odors.
Serenity Bladder Protection Pads	*Absorbency:* Light; regular; extra; extra plus; ultra. *Drylayer Plus* for drier protection and *Odasorb* system to help control odors.

Products listed are representative of currently available and widely distributed brands. Similar products, including regional and private label brands, may also exist.

PATIENT INFORMATION
Disposable Shields, Guards, and Undergarments

- Guards and shields are anchored to regular undergarments. Male patients should wear close-fitting undergarments; boxer shorts should not be worn with guards and shields.
- Disposable undergarments that fasten at the sides may come with velcro (straps or buttons). These fasteners may be reused; do not dispose of fasteners.
- Disposable undergarments that fasten at the sides may be preferred for immobile, bedridden patients because of ease of use.
- Patients should select products that best suit their needs. For example, patients with limited mobility may have difficulty using products with fasteners.
- Inspect skin daily for changes. Contact a health care provider immediately if changes in the skin occur.
- Diaper rash products may be used to treat noninfected skin irritations.
- Discard the soiled product according to product labeling. Discard nonflushable products in appropriate receptacles.
- Advise patients and caregivers that incontinence products may be covered by insurance.
- Patients should visit their health care providers regularly and discuss alternative therapies for the treatment of UI.

REUSABLE UNDERGARMENTS

▶ Actions

There are two types of reusable undergarments available. One type of reusable undergarment is used as a supplement for incontinence guards and pads. The undergarment secures the guard/pad into place by utilizing special fasteners (ie, velcro [pouch for pad insertion]). A second type of reusable undergarment is available, which is a replacement for conventional undergarments. An absorbent, nondegradable liner is sewn into place, eliminating the need for guards and pads. Reusable undergarments are generally constructed from sturdy fabrics are able to withstand high temperatures, strong detergents and bleach, and frequent washings.

▶ Indications

Reusable undergarments provide an additional barrier against leakage and aid in active management of light-to-moderate UI problems.

▶ Warnings

Urinary tract infections: Patients with UI (especially in combination with fecal incontinence) may be at increased risk for urinary tract infections. Caution should be taken to thoroughly clean the skin. Advise patients of the signs and symptoms of urinary tract infection.

Skin irritation: Consult a health care provider if skin becomes irritated. Only use normal saline skin cleansing products on open wounds.

▶ Adverse Reactions

Hypersensitivity reactions: Patients should be capable of following the product labeling for cleaning the garment. Garments should be washed in high temperatures and bleach should be used to eliminate bacteria on soiled undergarments. Some individuals may experience contact irritant dermatitis from the use of bleach.

▶ Guidelines for Use

Read and follow instructions for use and cleaning on the package labeling. Following labeling guidelines, wash undergarment prior to first wear. Promptly change soiled products. Only wear reusable undergarments that have been properly cleaned.

REUSABLE UNDERGARMENTS	
Trade name	Description
Compose Men's Washable Brief with 3 Disposable Guards	Full cut, brief style available in M, L, and XL. Made with *ComPly* fabric for very light protection. Added protection (light-to-moderate) when worn with bladder control disposable guards.
Compose Washable Panty with 5 Disposable Pads	Full cut, brief style available in M (5 to 7), L (8 to 9), and XL (10 to 12). Made with *ComPly* fabric for very light protection. Added protection (light-to-moderate) when worn with bladder control disposable pads.

Products listed are representative of currently available and widely distributed brands. Similar products, including regional and private label brands, may also exist.

PATIENT INFORMATION

Reusable Undergarments

- Reusable undergarments should be selected for the individual (ie, men's, women's, super absorbency).
- Many products have an added moisture-proof panel for additional moisture protection.
- Reusable undergarments that function as underwear replacement should be washed and changed following one soiling event.
- Guards and pads should fit the reusable undergarment properly.
- Garments should be thoroughly dried before wearing. Damp undergarments may irritate skin, especially when strong detergent or bleach has been used.
- Diaper rash products may be used to treat noninfected skin irritations.
- Discard the soiled guard/pad according to product labeling. Discard nonflushable products in appropriate receptacles.
- Advise patients and caregivers that incontinence products may be covered by insurance.
- Patients should visit their health care providers regularly and discuss alternative therapies for the treatment of UI.

UNDERPADS (BED PADS)

▶ Actions

Immobile or bedridden patients frequently use underpads. Pads should be changed frequently and patients should receive additional skin care to prevent irritation and pressure ulcers. Underpads generally contain three layers: 1) the top layer (next to the skin surface) is designed for skin protection against moisture; 2) the inner layer is constructed of highly absorbent rayon, cotton, or polyester fibers; 3) the outer layer is usually constructed of vinyl to protect the bed or furniture from moisture.

▶ Indications

Underpads are used to protect beds, chairs, and other surfaces and provide additional protection for patients who experience nighttime incontinence. These products are often used in institutional settings, especially with immobile or bedridden patients.

▶ Warnings

Skin infections and pressure ulcers: Immobile patients with UI should be checked frequently for signs of macerated skin and skin infections. Consult a health care professional if skin becomes irritated.

Suffocation Risk: Avoid use with babies and children. Underpads are not recommended for use in cribs, playpens, etc.

Flammable: These products do not retard flames. Avoid use near flames and other sources of ignition.

▶ Adverse Reactions

Hypersensitivity reactions: Many products utilize deodorants for odor control. Patients with sensitive skin may need to utilize fragrance-free products.

▶ Guidelines for Use

Read and follow instructions for use and cleaning on the package labeling. Unfold the clean, dry underpad and place lengthwise on a dry bed, chair, or other surface. Position the absorbent surface facing up and waterproof surface against the bed, chair, or other surface. Check the pad frequently for soiling. Promptly change soiled products to avoid skin irritation. Change the pad after each soiling event or every 2 to 4 hours. Dispose of soiled underpads in the appropriate receptacles. Do not flush disposable underpads.

UNDERPADS	
Trade name	**Description**
Depend Bed Size Underpads	Heavy absorbency. Three layers of absorbent material; stay-dry liner; waterproof backing.
Sure Care Underpads, Extra Large	Heavy absorbency.

Products listed are representative of currently available and widely distributed brands. Similar products, including regional and private label brands, may also exist.

PATIENT INFORMATION

Underpads

- Caregivers, relatives, and friends of patients in long-term care facilities should inquire about incontinence care guidelines. Check the patient for pressure sores and skin infections.
- Diaper rash products may be used to treat noninfected skin irritations.
- Discard the soiled product according to product labeling. Discard nonflushable products in appropriate receptacles.
- Advise patients and caregivers that incontinence products may be covered by insurance.
- Patients should visit their health care providers regularly and discuss alternative therapies for the treatment of UI.

MUSCULOSKELETAL CONDITIONS

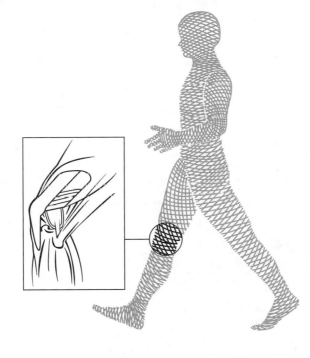

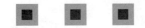

NONPRESCRIPTION DRUG THERAPY
TABLE OF CONTENTS

■ ■ ■

MUSCULOSKELETAL CONDITIONS

INTRODUCTION

Nearly every person has experienced some type of common musculoskeletal condition. Conditions such as aches and pains, sprains and strains, arthralgia, myalgia, and mysterious leg cramps are uncomfortable, painful, and often result in the inability to perform daily tasks. Prevention, acute care, and long-term treatment are all areas that can be discussed with patients who are experiencing or have experienced these conditions.

From accidents around the home or workplace to the weekend athlete, musculoskeletal conditions occur in a large number of patients but often go unreported or untreated (or are mistreated). Many patients are willing to simply "live with the pain." However, it is important to encourage patients to seek treatment or therapy, because there are several options available that can minimize the discomfort and help in recovery. Left untreated, some conditions can result in permanent impairment; therefore, patients need to understand the nature of the condition or injury to make an informed decision regarding the course of treatment. This may involve non-drug therapy such as ice or heat or stretching and exercise, the use of nonprescription analgesics or anti-inflammatories, or a visit to the physician with the potential for physical therapy.

Health care providers need to understand the nature of the condition and how the condition occurred. This is an important step in discussing the options with the patient. For example, differentiating strains and sprains, as well as differentiating the severity of the sprain or strain (ie, partial vs full tear of the muscle, tendon, or ligament) will determine the proper course of therapy. It is not always appropriate to recommend ice and analgesics to treat an injury. A full evaluation is necessary, because more severe conditions require referral, or in the case of osteoarthritis, the condition is chronic and needs to be handled with proper stretching, exercise, posture, and potentially, nonprescription or prescription drug therapy.

The general complaint of aches and pains can be a significant diagnostic and therapeutic challenge for health care providers. Often, the patient is unable to locate the exact source of the pain and may have trouble describing where the pain or discomfort is occurring. Sometimes a painful area is the result of pain radiating from an injury or condition in another part of the body. A classic example of this situation is pain, numbness, or tingling in the legs, which is the result of a lower back disorder. In addition, some patients cannot recall the specific situation that resulted in the pain. These issues pose a significant challenge when attempting to counsel a patient with non-specific complaints of pain or discomfort. The main goal is to ask proper questions and conduct an appropriate physical assessment to try to determine the proper course of treatment.

If it is determined that proper therapy for the musculoskeletal condition is the use of an OTC analgesic or anti-inflammatory agent, then the recommendation of the appropriate agent is the next crucial step in the process. Acetaminophen, salicylates (eg, aspirin), and nonsteroidal anti-inflammatory drugs (NSAIDs; ibuprofen, naproxen, and ketoprofen are the only agents from this class currently approved for OTC use) are available OTC that could be recommended based on the condition to be treated, as well as the patient's specific needs. While all 3 groups are analgesics and antipyretics, only the salicylates and NSAIDs are also anti-inflammatories. Each agent has a role in treating these conditions but must be chosen following a proper interview of the patient, taking into account concurrent conditions and medications. Although available without a prescription, these medications have adverse reactions and drug interaction potential that must be considered before a recommendation can be made. It is also important to note labeling restrictions pertaining to dosing and length of therapy.

Musculoskeletal conditions can range from mild to severe, but each situation must be handled individually, taking into account the age of the patient, the nature of the injury, the location, the situation that resulted in the condition, etc. An informed decision can be made with this data by both the health care provider and the patient in regard to the most appropriate course of therapy. Treat each and every occurrence as a unique situation that has no standard course of treatment. Pain tolerance varies greatly from patient to patient, so a minor complaint by a person does not necessarily indicate a minor condition. Although musculoskeletal pain is one of the most challenging areas to diagnose and treat, the patient can benefit greatly by appropriate care and counseling.

ACHES AND PAINS

DEFINITION

Pain is defined as an unpleasant sensation that is localized to a particular area of the body. Pain complaints are the most common reason for visits to physicians.

ETIOLOGY

Acute pain is a biological signal of potential or actual tissue injury and is usually short-lived but can develop into chronic pain. Chronic pain is defined as pain lasting for 3 to 6 months or more. The cause may be a painful disease (eg, arthritis, cancer, migraine headaches, diabetic neuropathy) for which there is no cure.

INCIDENCE

Most individuals experience pain several times a year. It is estimated that more than 50 million Americans are either partially or totally disabled by pain.

PATHOPHYSIOLOGY

The pain process involves a complex series of afferent and efferent neuronal connections. The sensation of pain is initiated by the stimulation of nociceptors that synapse in the spinal cord and travel to the brain. The threshold for pain decreases, and the intensity of pain increases with anxiety, depression, fear, anger, or fatigue.

SIGNS/SYMPTOMS

Pain of moderate-to-severe intensity may often be associated with anxiety. A stress response (increased blood pressure and heart rate, pupil dilation) is commonly seen with acute pain. With chronic pain, the stress response is typically not seen and there are often vegetative signs (eg, sleep disturbances, decreased appetite, loss of taste for food, decreased libido, constipation); signs of depression are not uncommon.

DIAGNOSTIC PARAMETERS/PHYSICAL ASSESSMENT

Clinical Observation: To determine effective treatment, it is important to obtain a proper assessment, comprehensive history, and accurate diagnosis of the cause of pain. Examine the painful area for deep tenderness to determine if the pain is localized to the muscle, ligaments, or joints. Evaluate the patient for nerve damage (eg, sensory impairment, oversensitive skin, weakness, or muscle atrophy). The diagnosis of chronic pain is often a challenge; rule out depression in these patients. Physical pain is usually localized, well described, and relieved by proper treatment; this is not true with psychogenic pain.

Interview: To ensure the proper diagnosis and treatment, it may be beneficial to ask the patient about the following:

- Onset, duration, and location of the pain.
- Quality and nature of the pain.
- The severity of the pain using a 10-point rating scale where the patient quantifies the intensity of pain (0 = no pain to 10 = most intense pain).
- Factors that relieve or exacerbate the pain.
- Patient's medical history (including recent illness, injury, or surgery).
- Patient's medication profile.

TREATMENT

Approaches to therapy: The ideal approach to treating pain is to remove the cause, if possible. Managing chronic pain can be more challenging. There are a variety of non-drug techniques and pharmacotherapies that can be used to alleviate pain. Question the patient about therapies that have been tried and how effective they were.

Nondrug therapy: Relaxation, mental imagery, hypnosis, and biofeedback have all been used to relieve pain. Improved sleeping patterns can help alleviate chronic pain.

Pharmacotherapy: Drugs that are effective for relieving pain include aspirin, acetaminophen, and nonsteroidal anti-inflammatory drugs (NSAIDs).

SALICYLATES

▶ Actions

The anti-inflammatory and analgesic activity of salicylates may be mediated through inhibition of the prostaglandin synthetase complex.

▶ Indications

For the treatment of mild-to-moderate pain. These agents have other labeled indications as well.

▶ Contraindications

Hypersensitivity to salicylates or nonsteroidal anti-inflammatory drugs (NSAIDs). Use with extreme caution in patients with a history of adverse reactions to salicylates. Cross-sensitivity may exist between aspirin and other NSAIDs that inhibit prostaglandin synthesis, and between aspirin and tartrazine. Aspirin cross-sensitivity does not appear to occur with sodium salicylate, or salicylamide. Aspirin hypersensitivity is more prevalent in those with asthma, nasal polyposis, or chronic urticaria.

Also contraindicated in patients with hemophilia or bleeding ulcers, or those in hemorrhagic states. Magnesium salicylate is contraindicated in patients with advanced chronic renal insufficiency.

▶ Warnings

Concurrent medications: Many other medications, specifically multi-ingredient cough and cold products, also contain aspirin or acetaminophen. It is important to advise patients of this possibility, and to inquire about other medications they might be taking before recommending an analgesic.

Otic effects: Discontinue use if dizziness, ringing in ears (tinnitus), or impaired hearing occurs. Tinnitus probably represents blood salicylic acid levels reaching or exceeding the upper limit of the therapeutic range; therefore, it is a helpful guide to toxicity. Temporary hearing loss disappears gradually upon discontinuation of the drug.

Hypersensitivity: Do not use if there is a history of sensitivity to aspirin or NSAIDs. Aspirin intolerance, manifested by acute bronchospasm, generalized urticaria/angioedema, severe rhinitis, or shock occurs in 4% to 19% of asthmatics. Symptoms occur within 3 hours after ingestion.

Foods may contribute to a reaction. Some foods with high salicylate content include curry powder, paprika, licorice, Benedictine liqueur, prunes, raisins, tea, and gherkins. A typical American diet contains 10 to 200 mg/day salicylate.

Hepatic function impairment: Use with caution in patients with liver damage, preexisting hypoprothrombinemia, and vitamin K deficiency.

GI effects: Use with caution in patients who are intolerant to salicylates because of GI irritation, and in those with gastric ulcers, peptic ulcers, mild diabetes, gout, erosive gastritis, or bleeding tendencies.

Hematologic effects: Aspirin interferes with hemostasis. Avoid use in patients with severe anemia, history of blood coagulation defects, or who take anticoagulants.

Pregnancy: Category D (aspirin); *Category C* (salsalate, magnesium salicylate, other salicylates). Aspirin may produce adverse effects in the mother, such as anemia, ante- or postpartum hemorrhage, or prolonged gestation and labor. Salicylates readily cross the placenta. By inhibiting prostaglandin synthesis, salicylates may cause constriction of ductus arteriosus, and, possibly, other untoward fetal effects. Maternal aspirin use during later stages of pregnancy may cause adverse fetal effects, such as low birth weight, increased incidence of intracranial hemorrhage in premature infants, stillbirth, or neonatal death. Salicylates may be teratogens. Avoid use during pregnancy, especially in the third trimester.

Lactation: Salicylates are excreted in breast milk in low concentrations. Adverse effects on platelet function in the nursing infant are a potential risk. The American Academy of Pediatrics recommends that aspirin be used cautiously in nursing mothers.

Children: Administration of aspirin to children, including teenagers, with acute febrile illness due to chickenpox and influenza has been associated with the development of Reye syndrome.

▶ **Drug Interactions**

Salicylate Drug Interactions			
Precipitant drug	**Object drug***		**Description**
Charcoal, activated	Aspirin	↓	Coadministration decreases aspirin absorption, depending on charcoal dose and interval between ingestion.
Urinary acidifiers	Salicylates	↑	Ammonium chloride, ascorbic acid, and methionine decrease salicylate excretion.
Antacids, urinary alkalinizers	Salicylates	↓	Decreased pharmacologic effects of salicylates may occur. The magnitude of the antacid interaction depends on the agent, dose, and pretreatment urine pH.

Salicylate Drug Interactions			
Precipitant drug	Object drug*		Description
Carbonic anhydrase inhibitors	Salicylates	⟷	Salicylate intoxication has occurred after coadministration of these agents. However, salicylic acid renal elimination may be increased by these drugs if urine is kept alkaline. Conversely, salicylates may displace acetazolamide from protein-binding sites, resulting in toxicity. Further study is needed.
Corticosteroids	Salicylates	↓	Corticosteroids increase salicylate clearance and decrease salicylate serum levels.
Nizatidine	Salicylates	↑	Increased serum salicylate levels have occurred in patients receiving high doses (3.9 g/day) of aspirin and concurrent nizatidine.
Salicylates	Alcohol	↑	The risk of GI ulceration increases when salicylates are given concomitantly. Ingestion of alcohol during salicylate therapy may also prolong bleeding time.
Salicylates	Angiotensin-converting enzyme inhibitors	↓	Antihypertensive effectiveness of these agents may be decreased by concurrent salicylate administration, possibly due to prostaglandin inhibition. Consider discontinuing salicylates if problems occur.
Aspirin	Heparin	↑	Aspirin can increase the risk of bleeding in heparin anticoagulated patients.
Salicylates	Loop diuretics	↓	Loop diuretics may be less effective when given with salicylates in patients with compromised renal function or with cirrhosis with ascites; however, data conflict.
Salicylates	Methotrexate	↑	Salicylates increase drug levels, causing toxicity by interfering with protein binding and renal elimination of the antimetabolite.
Aspirin	Nitroglycerin	↑	Nitroglycerin, when taken with aspirin, may result in unexpected hypotension. Data are limited. If hypotension occurs, reduce the nitroglycerin dose.
Aspirin	NSAIDs	↓	Aspirin may decrease NSAID serum concentrations. Avoid concomitant use; it offers no therapeutic advantage and may significantly increase incidence of GI effects.
Salicylates	Probenecid, sulfinpyrazone	⟷	Salicylates antagonize the uricosuric effect. While salicylates in large doses (> 3 g/day) have a uricosuric effect, smaller amounts may reduce the uricosuric effect of these agents.
Salicylates	Spironolactone	↓	Salicylates may inhibit the diuretic effects; antihypertensive action does not appear altered. Effects depend on the dose of spironolactone.
Salicylates	Sulfonylureas, exogenous insulin	↑	Salicylates in doses > 2 g/day have a hypoglycemic action, perhaps by altering pancreatic beta-cell function. They may potentiate the glucose-lowering effect of these drugs.
Aspirin	Valproic acid	↑	Aspirin displaces valproic acid from its protein-binding sites and may decrease its total body clearance, thus increasing the pharmacological effects.

* ↑ = Object drug increased. ↓ = Object drug decreased. ⟷ = Undetermined clinical effect.

► **Adverse Reactions**

Adverse reactions can be seen in the following body systems: GI (nausea, dyspepsia, heartburn, epigastric discomfort), hematologic (prolonged bleeding time, leukopenia, thrombocytopenia, purpura, decreased plasma iron concentration, shortened erythrocyte survival time), and dermatologic (rash, hives, and angioedema may occur, especially in patients suffering from chronic urticaria). Additional miscellaneous adverse reactions that have occurred include fever, thirst, and dimness of vision.

Allergic and anaphylactic reactions have been noted when hypersensitive individuals took aspirin. Fatal anaphylactic shock, while not common, has been reported.

Aspirin has an irreversible effect on platelet aggregation for the life of the platelet (approximately 7 days).

▶ Overdosage

Symptoms: The approximate acute lethal dose for adults is 10 to 30 g, and for children, 4 g. Respiratory alkalosis is seen initially in acute salicylate ingestions. Hyperpnea and tachypnea occur as a result of increased CO_2 production and a direct stimulatory effect of salicylate on the respiratory center. Other symptoms may include nausea, vomiting, hypokalemia, tinnitus, neurologic abnormalities (eg, disorientation, irritability, hallucinations, lethargy, stupor, coma, seizures), dehydration, hyperthermia, hyperventilation, hyperactivity, thrombocytopenia, platelet dysfunction, hypoprothrombinemia, increased capillary fragility, and other hematologic abnormalities. Symptoms may progress quickly to depression, coma, respiratory failure and collapse. Chronic salicylate toxicity may occur when more than 100 mg/kg/day is ingested for 2 days or longer. It is more difficult to recognize than acute overdosage and is associated with increased morbidity and mortality. Compared with acute poisoning, hyperventilation, dehydration, systemic acidosis, and severe CNS manifestations occur more frequently.

Treatment: Initial treatment includes induction of emesis or gastric lavage to remove any unabsorbed drug from the stomach. Activated charcoal diminishes salicylate absorption most effectively if given within 2 hours after ingestion. It is important to contact a local poison control center or emergency room if overdosage is suspected.

ASPIRIN

▶ Administration and Dosage

Adults: 325 to 650 mg orally every 4 hours as needed. Some extra-strength products recommend 500 mg every 3 hours or 1000 mg every 6 hours.

Children: The oral analgesic/antipyretic dosage is 10 to 15 mg/kg/dose every 4 hours (see table), up to 60 to 80 mg/kg/day. Do not use in children or teenagers with chickenpox or "flu" symptoms due to the possibility of Reye syndrome. Dosage recommendations by age and weight are as follows:

Recommended Aspirin Dosage in Children					
Age (years)	Weight		Dosage (mg every 4 hours)	No. of 81 mg tablets (every 4 hours)	No. of 325 mg tablets (every 4 hours)
	lbs	kg			
2-3	24-35	10.6-15.9	162	2	½
4-5	36-47	16-21.4	243	3	N/A
6-8	48-59	21.5-26.8	324	4	1
9-10	60-71	26.9-32.3	405	5	N/A
11	72-95	32.4-43.2	486	6	1½
12-14	≥ 96	≥ 43.3	648	8	2

ASPIRIN PRODUCTS	
Trade name	Doseform
Original Bayer, Norwich Aspirin	**Tablets**: 325 mg
Bayer Children's Chewable Aspirin	**Tablets, chewable**: 81 mg. Dextrose, saccharin. Cherry and orange flavors.
Adult Low Strength Ecotrin, Halfprin 81[1]	**Tablets, enteric coated**: 81 mg. Talc.
Halfprin 162	**Tablets, enteric coated**: 162 mg. Lactose, talc.
Ecotrin Regular Strength	**Tablets, enteric coated**: 325 mg. Talc.
Norwich Maximum Strength	**Tablets, enteric coated**: 500 mg
Ecotrin Maximum Strength	**Tablets, enteric coated**: 500 mg. Talc.
Alka-Seltzer Original Effervescent Antacid and Pain Relief Medicine	**Tablets, effervescent**: 325 mg, 1000 mg citric acid, 1916 mg sodium bicarbonate
Bayer Women's Aspirin Plus Calcium	**Caplets**: 81 mg, 300 mg calcium. Lactose, mineral oil.
Original Bayer	**Caplets**: 325 mg
Extra Strength Bayer PM Aspirin Plus Sleep Aid	**Caplets**: 500 mg, 25 mg diphenhydramine HCl
Extra Strength Bayer Aspirin	**Caplets, coated**: 500 mg
Extra Strength Bayer Back and Body Pain	**Caplets, coated**: 500 mg, 32.5 mg caffeine
Extra Strength Bayer Arthritis Pain Regimen	**Caplets, enteric coated**: 500 mg
Original Bayer	**Gelcaps**: 325 mg. Parabens, sorbitol, glycerin.
Extra Strength Bayer Aspirin	**Gelcaps, coated**: 500 mg. Parabens, glycerin.
BUFFERED ASPIRIN PRODUCTS	
Adprin-B	**Tablets, coated**: 325 mg with calcium carbonate, magnesium carbonate, magnesium oxide
Regular Strength Ascriptin	**Tablets, coated**: 325 mg with 50 mg magnesium hydroxide, 50 mg aluminum hydroxide, calcium carbonate. Talc.
Bufferin	**Tablets, coated**: 325 mg with 158 mg calcium carbonate, 63 mg magnesium oxide, 34 mg magnesium carbonate. Mineral oil, sorbitol, citric acid.
Extra Strength Adprin-B	**Tablets, coated**: 500 mg with calcium carbonate, magnesium carbonate, magnesium oxide.
Bayer Adult Low Strength	**Caplets**: 81 mg, buffered with 250 mg calcium carbonate
Extra Strength Bayer Plus	**Caplets**: 500 mg with calcium carbonate, magnesium carbonate, magnesium oxide
Maximum Strength Ascriptin	**Caplets, coated**: 500 mg with 80 mg magnesium hydroxide, 80 mg aluminum hydroxide, calcium carbonate. Saccharin, sorbitol, talc.

Products listed are representative of currently available and widely distributed brands. Similar products, including regional and private label brands, may also exist.

[1] Also contains lactose.

PATIENT INFORMATION
Aspirin
- Severe or recurrent pain may indicate a serious illness. Consult a physician.
- Patient instructions accompany each product. Have the patient read these instructions carefully before use, preferably before leaving the pharmacy, in case of any questions.
- May cause GI upset; take with or after meals. Enteric coated products may prevent or reduce stomach/GI distress.
- Do not use in children or adolescents because of the potential development of Reye syndrome.
- Take with a full glass of water (240 mL) to reduce the risk of lodging the medication in the esophagus.
- Avoid taking antacids within 2 hours of taking enteric coated tablets.
- Have patients allergic to tartrazine dye avoid aspirin.
- Notify physician if rash, difficult breathing, ringing in the ears, or persistent GI pain occurs. Internal bleeding may occur with no GI symptoms and may be indicated by bloody or black stools.
- Inform physician or dentist of aspirin use before surgery or dental care.
- Do not use aspirin if it has a strong vinegar-like odor. This suggests deterioration of aspirin and loss of potency.

MAGNESIUM SALICYLATE

▶ **Actions**

Magnesium salicylate is a sodium-free salicylate derivative that may have a low incidence of GI upset.

▶ **Contraindications**

Magnesium salicylate is contraindicated in patients with advanced chronic renal insufficiency due to magnesium retention.

▶ **Warnings**

The possibility of magnesium toxicity exists in patients with renal insufficiency.

▶ **Administration and Dosage**

Product labeling and dosages are expressed as magnesium salicylate anhydrous.

Adults: Usual dose is 650 mg every 4 hours or 1 g every 6 hours up to 4 g/day.

Children: Safety and efficacy for use in children have not been established.

MAGNESIUM SALICYLATE PRODUCTS	
Trade name	Doseform
Regular Strength Doan's	**Caplets**: 377 mg
Extra Strength Doan's	**Caplets**: 580 mg
Extra Strength Doan's P.M.	**Caplets**: 580 mg, 25 mg diphenhydramine HCl. Talc.

Products listed are representative of currently available and widely distributed brands. Similar products, including regional and private label brands, may also exist.

PATIENT INFORMATION

Magnesium Salicylate

- Do not use these products if you have renal insufficiency.
- Severe or recurrent pain may indicate a serious illness. Consult a physician.
- Patient instructions accompany each product. Have the patient read these instructions carefully before use, preferably before leaving the pharmacy, in case of any questions.
- May cause GI upset; take with food or after meals.
- Do not use in children or adolescents because of the potential development of Reye syndrome.
- Notify physician if rash, difficult breathing, ringing in the ears, or persistent GI pain occurs. Internal bleeding may occur with no GI symptoms and may be indicated by bloody or black stools.

ACETAMINOPHEN (APAP)

▶ Actions

Generally, the antipyretic and analgesic effects of APAP and aspirin are comparable; however, the site and mechanism of the analgesic effect of acetaminophen are unclear.

▶ Indications

For the treatment of mild-to-moderate pain. Also used as an analgesic-antipyretic in the presence of aspirin allergy, and in patients with blood coagulation disorders who are being treated with oral anticoagulants, bleeding diatheses (eg, hemophilia), upper GI disease (eg, ulcer, gastritis, hiatal hernia), and gouty arthritis. This agent has other labeled indications as well.

▶ Contraindications

Hypersensitivity to acetaminophen.

▶ Warnings

Concurrent medications: Many other medications, specifically multi-ingredient cough and cold products, also contain aspirin or acetaminophen. It is important to advise patients of this possibility, and to inquire about other medications they might be taking before recommending an analgesic.

Hepatotoxicity: Hepatotoxicity and severe hepatic failure occurred in chronic alcoholics following therapeutic doses. The hepatotoxicity may be caused by induction of hepatic microsomal enzymes, resulting in an increase in toxic metabolites, or by the reduced amount of glutathione responsible for conjugating toxic metabolites. A safe dose for chronic alcohol abusers has not been determined. Caution chronic alcoholics and those consuming alcohol on a daily basis to limit acetaminophen intake to up to 2 g/day.

Pregnancy: Category B. Acetaminophen crosses the placenta, but has been routinely used in all stages of pregnancy. When used in therapeutic doses, it appears safe for short-term use.

Lactation: APAP is excreted in low amounts, but no adverse effects have been reported. The American Academy of Pediatrics considers acetaminophen to be compatible with breastfeeding.

Children: Consult a physician before using in children under 3 years of age.

▶ Drug Interactions

Acetaminophen Drug Interactions			
Precipitant drug	Object drug*		Description
Alcohol, ethyl	APAP	↑	Hepatotoxicity has occurred in chronic alcohol-ics following various dose levels (moderate-to-excessive) of acetaminophen.
Anticholinergics	APAP	↔	The onset of acetaminophen effect may be delayed or decreased slightly, but the ultimate pharmacological effect is not significantly affected by anticholinergics.
Beta-blockers, propranolol	APAP	↑	Propranolol appears to inhibit the enzyme systems responsible for glucuronidation and oxidation of acetaminophen. Therefore, the pharmacologic effects of acetaminophen may be increased.
Charcoal, activated	APAP	↓	Reduces acetaminophen absorption when administered as soon as possible after overdose.
Contraceptives, oral	APAP	↓	Increase in glucuronidation resulting in increased plasma clearance and a decreased half-life of acetaminophen.
Probenecid	APAP	↑	Probenecid may increase the therapeutic effectiveness of acetaminophen slightly.
APAP	Lamotrigine	↓	Serum lamotrigine concentrations may be reduced, producing a decrease in therapeutic effects.
APAP	Loop diuretics	↓	The effects of the loop diuretic may be decreased because APAP may decrease renal prostaglandin excretion and decrease plasma renin activity.
APAP	Zidovudine	↓	The pharmacologic effects of zidovudine may be decreased because of enhanced nonhepatic or renal clearance of zidovudine.

* ↑ = Object drug increased. ↓ = Object drug decreased. ↔ = Undetermined clinical effect.

The potential hepatotoxicity of acetaminophen may be increased by large doses or long-term administration of barbiturates, carbamazepine, hydantoins, rifampin, and sulfinpyrazone. The therapeutic effects of acetaminophen may also be decreased.

▶ Adverse Reactions

When used as directed, acetaminophen rarely causes severe toxicity or side effects. However, the following adverse reactions have been reported:

Hematologic: Hemolytic anemia; neutropenia; leukopenia; pancytopenia; thrombocytopenia.

Miscellaneous: Fever; hypoglycemia; jaundice; rash.

▶ Overdosage

Symptoms: Acute poisoning may be manifested by nausea, vomiting, drowsiness, confusion, liver tenderness, low blood pressure, cardiac arrhythmias, jaundice, and acute hepatic and renal failure. These occur within the first 24 hours and may persist for 1 week or longer. Death has occurred because of liver necrosis. Acute renal failure may also occur. However, there are often no specific early symptoms or signs. The course of acetaminophen poisoning is divided into 4 stages (postingestion time):

Stage 1 (12 to 24 hours) – Nausea, vomiting, diaphoresis, anorexia.

Stage 2 (24 to 48 hours) – Clinically improved; AST, bilirubin, and prothrombin levels begin to rise.

Stage 3 (72 to 96 hours) – Peak hepatotoxicity; AST of 20,000 not unusual.

Stage 4 (7 to 8 days) – Recovery.

Hepatotoxicity may result. The minimal toxic dose is 10 g (140 mg/kg), but liver damage has occurred with a single 5.85 g dose; doses of 20 to 25 g or more are potentially fatal. Children appear less susceptible to toxicity than adults because they have less capacity for glucuronidation metabolism. Initial signs of toxicity may include nausea, vomiting, anorexia, malaise, diaphoresis, abdominal pain, and diarrhea. Hepatotoxicity is usually not apparent for 48 to 72 hours. Hepatic failure may lead to encephalopathy, coma, and death.

Plasma acetaminophen levels over 300 mcg/mL at 4 hours postingestion were associated with hepatic damage in 90% of patients; minimal hepatic damage is anticipated if plasma levels at 4 hours are less than 120 mcg/mL or under 30 mcg/mL at 12 hours after ingestion.

Chronic excessive use (over 4 g/day) may lead to transient hepatotoxicity. The kidneys may undergo tubular necrosis; the myocardium may be damaged.

Treatment: Perform gastric lavage in all cases, preferably within 4 hours of ingestion. Refer also to General Management of Acute Overdosage. It is important to contact a local poison control center or emergency room if overdosage is suspected.

▶ Administration and Dosage

Adults: 325 to 650 mg orally every 4 hours, or 1 g 3 to 4 times daily as needed. Do not exceed 4 g daily for all formulations containing acetaminophen.

Children: The usual oral dose is 10 mg/kg/dose, which may be repeated 4 to 5 times daily as needed. Do not exceed 5 doses in 24 hours.

Acetaminophen Dosage for Children			
Age	Dosage (mg)	Age	Dosage (mg)
0-3 months	40	6-8 years	320
4-11 months	80	9-10 years	400
1- 2 years	120	11 years	480
2-3 years	160	12-14 years	640
4-5 years	240	> 14 years	650

Suppositories:

Adults – 650 mg every 4 to 6 hours; do not exceed 4 g in 24 hours.

Children (3 to 11 months of age) – 80 mg every 6 hours.

(1 to 3 years of age) – 80 mg every 4 hours.

(3 to 6 years of age) – 120 to 125 mg every 4 to 6 hours; do not exceed 720 mg in 24 hours.

(6 to 12 years of age) – 325 mg every 4 to 6 hours; do not exceed 2.6 g in 24 hours.

Storage: Store suppositories below 27°C (80°F) or refrigerate. Store tablets and oral solutions at 15° to 30°C (59° to 86°F).

ACETAMINOPHEN PRODUCTS

Trade name	Doseform
Junior Strength Tylenol	**Tablets**: 160 mg. Aspartame (6 mg phenylala-nine).
Regular Strength Tylenol	**Tablets**: 325 mg
Aspirin Free Anacin Maximum Strength, Extra Strength Tylenol[1], Panadol	**Tablets**: 500 mg
Tylenol Extended Relief	**Tablets**: 650 mg
Children's Panadol, Children's Tylenol, Children's Tylenol Soft Chews	**Tablets, chewable**: 80 mg
Junior Strength Tylenol	**Tablets, chewable**: 160 mg
Meda-Cap	**Capsules**: 500 mg
Extra Strength Tylenol	**Gelcaps**: 500 mg
Extra Strength Tylenol	**Geltabs**: 500 mg
Infants' FeverAll	**Suppositories**: 80 mg
Children's FeverAll	**Suppositories**: 120 mg
Junior Strength FeverAll	**Suppositories**: 325 mg
Acephen	**Suppositories**: 650 mg
Children's Silapap	**Elixir**: 80 mg/2.5 mL. Alcohol free.
Children's Tylenol[3]	**Elixir**: 80 mg/2.5 mL. Alcohol free.
Aceta	**Elixir**: 120 mg/5 mL
Infants' Tylenol Concentrated Drops[4]	**Liquid**: 80 mg/0.8 mL. Alcohol free.
Extra Strength Tylenol[5]	**Liquid**: 500 mg/15 mL. 7% alcohol.
Liquiprin Drops for Children	**Solution**: 80 mg/1.66 mL. Alcohol free.
Infants' Panadol Drops[2], Infants' Silapap Drops, Infants' Tylenol Drops[4]	**Solution**: 80 mg/0.8 mL. Alcohol free.
Children's Tylenol Liquid	**Suspension**: 80 mg/2.5 mL
Tempra	**Syrup**: 160 mg/5 mL

Products listed are representative of currently available and widely distributed brands. Similar products, including regional and private label brands, may also exist.

[1] Gelatin coated.
[2] Contains saccharin.
[3] Contains butylparaben, sorbitol, and sucrose.
[4] Contains butylparaben, saccharin, and sorbitol.
[5] Contains sorbitol and sucrose.

PATIENT INFORMATION

Acetaminophen

- Severe or recurrent pain may indicate a serious illness. Consult a physician.
- Patient instructions accompany each product. Have the patient read these instructions carefully before use, preferably before leaving the pharmacy, in case of any questions.
- Do not exceed the recommended dosage. Do not exceed a total dose of 4 g/day of acetaminophen in all formulations consumed (2 g/day in regular alcohol users).
- Consult a physician for use in a child under 3 years of age.
- Do not take acetaminophen for longer than 5 days (children) or longer than 10 days (adults) for pain relief. If symptoms persist, worsen, or if new symptoms develop, contact a physician.
- Avoid alcohol and aspirin while taking this drug.

NONSTEROIDAL ANTI-INFLAMMATORY DRUGS

► Actions

Nonsteroidal anti-inflammatory drugs (NSAIDs) have analgesic, anti-inflammatory, and antipyretic activities. Their exact mode of action is unknown. The major mechanism of action of NSAIDs is believed to be inhibition of cyclooxygenase (COX) activity and prostaglandin synthesis. Other mechanisms, such as inhibition of lipoxygenase, leukotriene synthesis, lysosomal enzyme release, neutrophil aggregation, and various cell-membrane functions, may exist as well.

NSAIDs are capable of inhibiting the enzyme COX. COX allows the conversion of arachidonic acid into prostaglandins, which are mediators of the inflammatory response. Prostaglandin inhibition peripherally at the site of injury can decrease the inflammatory response and pain. Prostaglandin inhibition centrally can also result in analgesia similar to other centrally acting drugs such as acetaminophen. NSAIDs may also have a direct inhibiting effect on inflammatory cells.

► Indications

For the treatment of mild-to-moderate pain. These agents have other labeled indications as well.

These agents are particularly helpful for pain associated with inflammation.

► Contraindications

NSAID hypersensitivity: Because of potential cross-sensitivity to other NSAIDs, do not give these agents to patients in whom aspirin, iodides, or other NSAIDs have induced symptoms of asthma, rhinitis, urticaria, nasal polyps, angioedema, bronchospasm, and other symptoms of allergic or anaphylactoid reactions.

► Warnings

Acute renal insufficiency: Patients with preexisting renal disease or compromised renal perfusion are at greatest risk. A form of renal toxicity seen in patients with prerenal conditions leads to reduced renal blood flow or blood volume. NSAID use may cause a dose-dependent reduction in prostaglandin formation and precipitate renal decompensation. Patients at greatest risk are the elderly, premature infants, those with heart failure, renal or hepatic dysfunction, systemic lupus erythematosus (SLE), chronic glomerulonephritis, and those taking diuretics. Recovery usually follows discontinuation.

Hypersensitivity: Severe hypersensitivity reactions with fever, rash, abdominal pain, headache, nausea, vomiting, signs of liver damage, and meningitis have occurred in patients taking ibuprofen, especially those with SLE or other collagen diseases. Anaphylactoid reactions have occurred in patients with aspirin hypersensitivity.

Renal function impairment: NSAID metabolites are eliminated primarily by the kidneys; use with caution in patients with renal impairment. Reduce dosage to avoid excessive accumulation.

Platelet aggregation: NSAIDs can inhibit platelet aggregation; the effect is quantitatively less and of shorter duration than that seen with aspirin. These agents prolong bleeding time (within normal range) in healthy subjects. This may be exaggerated in patients with underlying hemostatic defects; use with caution in people with intrinsic coagulation defects and in those on anticoagulant therapy.

Cardiovascular effects: May cause fluid retention and peripheral edema. Use caution in compromised cardiac function, hypertension, or other conditions predisposing to fluid retention. Agents may be associated with significant deterioration of circulatory hemodynamics in severe heart failure and hyponatremia, presumably due to inhibition of prostaglandin-dependent compensatory mechanisms.

Infection: NSAIDs may mask the usual signs of infection. Use with extra care in the presence of existing controlled infection.

Photosensitivity: Photosensitivity may occur; caution patients to take protective measures (eg, sunscreens, protective clothing) against UV or sunlight until tolerance is determined.

GI effects: GI toxicity (including NSAID-induced ulcers and GI bleeding disorders) can occur with or without warning with chronic use of NSAIDs. High-dose NSAIDs probably carry a greater risk of causing GI adverse effects. Patients with a history of GI lesions should consult a physician before using these products. GI effects are more likely to occur and may be more pronounced in elderly patients.

Pregnancy: Category B; Category D in 3rd trimester. Safety for use during pregnancy has not been established; use is not recommended. There are no adequate, well controlled studies in pregnant women. An increased incidence of dystocia, increased post implantation loss, and delayed parturition has occurred in animals. Agents that inhibit prostaglandin synthesis may cause closure of the ductus arteriosus and other untoward effects in the fetus. GI tract toxicity is increased in pregnant women in the last trimester. Some NSAIDs may prolong pregnancy if given before onset of labor. Avoid use during pregnancy, especially during the 3rd trimester.

Lactation: Most NSAIDs are excreted in breast milk in low concentrations. The American Academy of Pediatrics considers ibuprofen and naproxen to be compatible with breastfeeding. Data on the use of ketoprofen during nursing are lacking.

Children: The use of ibuprofen and naproxen is not recommended in children under 12 years of age unless directed by a physician. Ketoprofen is not recommended for use in children under 16 years of age.

Elderly: Age appears to increase the possibility of adverse reactions to NSAIDs. The risk of serious ulcer disease is increased in elderly patients (older than 65 years of age) taking NSAIDs; this risk appears to increase with dose. Use with greater care and begin with reduced dosages in this patient population.

▶ **Drug Interactions**

NSAID Drug Interactions			
Precipitant drug	**Object drug***		**Description**
NSAIDs	Anticoagulants	↑	Coadministration may prolong prothrombin time (PT). Also consider the effects NSAIDs have on platelet function and gastric mucosa. Monitor PT and patients closely, and instruct patients to watch for signs and symptoms of bleeding.
NSAIDs	Beta blockers	↓	The antihypertensive effect of beta blockers may be impaired. Naproxen did not affect atenolol.
NSAIDs	Cyclosporine	↑	Nephrotoxicity of both agents may be increased.
NSAIDs	Digoxin	↑	Ibuprofen may increase digoxin serum levels.
NSAIDs	Hydantoins	↑	Serum phenytoin levels may be increased, resulting in an increase in pharmacologic and toxic effects of phenytoin.
NSAIDs	Lithium	↑	Serum lithium levels may be increased.
NSAIDs	Loop diuretics	↓	Effects of loop diuretics may be decreased.

NSAID Drug Interactions			
Precipitant drug	Object drug*		Description
NSAIDs	Methotrexate	↑	The risks of methotrexate toxicity (eg, stomatitis, bone marrow suppression, nephrotoxicity) may be increased.
NSAIDs	Thiazide diuretics	↓	Decreased antihypertensive and diuretic action of thiazides may occur with concurrent naproxen.
Cimetidine	NSAIDs	↔	NSAID plasma concentrations may be increased or decreased by cimetidine; some studies report no effect.
Probenecid	NSAIDs	↑	Probenecid may increase the concentrations and possibly the toxicity of the NSAIDs.
Salicylates	NSAIDs	↓	Plasma concentrations of NSAIDs may be decreased by salicylates. Avoid concurrent use because it offers no therapeutic advantage and may significantly increase the incidence of GI effects.

* ↑ = Object drug increased.   ↓ = Object drug decreased.   ↔ = Undetermined clinical effect.

▶ **Adverse Reactions**

Cardiovascular: Edema; congestive heart failure.

CNS: Dizziness; drowsiness; headache; lightheadedness; vertigo.

Dermatologic: Erythema; pruritus; rash.

GI: Bleeding; diarrhea; dyspepsia; heartburn; nausea; vomiting.

Miscellaneous: Muscle cramps; thirst.

IBUPROFEN

▶ **Administration and Dosage**

Adults: 200 mg orally every 4 to 6 hours as needed. If pain does not respond to 200 mg, 400 mg may be used. Do not exceed 1.2 g in 24 hours. Do not take for pain for longer than 10 days unless directed by physician. If GI upset occurs, take with meals or milk.

Children (6 months to 12 years of age): 5 to 10 mg/kg/dose orally and repeated 3 to 4 times daily as needed. Maximum daily dose is 40 mg/kg.

IBUPROFEN PRODUCTS	
Trade name	Doseform
Junior Strength Advil, Junior Strength Motrin	**Tablets**: 100 mg
Advil,[1] *Maximum Strength Midol Cramp, Motrin IB*	**Tablets**: 200 mg
Children's Advil, Children's Motrin	**Tablets, chewable**: 50 mg
Junior Strength Advil, Junior Strength Motrin	**Tablets, chewable**: 100 mg
Advil Liqui-Gels, Motrin IB[2]	**Gelcaps**: 200 mg
Infants' Advil Concentrated Drops	**Liquid**: 50 mg/1.25 mL
Children's Advil,[1,3] *Children's Motrin*[1]	**Suspension**: 100 mg/5 mL

Products listed are representative of currently available and widely distributed brands. Similar products, including regional and private label brands, may also exist.

[1] Contains sucrose.
[2] Contains parabens.
[3] Contains sorbitol.

PATIENT INFORMATION
Ibuprofen
- *Adults*: Do not exceed 1.2 g/day.
- Severe or recurrent pain may indicate a serious illness. Consult a physician.
- Patient instructions accompany each product. Have the patient read these instructions carefully before use, preferably before leaving the pharmacy, in case of any questions.
- May cause GI upset; take with food or after meals.
- Take with a full glass of water (240 mL) to reduce the risk of the medication lodging in the esophagus.
- Do not take OTC NSAIDs for longer than 10 days for pain unless directed by a physician. If symptoms persist, worsen, or if new symptoms develop, contact a physician.
- Notify physician if skin rash, itching, visual disturbances, edema, black stools, or persistent headache occurs.
- Avoid alcohol and aspirin while taking this medication.

KETOPROFEN

► Administration and Dosage

Adults: 12.5 mg orally every 4 to 6 hours as needed. If pain persists more than 1 hour, follow with 12.5 mg. Do not exceed 25 mg in a 4- to 6-hour period or 75 mg in a 24-hour period. Use the smallest effective dose.

Children: Do not give to children younger than 16 years of age unless directed by a physician.

KETOPROFEN PRODUCTS	
Trade name	Doseform
Orudis KT	Tablets: 12.5 mg

Products listed are representative of currently available and widely distributed brands. Similar products, including regional and private label brands, may also exist.

PATIENT INFORMATION
Ketoprofen
- *Adults:* Do not exceed 75 mg/day.
- Severe or recurrent pain may indicate a serious illness. Consult a physician.
- Patient instructions accompany each product. Have the patient read these instructions carefully before use, preferably before leaving the pharmacy, in case of any questions.
- May cause GI upset; take with food or after meals.
- Take with a full glass of water (240 mL) to reduce the risk of the medication lodging in the esophagus.
- Do not take OTC NSAIDs for longer than 10 days for pain unless directed by a physician. If symptoms persist, worsen, or if new symptoms develop, contact a physician.
- Notify physician if rash, itching, visual disturbances, edema, black stools, or persistent headache occurs.
- Avoid alcohol and aspirin while taking this medication.

NAPROXEN

▶ **Administration and Dosage**

Adults: 200 mg orally every 8 to 12 hours as needed. Do not exceed 600 mg in 24 hours.

Children: Do not give to children younger than 12 years of age unless directed by a physician.

Elderly (older than 65 years of age): Do not exceed 200 mg in a 12-hour period.

NAPROXEN PRODUCTS	
Trade name	Doseform
Aleve	**Tablets, Caplets, and Gelcaps**: 200 mg (220 mg naproxen sodium)

Products listed are representative of currently available and widely distributed brands. Similar products, including regional and private label brands, may also exist.

PATIENT INFORMATION

Naproxen

- *Adults:* Do not exceed 600 mg/day.
- Severe or recurrent pain may indicate a serious illness. Consult a physician.
- Patient instructions accompany each product. Have the patient read these instructions carefully before use, preferably before leaving the pharmacy, in case of any questions.
- May cause GI upset; take with food or after meals.
- Take with a full glass of water (240 mL) to reduce the risk of the medication lodging in the esophagus.
- Do not take OTC NSAIDs for longer than 10 days for pain unless directed by a physician. If symptoms persist, worsen, or if new symptoms develop, contact a physician.
- Notify physician if rash, itching, visual disturbances, edema, black stools, or persistent headache occurs.
- Avoid alcohol and aspirin while taking this medication.

RUBS AND LINIMENTS

▶ **Indications**

These products are used for relief of pain of muscular aches, neuralgia, rheumatism, arthritis, sprains, and like conditions, when skin is intact.

Individual components include:

Counterirritants: Camphor, capsicum preparations (capsicum oleoresin, capsaicin), eucalyptus oil, menthol, methyl nicotinate, methyl salicylate, mustard oil, wormwood oil.

Antiseptics: Thymol.

Analgesics: Trolamine salicylate, methyl salicylate.

▶ **Contraindications**

Allergy to components of any formulation or to salicylates.

▶ **Warnings**

For external use only: Avoid contact with eyes, eyelids, and mucous membranes.

Apply to affected parts only: Do not apply to irritated skin; discontinue use if excessive irritation develops. Consult a physician if pain persists for longer than 7 to 10 days, or if redness is present, or in conditions affecting children younger than 10 years of age.

Heat therapy: Do not use an external source of high heat (eg, heating pad) with these agents because irritation and burning of the skin may occur.

Protective covering: Applying a tight bandage or wrap over these agents is not recommended because increased absorption may occur.

▶ **Drug Interactions**

Anticoagulants: An enhanced anticoagulant effect (eg, increased prothrombin time) occurred in several patients receiving an anticoagulant and using topical methyl salicylate concurrently.

▶ **Adverse Reactions**

If applied to large skin areas and used over a prolonged period of time, salicylate side effects (eg, tinnitus, nausea, vomiting) may occur.

Products may be toxic if ingested.

Counterirritants may cause local irritation, especially in patients with sensitive skin.

▶ **Administration and Dosage**

Apply to affected areas as needed.

RUBS AND LINIMENTS	
Trade name	Doseform
Icy Hot	**Balm:** 29% methyl salicylate, 7.6% menthol, white petrolatum
Epiderm	**Balm:** Isopropyl alcohol, parabens, ureas, menthol, EDTA
JointFlex	**Cream:** 3.1% camphor, lanolin, aloe, urea, EDTA, glycerin, peppermint oil
Capzasin-P	**Cream:** 0.025% capsaicin
ArthriCare for Women Silky Dry	**Cream:** 0.025% capsaicin, parabens, mineral oil
ArthriCare for Women Extra Moisturizing	**Cream:** 0.025% capsaicin, aloe vera gel, cetyl and stearyl alcohol, parabens
ArthriCare for Women Multi-Action	**Cream:** 0.025% capsaicin, 1.25% menthol, 0.25% methyl nicotinate, aloe vera gel, cetyl alcohol, parabens
Capzasin-HP	**Cream:** 0.075% capsaicin
ArthriCare for Women Ultra Strength	**Cream:** 0.075% capsaicin, 2% menthol, aloe vera gel, cetyl and stearyl alcohol, parabens
Vicks VapoRub	**Cream:** 2.8% menthol, 5.2% camphor, 1.2% eucalyptus oil, cedarleaf oil, cetyl and stearyl alcohol, EDTA, glycerin, urea, parabens, turpentine oil
BenGay S.P.A.	**Cream:** 10% menthol, cetyl alcohol, urea, EDTA, glycerin
Arthritic Hot	**Cream:** Methyl salicylate, menthol
Ziks	**Cream:** 12% methyl salicylate, 1% menthol, 0.025% capsaicin, cetyl alcohol, urea
Thera-Gesic	**Cream:** 15% methyl salicylate, 1% menthol, glycerin, parabens

RUBS AND LINIMENTS	
Trade name	Doseform
BenGay Greaseless	**Cream**: 15% methyl salicylate, 10% menthol, cetyl alcohol, glycerin
Pain Bust-R II	**Cream**: 17% methyl salicylate, 12% menthol, cetyl and stearyl alcohol
ArthriCare for Women Nighttime	**Cream**: 30% methyl salicylate, 1.25% menthol, 0.25% methyl nicotinate, glycerin, isopropyl alcohol
Arthritis Formula BenGay	**Cream**: 30% methyl salicylate, 8% menthol, lanolin
Icy Hot	**Cream**: 30% methyl salicylate, 10% menthol
Ultra Strength BenGay	**Cream**: 30% methyl salicylate, 10% menthol, 4% camphor, EDTA, lanolin
Panalgesic Gold	**Cream**: 35% methyl salicylate, 4% menthol, lanolin, cetyl and stearyl alcohol, mineral oil
Myoflex	**Cream**: 10% triethanolamine salicylate, cetyl and stearyl alcohol, EDTA
Myoflex Extra, Myoflex Arthritic	**Cream**: 15% triethanolamine salicylate
Sportscreme	**Cream**: 10% trolamine salicylate, cetyl alcohol, glycerin, parabens, mineral oil
Aspercreme	**Cream**: 10% trolamine salicylate, aloe vera gel, cetyl alcohol, glycerin, parabens, mineral oil
Mobisyl	**Cream**: 10% trolamine salicylate, aloe vera gel, cetyl alcohol, urea, glycerin, parabens, mineral oil, sweet almond oil, EDTA
Icy Hot Arthritis Therapy	**Gel**: 0.025% capsaicin, aloe vera gel, benzyl alcohol, urea, maleated soybean oil, parabens
Flexall Quik Gel	**Gel**: Menthol, methyl salicylate
Vanishing Scent BenGay	**Gel**: 2.5% menthol, urea, isopropyl alcohol
Vicks VapoRub	**Gel**: 2.6% menthol, 4.8% camphor, 1.2% eucalyptus oil, cedarleaf oil, nutmeg oil, petrolatum, turpentine oil
Flexall 454	**Gel**: 7% menthol, aloe vera gel, eucalyptus oil, glycerin, peppermint oil, thyme oil
Maximum Strength Flexall 454	**Gel**: 16% menthol, aloe vera gel, eucalyptus oil, glycerin, peppermint oil, thyme oil
Flexall Ultra Plus	**Gel**: 16% menthol, 10% methyl salicylate, 3.1% camphor, aloe vera gel, eucalyptus oil, glycerin, peppermint oil, thyme oil
Icy Hot Chill Stick	**Gel**: 30% methyl salicylate, 10% menthol, hydrogenated castor oil, stearyl alcohol
Myoflex Ice Cold Plus	**Gel**: 15% triethanolamine salicylate
Absorbine Jr Arthritis Strength	**Liquid**: Capsaicin, echinacea, calendula, and wormwood extracts
Absorbine Jr	**Liquid**: 1.27% menthol, echinacea, calendula, and wormwood extracts, wormwood oil
Extra Strength Absorbine Jr	**Liquid**: 4% menthol, echinacea, calendula, and wormwood extracts, wormwood oil
Yager's	**Liniment**: Camphor, turpentine oil, clove oil
Panalgesic Gold	**Liniment**: 55.01% methyl salicylate, 1.25% menthol, 3.1% camphor, emollient oils, alcohol
Banalg	**Lotion**: 4.9% methyl salicylate, 1% menthol, 2% camphor, parabens, eucalyptus oil

RUBS AND LINIMENTS	
Trade name	Doseform
Banalg Hospital Strength	**Lotion**: 14% methyl salicylate, 3% menthol, parabens
Aspercreme	**Lotion**: Trolamine salicylate
Eucalyptamint	**Ointment**: 16% menthol, eucalyptus oil, lanolin, mineral oil
Original Formula BenGay	**Ointment**: 18.3% methyl salicylate, 16% menthol, lanolin
Absorbine Jr	**Patch**: Menthol, camphor, eucalyptus
Absorbine Jr Deep Pain Relief	**Patch**: Menthol, glucosamine, MSM
Icy Hot	**Patch**: Methyl salicylate, menthol

Products listed are representative of currently available and widely distributed brands. Similar products, including regional and private label brands, may also exist.

PATIENT INFORMATION

Rubs and Liniments

- For external use only. Avoid contact with eyes, eyelids, and mucous membranes.
- Apply to affected areas only. Do not apply to irritated skin; discontinue use if excessive irritation develops.
- Consult a physician if pain persists for longer than 7 to 10 days, if redness is present, or in conditions affecting children younger than 10 years of age.
- Do not use an external source of high heat (eg, heating pad) with these agents because irritation and burning of the skin may occur.
- Do not apply tight bandages or wraps over these agents.
- Do not apply to broken skin.

ARTHRALGIA

DEFINITION

Arthralgia is defined as joint pain and is typically associated with osteoarthritis. Osteoarthritis is commonly known as degenerative joint disease. It is a progressive deterioration of articular cartilage.

ETIOLOGY

While the etiology of arthralgia-associated osteoarthritis (AAO) is largely unknown, it is known that osteoarthritis occurs in almost all vertebrates. Potential causes include acute or chronic trauma, genetic defects, or infectious, metabolic, endocrine, or neuropathic diseases. The primary risk factor is advanced age; major trauma, weight bearing, and repetitive use are also risk factors.

INCIDENCE

Arthralgia-associated osteoarthritis is the most common form of joint disorder, with the knee being the most commonly affected joint. Almost all individuals older than 40 years of age have some pathological changes in weight-bearing joints, although few are symptomatic. Men and women are affected equally.

PATHOPHYSIOLOGY

Normal joints have a low level of friction and typically do not wear out unless there is unusual trauma or overuse. The pathogenesis of AAO involves biomechanical forces and inflammatory, biochemical, and immunologic factors. The primary changes involve cartilage in the affected joint. Initially, there is increased water content and biochemical changes that result in the cartilage being unable to repair itself. As cartilage destruction progresses, pathological changes in bone occur. Increased activity by osteoclasts causes increased bone formation, resulting in stiffer and less compliant bone. Microfractures often result.

SIGNS/SYMPTOMS

Initially, AAO affects only one or a few joints, is noninflammatory, and causes pain, stiffness, and limitation of motion. The onset is usually subtle and gradual. Pain is often described as a deep ache localized in the involved joint that is worsened with use and improves with rest. With advanced AAO, there may also be nocturnal pain that can interfere with sleep. Late signs include tenderness with palpation and pain with passive motion.

DIAGNOSTIC PARAMETERS/PHYSICAL ASSESSMENT

Clinical Observation: The diagnosis of AAO is usually based on clinical signs and symptoms and radiological findings. With physical exam, there may be localized tenderness, bony or soft tissue swelling, and warmth over the joint. Rule out rheumatoid arthritis and other arthritic conditions.

Interview: To ensure the proper diagnosis and treatment, it may be beneficial to ask about the following:

- Onset, duration, and location of the pain
- Quality or nature of the pain
- Factors that relieve or exacerbate the pain
- The severity of the pain using a 10-point rating scale where the patient quantifies the intensity of the pain (0 = no pain to 10 = most intense pain)

TREATMENT

Approaches to therapy: It is best to begin management early to reduce pain, maintain mobility, and minimize disability. Question the patient about therapies that have been tried and their effectiveness. While no cure exists, exercises help maintain healthy cartilage, range of motion, and strength.

Nondrug therapy: Have patients conduct daily stretching and postural exercises, avoid sitting in soft chairs, sit without slumping, and sleep on a firm bed. Application of heat or cold to the affected joint may decrease pain and stiffness.

Pharmacotherapy: Drug therapy is symptomatic. Drugs effective for relieving pain include aspirin, acetaminophen, and nonsteroidal anti-inflammatory drugs (NSAIDs).

SALICYLATES

▶ Actions

The anti-inflammatory and analgesic activity of salicylates may be mediated through inhibition of the prostaglandin synthetase complex.

▶ Indications

For the treatment of mild to moderate pain. These agents have other labeled indications as well.

▶ Contraindications

Hypersensitivity to salicylates or NSAIDs. Use with extreme caution in patients with a history of adverse reactions to salicylates. Cross-sensitivity may exist between aspirin and other NSAIDs that inhibit prostaglandin synthesis, and between aspirin and tartrazine. Aspirin cross-sensitivity does not appear to occur with sodium salicylate, salicylamide, or choline salicylate. Aspirin hypersensitivity is more prevalent in those with asthma, nasal polyposis, or chronic urticaria.

Also contraindicated in patients with hemophilia or bleeding ulcers, or those in hemorrhagic states. Magnesium salicylate is contraindicated in patients with advanced chronic renal insufficiency.

Do not use aspirin in children or teenagers during episodes of fever-causing illnesses because of the possiblity of Reye syndrome.

▶ Warnings

Concurrent medications: Many other medications, specifically multi-ingredient cough and cold products, also contain aspirin or acetaminophen. It is important to advise patients of this possibility, and to inquire about other medications they might be taking before recommending an analgesic.

Otic effects: Discontinue use if dizziness, ringing in ears (tinnitus), or impaired hearing occurs. Tinnitus probably represents blood salicylic acid levels reaching or exceeding the upper limit of the therapeutic range; therefore, it is a helpful guide to toxicity. Temporary hearing loss disappears gradually upon discontinuation of the drug.

Hypersensitivity: Do not use if there is a history of sensitivity to aspirin or NSAIDs.

Aspirin intolerance, manifested by acute bronchospasm, generalized urticaria/angio-edema, severe rhinitis, or shock occurs in 4% to 19% of asthmatics. Symptoms occur within 3 hours after ingestion.

Foods may contribute to a reaction. Some foods with high salicylate content include curry powder, paprika, licorice, Benedictine liqueur, prunes, raisins, tea, and gherkins. A typical American diet contains 10 to 200 mg/day salicylate.

Hepatic function impairment: Use with caution in patients with liver damage, preexisting hypoprothrombinemia, and vitamin K deficiency.

GI effects: Use with caution in patients who are intolerant to salicylates because of GI irritation, and in those with gastric ulcers, peptic ulcers, mild diabetes, gout, erosive gastritis, or bleeding tendencies.

Hematologic effects: Aspirin interferes with hemostasis. Avoid use in patients with severe anemia or a history of blood coagulation defects, or in those who take anticoagulants.

Pregnancy: Category D (aspirin); *Category C* (salsalate, magnesium salicylate, other salicylates). Aspirin may produce adverse effects in the mother, such as anemia, ante- or postpartum hemorrhage, or prolonged gestation and labor. Salicylates readily cross the placenta. By inhibiting prostaglandin synthesis, salicylates may cause constriction of ductus arteriosus, and, possibly, other untoward fetal effects. Maternal aspirin use during later stages of pregnancy may cause adverse fetal effects, such as low birth weight, increased incidence of intracranial hemorrhage in premature infants, stillbirth, or neonatal death. Salicylates may be teratogens. Avoid use during pregnancy, especially in the third trimester.

Lactation: Salicylates are excreted in breast milk in low concentrations. Adverse effects on platelet function in the nursing infant are a potential risk. The American Academy of Pediatrics recommends that aspirin be used cautiously in nursing mothers.

▶ Drug Interactions

Salicylate Drug Interactions			
Precipitant drug	**Object drug***		**Description**
Antacids, urinary alkalinizers	Salicylates	↓	Decreased pharmacologic effects of salicylates may occur. The magnitude of the antacid interaction depends on the agent, dose, and pretreatment urine pH.
Aspirin	Anticoagulants	↑	Aspirin can increase the risk of bleeding in anticoagulated patients.
Aspirin	Nitroglycerin	↑	Nitroglycerin, when taken with aspirin, may result in unexpected hypotension. Data are limited. If hypotension occurs, reduce the nitroglycerin dose.
Aspirin	NSAIDs	↓	Aspirin may decrease NSAID serum concentrations. Avoid concomitant use; it offers no therapeutic advantage and may significantly increase incidence of GI effects.

Salicylate Drug Interactions			
Precipitant drug	**Object drug***		**Description**
Aspirin	Valproic acid	↑	Aspirin displaces valproic acid from its protein-binding sites and may decrease its total body clearance, thus increasing pharmacological effects.
Carbonic anhy-drase inhibitors	Salicylates	↔	Salicylate intoxication has occurred after coadministration of these agents. However, salicylic acid renal elimination may be increased by these drugs if urine is kept alkaline. Conversely, salicylates may displace acetazolamide from protein-binding sites, resulting in toxicity. Further study is needed.
Charcoal, activated	Aspirin	↓	Coadministration decreases aspirin absorption, depending on charcoal dose and interval between ingestion.
Corticosteroids	Salicylates	↓	Corticosteroids increase salicylate clearance and decrease salicylate serum levels.
Nizatidine	Salicylates	↑	Increased serum salicylate levels have occurred in patients receiving high doses (3.9 g/day) of aspirin and concurrent nizatidine.
Salicylates	Alcohol	↑	The risk of GI ulceration increases when salicylates are given concomitantly. Ingestion of alcohol during salicylate therapy may also prolong bleeding time.
Salicylates	Angiotensin-converting enzyme inhibitors	↓	Antihypertensive effectiveness of these agents may be decreased by concurrent salicylate administration, possibly due to prostaglandin inhibition. Consider discontinuing salicylates if problems occur.
Salicylates	Loop diuretics	↓	Loop diuretics may be less effective when given with salicylates in patients with compromised renal function or with cirrhosis with ascites; however, data conflict.
Salicylates	Methotrexate	↑	Salicylates increase drug levels, causing toxicity by interfering with protein binding and renal elimination of the antimetabolite.
Salicylates	Probenecid, sulfinpyrazone	↔	Salicylates antagonize the uricosuric effect. While salicylates in large doses (> 3 g/day) have a uricosuric effect, smaller amounts may reduce the uricosuric effect of these agents.
Salicylates	Spironolactone	↓	Salicylates may inhibit the diuretic effects; antihypertensive action does not appear altered. Effects depend on the dose of spironolactone.
Salicylates	Sulfonylureas, exogenous insulin	↑	Salicylates in doses > 2 g/day have a hypoglycemic action, perhaps by altering pancreatic beta-cell function. They may potentiate the glucose-lowering effect of these drugs.
Urinary acidifiers	Salicylates	↑	Ammonium chloride, ascorbic acid, and methionine decrease salicylate excretion.

* ↑ = Object drug increased. ↓ = Object drug decreased. ↔ = Undetermined clinical effect.

▶ **Adverse Reactions**

Adverse reactions can be seen in the following body systems: GI (nausea, dyspepsia, heartburn, epigastric discomfort), hematologic (prolonged bleeding time, leukopenia, thrombocytopenia, purpura, decreased plasma iron concentration, shortened erythrocyte survival time), and dermatologic (rash, hives, and angioedema may occur, especially in patients suffering from chronic urticaria). Additional miscellaneous adverse reactions that have occurred include fever, thirst, and dimness of vision.

Allergic and anaphylactic reactions have been noted when hypersensitive individuals took aspirin. Fatal anaphylactic shock, while not common, has been reported.

Aspirin has an irreversible effect on platelet aggregation for the life of the platelet (approximately 7 days).

▶ Overdosage

Symptoms: The acute lethal dose for adults is approximately 10 to 30 g, and for children, approximately 4 g. Respiratory alkalosis is seen initially in acute salicylate ingestions. Hyperpnea and tachypnea occur as a result of increased CO_2 production and a direct stimulatory effect of salicylate on the respiratory center. Other symptoms may include nausea, vomiting, hypokalemia, tinnitus, neurologic abnormalities (eg, disorientation, irritability, hallucinations, lethargy, stupor, coma, seizures), dehydration, hyperthermia, hyperventilation, hyperactivity, thrombocytopenia, platelet dysfunction, hypoprothrombinemia, increased capillary fragility, and other hematologic abnormalities. Symptoms may progress quickly to depression, coma, or respiratory failure and collapse. Chronic salicylate toxicity may occur when more than 100 mg/kg/day is ingested for 2 or more days. It is more difficult to recognize than acute overdosage and is associated with increased morbidity and mortality. Compared with acute poisoning, hyperventilation, dehydration, systemic acidosis, and severe CNS manifestations occur more frequently.

Treatment: Initial treatment includes induction of emesis or gastric lavage to remove any unabsorbed drug from the stomach. Activated charcoal diminishes salicylate absorption most effectively if given within 2 hours after ingestion. Contact a local poison control center or emergency room if overdosage is suspected.

ASPIRIN

▶ Administration and Dosage

Adults: 325 to 650 mg orally every 4 hours as needed. Some extra-strength products recommend 500 mg every 3 hours or 1000 mg every 6 hours.

Children: The oral analgesic/antipyretic dosage is 10 to 15 mg/kg/dose every 4 hours (see table), up to 60 to 80 mg/kg/day. Do not use in children or teenagers during episodes of fever-causing illnesses because of the possibility of Reye syndrome. Dosage recommendations by age and weight are as follows:

Recommended Aspirin Dosage in Children					
Age (years)	Weight		Dosage (mg every 4 hours)	No. of 81 mg tablets (every 4 hours)	No. of 325 mg tablets (every 4 hours)
	lbs	kg			
2-3	24-35	10.6-15.9	162	2	½
4-5	36-47	16-21.4	243	3	N/A
6-8	48-59	21.5-26.8	324	4	1
9-10	60-71	26.9-32.3	405	5	N/A
11	72-95	32.4-43.2	486	6	1½
12-14	≥ 96	≥ 43.3	648	8	2

ASPIRIN PRODUCTS

Trade name	Doseform
Original Bayer, Norwich Aspirin	**Tablets**: 325 mg
Bayer Children's Chewable Aspirin	**Tablets, chewable**: 81 mg. Dextrose, saccharin. Cherry and orange flavors.
Adult Low Strength Ecotrin, Halfprin 81[1]	**Tablets, enteric coated**: 81 mg. Talc.
Halfprin 162	**Tablets, enteric coated**: 162 mg. Lactose, talc.
Ecotrin Regular Strength	**Tablets, enteric coated**: 325 mg. Talc.
Norwich Maximum Strength	**Tablets, enteric coated**: 500 mg
Ecotrin Maximum Strength	**Tablets, enteric coated**: 500 mg. Talc.
Alka-Seltzer Original Effervescent Antacid and Pain Relief Medicine	**Tablets, effervescent**: 325 mg, 1000 mg citric acid, 1916 mg sodium bicarbonate
Bayer Women's Aspirin Plus Calcium	**Caplets**: 81 mg, 300 mg calcium. Lactose, mineral oil.
Original Bayer	**Caplets**: 325 mg
Extra Strength Bayer PM Aspirin Plus Sleep Aid	**Caplets**: 500 mg, 25 mg diphenhydramine HCl
Extra Strength Bayer Aspirin	**Caplets, coated**: 500 mg
Extra Strength Bayer Back and Body Pain	**Caplets, coated**: 500 mg, 32.5 mg caffeine
Extra Strength Bayer Arthritis Pain Regimen	**Caplets, enteric coated**: 500 mg
Original Bayer	**Gelcaps**: 325 mg. Parabens, sorbitol, glycerin.
Extra Strength Bayer Aspirin	**Gelcaps, coated**: 500 mg. Parabens, glycerin.

BUFFERED ASPIRIN PRODUCTS

Adprin-B	**Tablets, coated**: 325 mg with calcium carbonate, magnesium carbonate, magnesium oxide
Regular Strength Ascriptin	**Tablets, coated**: 325 mg with 50 mg magnesium hydroxide, 50 mg aluminum hydroxide, calcium carbonate. Talc.
Bufferin	**Tablets, coated**: 325 mg with 158 mg calcium carbonate, 63 mg magnesium oxide, 34 mg magnesium carbonate. Mineral oil, sorbitol, citric acid.
Extra Strength Adprin-B	**Tablets, coated**: 500 mg with calcium carbonate, magnesium carbonate, magnesium oxide.
Bayer Adult Low Strength	**Caplets**: 81 mg, buffered with 250 mg calcium carbonate
Extra Strength Bayer Plus	**Caplets**: 500 mg with calcium carbonate, magnesium carbonate, magnesium oxide
Maximum Strength Ascriptin	**Caplets, coated**: 500 mg with 80 mg magnesium hydroxide, 80 mg aluminum hydroxide, calcium carbonate. Saccharin, sorbitol, talc.

Products listed are representative of currently available and widely distributed brands. Similar products, including regional and private label brands, may also exist.

[1] Also contains lactose.

PATIENT INFORMATION
Aspirin

- Patient instructions accompany each product. Have the patient read instructions carefully before use, preferably before leaving the pharmacy, in case of questions.
- May cause GI upset; take with food or after meals. Enteric-coated products may prevent or reduce stomach/GI distress.
- Take with a full glass of water (240 mL) to reduce the risk of the medication lodging in the esophagus.
- Have patients allergic to tartrazine dye avoid aspirin.
- Severe or recurrent pain may indicate a serious illness. Consult a physician.
- Notify a physician if rash, difficult breathing, ringing in the ears, or persistent GI pain occurs. Internal bleeding may occur with no GI symptoms and may be indicated by bloody or black stools.
- Do not use in children or adolescents during episodes of fever-causing illnesses because of the possibility of Reye syndrome.
- Do not use aspirin if it has a strong vinegar-like odor. This suggests deterioration of aspirin and loss of potency.
- Inform a physician or dentist of aspirin use at least 7 days before surgery or dental care.
- Avoid taking antacids within 2 hours of taking enteric-coated tablets.

MAGNESIUM SALICYLATE

▶ Actions

Magnesium salicylate is a sodium-free salicylate derivative that may have a low incidence of GI upset.

▶ Contraindications

Magnesium salicylate is contraindicated in patients with advanced chronic renal insufficiency due to magnesium retention.

▶ Warnings

The possibility of magnesium toxicity exists in patients with renal insufficiency.

▶ Administration and Dosage

Product labeling and dosages are expressed as magnesium salicylate anhydrous.

Adults: Usual dose is 650 mg every 4 hours as needed or 1 g every 6 hours as needed up to 4 g/day.

Children: Safety and efficacy for use in children have not been established.

MAGNESIUM SALICYLATE PRODUCTS	
Trade name	Doseform
Regular Strength Doan's	**Caplets:** 377 mg
Extra Strength Doan's	**Caplets:** 580 mg
Extra Strength Doan's P.M.	**Caplets:** 580 mg, 25 mg diphenhydramine HCl. Talc.

Products listed are representative of currently available and widely distributed brands. Similar products, including regional and private label brands, may also exist.

PATIENT INFORMATION
Magnesium Salicylate

- Patient instructions accompany each product. Have the patient read instructions carefully before use, preferably before leaving the pharmacy, in case of any questions.
- May cause GI upset; take with food or after meals.
- Do not use these products if you have diagnosed renal insufficiency.
- Severe or recurrent pain may indicate a serious illness. Consult a physician.
- Notify physician if rash, difficult breathing, ringing in the ears, or persistent GI pain occurs. Internal bleeding may occur with no GI symptoms and may be indicated by bloody or black stools.
- Do not use in children or adolescents during episodes of fever-causing illnesses because of the possibility of Reye syndrome.

ACETAMINOPHEN (APAP)

▶ Actions
Generally, the antipyretic and analgesic effects of APAP and aspirin are comparable; however, the site and mechanism of the analgesic effect of acetaminophen are unclear.

▶ Indications
For the treatment of mild to moderate pain. Also used as an analgesic-antipyretic in the presence of aspirin allergy, and in patients with blood coagulation disorders who are being treated with oral anticoagulants, bleeding diatheses (eg, hemophilia), upper GI disease (eg, ulcer, gastritis, hiatal hernia), and gouty arthritis.

▶ Contraindications
Hypersensitivity to acetaminophen.

▶ Warnings
Concurrent medications: Many other medications, specifically multi-ingredient cough and cold products, also contain aspirin or acetaminophen. It is important to advise patients of this possibility, and to inquire about other medications they might be taking before recommending an analgesic.

Hepatotoxicity: Hepatotoxicity and severe hepatic failure occurred in chronic alcoholics following therapeutic doses. The hepatotoxicity may be caused by induction of hepatic microsomal enzymes, resulting in an increase in toxic metabolites, or by the reduced amount of glutathione responsible for conjugating toxic metabolites. A safe dose for chronic alcohol abusers has not been determined. Caution chronic alcoholics and those consuming alcohol on a daily basis to limit acetaminophen intake to 2 g/day or less.

Pregnancy: Category B. Acetaminophen crosses the placenta, but has been routinely used in all stages of pregnancy. When used in therapeutic doses, it appears safe for short-term use.

Lactation: APAP is excreted in breast milk in low amounts, but no adverse effects have been reported. The American Academy of Pediatrics considers acetaminophen to be compatible with breastfeeding.

Children: Consult a physician before using in children younger than 3 years of age.

► **Drug Interactions**

Acetaminophen Drug Interactions			
Precipitant drug	**Object drug***		**Description**
Alcohol, ethyl	APAP	↑	Hepatotoxicity has occurred in chronic alcoholics following various dose levels (moderate to excessive) of acetaminophen.
Anticholinergics	APAP	↔	The onset of acetaminophen effect may be delayed or decreased slightly, but the ultimate pharmacological effect is not significantly affected by anticholinergics.
Beta blockers, propranolol	APAP	↑	Propranolol appears to inhibit the enzyme systems responsible for glucuronidation and oxidation of acetaminophen. Therefore, the pharmacologic effects of acetaminophen may be increased.
Charcoal, activated	APAP	↓	Reduces acetaminophen absorption when administered as soon as possible after overdose.
Contraceptives, oral	APAP	↓	Increase in glucuronidation resulting in increased plasma clearance and a decreased half-life of acetaminophen.
Probenecid	APAP	↑	Probenecid may slightly increase the therapeutic effectiveness of acetaminophen.
APAP	Lamotrigine	↓	Serum lamotrigine concentrations may be reduced, producing a decrease in therapeutic effects.
APAP	Loop diuretics	↓	The effects of the loop diuretic may be decreased because APAP may decrease renal prostaglandin excretion and decrease plasma renin activity.
APAP	Zidovudine	↓	The pharmacologic effects of zidovudine may be decreased because of enhanced nonhepatic or renal clearance of zidovudine.

* ↑ = Object drug increased. ↓ = Object drug decreased. ↔ = Undetermined clinical effect.

The potential hepatotoxicity of acetaminophen may be increased by large doses or long-term administration of barbiturates, carbamazepine, hydantoins, rifampin, and sulfinpyrazone. The therapeutic effects of acetaminophen may also be decreased.

► **Adverse Reactions**

When used as directed, acetaminophen rarely causes severe toxicity or side effects. However, the following adverse reactions have been reported:

Hematologic: Hemolytic anemia; neutropenia; leukopenia; pancytopenia; thrombocytopenia.

Miscellaneous: Fever; hypoglycemia; jaundice; rash.

► **Overdosage**

Symptoms: Acute poisoning may be manifested by nausea, vomiting, drowsiness, confusion, liver tenderness, low blood pressure, cardiac arrhythmias, jaundice, and acute hepatic and renal failure. These occur within the first 24 hours and may persist for 1 week or longer. Death has occurred because of liver necrosis. Acute renal failure may also occur; however, there are often no specific early symptoms or signs. The course of acetaminophen poisoning is divided into 4 stages (postingestion time):

Stage 1 (12 to 24 hours) – Nausea, vomiting, diaphoresis, anorexia.

Stage 2 (24 to 48 hours) – Clinically improved; AST, bilirubin, and prothrombin levels begin to rise.

Stage 3 (72 to 96 hours) – Peak hepatotoxicity; AST of 20,000 not unusual.

Stage 4 (7 to 8 days) – Recovery.

Hepatotoxicity may result. The minimal toxic dose is 10 g (140 mg/kg), but liver damage has occurred with a single 5.85 g dose; doses of 20 to 25 g or more are potentially fatal. Children appear less susceptible to toxicity than adults because they have less capacity for glucuronidation metabolism. Initial signs of toxicity may include nausea, vomiting, anorexia, malaise, diaphoresis, abdominal pain, and diarrhea. Hepatotoxicity is usually not apparent for 48 to 72 hours. Hepatic failure may lead to encephalopathy, coma, and death.

Plasma acetaminophen levels over 300 mcg/mL at 4 hours postingestion were associated with hepatic damage in 90% of patients; minimal hepatic damage is anticipated if plasma levels at 4 hours are less than 120 mcg/mL or less than 30 mcg/mL at 12 hours after ingestion.

Chronic excessive use (more than 4 g/day) may lead to transient hepatotoxicity. The kidneys may undergo tubular necrosis; the myocardium may be damaged.

Treatment: Perform gastric lavage in all acute overdosage cases, preferably within 4 hours of ingestion. Refer also to General Management of Acute Overdosage. It is important to contact a local poison control center or emergency room if overdosage is suspected.

▶ **Administration and Dosage**

Adults: 325 to 650 mg orally every 4 hours as needed or 1 g 3 to 4 times daily as needed. Do not exceed 4 g daily for all formulations containing acetaminophen.

Children: The usual oral dose is 10 mg/kg/dose, which may be repeated 4 to 5 times daily as needed. Do not exceed 5 doses in 24 hours.

Acetaminophen Dosage for Children			
Age	Dosage (mg)	Age	Dosage (mg)
0-3 months	40	6-8 years	320
4-11 months	80	9-10 years	400
1- 2 years	120	11 years	480
2-3 years	160	12-14 years	640
4-5 years	240	> 14 years	650

Suppositories:

Adults – 650 mg every 4 to 6 hours as needed; do not exceed 4 g in 24 hours.

Children (3 to 11 months of age) – 80 mg every 6 hours as needed.

Children (1 to 3 years of age) – 80 mg every 4 hours as needed.

Children (3 to 6 years of age) – 120 to 125 mg every 4 to 6 hours as needed; do not exceed 5 doses in 24 hours.

Children (6 to 12 years of age) – 325 mg every 4 to 6 hours as needed; do not exceed 5 doses in 24 hours.

Storage: Store suppositories below 27°C (80°F) or refrigerate. Store tablets and oral solutions at 15° to 30°C (59° to 86°F).

ACETAMINOPHEN PRODUCTS

Trade name	Doseform
Regular Strength Tylenol	**Tablets**: 325 mg
Aspirin Free Anacin Extra Strength, Extra Strength Tylenol	**Tablets**: 500 mg
Tylenol 8-Hour Extended Release	**Tablets**: 650 mg. Benzyl alcohol, parabens, castor oil.
Children's Tylenol	**Tablets, chewable**: 80 mg. Aspartame. Grape,[1] fruit[1] and bubble gum[2] flavors.
Junior Strength Tylenol Soft Chews	**Tablets, chewable**: 160 mg. Aspartame, 6 mg pheylalanine. Fruit and grape flavors.
Aspirin Free Anacin Maximum Strength	**Caplets**: 500 mg
Aspirin Free Anacin P.M.	**Caplets**: 500 mg, 25 mg diphenhydramine HCl
Tylenol Arthritis Pain Extended Relief	**Caplets**: 650 mg
Extra Strength Tylenol	**Gelcaps**: 500 mg. Benzyl alcohol, parabens, castor oil. EDTA.
Extra Strength Tylenol	**Geltabs**: 500 mg. Benzyl alcohol, parabens, castor oil. EDTA.
Infants' FeverAll	**Suppositories**: 80 mg. Hydrogenated vegetable oil.
Children's FeverAll, Acephen	**Suppositories**: 120 mg. Hydrogenated vegetable oil.
Jr. Strength FeverAll, Acephen	**Suppositories**: 325 mg. Hydrogenated vegetable oil.
Adults' FeverAll, Acephen	**Suppositories**: 650 mg. Hydrogenated vegetable oil.
Children's Silapap	**Elixir**: 80 mg/2.5 mL. Alcohol and sugar free.
Children's Tylenol	**Elixir**: 80 mg/2.5 mL. Saccharin. Alcohol free.
Dolono	**Flixir**: 80 mg/2.5 mL. Sorbitol, sucrose.
Aceta	**Elixir**: 120 mg/5 mL
Infants' Tylenol Concentrated Drops	**Liquid**: 80 mg/0.8 mL. Corn syrup, glycerin, sorbitol, butylparaben. Cherry and grape flavors.
Liquiprin Drops for Children	**Solution**: 120 mg/2.5 mL. Alcohol free.
Infants' Silapap Drops	**Solution**: 80 mg/0.8 mL. Alcohol free.
Infants' Tylenol Drops	**Suspension**: 80 mg/0.8 mL. Butylparaben, sorbitol, and sucrose. Alcohol free.
Children's Tylenol Liquid	**Suspension**: 160 mg/5 mL. Corn syrup, glycerin, sorbitol, butylparaben. Cherry, grape and bubble gum flavors.

Products listed are representative of currently available and widely distributed brands. Similar products, including regional and private label brands, may also exist.

[1] Contains 3 mg phenylalanine per tablet.
[2] Contains 6 mg phenylalanine per tablet.

PATIENT INFORMATION

Acetaminophen

- Patient instructions accompany each product. Have the patient read instructions carefully before use, preferably before leaving the pharmacy, in case of any questions.
- Severe or recurrent pain may indicate a serious illness. Consult a physician.
- Do not exceed the recommended dosage. Do not exceed a total dose of 4 g/day of acetaminophen in adults of all formulations consumed (2 g/day in regular alcohol users). Do not exceed 5 doses in 24 hours in children 6 to 12 years of age or 5 doses in 24 hours in children 3 to 6 years of age.
- Consult a physician for use in a child younger than 3 years of age.
- Do not take acetaminophen for longer than 5 days (children) or longer than 10 days (adults) for pain relief. If symptoms persist, worsen, or if new symptoms develop, contact a physician.
- Avoid alcohol and aspirin while taking this drug.

NONSTEROIDAL ANTI-INFLAMMATORY DRUGS

▶ **Actions**

NSAIDs have analgesic, anti-inflammatory, and antipyretic activities. Their exact mode of action is unknown. The major mechanism of action of NSAIDs is believed to be inhibition of cyclooxygenase (COX) activity and prostaglandin synthesis. Other mechanisms, such as inhibition of lipoxygenase, leukotriene synthesis, lysosomal enzyme release, neutrophil aggregation, and various cell-membrane functions, may exist as well.

NSAIDs are capable of inhibiting the enzyme COX. COX allows the conversion of arachidonic acid into prostaglandins, which are mediators of the inflammatory response. Prostaglandin inhibition peripherally at the site of injury can decrease the inflammatory response and pain. Prostaglandin inhibition centrally can also result in analgesia similar to other centrally acting drugs such as acetaminophen. NSAIDs may also have a direct inhibitory effect on inflammatory cells.

▶ **Indications**

For the treatment of mild to moderate pain. These agents have other labeled indications and are particularly helpful for pain associated with inflammation.

▶ **Contraindications**

NSAID hypersensitivity: Because of potential cross-sensitivity to other NSAIDs, do not give these agents to patients in whom aspirin, iodides, or other NSAIDs have induced symptoms of asthma, rhinitis, urticaria, nasal polyps, angioedema, bronchospasm, and other symptoms of allergic or anaphylactoid reactions.

▶ **Warnings**

Acute renal insufficiency: Patients with preexisting renal disease or compromised renal perfusion are at greatest risk. A form of renal toxicity seen in patients with prerenal conditions leads to reduced renal blood flow or blood volume. NSAID use may cause a dose-dependent reduction in prostaglandin formation and precipitate renal decompensation. Patients at greatest risk are the elderly, premature infants, those with heart failure, renal or hepatic dysfunction, systemic lupus erythematosus (SLE), chronic glomerulonephritis, dehydration, diabetes mellitus, septicemia, pyelonephritis, extracellular volume depletion from any cause, or impaired renal function, or those taking ACE inhibitors, any nephrotoxic drug, or diuretics. Recovery usually follows discontinuation.

Hypersensitivity: Severe hypersensitivity reactions with fever, rash, abdominal pain, headache, nausea, vomiting, signs of liver damage, and meningitis have occurred rarely in patients taking ibuprofen, especially those with SLE or other collagen diseases. Anaphylactoid reactions have occurred in patients with aspirin hypersensitivity.

Renal function impairment: NSAID metabolites are eliminated primarily by the kidneys; use with caution in patients with renal impairment. Reduce dosage to avoid excessive accumulation.

Platelet aggregation: NSAIDs can inhibit platelet aggregation; the effect is reversible, quantitatively less, and of shorter duration than that seen with aspirin. These agents prolong bleeding time (within normal range) in healthy subjects. This may be exaggerated in patients with underlying hemostatic defects; use with caution in people with intrinsic coagulation defects and in those on anticoagulant therapy.

Cardiovascular effects: May cause fluid retention and peripheral edema. Use caution in patients with compromised cardiac function (eg, heart failure), hypertension, or other conditions predisposing to fluid retention, and in those on chronic diuretic therapy. Agents may be associated with significant deterioration of circulatory hemodynamics in severe heart failure and hyponatremia, presumably due to inhibition of prostaglandin-dependent compensatory mechanisms.

Infection: NSAIDs may mask the usual signs of infection (eg, fever, myalgia, arthralgia). Use with extra care in the presence of existing controlled infection.

Photosensitivity: Photosensitivity may occur; caution patients to take protective measures (eg, sunscreens, protective clothing) against UV or sunlight until tolerance is determined.

GI effects: GI toxicity (including NSAID-induced ulcers and GI bleeding disorders) can occur at any time with or without warning with chronic use of NSAIDs. High-dose NSAIDs probably carry a greater risk of causing GI adverse effects. Have patients with a history of GI lesions consult a physician before using these products. GI adverse effects are more likely to occur and may be more pronounced in elderly patients.

Ibuprofen: Do not take for longer than 3 days for fever. If symptoms persist, worsen, or if new symptoms develop, contact a physician.

Pregnancy: Category B; Category D in 3rd trimester. Safety for use during pregnancy has not been established; use is not recommended. There are no adequate, well-controlled studies in pregnant women. An increased incidence of dystocia, increased postimplantation loss, and delayed parturition has occurred in animals. Agents that inhibit prostaglandin synthesis may cause closure of the ductus arteriosus and other untoward effects in the fetus. GI tract toxicity is increased in pregnant women in the last trimester. Some NSAIDs may prolong pregnancy if given before onset of labor. Avoid use during pregnancy, especially during the 3rd trimester.

Lactation: Most NSAIDs are excreted in breast milk in low concentrations. The American Academy of Pediatrics considers ibuprofen and naproxen to be compatible with breastfeeding. Data on the use of ketoprofen during nursing are lacking.

Children: The use of naproxen is not recommended in children younger than 12 years of age unless directed by a physician. Ketoprofen is not recommended for use in children younger than 16 years of age.

Elderly: Age appears to increase the possibility of adverse reactions to NSAIDs. The risk of serious ulcer disease is increased in elderly patients (older than 65 years of age) taking NSAIDs chronically; this risk appears to increase with dose. Use with greater care and begin with lower dosages in this patient population.

▶ **Drug Interactions**

NSAID Drug Interactions			
Precipitant drug	**Object drug***		**Description**
NSAIDs	ACE inhibitors	↓	NSAIDs may diminish the antihypertensive effect of ACE inhibitors.
NSAIDs	Aminoglycosides	↑	Aminoglycoside plasma concentrations may be elevated in premature infants because of NSAIDs, reducing the glomerular filtration rate. Reduce aminoglycoside dose prior to NSAID initiation and monitor serum aminoglycoside levels and renal function.
NSAIDs	Anticoagulants	↑	Coadministration may prolong prothrombin time (PT). Also consider the effects NSAIDs have on platelet function and gastric mucosa. Monitor PT and patients closely, especially during the first few days of therapy, and instruct patients to watch for signs and symptoms of bleeding.
NSAIDs	Beta blockers	↓	The antihypertensive effect of beta blockers may be impaired. Avoid using this combination if possible.
NSAIDs	Cyclosporine	↑	Nephrotoxicity of both agents may be increased.
NSAIDs	Digoxin	↑	Ibuprofen may increase digoxin serum levels.
NSAIDs	Hydantoins	↑	Serum phenytoin levels may be increased, resulting in an increase in pharmacologic and toxic effects of phenytoin.
NSAIDs	Lithium	↑	Serum lithium levels may be increased.
NSAIDs	Loop diuretics	↓	Effects of diuretics may be decreased.
NSAIDs	Methotrexate	↑	The risks of methotrexate toxicity (eg, stomatitis, bone marrow suppression, nephrotoxicity) may be increased.
NSAIDs	Thiazide diuretics	↓	Decreased antihypertensive and diuretic action of thiazides may occur with concurrent naproxen.
Bisphosphonates	NSAIDS	↑	Risk of gastric ulceration may be increased. Use cautiously.
Cholestyramine	NSAIDs	↓	The effects of NSAIDs may be decreased.
Cimetidine	NSAIDs	↔	NSAID plasma concentrations may be increased or decreased by cimetidine; some studies report no effect.
Probenecid	NSAIDs	↑	Probenecid may increase the concentrations and possibly the toxicity of the NSAIDs.
Salicylates	NSAIDs	↓	Plasma concentrations of NSAIDs may be decreased by salicylates. Avoid concurrent use because it offers no therapeutic advantage and may significantly increase the incidence of GI adverse effects.

* ↑ = Object drug increased. ↓ = Object drug decreased. ↔ = Undetermined clinical effect.

▶ **Adverse Reactions**

Cardiovascular: Edema; congestive heart failure; hypertension; tachycardia.

CNS: Dizziness; drowsiness; headache; light-headedness; vertigo.

Dermatologic: Erythema; pruritus; rash; increased sweating; urticaria; photosensitivity; eczema.

GI: Bleeding; diarrhea; dyspepsia; heartburn; nausea; vomiting; abdominal pain or cramps; constipation; flatulence; ulcer bleed; gastritis; melena; epigastric/GI pain; abdominal/GI distress; bloating; GI fullness; stomatitis; anorexia; dry mouth; peptic ulcer; jaundice; pancreatitis; colitis; hematemesis; appetite increase; eructation; rectal bleeding/hemorrhage.

GU: Urinary frequency; renal function impairment; hematuria; interstitial nephritis; renal failure; cystitis; menstrual disorder; azotemia; nephrotic syndrome; papillary necrosis.

Respiratory: Dyspnea; rhinitis; pharyngitis; epitaxis; bronchospasm.

Miscellaneous: Muscle cramps; thirst; purpura; anemia; thrombocytopenia; eosinophilia; liver test abnormalities; BUN increased; hemoglobin and hematocrit decreases; fluid retention; body weight changes; hyperglycemia; hyperkalemia; myalgia; muscle weakness; hearing disturbances; visual disturbances; taste disorder; chills; fever.

IBUPROFEN

▶ **Administration and Dosage**

Adults: 200 mg orally every 4 to 6 hours as needed. If pain does not respond to 200 mg, 400 mg may be used. Do not exceed 1.2 g in 24 hours. Do not take for pain for longer than 10 days unless directed by physician. If GI upset occurs, take with meals or milk.

Children (6 months to 12 years of age): 5 to 10 mg/kg/dose orally and repeated 3 to 4 times daily as needed. Maximum daily dose is 40 mg/kg.

IBUPROFEN PRODUCTS	
Trade name	**Doseform**
Advil,[1] Maximum Strength Midol, Motrin IB	**Tablets**: 200 mg
Junior Strength Advil	**Tablets, coated**: 100 mg. Parabens, sucrose.
Children's Advil,[2] Children's Motrin[3]	**Tablets, chewable**: 50 mg. Aspartame.
Junior Strength Advil,[4] Junior Strength Motrin[5]	**Tablets, chewable**: 100 mg. Aspartame.
Advil Liqui-Gels	**Capsules**: 200 mg. Sorbitol.
Junior Strength Motrin	**Caplets**: 100 mg
Motrin IB	**Caplets**: 200 mg
Advil [6]	**Gelcaps**: 200 mg
Motrin IB	**Gelcaps**: 200 mg. Benzyl alcohol, parabens, castor oil, and EDTA.
Infants' Advil Concentrated Drops,[7] Infants' Motrin Concentrated Drops[8]	**Liquid**: 50 mg/1.25 mL. Glycerin, sorbitol, sucrose.

IBUPROFEN PRODUCTS

Trade name	Doseform
Children's Advil,[9] Children's Motrin[10]	**Suspension**: 100 mg/5 mL. Glycerin, sucrose.

Products listed are representative of currently available and widely distributed brands. Similar products, including regional and private label brands, may also exist.

[1] Contains parabens and sucrose.
[2] Fruit and grape flavors.
[3] Orange flavor.
[4] Contains 2.1 mg phenylalanine. Fruit and grape flavors.
[5] Contains 2.8 mg phenylalanine. Orange and grape flavors.
[6] Also contains glycerin and simethicone.
[7] Fruit and grape flavors. Contains EDTA.
[8] Berry and berry dye-free flavors.
[9] Fruit, grape, and blue raspberry flavors. Also contains sorbitol and EDTA.
[10] Grape, berry, bubble gum, and dye-free berry flavors.

PATIENT INFORMATION

Ibuprofen

- *Adults:* Do not exceed 1.2 g/day.
- Patient instructions accompany each product. Have the patient read these instructions carefully before use, preferably before leaving the pharmacy, in case of any questions.
- May cause GI upset; take with food or after meals.
- Take with a full glass of water (240 mL) to reduce the risk of the medication lodging in the esophagus.
- Severe or recurrent pain may indicate a serious illness. Consult a physician.
- Do not take OTC NSAIDs for longer than 10 days for pain unless directed by a physician. If symptoms persist, worsen, or if new symptoms develop, contact a physician.
- Notify physician if rash, itching, visual disturbances, edema, black stools, or persistent headache occur.
- If the patient consumes 3 or more alcoholic drinks every day, taking ibuprofen or other pain relievers or fever reducers may cause stomach bleeding.
- Avoid aspirin while taking this medication.

KETOPROFEN

▶ Administration and Dosage

Adults: 12.5 mg every 4 to 6 hours as needed. If pain persists longer than 1 hour, follow with 12.5 mg. Do not exceed 25 mg in a 4- to 6-hour period or 75 mg in a 24-hour period. Use the smallest effective dose.

Children: Do not give to children younger than 16 years of age unless directed by a physician.

KETOPROFEN PRODUCTS

Trade name	Doseform
Orudis KT	**Tablets**: 12.5 mg

Products listed are representative of currently available and widely distributed brands. Similar products, including regional and private label brands, may also exist.

PATIENT INFORMATION

Ketoprofen

- *Adults:* Do not exceed 75 mg/day.
- Patient instructions accompany each product. Have the patient read these instructions carefully before use, preferably before leaving the pharmacy, in case of any questions.
- May cause GI upset; take with food or after meals.
- Take with a full glass of water (240 mL) to reduce the risk of the medication lodging in the esophagus.
- Severe or recurrent pain may indicate a serious illness. Consult a physician.
- Do not take OTC NSAIDs for longer than 10 days for pain unless directed by a physician. If symptoms persist, worsen, or if new symptoms develop, contact a physician.
- Notify physician if rash, itching, visual disturbances, edema, black stools, or persistent headache occur.
- Avoid alcohol and aspirin while taking this medication.

NAPROXEN

▶ Administration and Dosage

Adults: 200 mg with a full glass of liquid every 8 to 12 hours as needed. With experience, some patients may find an initial dose of 400 mg followed by 200 mg 12 hours later, if necessary, will give better relief. Do not exceed 600 mg in 24 hours unless otherwise directed. Use the smallest effective dose.

Children: Do not give to children younger than 12 years of age unless directed by a physician.

Elderly (older than 65 years of age): Do not take more than 200 mg in a 12-hour period.

NAPROXEN PRODUCTS	
Trade name	Doseform
Aleve	**Tablets:** 200 mg (220 mg naproxen sodium)
Aleve	**Caplets:** 200 mg (220 mg naproxen sodium)
Aleve	**Gelcaps:** 200 mg (220 mg naproxen sodium). EDTA, glycerin.

Products listed are representative of currently available and widely distributed brands. Similar products, including regional and private label brands, may also exist.

PATIENT INFORMATION

Naproxen

- *Adults:* Do not exceed 600 mg/day.
- Patient instructions accompany each product. Have the patient read these instructions carefully before use, preferably before leaving the pharmacy, in case of any questions.
- May cause GI upset; take with food or after meals.
- Take with a full glass of water (240 mL) to reduce the risk of the medication lodging in the esophagus.
- Severe or recurrent pain may indicate a serious illness. Consult a physician.
- Do not take OTC NSAIDs for longer than 10 days for pain unless directed by a physician. If symptoms persist, worsen, or if new symptoms develop, contact a physician.
- Notify physician if rash, itching, visual disturbances, edema, black stools, or persistent headache occur.
- If the patient consumes 3 or more alcoholic drinks every day, taking naproxen or other NSAID pain relievers or fever reducers may cause stomach bleeding.
- Avoid aspirin while taking this medication.

RUBS AND LINIMENTS

▶ Indications

These products are used for relief of pain of muscular aches, neuralgia, rheumatism, arthritis, sprains, and like conditions, when skin is intact.

Individual components include:

Counterirritants: Camphor, capsicum preparations (capsicum oleoresin, capsaicin), eucalyptus oil, menthol, methyl nicotinate, methyl salicylate, mustard oil, wormwood oil.

Antiseptics: Thymol.

Analgesics: Trolamine salicylate, methyl salicylate.

▶ Contraindications

Allergy to components of any formulation or to salicylates.

▶ Warnings

For external use only: Avoid contact with eyes, eyelids, and mucous membranes.

Apply to affected parts only: Do not apply to irritated skin; discontinue use if excessive irritation develops. Consult a physician if pain persists for longer than 7 to 10 days, or if redness is present, or in conditions affecting children younger than 10 years of age.

Heat therapy: Do not use an external source of high heat (eg, heating pad) with these agents because irritation and burning of the skin may occur.

Protective covering: Applying a tight bandage or wrap over these agents is not recommended because increased absorption may occur.

▶ Drug Interactions

Anticoagulants: An enhanced anticoagulant effect (eg, increased prothrombin time) occurred in several patients receiving an anticoagulant and using topical methyl salicylate concurrently.

► **Adverse Reactions**

If applied to large skin areas and used over a prolonged period of time, salicylate side effects (eg, tinnitus, nausea, vomiting) may occur.

Products may be toxic if ingested.

Counterirritants may cause local irritation, especially in patients with sensitive skin.

► **Administration and Dosage**

Apply to affected areas as needed.

RUBS AND LINIMENTS	
Trade name	Doseform
Icy Hot	**Balm**: 29% methyl salicylate, 7.6% menthol, white petrolatum
Epiderm	**Balm**: Isopropyl alcohol, parabens, ureas, menthol, EDTA
JointFlex	**Cream**: 3.1% camphor, lanolin, aloe, urea, EDTA, glycerin, peppermint oil
Capzasin-P	**Cream**: 0.025% capsaicin
ArthriCare for Women Silky Dry	**Cream**: 0.025% capsaicin, parabens, mineral oil
ArthriCare for Women Extra Moisturizing	**Cream**: 0.025% capsaicin, aloe vera gel, cetyl and stearyl alcohol, parabens
ArthriCare for Women Multi-Action	**Cream**: 0.025% capsaicin, 1.25% menthol, 0.25% methyl nicotinate, aloe vera gel, cetyl alcohol, parabens
Capzasin-HP	**Cream**: 0.075% capsaicin
ArthriCare for Women Ultra Strength	**Cream**: 0.075% capsaicin, 2% menthol, aloe vera gel, cetyl and stearyl alcohol, parabens
Vicks VapoRub	**Cream**: 2.8% menthol, 5.2% camphor, 1.2% eucalyptus oil, cedarleaf oil, cetyl and stearyl alcohol, EDTA, glycerin, urea, parabens, turpentine oil
BenGay S.P.A.	**Cream**: 10% menthol, cetyl alcohol, urea, EDTA, glycerin
Arthritic Hot	**Cream**: Methyl salicylate, menthol
Ziks	**Cream**: 12% methyl salicylate, 1% menthol, 0.025% capsaicin, cetyl alcohol, urea
Thera-Gesic	**Cream**: 15% methyl salicylate, 1% menthol, glycerin, parabens
BenGay Greaseless	**Cream**: 15% methyl salicylate, 10% menthol, cetyl alcohol, glycerin
Pain Bust-R II	**Cream**: 17% methyl salicylate, 12% menthol, cetyl and stearyl alcohol
ArthriCare for Women Nighttime	**Cream**: 30% methyl salicylate, 1.25% menthol, 0.25% methyl nicotinate, glycerin, isopropyl alcohol
Arthritis Formula BenGay	**Cream**: 30% methyl salicylate, 8% menthol, lanolin
Icy Hot	**Cream**: 30% methyl salicylate, 10% menthol
Ultra Strength BenGay	**Cream**: 30% methyl salicylate, 10% menthol, 4% camphor, EDTA, lanolin
Panalgesic Gold	**Cream**: 35% methyl salicylate, 4% menthol, lanolin, cetyl and stearyl alcohol, mineral oil
Myoflex	**Cream**: 10% triethanolamine salicylate, cetyl and stearyl alcohol, EDTA

RUBS AND LINIMENTS

Trade name	Doseform
Myoflex Extra, Myoflex Arthritic	**Cream**: 15% triethanolamine salicylate
Sportscreme	**Cream**: 10% trolamine salicylate, cetyl alcohol, glycerin, parabens, mineral oil
Aspercreme	**Cream**: 10% trolamine salicylate, aloe vera gel, cetyl alcohol, glycerin, parabens, mineral oil
Mobisyl	**Cream**: 10% trolamine salicylate, aloe vera gel, cetyl alcohol, urea, glycerin, parabens, mineral oil, sweet almond oil, EDTA
Icy Hot Arthritis Therapy	**Gel**: 0.025% capsaicin, aloe vera gel, benzyl alcohol, urea, maleated soybean oil, parabens
Flexall Quik Gel	**Gel**: Menthol, methyl salicylate
Vanishing Scent BenGay	**Gel**: 2.5% menthol, urea, isopropyl alcohol
Vicks VapoRub	**Gel**: 2.6% menthol, 4.8% camphor, 1.2% eucalyptus oil, cedarleaf oil, nutmeg oil, petrolatum, turpentine oil
Flexall 454	**Gel**: 7% menthol, aloe vera gel, eucalyptus oil, glycerin, peppermint oil, thyme oil
Maximum Strength Flexall 454	**Gel**: 16% menthol, aloe vera gel, eucalyptus oil, glycerin, peppermint oil, thyme oil
Flexall Ultra Plus	**Gel**: 16% menthol, 10% methyl salicylate, 3.1% camphor, aloe vera gel, eucalyptus oil, glycerin, peppermint oil, thyme oil
Icy Hot Chill Stick	**Gel**: 30% methyl salicylate, 10% menthol, hydrogenated castor oil, stearyl alcohol
Myoflex Ice Cold Plus	**Gel**: 15% triethanolamine salicylate
Absorbine Jr Arthritis Strength	**Liquid**: Capsaicin, echinacea, calendula, and wormwood extracts
Absorbine Jr	**Liquid**: 1.27% menthol, echinacea, calendula, and wormwood extracts, wormwood oil
Extra Strength Absorbine Jr	**Liquid**: 4% menthol, echinacea, calendula, and wormwood extracts, wormwood oil
Yager's	**Liniment**: Camphor, turpentine oil, clove oil
Panalgesic Gold	**Liniment**: 55.01% methyl salicylate, 1.25% menthol, 3.1% camphor, emollient oils, alcohol
Banalg	**Lotion**: 4.9% methyl salicylate, 1% menthol, 2% camphor, parabens, eucalyptus oil
Banalg Hospital Strength	**Lotion**: 14% methyl salicylate, 3% menthol, parabens
Aspercreme	**Lotion**: Trolamine salicylate
Eucalyptamint	**Ointment**: 16% menthol, eucalyptus oil, lanolin, mineral oil
Original Formula BenGay	**Ointment**: 18.3% methyl salicylate, 16% menthol, lanolin
Absorbine Jr	**Patch**: Menthol, camphor, eucalyptus
Absorbine Jr Deep Pain Relief	**Patch**: Menthol, glucosamine, MSM
Icy Hot	**Patch**: Methyl salicylate, menthol

Products listed are representative of currently available and widely distributed brands. Similar products, including regional and private label brands, may also exist.

PATIENT INFORMATION
Rubs and Liniments

- For external use only. Avoid contact with eyes, eyelids, and mucous membranes.
- Apply to affected areas only. Do not apply to irritated skin; discontinue use if excessive irritation develops.
- Consult a physician if pain persists for longer than 7 to 10 days, if redness is present, or in conditions affecting children younger than 10 years of age.
- Do not use an external source of high heat (eg, heating pad) with these agents because irritation and burning of the skin may occur.
- Do not apply tight bandages or wraps over these agents.
- Do not apply to broken skin.

BACK PAIN (LOWER)

DEFINITION

Lower (lumbar region) back pain is a common disorder experienced by many patients, and it is the most common of all chronic musculoskeletal pains. Depending on duration, back pain is classified as acute (lasting less than 3 months) or chronic (lasting longer than 3 to 6 months). Acute back pain generally follows overuse of or injury to the soft tissues of the back, such as ligaments or muscles, but may involve the intervertebral discs, bones, or joints of the back. A painful and often debilitating condition, lower back pain can affect the quality of life of many patients.

ETIOLOGY

Although the exact cause of lower back pain is often a mystery, it is generally due to 1 of the following causes: Mechanical problems (eg, muscle sprains and strains, herniated discs), trauma (acute and cumulative), infections (eg, meningitis), inflammation (including arthritis), metabolic disorders, neoplasms, and referred pain (pain originating from somewhere other than the back, such as abdominal or kidney disease). Mechanical problems are the most common cause of lower back pain and will be discussed in this mono graph. The other causes of lower back pain require specific treatments by physicians. In up to 97% of cases of lower back pain, there is no medical cause that can be determined; therefore, the condition is referred to as nonspecific back pain.

Some of the causes of mechanical problems resulting in lower back pain include, but are not limited to, the following: Poor posture (standing, sitting, and sleeping); obesity; improper lifting; abrupt movement; unaccustomed activity such as shoveling, digging, or raking; sedentary lifestyle; improper use of exercise equipment; improper shoes; pregnancy; age (back pain is more common in older patients); and height (taller patients experience a higher incidence of lower back pain).

INCIDENCE

An estimated 80% of American adults will experience low back pain at some point in their lifetime; some reports suggest a range of 60% to 90%. Of these patients, 5% to 10% will develop chronic back pain. These figures are staggering, especially considering that this condition is associated with estimated annual direct and indirect costs of $50 billion to $100 billion. In addition, an estimated 550 million workdays are lost annually because of back pain, resulting in $60 billion in lost productivity. Up to 2% of the population is totally disabled because of this condition, with 5% partially disabled. Considered rare in children, the peak incidence of back pain occurs in patients 30 to 50 years of age. Women are more likely to develop back pain, although this may be due to the fact that many pregnant women experience back pain.

As might be expected, patients who are less physically fit are more likely to develop back problems. Most patients recover from acute back pain (33% asymptomatic in 1 week, resolution in 90% within 6 weeks) and are able to return to work or other activities with proper treatment. Unfortunately, the rate of recurrence is high.

PATHOPHYSIOLOGY

The spine is a complex system of muscles, ligaments, tendons, joints, intervertebral discs, cartilage, and nerves; any one of these components can be affected and cause discomfort or pain. Most cases of lower back pain involve the lumbar region of the spine (see Figure 1). These vertebrae are larger and heavier than the vertebrae above them (thoracic), bear more weight, and allow for forward and backward motion. The healthy spine also has 4 normal curves, with pressure evenly distributed throughout. Poor posture, muscle spasms, etc., can "flatten" these curves, causing pain and dysfunction. If any of the muscle groups that run the length of the spine becomes injured, is unconditioned, or atrophies, the other muscle groups must

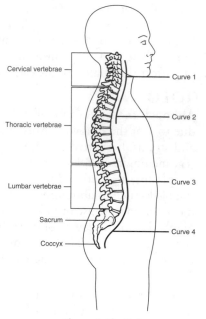

Figure 1. The Spine

work harder to compensate, thus becoming weak, fatigued, and more injury prone. Patients with chronic back pain tend to hold the injured muscles immobile, shifting pressure, weight, and work to the other muscles. These patients will often have a bent or otherwise awkward posture. The ligaments, which can also become injured, help hold the vertebrae together.

The discs, which contain a gelatinous fluid called the nucleus pulposus, are found between each vertebrae, acting as shock absorbers for the spine (see Figure 2). Discs can cause pain by bulging out and pressing on the nerves in the spinal column. This is sometimes caused by extreme compression from, for example, heavy lifting, but can also be caused by something as simple as sneezing. This condition is referred to by many names, including herniated, ruptured, slipped, bulging, prolapsed, or protruding disc. Basically, the disc wall is torn or deteriorated, allowing the fluid to bulge out. This condition is most likely to occur in the lumbar region, between the fifth lumbar and first sacral vertebrae, with decreasing frequency as you move up the lumbar region, and also in the cervical region. A common pain involved with this condition is called sciatica, which is due to disc pressure on the sciatic nerve, a large nerve formed from the convergence of specific nerve roots that run out of the pelvis below the sacrum and down both legs. It is interesting to note that some patients (up to 60%) have bulging discs with no pain at all, suggesting the condition may be normal and does not necessarily indicate a serious back problem. Another disc-related condition is degenerative disc disease. This condition involves the accelerated degeneration of the disc, leading to a narrowing of the space between the vertebrae. Usually there is no nerve involvement, so the pain tends to be localized to the lower back region.

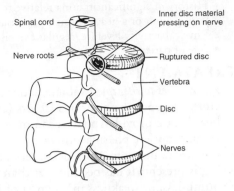

Figure 2. Disc Anatomy/Ruptured Disc

SIGNS/SYMPTOMS

As with any ache or pain, there is no single set of symptoms that accurately describes lower back pain in all patients. In addition, pain may not be localized in the lower back region. Symptoms may include the following: General pain; stiffness, dull, aching pain; sharp pain; pain in buttocks or legs; burning; numbness; weakness; intermittent pain; and constant pain. Outward signs of lower back pain may include holding the body at an awkward position, bending at the waist, and the inability to stand, sit, or walk without discomfort or pain.

DIAGNOSTIC PARAMETERS/PHYSICAL ASSESSMENT

Clinical Observation: To determine effective treatment for acute lower back pain, it is important to obtain a proper assessment and a comprehensive history from the patient. For the most part, the patient can determine whether the pain is localized to the lower back and can usually describe what occurred prior to the onset of pain. The patient may be holding his or her body in an awkward position in an attempt to lessen the pain or discomfort. Pain in the buttocks or legs becomes more challenging to diagnose, because it may or may not be referred pain from the lower back.

Interview: To help the patient determine if physician referral or self-treatment is warranted, it may be beneficial to ask about the following:

- Onset, duration, and location of the pain.
- Event(s) that precipitate the pain.
- Quality and nature of the pain.
- The severity of the pain using a 10-point rating scale where the patient quantifies the intensity of the pain (0 = no pain to 10 = most intense pain). If pain is intermittent, ask the patient to rate how they feel most of the time.
- Factors that relieve or exacerbate the pain.
- Response to previous therapy.
- Patient's medical history (including recent illness or surgery).

- History of significant trauma relative to age (eg, a fall from an elevation in a young adult or a heavy lift in a potentially osteoporotic older adult).
- Physical activity level (ie, regular exercise, occupation).
- Age of patient.

TREATMENT

Approaches to therapy: Evaluate patients using the previous diagnostic parameters. Depending on various factors (eg, symptoms, duration, recurrence), health care providers may recommend either (1) a nondrug approach, (2) appropriate pharmacotherapy, or (3) immediate referral to a physician for medical evaluation. A physician referral is necessary if any one of the following is present: It has been longer than 10 days since the pain began; tingling, numbness, or weakness in any part of the body; radiating pain into the buttocks, back of the thigh, and lower leg; pain worsens at night or when lying down; patient is younger than 20 years of age or older than 55 years of age; chronic back pain is present (longer than 3 to 6 months duration); the patient is immunosuppressed.

Nondrug therapy: There are many nondrug therapy options that may or may not be useful for treatment of lower back pain or prevention of future episodes. What may be helpful for the patient with acute back pain may not be helpful for the patient with chronic back pain. In most cases, refer chronic cases to a physician for full evaluation.

At one time it was thought that bed rest was beneficial in helping the patient recover. In fact, prolonged bed rest (longer than 3 days) may be counterproductive. Short-term bed rest (less than 2 days) or no bed rest at all is preferred, because normal physical activity and moderate exercises are useful for most patients and should be started immediately. At the other end of the extreme is over-exercising or over-stretching, which may slow recovery. The proper activities and exercises may need to be developed by a physician or physical therapist in conjunction with the patient.

Thermotherapy (heat) or cryotherapy (cold) or alternating heat and cold may be beneficial for some patients. Both may be used concurrently with systemic analgesics; however, the use of topical counterirritants is contraindicated with thermotherapy. Thermotherapy (eg, heating pad, hot water bottle, clay/gel pack, liquid sodium acetate containers) may quicken recovery. Do not use on insensitive skin, on areas with compromised blood flow, during sleep, on diabetics, or on infants because of the potential for burns. In addition, do not use on any areas that have been recently operated on because of the possibility of decreased blood flow. Cryotherapy devices (eg, gel packs) that are cooled in the refrigerator prior to application and used with a cover do not pose any danger to tissues when applied for up to 10 minutes. Avoid freezing these devices and then applying them to the skin, because they may freeze tissue.

Other nondrug measures include massage, acupuncture, and chiropractic manipulation. For chronic pain, relaxation training, biofeedback, yoga, and hypnosis have been used. The use of supportive belts, braces, corsets, etc., may be helpful in some patients but should be used only in the short term, if at all, because muscle tone can be reduced.

In patients who recover from acute back pain, preventive therapy is recommended. This includes a regular regimen of stretching and exercise, learning and using proper posture when standing and sitting, using proper positions when sleeping (on one's side in the fetal position with thin pillow between the knees, or on the back with a pillow under the knees, but never on the stomach), learning to lift and carry properly, and in general paying attention to how regular household chores and other movements are accomplished. These tasks are also important for the patient with chronic back pain.

Guidelines on lifting and carrying loads:

- Have a tight grip on the object before lifting it.
- Use slow and smooth movements while lifting. Avoid using hurried, jerky movements, which can strain back muscles.
- Face the object while lifting. Do not twist while lifting.
- Keep the load close to your body.
- Lift with your legs only when you can straddle the load. This is done by bending your knees and not your back. Keep your back straight.
- Carry the load in the area between your shoulder and waist to put less strain on your back.
- Test every load for heaviness before lifting by pushing the object lightly to see how easily it moves.

Pharmacotherapy: Discuss the use of OTC medications for long-term treatment of chronic back pain with a physician because no OTC analgesic should be used for a long period of time (longer than 10 days) without physician approval.

For treatment of acute lower back pain, salicylates, acetaminophen, and nonsteroidal anti-inflammatory drugs (NSAIDs) may be effective. Combination products containing these agents are also available. Rubs and liniments may be beneficial in some patients, but should not be used in conjunction with heat therapy (eg, a heating pad).

SALICYLATES

▶ **Actions**

The anti-inflammatory and analgesic activity of salicylates may be mediated through inhibition of the prostaglandin synthetase complex.

▶ **Indications**

For the treatment of mild-to-moderate pain. These agents have other labeled indications as well.

▶ **Contraindications**

Hypersensitivity to salicylates or nonsteroidal anti-inflammatory drugs (NSAIDs). Use with extreme caution in patients with a history of adverse reactions to salicylates. Cross-sensitivity may exist between aspirin and other NSAIDs that inhibit prostaglandin synthesis and between aspirin and tartrazine. Aspirin cross-sensitivity does not appear to occur with sodium salicylate, or salicylamide. Aspirin hypersensitivity is more prevalent in those with asthma, nasal polyposis, or chronic urticaria.

Also contraindicated in patients with hemophilia or bleeding ulcers, or those in hemorrhagic states. Magnesium salicylate is contraindicated in patients with advanced chronic renal insufficiency.

▶ **Warnings**

Concurrent medications: Many other medications, specifically multi-ingredient cough and cold products, also contain aspirin or acetaminophen. Advise patients of this possibility and to inquire about other medications they might be taking before recommending an analgesic.

Otic effects: Discontinue use if dizziness, ringing in ears (tinnitus), or impaired hearing occurs. Tinnitus probably represents blood salicylic acid levels reaching or exceeding the upper limit of the therapeutic range; therefore, it is a helpful guide to toxicity. Temporary hearing loss disappears gradually upon discontinuation of the drug.

Hypersensitivity: Do not use if there is a history of sensitivity to aspirin or NSAIDs.

Aspirin intolerance, manifested by acute bronchospasm, generalized urticaria/angioedema, severe rhinitis, or shock occurs in 4% to 19% of asthmatics. Symptoms generally occur within 3 hours after ingestion.

Foods may contribute to a reaction. Some foods with high salicylate content include curry powder, paprika, licorice, Benedictine liqueur, prunes, raisins, tea, and gherkins. A typical American diet contains 10 to 200 mg/day salicylate.

Hepatic function impairment: Use with caution in patients with liver damage, preexisting hypoprothrombinemia, and vitamin K deficiency.

GI effects: Use with caution in patients who are intolerant to salicylates because of GI irritation, and in those with gastric ulcers, peptic ulcers, mild diabetes, gout, erosive gastritis, or bleeding tendencies.

Surgical procedures: Aspirin should not be consumed within 7 days of a medical or dental surgical procedure.

Hematologic effects: Aspirin interferes with hemostasis. Avoid use in patients who take anticoagulants (eg, warfarin, heparin) and in those with severe anemia or a history of blood coagulation defects.

Pregnancy: Category D (aspirin); *Category C* (salsalate, magnesium salicylate, other salicylates). Aspirin may produce adverse effects in the mother, such as anemia, ante- or postpartum hemorrhage, or prolonged gestation and labor. Salicylates readily cross the placenta. By inhibiting prostaglandin synthesis, salicylates may cause constriction of ductus arteriosus and, possibly, other untoward fetal effects. Maternal aspirin use during later stages of pregnancy may cause adverse fetal effects, such as low birth weight, increased incidence of intracranial hemorrhage in premature infants, stillbirth, or neonatal death. Salicylates may be teratogens. Avoid use during pregnancy, especially in the third trimester.

Lactation: Salicylates are excreted in breast milk in low concentrations. Adverse effects on platelet function in the nursing infant are a potential risk. The American Academy of Pediatrics recommends that aspirin be used cautiously in nursing mothers.

Children: Administration of aspirin to children, including teenagers, with acute febrile illness due to chickenpox and influenza has been associated with the development of Reye syndrome.

▶ Drug Interactions

Salicylate Drug Interactions			
Precipitant drug	**Object drug***		**Description**
Salicylates	Alcohol	↑	The risk of GI ulceration increases when salicylates are given concomitantly. Ingestion of alcohol during salicylate therapy may also prolong bleeding time.
Salicylates	Angiotensin-converting enzyme inhibitors	↓	Antihypertensive effectiveness of these agents may be decreased by concurrent salicylate administration, possibly because of prostaglandin inhibition. Consider discontinuing salicylates if problems occur.
Salicylates	Anticoagulants	↑	Therapeutic aspirin has an additive hypoprothrombinemic effect. Bleeding time may be prolonged due to impaired platelet function. Use caution.
Salicylates	Heparin	↑	Aspirin can increase the risk of bleeding in heparin-anticoagulated patients.
Salicylates	Loop diuretics	↓	Loop diuretics may be less effective when given with salicylates in patients with compromised renal function or with cirrhosis with ascites; however, data conflict.
Salicylates	Methotrexate	↑	Salicylates increase drug levels, causing toxicity by interfering with protein binding and renal elimination of the antimetabolite.
Salicylates	Nitroglycerin	↑	Nitroglycerin, when taken with aspirin, may result in unexpected hypotension. Data are limited. If hypotension occurs, reduce the nitroglycerin dose.
Salicylates	NSAIDs	↓	Aspirin may decrease NSAID serum concentrations. Avoid concomitant use; it offers no therapeutic advantage and may significantly increase the incidence of GI effects.
Salicylates	Probenecid, sulfinpyrazone	⟷	Salicylates antagonize the uricosuric effect. While salicylates in large doses (> 3 g/day) have a uricosuric effect, smaller amounts may reduce the uricosuric effect of these agents.
Salicylates	Spironolactone	↓	Salicylates may inhibit the diuretic effects; antihypertensive action does not appear altered. Effects depend on the dose of spironolactone.
Salicylates	Sulfonylureas, exogenous insulin	↑	Salicylates in doses > 2 g/day have a hypoglycemic action, perhaps by altering pancreatic beta-cell function. They may potentiate the glucose-lowering effect of these drugs.
Salicylates	Valproic acid	↑	Aspirin displaces valproic acid from its protein-binding sites and may decrease its total body clearance, thus increasing the pharmacologic effects.
Antacids, urinary alkalinizers	Salicylates	↓	Decreased pharmacologic effects of salicylates may occur. The magnitude of the antacid interaction depends on the agent, dose, and pretreatment urine pH.
Carbonic anhydrase inhibitors	Salicylates	⟷	Salicylate intoxication has occurred after coadministration of these agents. However, salicylic acid renal elimination may be increased by these drugs if urine is kept alkaline. Conversely, salicylates may displace acetazolamide from protein-binding sites, resulting in toxicity. Further study is needed.

Salicylate Drug Interactions			
Precipitant drug	Object drug*		Description
Charcoal, activated	Salicylates	↓	Coadministration decreases aspirin absorption, depending on charcoal dose and interval between ingestion.
Corticosteroids	Salicylates	↓	Corticosteroids increase salicylate clearance and decrease salicylate serum levels.
Nizatidine	Salicylates	↑	Increased serum salicylate levels have occurred in patients receiving high doses (3.9 g/day) of aspirin and concurrent nizatidine.
Urinary acidifiers	Salicylates	↑	Ammonium chloride, ascorbic acid, and methionine decrease salicylate excretion.

* ↑ = Object drug increased. ↓ = Object drug decreased. ↔ = Undetermined clinical effect.

▶ **Adverse Reactions**

Adverse reactions can be seen in the following body systems: GI (nausea, dyspepsia, heartburn, epigastric discomfort); hematologic (prolonged bleeding time, leukopenia, thrombocytopenia, purpura, decreased plasma iron concentration, shortened erythrocyte survival time); and dermatologic (rash, hives, and angioedema may occur, especially in patients with chronic urticaria). Additional miscellaneous adverse reactions include fever, thirst, and dimness of vision.

Allergic and anaphylactic reactions have been noted when hypersensitive individuals took aspirin. Fatal anaphylactic shock, while not common, has been reported.

Aspirin has a reversible effect on platelet aggregation.

▶ **Overdosage**

Symptoms: The approximate acute lethal dose for adults is 10 to 30 g, and for children, 4 g. Respiratory alkalosis is seen initially in acute salicylate ingestions. Hyperpnea and tachypnea occur as a result of increased CO_2 production and a direct stimulatory effect of salicylate on the respiratory center. Other symptoms may include nausea, vomiting, hypokalemia, tinnitus, neurologic abnormalities (eg, disorientation, irritability, hallucinations, lethargy, stupor, coma, seizures), dehydration, hyperthermia, hyperventilation, hyperactivity, thrombocytopenia, platelet dysfunction, hypoprothrombinemia, increased capillary fragility, and other hematologic abnormalities. Symptoms may progress quickly to depression, coma, and respiratory failure and collapse. Chronic salicylate toxicity may occur when more than 100 mg/kg/day is ingested for 2 days or more. It is more difficult to recognize than acute overdosage and is associated with increased morbidity and mortality. Compared with acute poisoning, hyperventilation, dehydration, systemic acidosis, and severe CNS manifestations occur more frequently.

Treatment: Initial treatment includes induction of emesis or gastric lavage to remove any unabsorbed drug from the stomach. Activated charcoal diminishes salicylate absorption most effectively if given within 2 hours after ingestion. It is important to contact a local poison control center or emergency room if overdosage is suspected.

ASPIRIN

▶ **Administration and Dosage**

Adults: 325 to 650 mg orally every 4 hours as needed. Some extra-strength products recommend 500 mg every 3 hours or 1000 mg every 6 hours as needed.

Children: The oral analgesic/antipyretic dosage is 10 to 15 mg/kg/dose every 4 hours as needed (see table), up to 60 to 80 mg/kg/day. Do not use in children or teenagers with chickenpox or "flu" symptoms because of the possibility of Reye syndrome. Dosage recommendations by age and weight are as follows:

Recommended Aspirin Dosage in Children					
Age (years)	Weight		Dosage (mg every 4 hours)	No. of 81 mg tablets (every 4 hours)	No. of 325 mg tablets (every 4 hours)
	lbs	kg			
2-3	24-35	10.6-15.9	162	2	½
4-5	36-47	16-21.4	243	3	N/A
6-8	48-59	21.5-26.8	324	4	1
9-10	60-71	26.9-32.3	405	5	N/A
11	72-95	32.4-43.2	486	6	1½
12-14	≥ 96	≥ 43.3	648	8	2

ASPIRIN PRODUCTS	
Trade name	Doseform
Original Bayer, Norwich Aspirin	**Tablets**: 325 mg
Bayer Children's Chewable Aspirin	**Tablets, chewable**: 81 mg. Dextrose, saccharin. Cherry and orange flavors.
Adult Low Strength Ecotrin, Halfprin 81[1]	**Tablets, enteric coated**: 81 mg. Talc.
Halfprin 162	**Tablets, enteric coated**: 162 mg. Lactose, talc.
Ecotrin Regular Strength	**Tablets, enteric coated**: 325 mg. Talc.
Norwich Maximum Strength	**Tablets, enteric coated**: 500 mg
Ecotrin Maximum Strength	**Tablets, enteric coated**: 500 mg. Talc.
Alka-Seltzer Original Effervescent Antacid and Pain Relief Medicine	**Tablets, effervescent**: 325 mg, 1000 mg citric acid, 1916 mg sodium bicarbonate
Bayer Women's Aspirin Plus Calcium	**Caplets**: 81 mg, 300 mg calcium. Lactose, mineral oil.
Original Bayer	**Caplets**: 325 mg
Extra Strength Bayer PM Aspirin Plus Sleep Aid	**Caplets**: 500 mg, 25 mg diphenhydramine HCl
Extra Strength Bayer Aspirin	**Caplets, coated**: 500 mg
Extra Strength Bayer Back and Body Pain	**Caplets, coated**: 500 mg, 32.5 mg caffeine
Extra Strength Bayer Arthritis Pain Regimen	**Caplets, enteric coated**: 500 mg
Original Bayer	**Gelcaps**: 325 mg. Parabens, sorbitol, glycerin.
Extra Strength Bayer Aspirin	**Gelcaps, coated**: 500 mg. Parabens, glycerin.

BUFFERED ASPIRIN PRODUCTS	
Trade name	Doseform
Adprin-B	**Tablets, coated**: 325 mg with calcium carbonate, magnesium carbonate, magnesium oxide
Regular Strength Ascriptin	**Tablets, coated**: 325 mg with 50 mg magnesium hydroxide, 50 mg aluminum hydroxide, calcium carbonate. Talc.

BUFFERED ASPIRIN PRODUCTS	
Trade name	Doseform
Bufferin	**Tablets, coated**: 325 mg with 158 mg calcium carbonate, 63 mg magnesium oxide, 34 mg magnesium carbonate. Mineral oil, sorbitol, citric acid.
Extra Strength Adprin-B	**Tablets, coated**: 500 mg with calcium carbonate, magnesium carbonate, magnesium oxide.
Bayer Adult Low Strength	**Caplets**: 81 mg, buffered with 250 mg calcium carbonate
Extra Strength Bayer Plus	**Caplets**: 500 mg with calcium carbonate, magnesium carbonate, magnesium oxide
Maximum Strength Ascriptin	**Caplets, coated**: 500 mg with 80 mg magnesium hydroxide, 80 mg aluminum hydroxide, calcium carbonate. Saccharin, sorbitol, talc.

Products listed are representative of currently available and widely distributed brands. Similar products, including regional and private label brands, may also exist.

[1] Also contains lactose.

PATIENT INFORMATION
Aspirin

- Severe or recurrent low back pain may indicate a serious illness or injury. Consult a physician.
- Patient instructions accompany each product. Have the patient read these instructions carefully before use, preferably before leaving the pharmacy, in case of any questions.
- May cause GI upset; take with or after meals. Enteric-coated products may prevent or reduce stomach/GI distress.
- Do not use in children or adolescents because of the potential development of Reye syndrome.
- Take with a full glass of water (240 mL) to reduce the risk of the medication lodging in the esophagus.
- Avoid taking antacids within 2 hours of taking enteric-coated tablets.
- Have patients allergic to tartrazine dye avoid aspirin.
- Notify physician if rash, difficult breathing, ringing in the ears, unusual bruising or bleeding, or persistent GI pain occurs. Internal bleeding may occur with no GI symptoms and may be indicated by bloody or black stools.
- Inform physician or dentist of aspirin use before surgery or dental care.
- Do not use aspirin if it has a strong vinegar-like odor. This suggests deterioration of aspirin and loss of potency.

MAGNESIUM SALICYLATE

▶ Actions

Magnesium salicylate is a sodium-free salicylate derivative that may have a low incidence of GI upset.

▶ Contraindications

Magnesium salicylate is contraindicated in patients with advanced chronic renal insufficiency because of magnesium retention.

▶ Warnings

The possibility of magnesium toxicity exists in patients with renal insufficiency.

▶ **Administration and Dosage**

Product labeling and dosages are expressed as magnesium salicylate anhydrous.

Adults: Usual dose is 650 mg every 4 hours or 1 g every 6 hours as needed up to 4 g/day.

Children: Safety and efficacy for use in children have not been established.

MAGNESIUM SALICYLATE PRODUCTS	
Trade name	Doseform
Regular Strength Doan's	**Caplets:** 377 mg
Extra Strength Doan's	**Caplets:** 580 mg
Extra Strength Doan's P.M.	**Caplets:** 580 mg, 25 mg diphenhydramine HCl. Talc.

Products listed are representative of currently available and widely distributed brands. Similar products, including regional and private label brands, may also exist.

PATIENT INFORMATION

Magnesium Salicylate

- Do not use these products if you have renal insufficiency.
- Severe or recurrent low back pain may indicate a serious illness or injury. Consult a physician.
- Patient instructions accompany each product. Have the patient read these instructions carefully before use, preferably before leaving the pharmacy, in case of any questions.
- May cause GI upset; take with food or after meals.
- Do not use in children or adolescents because of the potential development of Reye syndrome.
- Notify physician if rash, difficult breathing, ringing in the ears, unusual bruising or bleeding, or persistent GI pain occurs. Internal bleeding may occur with no GI symptoms and may be indicated by bloody or black stools.

ACETAMINOPHEN (APAP)

▶ **Actions**

Generally, the antipyretic and analgesic effects of APAP and aspirin are comparable; however, the site and mechanism of the analgesic effect of acetaminophen are unclear.

▶ **Indications**

For the treatment of mild-to-moderate low back pain. Also used as an analgesic-antipyretic in the presence of aspirin allergy, and in patients with blood coagulation disorders who are being treated with oral anticoagulants, bleeding diatheses (eg, hemophilia), upper GI disease (eg, ulcer, gastritis, hiatal hernia), and gouty arthritis. This agent has other labeled indications as well.

▶ **Contraindications**

Hypersensitivity to acetaminophen.

▶ **Warnings**

Concurrent medications: Many medications, specifically multi-ingredient cough and cold products, contain aspirin or acetaminophen. It is important to advise patients of this, and to inquire about other medications they might be taking before recommending an analgesic.

Hepatotoxicity: Hepatotoxicity and severe hepatic failure have occurred in chronic alcoholics following therapeutic doses. The hepatotoxicity may be caused by induction of hepatic microsomal enzymes, resulting in an increase in toxic metabolites, or by the reduced amount of glutathione responsible for conjugating toxic metabolites. A safe dose for chronic alcohol abusers has not been determined. Caution chronic alcoholics and those consuming alcohol on a daily basis to limit acetaminophen intake to 2 g/day or less.

Pregnancy: Category B. Acetaminophen crosses the placenta, but has been routinely used in all stages of pregnancy. When used in therapeutic doses, it appears safe for short-term use.

Lactation: APAP is excreted in low amounts, but no adverse effects have been reported. The American Academy of Pediatrics considers acetaminophen to be compatible with breastfeeding.

Children: Consult a physician before using in children younger than 3 years of age.

▶ **Drug Interactions**

Acetaminophen Drug Interactions			
Precipitant drug	**Object drug***		**Description**
Alcohol, ethyl	APAP	↑	Hepatotoxicity has occurred in chronic alcoholics following various dose levels (moderate-to-high) of acetaminophen.
Anticholinergics	APAP	⟷	The onset of acetaminophen effect may be delayed or decreased slightly, but the ultimate pharmacologic effect is not significantly affected by anticholinergics.
Beta blockers, propranolol	APAP	↑	Propranolol appears to inhibit the enzyme systems responsible for glucuronidation and oxidation of acetaminophen. Therefore, the pharmacologic effects of acetaminophen may be increased.
Charcoal, activated	APAP	↓	Reduces acetaminophen absorption when administered as soon as possible after overdose.
Contraceptives, oral	APAP	↓	Increase in glucuronidation resulting in increased plasma clearance and a decreased half-life of acetaminophen.
Probenecid	APAP	↑	Probenecid may increase the therapeutic effectiveness of acetaminophen slightly.
APAP	Lamotrigine	↓	Serum lamotrigine concentrations may be reduced, producing a decrease in therapeutic effects.
APAP	Loop diuretics	↓	The effects of the loop diuretic may be decreased because APAP may decrease renal prostaglandin excretion and decrease plasma renin activity.
APAP	Zidovudine	↓	The pharmacologic effects of zidovudine may be decreased because of enhanced nonhepatic or renal clearance of zidovudine.

* ↑ = Object drug increased. ↓ = Object drug decreased. ⟷ = Undetermined clinical effect.

The potential hepatotoxicity of acetaminophen may be increased by large doses or long-term administration of barbiturates, carbamazepine, hydantoins, rifampin, and sulfinpyrazone. The therapeutic effects of acetaminophen may also be decreased.

▶ **Adverse Reactions**

When used as directed, acetaminophen rarely causes severe toxicity or side effects. However, the following adverse reactions have been reported:

Hematologic: Hemolytic anemia; neutropenia; leukopenia; pancytopenia; thrombocytopenia.

Miscellaneous: Fever; hypoglycemia; jaundice; rash.

▶ **Overdosage**

Symptoms: Acute poisoning may be manifested by nausea, vomiting, drowsiness, confusion, liver tenderness, low blood pressure, cardiac arrhythmias, jaundice, and acute hepatic and renal failure. These occur within the first 24 hours and may persist for 1 week or longer. Death has occurred because of liver necrosis. Acute renal failure may also occur. There are often no specific early symptoms or signs. There are 4 stages in the course of acetaminophen poisoning (postingestion):

Stage 1 (12 to 24 hours) – Nausea, vomiting, diaphoresis, anorexia.

Stage 2 (24 to 48 hours) – AST, bilirubin, and prothrombin levels begin to rise.

Stage 3 (72 to 96 hours) – Peak hepatotoxicity; AST of 20,000 not unusual.

Stage 4 (7 to 8 days) – Recovery.

Hepatotoxicity may result. The minimal toxic dose is 10 g (140 mg/kg), but liver damage has occurred with a single 5.85 g dose; doses of 20 to 25 g or more are potentially fatal. Children appear less susceptible to toxicity than adults because they have less capacity for glucuronidation metabolism. Initial signs of toxicity may include nausea, vomiting, anorexia, malaise, diaphoresis, abdominal pain, and diarrhea. Hepatotoxicity is usually not apparent for 48 to 72 hours. Hepatic failure may lead to encephalopathy, coma, and death.

Plasma acetaminophen levels greater than 300 mcg/mL at 4 hours postingestion were associated with hepatic damage in 90% of patients; minimal hepatic damage is anticipated if plasma levels are lower than 120 mcg/mL at 4 hours or lower than 30 mcg/mL at 12 hours after ingestion.

Chronic excessive use (over 4 g/day) may lead to transient hepatotoxicity. The kidneys may undergo tubular necrosis; the myocardium may be damaged.

Treatment: Perform gastric lavage in all cases, preferably within 4 hours of ingestion. Refer also to General Management of Acute Overdosage. It is important to contact a local poison control center or emergency room if overdosage is suspected.

▶ **Administration and Dosage**

Adults: 325 to 650 mg orally every 4 hours, or 1 g 3 to 4 times daily as needed. Do not exceed 4 g/day for all formulations containing acetaminophen. Do not exceed 2 g/day in chronic alcoholism.

Children: The usual oral dose is 10 mg/kg/dose, which may be repeated 4 to 5 times daily as needed. Do not exceed 5 doses in 24 hours.

Acetaminophen Dosage for Children			
Age	Dosage (mg)	Age	Dosage (mg)
0-3 months	40	6-8 years	320
4-11 months	80	9-10 years	400
1- 2 years	120	11 years	480
2-3 years	160	12-14 years	640
4-5 years	240	> 14 years	650

Suppositories:

Adults – 650 mg every 4 to 6 hours as needed; do not exceed 4 g in 24 hours.

Children (3 to 11 months of age) – 80 mg every 6 hours as needed.

(1 to 3 years of age) – 80 mg every 4 hours as needed.

(3 to 6 years of age) – 120 to 125 mg every 4 to 6 hours as needed; do not exceed 720 mg in 24 hours.

(6 to 12 years of age) – 325 mg every 4 to 6 hours as needed; do not exceed 2.6 g in 24 hours.

Storage: Store suppositories below 27°C (80°F) or refrigerate. Store tablets and oral solutions at 15° to 30°C (59° to 86°F).

ACETAMINOPHEN PRODUCTS	
Trade name	Doseform
Maranox, Tylenol Regular Strength	Tablets: 325 mg
Aspirin Free Anacin, Tylenol Extra Strength	Tablets: 500 mg
Tylenol Arthritis Pain Extended Relief	Tablets: 650 mg
Children's Tylenol	Tablets, chewable: 80 mg. Aspartame, mannitol.
Junior Strength Tylenol	Tablets, chewable: 160 mg. Aspartame, mannitol.
Tylenol Extra Strength	Gelcaps: 500 mg. Parabens.
Tylenol Extra Strength	Geltabs: 500 mg. Parabens.
Infants' FeverAll	Suppositories: 80 mg
Acephen, Children's FeverAll	Suppositories: 120 mg
Acephen, Jr. Strength FeverAll	Suppositories: 325 mg
Acephen, Adults' FeverAll	Suppositories: 650 mg
Aceta	Elixir: 120 mg/5 mL
Children's Silapap	Elixir: 80 mg/2.5 mL. Alcohol and sugar free.
Dolono	Elixir: 80 mg/2.5 mL. Sorbitol, sucrose. Alcohol free.
Infants' Tylenol Concentrated Drops	Liquid: 160 mg/1.6 mL. Parabens, corn syrup, sorbitol. Alcohol free.
Infants' Silapap Drops	Solution: 80 mg/0.8 mL. Alcohol free.
Children's Tylenol Suspension Liquid	Suspension: 160 mg/5 mL. Parabens, corn syrup, sorbitol.

Products listed are representative of currently available and widely distributed brands. Similar products, including regional and private label brands, may also exist.

PATIENT INFORMATION
Acetaminophen

- Severe or recurrent lower back pain may indicate a serious illness or injury. Consult a physician.
- Patient instructions accompany each product. Have the patient read these instructions carefully before use, preferably before leaving the pharmacy, in case of any questions.
- Do not exceed the recommended adult dosage. Do not exceed a total adult dose of 4 g/day of acetaminophen in all formulations consumed (2 g/day in regular alcohol users).
- Consult a physician for use in a child younger than 3 years of age.
- Do not take acetaminophen for longer than 5 consecutive days (children) or longer than 10 consecutive days (adults) for pain relief. If symptoms persist, worsen, or if new symptoms develop, contact a physician.
- Avoid alcohol and aspirin while taking this drug.

NONSTEROIDAL ANTI-INFLAMMATORY DRUGS

▶ **Actions**

NSAIDs have analgesic, anti-inflammatory, and antipyretic activities. Their exact mode of action is unknown. The major mechanism of action of NSAIDs is believed to be inhibition of cyclooxygenase (COX) activity and prostaglandin synthesis. Other mechanisms, such as inhibition of lipoxygenase, leukotriene synthesis, lysosomal enzyme release, neutrophil aggregation, and various cell-membrane functions, may exist as well.

NSAIDs inhibit the enzyme COX. COX allows the conversion of arachidonic acid into prostaglandins, which mediate the inflammatory response. Prostaglandin inhibition peripherally at the site of injury can decrease the inflammatory response and pain. Prostaglandin inhibition centrally can also result in analgesia similar to other centrally acting drugs such as acetaminophen. NSAIDs may also have a direct inhibiting effect on inflammatory cells.

▶ **Indications**

For the treatment of mild to moderate pain. These agents have other labeled indications and are particularly helpful for pain associated with inflammation.

▶ **Contraindications**

NSAID hypersensitivity: Because of potential cross-sensitivity to other NSAIDs, do not give these agents to patients in whom aspirin or other NSAIDs have induced symptoms of asthma, rhinitis, urticaria, nasal polyps, angioedema, bronchospasm, and other symptoms of allergic or anaphylactoid reactions.

▶ **Warnings**

Acute renal insufficiency: Patients with preexisting renal disease or compromised renal perfusion are at greatest risk. A form of renal toxicity seen in patients with prerenal conditions leads to reduced renal blood flow or blood volume. NSAID use may cause a dose-dependent reduction in prostaglandin formation and precipitate renal decompensation. Patients at greatest risk are the elderly, premature infants, those with heart failure, renal or hepatic dysfunction, systemic lupus erythematosus (SLE), chronic glomerulonephritis, dehydration, diabetes mellitus, septicemia, pyelonephritis, extracellular volume depletion from any cause, or impaired renal function, or those taking ACE inhibitors, any nephrotoxic drug, or diuretics. Recovery usually follows discontinuation.

Hypersensitivity: Severe hypersensitivity reactions with fever, rash, abdominal pain, headache, nausea, vomiting, signs of liver damage, and meningitis have occurred rarely in patients taking ibuprofen, especially those with SLE or other collagen diseases. Anaphylactoid reactions have occurred in patients with aspirin hypersensitivity.

Renal function impairment: NSAID metabolites are eliminated primarily by the kidneys; use with caution in patients with renal impairment. Reduce dosage to avoid excessive accumulation.

Platelet aggregation: NSAIDs can inhibit platelet aggregation; the effect is reversible, quantitatively less, and of shorter duration than that seen with aspirin. These agents prolong bleeding time (within normal range) in healthy subjects. This may be exaggerated in patients with underlying hemostatic defects; use with caution in people with intrinsic coagulation defects and in those on anticoagulant therapy.

Cardiovascular effects: May cause fluid retention and peripheral edema. Use with caution in patients with compromised cardiac function (eg, heart failure, hypertension, or other conditions predisposing to fluid retention, and in those on chronic diuretic therapy. Agents may be associated with significant deterioration of circulatory hemodynamics in severe heart failure and hyponatremia, presumably due to inhibition of prostaglandin-dependent compensatory mechanisms.

Infection: NSAIDs may mask the usual signs of infection (eg, fever, myalgia, arthralgia). Use with extra care in the presence of existing controlled infection.

Photosensitivity: Photosensitivity may occur; caution patients to take protective measures (eg, sunscreens, protective clothing) against UV or sunlight until tolerance is determined.

GI effects: GI toxicity (including NSAID-induced ulcers and GI bleeding disorders) can occur at any time with or without warning with chronic use of NSAIDs. High-dose NSAIDs probably carry a greater risk of causing GI adverse effects. Have patients with a history of GI lesions consult a physician before using these products. GI adverse effects are more likely to occur and may be more pronounced in elderly patients.

Pregnancy: Category B; Category D in 3rd trimester. Safety for use during pregnancy has not been established; use is not recommended. There are no adequate, well-controlled studies in pregnant women. An increased incidence of dystocia, increased postimplantation loss, and delayed parturition has occurred in animals. Agents that inhibit prostaglandin synthesis may cause closure of the ductus arteriosus and other untoward effects in the fetus. GI tract toxicity is increased in pregnant women in the last trimester. Some NSAIDs may prolong pregnancy if given before onset of labor. Avoid use during pregnancy, especially during the 3rd trimester.

Lactation: Most NSAIDs are excreted in breast milk in low concentrations. The American Academy of Pediatrics considers ibuprofen and naproxen to be compatible with breastfeeding. Data on the use of ketoprofen during breastfeeding are lacking.

Children: The use of naproxen is not recommended in children younger than 12 years of age unless directed by a physician. Ketoprofen is not recommended for use in children younger than 16 years of age.

Elderly: Age appears to increase the possibility of adverse reactions to NSAIDs. The risk of serious ulcer disease is increased in elderly patients (older than 65 years of age) taking NSAIDs chronically; this risk appears to increase with dose. Use with greater care and begin with lower dosages in this patient population.

▶ Drug Interactions

NSAID Drug Interactions			
Precipitant drug	**Object drug***		**Description**
NSAIDs	ACE Inhibitors	↓	NSAIDs may diminish the antihypertensive effect of ACE inhibitors.
NSAIDs	Aminoglycosides	↑	Aminoglycoside plasma concentrations may be elevated in premature infants because of NSAIDs, reducing the glomerular filtration rate. Reduce aminoglycoside dose prior to NSAID initiation and monitor serum aminoglycoside levels and renal function.
NSAIDs	Anticoagulants	↑	Coadministration may prolong prothrombin time (PT). Also consider the effects NSAIDs have on platelet function and gastric mucosa. Monitor PT and patients closely, especially during the first few days of therapy, and instruct patients to watch for signs and symptoms of bleeding.
NSAIDs	Beta blockers	↓	The antihypertensive effect of beta blockers may be impaired. Avoid using this combination if possible.
NSAIDs	Cyclosporine	↑	Nephrotoxicity of both agents may be increased.
NSAIDs	Digoxin	↑	Ibuprofen may increase digoxin serum levels.
NSAIDs	Hydantoins	↑	Serum phenytoin levels may be increased, resulting in an increase in pharmacologic and toxic effects of phenytoin.
NSAIDs	Lithium	↑	Serum lithium levels may be increased.
NSAIDs	Diuretics	↓	Effects of diuretics may be decreased.
NSAIDs	Methotrexate	↑	The risks of methotrexate toxicity (eg, stomatitis, bone marrow suppression, nephrotoxicity) may be increased.
NSAIDs	Thiazide diuretics	↔	Decreased antihypertensive and diuretic action of thiazides may occur with concurrent naproxen.
Bisphosphonates	NSAIDs	↑	Risk of gastric ulceration may be increased. Use cautiously.
Cholestyramine	NSAIDs	↓	The effects of NSAIDs may be decreased.
Cimetidine	NSAIDs	↔	NSAID plasma concentrations may be increased or decreased by cimetidine; some studies report no effect.
Probenecid	NSAIDs	↑	Probenecid may increase the concentrations and possibly the toxicity of the NSAIDs.
Salicylates	NSAIDs	↓	Plasma concentrations of NSAIDs may be decreased by salicylates. Avoid concurrent use because it offers no therapeutic advantage and may significantly increase the incidence of GI effects.

* ↑ = Object drug increased.   ↓ = Object drug decreased.   ↔ = Undetermined clinical effect.

▶ Adverse Reactions

Cardiovascular: Edema; congestive heart failure; hypertension; tachycardia.

CNS: Dizziness; drowsiness; headache; light-headedness; vertigo.

Dermatologic: Erythema; pruritus; rash; increased sweating; urticaria; photosensitivity; eczema.

GI: Bleeding; diarrhea; dyspepsia; heartburn; nausea; vomiting; abdominal pain or cramps; constipation; flatulence; ulcer bleed; gastritis; melena; epigastric/GI pain; abdominal/GI distress; bloating; GI fullness; stomatitis; anorexia; dry mouth; peptic ulcer; jaundice; pancreatitis; colitis; hematemesis; appetite increase; eructation; rectal bleeding/hemorrhage.

GU: Urinary frequency; renal function impairment; hematuria; interstitial nephritis; renal failure; cystitis; menstrual disorder; azotemia; nephrotic syndrome; papillary necrosis.

Respiratory: Dyspnea; rhinitis; pharyngitis; epistaxis; bronchospasm.

Miscellaneous: Muscle cramps; thirst; purpura; anemia; thrombocytopenia; eosinophilia; liver test abnormalities; BUN increased; hemoglobin and hematocrit decreases; fluid retention; body weight changes; hyperglycemia; hyperkalemia; myalgia; muscle weakness; hearing disturbances; visual disturbances; taste disorder; chills; fever.

IBUPROFEN

▶ Administration and Dosage

Adults: 200 mg orally every 4 to 6 hours as needed. If pain does not respond to 200 mg, 400 mg may be used. Do not exceed 1.2 g in 24 hours. Do not take for pain for longer than 10 days unless directed by physician. If GI upset occurs, take with meals or milk.

Children younger than 12 years of age: Ibuprofen is not approved for the treatment of lower back pain in children. For dosing information in this age group, see individual product labeling.

IBUPROFEN PRODUCTS	
Trade name	**Doseform**
Junior Strength Advil, Junior Strength Motrin	**Tablets**: 100 mg
Advil,[1] *Maximum Strength Midol Cramp, Motrin IB*	**Tablets**: 200 mg
Children's Advil, Children's Motrin	**Tablets, chewable**: 50 mg
Junior Strength Advil, Junior Strength Motrin	**Tablets, chewable**: 100 mg
Advil Liqui-Gels, Motrin IB[2]	**Gelcaps**: 200 mg
Infants' Advil Concentrated Drops	**Liquid**: 50 mg/1.25 mL
Children's Advil,[1,3] *Children's Motrin*[1]	**Suspension**: 100 mg/5 mL

Products listed are representative of currently available and widely distributed brands. Similar products, including regional and private label brands, may also exist.

[1] Contains sucrose.
[2] Contains parabens.
[3] Contains sorbitol.

PATIENT INFORMATION
Ibuprofen

- *Adults:* Do not exceed 1.2 g/day.
- Severe or recurrent pain may indicate a serious illness. Consult a physician.
- Patient instructions accompany each product. Have the patient read these instructions carefully before use, preferably before leaving the pharmacy, in case of any questions.
- May cause GI upset; take with food or after meals.
- Take with a full glass of water (240 mL) to reduce the risk of the medication lodging in the esophagus.
- Do not take OTC NSAIDs for longer than 10 days for pain unless directed by a physician. If symptoms persist, worsen, or if new symptoms develop, contact a physician.
- Notify physician if rash, itching, visual disturbances, edema, black stools, or persistent headache occur.
- If the patient consumes 3 or more alcoholic drinks every day, taking ibuprofen or other pain relievers or fever reducers may cause stomach bleeding.
- Avoid aspirin while taking this medication.

KETOPROFEN

▶ Administration and Dosage

Adults: 12.5 mg with a full glass of liquid every 4 to 6 hours as needed. If pain persists longer than 1 hour, follow with 12.5 mg. Do not exceed 25 mg in a 4- to 6-hour period or 75 mg in a 24-hour period. Use the smallest effective dose.

Children: Do not give to children younger than 16 years of age unless directed by a physician.

KETOPROFEN PRODUCTS	
Trade name	**Doseform**
Orudis KT	**Tablets:** 12.5 mg

Products listed are representative of currently available and widely distributed brands. Similar products, including regional and private label brands, may also exist.

PATIENT INFORMATION
Ketoprofen

- *Adults:* Do not exceed 75 mg/day.
- Severe or recurrent pain may indicate a serious illness. Consult a physician.
- Patient instructions accompany each product. Have the patient read these instructions carefully before use, preferably before leaving the pharmacy, in case of any questions.
- May cause GI upset; take with food or after meals.
- Take with a full glass of liquid (240 mL) to reduce the risk of the medication lodging in the esophagus.
- Do not take OTC NSAIDs for longer than 10 days for pain unless directed by a physician. If symptoms persist, worsen, or if new symptoms develop, contact a physician.
- Notify physician if rash, itching, visual disturbances, edema, black stools, or persistent headache occur.
- Avoid alcohol and aspirin while taking this medication.

NAPROXEN

▶ **Administration and Dosage**

Adults: 200 mg with a full glass of liquid every 8 to 12 hours as needed. With experience, some patients may find an initial dose of 400 mg followed by 200 mg 12 hours later, if necessary, will give better relief. Do not exceed 600 mg in 24 hours unless otherwise directed. Use the smallest effective dose.

Children: Do not give to children younger than 12 years of age unless directed by a physician.

Elderly (older than 65 years of age): Do not take over 200 mg in a 12-hour period.

NAPROXEN PRODUCTS	
Trade name	Doseform
Aleve	**Tablets, Caplets, and Gelcaps**: 200 mg (220 mg naproxen sodium)

Products listed are representative of currently available and widely distributed brands. Similar products, including regional and private label brands, may also exist.

PATIENT INFORMATION

Naproxen

- *Adults:* Do not exceed 600 mg/day.
- Severe or recurrent pain may indicate a serious illness. Consult a physician.
- Patient instructions accompany each product. Have the patient read these instructions carefully before use, preferably before leaving the pharmacy, in case of any questions.
- May cause GI upset; take with food or after meals.
- Take with a full glass of liquid (240 mL) to reduce the risk of medication lodging in the esophagus.
- Do not take OTC NSAIDs for longer than 10 days for pain unless directed by a physician. If symptoms persist, worsen, or if new symptoms develop, contact a physician.
- Notify physician if rash, itching, visual disturbances, edema, black stools, or persistent headache occur.
- If the patient consumes 3 or more alcoholic drinks every day, taking naproxen or other NSAID pain relievers or fever reducers may cause stomach bleeding.
- Avoid aspirin while taking this medication.

RUBS AND LINIMENTS

▶ Indications

These products are used for relief of pain of muscular aches, neuralgia, rheumatism, arthritis, sprains, and like conditions, when skin is intact.

Individual components include:

Counterirritants: Camphor, capsicum preparations (capsicum oleoresin, capsaicin), eucalyptus oil, menthol, methyl nicotinate, methyl salicylate, mustard oil, wormwood oil.

Antiseptics: Thymol.

Analgesics: Trolamine salicylate, methyl salicylate.

▶ Contraindications

Allergy to components of any formulation or to salicylates.

▶ Warnings

For external use only: Avoid contact with eyes, eyelids, and mucous membranes.

Apply to affected parts only: Do not apply to irritated skin; discontinue use if excessive irritation develops. Consult a physician if pain persists for longer than 7 to 10 days, or if redness is present, or in conditions affecting children younger than 10 years of age.

Heat therapy: Do not use an external source of high heat (eg, heating pad) with these agents because irritation and burning of the skin may occur.

Protective covering: Applying a tight bandage or wrap over these agents is not recommended because increased absorption may occur.

▶ Drug Interactions

Anticoagulants: An enhanced anticoagulant effect (eg, increased prothrombin time) occurred in several patients receiving an anticoagulant and using topical methyl salicylate concurrently.

▶ **Adverse Reactions**

If applied to large skin areas and used over a prolonged period of time, salicylate side effects (eg, tinnitus, nausea, vomiting) may occur.

Products may be toxic if ingested.

Counterirritants may cause local irritation, especially in patients with sensitive skin.

▶ **Administration and Dosage**

Apply to affected areas as needed.

RUBS AND LINIMENTS	
Trade name	**Doseform**
Icy Hot	**Balm**: 29% methyl salicylate, 7.6% menthol, white petrolatum
Epiderm	**Balm**: Isopropyl alcohol, parabens, ureas, menthol, EDTA
JointFlex	**Cream**: 3.1% camphor, lanolin, aloe, urea, EDTA, glycerin, peppermint oil
Capzasin-P	**Cream**: 0.025% capsaicin
ArthriCare for Women Silky Dry	**Cream**: 0.025% capsaicin, parabens, mineral oil
ArthriCare for Women Extra Moisturizing	**Cream**: 0.025% capsaicin, aloe vera gel, cetyl and stearyl alcohol, parabens
ArthriCare for Women Multi-Action	**Cream**: 0.025% capsaicin, 1.25% menthol, 0.25% methyl nicotinate, aloe vera gel, cetyl alcohol, parabens
Capzasin-HP	**Cream**: 0.075% capsaicin
ArthriCare for Women Ultra Strength	**Cream**: 0.075% capsaicin, 2% menthol, aloe vera gel, cetyl and stearyl alcohol, parabens
Vicks VapoRub	**Cream**: 2.8% menthol, 5.2% camphor, 1.2% eucalyptus oil, cedarleaf oil, cetyl and stearyl alcohol, EDTA, glycerin, urea, parabens, turpentine oil
BenGay S.P.A.	**Cream**: 10% menthol, cetyl alcohol, urea, EDTA, glycerin
Arthritic Hot	**Cream**: Methyl salicylate, menthol
Ziks	**Cream**: 12% methyl salicylate, 1% menthol, 0.025% capsaicin, cetyl alcohol, urea
Thera-Gesic	**Cream**: 15% methyl salicylate, 1% menthol, glycerin, parabens
BenGay Greaseless	**Cream**: 15% methyl salicylate, 10% menthol, cetyl alcohol, glycerin
Pain Bust-R II	**Cream**: 17% methyl salicylate, 12% menthol, cetyl and stearyl alcohol
ArthriCare for Women Nighttime	**Cream**: 30% methyl salicylate, 1.25% menthol, 0.25% methyl nicotinate, glycerin, isopropyl alcohol
Arthritis Formula BenGay	**Cream**: 30% methyl salicylate, 8% menthol, lanolin
Icy Hot	**Cream**: 30% methyl salicylate, 10% menthol
Ultra Strength BenGay	**Cream**: 30% methyl salicylate, 10% menthol, 4% camphor, EDTA, lanolin
Panalgesic Gold	**Cream**: 35% methyl salicylate, 4% menthol, lanolin, cetyl and stearyl alcohol, mineral oil
Myoflex	**Cream**: 10% triethanolamine salicylate, cetyl and stearyl alcohol, EDTA

RUBS AND LINIMENTS

Trade name	Doseform
Myoflex Extra, Myoflex Arthritic	**Cream**: 15% triethanolamine salicylate
Sportscreme	**Cream**: 10% trolamine salicylate, cetyl alcohol, glycerin, parabens, mineral oil
Aspercreme	**Cream**: 10% trolamine salicylate, aloe vera gel, cetyl alcohol, glycerin, parabens, mineral oil
Mobisyl	**Cream**: 10% trolamine salicylate, aloe vera gel, cetyl alcohol, urea, glycerin, parabens, mineral oil, sweet almond oil, EDTA
Icy Hot Arthritis Therapy	**Gel**: 0.025% capsaicin, aloe vera gel, benzyl alcohol, urea, maleated soybean oil, parabens
Flexall Quik Gel	**Gel**: Menthol, methyl salicylate
Vanishing Scent BenGay	**Gel**: 2.5% menthol, urea, isopropyl alcohol
Vicks VapoRub	**Gel**: 2.6% menthol, 4.8% camphor, 1.2% eucalyptus oil, cedarleaf oil, nutmeg oil, petrolatum, turpentine oil
Flexall 454	**Gel**: 7% menthol, aloe vera gel, eucalyptus oil, glycerin, peppermint oil, thyme oil
Maximum Strength Flexall 454	**Gel**: 16% menthol, aloe vera gel, eucalyptus oil, glycerin, peppermint oil, thyme oil
Flexall Ultra Plus	**Gel**: 16% menthol, 10% methyl salicylate, 3.1% camphor, aloe vera gel, eucalyptus oil, glycerin, peppermint oil, thyme oil
Icy Hot Chill Stick	**Gel**: 30% methyl salicylate, 10% menthol, hydrogenated castor oil, stearyl alcohol
Myoflex Ice Cold Plus	**Gel**: 15% triethanolamine salicylate
Absorbine Jr Arthritis Strength	**Liquid**: Capsaicin, echinacea, calendula, and wormwood extracts
Absorbine Jr	**Liquid**: 1.27% menthol, echinacea, calendula, and wormwood extracts, wormwood oil
Extra Strength Absorbine Jr	**Liquid**: 4% menthol, echinacea, calendula, and wormwood extracts, wormwood oil
Yager's	**Liniment**: Camphor, turpentine oil, clove oil
Panalgesic Gold	**Liniment**: 55.01% methyl salicylate, 1.25% menthol, 3.1% camphor, emollient oils, alcohol
Banalg	**Lotion**: 4.9% methyl salicylate, 1% menthol, 2% camphor, parabens, eucalyptus oil
Banalg Hospital Strength	**Lotion**: 14% methyl salicylate, 3% menthol, parabens
Aspercreme	**Lotion**: Trolamine salicylate
Eucalyptamint	**Ointment**: 16% menthol, eucalyptus oil, lanolin, mineral oil
Original Formula BenGay	**Ointment**: 18.3% methyl salicylate, 16% menthol, lanolin
Absorbine Jr	**Patch**: Menthol, camphor, eucalyptus
Absorbine Jr Deep Pain Relief	**Patch**: Menthol, glucosamine, MSM
Icy Hot	**Patch**: Methyl salicylate, menthol

Products listed are representative of currently available and widely distributed brands. Similar products, including regional and private label brands, may also exist.

PATIENT INFORMATION

Rubs and Liniments

- For external use only. Avoid contact with eyes, eyelids, and mucous membranes.
- Apply to affected areas only. Do not apply to irritated skin; discontinue use if excessive irritation develops.
- Consult a physician if pain persists for longer than 7 to 10 days, if redness is present, or in conditions affecting children younger than 10 years of age.
- Do not use an external source of high heat (eg, heating pad) with these agents because irritation and burning of the skin may occur.
- Do not apply tight bandages or wraps over these agents.
- Do not apply to broken skin.

DEFINITION

Myalgia is defined as muscle pain that may or may not be associated with fatigue or weakness. Fibromyalgia is defined as pain and tenderness of the muscle and the adjacent connective tissue.

ETIOLOGY

Any vigorous activity can lead to muscle tears that can cause pain, tenderness, swelling, and weakness. Overuse of muscle is the most common cause of injury. Muscle pain without weakness can be seen with acute infections (eg, influenza, coxsackievirus). Fibromyalgia occurs more commonly in females, and symptoms can be induced or intensified by physical or emotional stress, poor sleep, trauma, or exposure to damp cold.

INCIDENCE

Musculoskeletal disorders are one of the most commonly reported causes of impairment in the US adult population. It is estimated that in the US, over 7 million people are unable to perform some or all of their major activities because of musculoskeletal conditions.

PATHOPHYSIOLOGY

When muscles are stressed, some of the fibers are injured and others use all of their available glycogen stores, their main energy source. With repeated injury or overuse of the muscle, fewer muscle fibers are available to produce the same work. It takes at least 48 hours for muscle fibers to heal. Muscles can also be injured when they are too weak for the activity.

SIGNS/SYMPTOMS

Muscle pain can be the primary symptom of inflammatory, metabolic, endocrine, or toxic myopathies. The onset is often gradual with diffuse stiffness and pain. Muscle tears, commonly seen in athletes, are usually associated with acute pain, swelling, and tenderness. Fibromyalgia is often associated with fatigue, insomnia, and depression.

DIAGNOSTIC PARAMETERS/PHYSICAL ASSESSMENT

Clinical Observation: Myalgias are present as local muscle tightness or muscle spasms. Inflammation is usually not present.

Interview: To ensure the proper diagnosis and treatment, it may be beneficial to ask the patient about the following:

- Onset, duration, and location of the pain
- Quality or nature of the pain
- Factors that relieve or exacerbate the pain
- The severity of the pain using a 10-point rating scale where the patient qualifies the intensity of the pain (0 = no pain to 10 = most intense pain)

TREATMENT

Approaches to therapy: The pain associated with myalgias can be best relieved by resting the injured muscle. Anti-inflammatory agents may also provide some relief. Question the patient about therapies that have been tried and how effective they were.

Nondrug therapy: Pain from myalgias may be relieved by applying localized heat, gentle massage, stretching exercises, and rest.

Pharmacotherapy: Drugs that are effective for relieving pain associated with myalgias include aspirin, acetaminophen, and nonsteroidal anti-inflammatory drugs (NSAIDs).

SALICYLATES

▶ **Actions**

The anti-inflammatory and analgesic activity of salicylates may be mediated through inhibition of the prostaglandin synthetase complex.

▶ **Indications**

For the treatment of mild-to-moderate pain. These agents have other labeled indications as well.

▶ **Contraindications**

Hypersensitivity to salicylates or nonsteroidal anti-inflammatory drugs (NSAIDs). Use with extreme caution in patients with a history of adverse reactions to salicylates. Cross-sensitivity may exist between aspirin and other NSAIDs that inhibit prostaglandin synthesis, and between aspirin and tartrazine. Aspirin cross-sensitivity does not appear to occur with sodium salicylate, or salicylamide. Aspirin hypersensitivity is more prevalent in those with asthma, nasal polyposis, or chronic urticaria.

Also contraindicated in patients with hemophilia or bleeding ulcers, or those in hemorrhagic states. Magnesium salicylate is contraindicated in patients with advanced chronic renal insufficiency.

▶ **Warnings**

Concurrent medications: Many other medications, specifically multi-ingredient cough and cold products, also contain aspirin or acetaminophen. It is important to advise patients of this possibility, and to inquire about other medications they might be taking before recommending an analgesic.

Otic effects: Discontinue use if dizziness, ringing in ears (tinnitus), or impaired hearing occurs. Tinnitus probably represents blood salicylic acid levels reaching or exceeding the upper limit of the therapeutic range; therefore, it is a helpful guide to toxicity. Temporary hearing loss disappears gradually upon discontinuation of the drug.

Hypersensitivity: Do not use if there is a history of sensitivity to aspirin or NSAIDs.

Aspirin intolerance, manifested by acute bronchospasm, generalized urticaria/angioedema, severe rhinitis, or shock occurs in 4% to 19% of asthmatics. Symptoms occur within 3 hours after ingestion.

Foods may contribute to a reaction. Some foods with high salicylate content include curry powder, paprika, licorice, Benedictine liqueur, prunes, raisins, tea, and gherkins. A typical American diet contains 10 to 200 mg/day salicylate.

Hepatic function impairment: Use with caution in patients with liver damage, preexisting hypoprothrombinemia, and vitamin K deficiency.

GI effects: Use with caution in patients who are intolerant to salicylates because of GI irritation, and in those with gastric ulcers, peptic ulcers, mild diabetes, gout, erosive gastritis, or bleeding tendencies.

Hematologic effects: Aspirin interferes with hemostasis. Avoid use in patients with severe anemia, history of blood coagulation defects, or who take anticoagulants.

Pregnancy: Category D (aspirin); *Category C* (salsalate, magnesium salicylate, other salicylates). Aspirin may produce adverse effects in the mother, such as anemia, ante- or postpartum hemorrhage, or prolonged gestation and labor. Salicylates readily cross the placenta. By inhibiting prostaglandin synthesis, salicylates may cause constriction of ductus arteriosus, and, possibly, other untoward fetal effects. Maternal aspirin use during later stages of pregnancy may cause adverse fetal effects, such as low birth weight, increased incidence of intracranial hemorrhage in premature infants, stillbirth, or neonatal death. Salicylates may be teratogens. Avoid use during pregnancy, especially in the third trimester.

Lactation: Salicylates are excreted in breast milk in low concentrations. Adverse effects on platelet function in the nursing infant are a potential risk. The American Academy of Pediatrics recommends that aspirin be used cautiously in nursing mothers.

Children: Administration of aspirin to children, including teenagers, with acute febrile illness due to chickenpox and influenza has been associated with the development of Reye syndrome.

▶ Drug Interactions

Salicylate Drug Interactions			
Precipitant drug	**Object drug***		**Description**
Charcoal, activated	Aspirin	↓	Coadministration decreases aspirin absorption, depending on charcoal dose and interval between ingestion.
Urinary acidifiers	Salicylates	↑	Ammonium chloride, ascorbic acid, and methionine decrease salicylate excretion.
Antacids, urinary alkalinizers	Salicylates	↓	Decreased pharmacologic effects of salicylates may occur. The magnitude of the antacid interaction depends on the agent, dose, and pretreatment urine pH.
Carbonic anhydrase inhibitors	Salicylates	↔	Salicylate intoxication has occurred after coadministration of these agents. However, salicylic acid renal elimination may be increased by these drugs if urine is kept alkaline. Conversely, salicylates may displace acetazolamide from protein-binding sites, resulting in toxicity. Further study is needed.
Corticosteroids	Salicylates	↓	Corticosteroids increase salicylate clearance and decrease salicylate serum levels.
Nizatidine	Salicylates	↑	Increased serum salicylate levels have occurred in patients receiving high doses (3.9 g/day) of aspirin and concurrent nizatidine.
Salicylates	Alcohol	↑	The risk of GI ulceration increases when salicylates are given concomitantly. Ingestion of alcohol during salicylate therapy may also prolong bleeding time.

Salicylate Drug Interactions			
Precipitant drug	Object drug*		Description
Salicylates	Angiotensin-converting enzyme inhibitors	↓	Antihypertensive effectiveness of these agents may be decreased by concurrent salicylate administration, possibly due to prostaglandin inhibition. Consider discontinuing salicylates if problems occur.
Aspirin	Heparin	↑	Aspirin can increase the risk of bleeding in heparin anticoagulated patients.
Salicylates	Loop diuretics	↓	Loop diuretics may be less effective when given with salicylates in patients with compromised renal function or with cirrhosis with ascites; however, data conflict.
Salicylates	Methotrexate	↑	Salicylates increase drug levels, causing toxicity by interfering with protein binding and renal elimination of the antimetabolite.
Aspirin	Nitroglycerin	↑	Nitroglycerin, when taken with aspirin, may result in unexpected hypotension. Data are limited. If hypotension occurs, reduce the nitroglycerin dose.
Aspirin	NSAIDs	↓	Aspirin may decrease NSAID serum concentrations. Avoid concomitant use; it offers no therapeutic advantage and may significantly increase incidence of GI effects.
Salicylates	Probenecid, Sulfinpyrazone	↔	Salicylates antagonize the uricosuric effect. While salicylates in large doses (> 3 g/day) have a uricosuric effect, smaller amounts may reduce the uricosuric effect of these agents.
Salicylates	Spironolactone	↓	Salicylates may inhibit the diuretic effects; antihypertensive action does not appear altered. Effects depend on the dose of spironolactone.
Salicylates	Sulfonylureas, exogenous insulin	↑	Salicylates in doses > 2 g/day have a hypoglycemic action, perhaps by altering pancreatic beta-cell function. They may potentiate the glucose-lowering effect of these drugs.
Aspirin	Valproic acid	↑	Aspirin displaces valproic acid from its protein-binding sites and may decrease its total body clearance, thus increasing pharmacological effects.

* ↑ = Object drug increased. ↓ = Object drug decreased. ↔ = Undetermined clinical effect.

▶ **Adverse Reactions**

Adverse reactions can be seen in the following body systems: GI (nausea, dyspepsia, heartburn, epigastric discomfort), hematologic (prolonged bleeding time, leukopenia, thrombocytopenia, purpura, decreased plasma iron concentration, shortened erythrocyte survival time), and dermatologic (rash, hives, and angioedema may occur, especially in patients suffering from chronic urticaria). Additional miscellaneous adverse reactions that have occurred include fever, thirst, and dimness of vision.

Allergic and anaphylactic reactions have been noted when hypersensitive individuals took aspirin. Fatal anaphylactic shock, while not common, has been reported.

Aspirin has a reversible effect on platelet aggregation.

▶ **Overdosage**

Symptoms: The approximate acute lethal dose for adults is 10 to 30 g, and for children, 4 g. Respiratory alkalosis is seen initially in acute salicylate ingestions. Hyperpnea and tachypnea occur as a result of increased CO_2 production and a direct stimulatory effect of salicylate on the respiratory center. Other symptoms may include nausea, vomiting, hypokalemia, tinnitus, neurologic abnormalities (eg, disorientation, irritability, hallucinations, lethargy, stupor, coma, seizures), dehydration, hyperthermia, hyperventilation, hyperactivity, thrombocytopenia, platelet dysfunction, hypoprothrombinemia, increased capillary fragility, and other hematologic abnormalities. Symptoms may progress quickly to depression, coma, respiratory failure and collapse. Chronic salicylate toxicity may occur when more than 100 mg/kg/day is ingested for 2 or more days. It is more difficult to recognize than acute overdosage and is associated with increased morbidity and mortality. Compared with acute poisoning, hyperventilation, dehydration, systemic acidosis, and severe CNS manifestations occur more frequently.

Treatment: Initial treatment includes induction of emesis or gastric lavage to remove any unabsorbed drug from the stomach. Activated charcoal diminishes salicylate absorption most effectively if given within 2 hours after ingestion. It is important to contact a local poison control center or emergency room if overdosage is suspected.

ASPIRIN

▶ Administration and Dosage

Adults: 325 to 650 mg orally every 4 hours as needed. Some extra-strength products recommend 500 mg every 3 hours or 1000 mg every 6 hours.

Children: The oral analgesic/antipyretic dosage is 10 to 15 mg/kg/dose every 4 hours (see table), up to 60 to 80 mg/kg/day. Do not use in children or teenagers with chickenpox or "flu" symptoms due to the possibility of Reye syndrome. Dosage recommendations by age and weight are as follows:

Recommended Aspirin Dosage in Children					
Age (years)	Weight		Dosage (mg every 4 hours)	No. of 81 mg tablets (every 4 hours)	No. of 325 mg tablets (every 4 hours)
	lbs	kg			
2-3	24-35	10.6-15.9	162	2	½
4-5	36-47	16-21.4	243	3	N/A
6-8	48-59	21.5-26.8	324	4	1
9-10	60-71	26.9-32.3	405	5	N/A
11	72-95	32.4-43.2	486	6	1½
12-14	≥ 96	≥ 43.3	648	8	2

ASPIRIN PRODUCTS	
Trade name	Doseform
Original Bayer, Norwich Aspirin	**Tablets**: 325 mg
Bayer Children's Chewable Aspirin	**Tablets, chewable**: 81 mg. Dextrose, saccharin. Cherry and orange flavors.
Adult Low Strength Ecotrin, Halfprin 81[1]	**Tablets, enteric coated**: 81 mg. Talc.
Halfprin 162	**Tablets, enteric coated**: 162 mg. Lactose, talc.
Ecotrin Regular Strength	**Tablets, enteric coated**: 325 mg. Talc.
Norwich Maximum Strength	**Tablets, enteric coated**: 500 mg
Ecotrin Maximum Strength	**Tablets, enteric coated**: 500 mg. Talc.
Alka-Seltzer Original Effervescent Antacid and Pain Relief Medicine	**Tablets, effervescent**: 325 mg, 1000 mg citric acid, 1916 mg sodium bicarbonate
Bayer Women's Aspirin Plus Calcium	**Caplets**: 81 mg, 300 mg calcium. Lactose, mineral oil.
Original Bayer	**Caplets**: 325 mg

ASPIRIN PRODUCTS	
Trade name	Doseform
Extra Strength Bayer PM Aspirin Plus Sleep Aid	**Caplets**: 500 mg, 25 mg diphenhydramine HCl
Extra Strength Bayer Aspirin	**Caplets, coated**: 500 mg
Extra Strength Bayer Back and Body Pain	**Caplets, coated**: 500 mg, 32.5 mg caffeine
Extra Strength Bayer Arthritis Pain Regimen	**Caplets, enteric coated**: 500 mg
Original Bayer	**Gelcaps**: 325 mg. Parabens, sorbitol, glycerin.
Extra Strength Bayer Aspirin	**Gelcaps, coated**: 500 mg. Parabens, glycerin.
BUFFERED ASPIRIN PRODUCTS	
Adprin-B	**Tablets, coated**: 325 mg with calcium carbonate, magnesium carbonate, magnesium oxide
Regular Strength Ascriptin	**Tablets, coated**: 325 mg with 50 mg magnesium hydroxide, 50 mg aluminum hydroxide, calcium carbonate. Talc.
Bufferin	**Tablets, coated**: 325 mg with 158 mg calcium carbonate, 63 mg magnesium oxide, 34 mg magnesium carbonate. Mineral oil, sorbitol, citric acid.
Extra Strength Adprin-B	**Tablets, coated**: 500 mg with calcium carbonate, magnesium carbonate, magnesium oxide.
Bayer Adult Low Strength	**Caplets**: 81 mg, buffered with 250 mg calcium carbonate
Extra Strength Bayer Plus	**Caplets**: 500 mg with calcium carbonate, magnesium carbonate, magnesium oxide
Maximum Strength Ascriptin	**Caplets, coated**: 500 mg with 80 mg magnesium hydroxide, 80 mg aluminum hydroxide, calcium carbonate. Saccharin, sorbitol, talc.

Products listed are representative of currently available and widely distributed brands. Similar products, including regional and private label brands, may also exist.

[1] Also contains lactose.

PATIENT INFORMATION
Aspirin

- Severe or recurrent pain may indicate a serious illness. Consult a physician.
- Patient instructions accompany each product. Have the patient read these instructions carefully before use, preferably before leaving the pharmacy, in case of any questions.
- May cause GI upset; take with or after meals. Enteric coated products may prevent or reduce stomach/GI distress.
- Do not use in children or adolescents because of the potential risk of Reye syndrome.
- Take with a full glass of water (240 mL) to reduce the risk of lodging the medication in the esophagus.
- Avoid taking antacids within 2 hours of taking enteric coated tablets.
- Have patients allergic to tartrazine dye avoid aspirin.
- Notify physician if rash, difficult breathing, ringing in the ears, or persistent GI pain occurs. Internal bleeding may occur with no GI symptoms and may be indicated by bloody or black stools.
- Inform physician or dentist of aspirin use before surgery or dental care.
- Do not use aspirin if it has a strong vinegar-like odor. This suggests deterioration of aspirin and loss of potency.

MAGNESIUM SALICYLATE

▶ **Actions**

Magnesium salicylate is a sodium-free salicylate derivative that may have a low incidence of GI upset.

▶ **Contraindications**

Magnesium salicylate is contraindicated in patients with advanced chronic renal insufficiency due to magnesium retention.

▶ **Warnings**

The possibility of magnesium toxicity exists in patients with renal insufficiency.

▶ **Administration and Dosage**

Product labeling and dosages are expressed as magnesium salicylate anhydrous.

Adults: Usual dose is 650 mg every 4 hours to 1 g every 6 hours up to 4 g/day.

Children: Safety and efficacy for use in children have not been established.

MAGNESIUM SALICYLATE PRODUCTS	
Trade name	Doseform
Regular Strength Doan's	**Caplets**: 377 mg
Extra Strength Doan's	**Caplets**: 580 mg
Extra Strength Doan's P.M.	**Caplets**: 580 mg, 25 mg diphenhydramine HCl. Talc.

Products listed are representative of currently available and widely distributed brands. Similar products, including regional and private label brands, may also exist.

PATIENT INFORMATION

Magnesium Salicylate

- Do not use these products if you have renal insufficiency.
- Severe or recurrent pain may indicate a serious illness. Consult a physician.
- Patient instructions accompany each product. Have the patient read these instructions carefully before use, preferably before leaving the pharmacy, in case of any questions.
- May cause GI upset; take with food or after meals.
- Do not use in children or adolescents because of the potential risk of Reye syndrome.
- Notify physician if rash, difficult breathing, ringing in the ears, or persistent GI pain occurs. Internal bleeding may occur with no GI symptoms and may be indicated by bloody or black stools.

ACETAMINOPHEN (APAP)

▶ **Actions**

Generally, the antipyretic and analgesic effects of APAP and aspirin are comparable; however, the site and mechanism of the analgesic effect of acetaminophen are unclear.

▶ **Indications**

For the treatment of mild-to-moderate pain. Also used as an analgesic-antipyretic in the presence of aspirin allergy, and in patients with blood coagulation disorders who are being treated with oral anticoagulants, bleeding diatheses (eg, hemophilia), upper GI disease (eg, ulcer, gastritis, hiatal hernia), and gouty arthritis. This agent has other labeled indications as well.

► **Contraindications**

Hypersensitivity to acetaminophen.

► **Warnings**

Concurrent medications: Many other medications, specifically multi-ingredient cough and cold products, also contain aspirin or acetaminophen. It is important to advise patients of this possibility, and to inquire about other medications they might be taking before recommending an analgesic.

Hepatotoxicity: Hepatotoxicity and severe hepatic failure occurred in chronic alcoholics following therapeutic doses. The hepatotoxicity may be caused by induction of hepatic microsomal enzymes, resulting in an increase in toxic metabolites, or by the reduced amount of glutathione responsible for conjugating toxic metabolites. A safe dose for chronic alcohol abusers has not been determined. Caution chronic alcoholics and those consuming alcohol on a daily basis to limit acetaminophen intake to 2 g/day or less.

Pregnancy: Category B. Acetaminophen crosses the placenta, but has been routinely used in all stages of pregnancy. When used in therapeutic doses, it appears safe for short-term use.

Lactation: APAP is excreted in low amounts, but no adverse effects have been reported. The American Academy of Pediatrics considers acetaminophen to be compatible with breastfeeding.

Children: Consult a physician before using in children younger than 3 years of age.

► **Drug Interactions**

Acetaminophen Drug Interactions			
Precipitant drug	**Object drug***		**Description**
Alcohol, ethyl	APAP	↑	Hepatotoxicity has occurred in chronic alcoholics following various dose levels (moderate-to-excessive) of acetaminophen.
Anticholinergics	APAP	↔	The onset of acetaminophen effect may be delayed or decreased slightly, but the ultimate pharmacological effect is not significantly affected by anticholinergics.
Beta blockers, propranolol	APAP	↑	Propranolol appears to inhibit the enzyme systems responsible for glucuronidation and oxidation of acetaminophen. Therefore, the pharmacologic effects of acetaminophen may be increased.
Charcoal, activated	APAP	↓	Reduces acetaminophen absorption when administered as soon as possible after overdose.
Contraceptives, oral	APAP	↓	Increase in glucuronidation resulting in increased plasma clearance and a decreased half-life of acetaminophen.
Probenecid	APAP	↑	Probenecid may increase the therapeutic effectiveness of acetaminophen slightly.
APAP	Lamotrigine	↓	Serum lamotrigine concentrations may be reduced, producing a decrease in therapeutic effects.
APAP	Loop diuretics	↓	The effects of the loop diuretic may be decreased because APAP may decrease renal prostaglandin excretion and decrease plasma renin activity.

Acetaminophen Drug Interactions			
Precipitant drug	**Object drug***		**Description**
APAP	Zidovudine	↓	The pharmacologic effects of zidovudine may be decreased because of enhanced nonhepatic or renal clearance of zidovudine.

* ↑ = Object drug increased. ↓ = Object drug decreased. ↔ = Undetermined clinical effect.

The potential hepatotoxicity of acetaminophen may be increased by large doses or long-term administration of barbiturates, carbamazepine, hydantoins, rifampin, and sulfinpyrazone. The therapeutic effects of acetaminophen may also be decreased.

▶ **Adverse Reactions**

When used as directed, acetaminophen rarely causes severe toxicity or side effects. However, the following adverse reactions have been reported:

Hematologic: Hemolytic anemia; neutropenia; leukopenia; pancytopenia; thrombocytopenia.

Miscellaneous: Fever; hypoglycemia; jaundice; skin rash.

▶ **Overdosage**

Symptoms: Acute poisoning may be manifested by nausea, vomiting, drowsiness, confusion, liver tenderness, low blood pressure, cardiac arrhythmias, jaundice, and acute hepatic and renal failure. These occur within the first 24 hours and may persist for 1 week or longer. Death has occurred because of liver necrosis. Acute renal failure may also occur. However, there are often no specific early symptoms or signs. The course of acetaminophen poisoning is divided into 4 stages (postingestion time):

Stage 1 (12 to 24 hours) – Nausea, vomiting, diaphoresis, anorexia.

Stage 2 (24 to 48 hours) – Clinically improved; AST, bilirubin, and prothrombin levels begin to rise.

Stage 3 (72 to 96 hours) – Peak hepatotoxicity; AST of 20,000 not unusual.

Stage 4 (7 to 8 days) – Recovery.

Hepatotoxicity may result. The minimal toxic dose is 10 g (140 mg/kg), but liver damage has occurred with a single 5.85 g dose; doses 20 to 25 g or larger are potentially fatal. Children appear less susceptible to toxicity than adults because they have less capacity for glucuronidation metabolism. Initial signs of toxicity may include nausea, vomiting, anorexia, malaise, diaphoresis, abdominal pain, and diarrhea. Hepatotoxicity is usually not apparent for 48 to 72 hours. Hepatic failure may lead to encephalopathy, coma, and death.

Plasma acetaminophen levels over 300 mcg/mL at 4 hours postingestion were associated with hepatic damage in 90% of patients; minimal hepatic damage is anticipated if plasma levels at 4 hours are less than 120 mcg/mL or less than 30 mcg/mL at 12 hours after ingestion.

Chronic excessive use (over 4 g/day) may lead to transient hepatotoxicity. The kidneys may undergo tubular necrosis; the myocardium may be damaged.

Treatment: Perform gastric lavage in all cases, preferably within 4 hours of ingestion. Refer also to General Management of Acute Overdosage. It is important to contact a local poison control center or emergency room if overdosage is suspected.

▶ **Administration and Dosage**

Adults: 325 to 650 mg orally every 4 hours, or 1 g 3 to 4 times daily as needed. Do not exceed 4 g daily for all formulations containing acetaminophen.

Children: The usual oral dose is 10 mg/kg/dose, which may be repeated 4 to 5 times daily as needed. Do not exceed 5 doses in 24 hours.

Acetaminophen Dosage for Children			
Age	Dosage (mg)	Age	Dosage (mg)
0-3 months	40	6-8 years	320
4-11 months	80	9-10 years	400
1- 2 years	120	11 years	480
2-3 years	160	12-14 years	640
4-5 years	240	> 14 years	650

Suppositories:

   Adults – 650 mg every 4 to 6 hours; do not exceed 4 g in 24 hours.

   Children (3 to 11 months of age) – 80 mg every 6 hours.

   (1 to 3 years of age) – 80 mg every 4 hours.

   (3 to 6 years of age) – 120 to 125 mg every 4 to 6 hours; do not exceed 720 mg in 24 hours.

   (6 to 12 years of age) – 325 mg every 4 to 6 hours; do not exceed 2.6 g in 24 hours.

Storage: Store suppositories below 27°C (80°F) or refrigerate. Store tablets and oral solutions at 15° to 30°C (59° to 86°F).

ACETAMINOPHEN PRODUCTS	
Trade name	Doseform
Junior Strength Tylenol	**Tablets:** 160 mg. Aspartame (6 mg phenylalanine).
Regular Strength Tylenol	**Tablets:** 325 mg
Aspirin Free Anacin Maximum Strength, Extra Strength Tylenol[1], *Panadol*	**Tablets:** 500 mg
Tylenol Extended Relief	**Tablets:** 650 mg
Children's Panadol, Children's Tylenol, Children's Tylenol Soft Chews	**Tablets, chewable:** 80 mg
Junior Strength Tylenol	**Tablets, chewable:** 160 mg
Meda-Cap	**Capsules:** 500 mg
Extra Strength Tylenol	**Gelcaps:** 500 mg
Extra Strength Tylenol	**Geltabs:** 500 mg
Infants' FeverAll	**Suppositories:** 80 mg
Children's FeverAll	**Suppositories:** 120 mg
Junior Strength FeverAll	**Suppositories:** 325 mg
Acephen	**Suppositories:** 650 mg
Children's Silapap	**Elixir:** 80 mg/2.5 mL. Alcohol free
Children's Tylenol[3]	**Elixir:** 80 mg/2.5 mL. Alcohol free.
Aceta	**Elixir:** 120 mg/5 mL
Infants' Tylenol Concentrated Drops[4]	**Liquid:** 80 mg/0.8 mL. Alcohol free.
Extra Strength Tylenol[5]	**Liquid:** 500 mg/15 mL. 7% alcohol.
Liquiprin Drops for Children	**Solution:** 80 mg/1.66 mL. Alcohol free.

ACETAMINOPHEN PRODUCTS	
Trade name	Doseform
Infants' Panadol Drops,[2] Infants' Silapap Drops, Infants' Tylenol Drops[4]	**Solution**: 80 mg/0.8 mL. Alcohol free.
Children's Tylenol Liquid	**Suspension**: 80 mg/2.5 mL
Tempra	**Syrup**: 160 mg/5 mL

Products listed are representative of currently available and widely distributed brands. Similar products, including regional and private label brands, may also exist.

[1] Gelatin coated.
[2] Contains saccharin.
[3] Contains butylparaben, sorbitol, and sucrose.
[4] Contains butylparaben, saccharin, and sorbitol.
[5] Contains sorbitol and sucrose.

PATIENT INFORMATION

Acetaminophen

- Severe or recurrent pain may indicate a serious illness. Consult a physician.
- Patient instructions accompany each product. Have the patient read these instructions carefully before use, preferably before leaving the pharmacy, in case of any questions.
- Do not exceed the recommended adult dosage. Do not exceed a total adult dose of 4 g/day of acetaminophen in all formulations consumed (2 g/day in regular alcohol users).
- Consult a physician for use in a child younger than 3 years of age.
- Do not take acetaminophen for longer than 5 days (children) or longer than 10 days (adults) for pain relief. If symptoms persist, worsen, or if new symptoms develop, contact a physician.
- Avoid alcohol and aspirin while taking this drug.

NONSTEROIDAL ANTI-INFLAMMATORY DRUGS

▶ Actions

Nonsteroidal anti-inflammatory drugs (NSAIDs) have analgesic, anti-inflammatory, and antipyretic activities. Their exact mode of action is unknown. The major mechanism of action of NSAIDs is believed to be inhibition of cyclooxygenase (COX) activity and prostaglandin synthesis. Other mechanisms, such as inhibition of lipoxygenase, leukotriene synthesis, lysosomal enzyme release, neutrophil aggregation, and various cell-membrane functions, may exist as well.

NSAIDs are capable of inhibiting the enzyme COX. COX allows the conversion of arachidonic acid into prostaglandins, which are mediators of the inflammatory response. Prostaglandin inhibition peripherally at the site of injury can decrease the inflammatory response and pain. Prostaglandin inhibition centrally can also result in analgesia similar to other centrally acting drugs such as acetaminophen. NSAIDs may also have a direct inhibiting effect on inflammatory cells.

▶ Indications

For the treatment of mild to moderate pain. These agents have other labeled indications as well and are particularly helpful for pain associated with inflammation.

▶ Contraindications

NSAID hypersensitivity: Because of potential cross-sensitivity to other NSAIDs, do not give these agents to patients in whom aspirin or other NSAIDs have induced symptoms of asthma, rhinitis, urticaria, nasal polyps, angioedema, bronchospasm, and other symptoms of allergic or anaphylactoid reactions.

▶ Warnings

Acute renal insufficiency: Patients with preexisting renal disease or compromised renal perfusion are at greatest risk. A form of renal toxicity seen in patients with prerenal conditions leads to reduced renal blood flow or blood volume. NSAID use may cause a dose-dependent reduction in prostaglandin formation and precipitate renal decompensation. Patients at greatest risk are the elderly, premature infants, those with heart failure, renal or hepatic dysfunction, systemic lupus erythematosus (SLE), chronic glomerulonephritis, dehydration, diabetes mellitus, septicemia, pyelonephritis, extracellular volume depletion from any cause, or impaired renal function, or those taking ACE inhibitors, any nephrotoxic drug, or diuretics. Recovery usually follows discontinuation.

Hypersensitivity: Severe hypersensitivity reactions with fever, rash, abdominal pain, headache, nausea, vomiting, signs of liver damage, and meningitis have occurred rarely in patients taking ibuprofen, especially those with SLE or other collagen diseases. Anaphylactoid reactions have occurred in patients with aspirin hypersensitivity.

Renal function impairment: NSAID metabolites are eliminated primarily by the kidneys; use with caution in patients with renal impairment. Reduce dosage to avoid excessive accumulation.

Platelet aggregation: NSAIDs can inhibit platelet aggregation; the effect is reversible, quantitatively less, and of shorter duration than that seen with aspirin. These agents prolong bleeding time (within normal range) in healthy subjects. This may be exaggerated in patients with underlying hemostatic defects; use with caution in people with intrinsic coagulation defects and in those on anticoagulant therapy.

Cardiovascular effects: May cause fluid retention and peripheral edema. Use with caution in patients with compromised cardiac function (eg, heart failure), hypertension, or other conditions predisposing to fluid retention, and in those on chronic diuretic therapy. Agents may be associated with significant deterioration of circulatory hemodynamics in severe heart failure and hyponatremia, presumably due to inhibition of prostaglandin-dependent compensatory mechanisms.

Infection: NSAIDs may mask the usual signs of infection (eg, fever, myalgia, arthralgia). Use with extra care in the presence of existing controlled infection.

Photosensitivity: Photosensitivity may occur; caution patients to take protective measures (eg, sunscreens, protective clothing) against UV or sunlight until tolerance is determined.

GI effects: GI toxicity (including NSAID-induced ulcers and GI bleeding disorders) can occur at any time with or without warning with chronic use of NSAIDs. High-dose NSAIDs probably carry a greater risk of causing GI adverse effects. Have patients with a history of GI lesions consult a physician before using these products. GI adverse effects are more likely to occur and may be more pronounced in elderly patients.

Pregnancy: Category B; Category D in 3rd trimester. Safety for use during pregnancy has not been established; use is not recommended. There are no adequate, well-controlled studies in pregnant women. An increased incidence of dystocia, increased postimplantation loss, and delayed parturition has occurred in animals. Agents that inhibit prostaglandin synthesis may cause closure of the ductus arteriosus and other untoward effects in the fetus. GI tract toxicity is increased in pregnant women in the last trimester. Some NSAIDs may prolong pregnancy if given before onset of labor. Avoid use during pregnancy, especially during the 3rd trimester.

Lactation: Most NSAIDs are excreted in breast milk in low concentrations. The American Academy of Pediatrics considers ibuprofen and naproxen to be compatible with breastfeeding. Data on the use of ketoprofen during breastfeeding are lacking.

Children: The use of naproxen is not recommended in children younger than 12 years of age unless directed by a physician. Ketoprofen is not recommended for use in children younger than 16 years of age.

Elderly: Age appears to increase the possibility of adverse reactions to NSAIDs. The risk of serious ulcer disease is increased in elderly patients (older than 65 years of age) taking NSAIDs chronically; this risk appears to increase with dose. Use with greater care and begin with lower dosages in this patient population.

▶ **Drug Interactions**

NSAID Drug Interactions			
Precipitant drug	**Object drug***		**Description**
NSAIDs	ACE Inhibitors	↓	NSAIDs may diminish the antihypertensive effect of ACE inhibitors.
NSAIDs	Aminoglycosides	↑	Aminoglycoside plasma concentrations may be elevated in premature infants because of NSAIDs, reducing the glomerular filtration rate. Reduce aminoglycoside dose prior to NSAID initiation and monitor serum aminoglycoside levels and renal function.
NSAIDs	Anticoagulants	↑	Coadministration may prolong prothrombin time (PT). Also consider the effects NSAIDs have on platelet function and gastric mucosa. Monitor PT and patients closely, especially during the first few days of therapy, and instruct patients to watch for signs and symptoms of bleeding.
NSAIDs	Beta blockers	↓	The antihypertensive effect of beta blockers may be impaired. Avoid using this combination if possible.
NSAIDs	Cyclosporine	↑	Nephrotoxicity of both agents may be increased.
NSAIDs	Digoxin	↑	Ibuprofen may increase digoxin serum levels.
NSAIDs	Hydantoins	↑	Serum phenytoin levels may be increased, resulting in an increase in pharmacologic and toxic effects of phenytoin.
NSAIDs	Lithium	↑	Serum lithium levels may be increased.
NSAIDs	Diuretics	↓	Effects of diuretics may be decreased.
NSAIDs	Methotrexate	↑	The risks of methotrexate toxicity (eg, stomatitis, bone marrow suppression, nephrotoxicity) may be increased.
NSAIDs	Thiazide diuretics	↔	Decreased antihypertensive and diuretic action of thiazides may occur with concurrent naproxen.
Bisphosphonates	NSAIDs	↑	Risk of gastric ulceration may be increased. Use cautiously.
Cholestyramine	NSAIDs	↓	The effects of NSAIDs may be decreased.
Cimetidine	NSAIDs	↔	NSAID plasma concentrations may be increased or decreased by cimetidine; some studies report no effect.

NSAID Drug Interactions			
Precipitant drug	Object drug*		Description
Probenecid	NSAIDs	↑	Probenecid may increase the concentrations and possibly the toxicity of the NSAIDs.
Salicylates	NSAIDs	↓	Plasma concentrations of NSAIDs may be decreased by salicylates. Avoid concurrent use because it offers no therapeutic advantage and may significantly increase the incidence of GI effects.

* ↑ = Object drug increased.   ↓ = Object drug decreased.   ↔ = Undetermined clinical effect.

▶ **Adverse Reactions**

Cardiovascular: Edema; congestive heart failure; hypertension; tachycardia.

CNS: Dizziness; drowsiness; headache; light-headedness; vertigo.

Dermatologic: Erythema; pruritus; rash; increased sweating; urticaria; photosensitivity; eczema.

GI: Bleeding; diarrhea; dyspepsia; heartburn; nausea; vomiting; abdominal pain or cramps; constipation; flatulence; ulcer bleed; gastritis; melena; epigastric/GI pain; abdominal/GI distress; bloating; GI fullness; stomatitis; anorexia; dry mouth; peptic ulcer; jaundice; pancreatitis; colitis; hematemesis; appetite increase; eructation; rectal bleeding/hemorrhage.

GU: Urinary frequency; renal function impairment; hematuria; interstitial nephritis; renal failure; cystitis; menstrual disorder; azotemia; nephrotic syndrome; papillary necrosis.

Respiratory: Dyspnea; rhinitis; pharyngitis; epistaxis; bronchospasm.

Miscellaneous: Muscle cramps; thirst; purpura; anemia; thrombocytopenia; eosinophilia; liver test abnormalities; BUN increased; hemoglobin and hematocrit decreases; fluid retention; body weight changes; hyperglycemia; hyperkalemia; myalgia; muscle weakness; hearing disturbances; visual disturbances; taste disorder; chills; fever.

IBUPROFEN

▶ **Administration and Dosage**

Adults: 200 mg orally every 4 to 6 hours as needed. If pain does not respond to 200 mg, 400 mg may be used. Do not exceed 1.2 g in 24 hours. Do not take for pain for longer than 10 days unless directed by physician. If GI upset occurs, take with meals or milk.

Children younger than 12 years of age: Ibuprofen is not approved for the treatment of myalgia in children. For dosing information in this age group, see individual product labeling.

IBUPROFEN PRODUCTS	
Trade name	Doseform
Junior Strength Advil, Junior Strength Motrin	**Tablets:** 100 mg
Advil,[1] *Maximum Strength Midol Cramp, Motrin IB*	**Tablets:** 200 mg
Children's Advil, Children's Motrin	**Tablets, chewable:** 50 mg
Junior Strength Advil, Junior Strength Motrin	**Tablets, chewable:** 100 mg
Advil Liqui-Gels, Motrin IB[2]	**Gelcaps:** 200 mg

IBUPROFEN PRODUCTS	
Trade name	Doseform
Infants' Advil Concentrated Drops	Liquid: 50 mg/1.25 mL
Children's Advil,[1,3] Children's Motrin[1]	Suspension: 100 mg/5 mL

Products listed are representative of currently available and widely distributed brands. Similar products, including regional and private label brands, may also exist.

[1] Contains sucrose.
[2] Contains parabens.
[3] Contains sorbitol.

PATIENT INFORMATION
Ibuprofen

- *Adults:* Do not exceed 1.2 g/day.
- Severe or recurrent pain may indicate a serious illness. Consult a physician.
- Patient instructions accompany each product. Have the patient read these instructions carefully before use, preferably before leaving the pharmacy, in case of any questions.
- May cause GI upset; take with food or after meals.
- Take with a full glass of water (240 mL) to reduce the risk of the medication lodging in the esophagus.
- Do not take OTC NSAIDs for longer than 10 days for pain unless directed by a physician. If symptoms persist, worsen, or if new symptoms develop, contact a physician.
- Notify physician if rash, itching, visual disturbances, edema, black stools, or persistent headache occur.
- If the patient consumes 3 or more alcoholic drinks every day, taking ibuprofen or other pain relievers or fever reducers may cause stomach bleeding.
- Avoid aspirin while taking this medication.

KETOPROFEN

▶ Administration and Dosage

Adults: 12.5 mg with a full glass of liquid every 4 to 6 hours as needed. If pain persists longer than 1 hour, follow with 12.5 mg. Do not exceed 25 mg in a 4- to 6-hour period or 75 mg in a 24-hour period. Use the smallest effective dose.

Children: Do not give to children younger than 16 years of age unless directed by a physician.

KETOPROFEN PRODUCTS	
Trade name	Doseform
Orudis KT	Tablets: 12.5 mg

Products listed are representative of currently available and widely distributed brands. Similar products, including regional and private label brands, may also exist.

PATIENT INFORMATION
Ketoprofen

- *Adults:* Do not exceed 75 mg/day.
- Severe or recurrent pain may indicate a serious illness. Consult a physician.
- Patient instructions accompany each product. Have the patient read these instructions carefully before use, preferably before leaving the pharmacy, in case of any questions.
- May cause GI upset; take with food or after meals.
- Take with a full glass of liquid (240 mL) to reduce the risk of the medication lodging in the esophagus.
- Do not take OTC NSAIDs for longer than 10 days for pain unless directed by a physician. If symptoms persist, worsen, or if new symptoms develop, contact a physician.
- Notify physician if rash, itching, visual disturbances, edema, black stools, or persistent headache occur.
- Avoid alcohol and aspirin while taking this medication.

NAPROXEN

▶ Administration and Dosage

Adults: 200 mg with a full glass of liquid every 8 to 12 hours as needed. With experience, some patients may find an initial dose of 400 mg followed by 200 mg 12 hours later, if necessary, will give better relief. Do not exceed 600 mg in 24 hours unless otherwise directed. Use the smallest effective dose.

Children: Do not give to children younger than 12 years of age unless directed by a physician.

Elderly (older than 65 years of age): Do not take over 200 mg in a 12-hour period.

NAPROXEN PRODUCTS	
Trade name	Doseform
Aleve	**Tablets, Caplets, and Gelcaps**: 200 mg (220 mg naproxen sodium)

Products listed are representative of currently available and widely distributed brands. Similar products, including regional and private label brands, may also exist.

PATIENT INFORMATION

Naproxen

- *Adults:* Do not exceed 600 mg/day.
- Severe or recurrent pain may indicate a serious illness. Consult a physician.
- Patient instructions accompany each product. Have the patient read these instructions carefully before use, preferably before leaving the pharmacy, in case of any questions.
- May cause GI upset; take with food or after meals.
- Take with a full glass of liquid (240 mL) to reduce the risk of medication lodging in the esophagus.
- Do not take OTC NSAIDs for longer than 10 days for pain unless directed by a physician. If symptoms persist, worsen, or if new symptoms develop, contact a physician.
- Notify physician if rash, itching, visual disturbances, edema, black stools, or persistent headache occur.
- If the patient consumes 3 or more alcoholic drinks every day, taking naproxen or other NSAID pain relievers or fever reducers may cause stomach bleeding.
- Avoid aspirin while taking this medication.

RUBS AND LINIMENTS

▶ **Indications**

These products are used for relief of pain of muscular aches, neuralgia, rheumatism, arthritis, sprains, and like conditions, when skin is intact.

Individual components include:

Counterirritants: Camphor, capsicum preparations (capsicum oleoresin, capsaicin), eucalyptus oil, menthol, methyl nicotinate, methyl salicylate, mustard oil, wormwood oil.

Antiseptics: Thymol.

Analgesics: Trolamine salicylate, methyl salicylate.

▶ **Contraindications**

Allergy to components of any formulation or to salicylates.

▶ **Warnings**

For external use only: Avoid contact with eyes, eyelids, and mucous membranes.

Apply to affected parts only: Do not apply to irritated skin; discontinue use if excessive irritation develops. Consult a physician if pain persists for longer than 7 to 10 days, or if redness is present, or in conditions affecting children younger than 10 years of age.

Heat therapy: Do not use an external source of high heat (eg, heating pad) with these agents because irritation and burning of the skin may occur.

Protective covering: Applying a tight bandage or wrap over these agents is not recommended because increased absorption may occur.

▶ **Drug Interactions**

Anticoagulants: An enhanced anticoagulant effect (eg, increased prothrombin time) occurred in several patients receiving an anticoagulant and using topical methyl salicylate concurrently.

▶ **Adverse Reactions**

If applied to large skin areas and used over a prolonged period of time, salicylate side effects (eg, tinnitus, nausea, vomiting) may occur.

Products may be toxic if ingested.

Counterirritants may cause local irritation, especially in patients with sensitive skin.

▶ **Administration and Dosage**

Apply to affected areas as needed.

RUBS AND LINIMENTS	
Trade name	Doseform
Icy Hot	**Balm**: 29% methyl salicylate, 7.6% menthol, white petrolatum
Epiderm	**Balm**: Isopropyl alcohol, parabens, ureas, menthol, EDTA
JointFlex	**Cream**: 3.1% camphor, lanolin, aloe, urea, EDTA, glycerin, peppermint oil
Capzasin-P	**Cream**: 0.025% capsaicin
ArthriCare for Women Silky Dry	**Cream**: 0.025% capsaicin, parabens, mineral oil
ArthriCare for Women Extra Moisturizing	**Cream**: 0.025% capsaicin, aloe vera gel, cetyl and stearyl alcohol, parabens
ArthriCare for Women Multi-Action	**Cream**: 0.025% capsaicin, 1.25% menthol, 0.25% methyl nicotinate, aloe vera gel, cetyl alcohol, parabens
Capzasin-HP	**Cream**: 0.075% capsaicin
ArthriCare for Women Ultra Strength	**Cream**: 0.075% capsaicin, 2% menthol, aloe vera gel, cetyl and stearyl alcohol, parabens
Vicks VapoRub	**Cream**: 2.8% menthol, 5.2% camphor, 1.2% eucalyptus oil, cedarleaf oil, cetyl and stearyl alcohol, EDTA, glycerin, urea, parabens, turpentine oil
BenGay S.P.A.	**Cream**: 10% menthol, cetyl alcohol, urea, EDTA, glycerin
Arthritic Hot	**Cream**: Methyl salicylate, menthol
Ziks	**Cream**: 12% methyl salicylate, 1% menthol, 0.025% capsaicin, cetyl alcohol, urea
Thera-Gesic	**Cream**: 15% methyl salicylate, 1% menthol, glycerin, parabens
BenGay Greaseless	**Cream**: 15% methyl salicylate, 10% menthol, cetyl alcohol, glycerin
Pain Bust-R II	**Cream**: 17% methyl salicylate, 12% menthol, cetyl and stearyl alcohol
ArthriCare for Women Nighttime	**Cream**: 30% methyl salicylate, 1.25% menthol, 0.25% methyl nicotinate, glycerin, isopropyl alcohol
Arthritis Formula BenGay	**Cream**: 30% methyl salicylate, 8% menthol, lanolin
Icy Hot	**Cream**: 30% methyl salicylate, 10% menthol
Ultra Strength BenGay	**Cream**: 30% methyl salicylate, 10% menthol, 4% camphor, EDTA, lanolin
Panalgesic Gold	**Cream**: 35% methyl salicylate, 4% menthol, lanolin, cetyl and stearyl alcohol, mineral oil
Myoflex	**Cream**: 10% triethanolamine salicylate, cetyl and stearyl alcohol, EDTA

RUBS AND LINIMENTS

Trade name	Doseform
Myoflex Extra, Myoflex Arthritic	**Cream**: 15% triethanolamine salicylate
Sportscreme	**Cream**: 10% trolamine salicylate, cetyl alcohol, glycerin, parabens, mineral oil
Aspercreme	**Cream**: 10% trolamine salicylate, aloe vera gel, cetyl alcohol, glycerin, parabens, mineral oil
Mobisyl	**Cream**: 10% trolamine salicylate, aloe vera gel, cetyl alcohol, urea, glycerin, parabens, mineral oil, sweet almond oil, EDTA
Icy Hot Arthritis Therapy	**Gel**: 0.025% capsaicin, aloe vera gel, benzyl alcohol, urea, maleated soybean oil, parabens
Flexall Quik Gel	**Gel**: Menthol, methyl salicylate
Vanishing Scent BenGay	**Gel**: 2.5% menthol, urea, isopropyl alcohol
Vicks VapoRub	**Gel**: 2.6% menthol, 4.8% camphor, 1.2% eucalyptus oil, cedarleaf oil, nutmeg oil, petrolatum, turpentine oil
Flexall 454	**Gel**: 7% menthol, aloe vera gel, eucalyptus oil, glycerin, peppermint oil, thyme oil
Maximum Strength Flexall 454	**Gel**: 16% menthol, aloe vera gel, eucalyptus oil, glycerin, peppermint oil, thyme oil
Flexall Ultra Plus	**Gel**: 16% menthol, 10% methyl salicylate, 3.1% camphor, aloe vera gel, eucalyptus oil, glycerin, peppermint oil, thyme oil
Icy Hot Chill Stick	**Gel**: 30% methyl salicylate, 10% menthol, hydrogenated castor oil, stearyl alcohol
Myoflex Ice Cold Plus	**Gel**: 15% triethanolamine salicylate
Absorbine Jr Arthritis Strength	**Liquid**: Capsaicin, echinacea, calendula, and wormwood extracts
Absorbine Jr	**Liquid**: 1.27% menthol, echinacea, calendula, and wormwood extracts, wormwood oil
Extra Strength Absorbine Jr	**Liquid**: 4% menthol, echinacea, calendula, and wormwood extracts, wormwood oil
Yager's	**Liniment**: Camphor, turpentine oil, clove oil
Panalgesic Gold	**Liniment**: 55.01% methyl salicylate, 1.25% menthol, 3.1% camphor, emollient oils, alcohol
Banalg	**Lotion**: 4.9% methyl salicylate, 1% menthol, 2% camphor, parabens, eucalyptus oil
Banalg Hospital Strength	**Lotion**: 14% methyl salicylate, 3% menthol, parabens
Aspercreme	**Lotion**: Trolamine salicylate
Eucalyptamint	**Ointment**: 16% menthol, eucalyptus oil, lanolin, mineral oil
Original Formula BenGay	**Ointment**: 18.3% methyl salicylate, 16% menthol, lanolin
Absorbine Jr	**Patch**: Menthol, camphor, eucalyptus
Absorbine Jr Deep Pain Relief	**Patch**: Menthol, glucosamine, MSM
Icy Hot	**Patch**: Methyl salicylate, menthol

Products listed are representative of currently available and widely distributed brands. Similar products, including regional and private label brands, may also exist.

PATIENT INFORMATION

Rubs and Liniments

- For external use only. Avoid contact with eyes, eyelids, and mucous membranes.
- Apply to affected areas only. Do not apply to irritated skin; discontinue use if excessive irritation develops.
- Consult a physician if pain persists for longer than 7 to 10 days, if redness is present, or in conditions affecting children younger than 10 years of age.
- Do not use an external source of high heat (eg, heating pad) with these agents because irritation and burning of the skin may occur.
- Do not apply tight bandages or wraps over these agents.
- Do not apply to broken skin.

OSTEOPOROSIS

DEFINITION

Osteoporosis, Latin for "porous bone," is the most common bone disorder seen in clinical practice and is a worldwide health problem afflicting both sexes. Rather than characterizing osteoporosis as a normal part of aging (because some bone loss is expected as people age), the condition may be best described as a systemic skeletal disease characterized by the erosion of the microarchitecture of bone tissue and by low bone density or mass. These factors contribute to poor bone quality and increased skeletal fragility, which often result in fractures.

Osteoporosis may be stratified according to etiology (primary and secondary) and the bone tissue affected (primary type 1 vs primary type 2). The type of osteoporosis most familiar to the public is primary type 1 osteoporosis, also known as postmenopausal osteoporosis. Seen most frequently in postmenopausal women or women who have had oophorectomies, but also seen in men (female-to-male ratio is 6:1), type 1 is characterized by increased osteoclast activity (leading to bone breakdown), which compromises the integrity of the spongy inner bone, called the trabecular matrix. Type 2 (age-related or senile) osteoporosis occurs in both sexes at approximately 70 to 75 years of age. Women also are more likely than men (2:1 ratio) to develop type 2 osteoporosis, which is characterized by a generalized decrease in osteoblast (bone-building) activity. As a result, decreased cortical bone (the hard, outer surface of bone) and trabecular bone density develop in roughly equal proportions. Finally, secondary osteoporosis (also called type 3 osteoporosis) is drug- or disease-induced, afflicting both sexes equally.

ETIOLOGY

Osteoporosis is the result of an imbalance of osteoclast (bone-resorbing cells) and osteoblast activity, which would otherwise maintain a constant, healthy equilibrium of bone remodeling.

INCIDENCE

Approximately 28 million Americans are threatened by the consequences of osteoporosis. In 1998 alone, 10 million Americans were diagnosed with the disease and over 18 million others were found to have subclinical, low bone density. Overall, women are 4 times more likely than men to develop osteoporosis and account for 80% of those people diagnosed with the disease. One in 8 men and 1 in 2 women older than 50 years of age develop bone fractures as a result of osteoporosis.

PATHOPHYSIOLOGY

In humans, peak bone mass is achieved 2 to 3 years after linear bone growth stops. Bone remodeling is the dynamic process in which damaged or fatigued bone and calcium are removed by osteoclasts (a process called resorption) and replaced with new bone by osteoblasts. Bone remodeling maintains bone mass and is generally efficient until the third decade of life, when, at some point, bone mineral density slowly starts to decline.

High turnover bone loss can be a result of decreased serum estrogen concentrations after menopause. In type 1 osteoporosis, the resorptive cavities are deepened because of increased osteoclast activity in the face of unchanged osteoblast activity. Low turnover bone loss occurs when the osteoclast activity is steady, but osteoblast activity declines because of age (type 2 osteoporosis).

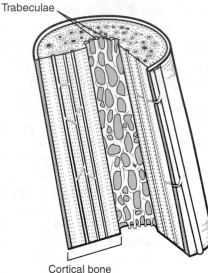 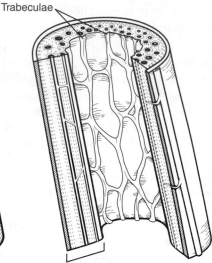

Trabeculae

Cortical bone

Figure 1. Normal Bone

Trabeculae

Cortical bone

Figure 2. Osteoporotic Bone

SIGNS/SYMPTOMS

Osteoporosis often is referred to as a silent disease. Patients are usually asymptomatic until fracture occurs, often causing immobility and severe pain. Shortened stature and "dowager's hump" (collapsing spinal vertebrae) also are likely.

Vertebral fractures are the most common in osteoporosis, followed by hip and wrist fractures. Fractures also may occur in other bony areas. In osteoporotic patients, bones may break during simple, daily activities (eg, stepping from a curb, hugging, sneezing, lifting).

Risk Factors		
Endogenous	**Exogenous***	**Secondary**
Genetic predisposition	Suboptimal dietary calcium	*Medications:*
Age	Insufficient vitamin D	Anticonvulsant therapy (long-term)
Female gender	Lack of exercise	Corticosteroids
White or Asian race	Lack of outdoor activities	Aluminum-containing
Small frame	Immobility	antacids (long-term)
Low body weight or BMI	Cigarette smoking	Levothyroxine (excessive)
Menopause or oophorectomy	Alcohol consumption	Furosemide
Small bone structure/tall stature	(excessive)	High-dose heparin (long-term)
	Caffeine consumption	*Concurrent disease states:*
	(chronic, excessive)	Chronic liver or renal disease
		Gastrointestinal diseases
		(eg, malabsorption syndrome)
		Endocrinopathies
		Hyperthyroidism
		Estrogen deficiency
		Cushing syndrome
		Primary hyperparathyroidism

* Risk factors that may be modified via lifestyle practices.

DIAGNOSTIC PARAMETERS/PHYSICAL ASSESSMENT

Clinical Observation: Because of the nature of the disease, diagnosis is unlikely prior to fracture unless the patient undergoes a screening. Advise patients at risk for osteoporosis to discuss the disease with their physician. There are several tests or scans available that detect osteoporosis and assess the risk for future fractures. The dual energy x-ray absorptiometry (DEXA) scan is usually the procedure of choice because it offers accurate, low-cost bone mineral density measurements where fractures are most likely to occur (ie, lumbar spine, upper femur, wrist) and poses minimal radiation exposure.

Interview: The patient interview can help identify risk factors for osteoporosis. Pharmacists may recommend products and appropriate lifestyle practices to help prevent or delay onset of disease. Performing a patient assessment and history prior to recommending products or behavior modifications may aid in preventing fractures. The interview should contain, but not be limited to, inquiries concerning the following:

- Hereditary predisposition
- Age and menstrual status
- Dietary/nutritional status
- Concurrent disease states
- Current medications
- Exercise regimen and degree of mobility
- Caffeine and alcohol consumption
- Smoking
- Outdoor activity

TREATMENT

Approaches to therapy: There is no cure for osteoporosis. Thus, prevention of osteoporosis is the primary goal of therapy and should begin during adolescence. Recent estimates predict that adolescents who achieve a 5% gain in bone mass may decrease their risk of osteoporosis by 40%. Behavior modification directed toward building and maintaining bone is important for both sexes and all age groups. However, lifestyle practices incorporated during the adolescent years appear to be most beneficial.

All patients should be educated about the presence and absence of risk factors. The presence of risk factors does not necessarily indicate that the patient will develop the disease nor is the lack of risk factors indicative of absence of disease. Osteoporosis prevention programs should begin early in life, preferably before bone loss begins.

Nondrug therapy: A nondrug therapy approach is perhaps the optimal method of preventing osteoporosis. Patients previously diagnosed with the disease may incorporate behavioral modifications into their daily routines to help minimize and deter the progression of osteoporosis. The following guidelines are recommended:

- **Proper nutrition** is essential for developing and maintaining strong bones. Dietary calcium is the preferred source of calcium. Dairy products, dark green leafy vegetables, shellfish, and tofu are good sources of calcium. However, many patients ingest suboptimal amounts of dietary calcium and should enhance their daily intake with calcium supplementation (see Calcium Administration & Dosage for Recommended Daily Intake). Dietary sources of vitamin D include fish, fish liver oils, and fortified milk.
- **Weight-bearing exercises** (eg, walking, climbing stairs) are preferred to build stronger bones. Urge patients to avoid exercises that jar the body and to participate in activities that minimize the risk of falls, especially if a previous diagnosis of bone loss or osteoporosis exists.
- **Adequate exposure to sunlight** may be accomplished by a brisk, daily 15-minute walk outdoors, which is usually sufficient for the body to produce enough vitamin D to absorb calcium properly.
- **Limited caffeine and alcohol consumption**.
- **Discontinuation of smoking**.

Pharmacotherapy: Several agents are available for the prevention and treatment of osteoporosis when calcium and vitamin D consumption are inadequate. Recommend OTC calcium supplements (unless otherwise contraindicated) for patients who do not attain sufficient calcium intake from dietary sources. Add vitamin D supplementation when dietary intake is low or when the patient is confined indoors and does not receive adequate sunlight.

Prescription drug therapy includes hormonal and nonhormonal agents. Estrogen replacement therapy may be recommended for some postmenopausal women or estrogen-deficient patients, unless the substance is contraindicated because of current or previous disease (eg, breast cancer) or risks of estrogen replacement therapy exceed potential benefits. Raloxifene (*Evista*) is a selective estrogen receptor modulator approved for the prevention of osteoporosis without increasing a woman's risk for certain estrogen-dependent cancers (eg, breast cancer). Calcitonin (*Miacalcin*) is a hormonal agent that may aid in reversing bone loss and relieving pain associated with fractured bones. Alendronate (*Fosamax*) and risedronate (*Actonel*) help rebuild bone and may be used for the prevention and treatment of osteoporosis.

Women and men should discuss concerns regarding therapy with both physicians and pharmacists. Patients should be given information that will empower them to take active roles in drug and nondrug prevention and therapy.

CALCIUM SUPPLEMENTS

▶ **Indications**

(Refer to the Vitamin and Non-Vitamin Deficiency monographs in the Nutrition Chapter for details concerning calcium and vitamin D supplementation not applicable to osteoporosis.)

Calcium: Dietary calcium is the preferred source of calcium. Use calcium supplements when dietary calcium consumption is insufficient for an individual to maximize peak adult bone mass, maintain adult bone mass, or minimize bone loss as one ages.

Vitamin D: Vitamin D supplementation is useful for patients who have low dietary intake of vitamin D or insufficient exposure to sunlight, which is necessary to produce the adequate amount of endogenous vitamin D needed to absorb calcium properly.

▶ **Contraindications**

Calcium: Hypercalcemia; ventricular fibrillation.

Vitamin D: Hypercalcemia; vitamin D toxicity; malabsorption syndrome; abnormal sensitivity to the effects of vitamin D; decreased renal function.

▶ **Warnings**

Calcium: Calcium salts may be mildly irritating to the gastrointestinal tract when administered orally and also may cause constipation. Hypercalcemia may occur when large doses of calcium are administered to patients with chronic renal failure. Recent evidence shows that high dietary intake of calcium decreases the risk of symptomatic renal calculi, while intake of supplemental calcium may increase the risk of symptomatic stones. Use calcium supplements cautiously in patients with sarcoidosis, cardiac or renal disease, and in patients receiving cardiac glycosides. Avoid concurrent use of calcium citrate and aluminum-containing antacids in patients with renal function impairment. Inform phenylketonuric patients that some of these products contain phenylalanine.

Vitamin D: Use with caution in patients with coronary artery disease, impaired renal function, and arteriosclerosis, and especially in elderly patients. Assess vitamin D attained from fortified foods, nutritional supplements, and sun exposure; it may be necessary to limit dietary vitamin D and its derivatives during treatment. Because of the effect on serum calcium, administer to patients with renal stones only when potential benefits outweigh possible risks. Patients with hypoparathyroidism may need calcium, parathyroid hormone, or dihydrotachysterol.

Pregnancy:

    Calcium – Category C. It is not known whether this drug can cause fetal harm. Use only when clearly needed and according to federal guidelines on recommended daily intake.

    Vitamin D – Category A (Category D in doses exceeding 400 units per day).

Lactation:

Calcium – It is not known if calcium is excreted in breast milk. Exercise caution when administering to a nursing woman. Follow federal guidelines on recommended daily intake.

Vitamin D – Vitamin D is excreted in breast milk in limited amounts. Exercise caution when administering to a nursing mother.

Children:

Calcium – Safety and efficacy in children have not been established. Follow federal guidelines on recommended daily intake.

Vitamin D – Safety and efficacy of vitamin D doses over 400 units/day in children have not been established. Pediatric doses must be individualized and monitored under close medical supervision.

Tartrazine sensitivity: Some of these products contain tartrazine, which may cause allergic-type reactions (including bronchial asthma) in susceptible individuals. Although the incidence of sensitivity is low, it is seen frequently in patients who have aspirin hypersensitivity. Specific products containing tartrazine are identified in the product listings.

▶ Drug Interactions

Calcium:

Calcium Drug Interactions			
Precipitant drug	**Object drug***		**Description**
Thiazide diuretics	Calcium salts	↑	Hypercalcemia resulting from renal tubular reabsorption or bone release of calcium by thiazides may be amplified by exogenous calcium.
Calcium carbonate	Quinolones	↓	GI absorption of quinolones may be decreased. The bioavailability of norfloxacin may be reduced; lomefloxacin and ofloxacin do not appear to be affected.
Calcium salts	Atenolol	↓	Mean peak plasma levels and bioavailability of atenolol may be decreased, possibly resulting in decreased beta blockade.
Calcium salts	Digitalis glycosides	↑	Inotropic and toxic effects are synergistic; arrhythmias may occur, especially if calcium is given IV. Avoid IV calcium in patients on digitalis glycosides; if necessary, give slowly in small amounts.
Calcium salts	Iron salts	↓	GI absorption of iron may be reduced. In order to avoid a possible interaction, separate administration times whenever possible.
Calcium salts	Sodium polystyrene sulfonate	↓	Coadministration in patients with renal impairment may result in an unanticipated metabolic alkalosis and a reduction of the resin's binding of potassium.
Calcium salts	Tetracyclines	↓	The absorption and serum levels of tetracyclines are decreased; a decreased anti-infective response may occur.
Calcium salts	Verapamil	↓	Clinical effects and toxicities of verapamil may be reversed.

* ↑ = Object drug increased. ↓ = Object drug decreased.

Food – Diets that consist of large amounts of animal protein and sodium may increase urinary calcium excretion. Diets that include large amounts of wheat bran may significantly decrease calcium absorption. Other sources of dietary fiber have not been shown to affect calcium absorption.

Vitamin D:

Vitamin D Drug Interactions			
Precipitant drug	**Object drug***		**Description**
Vitamin D	Antacids, magnesium-containing	↑	Hypermagnesemia may develop in patients on chronic renal dialysis.
Vitamin D	Digitalis glycosides	↑	Hypercalcemia in patients on digitalis glycosides may precipitate cardiac arrhythmias.
Vitamin D	Verapamil	↑	Atrial fibrillation has recurred when supplemental calcium and calciferol have induced hypercalcemia.
Cholestyramine	Vitamin D	↓	Intestinal absorption of vitamin D may be reduced.
Ketoconazole	Vitamin D	↓	Ketoconazole may inhibit synthetic and catabolic enzymes of calcitriol. Reductions in serum endogenous calcitriol concentrations have been observed following the administration of 300 to 1,200 mg/day ketoconazole for a week to healthy men.
Mineral oil	Vitamin D	↓	Absorption of vitamin D is reduced with prolonged use of mineral oil.
Phenytoin, Barbiturates	Vitamin D	↓	Half-life of vitamin D may be decreased.
Thiazide diuretics	Vitamin D	↑	Hypoparathyroid patients on vitamin D may develop hypercalcemia because of thiazide diuretics.

* ↑ = Object drug increased ↓ = Object drug decreased.

▶ **Adverse Reactions**

Calcium: May cause constipation. Mild hypercalcemia may manifest as headache, anorexia, nausea, or vomiting. More severe hypercalcemia is associated with confusion, delirium, stupor, and coma.

Vitamin D: Adverse reactions are mainly caused by induced hypercalcemia and are the same as those listed for calcium.

▶ **Overdosage**

Excessive use of calcium or vitamin D supplements can cause severe hypercalcemia (see Adverse Reactions). Severe hypercalcemia can be treated with acute hemodialysis and by discontinuing therapy.

▶ **Administration and Dosage**

Calcium: The Dietary Reference Intake (DRI) for calcium establishes the amount needed to protect against nutrient deficiency; this is intended to help optimize health and minimize the risk of chronic disease. However, calcium requirements for prevention of osteoporosis are greater than those noted in the DRIs. Therefore, the following table provides the Recommended Daily Intake (RDI), a guideline for optimal daily elemental calcium intake from the diet plus calcium supplements. (For a complete listing of RDIs and DRIs, see the tables at the beginning of the Nutrition chapter.) A total **elemental** calcium intake of 2,000 mg/day appears to be safe in most individuals. All calcium supplements are available in salt form (eg, citrate, carbonate, lactate, phosphate, gluconate). Read labels carefully to determine the calcium content of these products.

Dietary Reference Intakes for Calcium*		
Age	Adequate Intake† (mg/d)	UL‡ (mg/d)
Infants		
0 to 6 mo	210	ND**
7 mo to 12 mo	270	ND
Children		
1 to 3 y	500	2,500
4 to 8 y	800	2,500
Men/Women		
9 to 13 y	1,300	2,500
14 to 18 y	1,300	2,500
19 to 30 y	1,000	2,500
31 to 50 y	1,000	2,500
50 to 70 y	1,200	2,500
> 70 y	1,200	2,500
Pregnancy/Lactation		
≤ 18 y	1,300	2,500
19 to 30 y	1,000	2,500
31 to 50 y	1,000	2,500

* Table adapted from: *Dietary Reference Intakes Tables*. Institute of Medicine of the National Academies, Food and Nutrition Board. (http://www.iom.edu/fnb). Last accessed November 2004.
† AIs may be used as goals for individual intake. For healthy breastfed infants, AI is the mean intake. The AI for other life stage and gender groups is believed to cover the needs of all individuals in the group, but lack of data prevents the ability to specify with confidence the percentage of individuals covered by this intake.
‡ UL = The maximum level of daily nutrient intake that is likely to pose no risk of adverse effects. The UL represents total intake from food, water, and supplements.
** ND = Not determinable because of lack of adverse effects data in this age group and concern with regard to lack of ability to handle excess amounts. Source of intake should be from food only to prevent high levels of intake.

Conversion of Calcium Salts to Elemental Calcium			
Calcium salt	Elemental calcium (%)	Calcium salt (mg)	Elemental calcium (mg)
Calcium carbonate	40	500	200
Calcium citrate	21	500	105
Calcium gluconate	9	650	58.5
Calcium lactate	13	650	84.5
Dibasic calcium phosphate	23	500	115
Tribasic calcium phosphate	39	600	234

Calcium cannot be absorbed from tablets that do not disintegrate properly; several studies have documented solubility problems with calcium carbonate tablets. When recommending products containing calcium carbonate, pharmacists should choose products with "USP" on the package labeling or products that have been tested previously for dissolution (a calcium carbonate tablet should dissolve within 30 minutes in a glass of water).

Vitamin D: Daily exposure to sunlight is the optimal source of vitamin D. However, patients receiving limited exposure to sunlight may use dietary supplements. The RDI for those with limited sunlight exposure is 600 to 800 units/day.

CALCIUM PRODUCTS

Trade name	Doseform	Elemental Calcium (mg)
Calcium Gluconate	**Tablets**: 648 mg (10 grain) calcium gluconate	60
Calcium Lactate (sf)	**Tablets**: 650 mg calcium lactate	84
Calcium Gluconate	**Tablets**: 972 mg (15 grain) calcium gluconate	90
Florical	**Tablets**: 364 mg calcium carbonate, 3.75 mg fluoride	145
Titralac (sf)	**Tablets**: 420 mg calcium carbonate	168
Monocal	**Tablets**: 625 mg calcium carbonate, 3 mg fluoride	250
Titralac Extra Strength (sf)	**Tablets**: 750 mg calcium carbonate	300
Oysco 500	**Tablets**: 500 mg calcium (from oyster shell). Tartrazine.	500
Caltrate 600, Nephro-Calci	**Tablets**: 1.5 g calcium carbonate	600
Citracal Ultradense, Citrus Calcium	**Tablets, coated**: 200 mg calcium (as calcium citrate). Lactose free.	200
Amitone	**Tablets, chewable**: 350 mg calcium carbonate	140
Titralac Plus (sf)	**Tablets, chewable**: 420 mg calcium carbonate, 21 mg simethicone. Saccharin. Spearmint flavor.	168
Tums Regular Strength	**Tablets, chewable**: 500 mg calcium carbonate. Sucrose. Peppermint flavor.	200
Cal-Mint (sf)	**Tablets, chewable**: 650 mg calcium carbonate. Mannitol, sorbitol. Peppermint flavor.	260
Tums E•X	**Tablets, chewable**: 750 mg calcium carbonate. Sucrose, tartrazine. Assorted fruit flavors.	300
Tums Sugar Free Extra Strength (sf)	**Tablets, chewable**: 750 mg calcium carbonate. Sorbitol, aspartame. Orange cream flavor.	300
Tums Smooth Dissolve	**Tablets, chewable**: 750 mg calcium carbonate. Sorbitol, dextrose, sucrose, tartrazine. Assorted fruit flavors.	300
Alka-Mints	**Tablets, chewable**: 850 mg calcium carbonate. Sugar, sorbitol. Assorted and spearmint flavors.	340
Tums Ultra	**Tablets, chewable**: 1 g calcium carbonate. Sucrose, tartrazine. Assorted fruit and peppermint flavors.	400
Calci-Chew	**Tablets, chewable**: 1.25 g calcium carbonate. Sugar. Cherry, lemon, and orange flavors.	500
Os-Cal	**Tablets, chewable**: 1.25 g calcium carbonate. Dextrose monohydrate.	500
Tums Calcium for Life Bone Health	**Tablets, chewable**: 1.25 g calcium carbonate. Sucrose.	500
Citracal Effervescent Liquitabs	**Tablets, effervescent**: 500 mg calcium (as calcium citrate). Phenylalanine, aspartame. Orange flavor.	500
Cal-GLU (sf)	**Capsules**: 50 mg calcium (calcium gluconate)	50
Florical	**Capsules**: 364 mg calcium carbonate (as oyster shell), 3.75 mg fluoride	145
Cal-Citrate 225 (sf)	**Capsules**: 225 mg calcium (calcium citrate)	225
Calci-Mix	**Capsules**: 1.25 g calcium carbonate	500
Chooz (sf)	**Gum**: 500 mg calcium carbonate. Aspartame, 2.4 mg phenylalanine, sorbitol. Mint flavor.	200
Calcium Gluconate (sf)	**Powder**: 3.9 g calcium gluconate/tbsp. Lactose free.	347

CALCIUM PRODUCTS WITH VITAMIN D

Trade name	Doseform	Elemental Calcium (mg)
Calcimate 400 (sf)	**Tablets**: 133 mg (as calcium citrate malate), 67 units vitamin D	133
Calcimate Plus 800 (sf)	**Tablets**: 200 mg (as calcium citrate malate), 50 units vitamin D, 25 mg magnesium, 25 mg potassium	200
Oyst-Cal-D (sf)	**Tablets**: 250 mg calcium (from oyster shell), 125 units vitamin D. Tartrazine.	250
Calcium Plus 1000 (sf)	**Tablets**: 333 mg calcium (as calcium carbonate), 133 units vitamin D, 1,333 units vitamin A, 33 mg vitamin C, 3 mg iron, 166 mg magnesium. Rose hips powder.	333
Os-Cal 500 + D	**Tablets**: 1.25 g calcium carbonate, 200 units vitamin D	500
Caltrate 600+D	**Tablets**: 1.5 g calcium carbonate, 200 units vitamin D. Sucrose.	600
Caltrate 600 PLUS	**Tablets**: 1.5 g calcium carbonate, 200 units vitamin D, 40 mg magnesium, 7.5 mg zinc, 1 mg copper, 1.8 mg manganese, 250 mcg boron. Sucrose.	600
Calcarb 600 with Vitamin D	**Tablets**: 1.5 g calcium carbonate, 200 units vitamin D	600
Posture-D	**Tablets**: 600 mg calcium (as tricalcium phosphate), 125 units vitamin D, 266 mg phosphorus	600
Os-Cal Ultra	**Tablets**: 1.5 g calcium carbonate, 200 units vitamin D, magnesium, manganese, boron, zinc, copper, vitamins E and C	600
Calcium Citrate Plus (sf)	**Tablets**: 200 mg calcium (as calcium citrate), 25 units vitamin D, 100 mg magnesium, 18.75 mg casein phosphopeptide	200
Calcium Plus Vitamin D	**Tablets, film coated**: 1.5 g calcium carbonate, 125 units vitamin D	600
Caltrate 600 PLUS	**Tablets, chewable**: 1.5 g calcium carbonate, 200 units vitamin D, 40 mg magnesium, 7.5 mg zinc, 1 mg copper, 1.8 mg manganese, 250 mcg boron. Dextrose, sucrose. Assorted fruit flavors.	600
Citracal Caplets +D (sf)	**Caplets**: 315 mg calcium (as calcium citrate), 200 units vitamin D_3	315
Calcium Plus Vitamin D	**Softgels**: 1.25 g calcium carbonate, 50 units vitamin D. Gelatin.	500
Calcium Plus Vitamin D	**Softgels**: 1.5 g calcium carbonate, 100 units vitamin D. Gelatin.	600
Calcium Plus Vitamin D	**Wafers**: 140 mg calcium (as calcium carbonate and dicalcium phosphate), 100 units vitamin D, 25 mg phosphorous. Sucrose, dextrose.	140
VIACTIV	**Soft chews**: 1.25 g calcium carbonate, 100 units vitamin D_3, 40 mcg vitamin K_1. Corn syrup, non-fat milk, 3 g sugars, may contain tartrazine. Milk chocolate, caramel, chocolate mint, orange creme, and strawberry creme flavors.	500
Flintstones Bone Building Calcium Chews	**Soft chews**: 1.25 g calcium carbonate, 200 units vitamin D. Corn syrup, lactose, sugar. Chocolate flavor.	500

Products listed are representative of currently available and widely distributed brands. Similar products, including regional and private label brands, may also exist.

sf = Sugar free.

PATIENT INFORMATION
Calcium Supplements

- Do not take calcium supplements within 1 to 2 hours of interacting medications.
- Do not exceed the recommended dosage.
- Eating a well-balanced diet and obtaining periodic sun exposure usually satisfies vitamin D requirements necessary for adequate calcium absorption. Do not use vitamin D and calcium supplements as substitutes for a well-balanced diet.
- When determining calcium content of a product in reference to RDI or RDA, use the amount of elemental calcium contained in the product (not the total amount of calcium salt).
- Calcium is absorbed poorly. Thus, limit each dose to 500 mg elemental calcium.
- Avoid tobacco products and excessive consumption of alcohol and caffeine (more than 8 cups of coffee/day, or the caffeine equivalent), which increase your risk of developing osteoporosis.
- Chewable calcium tablets should be chewed thoroughly before swallowing.
- Drink a full glass of water with each dose.
- Take with or following meals to enhance absorption
- Discontinue use and notify your physician if you experience appetite loss, nausea, vomiting, constipation, stomach pain, dry mouth, thirst, or excessive urination.
- Some of these products contain phenylalanine. Read the package labeling carefully and consult your physician.
- Individuals with decreased gastric acid production (eg, the elderly, patients taking certain nonprescription and prescription H_2 antagonists and proton pump inhibitors) may derive maximum benefits from calcium citrate supplements.
- Avoid products made from bone meal or dolomite because of possible product contamination with lead, mercury, or arsenic. Calcium carbonate supplements, from oyster shell or "natural source," may contain lead and aluminum. To ensure federal standards regarding purity and quality are met, look for "USP" on the package labeling.
- If being treated for hypocalcemia, avoid taking calcium within 1 to 2 hours of eating large amounts of fiber-containing foods such as bran and whole-grain cereals or breads.
- Do not take other medicines or dietary supplements containing large amounts of calcium, phosphates, magnesium, or vitamin D without checking with your physician.

BENIGN LEG CRAMPS

DEFINITION

Benign leg cramps (idiopathic or nocturnal leg cramps), commonly referred to as charley horses, are involuntary contractions of the skeletal muscle. Benign leg cramps usually present as involuntary, localized, painful contractions that most often involve the calf muscles. Although normally localized to the calf, these cramps can occur in other areas of the leg.

ETIOLOGY

The underlying causes of benign leg cramps have not been determined. Because the condition is benign, little research has been done to investigate its causes. However, several hypotheses have been developed to explain the mechanism of the condition (see Pathophysiology).

INCIDENCE

Although leg cramps are a frequent occurrence, there is little mention of the affliction in the medical literature. Reported incidence of benign leg cramps ranges from 35% to 95% of the general adult population. Leg cramps occur at all ages, but are most commonly experienced in the elderly population. One survey targeting the general medicine clinic of a Veterans Administration Medical Center found that at least 50% of patients questioned reported at least 1 leg cramp in the previous month.

Leg cramps are reported by athletes, children experiencing rapid longitudinal growth, and in 5% to 30% of all pregnant women. In pregnancy, the cramps typically manifest in the later months of pregnancy. No relationship between either additional complications or unfavorable fetal outcomes has been established.

PATHOPHYSIOLOGY

The precise mechanism responsible for idiopathic leg cramps has not been established. However, several hypotheses have been proposed to explain the underlying pathogenesis. It has been suggested that stimulation of the reflex arc results in muscle cramps. Although most explanations are rooted in mechanical factors, hyperexcitation of the motor neurons in leg nerves and the spinal cord may also contribute.

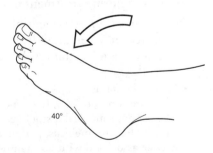

Figure 1. Plantar Flexion Position

Researchers have proposed that nocturnal leg cramps occur when maximally contracted calf muscles are stimulated, causing the muscle to shorten beyond physiological limit into a cramp. When an individual is lying prone or supine, the foot assumes a plantar flexion position (see figure 1), which leads to the sudden contraction of the calf muscles. This may explain the tendency of leg cramps to occur at night.

SIGNS/SYMPTOMS

Most patients describe benign leg cramps as involuntary painful contractions localized in the calf muscles (gastrocnemius or soleus). The sole of the foot is also a frequent site of cramps. Such cramps often occur at night and are sporadic and short-lived (usually lasting no more than a few minutes). Although leg cramps commonly occur at night, particularly after unusually strenuous activity, they may not present with any set pattern of frequency or duration.

Several considerations should be included in the differential diagnosis (see table).

Differential Diagnosis of Benign (Idiopathic) Leg Cramps	
Condition	Characteristics
Idiopathic leg cramps	Often in calf; associated with plantar flexion.
Peripheral neuropathy	Numbness, tingling, burning; frequently seen in diabetic patients.
Restless legs syndrome (RLS)	Creeping sensation; usually at night, relieved by walking.
Claudication	Leg pain, which may occur day or night; frequently seen in cardiac patients.
Hypnic jerks	Generalized body movement when falling asleep; considered normal.

DIAGNOSTIC PARAMETERS/PHYSICAL ASSESSMENT

Many medical conditions, including fluid and electrolyte disturbances, diabetes mellitus, peripheral vascular disease, and liver cirrhosis can be associated with leg cramps; therefore, it is important to eliminate these factors prior to exploring treatment options.

Interview: A thorough medical history can exclude many of the conditions considered in differential diagnosis. To aid in the proper diagnosis and treatment of benign leg cramps, it may be helpful to ask about the following:

- Patient's age
- Pregnancy status
- The duration, intensity, frequency, and location of symptoms
- The patient's medical history (ask specifically about fluid and electrolyte disturbances, diabetes mellitus, peripheral vascular disease, and liver cirrhosis, which may be associated with leg cramps)
- The patient's current medication profile
- Number of alcoholic drinks consumed per week by the patient
- Type of work/exercise in which the patient engages

TREATMENT

Approaches to therapy: Most leg cramps will resolve spontaneously, but some cases will require some form of treatment. Once other medical conditions have been dismissed, base decisions about treatment upon based on the severity or frequency of the muscle cramps. Have patients experiencing frequent leg cramps consider prophylactic therapy. Prudent judgment calls for an initial trial of nondrug prophylaxis utilizing stretching techniques, as well as non-pharmacologic treatment of acute attacks. For patients who do not respond to nondrug therapy, pharmacologic treatment may be indicated. Although several products have anecdotal experience as well as some limited data, little conclusive clinical evidence exists for the use of pharmacologic agents in the treatment of benign leg cramps.

Nondrug therapy: Non-pharmacologic therapy is recommended as first-line treatment in benign leg cramps. Preventive measures, including stretching exercises and appropriate sleep positioning, are among the most effective strategies for decreasing the incidence of idiopathic cramps. Either placing the foot in dorsiflexion (see figure 2) or stretching the calves by standing 2 feet from a wall and leaning forward while keeping the heels on the floor may help

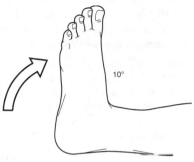

Figure 2. Dorsiflexion of the Foot

prevent leg cramps if performed 2 to 4/day. Using a footboard while sleeping to avoid plantar flexion, hanging the feet over the bed, or raising the foot of the bed may also help prevent the occurrence of muscle cramps. For acute cramping, massage of the calf muscle and dorsiflexion of the foot should relieve pain.

Pharmacotherapy: For many years, quinine sulfate had been the prophylactic agent of choice. Quinine causes increased muscle refractory periods and decreased motor end-plate excitability, which is thought to contribute to its action on leg cramps. Although still available by prescription, the OTC status was removed by the Food and Drug Administration (FDA) in February 1995. Citing insufficient evidence for the efficacy of quinine and safety concerns secondary to the potential for fatal hypersensitivity reactions and thrombocytopenia, the FDA stated that quinine should not generally be recognized as safe and effective for prophylactic treatment of leg cramps.

Other agents, both OTC and prescription, have been reported to be beneficial in the treatment of leg cramps. These include diphenhydramine, verapamil, nifedipine, phenytoin, carbamazepine, procainamide, calcium, and magnesium. Some people have reported benefit from drinking tonic water. However, there is no conclusive clinical evidence to support the use of any of these products. Before any of these products are considered, have the patient consult their physician.

The idea of using vitamin E (alpha-tocopherol) in leg cramps was considered after patients incidentally taking the vitamin experienced relief of cramping. Efficacy of vitamin E in prevention of leg cramps has been suggested in

small trials, although there is no conclusive evidence to date that supports
this practice. However, beneficial effects continue to be reported anecdotally.

VITAMIN E

▶ **Actions**

Although the exact biochemical mechanisms of vitamin E utilization by the body are
unclear, it is an essential element of human nutrition. Many of its actions are related
to its antioxidant properties. Vitamin E may protect cellular constituents from oxidation and prevent the formation of toxic oxidation products; it preserves red blood
cell (RBC) wall integrity and protects them against hemolysis; it may act as a cofactor in enzyme systems. Enhancement of vitamin A utilization and suppression of platelet aggregation have also been attributed to vitamin E.

Clinical deficiency of vitamin E is rare because adequate amounts are supplied in the
normal diet. Sources of vitamin E include vegetable oils, vegetable shortening, and
margarine. Other food sources include leafy vegetables, milk, eggs, and meats. Absorption depends on the ability to digest and absorb fat; bile is essential. There is no single
storage organ, but adipose tissue, liver, and muscle account for most of the body's
tocopherol storage.

Low tocopherol levels have been noted in the following: Premature infants; severe protein-calorie malnourished infants with macrocytic megaloblastic anemia; prolonged
fat malabsorption (eg, cystic fibrosis, hepatic cirrhosis, sprue); malabsorption syndromes (eg, celiac disease, GI resections); acanthocytosis; patients with abetalipoproteinemia. Low levels of vitamin E make the erythrocyte more susceptible to
destruction by oxidants. Vitamin E deficiency may result in hemolysis; also consider
the possibility of deficiency in spinocerebellar syndromes.

Vitamin E requirements: The daily vitamin E requirement is related to the dietary
intake of polyunsaturated fatty acids (PUFA), primarily linoleic acid. Vitamin E
requirements may be increased in patients taking large doses of iron; diets containing
selenium, sulfuramino acids, or antioxidants may decrease the daily requirement.

▶ **Indications**

Unlabeled uses: Vitamin E has been used in nocturnal leg cramps. However, data does
not conclusively support use of vitamin E for this condition.

▶ **Contraindications**

Vitamin E should not be administered IV.

▶ **Drug Interactions**

Oral anticoagulants: Hypoprothrombinemic effects may be increased, possibly with
bleeding.

▶ **Adverse Reactions**

Hypervitaminosis E symptoms include fatigue, weakness, nausea, headache, blurred
vision, flatulence, and diarrhea.

▶ **Administration and Dosage**

In studies, vitamin E in doses of 400 to 800 IU/day at bedtime have been used with
varying degrees of success.

Swallow capsules whole; do not crush or chew.

VITAMIN E PRODUCTS[1]	
Trade name	Doseform
Aquasol E	**Capsules**: 73.5 mg[2]
E-200 I.U. Softgels	**Capsules**: 147 mg[2]
E-Vitamin Succinate, Amino-Opti-E	**Capsules**: 165 mg[3]
Aquasol E, E-400 I.U. in a Water Soluble Base, Vita-Plus E Softgels	**Capsules**: 400 IU[4]
E-Vitamin Succinate	**Capsules**: 330 mg[2]
E-Complex-600	**Capsules**: 600 IU[4]
E-1000 I.U. Softgels	**Capsules**: 1000 IU[4]
Aquasol E	**Drops**: 50 mg/mL[5]

Products listed are representative of currently available and widely distributed brands. Similar products, including regional and private label brands, may also exist.

[1] Some products may be available in sugar-free formulations.
[2] As d-alpha tocopheryl acetate.
[3] As d-alpha tocopheryl acid succinate.
[4] Form of vitamin E unknown; content given in IU.
[5] As dl-alpha tocopheryl sulfate.

PATIENT INFORMATION

Vitamin E

- Have patients who experience leg cramps on a recurring basis consult their physician for a medical examination, complete with thorough history, to eliminate the possibility of any medical conditions that are contributing to the cramping.
- Employ daily stretching exercises to assist in prevention of nocturnal leg cramps. Methods that raise the feet during sleep are also of benefit.
- Monitor patients prescribed quinine by their physician closely for any signs of adverse effects.
- Advise patients taking vitamin E to swallow capsules whole, without crushing or chewing.
- Have patients taking other OTC medications for leg cramps inform their physician and pharmacist to ensure no drug interactions occur with prescription medications they may be taking.
- Have patients who experience changes in leg cramp intensity, frequency, or duration contact their physician.

Sprains and Strains

DEFINITION

Sprains and strains encompass all acute, traumatic injuries that affect ligaments, tendons, and muscles. Ligaments are strong fibrous bands that hold joints together. Tendons are bands that connect muscles to bone. These soft tissue structures are generally injured because of excessive force. The excessive force causes the soft tissue to tear, either partially or completely. Ligament tears are called sprains, whereas muscle and tendon tears are called strains.

ETIOLOGY

Strains and sprains are generally caused by traumatic accidents at the workplace, during sports, and during routine daily activities. A fall, mistep, collision with another object, or many other situations can place sudden mechanical stress on ligaments, tendons, and muscles. If this stress, usually caused by a stretching force, exceeds the mechanical strength of the soft tissue a strain or sprain will occur.

INCIDENCE

The exact incidence of strains and sprains is difficult to assess because many of these injuries go unreported. Workmen's Compensation data and sports injury surveillance studies suggest that sprains and strains are the most common acute musculoskeletal injury associated with sports and the workplace.

PATHOPHYSIOLOGY

Tearing of soft tissues such as ligaments, tendons, and muscles initially results in bleeding and swelling at the site of injury. This is rapidly followed by an intense inflammatory response. This initial phase often peaks at 48 to 72 hours. Following the inflammatory reaction, new cells migrate into the area and begin to repair the injured tissue. This is generally called the proliferative phase. In the final phase, maturation, the new repair tissue strengthens and matures. The entire pathophysiologic process often takes at least 4 to 6 weeks to complete.

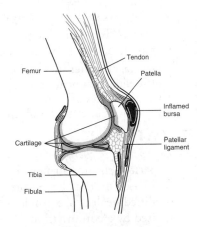

Figure 1. Inflamed Knee Joint

SIGNS/SYMPTOMS

Many patients will notice a painful snap or pop at the time of injury. If it is a complete tear, the pain following the initial injury may not be severe. Partial tears are more common and generally followed by more pain. Within hours, the swelling and pain becomes pronounced in all patients. The swelling and associated pain usually peaks at 48 to 72 hours. In the ensuing weeks, the pain gradually subsides. In complete ligament tears, patients may start noticing that the involved joint feels unstable. In complete muscle and tendon tears, the patients may notice weakness and atrophy of the involved muscle.

DIAGNOSTIC PARAMETERS/PHYSICAL ASSESSMENT

Clinical Observation: In cases of sprains (ligament tears around a joint) the affected area is visibly swollen. Bleeding from the torn ligament can often be seen after 24 to 48 hours as hemorrhagic areas around the joint. Pain with any use of the joint is common. Strains (tendon or muscle tears) are generally less obvious. The swelling may not be pronounced. Hematomas can been seen after several days as the blood migrates closer to the skin. Pain, however, is invariably present with attempted use of the muscle or tendon.

In patients with sprains (ligament tears) around a joint, it is important to determine which joint is affected. Ankle sprains are very common and usually recover well without specific intervention. Knee sprains are more unpredictable depending on the ligament that is involved. Have knee sprains with painful swelling and disability evaluated by a physician. Shoulder sprains are less common but may represent an actual dislocation and should be evaluated if any deformity is present. Strains (muscle and tendon tears) are usually partial tears and are common in the calf, thigh, and low back area. Only complete tears need urgent intervention. Complete tears are relatively common in the Achilles tendon near the heel and rotator cuff tendons of the shoulder. Further evaluate any injury in this area with complaints of weakness.

Interview: To determine proper diagnosis and treatment of sprains and strains, it may be beneficial to ask about the following:

- General characteristics of the condition (eg, location/intensity of pain, amount of swelling/hemorrhage, etc)
- Circumstances of accident or event that caused the injury
- Previous injuries to the affected area

TREATMENT

Approaches to therapy: Complete ligament, muscle, and tendon tears can result in permanent impairment if not treated appropriately. They can be identified based on the above noted parameters and should be further evaluated by qualified health care providers. Partial tears generally heal well. They can be treated by a combination of non-drug therapy and pharmacotherapy.

Nondrug therapy: In the first 24 to 72 hours following the injury, several nondrug measures can be helpful in diminishing the pain and swelling of the initial inflammatory response. Rest, ice, compression, and elevation (RICE) are routinely recommended for strains and sprains. Rest can include total inactivity (eg, bedrest) or relative inactivity such as the use of crutches, splints, or braces. Application of icebags for 15 to 25 minutes at a time, several times during the day, may alleviate pain and swelling. Compression may also alleviate some swelling and is generally accomplished by wrapping the affected joint snugly with an elastic bandage. Avoid tight bandages that actually cut off circulation in the extremity. Elevate the affected extremity at or above the level of the heart for extended periods of time to allow the swelling to drain by gravity. Following the initial RICE treatment of the injury, rehabilitation with a graduated exercise program is generally recommended to promote healing and avoid re-injury.

Pharmacotherapy: Nonprescription treatment for strains and sprains includes acetaminophen as an analgesic and nonsteroidal anti-inflammatory drugs (NSAIDs). Although topical OTC agents are available for sprains and strains, there is no scientific literature to indicate that they are of any significant benefit.

NONSTEROIDAL ANTI-INFLAMMATORY DRUGS

▶ Actions

Nonsteroidal anti-inflammatory drugs (NSAIDs) have analgesic, anti-inflammatory, and antipyretic activities. Their exact mode of action is unknown. The major mechanism of action of NSAIDs is believed to be inhibition of cyclooxygenase (COX) activity and prostaglandin synthesis. Other mechanisms, such as inhibition of lipoxygenase, leukotriene synthesis, lysosomal enzyme release, neutrophil aggregation, and various cell-membrane functions, may exist as well.

NSAIDs are capable of inhibiting the enzyme COX. COX allows the conversion of arachidonic acid into prostaglandins, which are mediators of the inflammatory response. Prostaglandin inhibition peripherally at the site of injury can decrease the inflammatory response and pain. Prostaglandin inhibition centrally can also result in analgesia similar to other centrally acting drugs such as acetaminophen. NSAIDs may also have a direct inhibiting effect on inflammatory cells.

▶ Indications

Treatment of mild-to-moderate pain. These agents have other labeled indications as well.

These agents are particularly helpful for pain associated with inflammation.

▶ Contraindications

NSAID hypersensitivity: Because of potential cross-sensitivity to other NSAIDs, do not give these agents to patients in whom aspirin, iodides, or other NSAIDs have induced symptoms of asthma, rhinitis, urticaria, nasal polyps, angioedema, bronchospasm, and other symptoms of allergic or anaphylactoid reactions.

▶ Warnings

Acute renal insufficiency: Patients with preexisting renal disease or compromised renal perfusion are at greatest risk. A form of renal toxicity seen in patients with prerenal conditions leads to reduced renal blood flow or blood volume. NSAID use may cause a dose-dependent reduction in prostaglandin formation and precipitate renal decompensation. Patients at greatest risk are the elderly, premature infants, those with heart failure, renal or hepatic dysfunction, systemic lupus erythematosus (SLE), chronic glomerulonephritis, and those on diuretics. Recovery usually follows discontinuation.

Hypersensitivity: Severe hypersensitivity reactions with fever, rash, abdominal pain, headache, nausea, vomiting, signs of liver damage, and meningitis have occurred in ibuprofen patients, especially those with SLE or other collagen diseases. Anaphylactoid reactions have occurred in patients with aspirin hypersensitivity.

Renal function impairment: NSAID metabolites are eliminated primarily by the kidneys; use with caution in patient with renal impairment. Reduce dosage to avoid excessive accumulation.

Platelet aggregation: NSAIDs can inhibit platelet aggregation; the effect is quantitatively less and of shorter duration than that seen with aspirin. These agents prolong bleeding time (within normal range) in healthy subjects. This may be exaggerated in patients with underlying hemostatic defects; use with caution in people with intrinsic coagulation defects and in those on anticoagulant therapy.

Cardiovascular effects: May cause fluid retention and peripheral edema. Use caution in compromised cardiac function, hypertension, or other conditions predisposing to fluid retention. Agents may be associated with significant deterioration of circulatory hemodynamics in severe heart failure and hyponatremia, presumably due to inhibition of prostaglandin-dependent compensatory mechanisms.

Infection: NSAIDs may mask the usual signs of infection. Use with extra care in the presence of existing controlled infection.

Photosensitivity: Photosensitivity may occur; caution patients to take protective measures (eg, sunscreens, protective clothing) against UV or sunlight until tolerance is determined.

GI effects: GI toxicity can occur with or without warning with chronic use of NSAIDs. High-dose NSAIDs probably carry a greater risk of causing GI adverse effects. In patients with a history of GI lesions, patients should consult a physician before using these products. These effects may be more pronounced in elderly patients.

Pregnancy: Category B; Category D in 3rd trimester. Safety for use during pregnancy has not been established; use is not recommended. There are no adequate, well-controlled studies in pregnant women. An increased incidence of dystocia, increased post implantation loss, and delayed parturition has occurred in animals. Agents that inhibit prostaglandin synthesis may cause closure of the ductus arteriosus and other untoward effects in the fetus. GI tract toxicity is increased in pregnant women in the last trimester. Some NSAIDs may prolong pregnancy if given before onset of labor. Avoid use during pregnancy, especially during the 3rd trimester.

Lactation: Most NSAIDs are excreted in breast milk in low concentrations. The American Academy of Pediatrics considers ibuprofen and naproxen to be compatible with breastfeeding. Data on the use of ketoprofen during nursing are lacking.

Children: The use of ibuprofen and naproxen is not recommended in children younger than 12 years of age unless directed by a physician. Ketoprofen is not recommended for use in children younger than 16 years of age.

Elderly: Age appears to increase the possibility of adverse reactions to NSAIDs. The risk of serious ulcer disease is increased in elderly patients (older than 65 years of age) taking NSAIDs; this risk appears to increase with dose. Use with greater care and begin with reduced dosages in this patient population.

▶ **Drug Interactions**

NSAID Drug Interactions			
Precipitant drug	**Object drug***		**Description**
NSAIDs	Anticoagulants	↑	Coadministration may prolong prothrombin time (PT). Also consider the effects NSAIDs have on platelet function and gastric mucosa. Monitor PT and patients closely, and instruct patients to watch for signs and symptoms of bleeding.
NSAIDs	Beta blockers	↓	The antihypertensive effect of beta blockers may be impaired. Naproxen did not affect atenolol.
NSAIDs	Cyclosporine	↑	Nephrotoxicity of both agents may be increased.
NSAIDs	Digoxin	↑	Ibuprofen may increase digoxin serum levels.
NSAIDs	Hydantoins	↑	Serum phenytoin levels may be increased, resulting in an increase in pharmacologic and toxic effects of phenytoin.
NSAIDs	Lithium	↑	Serum lithium levels may be increased.
NSAIDs	Loop diuretics	↓	Effects of loop diuretics may be decreased.
NSAIDs	Methotrexate	↑	The risks of methotrexate toxicity (eg, stomatitis, bone marrow suppression, nephrotoxicity) may be increased.
NSAIDs	Thiazide diuretics	↓	Decreased antihypertensive and diuretic action of thiazides may occur with concurrent naproxen.
Cimetidine	NSAIDs	↔	NSAID plasma concentrations may be increased or decreased by cimetidine; some studies report no effect.
Probenecid	NSAIDs	↑	Probenecid may increase the concentrations and possibly the toxicity of the NSAIDs.
Salicylates	NSAIDs	↓	Plasma concentrations of NSAIDs may be decreased by salicylates. Avoid concurrent use because it offers no therapeutic advantage and may significantly increase the incidence of GI effects.

* ↑ = Object drug increased.   ↓ = Object drug decreased.   ↔ = Undetermined clinical effect.

▶ **Adverse Reactions**

Cardiovascular: Edema; congestive heart failure.

CNS: Dizziness; drowsiness; headache; lightheadedness; vertigo.

Dermatologic: Erythema; pruritus; rash.

GI: Bleeding; diarrhea; dyspepsia; heartburn; nausea; vomiting.

Miscellaneous: Muscle cramps; thirst.

▶ **Administration and Dosage**

Although no controlled studies are available, most laboratory data suggest that NSAIDs are more effective in their anti-inflammatory action if given shortly after the injury and before a full-blown inflammatory response develops. Its central analgesic effect may be independent of the time of injury. Most NSAIDs appear to have an analgesic effect in a low dose and an additional anti-inflammatory effect at a higher dose. If an anti-inflammatory effect and analgesic effect is desired, use the higher dose. However, the risk of some side effects may also be dose-dependent. Most strains and sprains appear to benefit from continuous NSAID use for the first 7 to 14 days following the injury; however, OTC use for longer than 7 days is not recommended without consulting a physician. Appropriate dosing is listed in the following section.

IBUPROFEN

▶ **Administration and Dosage**

Analgesic dose: 200 to 400 mg orally 3 times/day as needed.

Anti-inflammatory dose: 600 to 800 mg orally 3 times/day as needed.

IBUPROFEN PRODUCTS	
Trade name	Doseform
Junior Strength Advil, Junior Strength Motrin	**Tablets:** 100 mg
Advil,[1] *Maximum Strength Midol Cramp, Motrin IB*	**Tablets:** 200 mg
Children's Advil, Children's Motrin	**Tablets, chewable:** 50 mg
Junior Strength Advil, Junior Strength Motrin	**Tablets, chewable:** 100 mg
Advil Liqui-Gels, Motrin IB[2]	**Gelcaps:** 200 mg
Infants' Advil Concentrated Drops	**Liquid:** 50 mg/1.25 mL
Children's Advil,[1,3] *Children's Motrin*[1]	**Suspension:** 100 mg/5 mL

Products listed are representative of currently available and widely distributed brands. Similar products, including regional and private label brands, may also exist.

[1] Contains sucrose.
[2] Contains parabens.
[3] Contains sorbitol.

PATIENT INFORMATION
Ibuprofen

- During the first 24 to 48 hours following a soft tissue injury, treat the injury with rest, ice, compression, and elevation. Minimize the use of the injured area by using crutches, sling, brace, or by complete bedrest. Application of icebags for 15 to 20 minutes at a time, several times during the day, may alleviate pain and swelling. During rest, elevate the involved extremity above the level of the heart to allow swelling to subside. A snug, compressive wrap may alleviate some swelling. Avoid tight bandages that cut off circulation in the extremity.
- If the medical condition allows, use NSAIDs like ibuprofen, ketoprofen, and naproxen to combat inflammation and pain. These drugs, as OTC agents, can be taken throughout the first 7 days of an injury. If NSAIDs are not tolerated, use acetaminophen for pain relief.
- If symptoms of instability, weakness, or deformity are present, consult a physician as soon as possible.
- As the initial pain and swelling subside, activities may be resumed gradually. A rehabilitative exercise program is generally recommended to promote healing and avoid re-injury.
- *Adults:* Do not exceed 1.2 g/day.
- May cause GI upset; take with food or after meals.
- Take with a full glass of water (240 mL) to reduce the risk of the medication lodging in the esophagus.
- Do not take OTC NSAIDs for longer than 7 days for pain unless directed by a physician. If symptoms persist, worsen, or if new symptoms develop, contact a physician.
- Avoid alcohol and aspirin while taking this medication.

KETOPROFEN

▶ Administration and Dosage

Analgesic dose: 12.5 to 25 mg orally 3 times/day as needed.

Anti-inflammatory dose: 50 to 75 mg orally 3 times/day as needed.

KETOPROFEN PRODUCTS	
Trade name	Doseform
Orudis KT	Tablets: 12.5 mg

Products listed are representative of currently available and widely distributed brands. Similar products, including regional and private label brands, may also exist.

PATIENT INFORMATION

Ketoprofen

- During the first 24 to 48 hours following a soft tissue injury, treat the injury with rest, ice, compression, and elevation. Minimize the use of the injured area by using crutches, sling, brace, or by complete bedrest. Application of icebags for 15 to 20 minutes at a time, several times during the day, may alleviate pain and swelling. During rest, elevate the involved extremity above the level of the heart to allow swelling to subside. A snug, compressive wrap may alleviate some swelling. Avoid tight bandages that cut off circulation in the extremity.
- If the medical condition allows, use NSAIDs like ibuprofen, ketoprofen, and naproxen to combat inflammation and pain. These drugs, as OTC agents, can be taken throughout the first 7 days of an injury. If NSAIDs are not tolerated, use acetaminophen for pain relief.
- If symptoms of instability, weakness, or deformity are present, consult a physician as soon as possible
- As the initial pain and swelling subside, activities may be resumed gradually. A rehabilitative exercise program is generally recommended to promote healing and avoid re-injury.
- May cause GI upset; take with food or after meals.
- Take with a full glass of water (240 mL) to reduce the risk of the medication lodging in the esophagus.
- Do not take OTC NSAIDs for longer than 7 days for pain. If symptoms persist, worsen, or if new symptoms develop, contact a physician.
- Avoid alcohol and aspirin while taking this medication.

NAPROXEN

▶ Administration and Dosage

Analgesic dose: 200 to 400 mg orally 3 times/day as needed.

Anti-inflammatory dose: 600 to 800 mg orally 3 times/day as needed.

NAPROXEN PRODUCTS	
Trade name	Doseform
Aleve	Tablets, Caplets, and Gelcaps: 200 mg (220 mg naproxen sodium)

Products listed are representative of currently available and widely distributed brands. Similar products, including regional and private label brands, may also exist.

PATIENT INFORMATION
Naproxen

- During the first 24 to 48 hours following a soft tissue injury, treat the injury with rest, ice, compression, and elevation. Minimize the use of the injured area by using crutches, sling, brace, or by complete bedrest. Application of icebags for 15 to 20 minutes at a time, several times during the day, may alleviate pain and swelling. During rest, elevate the involved extremity above the level of the heart to allow swelling to subside. A snug, compressive wrap may alleviate some swelling. Avoid tight bandages that cut off circulation in the extremity.
- If the medical condition allows, use NSAIDs like ibuprofen, ketoprofen, and naproxen to combat inflammation and pain. These drugs, as OTC agents, can be taken throughout the first 7 days of an injury. If NSAIDs are not tolerated, use acetaminophen for pain relief.
- If symptoms of instability, weakness, or deformity are present, consult a physician as soon as possible.
- As the initial pain and swelling subside, activities may be resumed gradually. A rehabilitative exercise program is generally recommended to promote healing and avoid re-injury.
- May cause GI upset; take with food or after meals.
- Take with a full glass of water (240 mL) to reduce the risk of the medication lodging in the esophagus.
- Do not take OTC NSAIDs for longer than 7 days for pain. If symptoms persist, worsen, or if new symptoms develop, contact a physician.
- Avoid alcohol and aspirin while taking this medication.

ACETAMINOPHEN (APAP)

▶ Actions

Generally, the antipyretic and analgesic effects of APAP and aspirin are comparable; however, the site and mechanism of the analgesic effect of acetaminophen are unclear.

▶ Indications

For the treatment of mild-to-moderate pain associated with sprains and strains, especially in patients in whom NSAIDs are contraindicated. Initial therapy of sprains and strains with NSAIDs is preferred because they produce an anti-inflammatory as well as analgesic effect. Acetaminophen possesses no significant anti-inflammatory activity. Also used as an analgesic-antipyretic in the presence of aspirin allergy, and in patients with blood coagulation disorders who are being treated with oral anticoagulants, bleeding diatheses (eg, hemophilia), upper GI disease (eg, ulcer, gastritis, hiatal hernia), and gouty arthritis. This agent has other labeled indications as well.

▶ Contraindications

Hypersensitivity to acetaminophen.

▶ Warnings

Concurrent medications: Many other medications, specifically multi-ingredient cough and cold products, also contain aspirin or acetaminophen. It is important to advise patients of this possibility, and to inquire about other medications they might be taking before recommending an analgesic.

Hepatotoxicity: Hepatotoxicity and severe hepatic failure occurred in chronic alcoholics following therapeutic doses. The hepatotoxicity is may be caused by induction of hepatic microsomal enzymes, resulting in an increase in toxic metabolites or by the reduced amount of glutathione responsible for conjugating toxic metabolites. A safe dose for chronic alcohol abusers has not been determined. Caution chronic alcoholics or those who consume alcohol on a daily basis to limit acetaminophen intake to 2 g/day or less.

Pregnancy: Category B. Acetaminophen crosses the placenta. It is routinely used during all stages of pregnancy; when used in therapeutic doses, it appears safe for short-term use.

Lactation: APA is excreted in low amounts, but no adverse effects have been reported. The American Academy of Pediatrics considers acetaminophen to be compatible with breastfeeding.

Children: Consult a physician before using in children younger than 3 years of age.

▶ **Drug Interactions**

Acetaminophen Drug Interactions			
Precipitant drug	**Object drug***		**Description**
Alcohol, ethyl	APAP	↑	Hepatotoxicity has occurred in chronic alcoholics following various dose levels (moderate-to-excessive) of acetaminophen.
Anticholinergics	APAP	↔	The onset of acetaminophen effect may be delayed or decreased slightly, but the ultimate pharmacological effect is not significantly affected by anticholinergics.
Beta blockers, propranolol	APAP	↑	Propranolol appears to inhibit the enzyme systems responsible for glucuronidation and oxidation of acetaminophen. Therefore, the pharmacologic effects of acetaminophen may be increased.
Charcoal, activated	APAP	↓	Reduces acetaminophen absorption when administered as soon as possible after overdose.
Contraceptives, oral	APAP	↓	Increase in glucuronidation resulting in increased plasma clearance and a decreased half-life of acetaminophen.
Probenecid	APAP	↑	Probenecid may increase the therapeutic effectiveness of acetaminophen slightly.
APAP	Lamotrigine	↓	Serum lamotrigine concentrations may be reduced, producing a decrease in therapeutic effects.
APAP	Loop diuretics	↓	The effects of the loop diuretic may be decreased because APAP may decrease renal prostaglandin excretion and decrease plasma renin activity.
APAP	Zidovudine	↓	The pharmacologic effects of zidovudine may be decreased because of enhanced nonhepatic or renal clearance of zidovudine.

* ↑ = Object drug increased. ↓ = Object drug decreased. ↔ = Undetermined clinical effect.

The potential hepatotoxicity of acetaminophen may be increased by large doses or long-term administration of barbiturates, carbamazepine, hydantoins, rifampin, and sulfinpyrazone. The therapeutic effects of acetaminophen may also be decreased by these drugs.

▶ Adverse Reactions

When used as directed, acetaminophen rarely causes severe toxicity or side effects. However, the following adverse reactions have been reported:

Hematologic: Hemolytic anemia; neutropenia; leukopenia; pancytopenia; thrombocytopenia.

Miscellaneous: Fever; hypoglycemia; jaundice; rash.

▶ Overdosage

Symptoms: Acute poisoning may be manifested by nausea, vomiting, drowsiness, confusion, liver tenderness, low blood pressure, cardiac arrhythmias, jaundice, and acute hepatic and renal failure. These occur within the first 24 hours and may persist for 1 week or longer. Death has occurred because of liver necrosis. Acute renal failure may also occur. However, there are often no specific early symptoms or signs. The course of acetaminophen poisoning is divided into 4 stages (postingestion time):

Stage 1 (12 to 24 hours) – Nausea, vomiting, diaphoresis, anorexia.

Stage 2 (24 to 48 hours) – Clinically improved; AST, AST, bilirubin, and prothrombin levels begin to rise.

Stage 3 (72 to 96 hours) – Peak hepatotoxicity; AST of 20,000 not unusual.

Stage 4 (7 to 8 days) – Recovery.

Hepatotoxicity may result. The minimal toxic dose is 10 g (140 mg/kg), but liver damage has occurred with a single 5.85 g dose; doses 20 to 25 g or more are potentially fatal. Children appear less susceptible to toxicity than adults because they have less capacity for glucuronidation metabolism. Initial signs of toxicity may include nausea, vomiting, anorexia, malaise, diaphoresis, abdominal pain, and diarrhea. Hepatotoxicity is usually not apparent for 48 to 72 hours. Hepatic failure may lead to encephalopathy, coma, and death.

Plasma acetaminophen levels over 300 mcg/mL at 4 hours postingestion were associated with hepatic damage in 90% of patients; minimal hepatic damage is anticipated if plasma levels at 4 hours are under 120 mcg/mL or under 30 mcg/mL at 12 hours after ingestion.

Chronic excessive use (over 4 g/day) eventually may lead to transient hepatotoxicity. The kidneys may undergo tubular necrosis; the myocardium may be damaged.

Treatment: Perform gastric lavage in all cases, preferably within 4 hours of ingestion. Refer also to General Management of Acute Overdosage. It is important to contact a local poison control center or emergency room if overdosage is suspected.

▶ Administration and Dosage

Adults: 325 to 650 mg orally every 4 to 6 hours or 1 g 3 to 4 times daily as needed for pain. Do not exceed 4 g daily for all formulations containing acetaminophen.

Children: The usual oral dose is 10 mg/kg/dose, which may be repeated 4 to 5 times daily as needed. Do not exceed 5 doses in 24 hours.

Acetaminophen Dosage for Children			
Age	Dosage (mg)	Age	Dosage (mg)
0-3 months	40	6-8 years	320
4-11 months	80	9-10 years	400
1- 2 years	120	11 years	480
2-3 years	160	12-14 years	640
4-5 years	240	> 14 years	650

Suppositories:

Adults – 650 mg every 4 to 6 hours as needed. Give no more than 4 g in 24 hours.

Children (3 to 11 months of age) – 80 mg every 6 hours as needed.

(1 to 3 years of age) – 80 mg every 4 hours as needed.

(3 to 6 years of age) – 120 to 125 mg every 4 to 6 hours as needed. Give 720 mg or less in 24 hours.

(6 to 12 years of age) – 325 mg every 4 to 6 hours as needed. Give 2.6 g or less in 24 hours.

Storage: Store suppositories below 27°C (80°F) or refrigerate. Store tablets and oral solutions at 15° to 30°C (59° to 86°F).

ACETAMINOPHEN PRODUCTS	
Trade name	Doseform
Junior Strength Tylenol	**Tablets:** 160 mg. Aspartame (6 mg phenylalanine).
Regular Strength Tylenol	**Tablets:** 325 mg
Aspirin Free Anacin Maximum Strength, Extra Strength Tylenol[1], Panadol	**Tablets:** 500 mg
Tylenol Extended Relief	**Tablets:** 650 mg
Children's Panadol, Children's Tylenol, Children's Tylenol Soft Chews	**Tablets, chewable:** 80 mg
Junior Strength Tylenol	**Tablets, chewable:** 160 mg
Meda Cap	**Capsules:** 500 mg
Extra Strength Tylenol	**Gelcaps:** 500 mg
Extra Strength Tylenol	**Geltabs:** 500 mg
Infants' FeverAll	**Suppositories:** 80 mg
Children's FeverAll	**Suppositories:** 120 mg
Junior Strength FeverAll	**Suppositories:** 325 mg
Acephen	**Suppositories:** 650 mg
Children's Silapap	**Elixir:** 80 mg/2.5 mL. Alcohol free.
Children's Tylenol[3]	**Elixir:** 80 mg/2.5 mL. Alcohol free.
Aceta	**Elixir:** 120 mg/5 mL
Infants' Tylenol Concentrated Drops[4]	**Liquid:** 80 mg/0.8 mL. Alcohol free.
Extra Strength Tylenol[5]	**Liquid:** 500 mg/15 mL. 7% alcohol.
Liquiprin Drops for Children	**Solution:** 80 mg/1.66 mL. Alcohol free.
Infants' Panadol Drops[2], Infants' Silapap Drops, Infants' Tylenol Drops[4]	**Solution:** 80 mg/0.8 mL. Alcohol free.
Children's Tylenol Liquid	**Suspension:** 80 mg/2.5 mL
Tempra	**Syrup:** 160 mg/5 mL

Products listed are representative of currently available and widely distributed brands. Similar products, including regional and private label brands, may also exist.

[1] Gelatin coated.
[2] Contains saccharin.
[3] Contains butylparaben, sorbitol, and sucrose.
[4] Contains butylparaben, saccharin, and sorbitol.
[5] Contains and sorbitol and sucrose.

PATIENT INFORMATION
Acetaminophen

- Severe or recurrent pain may indicate a serious illness. Consult a physician.
- During the first 24 to 48 hours following a soft tissue injury, treat the injury with rest, ice, compression, and elevation. Minimize the use of the injured area by using crutches, sling, brace, or by complete bedrest. Application of icebags for 15 to 20 minutes at a time, several times during the day, may alleviate pain and swelling. During rest, elevate the involved extremity above the level of the heart to allow swelling to subside. A snug, compressive wrap may alleviate some swelling. Avoid tight bandages that cut off circulation in the extremity.
- Use NSAIDs such as ibuprofen, ketoprofen, and naproxen initially to treat sprains and strains to combat inflammation and pain. These drugs can be taken throughout the first 5 to 7 days of an injury. If NSAIDs are not tolerated, use acetaminophen for pain relief.
- If symptoms of instability, weakness, or deformity are present, consult a physician as soon as possible.
- As the initial pain and swelling subside, activities may be resumed gradually. A rehabilitative exercise program is generally recommended to promote healing and avoid re-injury.
- Do not exceed the recommended dosage. Do not exceed a total dose of 4 g/day of acetaminophen in all formulations consumed (2 g/day in regular alcohol users).
- Consult a physician for use in a child younger than 3 years old.
- Do not take acetaminophen for longer than 5 days for children or longer than 10 days for adults for pain relief. If symptoms persist, worsen, or if new symptoms develop, contact a physician.
- Avoid alcohol and aspirin while taking this drug.

SALICYLATES

▶ **Actions**

The anti-inflammatory and analgesic activity of salicylates may be mediated through inhibition of the prostaglandin synthetase complex.

▶ **Indications**

For the treatment of mild-to-moderate pain. These agents have other labeled indications as well.

▶ **Contraindications**

Hypersensitivity to salicylates or nonsteroidal anti-inflammatory drugs (NSAIDs). Use with extreme caution in patients with a history of adverse reactions to salicylates. Cross-sensitivity may exist between aspirin and other NSAIDs that inhibit prostaglandin synthesis, and between aspirin and tartrazine. Aspirin cross-sensitivity does not appear to occur with sodium salicylate, or salicylamide. Hypersensitivity is more prevalent in those with asthma, nasal polyposis, or chronic urticaria.

Also contraindicated in patients with hemophilia or bleeding ulcers, or those in hemorrhagic states. Magnesium salicylate is contraindicated in patients with advanced chronic renal insufficiency.

▶ Warnings

Concurrent medications: Many other medications, specifically multi-ingredient cough and cold products, also contain aspirin or acetaminophen. It is important to advise patients of this possibility, and to inquire about other medications they might be taking before recommending an analgesic.

Otic effects: Discontinue use if dizziness, ringing in ears (tinnitus), or impaired hearing occurs. Tinnitus probably represents blood salicylic acid levels reaching or exceeding the upper limit of the therapeutic range; therefore, it is a helpful guide to toxicity. Temporary hearing loss disappears gradually upon discontinuation of the drug.

Hypersensitivity: Do not use if there is a history of sensitivity to aspirin or NSAIDs.

Aspirin intolerance, manifested by acute bronchospasm, generalized urticaria/angioedema, severe rhinitis, or shock occurs in 4% to 19% of asthmatics. Symptoms occur within 3 hours after ingestion.

Foods may contribute to a reaction. Some foods with high salicylate content include curry powder, paprika, licorice, Benedictine liqueur, prunes, raisins, tea, and gherkins. A typical American diet contains 10 to 200 mg/day salicylate.

Hepatic function impairment: Use caution in patients with liver damage, preexisting hypoprothrombinemia, and vitamin K deficiency.

GI effects: Use caution in patients who are intolerant to salicylates because of GI irritation, and in those with gastric ulcers, peptic ulcers, mild diabetes, gout, erosive gastritis, or bleeding tendencies.

Hematologic effects: Aspirin interferes with hemostasis. Avoid use in patients with severe anemia, history of blood coagulation defects, or who take anticoagulants.

Pregnancy: Category D (aspirin); *Category C* (salsalate, magnesium salicylate, other salicylates). Aspirin may produce adverse effects in the mother, such as anemia, ante- or postpartum hemorrhage, or prolonged gestation and labor. Salicylates readily cross the placenta. By inhibiting prostaglandin synthesis, salicylates may cause constriction of ductus arteriosus, and, possibly, other untoward fetal effects. Maternal aspirin use during later stages of pregnancy may cause adverse fetal effects, such as low birth weight, increased incidence of intracranial hemorrhage in premature infants, stillbirth, or neonatal death. Salicylates may be teratogens. Avoid use during pregnancy, especially in the third trimester.

Lactation: Salicylates are excreted in breast milk in low concentrations. Adverse effects on platelet function in the nursing infant are a potential risk. The American Academy of Pediatrics recommends that aspirin be used cautiously in nursing mothers.

Children: Administration of aspirin to children, including teenagers, with acute febrile illness due to chickenpox and influenza has been associated with the development of Reye syndrome.

▶ Drug Interactions

Salicylate Drug Interactions			
Precipitant drug	**Object drug***		**Description**
Activated charcoal	Aspirin	↓	Coadministration decreases aspirin absorption, depending on charcoal dose and interval between ingestion.
Urinary acidifiers	Salicylates	↑	Ammonium chloride, ascorbic acid, and methionine decrease salicylate excretion.

Salicylate Drug Interactions			
Precipitant drug	**Object drug***		**Description**
Antacids, urinary alkalinizers	Salicylates	↓	Decreased pharmacologic effects of salicylates may occur. The magnitude of the antacid interaction depends on the agent, dose, and pretreatment urine pH.
Carbonic anhydrase inhibitors	Salicylates	↔	Salicylate intoxication has occurred after coadministration of these agents. However, salicylic acid renal elimination may be increased by these drugs if urine is kept alkaline. Conversely, salicylates may displace acetazolamide from protein-binding sites, resulting in toxicity. Further study is needed.
Corticosteroids	Salicylates	↓	Corticosteroids increase salicylate clearance and decrease salicylate serum levels.
Nizatidine	Salicylate	↑	Increased serum salicylate levels have occurred in patients receiving high doses (3.9 g/day) of aspirin and concurrent nizatidine.
Salicylates	Alcohol	↑	The risk of GI ulceration increases when salicylates are given concomitantly. Ingestion of alcohol during salicylate therapy may also prolong bleeding time.
Salicylates	Angiotensin-converting enzyme inhibitors	↓	Antihypertensive effectiveness of these agents may be decreased by concurrent salicylate administration, possibly due to prostaglandin inhibition. Consider discontinuing salicylates if problems occur.
Aspirin	Heparin	↑	Aspirin can increase the risk of bleeding in heparin anticoagulated patients.
Salicylates	Loop diuretics	↓	Loop diuretics may be less effective when given with salicylates in patients with compromised renal function or with cirrhosis with ascites; however, data conflict.
Salicylates	Methotrexate	↑	Salicylates increase drug levels, causing toxicity by interfering with protein binding and renal elimination of the antimetabolite.
Aspirin	Nitroglycerin	↑	Nitroglycerin, when taken with aspirin, may result in unexpected hypotension. Data are limited. If hypotension occurs, reduce the nitroglycerin dose.
Aspirin	NSAIDs	↓	Aspirin may decrease NSAID serum concentrations. Avoid concomitant use; it offers no therapeutic advantage and may significantly increase incidence of GI effects.
Salicylates	Probenecid, Sulfinpyrazone	↔	Salicylates antagonize the uricosuric effect. While salicylates in large doses (> 3 g/day) have a uricosuric effect, smaller amounts may reduce the uricosuric effect of these agents.
Salicylates	Spironolactone	↓	Salicylates may inhibit the diuretic effects; antihypertensive action does not appear altered. Effects depend on the dose of spironolactone.
Salicylates	Sulfonylureas, exogenous insulin	↑	Salicylates in doses > 2 g/day have a hypoglycemic action, perhaps by altering pancreatic beta-cell function. They may potentiate the glucose-lowering effect of these drugs.
Aspirin	Valproic acid	↑	Aspirin displaces valproic acid from its protein-binding sites and may decrease its total body clearance, thus increasing pharmacological effects.

* ↑ = Object drug increased. ↓ = Object drug decreased. ↔ = Undetermined clinical effect.

▶ Adverse Reactions

Adverse reactions can be seen in the following body systems: GI (nausea, dyspepsia, heartburn, epigastric discomfort), hematologic (prolonged bleeding time, leukopenia, thrombocytopenia, purpura, decreased plasma iron concentration, shortened erythrocyte survival time), and dermatologic (rash, hives, and angioedema may occur, especially in patients suffering from chronic urticaria). Additional miscellaneous adverse reactions that have occurred include fever, thirst, and dimness of vision.

Allergic and anaphylactic reactions have been noted when hypersensitive individuals took aspirin. Fatal anaphylactic shock, while not common, has been reported.

Aspirin has a reversible effect on platelet aggregation.

▶ Overdosage

Symptoms: The approximate acute lethal dose for adults is 10 to 30 g, and for children, 4 g. Respiratory alkalosis is seen initially in acute salicylate ingestions. Hyperpnea and tachypnea occur as a result of increased CO_2 production and a direct stimulatory effect of salicylate on the respiratory center. Other symptoms may include nausea, vomiting, hypokalemia, tinnitus, neurologic abnormalities (eg, disorientation, irritability, hallucinations, lethargy, stupor, coma, seizures), dehydration, hyperthermia, hyperventilation, hyperactivity, thrombocytopenia, platelet dysfunction, hypoprothrombinemia, increased capillary fragility, and other hematologic abnormalities. Symptoms may progress quickly to depression, coma, respiratory failure and collapse. Chronic salicylate toxicity may occur when over 100 mg/kg/day is ingested for 2 days or longer. It is more difficult to recognize than acute overdosage and is associated with increased morbidity and mortality. Compared with acute poisoning, hyperventilation, dehydration, systemic acidosis, and severe CNS manifestations occur more frequently.

Treatment: Initial treatment includes induction of emesis or gastric lavage to remove any unabsorbed drug from the stomach. Activated charcoal diminishes salicylate absorption most effectively if given within 2 hours after ingestion. It is important to contact a local poison control center or emergency room if overdosage is suspected.

ASPIRIN

▶ Administration and Dosage

Analgesic dose: 325 mg 4 times/day as needed.

Anti-inflammatory dose: 650 to 1000 mg 4 times/day as needed.

ASPIRIN PRODUCTS	
Trade name	Doseform
Original Bayer, Norwich Aspirin	**Tablets**: 325 mg
Bayer Children's Chewable Aspirin	**Tablets, chewable**: 81 mg. Dextrose, saccharin. Cherry and orange flavors.
Adult Low Strength Ecotrin, Halfprin 81[1]	**Tablets, enteric coated**: 81 mg. Talc.
Halfprin 162	**Tablets, enteric coated**: 162 mg. Lactose, talc.
Ecotrin Regular Strength	**Tablets, enteric coated**: 325 mg. Talc.
Norwich Maximum Strength	**Tablets, enteric coated**: 500 mg
Ecotrin Maximum Strength	**Tablets, enteric coated**: 500 mg. Talc.
Alka-Seltzer Original Effervescent Antacid and Pain Relief Medicine	**Tablets, effervescent**: 325 mg, 1000 mg citric acid, 1916 mg sodium bicarbonate
Bayer Women's Aspirin Plus Calcium	**Caplets**: 81 mg, 300 mg calcium. Lactose, mineral oil.

ASPIRIN PRODUCTS	
Trade name	**Doseform**
Original Bayer	**Caplets**: 325 mg
Extra Strength Bayer PM Aspirin Plus Sleep Aid	**Caplets**: 500 mg, 25 mg diphenhydramine HCl
Extra Strength Bayer Aspirin	**Caplets, coated**: 500 mg
Extra Strength Bayer Back and Body Pain	**Caplets, coated**: 500 mg, 32.5 mg caffeine
Extra Strength Bayer Arthritis Pain Regimen	**Caplets, enteric coated**: 500 mg
Original Bayer	**Gelcaps**: 325 mg. Parabens, sorbitol, glycerin.
Extra Strength Bayer Aspirin	**Gelcaps, coated**: 500 mg. Parabens, glycerin.
BUFFERED ASPIRIN PRODUCTS	
Adprin-B	**Tablets, coated**: 325 mg with calcium carbonate, magnesium carbonate, magnesium oxide
Regular Strength Ascriptin	**Tablets, coated**: 325 mg with 50 mg magnesium hydroxide, 50 mg aluminum hydroxide, calcium carbonate. Talc.
Bufferin	**Tablets, coated**: 325 mg with 158 mg calcium carbonate, 63 mg magnesium oxide, 34 mg magnesium carbonate. Mineral oil, sorbitol, citric acid.
Extra Strength Adprin-B	**Tablets, coated**: 500 mg with calcium carbonate, magnesium carbonate, magnesium oxide.
Bayer Adult Low Strength	**Caplets**: 81 mg, buffered with 250 mg calcium carbonate
Extra Strength Bayer Plus	**Caplets**: 500 mg with calcium carbonate, magnesium carbonate, magnesium oxide
Maximum Strength Ascriptin	**Caplets, coated**: 500 mg with 80 mg magnesium hydroxide, 80 mg aluminum hydroxide, calcium carbonate. Saccharin, sorbitol, talc.

Products listed are representative of currently available and widely distributed brands. Similar products, including regional and private label brands, may also exist.

[1] Also contains lactose.

PATIENT INFORMATION
Aspirin
- During the first 24 to 48 hours following a soft tissue injury, treat the injury with rest, ice, compression, and elevation. Minimize the use of the injured area by using crutches, sling, brace, or by complete bedrest. Application of icebags for 15 to 20 minutes at a time, several times during the day, may alleviate pain and swelling. During rest, elevate the involved extremity above the level of the heart to allow swelling to subside. A snug, compressive wrap may alleviate some swelling. Avoid tight bandages that cut off circulation in the extremity.
- If the medical condition allows, use nonsteroidal anti-inflammatory drugs (NSAIDs) like ibuprofen, ketoprofen, and naproxen to combat inflammation and pain. If NSAIDs are not tolerated, use acetaminophen or salicylates for pain relief.
- If symptoms of instability, weakness or deformity are present, consult a physician as soon as possible.
- As the initial pain and swelling subside, activities may be resumed gradually. A rehabilitative exercise program is generally recommended to promote healing and avoid re-injury.
- May cause GI upset; take with food or after meals.
- Do not use in children because of the potential development of Reye syndrome.
- Take with a full glass of water (240 mL) to reduce the risk of lodging the medication in the esophagus.
- Have patients allergic to tartrazine dye avoid aspirin.
- Notify physician if ringing in the ears or persistent GI pain occurs. (Internal bleeding may occur with no GI symptoms and may be indicated by bloody or black stools.)
- Do not use aspirin if it has a strong vinegar-like odor.

MAGNESIUM SALICYLATE

▶ **Actions**

Magnesium salicylate is a sodium-free salicylate derivative that may have a low incidence of GI upset.

▶ **Contraindications**

Magnesium salicylate is contraindicated in patients with advanced chronic renal insufficiency due to magnesium retention.

▶ **Warnings**

The possibility of magnesium toxicity exists in patients with renal insufficiency.

▶ **Administration and Dosage**

Product labeling and dosages are expressed as magnesium salicylate anhydrous.

Adults: Usual dose is 650 mg every 4 hours to 1 g every 6 hours, up to 4 g/day.

Children: Safety and efficacy for use in children have not been established.

MAGNESIUM SALICYLATE PRODUCTS	
Trade name	Doseform
Regular Strength Doan's	Caplets: 377 mg
Extra Strength Doan's	Caplets: 580 mg
Extra Strength Doan's P.M.	Caplets: 580 mg, 25 mg diphenhydramine HCl. Talc.

Products listed are representative of currently available and widely distributed brands. Similar products, including regional and private label brands, may also exist.

PATIENT INFORMATION
Magnesium Salicylate

- Do not use these products if you have renal insufficiency.
- Severe or recurrent pain may indicate a serious illness. Consult a physician.
- During the first 24 to 48 hours following a soft tissue injury, treat the injury with rest, ice, compression, and elevation. Minimize the use of the injured area by using crutches, sling, brace, or by complete bedrest. Application of icebags for 15 to 20 minutes at a time, several times during the day, may alleviate pain and swelling. During rest, elevate the involved extremity above the level of the heart to allow swelling to subside. A snug, compressive wrap may alleviate some swelling. Avoid tight bandages that cut off circulation in the extremity.
- If the medical condition allows, use NSAIDs such as ibuprofen, ketoprofen, and naproxen to combat inflammation and pain. If NSAIDs are not tolerated, use acetaminophen or salicylates for pain relief.
- May cause GI upset; take with food or after meals.
- Do not use in children because of the potential development of Reye syndrome.
- Notify physician if ringing in the ears or persistent GI pain occurs. Internal bleeding may occur with no GI symptoms and may be indicated by bloody or black stools.

RUBS AND LINIMENTS

▶ Indications

These products are used for relief of pain of muscular aches, neuralgia, rheumatism, arthritis, sprains, and like conditions, when skin is intact.

Individual components include:

Counterirritants: Camphor, capsicum preparations (capsicum oleoresin, capsaicin), eucalyptus oil, menthol, methyl nicotinate, methyl salicylate, mustard oil, wormwood oil.

Antiseptics: Thymol.

Analgesics: Trolamine salicylate, methyl salicylate.

▶ Contraindications

Allergy to components of any formulation or to salicylates.

▶ Warnings

For external use only: Avoid contact with eyes, eyelids, and mucous membranes.

Apply to affected parts only: Do not apply to irritated skin; discontinue use if excessive irritation develops. Consult a physician if pain persists for longer than 7 to 10 days, or if redness is present, or in conditions affecting children younger than 10 years of age.

Heat therapy: Do not use an external source of high heat (eg, heating pad) with these agents because irritation and burning of the skin may occur.

Protective covering: Applying a tight bandage or wrap over these agents is not recommended because increased absorption may occur.

▶ **Drug Interactions**

Anticoagulants: An enhanced anticoagulant effect (eg, increased prothrombin time) occurred in several patients receiving an anticoagulant and using topical methyl salicylate concurrently.

▶ **Adverse Reactions**

If applied to large skin areas and used over a prolonged period of time, salicylate side effects (eg, tinnitus, nausea, vomiting) may occur.

Products may be toxic if ingested.

Counterirritants may cause local irritation, especially in patients with sensitive skin.

▶ **Administration and Dosage**

Apply to affected areas as needed.

RUBS AND LINIMENTS	
Trade name	**Doseform**
Icy Hot	**Balm:** 29% methyl salicylate, 7.6% menthol, white petrolatum
Epiderm	**Balm:** Isopropyl alcohol, parabens, ureas, menthol, EDTA
JointFlex	**Cream:** 3.1% camphor, lanolin, aloe, urea, EDTA, glycerin, peppermint oil
Capzasin-P	**Cream:** 0.025% capsaicin
ArthriCare for Women Silky Dry	**Cream:** 0.025% capsaicin, parabens, mineral oil
ArthriCare for Women Extra Moisturizing	**Cream:** 0.025% capsaicin, aloe vera gel, cetyl and stearyl alcohol, parabens
ArthriCare for Women Multi-Action	**Cream:** 0.025% capsaicin, 1.25% menthol, 0.25% methyl nicotinate, aloe vera gel, cetyl alcohol, parabens
Capzasin-HP	**Cream:** 0.075% capsaicin
ArthriCare for Women Ultra Strength	**Cream:** 0.075% capsaicin, 2% menthol, aloe vera gel, cetyl and stearyl alcohol, parabens
Vicks VapoRub	**Cream:** 2.8% menthol, 5.2% camphor, 1.2% eucalyptus oil, cedarleaf oil, cetyl and stearyl alcohol, EDTA, glycerin, urea, parabens, turpentine oil
BenGay S.P.A.	**Cream:** 10% menthol, cetyl alcohol, urea, EDTA, glycerin
Arthritic Hot	**Cream:** Methyl salicylate, menthol
Ziks	**Cream:** 12% methyl salicylate, 1% menthol, 0.025% capsaicin, cetyl alcohol, urea
Thera-Gesic	**Cream:** 15% methyl salicylate, 1% menthol, glycerin, parabens
BenGay Greaseless	**Cream:** 15% methyl salicylate, 10% menthol, cetyl alcohol, glycerin
Pain Bust-R II	**Cream:** 17% methyl salicylate, 12% menthol, cetyl and stearyl alcohol

RUBS AND LINIMENTS

Trade name	Doseform
ArthriCare for Women Nighttime	**Cream**: 30% methyl salicylate, 1.25% menthol, 0.25% methyl nicotinate, glycerin, isopropyl alcohol
Arthritis Formula BenGay	**Cream**: 30% methyl salicylate, 8% menthol, lanolin
Icy Hot	**Cream**: 30% methyl salicylate, 10% menthol
Ultra Strength BenGay	**Cream**: 30% methyl salicylate, 10% menthol, 4% camphor, EDTA, lanolin
Panalgesic Gold	**Cream**: 35% methyl salicylate, 4% menthol, lanolin, cetyl and stearyl alcohol, mineral oil
Myoflex	**Cream**: 10% triethanolamine salicylate, cetyl and stearyl alcohol, EDTA
Myoflex Extra, Myoflex Arthritic	**Cream**: 15% triethanolamine salicylate
Sportscreme	**Cream**: 10% trolamine salicylate, cetyl alcohol, glycerin, parabens, mineral oil
Aspercreme	**Cream**: 10% trolamine salicylate, aloe vera gel, cetyl alcohol, glycerin, parabens, mineral oil
Mobisyl	**Cream**: 10% trolamine salicylate, aloe vera gel, cetyl alcohol, urea, glycerin, parabens, mineral oil, sweet almond oil, EDTA
Icy Hot Arthritis Therapy	**Gel**: 0.025% capsaicin, aloe vera gel, benzyl alcohol, urea, maleated soybean oil, parabens
Flexall Quik Gel	**Gel**: Menthol, methyl salicylate
Vanishing Scent BenGay	**Gel**: 2.5% menthol, urea, isopropyl alcohol
Vicks VapoRub	**Gel**: 2.6% menthol, 4.8% camphor, 1.2% eucalyptus oil, cedarleaf oil, nutmeg oil, petrolatum, turpentine oil
Flexall 454	**Gel**: 7% menthol, aloe vera gel, eucalyptus oil, glycerin, peppermint oil, thyme oil
Maximum Strength Flexall 454	**Gel**: 16% menthol, aloe vera gel, eucalyptus oil, glycerin, peppermint oil, thyme oil
Flexall Ultra Plus	**Gel**: 16% menthol, 10% methyl salicylate, 3.1% camphor, aloe vera gel, eucalyptus oil, glycerin, peppermint oil, thyme oil
Icy Hot Chill Stick	**Gel**: 30% methyl salicylate, 10% menthol, hydrogenated castor oil, stearyl alcohol
Myoflex Ice Cold Plus	**Gel**: 15% triethanolamine salicylate
Absorbine Jr Arthritis Strength	**Liquid**: Capsaicin, echinacea, calendula, and wormwood extracts
Absorbine Jr	**Liquid**: 1.27% menthol, echinacea, calendula, and wormwood extracts, wormwood oil
Extra Strength Absorbine Jr	**Liquid**: 4% menthol, echinacea, calendula, and wormwood extracts, wormwood oil
Yager's	**Liniment**: Camphor, turpentine oil, clove oil
Panalgesic Gold	**Liniment**: 55.01% methyl salicylate, 1.25% menthol, 3.1% camphor, emollient oils, alcohol
Banalg	**Lotion**: 4.9% methyl salicylate, 1% menthol, 2% camphor, parabens, eucalyptus oil
Banalg Hospital Strength	**Lotion**: 14% methyl salicylate, 3% menthol, parabens
Aspercreme	**Lotion**: Trolamine salicylate

RUBS AND LINIMENTS	
Trade name	**Doseform**
Eucalyptamint	**Ointment**: 16% menthol, eucalyptus oil, lanolin, mineral oil
Original Formula BenGay	**Ointment**: 18.3% methyl salicylate, 16% menthol, lanolin
Absorbine Jr	**Patch**: Menthol, camphor, eucalyptus
Absorbine Jr Deep Pain Relief	**Patch**: Menthol, glucosamine, MSM
Icy Hot	**Patch**: Methyl salicylate, menthol

Products listed are representative of currently available and widely distributed brands. Similar products, including regional and private label brands, may also exist.

PATIENT INFORMATION
Rubs and Liniments

- For external use only. Avoid contact with eyes, eyelids, and mucous membranes.
- Apply to affected areas only. Do not apply to irritated skin; discontinue use if excessive irritation develops.
- Consult a physician if pain persists for longer than 7 to 10 days, if redness is present, or in conditions affecting children younger than 10 years of age.
- Do not use an external source of high heat (eg, heating pad) with these agents because irritation and burning of the skin may occur.
- Do not apply tight bandages or wraps over these agents.
- Do not apply to broken skin.

NUTRITION

NONPRESCRIPTION DRUG THERAPY
TABLE OF CONTENTS

■ ■ ■

NUTRITION

INTRODUCTION

Nutrition is the process of building up tissue and liberating energy through the metabolism of food by living plants and animals. Malnutrition is defined as either lack of food, or an adequate diet but inefficient nutrient utilization related to chronic or acute diseases and treatment. Nutrition affects every metabolic and organ process in the body. Nutritional therapeutics involves management of the patient's nutritional state. Its purpose is to prevent, recognize, and manage malnutrition.

The body needs a constant source of proper fuel for growth and maintenance. Providing adequate nutrition is an essential component of health care for all patients, and it is especially important in children. Inadequate nutrition is associated with increased morbidity, delays in growth and development, and complications of acute and chronic disease states in infants and children. As people age, their risk of malnutrition increases. Aging is accompanied by economic, psychological, physiological, and social changes that may compromise good nutrition. Signs and symptoms of specific nutritional deficiencies are presented under individual monographs.

In addition to physical findings, laboratory tests may confirm malnutrition and the degree of malnutrition from a biochemical standpoint, and also reflect the end organ changes that occur in the body. These objective measures provide the basis for therapy to correct the malnutrition. Anthropometric measures (gross measurements of body cell mass) may assist medical professionals in the assessment of nutritional status. Height, weight, body mass index (BMI), limb size, skinfold thickness, and wrist circumference are common measurements used to compare individuals with the general population to indicate the response to nutritional intervention.

The link between poor diet and disease has been well documented. The overconsumption of fat contributes to the development of obesity, coronary artery disease, and atherosclerosis, which can lead to heart attack, stroke, and some types of cancer. Diets high in sodium may aggravate hypertension. Excess alcohol consumption can lead to weight gain, liver disease, and brain damage. Adolescent and adult men and women who do not have adequate calcium intake in their diets are unable to maintain optimal bone health and prevent age-related bone loss. Diet-related diseases cost more than $250 billion annually.

With OTC vitamins, health foods, and nutraceuticals becoming increasingly popular, the pharmacist must be educated to make contributions to the improvement of health care. Referrals to physicians, registered dieticians, or other related experts are often essential in providing good pharmaceutical care.

Based on evidence in a review published in the *Journal of the American Medical Association*, it is now recommended that all adults take a multivitamin. Pharmacists are in an excellent position to manage and educate consumers on the toxic effects of excessive intake and drug-nutrient interactions. Certain foods and drugs, when taken together, can cause a deleterious effect or alter the body's ability to utilize a food or drug. Interactions vary according to dosage, sex, age, and overall health of the patient. Drug-nutrient counseling should be incorporated into pharmaceutical care.

Recognizing the importance of a healthy diet, the National Academy of Sciences, the Food and Drug Administration (FDA), and the United States Department of Agriculture have established dietary guidelines for Americans. If a medical condition is diet related, it is easier to correct the problem with proper diet rather than nutritional supplements because nutrients are better absorbed from food than from supplements. The more patients learn about proper nutrition, the better equipped they are to maintain their health.

NUTRITIONAL REFERENCE VALUES

The following pages provide nutritional reference values established by the National Academy of Sciences and the FDA.

Table 1 presents the Recommended Dietary Allowances (RDAs) expressed as average daily intakes over time. These values are intended to provide for individual variations among most healthy people living in the United States under normal environmental stresses. RDAs are estimated to meet the needs of 97% to 98% of individuals. Diets should incorporate a variety of common foods to provide nutrients for which human requirements have been less well defined.

NUTRIENT VALUES FOR FOOD LABELING

The FDA created a less comprehensive set of values for food labeling. The new label reference value, Daily Value, comprises two sets of dietary standards: Daily Reference Values (DRVs) and Reference Daily Intakes (RDIs). Only the Daily Value term appears on the label, to make label reading less confusing.

DRVs have been established for macronutrients that are sources of energy (ie, fat, saturated fat, carbohydrates [including fiber], protein) and for cholesterol, sodium, and potassium, which do not contribute calories.

DRVs for energy-producing nutrients are based on the number of calories consumed per day. A daily intake of 2000 calories has been established as the reference. This level was chosen, in part, because it approximated the caloric requirements for postmenopausal women. This group has the highest risk for excessive intake of calories and fat.

DRVs for the energy-producing nutrients are calculated as follows:

- Fat: 30% of calories
- Saturated fat: 10% of calories
- Carbohydrates: 60% of calories
- Protein: 10% of calories (The DRV for protein applies only to adults and children older than 4 years of age. RDIs for protein for special groups have been established.)
- Fiber: 11.5 g/1000 calories

Because of current public health recommendations, DRVs for some nutrients represent the uppermost limit that is considered desirable. The DRVs for fats and sodium are as follows:

- Total fat: less than 65 g
- Saturated fat: less than 20 g
- Cholesterol: less than 300 mg
- Sodium: less than 2400 mg

RDI replaces the term "US RDA," which was introduced in 1973 as a label reference value for vitamins, minerals, and protein in voluntary nutrition labeling. The name change was sought because of confusion that existed over US RDAs, the values determined by the FDA and used on food labels, and RDAs (Recommended Dietary Allowances), the values determined by the National Academy of Sciences for various population groups and used by the FDA to figure the US RDAs. However, the values for new RDIs remain the same as the old US RDAs for the time being.

Table 1. Dietary Reference Intakes[1]

Patient Parameters	Macronutrients				Fat-Soluble Vitamins				Water-Soluble Vitamins							Minerals						
Age (years) or Condition	Carbohydrate	Fat	Fiber	Protein	Vitamin A	Vitamin D	Vitamin E	Vitamin K	Ascorbic Acid (C)	Thiamine (B₁)	Riboflavin (B₂)	Niacin (B₃)	Vitamin B₆	Folate (Folic Acid)	Cyanocobalamin (B₁₂)	Calcium	Phosphorus	Magnesium	Iron	Zinc	Iodine	Selenium
	g	g	g	g[2]	µg[3]	IU[4]	mg[5]	µg	mg	mg	mg	mg[6]	mg	µg[7]	µg	mg	mg	mg	mg	mg	µg	µg
Infants 0 to 6 mo	60*	31*	ND	9.1*	400*	200*	4*	2*	40*	0.2*	0.3*	2*	0.1*	65*	0.4*	210*	100*	30*	0.27*	2*	110*	15*
7 to 12 mo	95*	30*	ND	13.5	500*	200*	5*	2.5*	50*	0.3*	0.4*	4*	0.3*	80*	0.5*	270*	275*	75*	11	3	130*	20*
Children 1 to 3	130		19*	13	300	200*	6	30*	15	0.5	0.5	6	0.5	150	0.9	500*	460	80	7	3	90	20
4 to 8	130		25*	19	400	200*	7	55*	25	0.6	0.6	8	0.6	200	1.2	800*	500	130	10	5	90	30
Males 9 to 13	130		31*	34	600	200*	11	60*	45	0.9	0.9	12	1	300	1.8	1300*	1250	240	8	8	120	40
14 to 18	130		38*	52	900	200*	15	75*	75	1.2	1.3	16	1.3	400	2.4	1300*	1250	410	11	11	150	55
19 to 30	130		38*	56	900	200*	15	120*	90	1.2	1.3	16	1.3	400	2.4	1000*	700	400	8	11	150	55
31 to 50	130		38*	56	900	200*	15	120*	90	1.2	1.3	16	1.3	400	2.4	1000*	700	420	8	11	150	55
50 to 70	130		30*	56	900	400*	15	120*	90	1.2	1.3	16	1.7	400	2.4	1200*	700	420	8	11	150	55
70+	130		30*	56	900	600*	15	120*	90	1.2	1.3	16	1.7	400	2.4	1200*	700	420	8	11	150	55
Females 9 to 13	130		26*	34	600	200*	11	60*	45	0.9	0.9	12	1	300	1.8	1300*	1250	240	8	8	120	40
14 to 18	130		26*	46	700	200*	15	75*	65	1	1	14	1.2	400	2.4	1300*	1250	360	15	9	150	55
19 to 30	130		25*	46	700	200*	15	90*	75	1.1	1.1	14	1.3	400	2.4	1000*	700	310	18	8	150	55
31 to 50	130		25*	46	700	200*	15	90*	75	1.1	1.1	14	1.3	400	2.4	1000*	700	320	18	8	150	55
50 to 70	130		21*	46	700	400*	15	90*	75	1.1	1.1	14	1.5	400	2.4	1200*	700	320	8	8	150	55
70+	130		21*	46	700	600*	15	90*	75	1.1	1.1	14	1.5	400	2.4	1200*	700	320	8	8	150	55
Pregnancy ≤ 18	175		28*	71	750	200*	15	75*	80	1.4	1.4	18	1.9	600	2.6	1300*	1250	400	27	12	220	60
19 to 30	175		28*	71	770	200*	15	90*	85	1.4	1.4	18	1.9	600	2.6	1000*	700	350	27	11	220	60
31 to 50	175		28*	71	770	200*	15	90*	85	1.4	1.4	18	1.9	600	2.6	1000*	700	360	27	11	220	60
Lactation ≤ 18	210		29*	71	1200	200*	19	75*	115	1.4	1.6	17	2	500	2.8	1300*	1250	360	10	13	290	70
19 to 30	210		29*	71	1300	200*	19	90*	120	1.4	1.6	17	2	500	2.8	1000*	700	310	9	12	290	70
31 to 50	210		29*	71	1300	200*	19	90*	120	1.4	1.6	17	2	500	2.8	1000*	700	320	9	12	290	70

Adapted from *Dietary Reference Intakes* (table). Institute of Medicine of the National Academies, Food and Nutrition Board. (http://www.iom.edu/fnb) Accessed: November 2003.

[1] The table represents Recommended Dietary Allowances (RDAs) and Adequate Intakes (AIs). AIs are followed by an asterisk (*). Both RDAs and AIs may be used as goals for individual intake. RDAs are set to meet the needs of almost all (97% to 98%) individuals in a group. For healthy breastfed infants, AIs are the mean intake; for other life stage and gender groups it is believed to cover the needs of all individuals in the group, but lack of data prevent confident specifications of the percentage of individuals covered by this intake.

[2] Based on 1.5 g/kg/day for infants, 1.1 g/kg/day for 1 to 3 y, 0.95 g/kg/day for 4 to 13 y, 0.85 g/kg/day for 14 to 18 y, 0.8 g/kg/day for adults, and 1.1 g/kg/day for pregnant (using pregnancy weight) and lactating women.

[3] Given as retinol activity equivalents (RAEs). 1 RAE = 1 µg retinol, 12 µg beta-carotene, 24 µg alpha-carotene, or 24 µg beta-cryptoxanthin. To calculate RAEs from REs of provitamin A carotenoids in foods, divide the REs by 2. For preformed vitamin A in foods or supplements and for provitamin A carotenoids in supplements, 1 RE = 1 RAE.

[4] 1 µg calciferol = 40 IU vitamin D.

[5] α-Tocopherol equivalents (TE). 1 mg d-α-tocopherol = α-TE = 1.49 IU.

[6] Given as niacin equivalents (NE). 1 mg niacin = 60 mg tryptophan; 0 to 6 mo = preformed niacin (not NE).

[7] Given as dietary folate equivalents (DFE). 1 DFE = 1 µg food folate = 0.6 µg folate from fortified food or as a supplement consumed with food = 0.5 µg supplement taken on an empty stomach.

■ ■ ■

Table 2. Reference Daily Intakes (RDIs)[1]

	Unit	Infants	Children < 4 years of age	Adults and children ≥ 4 years of age	Pregnant and lactating women
Ascorbic acid (Vitamin C)	mg	35	40	60	60
Biotin	mg	0.05	0.15	0.3	0.3
Calcium	g	0.6	0.8	1	1.3
Copper	mg	0.6	1	2	2
Cyanocobalamin	mcg	2	3	6	8
Folic acid (Folate)	mg	0.1	0.2	0.4	0.8
Iodine	mcg	45	70	150	150
Iron	mg	15	10	18	18
Magnesium	mg	70	200	400	450
Manganese[2]	mg	0.5	1	4	4
Niacin	mg	8	9	20	20
Pantothenic acid	mg	3	5	10	10
Phosphorus	g	0.5	0.8	1	1.3
Protein	g	—	20 (28)[3]	45 (65)[3]	—
Pyridoxine	mg	0.4	0.7	2	2.5
Riboflavin	mg	0.6	0.8	1.7	2
Thiamine	mg	0.5	0.7	1.5	1.7
Vitamin A	IU	1500	2500	5000	8000
Vitamin D	IU	400	400	400	400
Vitamin E	IU	5	10	30	30
Zinc	mg	5	8	15	15

[1] Table adopted from: Handbook of Nonprescription Drugs. 12th ed. Washington, DC; American Pharmaceutical Association; 2000.
[2] Proposed US RDI.
[3] Values in parentheses are US RDIs when the protein efficiency ratio (PER) is less than that of casein. The other values are used when the PER is equal to or greater than that of casein. No claim may be made for a protein with a PER equal to or less than 20% that of casein.

Vitamin Deficiency

DEFINITION

Vitamins are micronutrients that have no caloric or energy value but are necessary for good health. These complex organic molecules are essential for biochemical transformation of energy and regulation of metabolism. Most vitamins cannot be synthesized in vivo, or at least not in adequate amounts for normal function; therefore, they or their precursors must be obtained from food or nutritional supplements. Vitamins can be divided into two groups: fat-soluble (vitamins A, D, E, and K) and water-soluble (vitamin C, thiamine, riboflavin, niacin, pantothenic acid, pyridoxine, folic acid, biotin, and cyanocobalamin). The lack of any of the known 13 vitamins may result in a specific vitamin deficiency with a syndrome of specific symptoms. While clinical deficiency diseases in the United States are uncommon, subclinical nutrient deficiencies affecting the development and progression of nondeficient diseases are common. The symptoms of these long-term marginal deficiencies are less dramatic than overt clinical disease, but their impact on health can be significant. Unbalanced nutrition can be a significant factor in the development or progression of some chronic, degenerative diseases including cardiovascular disease, cancer, diabetes mellitus, and obesity.

ETIOLOGY

For most Americans, the diet does not require routine broad-spectrum vitamin or mineral supplementation. In most healthy individuals, the food pyramid developed by the US Department of Agriculture is a good guide to follow to ensure sufficient intake of nutrients (see Figure 1). The pyramid displays the recommended number of daily servings from each of the six food groups. However, some individuals require supplementation with one or more

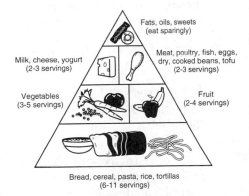

Figure 1. USDA Food Guide Pyramid

vitamins or minerals. The following list provides examples of conditions, situations, or patient groups that may require increased vitamin or mineral supplementation:

Conditions/Situations:

- Pregnancy
- Lactation
- Rapid growth (in pediatric patients)
- Malabsorption syndrome(s)

- Food allergies or intolerances
- Regular, strenuous physical activity (occupational or athletic)
- Neglect of diet (eg, elderly patients, food faddists, crash dieters, homeless patients, drug abusers, alcoholics, teens, those with dentition problems)
- Chronic drug ingestion (may increase vitamin requirements)
- Breastfed infants
- Premature infants
- Vegetarians
- Children receiving nonfortified skim milk
- Smokers
- Women with excessive menstrual flows

Acute or chronic hypermetabolic or catabolic illness:
- Chronic infection with long-term antibiotic use
- Surgery
- Burns
- Major trauma
- Cancer
- Cystic fibrosis
- Severe alcoholism
- Crohn disease
- Bulimia or anorexia nervosa

Several of these risk factors warrant further discussion:

Age – Age can be a risk factor for vitamin deficiencies. During certain years, dietary intake can be inadequate because of periods of rapid growth (adolescence), increased nutritional requirements or increased loss of nutrients (pregnancy and lactation, reproductive years in women), or decreased nutrient absorption or inability to attend to nutritional needs (advanced age).

Low socioeconomic status – Living below the poverty level has been shown to adversely affect nutritional status, especially in the elderly and ethnic minorities.

Dietary behaviors – Dietary behaviors can cause nutrient imbalances as a result of restrictive or unbalanced diets; such behaviors include anorexia, food allergies, fad diets, strict vegetarian diets, continual dieting for weight control, and diets with habitual, excessive amounts of substances such as fiber or caffeine. Other behavioral factors associated with nutritional deficiencies include cigarette smoking, exposure to secondhand smoke, alcohol abuse, drug abuse, bulimia, immobility, and heavy exercise. Skipping meals, eating alone, eating out frequently, and eating too many processed foods also have been shown to increase the risk of developing nutritional imbalances.

Pathologic conditions – Pathologic conditions or treatment of disease can affect vitamin and other nutritional needs. Interference with food consumption (eg, dentition problems, patients scheduled for surgery, disease requiring a restricted diet); interference with absorption, utilization, or storage of nutrients (eg, intestinal hypermotility, malabsorption disorders, liver dysfunction, hypothyroidism, drug therapy); increased destruction of tissues (eg, recovery from severe trauma); increased excretion or loss of nutrients (eg, lactation, burns, or chronic, excessive menstrual bleeding); and increased nutrient requirements (eg, fever, long-term antibiotic therapy, hyperthyroidism) are nondietary or conditional factors that interfere with a patient's nutritional status.

INCIDENCE

National surveys repeatedly show that many Americans and people in other westernized cultures consume suboptimal amounts of several nutrients including vitamin A, vitamin C, thiamine, riboflavin, pyridoxine, and folic acid. One study reported that 90% of Americans do not consume the recommended five daily servings of fruits and vegetables. The National Health and Nutrition Examination Survey indicated that on any given day, 46% of Americans eat no fruit, 18% eat no vegetables, and 24% go without a milk product, all of which are primary dietary sources for vitamin A, vitamin C, folic acid, and riboflavin.

PATHOPHYSIOLOGY

Fat-soluble vitamins:

Vitamin A – Vitamin A (retinol) helps maintain the integrity of epithelial membranes. Vitamin A deficiency can interfere with the proper functioning of many specialized tissues, including the cornea, mucous membranes, lining of the GI tract, lungs, vagina, urinary tract, bladder, and skin. Retinol (vitamin A aldehyde) is essential for the synthesis of rhodopsin and for normal functioning of the retina; deficiency interferes with visual dark adaptation.

Vitamin D – Vitamin D (calciferol) promotes calcium absorption from the intestinal tract, calcium resorption from the bone, calcium deposition into osseous tissue, and the resorption of phosphate in the renal tubule. A deficiency results in faulty mineralization and malformation of bone structures. Defective ossification leads to reduced rigidity in bones.

Vitamin E – Vitamin E (alpha tocopherol) interlocks with the main structural elements of cell membranes and serves as an antioxidant to protect cells, especially those with high levels of polyunsaturated fats, from oxidative deterioration by high-energy free radicals. In the absence of vitamin E, free radical damage to critical enzyme sites and structural membranes compromises cell membrane integrity and stability. It has been suggested that vitamin E prevents some cancers and atherosclerosis, possibly by preventing free radical and lipid peroxidation associated with tumor growth and atherogenesis, respectively. Tissues that accumulate polyunsaturated fats, such as the testes, are most sensitive and are the first to deteriorate when vitamin E is deficient. Diets high in polyunsaturated fatty acids are known to increase vitamin E requirements, while pancreatic insufficiencies or bile obstructions can decrease vitamin E absorption and lead to a deficiency.

Vitamin K – Vitamin K (phytonadione; menadiol) is necessary for gamma-carboxylation of glutamate in the synthesis of several factors in the blood-clotting cascade, including prothrombinogen and factors VII, IX, and X, as well as osteocalcin and matrix 4-carboxyglutamic acid (Gla) protein in bone.

Water-soluble vitamins:

Biotin – Biotin is essential for the metabolism of protein, fats, and carbohydrates. It functions within enzyme systems in the carboxylation and decarboxylation of intermediary molecules, catalyzing the deamination of amino acids and the synthesis of oleic acid. A deficiency could potentially affect multiple metabolic pathways and inhibit the incorporation of amino acids into protein, interfere with fatty acid synthesis, decrease energy derived from glucose, cause defects in pyrimidine and DNA synthesis, prevent conversion of folic acid to tetrahydrofolic acid, and even exacerbate symptoms of zinc deficiency.

Cyanocobalamin – Cyanocobalamin (B_{12}) participates in the metabolism of carbohydrates, proteins, and fats, but most significantly in the anabolism of DNA. Deficiency leads to dysfunctional DNA in all cells but most significantly affects the bone marrow, nervous system, and GI tract. Cyanocobalamin plays a secondary role in choline synthesis via its participation in the conversion of homocysteine to methionine. Interruption in this lipid pathway results in fatty liver disorders.

Folic acid – Folic acid (folacin, B_9) is converted in the body to its biologically active form, tetrahydrofolic acid (THFA). THFA, in conjunction with cyanocobalamin, catalyzes intermediary metabolic reactions of amino acids and methylation of choline, methionine, serine, and histidine. Folic acid deficiency is ultimately associated with defects in nucleotide, RNA, and DNA formation.

Niacin – Niacin (nicotinic acid) is an essential component of nicotinamide adenine dinucleotide (NAD+) and nicotinamide adenine dinucleotide phosphate (NADP+), two coenzymes involved in glycolysis, the conversion of pyruvic acid to acetyl coenzyme A, and Krebs cycle reactions. A deficiency affects the integrity and energy of all cells in the body. Endogenously, niacin is synthesized from tryptophan; 60 mg of dietary tryptophan is equivalent to 1 mg niacin.

Pantothenic acid – Pantothenic acid is incorporated into coenzyme A (CoA), an enzyme involved in the metabolism of carbohydrates, fats, and proteins. Deficiency can affect the synthesis of fatty acids, phospholipids, cholesterol, and by-products of cholesterol, including bile, vitamin D, and steroid hormones. Decreased levels of CoA also can disrupt the synthesis of acetylcholine and porphyrin, a heme-component of erythrocytes.

Pyridoxine – Pyridoxine (B_6) participates in the metabolism of carbohydrates, fats, and proteins but with emphasis in protein and amino acid metabolism. Fatty acid synthesis, conversion of linoleic acid to arachidonic acid, and cholesterol metabolism also are pyridoxine-dependent. Deficiency interferes with the synthesis of gamma amino butyric acid (GABA), norepinephrine, acetylcholine, and histamine, and the conversion of tryptophan to serotonin and niacin. Normal function and growth of erythrocytes also are affected by a lack of pyridoxine, including the synthesis of porphyrin, which is required for hemoglobin formation.

Riboflavin – Riboflavin (B_2) is a component of two enzyme systems that play significant roles in oxidation-reduction reactions responsible for the formation of ATP. These coenzymes, flavin mononucleotide (FMN) and flavin adenine dinucleotide (FAD), are essential for carbohydrate and amino acid metabolism. Cellular growth is inhibited in the absence of riboflavin.

Thiamine – Thiamine (B_1) participates in the decarboxylation, transketolation, and synthesis of alpha-keto acids essential for the production of energy from carbohydrates, fats, and amino acids. Thiamine also is believed to participate in the synthesis of acetylcholine. Therefore, a lack of thiamine can lead to decreased acetylcholine levels as well as an accumulation of intermediary products of metabolism.

Vitamin C – Vitamin C (ascorbic acid) is essential for fibroblast maturation related to intercellular collagen formation and wound healing. It is a coenzyme responsible for the hydroxylation of the amino acids proline and lysine, which help maintain collagen's tertiary structure. Lack of vitamin C affects collagen deposition in intervertebral discs, eustachian tubes, adipose tissue, bones, teeth, tendons, skin, scar tissue, and capillaries. In profound deficiency states, capillary walls become fragile, bones cease to grow and become brittle, hematopoiesis is impaired, iron absorption and utilization is altered, and structural changes occur in tooth enamel, cementum, and dentin. Vitamin C deficiency can impede the synthesis of some amino acids and neurotransmitters such as tyrosine, epinephrine, norepinephrine, and serotonin. Numerous studies suggest a protective effect (possibly as an antioxidant) of vitamin C against certain types of cancers (eg, esophageal, stomach, cervical).

SIGNS/SYMPTOMS

Fat-soluble vitamins:

Vitamin A – Vitamin A deficiency results in impaired dark adaptation, also known as "night-blindness." Vitamin A deficiency affects the epithelium of the eyes and the respiratory, GI, and GU tracts. Keratin deposits also can accumulate around the hair follicles and surfaces of the upper and lower extremities, creating hardened, pigmented goose bumps. However, the basal cells do not lose their function and can be restored to normal when vitamin A is replenished. Vitamin A is necessary in the formation and modeling of the endochondral tissue of long bones and in the normal spacing of teeth. Abnormalities of nerve and connective tissue occur in vitamin A deficient states. Severe, affected epithelial and connective tissues may become prime sites for infectious diseases caused by decreased bacterial resistance. Interference with wound healing occurs during vitamin A deficiency as a result of decreased collagen accumulation and formation of abnormal collagen. Because vitamin A is necessary for normal cell differentiation of epithelial stem cells, chronic deficiency has been associated with a variety of epithelial cancers.

Diabetic patients have a diminished capability to convert beta-carotene to retinol and can develop a low-grade deficiency if placed on a restricted diet without insulin.

Vitamin D – A deficiency of vitamin D, even in the presence of adequate calcium and phosphorus, results in faulty mineralization and malformation of bone structures referred to as rickets in children and osteomalacia in adults. In both conditions, defective ossification leads to reduced rigidity in bones and ultimately causes bones to become soft and pliable and to readily bend. Muscle weakness has resulted from vitamin D deficiency.

Vitamin E – No clearly defined vitamin E deficient disease is evident in humans; because of its wide distribution in food, clinical deficiency is uncommon. However, major tissues have been shown to be experimentally affected by inadequate vitamin E intake; these include the nervous system, reproductive system, muscle tissue, and erythrocytes. Hemorrhaging or hemolytic anemia (especially in premature infants) from oxidation of erythrocyte membranes has been demonstrated in humans; oxidative damage to lysosomal membranes of skeletal, cardiac, and smooth muscle tissue has resulted in a nutritional muscular dystrophy in animals; skeletal muscle can become ischemic and gritty, decreasing the ability to use creatine and leading to creatinuria (creatinuria in children with cystic fibrosis has been reduced with vitamin E therapy); oxidative damage to epithelial tissue of the lungs appears to potentiate pulmonary oxygen poisoning associated with air pollutants; and damaged neurological membranes have led to peripheral neuropathy in some patients.

Research regarding the effects of free radicals suggests that oxidative reactions play a role in the pathogenesis of many diseases such as cancer, arthritis, reperfusion injury during MI, cataracts, and atherosclerosis. However, more research is needed to determine the role that antioxidant vitamins, such as vitamin E, may play in the prevention or treatment of these disease states.

Vitamin K – A deficiency in vitamin K can interfere with the formation of clotting factors and reduce the clotting ability of the blood. In severe deficiencies, hypoprothrombinemia can lead to internal or external hemorrhaging that may develop either spontaneously or following tissue insult (injury or surgery). Vitamin K deficiency is uncommon in humans because of its wide distribution among plant and animal sources, as well as microbial synthesis within the intestinal lumen. Interference with the microbial synthesis of vitamin K in the intestinal wall (as seen with long-term, broad-spectrum antimicrobial therapy) is unlikely to create a deficiency.

Water-soluble vitamins:

Biotin – A specific biotin deficiency syndrome is not discernible in humans. Intestinal microbial synthesis is a significant source of biotin, and deficiency is uncommon unless intestinal absorption is inhibited. Some antibiotics, as well as diets high in avidin (a protein found in raw egg whites), can interfere with intestinal absorption of biotin. Biotin deficiency has resulted in vague symptoms, including a change in skin color, nonpruritic dermatitis, alopecia, hypercholesterolemia, ECG changes, anemia, anorexia, insomnia, lassitude, depression, muscle pain, and a slight change in lingual papillae of the tongue.

Cyanocobalamin – Prolonged deficiency of cyanocobalamin leads to the development of pernicious or megaloblastic anemia. This deficiency usually results from the lack of intrinsic factor, a glycoprotein secreted from gastric parietal cells essential for cyanocobalamin absorption.

Folic acid – Folic acid deficiency is one of the most common vitamin deficiencies. Utilization of folic acid requires a B_{12}-dependent pathway; thus folic acid and vitamin B_{12} deficiencies present similarly. Folic acid is very vulnerable to destruction, with significant losses occurring in cooking, storage, improper handling, exposure to light, and preparation of foods. Many medications and certain diseases also interfere with folic acid absorption and metabolism, creating several potential pathways for ensuing deficiencies. Deficient dietary intake results in megaloblastic anemia most commonly seen in people older than 65 years of age, people with malabsorption syndromes, women during the last trimester of pregnancy, and infants receiving unfortified formula or goat's milk. Deficiency also can cause irritability, weakness, weight loss, apathy, anorexia, dyspnea, sore tongue, headache, palpitations, forgetfulness, hostility, paranoid behavior, glossitis, and GI disturbances. Contrary to vitamin B_{12} deficiency, folic acid-deficient nerve damage is reversible. Inadequate folic acid intake (less than 400 mcg/day) before conception and during pregnancy has been linked to neural tube birth defects such as spina bifida and anencephaly.

Niacin – Classic niacin deficiency is known as pellagra. Tissues with rapid cellular proliferation, such as the skin, GI, and neurological systems, are more sensitive to deficient niacin levels. Early symptoms may include abdominal pain, nervousness, mental confusion, weight loss, anorexia, weakness, insomnia, headache, gastric achlorhydria, and glossitis. Severe deficiencies result in scaly, hyperpigmented dermatitis, moderate to severe diarrhea, and dementia; in advanced stages, hallucinations, catatonia, mania, and delirium may occur. Niacin deficiency rarely occurs alone and usually requires the simultaneous treatment of other vitamin B deficiencies.

Pantothenic acid – A naturally occurring pantothenic acid deficiency disease has not been identified in humans. The most significant source of this vitamin in humans is intestinal microbial synthesis, but pantothenic acid also is found in a wide variety of foods. A deficiency syndrome induced experimentally produced the following symptoms: fatigue, malaise, headache, insomnia, GI problems (eg, nausea, abdominal cramps, epigastric distress, vomiting, flatulence), neuromuscular disturbances (eg, paresthesia of hands and feet, leg cramps, dyskinesia), altered ACTH response, increased sensitivity to insulin, decreased antibody production, upper respiratory tract infections, depression.

Pyridoxine – No classic syndrome has been associated with pyridoxine deficiency, although symptoms similar to those of niacin and riboflavin deficiencies have been reported and include the following: weakness, mental confusion, irritability, nervousness, insomnia, decreased coordination in walking, hyperactivity, convulsions, abnormal EEG, leukocytopenia, anemia, dermatitis, skin lesions.

Riboflavin – No specific syndrome has been associated with riboflavin deficiency. Isolated deficiency is uncommon and usually is a component of multiple nutrient deficiencies. Several symptoms are associated with inadequate riboflavin intake: cheilosis (fissures at the corners of the mouth and reddening of the lips), inflammation of oral mucous membranes, purple-tinged glossitis, denuding of the tongue, seborrheic dermal lesions, impaired wound healing, ocular irritations (eg, reddening, itching, burning, lacrimation, photophobia), nerve damage, malformations, and retarded growth in infants and children.

Thiamine – Thiamine deficiency disease is referred to as beriberi. Symptoms characteristic of beriberi include polyneuritis (eg, loss of sensation in extremities, burning sensation in soles of feet, muscle weakness, muscle atrophy, calf muscle tenderness, paralysis of the extremities) and cardiac abnormalities (eg, bradycardia, cardiac hypertrophy, CHF) that are believed to be a result of impaired synthesis of acetylcholine. Early symptoms may include fatigue, anorexia, nystagmus, weight loss, GI disorders, and weakness, with memory loss, decreased attention span, irritability, confusion, and depression that develops later. Muscle atrophy may lead to reduced gastric tone causing constipation. Some cases of beriberi are associated with edema that can become fatal if excess fluid interferes with normal cardiac function. Thiamine deficiency usually occurs as part of a more complex nutrient-deficient state.

Vitamin C – The classic deficiency symptom is scurvy manifested as the following: petechial hemorrhages, anemia, joint tenderness and swelling, poor wound healing, weakness, defective skeletal calcification, hemorrhaging gums, tooth loss or loosening, gingivitis, oral ulcerations with occasional gangrene. Conjunctivitis with decreased tearing, dry mouth caused by decreased salivation, salivary gland enlargement, pathologic dryness of the skin, hyperpigmentation, ichthyosis, neuropathies, and depression also may occur.

DIAGNOSTIC PARAMETERS/PHYSICAL ASSESSMENT

Clinical Observation: Clinical observation should augment a thorough health and nutrition history to identify patients at increased risk for developing nutritional deficiencies. Refer suspected pathologic deficiencies to a physician for appropriate diagnosis and laboratory analysis.

In general, true nutritional deficiencies are uncommon in the United States and difficult to detect. However, prominent objective findings that can be readily observed in the outpatient setting are listed below. A systematic assessment of several systems, as well as overall appearance, should be included as part of the health and nutrition survey. The following checklist is a guide to help identify some signs that may be indicative of nutritional inadequacies/deficiencies; it is not intended to be used for diagnostic purposes:

General Appearance
- Cachexia, obesity
- Edema
- Signs of dehydration (eg, skin turgor test, sunken eyes, dry mucous membranes)

Skin and Mucous Membranes
- Thin, shiny, scaly, or hyperpigmented skin
- Ulcerations
- Abnormal bruising or petechiae
- Depressed wound healing
- Discoloration, inflammation, or bleeding of oral mucosa
- Glossitis
- Cheilosis
- Keratin deposits in hair follicles of upper arms or legs

Musculoskeletal System
- Bone pain or tenderness, epiphysial swelling
- Abnormal muscle mass
- Abnormal growth pattern

Neurologic System
- Nystagmus
- Dyskinesia, ataxia
- Irritability, confusion, depression
- Nervousness, hyperactivity

Hepatic Function
- Jaundice

Special Senses
- Redness, burning, itching, or tearing of eyes

Interview: The health and nutrition history is the most important tool for identifying patient risk factors that might lead to clinical or subclinical nutritional deficiencies. Assessment of patient-specific nutritional requirements, identification of risk factors that might compromise the patient's nutritional status, and a history of current nutrient supplementation is essential in the screening process. This assessment tool allows for the systematic identification of nutritional risk factors that help to define the health and nutritional status of each patient, as well as differentiating between patients in need of nutritional supplementation and those who need physician referral. The following checklist is a guide for identifying common risk factors that promote nutritional deficiencies; it should not be used to diagnose nutritional disease:

Age/Stage of Life
- Adolescence
- Pregnant, lactating
- Female of reproductive age
- Older than 50 years of age

Socioeconomic Status
- Living at or below the poverty level

Dietary Behaviors
- Anorexia
- Bulimia
- Food allergies or intolerances (eg, lactase deficiency)
- Fad diet
- Vegetarian diet
- Low-calorie (less than 1200 calories) diet
- Low-fat (less than 10% calories from fat) diet
- Less than 3 to 5 servings of fruits/vegetables daily
- High-fiber or high-caffeine diet
- Skip meals, eat alone
- Eat out frequently, diet high in processed foods

Nondietary Behaviors
- Smoking, exposure to secondhand smoke
- Alcohol abuse
- Drug abuse (illicit, prescription, or OTC drugs [eg, laxatives])
- Immobile, sedentary lifestyle
- Heavy exercise

Pathologic Conditions
- Dentition dysfunction or irritation
- GI dysfunction (eg, hypermotility, hypomotility, irritable bowel syndrome, short bowel syndrome, gastric or duodenal ulcer, malabsorption disorder, diarrhea, vomiting, constipation)
- Liver disease (cirrhosis)
- Thyroid dysfunction (hyperthyroid, hypothyroid)
- Recovery from severe trauma, burns
- Fever
- Chronic, excessive menstrual bleeding

Therapeutic Conditions/Drug Therapy
- Scheduled for surgery
- Antacids
- Antibiotics, long-term
- Anticonvulsants (phenytoin, phenobarbital)
- Antineoplastics

- Catabolic medications (steroids, immunosuppressants, radiation, chemo-therapy)
- Cathartics
- Cephalosporins with MTT side chain (cefotetan, cefamandole, cefmetazole, moxalactam)
- Cholestyramine
- Colchicine
- Contraceptives, oral (high-dose estrogen)
- Immunosuppressants
- Isoniazid
- Metformin
- Potassium chloride
- Primidone
- Salicylates, chronic

▶ **Dietary Recommendations**

Recommended Dietary Allowances (RDAs), developed by the Food and Nutrition Board of the National Academy of Sciences, should be considered a general reference point for average daily vitamin intake requirements. These values (presented at the beginning of this chapter in Table 1) are considered adequate to meet the known nutritional needs of most healthy people under usual environmental stresses. However, they are not absolute recommendations and do not meet the needs of seriously or chronically ill patients. In addition, RDAs do not account for nutrients lost in cooking or other handling procedures. A diet consisting of a variety of foods from all the food groups is the first and most appropriate source of nutrients. Consider vitamin or mineral supplementation if a change in the patient's diet alone cannot meet nutritional demands, the patient is unwilling or unable to make the necessary dietary changes, or the patient presents with a physical or therapeutic condition that places him or her at nutritional risk.

Reference Daily Intakes (RDIs) are values established for vitamins and minerals; these values represent average allowances based on the RDA. Daily Reference Values (DRVs) have been established for nutrients and food components (eg, fat, fiber, sodium) that may not have an established RDA. Together, RDIs and DRVs comprise the Daily Values used on food and vitamin supplement labeling for consumers. RDI (see Table 2 at the beginning of this chapter) and DRV values are discussed at the beginning of this chapter. These values are helpful in selecting an appropriate supplement product.

In 1989, the National Research Council (NRC), via their Food and Nutrition Board (FNB), published the 10th edition of the *Recommended Dietary Allowances* for most vitamins and minerals. RDA values are considered minimal daily requirements necessary to prevent a deficiency in the US population. RDAs allow for variations in individual requirements (eg, age, gender, height, weight, pregnancy, lactation status), but a variety of limitations in

RDAs should be acknowledged. Among the limitations of RDAs are:
1.) They are complex, making direct consumer use difficult.
2.) Ideal or optimal levels of intake are unstated.
3.) Data on some nutrients are limited.
4.) The individual's nutritional status is not taken into account.
5.) They do not take into account seriously ill, cachectic, or malnourished patients.

VITAMIN SUPPLEMENTATION

► Actions

A properly selected diet is the cornerstone of good nutrition. A low-fat, high-fiber, nutrient-dense diet containing a variety of fresh fruits, fresh or frozen plain vegetables, wholegrain breads and cereals, dried beans and peas, low-fat or nonfat milk and yogurt, small amounts of extra-lean meats, chicken, or fish, as well as minimal the amounts of processed foods is important for health and the prevention of disease. Epidemiologic studies indicate that people consuming large daily quantities of fruits, vegetables, and grains have a significantly lower risk of cardiovascular disease and cancer.

Patient nutritional assessment (see Interview) will help to quickly and systematically review the health and nutrition status of each patient to determine if supplementation is warranted. However, establishing an appropriate supplement regimen is contingent not only on successful nutrition assessment but also on the identification of nutritional products currently being used by the patient and determination of the patient's level of knowledge regarding the use of supplements. Patient education regarding appropriate dosages, toxicities, and proper product selection is necessary for proper supplementation and prevention of supplement misuse. To help patients ensure their own proper nutrition and, if necessary, supplementation, it may be beneficial for health care professionals to do the following:

- Recommend a diet consisting of diverse foods from a variety of food groups, and stress the importance of eating 3 to 5 servings of fruits and vegetables each day.
- Identify and try to eliminate conditional risk factors for poor nutrition such as smoking, excessive alcohol intake, fad diets, extremely low-calorie or low-fat diets, eating out frequently, and diets high in processed foods.
- Advise patients to maintain a healthy lifestyle, including regular exercise (20 to 30 minutes three times weekly), a desirable body weight (not exceeding 20% of ideal body weight), 7 to 8 hours of sleep each night, and effective stress management.
- Educate patients regarding medications that might alter eating behaviors or interfere with vitamin utilization.
- Educate patients regarding age, gender, and lifestyle factors that affect vitamin requirements.
- Warn patients about unsubstantiated advertising claims of dietary supplements.
- Help patients select appropriate supplements for their needs, without unnecessary inactive ingredients, that offer 50% to 100% of the RDA/DRV for each nutrient at a cost they can afford. A product expiration date should be visible. If children have potential access to supplements, child-resistant packaging should be a factor in product selection.
- Instruct patients taking supplements to take them with a meal (except for iron, which is best absorbed on an empty stomach) and without coffee or tea.

Factors affecting product selection include:
- Patient needs (single- vs multiple-nutrient requirements)
- Quality of supplement (eg, USP standardized ingredients)
- RDIs (or DRVs) provided by the supplement (balanced quantities between 50% to 100% of DRVs except for vitamins C and E, which may be 150% or more; avoid products with more than 100% DRV of vitamin A and D)
- Unnecessary inactive ingredients (eg, PABA, lecithin, fillers)
- Cost (compare product ingredients and cost; comparable ingredients may not always be comparable in cost)
- Packaging (eg, presence of expiration date, child-resistant packaging)

In general, products with balanced proportions of multiple vitamins and minerals are beneficial in filling the gaps of poor diet habits in healthy individuals. Products supplying 50% to 100% of RDAs are recommended, but research indicates higher levels of vitamins C and E are safe and may be beneficial. Avoid using products with unbalanced proportions of RDAs/DRVs; excessively high levels of one vitamin might negatively affect levels of another vitamin (eg, an intake of 50 times the RDA for pantothenic acid can increase niacin loss). Avoid products with more than 100% RDA/DRV of vitamins A and D because of the possibility of toxic effects. However, patient-specific needs should be determined and addressed with more specific products if a patient is at increased risk for developing a deficiency of a single vitamin (eg, vitamin C and smoking, vitamin D and anticonvulsants) or a group of vitamins (eg, fat-soluble vitamins, B vitamins).

▶ Administration and Dosage

To help reduce the risk of ingestion of toxic doses of vitamins, the table below presents minimum toxic doses of vitamins and selected signs and symptoms associated with toxicity.

		Vitamin Toxicities	
Vitamin	Minimum Toxic Dose[1]	Signs/Symptoms of Toxicity	Warning/Precaution
Biotin	50,000 mcg	Relatively nontoxic	None
Cyanocobalamin	not known	A 10,000-fold increase in daily doses has been taken without signs of toxicity	May reduce response to epoetin
Folic acid	400,000 mcg	A 1000-fold increase in daily doses can be taken without side effects, but large doses can mask B$_{12}$ deficiency with potential irreversible nerve damage	Doses ≥ 1000 mcg can mask B$_{12}$ deficiency; may reduce response to epoetin and phenytoin
Niacin	1,000 mg NE[2]	Cutaneous vasodilation, histamine release, stomach pain, nausea, diarrhea (nicotinic acid); hepatotoxicity with possible glucose intolerance and multiple enzyme changes (especially timed-release), uricosuria, glycosuria	Patients with peptic ulcer disease, asthma, gout
Pantothenic acid	1,000 mg	Relatively nontoxic	None
Pyridoxine	200 mg[3]	Muscle incoordination, peripheral neuropathy, fatigue, depression, nerve damage, paresthesia, mouth fissures	Doses > 10 mg/day can reverse effects of levodopa
Riboflavin	1,000 mg	Relatively nontoxic	None
Thiamine	300 mg	Headache, irritability, insomnia, tachycardia	None
Vitamin A	7,500 to 15,000 mcg RE[4]	Hydrocephalus, vomiting, weight loss, joint pain, stunted growth, abdominal pain, irritability, bone abnormalities, amenorrhea, nausea, itching, headache, anorexia, cracking/drying/scaling/bleeding of lips, mouth fissures, spleen/liver/lymph node enlargement, hair loss, fetal birth defects	More pronounced in children; potentiates side effects of analogues (eg, isotretinoin)
Vitamin C	1,000 to 5,000 mg	Nausea, diarrhea, increased hemolysis, decreased leukocyte bactericidal activity, increased susceptibility to kidney stones, false-positive diabetes and hemoglobin tests	Children; patients with kidney disease; may increase oral estrogen contraceptive coagulation; may affect warfarin and iron therapy

Vitamin Toxicities

Vitamin	Minimum Toxic Dose[1]	Signs/Symptoms of Toxicity	Warning/Precaution
Vitamin D	1250 mcg[5] (threshold: 500 to 600 mcg/kg/day)	Nausea, anorexia, weakness, headache, polyuria, mental retardation, constipation, irreversible calcification of kidneys/vasculature/heart/lungs/joints, dermatitis, tissue lipid oxidation, hypercalcemia, and hypermagnesemia	More common in infants and young children, patients with chronic renal failure, or those on thiazide diuretics
Vitamin E	not known (mg α-TE)[6]	GI problems, anticoagulation with extremely high doses (≤3000 mg/day in humans has resulted in few or no side effects)	Doses > 533 mg/day (800 IU/day) may potentiate effects of warfarin
Vitamin K	not known	Hemolytic anemia (not with vitamin K₁)	Low birth-weight infants; antagonizes effects of warfarin

[1] Minimum toxic daily dose reported; higher doses of some vitamins have been consumed without adverse effects.
[2] Niacin equivalents. 1 NE = 1 mg niacin or 60 mg tryptophan.
[3] Some reports indicate a minimum toxic dose to be as high as 2000 mg of pyridoxine. Toxicity may occur at lower doses in children and smaller adults.
[4] Retinol equivalents. 1 RE = 1 mcg retinol, 6 mcg beta-carotene; 1 RE = 3.3 IU vitamin A.
[5] As cholecalciferol. 10 mcg = 400 IU vitamin D.
[6] Alpha tocopherol equivalents. 1 α-TE = 1 mg d-alpha-tocopherol = 1.5 IU vitamin E.

VITAMIN A

▶ **Actions**

Vitamin A is found naturally in animal sources; it occurs in high concentrations in the liver of cod, halibut, tuna, and shark. It also is prepared synthetically.

Vitamin A activity is expressed as retinol activity equivalents (RAE). One RAE is equivalent to 1 mcg retinol or 12 mcg beta-carotene. Beta-carotene (provitamin A) is converted to retinol, primarily in the intestinal mucosa. In terms of vitamin activity, 0.6 mcg of dietary beta-carotene is equivalent to 0.3 mcg of vitamin A (retinol).

Vitamin A prevents night blindness and growth retardation, and preserves the integrity of epithelial cells. Deficiency is characterized by nyctalopia (night blindness), keratomalacia (corneal necrosis), keratinization and drying of skin, lowered resistance to infection, retardation of growth, thickening of bone, diminished production of cortical steroids, and fetal malformations.

Vitamin A is fat soluble; absorption requires bile salts, pancreatic lipase, and dietary fat.

The excretion pathways are uncertain; a major portion appears to be excreted in the bile, and a small amount is excreted in the urine.

▶ **Indications**

Treatment or prevention of vitamin A deficiency: Deficiencies occur rarely in well-nourished individuals; conditions that may cause vitamin A deficiency include the following: biliary tract or pancreatic disease, sprue, ulcerative colitis, hepatic cirrhosis, celiac disease, regional enteritis (eg, Crohn disease), extreme dietary inadequacy, partial gastrectomy, or cystic fibrosis.

▶ **Contraindications**

Hypervitaminosis A; oral use in malabsorption syndrome; hypersensitivity to vitamin A; IV use.

▶ **Warnings**

Prolonged administration: Closely supervise prolonged daily administration over 25,000 IU, and monitor for signs of vitamin A toxicity. Evaluate vitamin A intake from fortified foods, dietary supplements, self-administered drugs, and prescription drug sources.

Multiple vitamin deficiency: Single vitamin A deficiency is rare; multiple vitamin deficiency is expected in any dietary deficiency.

Acne: Efficacy of large systemic doses of vitamin A in the treatment of acne has not been established; in view of the potential for toxicity, avoid this use.

Renal function impairment: Vitamin A toxicity and elevated plasma calcium and alkaline phosphatase levels have been reported in chronic renal failure patients undergoing hemodialysis.

Pregnancy: Category A (Category X in doses exceeding the RDI). Safety of daily amounts over 5000 IU oral or 6000 IU parenteral during pregnancy has not been established. Avoid use of vitamin A in excess of the RDI (8000 IU) during normal pregnancy. Animal reproduction studies have shown fetal abnormalities associated with overdosage in several species.

Lactation: The US RDI of vitamin A is 4000 IU for nursing mothers. Human milk supplies sufficient vitamin A for infants unless maternal diet is inadequate.

▶ **Drug Interactions**

Cholestyramine: Cholestyramine may reduce absorption of vitamin A because of the reduced availability of fat-soluble bile salts.

Mineral oil: Chronic mineral oil use may interfere with the intestinal absorption of vitamin A.

Contraceptives, oral: Oral contraceptives significantly increase plasma vitamin A levels.

▶ **Overdosage**

Toxic manifestations depend on patient's age, dosage, duration of administration, retinol-binding protein (RBP) levels, and the liver's ability to store or eliminate vitamin A.

Acute toxicity: Signs of increased intracranial pressure develop in 8 to 12 hours; cutaneous desquamation follows in a few days.

> *Adults* – Doses over 2 million IU.

> *Infants* – Doses over 350,000 IU.

Chronic toxicity: 4000 IU/kg/day administered for 6 to 15 months.

> *Adults* – 1 million IU daily for 3 days, 50,000 IU daily for longer than 18 months, or 500,000 IU daily for 2 months.

> *Infants (3 to 6 months of age)* – 18,500 IU (water dispersed) daily for 1 to 3 months.

Hypervitaminosis A syndrome: Hypervitaminosis A syndrome generally manifests as a cirrhotic-like liver syndrome. The following have been reported as manifestations of chronic overuse:

> *Body as a whole* – Malaise; lethargy; night sweats; abdominal discomfort; jaundice; anorexia; vomiting.

> *CNS* – Irritability; headache; vertigo; increased intracranial pressure as manifested by bulging fontanelles, papilledema, and exophthalmos.

> *Dermatologic* – Lip fissures; drying and cracking of the skin; alopecia; scaling; massive desquamation; increased pigmentation; generalized pruritus; erythema; inflammation of the tongue, lips, and gums.

> *Musculoskeletal* – Slow growth; hard, tender cortical thickening over radius and tibia; migratory arthralgia; premature closure of epiphysis; bone pain.

> *Miscellaneous* – Hypomenorrhea; hepatosplenomegaly; edema; leukopenia; vitamin A plasma levels over 1200 IU/dL; polydipsia; polyuria; hypercalcemia.

Treatment: Discontinue vitamin A. Perform liver function tests; liver damage may be permanent.

▶ **Administration and Dosage**

Recommended dietary allowance (RDA): See Table 1 for dosage guidelines under various conditions of age, gender, and special circumstances (eg, pregnancy, lactation).

VITAMIN A PRODUCTS	
Trade name	**Doseform**
Palmitate-A 5000	**Tablets**: 5000 IU
Vitamin A Palmitate, Beta Carotene	**Tablets**: 10,000 IU
Palmitate-A	**Tablets**: 15,000 IU
Vitamin A & Beta Carotene	**Tablets**: 25,000 IU

VITAMIN A PRODUCTS	
Trade name	Doseform
Vitamin A	**Softgels**: 8000 IU, 10,000 IU. Fish liver oil, glycerin, soybean oil.
	Softgels: 10,000 IU, 25,000 IU. Glycerin, soybean oil.
Beta-Carotene, A-Caro-25	**Softgels**: 25,000 IU. Glycerin, soybean oil.

Products listed are representative of currently available and widely distributed brands. Similar products, including regional and private label brands, may also exist.

PATIENT INFORMATION

Vitamin A Supplements

- Common sources of vitamin A include liver, sweet potatoes, carrots, dark green, leafy vegetables, whole milk, butter, cheese, egg yolk, meat, fish, squash, and cantaloupes.
- Do not exceed recommended dosage.
- Consult a physician if you have, or have had, heart problems or liver disease.
- Discontinue use and consult a physician if headache, dry skin, hair loss, fatigue, bone or liver problems, or changes in blood lipid levels occur.
- Notify a physician if signs of overdosage (eg, nausea, vomiting, drowsiness, headache, dizziness/feeling of whirling motion, blurred vision) or bulging fontanelles in infants occur.
- Inform a physician if you are pregnant, become pregnant, plan on becoming pregnant, or are breastfeeding.
- Avoid prolonged use of mineral oil while taking this supplement.

VITAMIN D

▶ Actions

Vitamin D is a fat-soluble vitamin derived from natural sources such as fish liver oils or from conversion of provitamins (ergosterol and 7-dehydrocholesterol) derived from foodstuffs. One USP unit or 1 IU vitamin D activity is equal to 0.025 mcg vitamin D_3 (1 mg = 40,000 units). "Vitamin D" refers to both ergocalciferol (D_2) and cholecalciferol (D_3). Vitamin D_2, essentially a plant vitamin, is used in fortified milk and cereals. Natural supplies of vitamin D depend on ultraviolet light for conversion of 7-dehydrocholesterol to vitamin D_3 or ergosterol to vitamin D_2.

Vitamin D is hydroxylated by the hepatic microsomal enzymes to 25-hydroxy-vitamin D (25-]-D_3 or calcifediol). Calcifediol is hydroxylated, primarily in the kidney, to 1,25-dihydroxy-vitamin D (1, 25-]$_2$-D_3 or calcitriol). Calcitriol is believed to be the most active form of vitamin D_3 in stimulating intestinal calcium and phosphate transport.

Dihydrotachysterol is a synthetic reduction product of tachysterol, a close isomer of vitamin D. Dihydrotachysterol is hydroxylated in the liver to 25-hydroxydihydrotachysterol, the major circulating active form of the supplement. It does not undergo further hydroxylation by the kidney and, therefore, is the analog of 1,25-dihydroxy-vitamin D.

Physiological function: Vitamin D is considered a hormone. Although not a natural human hormone, vitamin D_2 apparently can substitute for D_3 in every metabolic step. Vitamin D regulates calcium homeostasis in conjunction with parathyroid hormone (PTH) and calcitonin. Vitamin D metabolites promote active absorption of calcium and phosphorus by the small intestine, increase rate of accretion and resorption of minerals in bone, and promote resorption of phosphate by renal tubules. Vitamin D also is involved in magnesium metabolism.

Severe vitamin D deficiency leads to progressive hearing loss, rickets in children, and osteomalacia in adults. Vitamin D reverses symptoms of nutritional rickets or osteomalacia unless permanent deformities have occurred.

Absorption: Vitamin D is readily absorbed from the small intestine. Vitamin D_3 may be absorbed more rapidly and more completely than vitamin D_2. Bile is essential for adequate absorption. Absorption is reduced in liver or biliary disease and steatorrhea.

Distribution: Stored chiefly in the liver, vitamin D also is found in fat, muscle, skin, and bone. In plasma, it is bound to alpha globulins and albumin.

Metabolism: There is a 10- to 24-hour lag between administration of ergocalciferol and onset of its action. Maximal hypercalcemic effects occur approximately 4 weeks after using a daily fixed dose; duration of action can be 2 months or more. Serum half-life of calcifediol is approximately 16 days. Elimination half-life of calcitriol is 3 to 6 hours; pharmacologic activity persists for 3 to 5 days. Dihydrotachysterol has a rapid onset of effect and is less persistent after treatment cessation.

Excretion: The primary route of excretion of vitamin D is bile; only a small percentage is found in the urine.

▶ **Indications**

Ergocalciferol: Treatment of refractory rickets (also known as vitamin D-resistant rickets), familial hypophosphatemia, and hypoparathyroidism.

Cholecalciferol: Dietary supplement, treatment and prevention of vitamin D deficiency.

▶ **Contraindications**

Hypercalcemia; evidence of vitamin D toxicity; malabsorption syndrome; hypervitaminosis D; hypersensitivity to vitamin D; decreased renal function.

▶ **Warnings**

Special risk patients: Use caution in patients with coronary artery disease, renal function impairment, or arteriosclerosis, especially in the elderly.

Concomitant vitamin D intake: Evaluate vitamin D ingested in fortified foods, dietary supplements, and other concomitantly administered drugs. It may be necessary to limit dietary vitamin D and its derivatives during treatment.

Hypoparathyroidism: May need calcium, parathyroid hormone, or dihydrotachysterol.

Hypersensitivity: Hypersensitivity to vitamin D may be an etiological factor in infants with idiopathic hypercalcemia. In these cases, severely restrict vitamin D intake.

Concomitant calcium administration: Adequate dietary calcium is necessary for clinical response to vitamin D therapy.

Monitoring: Dosage adjustment is required as soon as there is clinical improvement. Individualize dosage. Start therapy at the lowest possible dose and do not increase without careful monitoring of the serum calcium. Estimate daily dietary calcium intake and adjust the intake when indicated. Patients with normal renal function taking calcitriol should avoid dehydration. Maintain adequate fluid intake. In vitamin D-resistant rickets, the range between therapeutic and toxic doses is narrow. When high therapeutic doses are used, follow progress with frequent serum and urinary calcium, phosphate, and urea nitrogen determinations.

Periodically determine serum calcium, phosphate, magnesium, and alkaline phosphatase; monitor 24-hour urinary calcium and phosphate, especially in hypoparathyroid and dialysis patients. During the initial treatment phase, determine serum calcium levels twice weekly. Maintain serum calcium levels between 9 and 10 mg/dL.

Hypercalcemia: The product of serum calcium multiplied by phosphate (Ca × P) should not exceed 70; exceeding the solubility product may result in precipitation of calcium phosphate. Progressive hypercalcemia caused by overdosage may require emergency attention. Chronic hypercalcemia can lead to generalized vascular calcification, nephrocalcinosis, and other soft tissue calcification. Radiographic evaluation of suspect anatomical regions may be useful for early detection.

In patients with normal renal function, chronic hypercalcemia may be associated with an increase in serum creatinine. While this is usually reversible, it is important to pay careful attention to factors that may lead to hypercalcemia.

A fall in serum alkaline phosphatase levels usually precedes hypercalcemia and may indicate impending hypercalcemia. Discontinue the drug immediately if hypercalcemia develops. After achieving normal calcium levels, readminister at a lower dosage.

Renal function impairment: The kidneys of uremic patients cannot adequately synthesize calcitriol, the active hormone formed from precursor vitamin D. Resultant hypocalcemia and secondary hyperparathyroidism are the major causes of metabolic bone disease and renal failure. However, other bone-toxic substances that accumulate in uremia (eg, aluminum) also may contribute.

Because of the effect on serum calcium, administer to patients with renal stones only when potential benefits outweigh possible hazards.

Pregnancy: Category A (Category D in doses exceeding the RDI). Safety of amounts over 400 IU/day is not established. Avoid doses over 400 IU during a normal pregnancy. Animal studies have shown fetal abnormalities associated with hypervitaminosis D. Calcifediol and calcitriol are teratogenic in animals when given in doses several times the human dose. There are no adequate and well-controlled studies in pregnant women.

Lactation: Vitamin D is excreted in breast milk in limited amounts. In a mother given large doses of vitamin D, 25-hydroxycholecalciferol appeared in the milk and caused hypercalcemia in the child. Monitoring of the infant's serum calcium concentration was required. Exercise caution when giving to a nursing mother.

Children: Safety and efficacy have not been established in children undergoing dialysis or for doses over 400 IU. Individualize pediatric doses and monitor under close medical supervision.

Tartrazine sensitivity: Some of these products contain tartrazine, which may cause allergic-type reactions (including bronchial asthma) in susceptible individuals.

► **Drug Interactions**

Vitamin D Drug Interactions			
Precipitant drug	**Object drug***		**Description**
Vitamin D	Antacids, magnesium-containing	↑	Hypermagnesemia may develop in patients on chronic renal dialysis.
Vitamin D	Digitalis glycosides	↑	Hypercalcemia in patients on digitalis glycosides may precipitate cardiac arrhythmias.

Vitamin D Drug Interactions			
Precipitant drug	Object drug*		Description
Vitamin D	Verapamil	↑	Atrial fibrillation has recurred when supplemental calcium and calciferol have induced hypercalcemia.
Cholestyramine	Vitamin D	↓	Intestinal absorption of vitamin D may be reduced.
Ketoconazole	Vitamin D	↓	Ketoconazole may inhibit synthetic and catabolic enzymes of calcitriol. Reductions in serum endogenous calcitriol concentrations have been observed following the administration of 300 to 1200 mg/day ketoconazole for a week to healthy men.
Mineral oil	Vitamin D	↓	Absorption of vitamin D is reduced with prolonged use of mineral oil.
Phenytoin, Barbiturates	Vitamin D	↓	Half-life of vitamin D may be decreased.
Thiazide diuretics	Vitamin D	↑	Hypoparathyroid patients on vitamin D may develop hypercalcemia because of thiazide diuretics.

* ↑ = Object drug increased.   ↓ = Object drug decreased.

▶ **Adverse Reactions**

Early: Weakness; headache; somnolence; nausea; vomiting; dry mouth; constipation; muscle pain; bone pain; metallic taste.

Late: Polyuria; polydipsia; anorexia; irritability; weight loss; nocturia; mild acidosis; reversible azotemia; generalized vascular calcification; nephrocalcinosis; conjunctivitis (calcific); pancreatitis; photophobia; rhinorrhea; pruritus; hyperthermia; decreased libido; elevated BUN; albuminuria; hypercholesterolemia; elevated AST and ALT; ectopic calcification; hypertension; cardiac arrhythmias; overt psychosis (rare).

▶ **Overdosage**

Symptoms: Administration to patients in excess of their daily requirements can cause hypercalcemia, hypercalciuria, and hyperphosphatemia. Concomitant high intake of calcium and phosphate may lead to similar abnormalities.

Hypercalcemia leads to anorexia, nausea, weakness, weight loss, vague aches and stiffness, constipation, diarrhea, mental retardation, tinnitus, ataxia, hypotonia, depression, amnesia, disorientation, hallucinations, syncope, coma, anemia, and mild acidosis. Impairment of renal function may cause polyuria, nocturia, hypercalciuria, polydipsia, reversible azotemia, hypertension, nephrocalcinosis, generalized vascular calcification, irreversible renal insufficiency, or proteinuria. Widespread calcification of soft tissues, including heart, blood vessels, renal tubules, and lungs can occur. Bone demineralization (osteoporosis) may occur in adults; decline in average linear growth rate and increased bone mineralization may occur in infants and children (dwarfism). Effects can persist 2 months or longer after ergocalciferol treatment, 1 month after cessation of dihydrotachysterol therapy, 2 to 4 weeks for calcifediol, and 2 to 7 days for calcitriol. Death can result from cardiovascular or renal failure.

Treatment: Treatment of accidental overdosage consists of general supportive measures. Refer to General Management of Acute Overdosage. If ingestion is discovered within a short time, emesis or gastric lavage may be of benefit. Mineral oil may promote fecal elimination. Treat hypercalcemia as outlined above.

Treatment of hypervitaminosis D with hypercalcemia: Treatment of hypervitaminosis D with hypercalcemia consists of immediate withdrawal of the vitamin, a low-calcium diet, generous fluid intake, and urine acidification, along with symptomatic and supportive treatment.

Hypercalcemic crisis with dehydration, stupor, coma, and azotemia requires more vigorous treatment. The first step is hydration; a saline IV may quickly and significantly increase urinary calcium excretion. A loop diuretic (eg, furosemide) may be given with the saline infusion to further increase calcium excretion. Other measures include administration of citrates, sulfates, phosphates, corticosteroids, EDTA, and plicamycin. Persistent or markedly elevated serum calcium levels may be corrected by dialysis against a calcium-free dialysate. With appropriate therapy, and when no permanent damage has occurred, recovery is probable.

▶ Administration and Dosage

RDA: See Table 1 for dosage guidelines under various conditions of age, gender, and special circumstances (eg, pregnancy, lactation).

VITAMIN D PRODUCTS	
Trade name	**Doseform**
Vitamin D	**Tablets**: 400 IU vitamin D
Vitamin D$_2$	**Tablets**: 400 IU vitamin D$_2$
Delta-D3, Vitamin D-400	**Tablets**: 400 IU vitamin D$_3$
Vitamin D$_3$	**Tablets**: 1000 IU vitamin D$_3$
Calciferol Drops, Drisdol	**Liquid, drops**: 8000 IU vitamin D$_2$/mL

Products listed are representative of currently available and widely distributed brands. Similar products, including regional and private label brands, may also exist.

PATIENT INFORMATION

Vitamin D Supplements

- Common sources of vitamin D include fortified milk and milk products, eggs, fish liver oils, and livers of animals that eat fish.
- Compliance with dosage instructions, diet, and calcium supplementation is essential.
- Do not exceed recommended dosage.
- Swallow tablets whole; do not crush or chew.
- Eating a balanced diet and periodic exposure to sunlight usually satisfies normal vitamin D requirements. Never use vitamin supplements as a substitute for a balanced diet.
- Discontinue therapy and notify a physician if any of the following occurs: weakness, lethargy, headache, loss of appetite, weight loss, nausea, vomiting, abdominal cramps, diarrhea, constipation, vertigo, excessive thirst, excessive urine output, dry mouth, muscle or bone pain.
- Inform a physician if you are pregnant, become pregnant, plan on becoming pregnant, or are breastfeeding.
- Avoid concurrent, prolonged use of mineral oil. If on chronic renal dialysis, avoid magnesium-containing antacids while taking this drug (see Drug Interactions).

VITAMIN E

▶ **Actions**

Clinical deficiency of vitamin E is rare because adequate amounts are supplied in the normal diet. Sources of vitamin E include vegetable oils, vegetable shortening, and margarine. Other food sources include leafy vegetables, milk, eggs, and meats. Absorption depends on the ability to digest and absorb fat; bile is essential. There is no single storage organ, but adipose tissue, liver, and muscle account for most of the body's tocopherol.

Although the exact biochemical function of vitamin E (tocopherol) in the body is unclear, it is an essential element of human nutrition. Many of its actions are related to its antioxidant properties. Vitamin E may protect cellular constituents from oxidation and prevent the formation of toxic oxidation products; it preserves red blood cell (RBC) wall integrity and protects against hemolysis; it may act as a cofactor in enzyme systems. Enhancement of vitamin A utilization and suppression of platelet aggregation have been attributed to vitamin E.

Low tocopherol levels have been noted in the following: premature infants; severe protein-calorie malnourished infants with macrocytic megaloblastic anemia; prolonged fat malabsorption (eg, cystic fibrosis, hepatic cirrhosis, sprue); malabsorption syndromes (eg, celiac disease, GI resections); acanthocytosis; patients with abetalipoproteinemia. Low levels of vitamin E make the erythrocyte more susceptible to destruction by oxidants. Vitamin E deficiency may result in hemolysis.

Vitamin E is 20% to 50% absorbed by intestinal epithelial cells in the small intestine. Bile and pancreatic juice are needed for tocopherol absorption. Absorption is increased when administered with medium-chain triglycerides. Distribution to tissues via the lymphatic system occurs as a lipoprotein complex. High concentrations of vitamin E are found in the adrenals, pituitary, testes, and thrombocytes. Vitamin E is stored unmodified in tissues (principally the liver and adipose tissue) and excreted via the feces. Excess vitamin E is converted to a lactone, esterified to glucuronic acid, and subsequently excreted in the urine.

Vitamin E requirements: The daily vitamin E requirement is related to the dietary intake of polyunsaturated fatty acids (PUFA), primarily linoleic acid. Vitamin E requirements may be increased in patients taking large doses of iron; diets containing selenium, sulfur-amino acids, or antioxidants may decrease the daily requirement. Vitamin E supplementation has been effective in preventing hemolytic anemia and relieving edema and skin lesions that develop in low-birth-weight premature infants fed artificial formulas containing iron and high concentrations of PUFA. Commercial infant formulas that are currently available provide an adequate ratio of vitamin E to PUFA; formulas for premature infants have a lower level of iron to preclude interference with vitamin E use. Thus, there is no longer a need to routinely administer vitamin E supplementation to prevent anemia.

▶ **Indications**

Treatment or prevention of vitamin E deficiency.

▶ **Contraindications**

Do not administer vitamin E IV because its role in the deaths of 38 infants remains unclear.

▶ **Warnings**

Pregnancy: Category A (Category C in doses exceeding the RDI).

Lactation: Vitamin E is excreted into breast milk.

▶ **Drug Interactions**

Oral anticoagulants: Vitamin E in high doses (more than 4,000 IU) may increase the hypoprothrombinemic effects of oral anticoagulants.

Iron: Vitamin E may impair the hematologic response to iron therapy in children with iron-deficiency anemia.

▶ **Adverse Reactions**

Hypervitaminosis E symptoms include fatigue, weakness, nausea, headache, blurred vision, flatulence, intestinal cramps, and diarrhea.

▶ **Overdosage**

Doses greater than 2,000 IU are not likely to cause side effects. However, large doses (greater than 3,000 IU) have been noted to produce symptoms of hypervitaminosis E, which include nausea, weakness, intestinal cramps, headache, flatulence, diarrhea, thrombophlebitis, pulmonary embolism, severe fatigue syndrome, gynecomastia, breast tumors, increased cholesterol and triglycerides, decrease in serum thyroid hormone, and altered immunity. Doses less than 2,000 IU are unlikely to cause side effects. Sepsis and necrotizing enterocolitis have been reported when vitamin E levels are maintained at 5 mg/dL in low-birth-weight infants.

▶ **Administration and Dosage**

RDA: See Table 1 for dosage guidelines under various conditions of age, gender, and special circumstances (eg, pregnancy, lactation).

VITAMIN E PRODUCTS	
Trade name	**Doseform**
Vitamin E	**Tablets**: 100 IU[1], 200 IU[1], 400 IU[1], 500 IU[1], 800 IU[1]
Vitamin E with Mixed Tocopherols	**Tablets**: 100 IU[2], 5 mg apple pectin
	Tablets: 200 IU[2], 10 mg apple pectin
	Tablets: 400 IU[2], 60 mg calcium, 10 mg apple pectin
Alph-E Mixed	**Capsules**: 200 IU[2], 400 IU[2], 1000 IU[2]
Vitamin E-100 IU	**Softgels**: 100 IU[3]. Glycerin, soybean oil.
Vitamin E-200 IU	**Softgels**: 200 IU[3]. Glycerin, soybean oil.
Mixed E 400	**Softgels**: 400 IU[2]
Vita-Plus E	**Softgels**: 400 IU[3]
E-400 IU	**Softgels**: 400 IU[3]. Glycerin, soybean oil.
Vitamin E + CoQ₁₀	**Softgels**: 400 IU[4], 30 mg coenzyme Q_{10}. Glycerin, soybean oil.
Alph-E, Vitamin E, Vitamin E Water Soluble	**Softgels**: 100 IU[3], 200 IU[3], 400 IU[3]. Glycerin.
Vitamin E Natural	**Softgels**: 200 IU[4], 400 IU[4], 800 IU[4], 1000 IU[4]. Glycerin, soybean oil.
E-400 IU with Selenium	**Softgels**: 400 IU[3], 50 mcg selenium
Vitamin E-600 IU	**Softgels**: 600 IU[3]. Glycerin, soybean oil.
Mixed E 1000	**Softgels**: 1000 IU[2]
Vitamin E, Vitamin E Water Soluble	**Softgels**: 1000 IU[3]. Glycerin.
E-1000 IU, Vitamin E-1000 IU	**Softgels**: 1000 IU[3]. Glycerin, soybean oil.

VITAMIN E PRODUCTS	
Trade name	Doseform
Aquavit-E	**Liquid**: 15 IU/0.3 mL³
Vitamin E	**Liquid**: 1150 IU/1.25 mL⁴
Vitamin E	**Oil**: 28,000 IU/30 mL³

Products listed are representative of currently available and widely distributed brands. Similar products, including regional and private label brands, may also exist.

¹ As d-alpha tocopheryl acid succinate.
² As d-alpha tocopheryl acid succinate plus beta, gamma, and delta tocopherols.
³ As d-alpha tocopheryl acetate.
⁴ As d-alpha tocopheryl.

PATIENT INFORMATION
Vitamin E Supplements
- Common sources of vitamin E include vegetable oils, seeds, corn, soy, margarine, leafy vegetables, milk, eggs, meat, and nuts.
- Swallow capsules and softgels whole; do not crush or chew.
- Patients taking blood-thinning medication such as warfarin should use caution in taking high doses of vitamin E.
- Vitamin E supplementation should be stopped at least 4 weeks prior to surgery and may be resumed following surgery as recommended by a physician.

CYANOCOBALAMIN (B₁₂)

▶ **Actions**

Vitamin B_{12} is essential to growth, cell reproduction, hematopoiesis, and nucleic acid and myelin synthesis. Sources of vitamin B_{12} include liver, meat, fish, and dairy products (eg, milk and cheese). Vitamin B_{12} is not present in foods of plant origin. Deficiency may result in megaloblastic anemia or pernicious anemia. Ten to 30% of Americans older than 60 years of age experience atrophic gastritis, resulting in an inability to absorb vitamin B_{12} bound to food protein. Because of enterohepatic recycling, patients who do not absorb, or have a diet deficient in, vitamin B_{12} may not see signs of deficiency for 3 to 5 years.

The parietal cells of the stomach secrete intrinsic factor, which regulates the amount of vitamin B_{12} absorbed into the terminal ileum. Simple diffusion is responsible for absorption when more than 30 mcg vitamin B_{12} is ingested. Bioavailability of oral preparations is approximately 25%. Vitamin B_{12} is primarily stored in the liver. Enterohepatic circulation plays a key role in recycling vitamin B_{12} from bile and other intestinal secretions. If plasma-binding proteins are saturated, excess free vitamin B_{12} will be excreted in the kidney.

▶ **Indications**

Treatment and prevention of nutritional vitamin B_{12} deficiency (not caused by lack of intrinsic factor).

▶ **Contraindications**

Hypersensitivity to cyanocobalamin.

▶ **Warnings**

Cyanocobalamin works very closely with folic acid. A deficiency in vitamin B_{12} can cause a deficiency in folic acid if folic acid intake is not adequate.

Pregnancy: Category A (*Category C* in doses exceeding the RDI).

Lactation: Vitamin B_{12} is excreted into breast milk.

▶ **Overdosage**

Vitamin B_{12} is essentially nontoxic in humans. Allergic reactions and hypersensitivity have been reported.

▶ **Administration and Dosage**

RDA: See Table 1 for dosage guidelines under various conditions of age, gender, and special circumstances (eg, pregnancy, lactation).

Nutritional deficiency: 25 to 250 mcg/day.

CYANOCOBALAMIN PRODUCTS	
Trade name	**Doseform**
Vitamin B₁₂	**Tablets**: 100 mcg, 500 mcg
Vitamin B-12	**Tablets**: 250 mcg, 500 mcg, 1000 mcg
	Tablets, timed-release: 1000 mcg, 1500 mcg
Vitamin B¹²	**Tablets**: 500 mcg vitamin B_{12}, 55 mg calcium. Mannitol.
Vitamin B 12 and Folic Acid	**Tablets**: 500 mcg vitamin B_{12}, 400 mcg folic acid. Sorbitol.
Vitamin B₁₂ with Calcium	**Tablets**: 1000 mcg vitamin B_{12}, 88 mg calcium
Vitamin B 12	**Lozenges**: 50 mcg, 100 mcg, 250 mcg, 500 mcg. Mannitol, sorbitol.

Products listed are representative of currently available and widely distributed brands. Similar products, including regional and private label brands, may also exist.

PATIENT INFORMATION

Cyanocobalamin Supplements

- Common sources of vitamin B_{12} include meat and liver.
- A well-balanced diet is necessary. Strict vegetarian diets containing no animal products (including milk products and eggs) do not supply vitamin B_{12}. Vegetarians should take vitamin B_{12} supplements regularly.
- In some cases, vitamin B_{12} must be continued indefinitely to prevent the return of anemia and to prevent damage to the central nervous system.
- Folic acid is sometimes taken with vitamin B_{12} but is not a substitute for it. In pernicious anemia, folic acid may effectively return the blood profile to normal while nerve damage caused by vitamin B_{12} progresses.

FOLIC ACID (B₉)

▶ **Actions**

Folic acid (vitamin B_9) stimulates the production of red and white blood cells and platelets and is required for nucleoprotein synthesis and maintenance of normal erythropoiesis.

Folic acid is present in foods (eg, liver, dried beans, peas, asparagus, beets, broccoli, brussels sprouts, spinach, lentils, oranges, whole-wheat products), primarily as reduced folate polyglutamate. It must undergo hydrolysis, reduction, and methylation in the GI tract before it is absorbed and converted to tetrahydrofolic acid, which is involved as a cofactor for transformylation reactions in the biosynthesis of purines and thymidylates of nucleic acids. Impairment of thymidylate synthesis in patients with folic acid deficiency is believed to cause the defective DNA synthesis that leads to megalo-blast formation and megaloblastic and macrocytic anemias.

Folic acid appears in the plasma approximately 15 to 30 minutes after an oral dose with peak levels reached within 1 hour. After a single oral dose of 100 mcg folic acid in a limited number of healthy adults, only a trace amount of the drug appeared in the urine. However, a dose of 5 mg in one study and a dose of 40 mcg/kg in another study resulted in approximately 50% of the dose appearing in urine; up to 90% of the dose was recovered in urine after a dose of 15 mg. Small amounts of folic acid also have been recovered in the feces.

▶ Indications

Treatment of megaloblastic anemias caused by a deficiency of folic acid as seen in tropical or nontropical sprue, anemias of nutritional origin, pregnancy, infancy, or childhood.

▶ Contraindications

Treatment of pernicious anemia and other megaloblastic anemias for which vitamin B_{12} is not effective.

▶ Warnings

Pernicious anemia: Folic acid may obscure the diagnosis of pernicious anemia by alle-viating the hematologic manifestations of the disease while allowing the neurologic complications to progress. This may result in severe nervous system damage before the correct diagnosis is made. Vitamin B_{12} may prevent, halt, or improve the neuro-logic changes caused by anemia.

Benzyl alcohol: Benzyl alcohol, contained in some of these products as a preservative, has been associated with a fatal "gasping syndrome" in premature infants.

Pregnancy: Category A (Category C in doses exceeding the RDI). Studies in pregnant women have not shown that folic acid increases the risk of abnormalities if adminis-tered during pregnancy. The possibility of fetal harm appears remote. Because studies cannot rule out the possibility of harm, use folic acid during pregnancy only if clearly needed.

The US Public Health Service has recommended 0.4 mg folic acid per day in women of childbearing age to reduce the incidence of neural tube defects (NTDs). Several studies reported a greater than 50% reduced risk of NTDs in women who received 0.4 mg folic acid prior to conception and during early pregnancy.

Women who have had a prior NTD-affected pregnancy are at high risk of having a subsequent affected pregnancy. These women should consult their physicians for advice before planning to become pregnant.

Lactation: Folic acid is excreted in breast milk. During lactation, folic acid require-ments are increased; however, amounts present in human milk are adequate to fulfill infant requirements. Supplementation may be needed in low-birth-weight infants, in those who are breastfed by mothers with folic acid deficiency (50 mcg/day), or in those with infections or prolonged diarrhea. Consult your doctor before breastfeeding.

Children: Supplementation is not recommended in children.

▶ **Drug Interactions**

Aminosalicylic acid: Decreased serum folate levels may occur during concurrent use.

Contraceptives, oral: Oral contraceptives may impair folate metabolism and produce folate depletion.

Dihydrofolate reductase inhibitors: A dihydrofolate reductase deficiency caused by administration of folic acid antagonists may interfere with folic acid utilization.

Hydantoins: An increase in seizure frequency and a decrease in serum concentration to subtherapeutic levels have been reported in patients receiving folic acid (5 to 30 mg/day) with phenytoin. Phenytoin may cause a decrease in serum folate levels, producing symptoms of folic acid deficiency in patients on long-term therapy.

Sulfasalazine: Signs of folate deficiency have occurred with coadministration.

▶ **Adverse Reactions**

Rare instances of allergic responses to folic acid have occurred (eg, erythema, skin rash, itching, general malaise, bronchospasm). Patients receiving 15 mg daily reported altered sleep patterns, difficulty concentrating, irritability, hyperactivity, excitement, mental depression, confusion, impaired judgment, anorexia, nausea, abdominal distention, flatulence, and a bitter or bad taste. Decreased vitamin B_{12} serum levels may occur in patients receiving prolonged therapy.

▶ **Administration and Dosage**

RDA: See Table 1 for dosage guidelines under various conditions of age, gender, and special circumstances (eg, pregnancy, lactation).

Dietary deficiency: Administer up to 1 mg for all patients until symptoms have subsided, then use the following dosage: adults and children (older than 4 years of age), 0.4 mg; pregnancy and lactation, 0.8 mg; children (younger than 4 years of age), up to 0.3 mg; infants, 0.1 mg.

FOLIC ACID PRODUCTS	
Trade name	Doseform
Folic Acid	**Tablets**: 0.4 mg, 0.8 mg
	Tablets: 0.4 mg, 0.8 mg, 25 mg calcium

Products listed are representative of currently available and widely distributed brands. Similar products, including regional and private label brands, may also exist.

PATIENT INFORMATION
Folic Acid Supplements

• In the presence of alcoholism, hemolytic anemia, anticonvulsant therapy, or chronic infection, the maintenance dose may need to be increased.

• Except during pregnancy and lactation, do not take doses greater than 0.4 mg/day until pernicious anemia has been ruled out.

NIACIN (B₃)

▶ **Actions**

Niacin (vitamin B_3) is the common name for nicotinic acid. Nicotinic acid functions in the body as a component of two coenzymes: NAD (nicotinamide adenine dinucleotide, coenzyme I) and NADP (nicotinamide adenine dinucleotide phosphate, coenzyme II), which serve a role in oxidation-reduction reactions essential for tissue respiration. Nicotinic acid is present in NAD and NADP in its active form, nicotinamide (niacinamide). The niacin-deficient state *pellagra* is rare and is character-ized by mucous membrane, GI, and CNS manifestations, a triad often referred to as dermatitis, diarrhea, and dementia.

Although nicotinic acid and nicotinamide function identically as vitamins, their phar-macologic effects differ. In large doses (up to 6 g/day), nicotinic acid is effective in reduction of serum lipids (both LDL cholesterol and triglycerides). The mechanism of this action may involve decreased production of VLDL by the liver, inhibition of lipolysis in adipose tissue, decreased esterification of triglycerides by the liver, or increased action of lipoprotein lipase. In large doses, peripheral vasodilation is pro-duced, predominantly in the cutaneous vessels of the face, neck, and chest. Nicotinic acid causes a release of histamine, which acts directly on peripheral vessels, produc-ing vasodilation and increased blood flow. Nicotinamide does not affect blood lipid levels or the cardiovascular system.

Niacin is rapidly absorbed from the GI tract; peak serum concentrations usually occur within 45 minutes. Approximately 33% of an oral dose is excreted unchanged in the urine.

▶ **Indications**

The following prescribing information pertains primarily to therapeutic uses of niacin in doses exceeding basic nutritional intake.

Correction of niacin deficiency; prevention and treatment of pellagra; adjunctive therapy in patients with significant hyperlipidemia who do not respond adequately to diet, weight loss, and standard therapies (eg, statins).

▶ **Contraindications**

Hepatic dysfunction; active peptic ulcer; arterial bleeding; hypersensitivity to niacin.

▶ **Warnings**

Schizophrenia: There is no convincing evidence to support the use of megadoses of nicotinic acid in the treatment of schizophrenia as part of what is referred to as ortho-molecular psychiatry. Furthermore, high doses are associated with considerable tox-icity, including liver damage, hypotension, peptic ulceration, hyperglycemia, hyperuricemia, dermatoses, cardiac arrhythmias, tachycardia, heartburn, nausea, vom-iting, diarrhea, and other effects commonly seen with lower doses such as flushing and pruritus.

Monitoring: Frequently monitor liver function tests and blood glucose.

Closely observe patients with coronary artery disease, gallbladder disease, a history of jaundice, liver disease, peptic ulcer, or arterial bleeding.

Diabetes: Closely observe diabetic or potential diabetic patients for decreased glucose tolerance. Adjustment of diet or hypoglycemic therapy may be necessary.

Gout: Elevated uric acid levels have occurred; use caution in patients predisposed to gout.

Flushing: Flushing frequently appears with oral therapy and may occur within the first 2 hours of administration. This is transient and usually will subside with contin-ued therapy. The flush response can be attenuated with a prostaglandin inhibitor (eg, aspirin) administered at a dose of approximately 325 mg 30 minutes to 1 hour before niacin administration.

Pregnancy: Category A (Category C in doses exceeding the RDI). It is not known whether niacin at doses typically used for lipid disorders can cause fetal harm when administered to pregnant women. If a woman receiving nicotinic acid for primary hypercholesterolemia (types IIa or IIb) becomes pregnant, discontinue the drug. If a woman being treated with nicotinic acid for hypertriglyceridemia (types IV or V) conceives, assess the benefits and risks of continued drug therapy on an individual basis.

Lactation: Niacin is excreted in breast milk.

Children: Safety and efficacy in children have not been established in doses that exceed nutritional requirements.

Tartrazine sensitivity: Some of these products contain tartrazine, which may cause allergic-type reactions (including bronchial asthma) in susceptible individuals.

▶ **Drug Interactions**

HMG-CoA reductase inhibitors: Coadministration of niacin and HMG-CoA reductase inhibitors (eg, lovastatin) may result in myopathy and rhabdomyolysis.

Sulfinpyrazone: Sulfinpyrazone's uricosuric effect may be inhibited by nicotinic acid.

▶ **Adverse Reactions**

Flushing (see Warnings), pruritus, and GI distress appear frequently with nicotinic acid oral therapy.

Dermatologic: Severe generalized flushing; sensation of warmth; pruritus; rash; dry skin; itching; tingling.

GI: Activation of peptic ulcer; nausea; vomiting; abdominal pain; diarrhea; dyspepsia.

The hepatotoxicity of nicotinic acid (including cholestatic jaundice) has occurred with as little as 750 mg/day for less than 3 months. Hepatitis occurred with sustained-release nicotinic acid with as little as 500 mg/day for 2 months. Crystalline (nonsustained release) niacin may be less hepatotoxic.

Lab test abnormalities: Decreased glucose tolerance; abnormalities of hepatic function tests; hyperuricemia.

Miscellaneous: Toxic amblyopia; hypotension; transient headache; atrial fibrillation and other cardiac arrhythmias; cystoid macular edema; decreased glucose tolerance; orthostasis.

▶ **Administration and Dosage**

RDA: See Table 1 for dosage guidelines under various conditions of age, gender, and special circumstances (eg, pregnancy, lactation).

Oral: Begin therapy with small doses and increase in gradual increments, observing for adverse effects and efficacy.

Niacin deficiency – 100 mg/day or less.

Pellagra – 500 mg/day or less.

Hyperlipidemia – 1 to 2 grams 3 times daily. Do not exceed 6 g/day.

NIACIN PRODUCTS	
Trade name	Doseform
Niacin	**Tablets**: 50 mg, 100 mg, 125 mg, 250 mg, 500 mg, 750 mg
	Tablets, sustained-release: 500 mg
	Tablets, timed-release: 250 mg, 500 mg, 750 mg, 1000 mg
	Caplets: 500 mg
	Capsules, extended-release: 250 mg, 400 mg. Talc.
	Capsules, sustained-release: 125 mg
	Capsules, timed-release: 125 mg, 250 mg, 500 mg. Talc.
Niacinamide	**Tablets**: 100 mg, 250 mg, 500 mg
Slo-Niacin	**Tablets, controlled-release**: 250 mg, 500 mg, 750 mg
Flush-Free Niacin	**Capsules**: 400 mg niacin, 100 mg inositol
Niacin Flush-Free	**Capsules**: 590 mg

Products listed are representative of currently available and widely distributed brands. Similar products, including regional and private label brands, may also exist.

PATIENT INFORMATION

Niacin Supplements

- Some common sources of niacin include liver, meat, fish, chicken, nuts, legumes, green vegetables, potatoes, and wholegrain enriched cereals and breads.
- May cause GI upset; take with meals.
- Swallow extended-, sustained-, or timed-release products whole; do not break, crush, or chew.
- Cutaneous flushing and a sensation of warmth, especially in the area of the face, neck, and ears, may occur within the first 2 hours after administration. Itching or tingling and headache also may occur. These effects are transient and usually will subside with continued therapy. The flush response can be reduced by slowly increasing the dose, administering with food or milk, or by administering an NSAID or aspirin 1 hour prior to niacin administration.
- Stop taking and contact a physician immediately if any of the following occur: persistent, flu-like symptoms (nausea, vomiting, general not-well feeling), loss of appetite, decreased urine output associated with dark-colored urine, muscle discomfort (eg, tender swollen muscles, muscle weakness), irregular heartbeat, or cloudy or blurred vision.
- If dizziness (postural hypotension) occurs, avoid sudden changes in posture.

PYRIDOXINE HCL (B₆)

▶ Actions

Vitamin B_6 activity in natural substances, pyridoxine in plants, and pyridoxal or pyridoxamine in animals is converted to physiologically active forms of vitamin B_6, pyridoxal phosphate (codecarboxylase), and pyridoxamine phosphate.

Vitamin B_6 acts as a coenzyme in the metabolism of protein, carbohydrates, and fats. In protein metabolism, it participates in the decarboxylation of amino acids; conversion of tryptophan to niacin or serotonin (5-hydroxytryptamine); and deamination, transamination, and transulfuration of amino acids. In carbohydrate metabolism, it is responsible for the breakdown of glycogen to glucose-1-phosphate.

The need for pyridoxine increases with the amount of protein in the diet.

Pyridoxine is readily absorbed from the GI tract. Its biologic half-life appears to be 15 to 20 days. This metabolite is excreted in the urine.

▶ **Indications**

Treatment of pyridoxine deficiency, including inadequate diet; drug-induced deficiency (eg, isoniazid, hydralazine, oral contraceptives); inborn errors of metabolism (eg, B_6-dependent seizures, B_6-responsive anemia).

▶ **Contraindications**

Hypersensitivity to pyridoxine.

▶ **Warnings**

Pyridoxine deficiency: Pyridoxine deficiency alone is rare. Multiple vitamin deficiencies can be expected in any inadequate diet. Some drugs (eg, cycloserine, hydralazine, isoniazid, oral contraceptives, penicillamine) may result in increased pyridoxine requirements.

Pregnancy: Category A. Pyridoxine requirements are increased during pregnancy.

Lactation: Pyridoxine requirements are increased during lactation. Pyridoxine concentration in breast milk varies in response to changes in maternal intake of the vitamin. Use doses in excess of the RDI for lactating females with caution. Pyridoxine may inhibit lactation by prolactin suppression.

Children: Safety and efficacy have not been established.

▶ **Drug Interactions**

Pyridoxine Drug Interactions			
Precipitant drug	**Object drug***		**Description**
Pyridoxine	Levodopa	↓	Pyridoxine reduces levodopa's efficacy by increasing its peripheral metabolism; therefore, lower levels are available for CNS penetration. Avoid supplemental vitamins that contain more than 5 mg pyridoxine in the daily dose.
Pyridoxine	Phenobarbital	↓	Phenobarbital serum levels may be decreased.
Pyridoxine	Phenytoin	↓	Phenytoin serum levels may be decreased.

* ↓ = Object drug decreased.

▶ **Adverse Reactions**

Sensory neuropathic syndromes; unstable gait; numb feet; awkwardness of hands; perioral numbness; decreased sensation to touch, temperature, and vibration; paresthesia; somnolence; low serum folic acid levels.

▶ **Overdosage**

Ataxia and severe sensory neuropathy have occurred in patients who consumed pyridoxine (50 mg to 2 g) over a long period of time. When pyridoxine is discontinued, symptoms will lessen. It may take six months for sensation to normalize.

▶ **Administration and Dosage**

RDA: See Table 1 for dosage guidelines under various conditions of age, gender, and special circumstances (eg, pregnancy, lactation). Requirements are greater in people with certain genetic defects or those receiving isonicotinic acid hydrazide or oral contraceptives.

Dietary deficiency: 10 to 20 mg daily for 3 weeks. Follow-up treatment is recommended daily for several weeks with an oral therapeutic multivitamin containing 2 to 5 mg pyridoxine. Correct poor dietary habits and encourage an adequate, well-balanced diet.

Vitamin B_6 dependency syndrome: May require an initial therapeutic dosage of as much as 600 mg/day and 30 mg/day for life.

Deficiencies due to isoniazid: Some advocate pyridoxine prophylaxis for all isoniazid-treated patients; others advocate prophylaxis only for those predisposed to neuropathy. Recommended prophylactic doses range from 6 to 100 mg daily, but the lower doses appear more common. Treatment of established neuropathy requires 50 to 200 mg daily.

PYRIDOXINE PRODUCTS	
Trade name	**Doseform**
Nestrex	**Tablets**: 25 mg
Vitamin B^6	**Tablets**: 50 mg vitamin B$_6$, 45 mg calcium
	Tablets: 100 mg vitamin B$_6$, 37 mg calcium
Vitamin B-6	**Tablets**: 25 mg, 50 mg, 100 mg
	Tablets, sustained-release: 500 mg
Vitamin B 6	**Tablets**: 50 mg, 100 mg, 250 mg, 500 mg
Vitamin B-6 with Calcium	**Tablets**: 50 mg vitamin B $_6$, 58 mg calcium
Vitamin B$_6$ with Calcium	**Tablets**: 100 mg vitamin B$_6$, 73 mg calcium
Aminoxin	**Capsules**: 20 mg

Products listed are representative of currently available and widely distributed brands. Similar products, including regional and private label brands, may also exist.

PATIENT INFORMATION
Pyridoxine Supplements
- Common sources of pyridoxine include liver, eggs, meat, whole-grain breads and cereals, soybeans, vegetables, peanuts, walnuts, and corn.
- Do not cut, crush, or chew sustained-release tablets. Swallow whole with a glass of water.

RIBOFLAVIN (B$_2$)

▶ **Actions**

Riboflavin functions in the body as a coenzyme in the forms of flavin adenine dinucleotide (FAD) and flavin mononucleotide (FMN), which play a vital metabolic role in cellular integrity and cell growth. Symptoms of riboflavin deficiency include corneal vascularization, cheilosis, stomatitis, glossitis, and seborrheic dermatitis (especially in skin folds). Corneal vascularization usually is accompanied by itching and burning, blepharospasm, and photophobia.

▶ **Indications**

Treatment and prevention of riboflavin deficiency.

▶ **Warnings**

Riboflavin deficiency seldom occurs alone and often is associated with deficiency of other B vitamins and protein.

Pregnancy: Category A (Category C in doses exceeding the RDI).

Lactation: Riboflavin is excreted in breast milk.

▶ **Administration and Dosage**

RDA: See Table 1 for dosage guidelines under various conditions of age, gender, and special circumstances (eg, pregnancy, lactation).

Treatment of deficiency: 5 to 25 mg daily.

RIBOFLAVIN PRODUCTS	
Trade name	Doseform
Vitamin B 2	**Tablets**: 50 mg, 100 mg
Ribo-100	**Tablets**: 100 mg
Riboflavin	**Tablets**: 400 mg

Products listed are representative of currently available and widely distributed brands. Similar products, including regional and private label brands, may also exist.

PATIENT INFORMATION
Riboflavin Supplements

- Common sources of riboflavin include meats, poultry, fish, dairy products, broccoli, turnips, asparagus, spinach, enriched and fortified grains, and cereals.
- Riboflavin may cause a yellow/orange discoloration of the urine.

THIAMINE (B$_1$)

▶ **Actions**

Thiamine combines with adenosine triphosphate (ATP) to form thiamine pyrophosphate, a coenzyme. Its role in carbohydrate metabolism is the decarboxylation of pyruvic and alpha keto acids. An increase in serum pyruvic acid is a sign of the deficiency state. The need for thiamine is greater when the carbohydrate content of the diet is high. Significant vitamin B$_1$ depletion can occur within 3 weeks of total thiamine dietary absence.

Maximum oral absorption is 8 to 15 mg daily. Oral absorption may be increased by administering in divided doses with food. Tissue stores are saturated when intake exceeds minimal requirement (approximately 1 mg/day); excess thiamine is excreted in urine.

▶ **Indications**

Treatment or prevention of thiamine deficiency.

▶ **Contraindications**

Hypersensitivity to thiamine.

▶ **Warnings**

Sensitivity: Sensitivity reactions can occur. Deaths have resulted from IV use. An intradermal test dose is recommended in patients with suspected sensitivity.

Wernicke encephalopathy: Thiamine-deficient patients may experience a sudden onset or worsening of Wernicke encephalopathy following glucose administration. In suspected thiamine deficiency, administer thiamine before or along with dextrose-containing fluids.

Single vitamin B$_1$ deficiency: Single vitamin B$_1$ deficiency is rare.

Pregnancy: Category A (Category C in doses exceeding the RDI).

Lactation: Thiamine is excreted in breast milk.

▶ **Adverse Reactions**

Feeling of warmth; pruritus; urticaria; weakness; sweating; nausea; restlessness; tightness of the throat; angioneurotic edema; cyanosis; pulmonary edema; hemorrhage into the GI tract; cardiovascular collapse; death.

▶ **Administration and Dosage**

RDA: See Table 1 for dosage guidelines under various conditions of age, gender, and special circumstances (eg, pregnancy, lactation).

Beriberi: Give an oral therapeutic multivitamin containing 5 to 10 mg thiamine daily for 1 month to achieve body tissue saturation.

THIAMINE HYDROCHLORIDE PRODUCTS	
Trade name	Doseform
Thiamilate	**Tablets**: 20 mg
Vitamin B-1	**Tablets**: 100 mg
Vitamin B1 (sf)	**Tablets**: 100 mg, 250 mg, 500 mg
Vitamin B₁ (sf)	**Tablets**: 100 mg vitamin B_1, 80 mg calcium

Products listed are representative of currently available and widely distributed brands. Similar products, including regional and private label brands, may also exist.

sf – Sugar free.

PATIENT INFORMATION

Thiamine Supplements

• Common sources of thiamine include pork, liver, brewer's yeast, legumes, beef, milk, nuts, whole grains, and enriched flour.

• Do not exceed recommended dosages.

• It is unusual for thiamine deficiency to occur without other vitamin deficiencies. Consult a physician if you suspect you have a thiamine deficiency.

VITAMIN C (ASCORBIC ACID)

▶ **Actions**

Vitamin C is an essential vitamin in humans; however, its exact biological functions are not fully understood. It is essential for the formation and maintenance of intercellular ground substance and collagen, catecholamine biosynthesis, synthesis of carnitine and steroids, conversion of folic acid to folinic acid, and tyrosine metabolism.

The deficiency state scurvy is characterized by degenerative changes in the capillaries, bone, and connective tissues. Vitamin C deficiency symptoms may include faulty bone and tooth development, gingivitis, bleeding gums, and loosened teeth. Febrile states, chronic illness, and infection increase the need for ascorbic acid. Premature and immature infants require relatively large amounts of the vitamin. Hemovascular disorders, burns, and delayed fracture and wound healing are indications for an increase in daily intake.

Absorption of dietary ascorbate from the intestines is nearly complete. Vitamin C is readily available in citrus fruit, tomatoes, potatoes, and leafy vegetables.

▶ **Indications**

Treatment and prevention of scurvy. Parenteral administration is desirable in an acute deficiency.

▶ Warnings

Excessive vitamin C doses: Diabetic patients, patients prone to recurrent renal calculi, those undergoing stool occult blood tests, and those on sodium-restricted diets or anticoagulant therapy should not take excessive doses of vitamin C over an extended period of time.

Pregnancy: Category A (Category C in doses exceeding RDI). It is not known whether ascorbic acid can cause fetal harm or affect reproductive capacity. Give to pregnant women only if clearly needed.

Do not administer ascorbic acid to pregnant women in doses in excess of the amount recommended. The fetus may adapt to high levels of the vitamin, resulting in a scorbutic condition after birth when the intake drops to normal levels.

Lactation: Administer with caution to a nursing mother. Ascorbic acid is excreted in breast milk but does not necessarily increase in response to increasing doses.

Tartrazine sensitivity: Some of these products may contain tartrazine, which may cause allergic-type reactions (including bronchial asthma) in susceptible individuals.

Sulfite sensitivity: Some of these products may contain sulfites, which may cause allergic-type reactions in certain susceptible people.

▶ Drug Interactions

Oral contraceptives and estrogens: Ascorbic acid increases serum levels of estrogen and estrogen contained in oral contraceptives, possibly resulting in adverse reactions.

Warfarin: The anticoagulant action of warfarin may be reduced.

Drug-lab interactions: Large doses (over 500 mg) of vitamin C can cause false-negative urine glucose determinations.

No exogenous vitamin C should be ingested for 48 to 72 hours before conducting amine-dependent stool occult blood tests because false-negative results may occur.

▶ Adverse Reactions

Large doses may cause diarrhea and precipitation of cystine, oxalate, or urate renal stones if the urine becomes acidic during therapy. Doses of approximately 2 g will acidify urine in adults.

▶ Administration and Dosage

RDA: See Table 1 for dosage guidelines under various conditions of age, gender, and special circumstances (eg, pregnancy, lactation).

Infants: Average daily protective requirement is 30 mg. The usual curative dose of a severe deficiency is 100 to 300 mg daily, continued as long as clinical symptoms persist or until saturation, as indicated by excretion tests, has been attained.

Premature infants: May require 75 to 100 mg/day.

Adults: The average protective dose is 70 to 150 mg daily.

  Burns – Individualize dosage. For severe burns, daily doses of 1 to 2 g are recommended.

  Enhanced wound healing – Doses of 300 to 500 mg daily for 7 to 10 days both preoperatively and postoperatively are adequate, although considerably larger amounts have been recommended.

  Scurvy – 300 mg to 1 g daily is recommended.

In other conditions in which the need for vitamin C is increased, 3 to 5 times the daily optimum allowances appears adequate.

VITAMIN C PRODUCTS	
Trade name	**Doseform**
Ascorbic Acid Products	
Vitamin C (sf)	**Tablets**: 250 mg, 500 mg, 1000 mg
	Tablets, timed-release: 500 mg
	Caplets, timed-release: 500 mg
	Powder: 1060 mg/¼ tsp
Vitamin C with Rose Hips	**Tablets**: 500 mg, 1000 mg, 1500 mg
	Tablets, timed-release: 500 mg, 1000 mg
Pan-C 500 (sf)	**Tablets**: 500 mg vitamin C, 100 mg hesperidin, 100 mg citrus bioflavonoids
C Factors "1000" Plus (sf)	**Tablets**: 1000 mg vitamin C, 250 mg citrus bio-flavonoids, 25 mg rosehips, 50 mg rutin, 25 mg hesperidin. Vegetable glycerin.
Vitamin C Plus Rose Hips (sf)	**Tablets**: 1000 mg
Vitamin C Chewable	**Tablets, chewable**: 500 mg. Sugar, fructose, dextrose.
Fruit C	**Tablets, chewable**: 100 mg, 200 mg, 500 mg
Cevi-Bid (sf)	**Tablets, sustained-release**: 500 mg. Talc.
Vita-C (sf)	**Crystals**: 1000 mg/¼ tsp
Cecon	**Solution**: 100 mg/mL
Calcium Ascorbate Products	
Chewable C (sf)	**Tablets, chewable**: 100 mg vitamin C, 10 mg acerola, 10 mg citrus bioflavonoids, 10 mg rose hips. Mannitol, sorbitol.
	Tablets, chewable: 200 mg vitamin C, 20 mg acerola, 20 mg citrus bioflavonoids, 20 mg rose hips. Mannitol, sorbitol.
	Tablets, chewable: 500 mg vitamin C, 50 mg acerola, 50 mg citrus bioflavonoids, 50 mg rose hips. Mannitol, sorbitol.
Calcium Ascorbate (sf)	**Tablets**: 500 mg vitamin C, 75 mg calcium
	Powder: 814 mg, 100 mg calcium/¼ tsp
Ester-C Plus (sf)	**Tablets**: 1000 mg vitamin C, 125 mg calcium, 200 mg citrus bioflavonoids, 25 mg acerola, 25 mg rose hips, 25 mg rutin. Vegetable glycerin.
	Capsules: 500 mg vitamin C, 62 mg calcium, 25 mg citrus bioflavonoids, 10 mg acerola, 10 mg rose hips, 5 mg rutin. Vegetable glycerin.
Span C	**Tablets**: 200 mg vitamin C, 300 mg bioflavonoids
Ascorbic Acid Combination Products	
SunKist Vitamin C	**Tablets, chewable**: 250 mg (as sodium ascorbate and ascorbic acid). Fructose, sorbitol, lactose, sucrose, soybean oil, hydrogenated castor oil.
Vicks Vitamin C Drops	**Drops**: 25 mg (as sodium ascorbate and ascorbic acid). Sucrose, corn syrup, 5 mg sodium.

Products listed are representative of currently available and widely distributed brands. Similar products, including regional and private label brands, may also exist.

sf = Sugar free.

PATIENT INFORMATION
Vitamin C Supplements

- Common sources of vitamin C include strawberries, citrus fruit, tomatoes, potatoes, leafy vegetables, green cabbage, and melons.
- Consult your doctor before using these products if you have diabetes, a history of kidney stones, or are on a salt-restricted diet or anticoagulant therapy.
- Do not exceed recommended dosages.
- Do not cut, crush, or chew sustained-release products.

MULTIVITAMIN COMBINATIONS

► **Actions**

In addition to the products listed below, many other forms of combination vitamin products are available. Many of these products also contain recommended amounts of minerals. However, for the purposes of this monograph, only vitamin content has been provided.

MULTIVITAMIN PRODUCTS	
Trade name	**Doseform**
One-A-Day Women's Formula	**Tablets:** 2500 IU vitamin A, 400 IU vitamin D, 30 IU vitamin E[1], 1.5 mg vitamin B_1, 1.7 mg vitamin B_2, 10 mg vitamin B_3, 5 mg vitamin B_5, 2 mg vitamin B_6, 6 mcg vitamin B_{12}, 60 mg vitamin C, 0.4 mg folic acid
Centrum	**Tablets:** 3500 IU vitamin A, 400 IU vitamin D, 30 IU vitamin E[2], 1.5 mg vitamin B_1, 1.7 mg vitamin B_2, 20 mg vitamin B_3, 10 mg vitamin B_5, 2 mg vitamin B_6, 6 mcg vitamin B_{12}, 60 mg vitamin C, 0.4 mg folic acid, 25 mcg vitamin K. Sucrose, lactose.
One-A-Day Men's Health Formula	**Tablets:** 3500 IU vitamin A, 400 IU vitamin D, 45 IU vitamin E[2], 1.2 mg vitamin B_1, 1.7 mg vitamin B_2, 16 mg vitamin B_3, 5 mg vitamin B_5, 3 mg vitamin B_6, 18 mcg vitamin B_{12}, 90 mg vitamin C, 0.4 mg folic acid, 20 mcg vitamin K. Sucrose, mannitol, dextrose.
Centrum Silver	**Tablets:** 3500 IU vitamin A, 400 IU vitamin D, 45 IU vitamin E[2], 1.5 mg vitamin B_1, 1.7 mg vitamin B_2, 20 mg vitamin B_3, 10 mg vitamin B_5, 3 mg vitamin B_6, 25 mcg vitamin B_{12}, 60 mg vitamin C, 0.4 mg folic acid, 10 mcg vitamin K. Sucrose. May contain lactose.
Prenatal Vitamins	**Tablets:** 4000 IU vitamin A, 400 IU vitamin D, 11 IU vitamin E[2], 1.84 mg vitamin B_1, 1.7 mg vitamin B_2, 18 mg vitamin B_3, 2.6 mg vitamin B_6, 4 mcg vitamin B_{12}, 100 mg vitamin C, 0.8 mg folic acid
Dayalets Filmtabs, Dayalets Plus Iron Filmtabs	**Tablets:** 4500 IU vitamin A, 360 IU vitamin D, 27 IU vitamin E[2], 1.2 mg vitamin B_1, 1.53 mg vitamin B_2, 18 mg vitamin B_3, 1.6 mg vitamin B_6, 5.4 mcg vitamin B_{12}, 54 mg vitamin C, 0.36 mg folic acid
Optilets-500 Filmtabs, Optilets-M-500 Filmtabs	**Tablets:** 4500 IU vitamin A, 360 IU vitamin D, 27 IU vitamin E[2], 12.4 mg vitamin B_1, 9 mg vitamin B_2, 90.7 mg vitamin B_3, 16.6 mg vitamin B_5, 3.7 mg vitamin B_6, 10.8 mcg vitamin B_{12}, 500 mg vitamin C. Talc.

MULTIVITAMIN PRODUCTS

Trade name	Doseform
Unicap Sr. (sf)	**Tablets:** 5000 IU vitamin A, 200 IU vitamin D, 15 IU vitamin E[2], 1.2 mg vitamin B_1, 1.4 mg vitamin B_2, 16 mg vitamin B_3, 10 mg vitamin B_5, 2.2 mg vitamin B_6, 3 mcg vitamin B_{12}, 60 mg vitamin C, 0.4 mg folic acid. Sucrose, parabens.
Multi-Day with Beta Carotene	**Tablets:** 5000 IU vitamin A, 400 IU vitamin D, 10 IU vitamin E[2], 1.5 mg vitamin B_1, 1.7 mg vitamin B_2, 20 mg vitamin B_3, 10 mg vitamin B_5, 2 mg vitamin B_6, 6 mcg vitamin B_{12}, 60 mg vitamin C, 0.4 mg folic acid. Mannitol.
Multi-Day Plus Iron	**Tablets:** 5000 IU vitamin A, 400 IU vitamin D, 15 IU vitamin E[2], 1.5 mg vitamin B_1, 1.7 mg vitamin B_2, 20 mg vitamin B_3, 2 mg vitamin B_6, 6 mcg vitamin B_{12}, 60 mg vitamin C, 0.4 mg folic acid. Tartrazine, mannitol.
Sigtab	**Tablets:** 5000 IU vitamin A, 400 IU vitamin D, 15 IU vitamin E[2], 10.3 mg vitamin B_1, 10 mg vitamin B_2, 100 mg vitamin B_3, 20 mg vitamin B_5, 6 mg vitamin B_6, 18 mcg vitamin B_{12}, 333 mg vitamin C, 0.4 mg folic acid
Geri-Freeda[3] (sf)	**Tablets:** 5000 IU vitamin A, 400 IU vitamin D, 15 IU vitamin E[4], 15 mg vitamin B_1, 15 mg vitamin B_2, 50 mg vitamin B_3, 15 mg vitamin B_5, 15 mg vitamin B_6, 15 mcg vitamin B_{12}, 150 mg vitamin C, 0.4 mg folic acid
One-A-Day Essential, One-Tablet-Daily (sf), *Unicap M*[5] (sf)	**Tablets:** 5000 IU vitamin A, 400 IU vitamin D, 30 IU vitamin E[2], 1.5 mg vitamin B_1, 1.7 mg vitamin B_2, 20 mg vitamin B_3, 10 mg vitamin B_5, 2 mg vitamin B_6, 6 mcg vitamin B_{12}, 60 mg vitamin C, 0.4 mg folic acid
Freedavite (sf)	**Tablets:** 5000 IU vitamin A, 400 IU vitamin D, 30 IU vitamin E[4], 1.5 mg vitamin B_1, 1.7 mg vitamin B_2, 20 mg vitamin B_3, 10 mg vitamin B_5, 2 mg vitamin B_6, 6 mcg vitamin B_{12}, 60 mg vitamin C, 0.4 mg folic acid
One-A-Day Maximum Formula	**Tablets:** 5000 IU vitamin A, 400 IU vitamin D, 30 IU vitamin E[1], 1.5 mg vitamin B_1, 1.7 mg vitamin B_2, 20 mg vitamin B_3, 10 mg vitamin B_5, 2 mg vitamin B_6, 6 mcg vitamin B_{12}, 60 mg vitamin C, 0.4 mg folic acid, 25 mcg vitamin K
Multi-Day Plus Minerals	**Tablets:** 5000 IU vitamin A, 400 IU vitamin D, 30 IU vitamin E[2], 1.5 mg vitamin B_1, 1.7 mg vitamin B_2, 20 mg vitamin B_3, 10 mg vitamin B_5, 2 mg vitamin B_6, 6 mcg vitamin B_{12}, 60 mg vitamin C, 0.4 mg folic acid, 25 mcg vitamin K. Mannitol.
Therems, Theravim-M[6], *Therapeutic* (sf), *Therapeutic-M* (sf)[6]	**Tablets:** 5000 IU vitamin A, 400 IU vitamin D, 30 IU vitamin E[2], 3 mg vitamin B_1, 3.4 mg vitamin B_2, 20 mg vitamin B_3, 10 mg vitamin B_5, 3 mg vitamin B_6, 9 mcg vitamin B_{12}, 90 mg vitamin C, 0.4 mg folic acid
Yelets (sf)	**Tablets:** 5000 IU vitamin A, 400 IU vitamin D, 30 IU vitamin E[4], 10 mg vitamin B_1, 10 mg vitamin B_2, 25 mg vitamin B_3, 10 mg vitamin B_5, 10 mg vitamin B_6, 10 mcg vitamin B_{12}, 100 mg vitamin C, 0.4 mg folic acid

MULTIVITAMIN PRODUCTS

Trade name	Doseform
Hi-Kovite (sf)	**Tablets**: 5000 IU vitamin A, 400 IU vitamin D, 30 IU vitamin E[4], 10 mg vitamin B_1, 10 mg vitamin B_2, 100 mg vitamin B_3, 10 mg vitamin B_5, 10 mg vitamin B_6, 10 mcg vitamin B_{12}, 200 mg vitamin C, 0.4 mg folic acid. PABA.
Unicap T Stress Formula (sf)	**Tablets**: 5000 IU vitamin A, 400 IU vitamin D, 30 IU vitamin E[2], 10 mg vitamin B_1, 10 mg vitamin B_2, 100 mg vitamin B_3, 25 mg vitamin B_5, 6 mg vitamin B_6, 18 mcg vitamin B_{12}, 500 mg vitamin C, 0.4 mg folic acid. Tartrazine, sucrose, parabens.
Certagen Senior (sf)	**Tablets**: 5000 IU vitamin A, 400 IU vitamin D, 45 IU vitamin E[2], 1.5 mg vitamin B_1, 1.7 mg vitamin B_2, 20 mg vitamin B_3, 10 mg vitamin B_5, 3 mg vitamin B_6, 25 mcg vitamin B_{12}, 60 mg vitamin C, 0.4 mg folic acid, 10 mcg vitamin K. Mannitol.
Quintabs (sf), *Quintabs-M*[3] (sf), *Quintabs-M Iron Free*[3] (sf)	**Tablets**: 5000 IU vitamin A, 400 IU vitamin D, 50 IU vitamin E[4], 30 mg vitamin B_1, 30 mg vitamin B_2, 100 mg vitamin B_3, 30 mg vitamin B_5, 30 mg vitamin B_6, 30 mcg vitamin B_{12}, 300 mg vitamin C, 0.4 mg folic acid
One-A-Day 50 Plus Formula	**Tablets**: 5000 IU vitamin A, 400 IU vitamin D, 60 IU vitamin E[1], 4.5 mg vitamin B_1, 3.4 mg vitamin B_2, 20 mg vitamin B_3, 15 mg vitamin B_5, 6 mg vitamin B_6, 30 mcg vitamin B_{12}, 120 mg vitamin C, 0.4 mg folic acid, 20 mcg vitamin K
Ultra Freeda Iron Free (sf)	**Tablets**: 5000 IU vitamin A, 400 IU vitamin D, 200 IU vitamin E[4], 50 mg vitamin B_1, 50 mg vitamin B_2, 100 mg vitamin B_3, 100 mg vitamin B_5, 50 mg vitamin B_6, 100 mcg vitamin B_{12}, 1000 mg vitamin C, 0.8 mg folic acid
Oncovite	**Tablets**: 9000 IU vitamin A, 400 IU vitamin D, 100 IU vitamin E[4], 0.34 mg vitamin B_1, 0.5 mg vitamin B_2, 5 mg vitamin B_3, 2.3 mg vitamin B_5, 25 mg vitamin B_6, 1.6 mcg vitamin B_{12}, 500 mg vitamin C, 0.4 mg folic acid
Hexavitamin	**Tablets**: 5000 IU vitamin A, 400 IU vitamin D, 2 mg vitamin B_1, 3 mg vitamin B_2, 20 mg vitamin B_3, 75 mg vitamin C. Sucrose, parabens.
Oxi-Freeda (sf)	**Tablets**: 5000 IU vitamin A, 150 IU vitamin E[4], 20 mg vitamin B_1, 20 mg vitamin B_2, 40 mg vitamin B_3, 20 mg vitamin B_5, 20 mg vitamin B_6, 20 mcg vitamin B_{12}, 100 mg vitamin C
Os-Cal	**Tablets**: 125 IU vitamin D, 0.8 IU vitamin E[2], 1.7 mg vitamin B_1, 1.7 mg vitamin B_2, 15 mg vitamin B_3, 2 mg vitamin B_6, 50 mg vitamin C. Corn syrup, mineral oil, parabens, EDTA.
Ultra Freeda A-Free (sf)	**Tablets**: 400 IU vitamin D, 200 IU vitamin E[4], 50 mg vitamin B_1, 50 mg vitamin B_2, 100 mg vitamin B_3, 100 mg vitamin B_5, 50 mg vitamin B_6, 100 mcg vitamin B_{12}, 1000 mg vitamin C, 0.8 mg folic acid
Stress Formula Vitamins (sf), *Stress Formula with Iron* (sf), *Stress Formula with Zinc* (sf)	**Tablets**: 30 IU vitamin E[2], 10 mg vitamin B_1, 10 mg vitamin B_2, 100 mg vitamin B_3, 20 mg vitamin B_5, 5 mg vitamin B_6, 12 mcg vitamin B_{12}, 500 mg vitamin C, 0.4 mg folic acid

MULTIVITAMIN PRODUCTS

Trade name	Doseform
Nephro-Vite, Dialyvite 800, Dialyvite 800 with with Iron, Dialyvite 800 with Zinc 15	**Tablets:** 1.5 mg vitamin B_1, 1.7 mg vitamin B_2, 20 mg vitamin B_3, 10 mg vitamin B_5, 10 mg vitamin B_6, 6 mcg vitamin B_{12}, 60 mg vitamin C, 0.8 mg folic acid. Lactose.
Vitalets (sf)	**Tablets, chewable:** 2500 IU vitamin A, 200 IU vitamin D, 15 IU vitamin E^4, 0.75 mg vitamin B_1, 0.85 mg vitamin B_2, 10 mg vitamin B_3, 5 mg vitamin B_5, 1 mg vitamin B_6, 3 mcg vitamin B_{12}, 40 mg vitamin C, 0.2 mg folic acid. Mannitol, sorbitol.
One-A-Day Kids Scooby Doo Plus Calcium[7], My First Flintstones, Flintstones Plus Calcium[7], Flintstones Plus Iron, Poly-Vi-Sol, Poly-Vi-Sol with Iron	**Tablets, chewable:** 2500 IU vitamin A, 400 IU vitamin D, 15 IU vitamin E^1, 1.05 mg vitamin B_1, 1.2 mg vitamin B_2, 13.5 mg vitamin B_3, 1.05 mg vitamin B_6, 4.5 mcg vitamin B_{12}, 60 mg vitamin C, 0.3 mg folic acid
Fruity Chews[8], Fruity Chews with Iron[8]	**Tablets, chewable:** 2500 IU vitamin A, 400 IU vitamin D, 15 IU vitamin E^2, 1.05 mg vitamin B_1, 1.2 mg vitamin B_2, 13.5 mg vitamin B_3, 1.05 mg vitamin B_6, 4.5 mcg vitamin B_{12}, 60 mg vitamin C, 0.3 mg folic acid
Flintstones Plus Extra C Children's, One-A-Day Kids Bugs Bunny and Friends Plus Extra C[7] (sf)	**Tablets, chewable:** 2500 IU vitamin A, 400 IU vitamin D, 15 IU vitamin E^1, 1.05 mg vitamin B_1, 1.2 mg vitamin B_2, 13.5 mg vitamin B_3, 1.05 mg vitamin B_6, 4.5 mcg vitamin B_{12}, 250 mg vitamin C, 0.3 mg folic acid
Bounty Buddies Plus Extra C	**Tablets, chewable:** 2500 IU vitamin A, 400 IU vitamin D, 15 IU vitamin E^2, 1.05 mg vitamin B_1, 1.2 mg vitamin B_2, 13.5 mg vitamin B_3, 1.05 mg vitamin B_6, 4.5 mcg vitamin B_{12}, 250 mg vitamin C, 0.3 mg folic acid. Sucrose.
SunKist Children's Plus Extra C	**Tablets, chewable:** 2500 IU vitamin A, 400 IU vitamin D, 15 IU vitamin E^1, 1.1 mg vitamin B_1, 1.2 mg vitamin B_2, 14 mg vitamin B_3, 1 mg vitamin B_6, 5 mcg vitamin B_{12}, 235 mg vitamin C, 0.3 mg folic acid, 5 mcg vitamin K. Sorbitol, tartrazine, sucrose, lactose, aspartame.
Centrum Chewables	**Tablets, chewable:** 3500 IU vitamin A, 400 IU vitamin D, 30 IU vitamin E^2, 1.5 mg vitamin B_1, 1.7 mg vitamin B_2, 20 mg vitamin B_3, 10 mg vitamin B_5, 2 mg vitamin B_6, 6 mcg vitamin B_{12}, 60 mg vitamin C, 0.4 mg folic acid, 10 mcg vitamin K. Sucrose, lactose, dextrose, fructose, mannitol, aspartame.
Centrum Kids Extra Calcium	**Tablets, chewable:** 5000 IU vitamin A, 400 IU vitamin D, 15 IU vitamin E^2, 1.5 mg vitamin B_1, 1.7 mg vitamin B_2, 13.5 mg vitamin B_3, 1 mg vitamin B_6, 5 mcg vitamin B_{12}, 60 mg vitamin C, 0.3 mg folic acid. Sucrose, mannitol, lactose, fructose, dextrose, aspartame.
Centrum Kids with Extra C	**Tablets, chewable:** 5000 IU vitamin A, 400 IU vitamin D, 15 IU vitamin E^2, 1.5 mg vitamin B_1, 1.7 mg vitamin B_2, 13.5 mg vitamin B_3, 1 mg vitamin B_6, 5 mcg vitamin B_{12}, 250 mg vitamin C, 0.3 mg folic acid. Sucrose, mannitol, lactose, fructose, dextrose, aspartame.
Flintstones Complete[7], One-A-Day Kids Scooby Doo Complete	**Tablets, chewable:** 5000 IU vitamin A, 400 IU vitamin D, 30 IU vitamin E^1, 1.5 mg vitamin B_1, 1.7 mg vitamin B_2, 20 mg vitamin B_3, 10 mg vitamin B_5, 2 mg vitamin B_6, 6 mcg vitamin B_{12}, 60 mg vitamin C, 0.4 mg folic acid

MULTIVITAMIN PRODUCTS

Trade name	Doseform
Centrum Kids Complete	**Tablets, chewable**: 5000 IU vitamin A, 400 IU vitamin D, 30 IU vitamin E[2], 1.5 mg vitamin B_1, 1.7 mg vitamin B_2, 20 mg vitamin B_3, 10 mg vitamin B_5, 2 mg vitamin B_6, 6 mcg vitamin B_{12}, 60 mg vitamin C, 0.4 mg folic acid, 10 mcg vitamin K. Sucrose, fructose, mannitol, lactose, aspartame.
Theragran-M	**Caplets**: 5000 IU vitamin A, 400 IU vitamin D, 30 IU vitamin E[2], 3 mg vitamin B_1, 3.4 mg vitamin B_2, 20 mg vitamin B_3, 10 mg vitamin B_5, 3 mg vitamin B_6, 9 mcg vitamin B_{12}, 90 mg vitamin C, 0.4 mg folic acid. Lactose, sucrose.
Drops and Liquids[9]	
Certagen	**Liquid**: 2500 IU vitamin A, 400 IU vitamin D, 30 IU vitamin E[2], 1.5 mg vitamin B_1, 1.7 mg vitamin B_2, 20 mg vitamin B_3, 10 mg vitamin B_5, 2 mg vitamin B_6, 6 mcg vitamin B_{12}, 60 mg vitamin C/15 mL. Glycerin, orange oil, lemon oil.
Theravite	**Liquid**: 5000 IU vitamin A, 400 IU vitamin D, 10 mg vitamin B_1, 10 mg vitamin B_2, 100 mg vitamin B_3, 21.4 mg vitamin B_5, 4.1 mg vitamin B_6, 5 mcg vitamin B_{12}, 200 mg vitamin C/5 mL. Glycerin, methylparaben.
Geri-Vite	**Drops**: 5 mg vitamin B_1, 2.5 mg vitamin B_2, 50 mg vitamin B_3, 10 mg vitamin B_5, 1 mg vitamin B_6, 1 mcg vitamin B_{12}/30 mL. Glycerin, sorbitol, saccharin.
Baby Vitamin (sf)	**Drops**: 1500 IU vitamin A, 400 IU vitamin D, 5 IU vitamin E[4], 0.5 mg vitamin B_1, 0.6 mg vitamin B_2, 8 mg vitamin B_3, 0.4 mg vitamin B_6, 2 mcg vitamin B_{12}, 35 mg vitamin C/mL. Glycerin.
Poly-Vi-Sol, Poly-Vi-Sol with Iron	**Drops**: 1500 IU vitamin A, 400 IU vitamin D, 5 IU vitamin E[1], 0.5 mg vitamin B_1, 0.6 mg vitamin B_2, 8 mg vitamin B_3, 0.4 mg vitamin B_6, 2 mcg vitamin B_{12}, 35 mg vitamin C/mL. Glycerin, methylparaben, orange oil. Alcohol free.
Tri-Vi-Sol, Tri-Vi-Sol with Iron	**Drops**: 1500 IU vitamin A, 400 IU vitamin D, 35 mg vitamin C/mL. Glycerin.

Products listed are representative of currently available and widely distributed brands. Similar products, including regional and private label brands, may also exist.

sf = Sugar free.
[1] Form of vitamin E unknown.
[2] As dl-alpha tocopheryl acetate.
[3] Contains PABA.
[4] As d-alpha tocopheryl acid succinate.
[5] Contains sucrose, tartrazine, parabens.
[6] Contains mannitol.
[7] Contains aspartame.
[8] Contains sucrose, cottonseed oil.
[9] May contain alcohol.

PATIENT INFORMATION
Multivitamin Products
- Do not exceed recommended dosages.
- Swallow tablets whole; do not crush or chew.

MULTIVITAMIN/HERBAL COMBINATIONS

► Actions

In addition to the products listed below, many other forms of combination vitamin/herbal products are available. Many of these products also contain recommended amounts of minerals. However, for the purposes of this monograph, only vitamin and herbal content have been provided.

MULTIVITAMIN/HERBAL PRODUCTS	
Trade Name	Doseform
One-A-Day WeightSmart	**Tablets**: 2500 IU vitamin A, 400 IU vitamin D, 30 IU vitamin E[1], 1.9 mg vitamin B_1, 2.125 mg vitamin B_2, 25 mg vitamin B_3, 12.5 mg vitamin B_5, 2.5 mg vitamin B_6, 7.5 mcg vitamin B_{12}, 60 mg vitamin C, 0.4 mg folic acid, 80 mcg vitamin K, 27 mg green tea extract. Dextrose.
One-A-Day Today For Active Women 50 and Over	**Tablets**: 3000 IU vitamin A, 400 IU vitamin D, 33 IU vitamin E[2], 1.1 mg vitamin B_1, 1.7 mg vitamin B_2, 14 mg vitamin B_3, 5 mg vitamin B_5, 3 mg vitamin B_6, 18 mcg vitamin B_{12}, 75 mg vitamin C, 0.4 mg folic acid, 20 mcg vitamin K, 10 mg soy extract
Centrum Performance	**Tablets**: 3500 IU vitamin A, 400 IU vitamin D, 60 IU vitamin E[1], 4.5 mg vitamin B_1, 5.1 mg vitamin B_2, 40 mg vitamin B_3, 10 mg vitamin B_5, 6 mg vitamin B_6, 18 mcg vitamin B_{12}, 120 mg vitamin C, 0.4 mg folic acid, 25 mcg vitamin K, 50 mg ginseng root[3], 60 mg ginkgo biloba leaf. Lactose, sucrose.
One-A-Day Active Formula	**Tablets**: 5000 IU vitamin A, 400 IU vitamin D, 60 IU vitamin E[2], 4.5 mg vitamin B_1, 5.1 mg vitamin B_2, 40 mg vitamin B_3, 10 mg vitamin B_5, 6 mg vitamin B_6, 18 mcg vitamin B_{12}, 120 mg vitamin C, 0.4 mg folic acid, 25 mcg vitamin K, 55 mg ginseng extract[3]
One-A-Day Joint Health	**Tablets**: 30 mg vitamin C, 30 IU vitamin E[2], 500 mg glucosamine sulfate, 134 mg devil's claw extract
One-A-Day Energy Formula	**Tablets**: 2.25 mg vitamin B_1, 20 mg vitamin B_3, 10 mg vitamin B_5, 3 mg vitamin B_6, 200 mg ginseng root[3], 0.2 mg folic acid

Products listed are representative of currently available and widely distributed brands. Similar products, including regional and private label brands, may also exist.

[1] As dl-alpha tocopheryl acetate.
[2] Form of vitamin E unknown.
[3] As panax ginseng.

NON-VITAMIN DEFICIENCY
(Minerals, Electrolytes, and Trace Elements)

DEFINITION

Non-vitamin deficiencies are caused by a person's inability to utilize minerals, electrolytes, or trace elements because of a genetic defect, malabsorption dysfunction, or dietary deficiency.

ETIOLOGY

Many individuals have incorporated supplemental minerals, electrolytes, or trace elements into their health lifestyle. This is appropriate when the diet is neglected or nutritional needs require supplementation (eg, pregnancy, lactation, excessive menstrual flow, malabsorption, hypermetabolic or catabolic conditions, crash diets, alcoholism, dentition problems, rapid growth phases in children).

One of the great potential dangers of overreliance on vitamin, mineral, electrolyte, or trace element supplementation is that the individual may allow these supplements to supplant other nutrients in food, particularly protein, carbohydrates, and fat. Further, if vitamins, minerals, electrolytes, or trace elements are used to treat undiagnosed medical conditions, the delays in seeking appropriate medical attention can be extremely dangerous.

This monograph recognizes the essentiality of a variety of minerals, electrolytes, and trace elements (eg, iodine, manganese, copper, zinc, selenium, chromium, molybdenum) but will focus on the 5 agents most commonly associated with deficiency states: calcium, phosphorus, magnesium, potassium, and iron.

Minerals:

Calcium – Calcium, the most abundant mineral in the body, plays an important role in nerve and muscle function, is integral to the structure of teeth and bones, and is needed for blood to clot. Bones and teeth are 90% calcium. The small intestine controls calcium absorption. Calcium requirements may increase as protein consumption increases. Decreased calcium levels for prolonged periods of time may contribute significantly to growth retardation, bone deformities, fractures, and accelerated osteoporosis.

Phosphorus – Phosphorus helps to build bones and teeth. It is involved in the release of energy from fats, protein, and carbohydrates, and in the formation of genetic material, cell membranes, and many enzymes. Phosphate balance is maintained by the GI tract and the kidneys. Hypophosphatemia affects the central nervous, musculoskeletal, cardiac, respiratory, and hematopoietic systems. Most effects can be attributed to impaired cellular energy stores and tissue hypoxia.

Magnesium – Magnesium is a mineral used in building bones, manufacturing proteins, releasing energy from muscle storage, and regulating body temperature. Deficiency is related to decreased intake, decreased absorption, or an increased loss in the urine or GI fluids. Drugs also may cause increased magnesium loss.

Electrolytes:

Potassium – Potassium has 2 major functions in the body: participation in cell metabolism in such processes as protein and glycogen synthesis, and determination of resting potential across cell membranes. Under normal conditions, dietary deficiency of potassium does not occur. The most common cause of deficiency is excessive loss from prolonged vomiting, chronic diarrhea, laxative abuse, and diuretic use.

Trace elements:

Iron – Iron primarily functions as a carrier of oxygen in the body, both as a part of hemoglobin in the blood and myoglobin in the muscles. It plays an important role in the formation of red blood cells and a number of enzymes that work to build, repair, and maintain the body. Iron deficiency may occur in anyone consuming a diet deficient in iron. However, there are time periods and life stages when iron deficiency is most likely. These include the following:

- six months to 4 years of age
- early adolescence/rapid growth phases
- menstrual iron loss in female reproductive years (blood loss is typically 60 to 80 mL/cycle but may be as high as 200 mL)
- during or immediately after pregnancy

Donation of 1 unit (1 pint) of blood produces a loss of approximately 250 mg of iron. Drug-induced blood loss may occur with chronic use of salicylates, nonsteroidal anti-inflammatory drugs (NSAIDs), warfarin, and ulcerogenic drugs (eg, oral corticosteroids). Excessive blood loss also may be associated with gastrointestinal diseases such as gastric or duodenal ulcer, ulcerative colitis, Crohn disease, esophageal varices, diverticulitis, hemorrhoids, intestinal parasites, and cancer.

PATHOPHYSIOLOGY

Minerals: Minerals are essential in promoting growth and maintaining health. They are constituents of all body tissues and fluids, and they are important factors in maintaining many physiologic processes. Minerals act as catalysts in nerve response, muscle contraction, and metabolism of nutrients. They assist in regulating electrolyte balance and hormonal production, and strengthen skeletal structures. Mineral deficiencies are treated by adding the deficient mineral(s) to the diet through appropriate foods or dietary supplements.

Electrolytes: Principal electrolytes (potassium, sodium, and chloride) are essential dietary components. Electrolytes maintain water balance, encourage or prevent water flow across cell membranes (through osmosis), transmit electrical impulses across cell membranes, and play a role in enzyme and chemical reactions.

Trace elements: Trace elements (also known as microminerals) include arsenic, chromium, cobalt, copper, fluoride, iodine, iron, manganese, molybdenum, nickel, selenium, silicon, tin, vanadium, and zinc. Trace elements have varying uses in the body.

SIGNS/SYMPTOMS

Calcium: Calcium deficiency may lead to osteoporosis, growth retardation, bone deformities, or fractures. Osteoporosis is the gradual reduction in bone mass to a point where the skeleton is compromised, thus increasing fracture risk. For more information, see the Osteoporosis monograph in the Musculoskeletal Conditions chapter. The current RDA for calcium establishes the amount needed to protect against nutrient deficiency.

Phosphorus: Severe hypophosphatemia may be associated with generalized muscle weakness, paresthesia, acute respiratory failure, seizures, and coma.

Magnesium: Hypomagnesemia may cause neuromuscular changes, psychiatric effects, and adverse cardiac rhythm.

Potassium: Deficiency symptoms include muscle weakness, anorexia, nausea, muscle cramps, listlessness, apprehension, drowsiness, and irrational behavior. Severe hypokalemia may result in cardiac dysrhythmias.

Iron: Iron deficiency causes anemia. Symptoms of deficiency include fatigue, lethargy, pallor, shortness of breath, dizziness, palpitations, tachycardia, exhaustion, and decreased physical performance.

DIAGNOSTIC PARAMETERS/PHYSICAL ASSESSMENT

Clinical Observation: Serum concentrations of these agents can be tested by drawing and analyzing blood.

Calcium – The normal serum calcium concentration is 9 to 10.5 mg/dL.

Potassium – The normal serum potassium concentration is 3.5 to 5.5 mEq/L.

Phosphorus – The normal serum phosphorus concentration is 2.5 to 5 mg/dL.

Magnesium – The normal serum magnesium concentration is 1.3 to 2.2 mEq/L.

Iron – The normal iron concentration is 30 to 160 mcg/dL (women) and 45 to 160 mcg/dL (men).

Interview:

- Detect dietary habits that predispose to mineral, electrolyte, or trace element deficiency (eg, low consumption of dairy products and other calcium-rich foods).
- Investigate presence of signs and symptoms as listed above.
- Query about medical conditions that could predispose to mineral, electrolyte, or trace element deficiency.

TREATMENT

Nondrug therapy:

Calcium – Eating calcium-rich food replenishes calcium in bone. Milk, yogurt, cheese, tofu, dark green leafy vegetables, eggs, and fish contain the greatest concentration of dietary calcium.

Dietary sources rich in calcium include:

Dietary Product	Calcium Content
Yogurt, plain, low-fat	400 mg/cup (8 oz)
Milk, skim, low-fat, or whole	300 mg/cup (8 oz)
Collard greens	300 mg/cup (8 oz)
Cheese	200 mg/oz
Ice cream	200 mg/cup (8 oz)
Canned pink tuna	200 mg/3.5 oz
Broccoli	100 mg/cup (8 oz)
Navy beans	100 mg/cup (8 oz)

Phosphorus – Phosphorus is supplied in the diet from meat, poultry, fish, grain products, and milk.

Magnesium – All unprocessed foods contain magnesium in differing amounts. The highest concentrations are found in nuts, legumes, and unmilled grains. Magnesium also may be found in meat, poultry, and fish.

Potassium – Potassium is distributed widely in foods, with the richest sources being fruits and vegetables. Salt substitutes also are a source of potassium.

Iron – Dietary iron comes from meat, eggs, chicken, fish, green leafy vegetables, fruit, grain cereals, breads, nuts, and beans. The ability of the body to absorb and utilize iron from various food sources varies.

Pharmacotherapy: Mineral, electrolyte, and trace element supplements are used in individuals who do not obtain them in adequate amounts from their diet or when a significant deficiency exists.

In the following product tables, only single-agent mineral supplements are listed; however, patients should be aware that many multivitamin and mineral products also exist and certain recommended amounts of the minerals are discussed in this monograph.

CALCIUM

▶ **Actions**

Calcium is the fifth most abundant element in the body; the majority is found in bone. It is essential for the functional integrity of the central nervous and muscular systems, normal cardiac function, cell permeability, and blood coagulation. It also functions as an enzyme cofactor and affects the secretory activity of endocrine and exocrine glands.

Adequate calcium intake is particularly important during periods of bone growth in childhood and adolescence, during pregnancy and lactation, in postmenopausal women, and in men older than 50 years of age. An adequate supply of calcium is necessary in adults, especially those older than 40 years of age, to prevent a negative calcium balance that may contribute to the development of osteoporosis. (For more information, see the Osteoporosis monograph in the Musculoskeletal Conditions chapter.)

Patients with advanced renal insufficiency exhibit phosphate retention and some degree of hyperphosphatemia. The retention of phosphate plays a pivotal role in causing secondary hyperparathyroidism associated with osteodystrophy and soft tissue calcification.

Calcium must be in a soluble, ionized form to be absorbed. Solubility (except calcium lactate) is increased in an acidic pH. Different forms of supplemental calcium vary in the amount of elemental calcium they contain as indicated in the chart below:

Calcium Supplement	% Elemental Calcium
Calcium glubionate	6.5
Calcium gluconate	9.3
Calcium lactate	13
Calcium citrate	21
Calcium acetate	25
Tricalcium phosphate	39
Calcium carbonate	40

Calcium carbonate is the richest source of calcium and is recommended frequently. Calcium citrate is the most soluble source of calcium and is frequently recommended in patients receiving acid-secretory drugs such as H_2 antagonists (eg, famotidine, ranitidine) and proton pump inhibitors (eg, omeprazole, lansoprazole). Less soluble calcium supplements have their absorption impaired by H_2 antagonists and proton pump inhibitors.

An adequate amount of vitamin D is needed for proper absorption of calcium. Vitamin D supplementation is useful in patients who have low dietary intake of vitamin D or insufficient exposure to sunlight. Many calcium supplements contain vitamin D. For more information on vitamin D, see the Vitamin Deficiency monograph.

► Indications

As a dietary supplement when calcium intake may be inadequate. Conditions that may be associated with calcium deficiency include the following: vitamin D deficiency, sprue, pregnancy and lactation, achlorhydria, chronic diarrhea, hypoparathyroidism, steatorrhea, menopause, renal failure, pancreatitis, hyperphosphatemia, and alkalosis. Some diuretics and anticonvulsants may precipitate hypocalcemia, which may validate calcium replacement therapy. Calcium salt therapy should not preclude the use of other corrective measures intended to treat the underlying cause of calcium depletion.

Oral calcium also may be used in the treatment of osteoporosis, osteomalacia, rickets, and latent tetany.

Calcium taken daily may help reduce typical premenstrual syndrome (PMS) symptoms such as bloating, cramps, fatigue, and moodiness.

Unlabeled uses: Calcium supplementation may lower blood pressure in some hypertensive patients with indices suggesting calcium "deficiency." However, other hypertensive patients may experience a blood pressure-elevating response. Also, people with a high dietary intake of calcium may have a lower incidence of polyps in the colon and rectum (colorectal adenomas).

▶ **Contraindications**

Hypercalcemia; ventricular fibrillation.

▶ **Warnings**

GI effects: Calcium salts may be irritating to the GI tract when administered orally and also may cause constipation.

Hypercalcemia: Hypercalcemia may occur when large doses of calcium are administered to patients with chronic renal failure. Mild hypercalcemia may exhibit as nausea, vomiting, anorexia, or constipation, with mental changes such as stupor, delirium, coma, or confusion. By reducing calcium intake, mild hypercalcemia usually is controlled.

Renal calculi: Recent evidence from studies in men 40 to 75 years of age with no history of kidney stones and women 34 to 59 years of age show that high dietary intake of calcium decreases the risk of symptomatic renal calculi, while intake of supplemental calcium may increase the risk of symptomatic stones. This conflicts with the previous theory that high calcium intake contributes to the risk of renal calculi.

Special-risk patients: Use calcium salts cautiously in patients with sarcoidosis, cardiac or renal disease, and in patients receiving cardiac glycosides.

Calcium citrate:

  Renal function impairment – Avoid concurrent aluminum-containing antacids.

Phenylketonurics: Inform phenylketonuric patients that some of these products contain phenylalanine.

Tartrazine sensitivity: Some of these products may contain tartrazine, which may cause allergic-type reactions (including bronchial asthma) in susceptible individuals. Although the incidence of sensitivity is low, it is seen frequently in patients who have aspirin hypersensitivity. Specific products containing tartrazine are identified in the product listings.

▶ **Drug Interactions**

Calcium Drug Interactions			
Precipitant	**Object drug***		**Description**
Calcium carbonate	Quinolones	↓	GI absorption of quinolones may be decreased. The bioavailability of norfloxacin may be reduced; lomefloxacin and ofloxacin do not appear to be affected. Give antacids at least 6 hours before or 2 hours after the quinolone.
Calcium salts	Iron salts	↓	GI absorption of iron may be reduced. In order to avoid a possible interaction, separate administration times whenever possible.
Calcium salts	Sodium polystyrene sulfonate	↓	Coadministration in patients with renal impairment may result in an unanticipated metabolic alkalosis and a reduction of the resin's binding of potassium. Separate drugs by several hours.
Calcium salts	Tetracyclines	↓	The absorption and serum levels of tetracyclines are decreased; a decreased anti-infective response may occur. Avoid simultaneous administration. Separate administration by 3 to 4 hours.

Calcium Drug Interactions			
Precipitant	**Object drug***		**Description**
Calcium salts	Verapamil	↓	Clinical effects and toxicities of verapamil may be reversed.

* ↓ = Object drug decreased.

Food: Diets that consist of large amounts of animal protein and sodium may increase urinary calcium excretion. Diets that include large amounts of wheat bran may decrease calcium absorption. Other sources of dietary fiber have not been shown to affect calcium absorption.

► **Adverse Reactions**

GI disturbances are rare. Mild hypercalcemia (Ca^{++} greater than 10.5 mg/dL) may be asymptomatic or manifest as anorexia, nausea, vomiting, or constipation. More severe hypercalcemia (Ca^{++} greater than 12 mg/dL) may be associated with kidney stones, confusion, delirium, stupor, and coma.

► **Overdosage**

Excessive use of calcium supplements can cause severe hypercalcemia (see Adverse Reactions). Severe hypercalcemia can be treated with acute hemodialysis and by discontinuing therapy.

► **Administration and Dosage**

The previous RDA for calcium had been set at levels associated with maximum retention of body calcium. In new information, the DRI for calcium establishes the amount needed to protect against nutrient deficiency; this is intended to optimize health and minimize the risk of chronic disease. For a complete listing of RDAs and DRIs, see the tables at the beginning of this chapter.

Daily Reference Intakes (DRIs) for Calcium	
Age (years) or condition	**DRI (mg)**
0 to 6 months	210
7 months to 1 year	270
1 to 3 years	500
4 to 8 years	800
9 to 18 years	1300
Adults	1000-1300
Pregnant/Lactating women	1000-1300

Calcium carbonate is recommended as the initial choice. A calcium supplement that contains vitamin D may increase the absorption of calcium (for a representative list of calcium products that contain vitamin D, refer to the Osteoporosis monograph in the Musculoskeletal Conditions chapter). The usual daily dose of calcium is 500 mg 2 to 4 times daily; doses over 1500 mg/day are seldom recommended because of increased potential for adverse effects.

Calcium-containing antacids: Calcium-containing antacids also may be used; refer to the Heartburn and GERD monograph in the Gastrointestinal Conditions chapter for product information on calcium-containing antacids (eg, *Tums*).

CALCIUM PRODUCTS

Trade name	Doseform	Elemental Calcium (mg)
Calcium Gluconate	**Tablets**: 648 mg (10 grain) calcium gluconate	60
Calcium Lactate(sf)	**Tablets**: 650 mg calcium lactate	84
Calcium Gluconate	**Tablets**: 972 mg (15 grain) calcium gluconate	90
Florical	**Tablets**: 364 mg calcium carbonate, 3.75 mg fluoride	145
Titralac(sf)	**Tablets**: 420 mg calcium carbonate	168
Monocal	**Tablets**: 625 mg calcium carbonate, 3 mg fluoride	250
Titralac Extra Strength(sf)	**Tablets**: 750 mg calcium carbonate	300
Oysco 500	**Tablets**: 500 mg calcium (from oyster shell). Tartrazine.	500
Caltrate 600, Nephro-Calci	**Tablets**: 1.5 g calcium carbonate	600
Citracal Ultradense, Citrus Calcium	**Tablets, coated**: 200 mg calcium (as calcium citrate). Lactose free.	200
Amitone	**Tablets, chewable**: 350 mg calcium carbonate	140
Titralac Plus(sf)	**Tablets, chewable**: 420 mg calcium carbonate, 21 mg simethicone. Saccharin. Spearmint flavor.	168
Tums Regular Strength	**Tablets, chewable**: 500 mg calcium carbonate. Sucrose. Peppermint flavor.	200
Cal-Mint(sf)	**Tablets, chewable**: 650 mg calcium carbonate. Mannitol, sorbitol. Peppermint flavor.	260
Tums E•X	**Tablets, chewable**: 750 mg calcium carbonate. Sucrose, tartrazine. Assorted fruit flavors.	300
Tums Sugar Free Extra Strength(sf)	**Tablets, chewable**: 750 mg calcium carbonate. Sorbitol, aspartame. Orange cream flavor.	300
Tums Smooth Dissolve	**Tablets, chewable**: 750 mg calcium carbonate. Sorbitol, dextrose, sucrose, tartrazine. Assorted fruit flavors.	300
Alka-Mints	**Tablets, chewable**: 850 mg calcium carbonate. Sugar, sorbitol. Assorted and spearmint flavors.	340
Tums Ultra	**Tablets, chewable**: 1 g calcium carbonate. Sucrose, tartrazine. Assorted fruit and peppermint flavors.	400
Calci-Chew	**Tablets, chewable**: 1.25 g calcium carbonate. Sugar. Cherry, lemon, and orange flavors.	500
Os-Cal	**Tablets, chewable**: 1.25 g calcium carbonate. Dextrose monohydrate.	500
Tums Calcium for Life Bone Health	**Tablets, chewable**: 1.25 g calcium carbonate. Sucrose.	500
Citracal Effervescent Liqui-tabs	**Tablets, effervescent**: 500 mg calcium (as calcium citrate). Phenylalanine, aspartame. Orange flavor.	500
Cal-GLU(sf)	**Capsules**: 50 mg calcium (calcium gluconate)	50
Florical	**Capsules**: 364 mg calcium carbonate (as oyster shell), 3.75 mg fluoride	145
Cal-Citrate 225(sf)	**Capsules**: 225 mg calcium (calcium citrate)	225
Calci-Mix	**Capsules**: 1.25 g calcium carbonate	500
Chooz(sf)	**Gum**: 500 mg calcium carbonate. Aspartame, 2.4 mg phenylalanine, sorbitol. Mint flavor.	200
Calcium Gluconate(sf)	**Powder**: 3.9 g calcium gluconate/tbsp. Lactose free.	347

Products listed are representative of currently available and widely distributed brands. Similar products, including regional and private label brands, may also exist.

sf = Sugar free.

PATIENT INFORMATION
Calcium Supplements

- Do not take calcium supplements within 1 to 2 hours of interacting medications.
- Eating a well-balanced diet and obtaining periodic sun exposure usually satisfies vitamin D requirements necessary for adequate calcium absorption. Do not use vitamin D and calcium supplements as a substitute for a well-balanced diet.
- When determining calcium content of a product in reference to RDI or RDA, use the amount of elemental calcium contained in the product (not the amount of calcium salt).
- Calcium is poorly absorbed. Thus, limit each dose to 500 mg elemental calcium.
- Avoid tobacco products and excessive consumption of alcohol and caffeine (over 8 cups of coffee/day or the caffeine equivalent), which increase your risk of developing osteoporosis.
- Chewable calcium tablets should be chewed before swallowing.
- Take with or following meals to enhance absorption.
- Drink a full glass of water with each dose.
- Notify your doctor if you experience appetite loss, nausea, vomiting, constipation, stomach pain, dry mouth, thirst, or polyuria.
- Some of these products contain phenylalanine. Consult your doctor.
- Individuals with decreased gastric acid production (eg, the elderly, patients taking certain nonprescription H_2 antagonists and prescription H_2 antagonists and proton pump inhibitors) may derive maximum benefits from calcium citrate supplements.
- Avoid products made from bone meal or dolomite because of possible product contamination with lead, mercury, or arsenic. Calcium carbonate supplements from oyster shell or "natural sources" may contain lead and aluminum. To ensure federal standards regarding purity and quality are met, look for "USP" on the package labeling.
- If being treated for hypocalcemia, avoid taking calcium within 1 to 2 hours of eating large amounts of fiber-containing foods, such as bran and whole-grain cereals or breads.
- Do not take other medicines or dietary supplements containing large amounts of calcium, phosphates, magnesium, or vitamin D without checking with your doctor.

PHOSPHORUS

▶ **Actions**

Phosphorus is an important component of all cells in the body; 80% to 85% of body phosphorus is present in the skeletal system. The remainder functions intracellularly for: 1) Energy transport and production in the form of ATP and ADP; 2) phospholipids in cell membranes responsible for nutrient transport; 3) part of nucleic acids (RNA, DNA); and 4) buffering systems and calcium transport.

Phosphate administration may lower urinary calcium levels and increases urinary phosphate levels.

▶ Indications

For use as a dietary supplement of phosphorus, particularly if the diet is restricted or if nutritional needs are increased.

Neutra-Phos and *Neutra-Phos-K* are useful in the treatment of children and adults with conditions associated with excessive renal phosphate loss or inadequate GI absorption of phosphate. They are useful also as adjunct supplementation in the management of phosphate diabetes.

▶ Contraindications

Addison disease; hyperkalemia; acid urine in urinary stone disease; patients with infected urolithiasis or struvite stone formation; severely impaired renal function (less than 30% of normal); presence of hyperphosphatemia; hypersensitivity to active or inactive ingredients.

▶ Warnings

Monitoring: The following determinations are important in patient monitoring (other tests may be warranted in some patients): renal function; serum calcium; serum phosphorus; serum potassium; serum sodium. Monitor at periodic intervals during therapy.

Sodium/Potassium restriction: Use with caution if patient is on a sodium- or potassium-restricted diet. These products may provide significant amounts of sodium or potassium.

Special-risk patients: Use with caution when the following medical problems exist: cardiac disease (particularly in digitalized patients); acute dehydration; significant renal function impairment or chronic renal disease; extensive tissue breakdown; myotonia congenita; cardiac failure; cirrhosis of the liver or severe hepatic disease; peripheral and pulmonary edema; hypernatremia; hypertension; preeclampsia; hypoparathyroidism; osteomalacia; acute pancreatitis; rickets (rickets may benefit from phosphate therapy; however, use caution); severe adrenal insufficiency.

Kidney stones: Advise patients with kidney stones of the possibility of passing stones when phosphate therapy is started.

Potential GI problems: There have been reports in the literature of small bowel lesions with some long-acting and coated potassium tablets. Orthophosphates may cause dyspepsia in patients with a history of peptic ulcer; other modes of therapy may be necessary in such patients.

Pregnancy: Category C. It is not known whether this product can cause fetal harm or can affect reproductive capacity when administered to a pregnant woman. Use only when clearly needed.

Lactation: It is not known whether this drug is excreted in breast milk. Exercise caution when administering to a nursing woman.

Children: For pediatric patients younger than 4 years of age, use only as directed by your doctor.

► Drug Interactions

Phosphate Drug Interactions			
Precipitant drug	**Object drug***		**Description**
Antacids	Phosphates	↓	Antacids containing magnesium, aluminum, or calcium may bind to phosphate and prevent its absorption.
Calcium Vitamin D	Phosphates	↓	The effects of phosphates may be antagonized in the treatment of hypercalcemia.
Iron supplements	Phosphate	↓	Iron-containing medications have the ability to bind phosphate and form an insoluble complex, thus preventing absorption.
Androgens	Potassium and phosphate	↑	Androgens may cause retention of potassium and phosphate. Therefore, concurrent use with potassium phosphate may cause hyperkalemia or hyperphosphatemia.
Phosphate	Anorexiants	↓	Acidification of urine may increase elimination and decrease therapeutic effect of anorexiants.
Phosphate	Chlorpropamide (sulfonylurea)	↑	Acidification of urine may increase bioavailability of chlorpropamide and enhance the hypoglycemic actions.
Phosphate	Methadone	↓	Acidification of the urine increases renal clearance of methadone because of increased ionization.
Phosphate	Sympatho-mimetics	↓	Acidification of urine may increase elimination and decrease therapeutic effect of sympathomimetics.

* ↑ = Object drug increased.   ↓ = Object drug decreased.

► Adverse Reactions

Individuals may experience a mild laxative effect for the first few days. If this persists, reduce the daily intake until this effect subsides, take with food or soon after meals, or discontinue use if necessary.

GI upset (eg, diarrhea, nausea, stomach pain, vomiting, flatulence) may occur with phosphate therapy. The following side effects have been reported less frequently: headaches; dizziness; mental confusion; seizures; weakness or heaviness of legs; unusual tiredness or weakness; muscle cramps; numbness, tingling, pain, or weakness of hands or feet; numbness or tingling around lips; tachycardia; bradycardia; dyspnea; swelling of feet or lower legs; unusual weight gain; low urine output; unusual thirst; bone and joint pain (possible phosphate-induced osteomalacia). High serum phosphate levels may increase the incidence of extraskeletal calcification.

► Administration and Dosage

Dietary Reference Intakes (DRIs) for Phosphorus	
Age	**DRI (mg)**
0 to 6 months	100
7 months to 1 year	275
1 to 3 years	460
4 to 8 years	500
9 to 18 years	1250
Adults	700
Pregnant/Lactating women	700-1250

Phosphate supplementation should be used only upon the advice of a health care professional.

PHOSPHORUS PRODUCTS	
Trade name	Doseform
Neutra-Phos	**Powder**: 250 mg phosphorus, 278 mg potassium, 164 mg sodium/packet
PHOS-NaK	**Powder**: 250 mg phosphorus, 280 mg potassium, 160 mg sodium/packet. Mannitol.
Neutra-Phos-K	**Powder**: 250 mg phosphorus, 556 mg potassium/packet

Products listed are representative of currently available and widely distributed brands. Similar products, including regional and private label brands, may also exist.

PATIENT INFORMATION
Phosphorus Supplements

- Patients may experience a mild laxative effect for the first few days. If this persists, reduce the daily dose until the effect subsides, take with food or soon after meals, or discontinue use if necessary.
- *Powder concentrate:* Dissolve entire contents of 1 bottle in 3.8 L (1 gallon) of water or other desirable liquid. This solution should not be further diluted, but can be chilled to increase palatability and can be stored for up to 60 days.
- *Unit-dose packets:* Empty contents of 1 packet into ⅓ glassful of water (approximately 75 mL) or other liquid, such as juice, and stir well before taking.
- Discuss use with your doctor if you know your kidney function is decreased substantially or you have chronic kidney or liver disease.
- Wait 2 or more hours between taking a phosphorus supplement and an antacid containing magnesium, aluminum, or calcium.
- Use vitamin D supplements with caution if you are taking a phosphorus supplement.
- Soda drinks may contain significant amounts of phosphoric acid. This may lead to a calcium deficiency resulting in an increased risk of kidney stones, osteoporosis, and arteriosclerosis. Excess phosphorus intake can decrease vitamin D levels and reduce the absorption of iron, magnesium, and zinc.
- Patients should consult their doctor about oral hydration requirements while taking phosphorus supplements to reduce the risk of kidney stone formation.

MAGNESIUM

▶ Actions

Magnesium is a mineral that is necessary in a number of enzyme systems, phosphate transfer, muscular contraction, and nerve conduction. Magnesium deficiency may occur in the following conditions: malabsorption syndrome; prolonged diarrhea or steatorrhea; vomiting; pancreatitis; aldosteronism; renal tubular damage; chronic alcoholism; prolonged IV therapy with magnesium-free solutions; diuretic therapy; hemodialysis; disorders associated with hypokalemia and hypocalcemia; patients on digitalis therapy. While there are large stores of magnesium present intracellularly and in bone in adults, these stores often are not mobilized sufficiently to maintain plasma levels; therefore, serum levels may not reflect total magnesium stores.

Magnesium is eliminated by the kidney; individuals with significant renal insufficiency can accumulate magnesium if intake is not restricted.

► **Indications**

As a dietary supplement.

Unlabeled uses: A pyridoxine/magnesium oxide combination has been used to prevent recurrence of calcium oxalate kidney stones. Magnesium also may reduce hyperactivity and improve symptoms of chronic fatigue syndrome if magnesium levels are low.

Oral magnesium gluconate may be a cost-effective and clinically effective alternative to oral ritodrine as a tocolytic for continued inhibition of contractions following parenteral magnesium sulfate. Further study is needed.

► **Warnings**

Renal disease: Do not use without physician supervision because of the risk of potential accumulation.

Heart disease: Magnesium supplements may make this condition worse.

Excessive dosage: Excessive dosage may cause diarrhea and GI irritation.

Pregnancy: It is unknown whether magnesium supplementation will harm an unborn child or a breastfeeding child. Do not take this mineral without speaking to a physician if pregnant, planning a pregnancy, or breastfeeding.

► **Drug Interactions**

Magnesium Drug Interactions			
Precipitant drug	Object drug*		Description
Magnesium salts	Aminoquino-lones	↓	The absorption and therapeutic effect of the aminoquinolones (eg, chloroquine) may be decreased.
Magnesium salts	Nitrofurantoin	↓	Adsorption of nitrofurantoin onto magnesium salts may occur, decreasing the bioavailability and possibly the anti-infective effect of nitrofurantoin.
Magnesium salts	Penicillamine	↓	The GI absorption of penicillamine may be decreased, possibly decreasing its pharmacologic effects; however, this has only been reported for magnesium-containing antacids.
Magnesium salts	Tetracyclines	↓	The GI absorption and serum levels of tetracyclines may be decreased; a decreased antimicrobial response may occur.

* ↓ = Object drug decreased.

► **Adverse Reactions**

Diarrhea.

► **Overdosage**

It is possible to overdose on any mineral if large quantities are given; magnesium is no exception. Administer magnesium cautiously, especially to patients with decreased renal function. The most common symptom of overdose is diarrhea. At serum levels between 3 to 5 mEq/L, there is a propensity for hypotension because of peripheral dilation. Severe hypotension may be seen at higher levels. Facial flushing may be seen, associated with a feeling of warmth or thirst. Nausea and vomiting may occur but are not always present. Lethargy, dysarthria, and drowsiness can appear when levels reach 5 to 7 mEq/L. Deep tendon reflexes are lost when levels reach 7 mEq/L. Shallow respirations, irregular brief periods of apnea, and, finally, prolonged apnea are expected when levels exceed 10 mEq/L. Coma occurs when serum levels are between 12 and 15 mEq/L. Finally, when levels exceed 15 to 20 mEq/L, cardiac arrest may be expected.

Treatment: Terminate exposure. Calcium administration improves many toxic symptoms. Forced diuresis intensifies the elimination of magnesium; hemodialysis is extremely effective at magnesium removal but is infrequently necessary in the absence of renal failure.

► Administration and Dosage

Dietary Reference Intakes (DRIs) for Magnesium	
Age	DRI (mg)
0 to 6 months	30
7 months to 1 year	75
1 to 3 years	80
4 to 8 years	130
9 to 13 years	240
14 to 18 years	240-410
Adults	310-420
Pregnant/Lactating women	310-400

Magnesium-containing antacids also may be used; refer to the Heartburn and GERD monograph in the Gastrointestinal Conditions chapter.

Dietary supplement: 54 to 483 mg/day in divided doses. Refer to product labeling for specific instructions.

MAGNESIUM PRODUCTS	
Trade name	Doseform
Almora, Magonate	**Tablets**: 27 mg (as gluconate dihydrate)
Magnesium	**Tablets**: 27 mg (as chelated gluconate)
Magtrate	**Tablets**: 29.25 mg (as gluconate)
Mag-SR (sf)	**Tablets**: 64 mg (as chloride hexahydrate)
Mag-200	**Tablets**: 200 mg (as oxide)
Mag-Ox 400	**Tablets**: 240 mg (as oxide)
Slow-Mag	**Tablets, controlled-release, enteric-coated**: 64 mg magnesium (as chloral hexahydrate), 106 mg calcium
Uro-Mag	**Capsules**: 85 mg (as oxide)
Magonate Natal (sf)	**Liquid**: 3.52 mg/mL (as gluconate)
Magonate	**Liquid**: 54 mg/5 mL (as gluconate). Sorbitol.

Products listed are representative of currently available and widely distributed brands. Similar products, including regional and private label brands, may also exist.

sf = Sugar free.

PATIENT INFORMATION

Magnesium Supplements

- Excessive doses may cause diarrhea.
- Patients with significant renal impairment should consult a physician before beginning magnesium supplementation because of the risk of accumulation (hypermagnesemia).
- Magnesium-containing antacids also may be used as dietary supplements.
- Do not crush or chew sustained-release preparations.

POTASSIUM

▶ **Actions**

Potassium, the principal intracellular cation of most body tissues, participates in a number of essential physiological processes, such as maintenance of intracellular tonicity, transmission of nerve impulses, contraction of cardiac, skeletal, and smooth muscle, acid-base balance, and maintenance of normal renal function. The active ion transport system maintains this gradient across the plasma membrane.

Potassium homeostasis: The potassium concentration in extracellular fluid is normally 4 to 5 mEq/L; the concentration in intracellular fluid is approximately 150 to 160 mEq/L. Plasma concentration provides a useful clinical guide to disturbances in potassium balance. By producing large differences in the ratio of intracellular to extracellular potassium, relatively small absolute changes in extracellular concentration may have important effects on neuromuscular activity.

Despite wide variations in dietary intake of potassium (eg, 40 to 120 mEq/day), plasma potassium concentration normally is stabilized within the narrow range of 4 to 5 mEq/L by virtue of close renal regulation of potassium balance. Fecal excretion of potassium is normally only a few mEq/day and does not play a primary role in potassium homeostasis.

Natural potassium sources: Foods rich in potassium include beef, veal, ham, chicken, turkey, fish, milk, bananas, dates, prunes, raisins, avocados, watermelon, cantaloupe, apricots, molasses, beans, yams, broccoli, brussels sprouts, lentils, potatoes, and spinach.

Hypokalemia: Gradual potassium depletion may occur whenever the rate of potassium loss through renal excretion or GI loss exceeds the rate of potassium intake. Potassium depletion is usually a consequence of prolonged therapy with oral diuretics, primary or secondary hyperaldosteronism, diabetic ketoacidosis, severe diarrhea (especially if associated with vomiting), or inadequate replacement during prolonged parenteral nutrition. Potassium depletion because of these causes usually is accompanied by a concomitant deficiency of chloride and is manifested by hypokalemia, hypochloremia, and metabolic alkalosis.

The use of potassium salts in patients receiving diuretics for uncomplicated essential hypertension is often unnecessary when such patients have a normal diet. However, if hypokalemia occurs, dietary supplementation with potassium-containing foods may be adequate. In more severe cases, potassium salt supplementation may be indicated.

Potassium depletion sufficient to cause 1 mEq/L drop in serum potassium requires a loss of approximately 100 to 200 mEq potassium from the total body store.

   Symptoms of hypokalemia – Weakness; fatigue; ileus; cramping; polydipsia; flaccid paralysis; impaired ability to concentrate urine (in advanced cases). ECG may reveal atrial and ventricular ectopy, prolongation of QT interval, ST segment depression, conduction defects, broad or flat T waves, or appearance of U waves.

▶ **Indications**

Treatment of hypokalemia in the following conditions: with or without metabolic alkalosis; digitalis intoxication; familial periodic paralysis; diabetic acidosis; diarrhea and vomiting; surgical conditions accompanied by nitrogen loss, vomiting, suction drainage, diarrhea, and increased urinary excretion of potassium; certain cases of uremia; hyperadrenalism; starvation and debilitation; corticosteroid or diuretic therapy.

Prevention of potassium depletion when dietary intake is inadequate in the following conditions: patients receiving digitalis and diuretics for congestive heart failure; significant cardiac arrhythmias; hepatic cirrhosis with ascites; states of aldosterone excess with normal renal function; potassium-losing nephropathy; certain diarrheal states.

Use potassium chloride when hypokalemia is associated with alkalosis. When acidosis is present, use the bicarbonate, citrate, acetate, or gluconate potassium salts.

Unlabeled uses: In patients with mild hypertension, the use of potassium supplements (24 to 60 mmol/day) appears to result in a long-term reduction of blood pressure.

▶ Contraindications

Severe renal impairment with oliguria or azotemia; untreated Addison disease; hyperkalemia from any cause (eg, systemic acidosis, acute dehydration, extensive tissue breakdown); adynamia episodica hereditaria; acute dehydration; heat cramps; potassium-sparing diuretic treatment (spironolactone, triamterene, or amiloride) or aldosterone-inhibiting agent use.

Solid dosage forms of potassium supplements are contraindicated in any patient in whom there is cause for arrest or delay in tablet passage through the GI tract. Wax matrix potassium chloride preparations have produced esophageal ulceration in cardiac patients with esophageal compression caused by an enlarged left atrium; give potassium supplementation as a liquid preparation to these patients.

▶ Warnings

Hypokalemia: Hypokalemia ordinarily is diagnosed by demonstrating potassium depletion in a patient and by a careful clinical history.

The administration of concentrated dextrose or sodium bicarbonate may cause an intracellular potassium shift. This can cause hypokalemia, which may lead to serious cardiac arrhythmias.

Giving potassium to hypokalemic hypertensive patients may lower blood pressure.

Hyperkalemia: In patients with impaired potassium excretion, potassium salts can produce hyperkalemia or cardiac arrest. This occurs most commonly in patients given IV potassium but also may occur in patients given oral potassium. Potentially fatal hyperkalemia can develop rapidly and be asymptomatic.

Symptoms of hyperkalemia may include paresthesias, heaviness of legs or arms, muscle weakness and flaccid paralysis of the extremities, listlessness, mental confusion, decreased blood pressure, shock, cardiac arrhythmia, or heart block.

Renal function impairment: Renal function impairment requires careful monitoring of the serum potassium concentration and appropriate dosage adjustment.

Pregnancy: Category C. It is not known whether potassium salts can cause fetal harm when administered to a pregnant woman or can affect reproductive capacity. Give to a pregnant woman only if clearly needed.

Lactation: It is not known whether, or to what extent, supplemental potassium is excreted in breast milk. Exercise caution when administering to a nursing woman. The normal potassium content of breast milk is approximately 13 mEq/L. As long as body potassium is not excessive, the contribution of potassium salts should have little or no effect on the potassium level in breast milk.

Children: Safety and efficacy for use in children have not been established.

► **Drug Interactions**

Potassium Preparation Drug Interactions			
Precipitant drug	**Object drug***		**Description**
ACE inhibitors	Potassium preparations	↑	Concurrent use may result in elevated serum potassium concentrations in certain patients.
Potassium-sparing diuretics	Potassium preparations	↑	Potassium-sparing diuretics will increase potassium retention and can produce severe hyperkalemia.
Potassium preparations	Digitalis	↑	In patients receiving digoxin, hypokalemia may result in digoxin toxicity. Therefore, use caution if discontinuing a potassium preparation in patients maintained on digoxin.

* ↑ = Object drug increased

► **Adverse Reactions**

Nausea, vomiting, diarrhea, flatulence, and abdominal discomfort caused by GI irritation are best managed by diluting the preparation further, taking with meals, or reducing the dosage. Hyperkalemia, GI obstruction, bleeding, ulceration, or perforation are the most severe reactions that have occurred. Rash, bradycardia, weakness, and dyspnea also have occurred.

► **Overdosage**

Potentially life-threatening. Refer patient to an emergency department or poison control center for immediate evaluation.

► **Administration and Dosage**

Potassium supplementation should be used only on the advice of a health care professional.

The usual dietary intake of potassium ranges between 40 to 150 mEq/day.

Nonprescription products normally are not used to treat hypokalemia or as a preventative in high-risk patients.

Potassium intoxication may result from any therapeutic dosage.

POTASSIUM PRODUCTS	
Trade name	**Doseform**
Potassium Gluconate	**Tablets**: 80 mg, 99 mg
Chelated Potassium (sf)	**Tablets, timed-release**: 95 mg (as chelate)
K-99	**Capsules**: 99 mg (as gluconate)

Products listed are representative of currently available and widely distributed brands. Similar products, including regional and private label brands, may also exist.

sf = Sugar free.

PATIENT INFORMATION

Potassium Supplements

- May cause GI upset; take after meals or with food and with a full glass of water.
- Do not chew or crush tablets; swallow whole.
- Do not use salt substitutes concurrently, except on the advice of a physician.
- Notify physician if tingling of the hands and feet, unusual tiredness or weakness, a feeling of heaviness in the legs, severe nausea, vomiting, abdominal pain, or black stools (indicative of GI bleeding) occurs.

IRON

▶ **Actions**

Iron, a trace element, is a component of hemoglobin, myoglobin, and a number of enzymes (eg, cytochromes, catalase, peroxidase). The total body content of iron is approximately 50 mg/kg in men (3.5 g in the average 70 kg man) and 37 mg/kg in women. Iron is stored primarily as hemosiderin or aggregated ferritin, found in the reticuloendothelial cells of the liver, spleen, and bone marrow. Approximately 67% of total body iron is in the circulating red blood cell mass in hemoglobin, the major factor in oxygen transport.

Iron deficiency can affect muscle metabolism, heat production, and catecholamine metabolism and has been associated with behavioral or learning problems in children.

The average dietary intake of iron is 12 to 20 mg/day for men and 8 to 15 mg/day for women; however, only approximately 10% of this iron is absorbed (1 to 2 mg/ day) in individuals with adequate iron stores. Absorption is enhanced (20% to 30%) when storage iron is depleted or when erythropoiesis occurs at an increased rate.

Iron is primarily absorbed from the duodenum and upper jejunum by an active transport mechanism. The ferrous salt form is absorbed 3 times more readily than the ferric form. The common ferrous salts (sulfate, gluconate, fumarate) are absorbed almost on a milligram-for-milligram basis but differ in the content of elemental iron. Ferrous sulfate contains 20% elemental iron, while ferrous gluconate and ferrous fumarate contain 12% and 33% elemental iron, respectively. Sustained-release or enteric-coated preparations reduce the amount of available iron; absorption from these dosage forms is reduced because iron is transported beyond the duodenum. Dose also influences the amount of iron absorbed. The amount of iron absorbed increases progressively with larger doses; however, the percentage absorbed decreases. Food can decrease the absorption of iron by 40% to 66%; however, gastric intolerance may necessitate administering the drug with food.

Iron is transported via the blood and bound to transferrin. The daily loss of iron from urine, sweat, and sloughing of intestinal mucosal cells amounts to approximately 0.5 to 1 mg in healthy men; in menstruating women, approximately 1 to 2 mg is the normal daily loss (excluding menstruation).

▶ **Indications**

Iron deficiency: For the prevention and treatment of iron deficiency and iron deficiency anemias.

Iron supplement: As a dietary supplement for iron.

Unlabeled uses: Iron supplementation may be required by most patients receiving epoetin therapy. Failure to administer iron supplements (oral or IV) during epoetin therapy can impair the hematologic response to epoetin.

▶ **Contraindications**

Hemochromatosis; hemosiderosis; hemolytic anemias; known hypersensitivity to any ingredients.

▶ **Warnings**

Chronic iron intake: Individuals with normal iron balance should not take iron chronically.

Accidental overdose: Accidental overdose of iron-containing products is a leading cause of fatal poisoning in children younger than 6 years of age. Keep this product out of reach of children.

Intolerance: Discontinue use if symptoms of intolerance appear.

GI effects: Occasional GI discomfort, such as nausea, abdominal pain, and diarrhea may be minimized by taking with meals and slowly increasing to the recommended dosage.

Tartrazine sensitivity: Some of these products contain tartrazine, which may cause allergic-type reactions (including bronchial asthma) in susceptible individuals. Although the incidence of tartrazine sensitivity in the general population is low, it is frequently seen in patients who also have aspirin hypersensitivity.

Sulfite sensitivity: Some of the products contain sulfites, which may cause allergic-type reactions (eg, hives, itching, wheezing, anaphylaxis) in certain susceptible patients. Although the overall prevalence of sulfite sensitivity in the general population is probably low, it is seen more frequently in asthmatics or in atopic nonasthmatic patients.

▶ **Drug Interactions**

Iron Salts Drug Interactions			
Precipitant drug	**Object drug***		**Description**
Antacids	Iron salts	↓	GI absorption of iron may be reduced.
Ascorbic acid	Iron salts	↑	Ascorbic acid at doses 200 mg or more have been shown to enhance the absorption of iron 30% or more.
Chloramphenicol	Iron salts	↑	Serum iron levels may be increased.
Cimetidine	Iron salts	↓	GI absorption of iron may be reduced.
Iron salts	Levodopa	↓	Levodopa appears to form chelates with iron salts, decreasing levodopa absorption and serum levels.
Iron salts	Levothyroxine	↓	The efficacy of levothyroxine may be decreased, resulting in hypothyroidism. Avoid concomitant administration.
Iron salts	Methyldopa	↓	Extent of methyldopa absorption may be decreased, possibly resulting in decreased efficacy.
Iron salts	Penicillamine	↓	Marked reduction in GI absorption of penicillamine may occur, possibly because of chelation.
Iron salts	Quinolones	↓	GI absorption of quinolones may be decreased because of formation of ferric ion-quinolone complex.
Iron salts	Tetracyclines	↓	Concomitant use within 2 hours may decrease absorption and serum levels of tetracyclines. Absorption of iron salts also may be decreased.
Tetracyclines	Iron salts		

* ↑ = Object drug increased.   ↓ = Object drug decreased.

Drug-food interactions: Eggs and milk inhibit iron absorption. Coffee and tea consumed with a meal or 1 hour after a meal may significantly inhibit the absorption of dietary iron; clinical significance has not been determined. Administration of calcium and iron supplements with food can reduce ferrous sulfate absorption by 33%. If combined iron and calcium supplementation is required, iron absorption is not decreased if calcium carbonate is used and the supplements are taken between meals.

▶ Adverse Reactions

GI irritation; nausea; vomiting; constipation; abdominal cramps and diarrhea; epigastric pain. Stools may appear darker in color because of unabsorbed iron, but this is to be expected and is not cause for alarm.

Iron-containing liquids may temporarily stain the teeth. Dilute the liquid to reduce this possibility. When iron-containing drops are given to infants, the membrane covering the teeth may darken.

▶ Overdosage

Symptoms: The oral lethal dose of elemental iron is approximately 200 to 250 mg/kg; however, considerably less has been fatal. Symptoms may present when 30 to 60 mg/kg is ingested. Acute poisoning will produce symptoms in 4 stages:

1.) Within 1 to 6 hours: lethargy; nausea; vomiting; abdominal pain; tarry stools; weak-rapid pulse; hypotension; diminished tissue perfusion; metabolic acidosis; fever; leukocytosis; hyperglycemia; dyspnea; coma.
2.) If not immediately fatal, symptoms may subside for approximately 24 hours.
3.) Symptoms return 12 to 48 hours after ingestion and may include the following: diffuse vascular congestion; pulmonary edema; shock; metabolic acidosis; convulsions; anuria; hyperthermia; death.
4.) If the patient survives, pyloric or antral stenosis, hepatic cirrhosis, and CNS damage may be seen 2 to 6 weeks after ingestion.

Treatment: Maintain proper airway, respiration, and circulation. If the patient is a candidate for emesis, induce with syrup of ipecac; follow with gastric lavage using tepid water or 1% to 5% sodium bicarbonate to convert the ferrous sulfate to ferrous carbonate, which is poorly absorbed and less irritating. Systemic chelation therapy with deferoxamine generally is recommended for patients with serum iron levels greater than the total iron binding capacity (63 mcmol; 3.5 mg/L); IM therapy may suffice, but severe poisoning (eg, shock, coma) may require IV administration. Oral use of deferoxamine is controversial and generally discouraged. Saline cathartics may be used. Specific treatment for shock, convulsions, acidosis, and renal failure may be necessary. Treatment includes the usual supportive measures.

▶ Administration and Dosage

A good food source of iron (eg, veal, liver, beef, enriched bread, fish, green vegetables) contains a substantial amount of iron in relation to its calorie content and can contribute 10% or more of the RDA of iron in a serving.

| Dietary Reference Intakes (DRIs) for Iron ||
Age	DRI (mg)
Children	
0 to 6 months	0.27
7 months to 1 year	11
1 to 3 years	7
4 to 8 years	10
Men	
9 to 13 years	8
14 to 18 years	11
Adults	8
Women	
9 to 13 years	8
14 to 18 years	15
Adults	8-18
Pregnant	27
Lactating	9-10

Iron replacement therapy in deficiency states: Iron doses are given as elemental iron.

Premature infants – 2 to 4 mg/kg/day given in 1 to 2 divided doses. Maximum dose is 15 mg/day.

Children – 3 to 6 mg/kg/day given in 1 to 3 divided doses.

Adults – 150 to 300 mg/day given in 3 divided doses. Alternatively, 60 mg given 2 to 4 times/day may help to lessen GI effects.

The length of iron therapy depends upon the cause and severity of the iron deficiency. In general, approximately 4 to 6 months of oral iron therapy is required to reverse uncomplicated iron deficiency anemias.

Elemental Iron Content of Iron Salts	
Iron salt	% Iron
Ferrous sulfate	≈ 20
Ferrous sulfate exsiccated	≈ 30
Ferrous gluconate	≈ 12
Ferrous fumarate	≈ 33

IRON-CONTAINING PRODUCTS

Trade name	Doseform	Elemental Iron (mg)
Femiron	**Tablets:** 63 mg ferrous fumarate	20
Fergon	**Tablets:** 240 mg ferrous gluconate	27
Ferrous Gluconate	**Tablets:** 300 mg ferrous gluconate	35
Ferrous Gluconate	**Tablets:** 324 mg ferrous gluconate. Sucrose.	38
Feratab	**Tablets:** 300 mg ferrous sulfate heptahydrate, 40 mg calcium	60
Feosol	**Tablets:** 200 mg ferrous sulfate	65
Ferrous Sulfate	**Tablets:** 324 mg ferrous sulfate. Lactose, sucrose.	65
Vitron-C	**Tablets:** 200 mg ferrous fumarate, 125 mg vitamin C	66
Hemocyte	**Tablets:** 324 mg ferrous fumarate	106
Nephro-Fer	**Tablets:** 350 mg ferrous fumarate. Lactose.	115
Icar	**Tablets, chewable:** 15 mg iron (as carbonyl iron)	15
Feostat	**Tablets, chewable:** 100 mg ferrous fumarate	33
Fero-Grad-500	**Tablets, controlled-release:** 525 mg ferrous sulfate, 500 mg vitamin C	105
SlowFe Iron	**Tablets, slow-release:** 160 mg dried ferrous sulfate. Lactose.	50
SlowFe Iron + Folic Acid	**Tablets, slow-release:** 160 mg dried ferrous sulfate, 400 mcg folic acid. Lactose.	50
Feosol	**Caplets:** 250 mg ferrous sulfate	45
Fe-20	**Capsules:** 167 mg ferrous gluconate dihydrate	20
Niferex	**Capsules:** 40 mg Ferrochel®, 20 mg polysaccharide iron. Lactose.	60
Niferex-150	**Capsules:** 80 mg Ferrochel®, 70 mg polysaccharide iron, 50 mg vitamin C	150
Hytinic, Nu-Iron 150	**Capsules:** 150 mg iron (as polysaccharide-iron complex)	150
Icar	**Suspension, oral:** 15 mg iron (as carbonyl iron)/ 1.25 mL	15

IRON-CONTAINING PRODUCTS

Trade name	Doseform	Elemental Iron (mg)
Feosol, Ferrous Sulfate	**Elixir**: 220 mg ferrous sulfate/5 mL	44
Hytinic	**Elixir**: 100 mg polysaccharide-iron complex/ 5 mL. 10% alcohol.	100
Fer-gen-sol[1], *Fer-In-Sol*[1], Ferrous Sulfate	**Drops**: 75 mg ferrous sulfate/0.6 mL. 0.2% alcohol. Sorbitol, sugar.	15

Products listed are representative of currently available and widely distributed brands. Similar products, including regional and private label brands, may also exist.

[1] Contains sodium bisulfite.

PATIENT INFORMATION
Iron-Containing Products

- Take on an empty stomach; if GI upset occurs, take after meals or with food.
- Do not eat the following foods within 1 to 2 hours of taking iron: cheese and yogurt; eggs; milk; spinach; tea or coffee; whole-grain breads; cereals; bran.
- Do not take within 2 hours of antacids, tetracyclines, fluoroquinolones, or levothyroxine.
- Do not take large amounts of iron for more than 6 months without checking with your health care professional.
- Do not take iron, calcium supplements, or antacids at the same time. Space doses apart by 1 to 2 hours.
- Drink liquid iron preparations in water or juice and through a straw to prevent staining of teeth.
- Medication may cause black stools, constipation, or diarrhea. If iron causes constipation, concurrent use of stool softener (eg, docusate) may be appropriate.
- Do not crush or chew sustained-release preparations.
- Keep away from children.

PROTEIN CALORIE MALNUTRITION

DEFINITION

Protein calorie malnutrition (PCM) is defined as the physiological state that develops when energy or protein are inadequate to meet the body's needs. PCM is characterized by weight loss, depletion of visceral proteins, and decreased immune competence, impaired wound healing, and decreased functional ability/strength. PCM is also a cause of growth retardation in children.

ETIOLOGY

Protein calorie malnutrition may be caused by primary factors such as inadequate food intake, or secondary factors such as illnesses or diseases leading to inadequate food intake, decreased nutrient absorption/utilization, and increased nutritional needs.

Primary factors of PCM: The problem of simply consuming inadequate amounts of food is frequently related to social and economic factors such as poverty, ignorance, diet fads, and drug and alcohol addiction. In the elderly, PCM may occur because of social isolation or depression.

Secondary factors of PCM: Acute or chronic illnesses often result in depression of appetite that leads to poor nutritional intake and PCM. Physiologic changes associated with an illness can also cause decreased nutrient absorption/utilization and increased energy and protein requirements that make it difficult to maintain adequate nutritional intake.

INCIDENCE

In the US, PCM mainly affects certain subgroups of the population. A significant incidence of malnutrition has been documented in hospitalized patients and in the elderly. A number of studies have revealed an incidence of PCM ranging from 30% to 55% in hospitalized patients. It has been estimated that as many as 60% of hospitalized elderly patients have evidence of PCM, while as many as 30% of elderly patients admitted to long-term care facilities have PCM. The elderly within the community have also been identified as a group at risk for PCM. An evaluation of the Elderly Nutrition Program of the Older Americans Act has indicated an incidence of moderate-to-high nutritional risk among 67% to 88% of participants. Other segments of the general population that are also susceptible to the development of malnutrition include: Children of lower socioeconomic status; the chronically ill; and those with alcohol/drug addiction.

PATHOPHYSIOLOGY

PCM resulting from inadequate intake or starvation has a different physiologic course than does PCM resulting from the stresses of illness or disease.

Although there appear to be two different physiologic responses based on etiology, the two may be present concurrently and may interact.

PCM resulting from starvation develops over several weeks or months of inadequate nutritional intake. As energy intake decreases, the body adapts by decreasing energy expenditure. When a reduction in energy expenditure can no longer offset the inadequate intake, subcutaneous fat stores are mobilized for energy resulting in decreased adiposity and weight loss. Lean body mass decreases more slowly. This response, mediated by a decrease in serum glucose and amino acid concentrations, involves a decrease in serum insulin, and an increase in epinephrine, growth hormone, and somatomedin circulation. These endocrine changes work to spare visceral protein stores by decreasing synthesis and storage of glycogen, protein, and fat; increasing glycogen and fat breakdown; increasing amino acid recycling. In addition to efficient amino acid recycling, the body preferentially targets breakdown of peripheral muscle protein over visceral proteins to compensate for inadequate energy/protein intake.

When PCM develops in response to stress factors such as serious illnesses, infections, or injuries, the physiologic response is mediated by cytokines and results in an increase in resting energy expenditure and an exaggerated elevation of glucagon, epinephrine, glucocorticoids, and growth hormone. The elevation in these hormones again leads to increased fat and muscle protein breakdown, but in contrast to the starvation response, visceral protein stores are rapidly depleted.

Other physiologic changes that occur in starvation type PCM include a decrease in hemoglobin concentration and red blood cell mass secondary to a decrease in oxygen demands (decreased lean body mass and decreased energy expenditure). With prolonged starvation there tends to be a decrease in cardiac output, heart rate, and blood pressure. Cardiovascular changes result in postural hypotension and decreased venous return. Total body potassium is decreased with a reduction in muscle protein and intracellular potassium. GI function may be altered after prolonged starvation with a decreased production of gastric acid, pancreatic enzymes, and bile. Immunocompetence is also altered as the production of immunocompetent cells falls and the body's reaction to antigens is less efficient. The body becomes immunocompromised after prolonged or severe starvation, but this occurs more rapidly in the stressed form of malnutrition as a result of rapid visceral protein depletion.

SIGNS/SYMPTOMS

An initial symptom of inadequate energy/protein intake is a decrease in energy level and a generalized weakness and apathy. Other signs include leanness with a loss of subcutaneous fat, weight loss, and growth retardation/short stature in children.

More prolonged or severe starvation will present with muscle wasting, absence of subcutaneous fat; dry, thin, easily plucked hair; poor skin turgor; skin dyspigmentation. Decreased heart rate, blood pressure, and body temperature may also occur. In PCM caused by stress, clinical features may be more difficult to identify. Weight may remain relatively stable or may actually increase with fluid retention. Edema may be present. A sign of visceral protein depletion that may occur with prolonged starvation or stress-induced PCM is increased susceptibility to infections and poor wound healing.

DIAGNOSTIC PARAMETERS/PHYSICAL ASSESSMENT

Clinical Observation: PCM is simply classified as mild, moderate, or severe. Anthropometric, biochemical, clinical, and dietary parameters are used to diagnose PCM and its degree of severity.

Anthropometric assessment – Anthropometry is a series of simple measurements that provide an assessment of the body's calorie and protein reserves. Although simple to perform, anthropometric measurements can be unreliable secondary to instrument error, inaccurate interpretation of measurements, or alteration of measurements secondary to edema.

Anthropometric measurement of adults: The most commonly used measurement in nutritional assessment is weight. An individual's weight and height can be compared with that of an ideal using standard weight and height tables. Current weight should also be compared with usual weight and percent weight loss should be determined. Percent of ideal weight, percent of usual weight, and amount of recent weight loss correlate with varying degrees of PCM.

Wrist circumference is a measurement used to determine frame size. Comparison of actual weight to ideal weight should be based on frame size.

Triceps skinfold thickness (TSF) is a measurement made with calipers at the midpoint of the upper arm to determine body fat mass. An average of 3 measurements is compared with a standard. TSF values less than 90% of the standard suggest depletion of fat stores.

Mid Arm Muscle Circumference (MAMC) is a calculated measurement using the TSF value and a measurement of the mid-arm circumference. The measurement determines somatic protein mass and is again compared with a standard to determine adequacy of somatic protein stores.

Anthropometric measurement of children: In the pediatric population, measurements for weight and height/length are compared to reference standards. The reference standards are percentile curves developed by the National Center for Health Statistics (NCHS), which represent the physical growth of infants and children in the US. Serial measurements of weight and height/length are plotted over time on the NCHS growth changes to track growth. A deceleration in height growth suggests stunting related to PCM.

Head circumference is measured from birth to 3 years of age and is also compared with NCHS reference standards. Serial measurements over time are plotted on the NCHS growth charts for head circumference to track brain growth.

TSF and MAMC measurements can also be used in the pediatric population to estimate somatic fat and protein stores.

Biochemical assessment – The biochemical measurements used for adults are the same as for the pediatric population. Biochemical measurements most often assess visceral protein status and immune function. Albumin, transferrin, prealbumin, and total lymphocyte count are frequently used.

Serum albumin is one of the many proteins that the liver produces. Albumin functions as a carrier of many substances including hormones, enzymes, drugs, and metabolites. Serum concentrations of albumin depend on the rates of synthesis and catabolism, its distribution and excretion, and the degree of hydration. Its half-life is 10 to 20 days. Two factors that significantly impact albumin synthesis are liver function and nutritional status. Albumin levels are correlated with degree of malnutrition.

Serum transferrin is a globulin that binds and transports iron. Levels are also dependent upon the rates of synthesis, catabolism, distribution, excretion, and hydration. The half-life of serum transferrin is 8 to 11 days. Transferrin levels are correlated with degree of malnutrition. Its reliability as a marker of nutritional status is limited if iron deficiency is present.

Serum prealbumin is produced by the liver and is the carrier protein for retinol binding protein. It is useful as a marker not only for current nutritional status, but as an indicator of acute changes in nutritional status because of its relatively short half-life of 1 to 2 days. Serum prealbumin levels are correlated with degree of malnutrition.

Total lymphocyte count (TLC) is a measurement derived from a calculation using WBC and percent lymphocytes. It serves as an assessment of humoral and cell-mediated immunity, as well as an indicator of nutritional status. TLC is correlated with degree of malnutrition.

Clinical/Physical assessment – In mild-to-moderate PCM, a physical exam may reveal leaness with a decrease in SC fat. In more severe or prolonged cases of malnutrition, there may be an absence of SC fat with muscular wasting and cachexia. Other physical signs of PCM can be identified in examination of hair, eyes, face, lips, tongue, teeth, gums, skin, and nails. The changes in these physical features are related to specific vitamin and mineral deficiencies that accompany PCM. In PCM resulting from acute stress, clinical features may be more difficult to identify, and diagnosis is often confirmed by biochemical parameters.

Dietary assessment – An important part of the clinical assessment of PCM involves an evaluation of the selection and quantity of food actually consumed by an individual. This method of assessment is completed most often through an interview. Its reliability depends on the ability of the patient to relate his/her past diet intake. If the patient is unable to provide this information, a caretaker may be able to give an estimate of actual intake or describe the dietary habits.

Interview: It may be beneficial to ask the patient about the following:

- Recent changes in the nature/appearance of hair, eyes, face, lips, tongue, teeth, gums, skin, and nails.
- Dietary habits.
- Weight changes.
- Impaired wound healing.
- Decreased funtional ability/strength/energy.
- Recent illnesses or disease.
- Consumption of drugs or alcohol.

TREATMENT

Nondrug therapy: Prevention or treatment of PCM should be based on data from a complete nutrition assessment and diet history. The treatment options for restoring nutritional well-being include: A well-balanced diet rich in calories, protein, vitamins, and minerals; oral nutritional supplements; enteral tube feedings; total parenteral nutrition. Whenever possible, prevention of PCM or nutritional repletion should be accomplished by a healthy diet. In some cases (ie, mild PCM, risk for PCM), nutrition counseling with diet modification is sufficient to attain this goal. However, when inadequate diet intake persists, oral nutritional supplements, enteral tube feedings, or total parenteral nutrition may be indicated. Providing nutritional repletion through the GI tract (enteral nutrition) is preferred over the parenteral route when the GI tract is functional.

Pharmacotherapy:

Enteral products — Oral nutritional supplements and enteral tube feeding products – These products are indicated when diet intake is inadequate to sustain nutritional status and the GI tract is functional. They may be used in addition to a diet or as the sole source of nutrition. These products are now widely available in the commercial setting. In general, for the healthy population, a well-balanced diet should be adequate to meet nutritional needs, and well-balanced meals should not be replaced by liquid supplements.

In attempting to prevent PCM or in treating mild nutritional deficits, oral nutritional supplements may be given to add calories and protein to the diet. When addition of a supplement fails to significantly impact calorie and protein intake, then feedings directly into the GI tract may be instituted. Certain groups of individuals with poor diet intake may benefit from oral supplements or enteral tube feedings. They include individuals with neurological impairments, dysphagia, malnutrition, GI disease, cancer, HIV/AIDS, liver disease, COPD, and renal disease. Formula selection should be based on meeting an individual's nutritional needs within a reasonable cost range. Selection will also be influenced by an individual's GI function and clinical situation/disease process. Enteral products may be classified as polymeric, chemically defined, modular, and disease-specific. Although many companies provide a variety of these products, only a few examples from each category are mentioned here.

Polymeric formulas – Polymeric formulas contain macronutrients (protein, carbohydrate, and fat) in their whole, undigested form. Normal digestion and absorption capacity are required. These products may be designed for oral or tube feeding use. Caloric density generally ranges from 1 to 2 calories/mL. Osmolality ranges from isotonic, approximately 270 to 320 mOsm/kg, to hypertonic, approximately 400 to 700 mOsm/kg. Degree of osmolality increases as caloric density increases. The RDA for most vitamins and minerals can usually be met in 1 to 2 L of formula. Some of these products are milk-based and require lactose tolerance. However, a large number of enteral formulas, are lactose free. A few examples of these products include:

1.) 1 cal/mL: *Ensure* products by Ross Products, *Sustacal* products by Mead Johnson Nutritionals, *Resource* by Novartis. These formulas are appropriate for most individuals who require general dietary supplementation.

2.) 1.5 cal/mL: *Ensure Plus* by Ross Products, *Sustacal Plus* by Mead Johnson Nutritionals, *Resource Plus* by Novartis. These formulas are indicated when concentrated calories and protein are required in a limited volume.

3.) 2 cal/mL: *Deliver 2.0* by Mead Johnson Nutritionals, *TwoCal HN* by Ross Products. These formulas are designed to meet the nutritional needs of individuals who are fluid- and volume-restricted.

4.) Basic pediatric formulas: *Pediasure* by Ross Products, *Kindercal* by Mead Johnson Nutritionals. These formulas contain calorie protein levels and vitamin and mineral profiles suitable for children 1 to 10 years of age.

Chemically defined formulas – Chemically defined formulas contain macronutrients in a predigested, easily absorbable form. These formulas are lactose free and generally low in fat. They are usually unpalatable and have high osmolality. The RDA for vitamins and minerals can usually be met in 1 to 2 L of formula. Indications for use are limited digestive or absorptive capacities. A few examples of these products include: *Vital HN* and *Alitraq* by Ross Products, *Criticare HN* by Mead Johnson Nutritionals, *Vivonex Plus* and *Vivonex Pediatric* by Novartis.

Modular products – Modular products contain only 1 macronutrient, and can be added to the diet or to other enteral formulas to increase calorie or protein content. These products do not contain significant amounts of vitamins or minerals. A few examples of these products include:

1.) Protein modules: *Casec* by Mead Johnson Nutritionals, *ProMod Powder* by Ross Products.

2.) Carbohydrate modules: *Moducal* by Mead Johnson Nutritionals, *Polycose Powder* or *Liquid* by Ross Products.

3.) Fat modules: *MCT Oil* by Mead Johnson Nutritionals.

Disease-specific formulas – Disease-specific formulas contain macronutrient and micronutrient (vitamins and minerals) profiles that meet the special nutritional needs of individuals with certain clinical conditions. These formulas range in osmolality from isotonic to hypertonic, and in caloric den sity from 1 to 2 cal/mL. A few examples of these products include:

1.) Chronic obstructive pulmonary disease: *Pulmocare* by Ross Products, *Respalor* by Mead Johnson Nutritionals.

2.) Renal disease: *Deliver 2.0* by Mead Johnson Nutritionals, *Nepro* and *Suplena* by Ross Products, *Amin-Aid* by McGaw.

3.) Glucose intolerance/Diabetes mellitus: *Glucerna* by Ross Products, *Ultracal* by Mead Johnson Nutritionals, *Resource Diabetic* by Novartis.

4.) Hepatic disease: *Deliver 2.0* by Mead Johnson Nutritionals, *Hepatic-Aid* by McGaw.

5.) Trauma: *Perative* by Ross Products, *Traumacal* by Mead Johnson Nutritionals, *Impact* by Novartis, *Immun-Aid* by McGaw.

Of all the categories of products listed, the polymeric formulas tend to be the least costly and appropriate for the widest range of individuals. Chemically defined and disease-specific formulas are expensive and are used most often in the hospital setting.

Complications associated with enteral formula use are primarily metabolic or GI in nature. These complications can also often be related to the clinical condition of the individual or to medication use; therefore, clinical and pharmacological origins of these complications must also be investigated. Metabolic complications that may be associated with formula use include: Elevated blood urea nitrogen secondary to excess protein, inadequate free water and dehydration; elevated blood glucose secondary to excess caloric or carbohydrate or inadequate free water; elevated serum sodium secondary to inadequate free water or dehydration. GI complications that may be associated with formula use include diarrhea secondary to hyperosmolality of the formula or possibly lack of fiber; constipation secondary to lack of fiber or inadequate free water; and delayed gastric emptying with abdominal distention and possibly vomiting secondary to hyperosmolality or high-fat content of the formula.

Several companies manufacture a variety of these products, only a few are represented here. Many of these products have similar characteristics, but each is specialized in its own way. Tolerance and preference are always variable among individuals; therefore, formula selection should be individualized.

ENTERAL NUTRITIONAL THERAPY

PROTEIN PRODUCTS

▶ Administration and Dosage

See product information for individual dosing guidelines.

PROTEIN PRODUCTS	
Trade name	Doseform
Gevral Protein	**Powder**: Ca casseinate and sucrose. Each cup (≈ 26 g) contains: 15.6 g protein, 7.05 g carbohydrate, 0.52 g fat, < 50 mg Na, ≥ 13 mg K, and 95.3 calories. < 1% alcohol.

PROTEIN PRODUCTS	
Trade name	Doseform
ProMod	**Powder**: D-whey protein concentrate and soy lecithin. Each 26.4 g provides 20 g protein, 2.4 g fat, 2.68 g carbohydrate, 176 mg Ca, 60 mg Na, 260 mg K, 132 mg P, and 112 calories.
Propac	**Powder**: Each tablespoon (4 g) contains 3 g protein (from whey protein), 0.24 g carbohydrate from lactose, 0.32 g fat, 2 mg Cl, 20 mg K, 9 mg Na, 14 mg Ca, 12 mg P, 2 mg Mg, and 16 calories.

Products listed are representative of currently available and widely distributed brands. Similar products, including regional and private label brands, may also exist.

GLUCOSE POLYMERS

▶ Indications

Supplies calories in patients with increased caloric needs or patients unable to meet their caloric needs with usual food intake. Supplies carbohydrate calories in protein-, electrolyte-, and fat-restricted diets. Also used to increase the caloric density of traditional foods, liquid, and tube feedings.

▶ Administration and Dosage

Add to foods or beverages or mix in water. Small, frequent feedings are more desirable than large amounts given infrequently. May be used for extended periods with diets containing all other essential nutrients, or as an oral adjunct to IV administration of nutrients. Not a balanced diet; do not use as a sole source of nutrition.

Content given per 100 mL liquid or 100 g powder.

GLUCOSE POLYMER PRODUCTS	
Trade name	Doseform
Polycose	**Liquid**: 50 g carbohydrate, 200 calories, 70 mg sodium, 140 g chloride, 6 mg potassium, 20 mg calcium, 3 mg phosphorus
Polycose	**Powder**: 94 g carbohydrate, 380 calories, 110 mg sodium, 223 mg chloride, 10 mg potassium, 30 mg calcium, 5 mg phosphorus
Moducal[1]	**Powder**: 95[2] g carbohydrate, 380 calories, 70 mg sodium, 150 mg chloride, < 10 mg potassium
Sumacal[1]	**Powder**: 95[2] g carbohydrate, 380 calories, 100 mg sodium, 210 mg chloride, < 39 mg potassium, < 20 mg calcium, < 31 mg phosphorus

Products listed are representative of currently available and widely distributed brands. Similar products, including regional and private label brands, may also exist.

[1] Contains 0.4 g/100 g minerals (ash).
[2] Maltodextrin.

MEDIUM CHAIN TRIGLYCERIDES (MCT)

▶ Actions

Medium chain triglycerides (MCT) are more rapidly hydrolyzed than conventional food fat, require less bile acid for digestion, are carried by the portal circulation, and are not dependent on chylomicron formation or lymphatic transport. MCT does not provide essential fatty acids.

■ ■ ■

► **Indications**

A special dietary supplement for use in the nutritional management of patients who cannot efficiently digest and absorb conventional long chain food fats.

► **Warnings**

Hepatic cirrhosis: In patients with advanced cirrhosis, large amounts of MCT may elevate blood and spinal fluid levels of medium chain fatty acids (MDFA) due to impaired hepatic clearance of MCFA that are rapidly absorbed via the portal vein. These elevated levels have caused reversible coma and precoma in subjects with advanced cirrhosis, particularly with portacaval shunts. Use with caution in patients with hepatic cirrhosis and complications such as portacaval shunts or tendency to encephalopathy.

► **Administration and Dosage**

15 mL 3 to 4 times per day. Mix with fruit juices, use on salads and vegetables, incorporate into sauces, or use in cooking or baking. Do not use plastic containers or utensils.

MEDIUM CHAIN TRIGLYCERIDES PRODUCTS	
Trade name	Doseform
MCT	**Oil**: Lipid fraction of coconut oil consisting primarily of the triglycerides of C8 ($\approx$ 67%) and C10 ($\approx$ 23%) saturated fatty acids. Contains 115 calories/15 mL.

Products listed are representative of currently available and widely distributed brands. Similar products, including regional and private label brands, may also exist.

MILK-BASED FORMULAS

► **Administration and Dosage**

See product information for individual dosing guidelines.

MILK-BASED FORMULA PRODUCTS	
Trade name	Doseform
Nepro[1]	**Liquid**: 16.6 g protein, 51.1 g carbohydrates, 22.7 g fat, 197 mg Na, 251 mg K
Sustacal[2]	**Powder**: 87.5 g protein, 200 g carbohydrate, 2.9 g fat, 133 mg Na, 4042 mg K
Meritene[3]	**Powder**: 18 g protein, 31 g carbohydrate, 9 g fat, 280 mg Na, 730 mg K
Forta Shake[4]	**Powder**: 9 g protein, 26 g carbohydrate, < 1 g fat, 115 mg Na, 440 mg K
Sustacal[5]	**Pudding**: 6.8 g protein, 32 g carbohydrate, 9.5 g fat, 220 mg Na, 710 mg K
Lofenalac[5]	**Powder**: 15 g protein, 60 g carbohydrate, 18 g fat, 220 mg Na, 470 mg K
Sustagen[6]	**Powder**: 24 g protein, 66 g carbohydrate, 3.5 g fat, 220 mg Na, 710 mg K
Ensure[4]	**Pudding**: 6.8 g protein, 34 g carbohydrate, 9.7 g fat, 240 mg Na, 330 mg K

Products listed are representative of currently available and widely distributed brands. Similar products, including regional and private label brands, may also exist.

[1] Content given per 8 fluid ounces.
[2] Content given for powder mixed with skim milk.
[3] Content given for powder mixed with whole milk.
[4] Content given per serving (42 g mix).
[5] Content given per serving (150 g).
[6] Content given per serving (100 g).

SPECIALIZED FORMULAS

► Administration and Dosage

See product information for individual dosing guidelines.

SPECIALIZED FORMULA PRODUCTS	
Trade name	Doseform
Boost [2]	**Liquid**: 10 g protein, 40 g carbohydrate, 4 g fat, 130 mg Na, 400 mg K
Boost Plus	**Liquid**: 14 g protein, 45 g carbohydrate, 14 g fat, 200 mg Na, 350 mg K
Boost with Fiber[2]	**Liquid**: 11 g protein, 33 g carbohydrate, 8 g fat, 170 mg Na, 330 mg K
Epulor	**Liquid**: 4 g protein, 5 g carbohydrate, 31 g fat
Suplena	**Liquid**: 29.6 g protein, 252.5 g carbohydrate, 95 g fat, 775 mg Na, 1104 mg K
Glucerna	**Liquid**: 41 g protein, 93 g carbohydrate, 55 g fat, 917 mg Na, 1542 mg K
TraumaCal	**Liquid**: 83 g protein, 195 g carbohydrate, 69 g fat, 1200 mg Na, 1400 mg K
Pulmocare [6]	**Liquid**: 62 g protein, 104 g carbohydrate, 92 g fat, 1292 mg Na, 1708 mg K
Respalor	**Liquid**: 75 g protein, 146 g carbohydrate, 70 g fat, 1250 mg Na, 1458 mg K
Peptamen	**Liquid**: 40 g protein, 127.2 g carbohydrate, 39.2 g fat, 500 mg Na, 1252 mg K
Amin-Aid Instant [1]	**Powder**: 6.6 g protein, 124.3 g carbohydrate, 15.7 g fat, < 5 mEq Na
Travasorb Hepatic Diet	**Powder**: 29.4 g protein, 215.2 g carbohydrate, 14.7 g fat, 235 mg Na, 882 mg K
Hepatic-Aid II Instant Drink[3]	**Powder**: 15 g protein, 57.3 g carbohydrate, 12.3 g fat, < 5 mEq Na
Accupep HPF	**Powder**: 40 g protein, 188 g carbohydrate, 10 g fat, 680 mg Na, 1150 mg K
Cyclinex-2[4]	**Powder**: 15 g protein, 40 g carbohydrate, 20.7 g fat, 1175 mg Na, 1830 mg K
Glutarex-2,[4] Hominex-2,[4] I-Valex-2,[4] Ketonex-2,[4] Phenex-2,[4] Propimex-2,[4] Tyrex-2[4]	**Powder**: 30 g protein, 30 g carbohydrate, 15.5 g fat, 880 mg Na, 1370 g K
Immun-Aid[5]	**Powder**: 18.5 g protein, 60 g carbohydrate, 11 g fat, Na, K
Regain Medical Nutrition[7]	**Bar**: 15 g protein, 53 g carbohydrate, 7 g fat, 95 mg Na, 65 mg K
Boost Nutritional Energy[8]	**Bar**: 5 g protein, 30 g carbohydrate, 6 g fat, 50 mg Na, 115 mg K
Boost Nutritional[9]	**Pudding**: 7 g protein, 32 g carbohydrate, 9 g fat, 120 mg Na, 320 mg K

Products listed are representative of currently available and widely distributed brands. Similar products, including regional and private label brands, may also exist.

[1] Content given per 156 g package.
[2] Content given per 237 mL.
[3] Content given per approximately 93 g packets.
[4] Content given per 100 g.
[5] Content given per 123 g.
[6] Content given for vanilla flavor.
[7] Content given per 85 g bar.
[8] Content given per 176 g bar.
[9] Content given per 142 g can.

LACTOSE-FREE PRODUCTS

▶ Administration and Dosage

See product information for individualized dosing guidelines.

LACTOSE-FREE PRODUCTS	
Trade name	Doseform
Nepro	**Liquid**: 69.7 g, protein, 214.6 g carbohydrate, 95.3 g fat, 215 mg Na, 1054 mg K
Entrition 0.5	**Liquid**: 17.5 g protein, 68 g carbohydrate, 17.5 g fat, 350 mg Na, 600 mg K
Pre-Attain	**Liquid**: 20 g protein, 60 g carbohydrate, 20 g fat, 340 mg Na, 575 mg K
Choice dm	**Liquid**: 10.6 g protein, 25 g carbohydrate, 12 g fat, 702 mg Na, 1252 mg K
Vitaneed	**Liquid**: 40 g protein, 128 g carbohydrate, 40 g fat, 630 mg Na, 1250 mg K
Replete-Oral	**Liquid**: 62.5 g protein, 113.2 g carbohydrate, 34 g fat, 500 mg Na, 1560 mg K
Kindercal	**Liquid**: 34 g protein, 135 g carbohydrate, 44 g fat, 370 mg Na, 1310 mg K
Attain	**Liquid**: 40 g protein, 135 g carbohydrate, 35 g fat, 805 mg Na, 1600 mg K
Profiber	**Liquid**: 40 g protein, 132 g carbohydrate, 40 g fat, 730 mg Na, 1250 K
Impact	**Liquid**: 56 g protein, 130 g carbohydrate, 28 g fat, 1100 mg Na, 1300 mg K
Nutren 1.0	**Liquid**: 40 g protein, 127 g carbohydrate, 38 g fat, 500 mg Na, 1252 mg K
Sustacal	**Liquid**: 60.4 g protein, 128 g carbohydrate, 23 g fat, 1000 mg Na, 2042 mg K
TwoCal HN	**Liquid**: 83 g protein, 214.2 g carbohydrate, 90 g fat, 1292 mg Na, 1292 mg K
Entriton HN EntriPak	**Liquid**: 44 g protein, 114 g carbohydrate, 41 g fat, 645 mg Na, 1579 mg K
Criticare HN	**Liquid**: 38 g protein, 220 g carbohydrate, 5.3 g fat, 630 mg Na, 1320 mg K
Isocal	**Liquid**: 34 g protein, 135 g carbohydrate, 44 g fat, 530 mg Na, 1320 mg K
Isocal HN	**Liquid**: 44 g protein, 123 g carbohydrate, 45 g fat, 930 mg Na, 1610 mg K
Jevity	**Liquid**: 44 g protein, 150.8 g carbohydrate, 35 g fat, 917 mg Na, 1542 mg K
Resource	**Liquid**: 9 g protein, 40 g carbohydrate, 6 g fat, 220 mg Na, 350 mg K
Osmolite	**Liquid**: 37 g protein, 143 g carbohydrate, 37 g fat, 625 mg Na, 1000 mg K
Introlite	**Liquid**: 22.2 g protein, 70.5 g carbohydrate, 18.4 g fat, 930 mg Na, 1570 mg K
Osmolite HN	**Liquid**: 44 g protein, 140 g carbohydrate, 35 g fat, 917 mg Na, 1541 mg K
Sustacal Basic	**Liquid**: 37 g protein, 147 g carbohydrate, 35 g fat, 833 mg Na, 1583 mg K
Nutrilan	**Liquid**: 38 g protein, 143 g carbohydrate, 37 g fat, 632.5 mg Na, 1057 mg K
Ensure HN	**Liquid**: 44 g protein, 140 g carbohydrate, 35 g fat, 792 mg Na, 1042 mg K

LACTOSE-FREE PRODUCTS

Trade name	Doseform
Ultracal	**Liquid**: 44 g protein, 123 g carbohydrate, 45 g fat, 930 mg Na, 1610 mg K
Compleat Modified Formula	**Liquid**: 10.7 g protein, 35 g carbohydrate, 9.2 g fat, 250 mg Na, 350 mg K
Ensure Fiber with NutraFlora FOS	**Liquid**: 9 g protein, 42 g carbohydrate, 6 g fat, 200 mg Na, 370 mg K per 237 mL
Isosource	**Liquid**: 10.8 g protein, 42.5 g carbohydrate, 9.84 g fat, 267 mg Na, 417 mg K
Isosource HN	**Liquid**: 13.4 g protein, 39.9 g carbohydrate, 9.84 g fat, 267 mg Na, 417 mg K
Comply	**Liquid**: 60 g protein, 180 g carbohydrate, 60 g fat, 1100 mg Na, 1850 mg K
Nutren 1.5	**Liquid**: 60 g protein, 169.2 g carbohyrate, 67.6 g fat, 752 mg Na, 1872 mg K
Ensure Plus	**Liquid**: 54.2 g protein, 197.1 g carbohydrate, 53 g fat, 1042 mg Na, 1917 mg K
Resource Plus	**Liquid**: 13 g protein, 52 g carbohydrate, 11 g fat, 310 mg Na, 460 mg K
Sustacal Plus	**Liquid**: 61 g protein, 190 g carbohydrate, 58 g fat, 850 mg Na, 1480 mg K
Ensure Plus HN	**Liquid**: 62 g protein, 197 g carbohydrate, 49 g fat, 1167 mg Na, 1792 mg K
Advera	**Liquid**: 60 g protein, 215.8 g carbohydrate, 22.8 g fat, 1046 mg Na, 2827 mg K
Magnacal	**Liquid**: 70 g protein, 250 g carbohydrate, 80 g fat, 1000 mg Na, 1250 mg K
Isocal HCN	**Liquid**: 75 g protein, 200 g carbohydrate, 102 g fat, 800 mg Na, 1700 mg K
Nutren 2.0	**Liquid**: 80 g protein, 196 g carbohydrate, 106 g fat, 1000 mg Na, 2500 mg K
Neocate One +	**Liquid**: ≈ 2.5 g protein, 14.6 g carbohydrate, 3.5 g fat, 20 mg Na, 93 mg K per 100 mL
Isosource 1.5 Cal	**Liquid**: 16.9 g protein, 42 g carbohydrate, 16.2 g fat, 322 mg Na, 536 mg K
Isosource VHN	**Liquid**: 15.6 g protein, 32 g carbohydrate, 7.2 g fat, 320 mg Na, 400 mg K
Nutri-Drink	**Liquid**: 9 g protein, 40 g carbohydrate, 6 g fat, 200 mg Na, 410 mg K per 237 mL
Nutri-Drink Plus	**Liquid**: 13 g protein, 47 g carbohydrates, 13 g fat, 250 mg Na, 460 mg K per 237 mL
Ensure	**Liquid and Powder**: 37 g protein, 143 g carbohydrate, 37 g fat, 833 mg Na, 1542 mg K
Citrotein [1]	**Powder and Liquid**: 10.5 g protein, 31.1 g carbohydrate, 0.4 g fat, 170 mg Na, 140 mg K
Travasorb MCT	**Powder**: 49.6 g protein, 122.8 g carbohydrate, 33 g fat, 350 mg Na, 1000 K
Travasorb HN	**Powder**: 45 g protein, 175 g carbohydrate, 13 g fat, 921 mg Na, 1170 mg K
Travasorb STD	**Powder**: 30 g protein, 190 g carbohydrate, 14 g fat, 921 mg Na, 1170 mg K
Lipisorb	**Powder**: 35 g protein, 117 g carbohydrate, 48 g fat, 733 mg Na, 1250 mg K
Tolerex	**Powder**: 6.2 g protein, 68 g carbohydrate, 0.4 g fat, 141 mg Na, 350 mg K

LACTOSE-FREE PRODUCTS	
Trade name	Doseform
Vivonex T.E.N.	**Powder**: 38.2 g protein, 205 g carbohydrate, 2.77 g fat, 460 mg Na, 782 mg K
Portagen	**Powder**: 23.3 protein, 77 g carbohydrate, 32 g fat, 367 mg Na, 833 mg K
Vital High Nitrogen	**Powder**: 41.7 g protein, 10.8 g carbohydrate, 184.7 g fat, 566.7 mg Na, 1400 mg K
Isotein HN	**Powder**: 20 g protein, 46.7 g carbohydrate, 10 g fat, 183 mg Na, 317 mg K
Precision LR Diet	**Powder**: 7.5 g protein, 71 g carbohydrate, 0.45 g fat, 200 mg Na, 250 mg K
Resource Select	**Powder**: 12.5 g protein, 25.6 g carbohydrate, 8.2 g fat, 200 mg Na, 140 mg K
Forta Drink	**Powder**: 5 g protein, 15 g carbohydrate, < 1 g fat, 50 mg Na, 70 mg K
Neocate	**Powder**: $\approx$ 13 g protein, 49.3 g carbohydrate, 19.1 g fat, 157 mg Na, 653 mg K per 100 g
Neocate One +	**Powder**: $\approx$ 10 g protein, 58 g carbohydrate, 14 g fat, 80 mEq sodium, 372 mEq potassium per 100 g

Products listed are representative of currently available and widely distributed brands. Similar products, including regional and private label brands, may also exist.

[1] Content given per orange flavor.

PATIENT INFORMATION

Enteral Nutritional Products

- Decreased energy level, generalized weakness, and apathy may be initial symptoms of inadequate energy/protein intake. Be aware of this possibility if these symptoms occur.
- A balanced diet is encouraged for all patients; however, nutritional supplements may be necessary if inadequate diet intake persists.
- GI and metabolic complications may result from use of enteral nutritional therapy or may be due to the condition itself. Consider all factors if these symptoms appear/persist.
- Individualize formula selection, because tolerance and preference vary greatly among patients.
- Carefully follow the instructions with the product for specific mixing and dosing guidelines.
- Many products do not provide a balanced diet; do not use as the sole source of nutrition.

INFANT NUTRITION

DEFINITION

Infant formulas must meet standards set forth by the National Research Council of the United States Academy of Sciences to ensure adequate nutrition to support proper growth and development. Prior to the summer of 1997, these were called Recommended Daily Allowances (RDAs), but are now a part of a collective group referred to as the Dietary Reference Intakes (DRIs). DRI is a term that includes four nutrient-based dietary reference values for every life stage and gender group: (1) estimated average requirement, (2) RDA, (3) adequate intake (AI), and (4) tolerable upper intake level. The target intake for individuals is the RDA and is defined as the dietary intake level that meets the daily nutrient requirement of almost all (97% to 98%) of the individuals in a specific life stage and gender group. For healthy breastfed infants, AIs are the mean intake. For more information on RDA guidelines, see Table 1 in the chapter introduction.

Infants require 93 to 120 kcal/kg/day, the highest requirement in the life cycle, and must nurse (intake human milk or infant formula) several times during the day to meet these needs. In general, infant formulas must be lipid and carbohydrate rich. Energy for growth and development comes from carbohydrates, fat, and protein metabolism: 40% to 50% as carbohydrates, 45% to 50% as lipids, and 8% to 15% as protein. Although optimal protein intake is rather low, insufficient calories tend to cause protein to be alternatively used for energy to a higher extent. An essential nutrient cannot be synthesized by the body and must be obtained from an exogenous source to prevent abnormality. Necessary nutrients include the essential amino and fatty acids, as well as vitamins and minerals. Nutritional requirements for infants include:

Sources of Infant Energy/Nutrition	
Source	**Description**
Energy	The body uses energy for basal metabolism, growth, and activity. The mean RDA is 108 kcal/kg/day for infants up to 6 months of age and 98 kcal/kg/day for infants 6 to 12 months of age.
Protein	Protein provides 4 kcal of energy per gram. In addition to energy, protein is utilized by the body for the synthesis of new tissue, antibodies, and hormones. Protein is also a source of nitrogen and nine essential amino acids that cannot be synthesized from other precursors (eg, histidine, isoleucine, leucine, lysine, methionine or cysteine, phenylalanine or tyrosine, threonine, tryptophan, valine). The AI for infants up to 6 months of age is 9.1 g/day and for infants 7 to 12 months of age the RDA is 13.5 g/day.
Fats	Fats provide 9 kcal of energy per gram and are a high caloric source of energy storage. In addition, fat serves as a protective cushion for organs and an insulator against cold. Except for essential fatty acids (eg, linoleic, linolenic, arachidonic), the body can manufacture fats from carbohydrates and proteins. The fatty acids arachidonic acid (ARA) and docosahexaenoic acid (DHA) are being added to several infant formulas; these fats are found in breast milk and are promoted to help with growth and development particularly for eyesight and brain development.

Sources of Infant Energy/Nutrition	
Source	Description
Carbohy-drates	Carbohydrates provide 4 kcal of energy per gram and are classified as monosaccharides, disaccharides, and polysaccharides. They are the main source of energy and can be produced by the body from proteins and fats.
Water	All tissues contain water, and most chemical reactions in the body occur in an aqueous media. Water is supplied to the body from food, drink, and metabolism. Infants receive the majority of their fluid requirement from breast milk and formulas.
Minerals	Minerals are an essential component of body tissue. The majority of the body's minerals consist of calcium, magnesium, and phosphorus. Iron-fortified formulas often are recommended to prevent anemia.
Vitamins	Vitamins are necessary for tissue growth and development. They function as cofactors for a number of enzymatic metabolic reactions. Most are essential and, therefore, cannot be manufactured by the body. Except for vitamin D, breast milk can provide all the vitamins necessary to the infant.

ETIOLOGY

Pediatric patients require sufficient nutrition to meet the demands of growth and development. Most healthy, full-term infants will meet the AI of nutrients from breast milk or infant formulas. Premature or underdeveloped infants or those with certain metabolic disorders, infections, or acute or chronic illness will require an adjustment in their AI of nutrient intake. Special formulas with different amounts of protein, fat, carbohydrates, and caloric content are available for such purposes. It should be noted that certain formulas listed as "metabolic formulas" only should be used under medical supervision to prevent under- or overfeeding, and possibly further complications. Failure to meet the nutritional needs of the infant or to provide adequate essential nutrients can lead to abnormal physical and neurological growth and development, while providing an excess can result in obesity and toxicity.

INCIDENCE

Although there is considerable variation in the nutritional management of infants, most infants in the United States show normal growth and development from the intake of breast milk and/or infant formula.

PATHOPHYSIOLOGY

Failure to meet adequate nutritional requirements may result in recognized nutritional deficiencies that are reversed following correction of the nutrient deficiencies.

SIGNS/SYMPTOMS

Adequate nutrition usually will lead to normal growth, body structure, and integrity. Abnormal growth, impaired immune system, and neurologic deficits may occur when essential nutrients are not provided. If an excess is provided, obesity or toxicity may occur.

DIAGNOSTIC PARAMETERS/PHYSICAL ASSESSMENT

Clinical Observation: Because of the age of the patient, clinical assessment usually will occur by observation and interview with the parent. Abnormal body weight and growth rate are important assessment tools in the evaluation of an infant's nutritional status. Growth charts track body weight to measure nutritional status and detect malnutrition. Length and head circumference also are good measures. If the nutritional needs of the infant are not being met, or if there is an underlying abnormality or disease, nutritional support may be indicated—this requires physician referral.

Interview: To help determine whether the infant's nutritional needs are being met, ask parents about the following:

- Age, height, and weight of the infant
- Frequency of visits to the pediatrician
- Pediatrician recommendations
- Breastfeeding status
- Mother's feelings about breastfeeding
- Supplemental feedings with infant formula or other foods or liquids
- Feeding schedule
- Allergic history of the infant
- Medications, including fluoride, vitamins, and minerals
- Concomitant diseases
- Presence of vomiting, diarrhea, or constipation
- Consistency and appearance of the stool

TREATMENT

Approaches to therapy: Evaluate patients using the previous diagnostic parameters. Depending on various factors (eg, symptoms, duration, recurrence), recommend either: 1) a nondrug therapy—an alteration in nutritional intake using appropriate infant formula, 2) appropriate pharmacotherapy to correct a medical disorder or a vitamin or mineral deficiency, or 3) immediate referral to a pediatrician for further medical evaluation.

Nondrug therapy: Nutrition for infants 6 months of age or younger usually involves breastfeeding, supplementation feedings with infant formula, or infant formula alone. In children older than 6 months of age, the previous diet usually is supplemented with food. Cow's milk and baby food also can be used to supply adequate nutrition to children older than 6 months of age. Usually, adult table food is started at 1 year of age.

Advantages associated with breastfeeding compared with not breastfeeding:

- Less expensive than formula
- Correct consistency and temperature
- Lower incidence of GI disease, otitis media, and allergies
- No artificial ingredients or preservatives
- Maximum antibody protection against infections
- Curds are more easily digested than from formula

Disadvantages associated with breastfeeding:

- Contents of milk are determined by the mammary gland with no external control
- Inconvenience, engorgement, possible infections, and inflammation
- Necessary to avoid drugs that may be excreted in breast milk

FDA-approved infant (individuals 12 months of age and younger) formula is the only acceptable substitute for breast milk for those mothers who cannot or who choose not to breastfeed. Infant formula contains ingredients similar to breast milk and provides a full source of the RDA of nutrients for caloric needs. Mothers may use infant formulas for the sole nutrient source for infants or to supplement breastfed infants for enhanced nutrient intake to achieve normal growth and development. Nutrition for preterm infants and those with metabolic abnormalities should be provided based on instructions from and under the medical supervision of a pediatrician. A list of the most commonly available formulas used for infants with normal nutritional needs is provided in the following pages. In addition, some hypoallergenic formulas and formulas for special populations are also listed. Many products are fortified with iron (average, 1.8 mg/100 cal). It is advised that a pediatrician recommends an appropriate formula based on the infant's specific needs. Weaning usually occurs between 6 and 15 months of age. When weaning occurs before the twelfth month, cow milk-based formula may be used. Because skim milk provides excess protein and insufficient amounts of calories and essential fatty acids, it should be avoided in infants younger than 2 years of age. Infant formulas are marketed in the United States in three forms, as powdered, liquid concentrate, and liquid ready-to-feed products.

INFANT FOODS

▶ **Actions**

Most commercial infant formulas are modified whole cow milk, approximating human breast milk. Their content of carbohydrates, protein, and fats is similar to human breast milk. Other commercial sources of protein include soybeans and soy. Formulas contain vitamins and minerals while supplying a known amount of calories (eg, standard infant formulas supply 20 kcal/oz). Special formulations are available for infants who have a higher caloric requirement, are intolerant to cow's milk, or have malabsorption or metabolic disorders. Protein hydrolysate formulas are available for infants allergic to cow's milk- or soy-based formulas. The primary source of carbohydrates in infant formulas is lactose. Corn syrup is available as the carbohydrate source in lactose-free formulas. Vegetable oil blends are the primary source of fat in infant formulas; they contain little or no cholesterol and substantial amounts of essential fatty acids. Infant formulas reformulated to more closely resemble breast milk now contain arachidonic acid (ARA) and docosahexaenoic acid (DHA) derived from *Mortierella alpina* oil and *Crypthecodinium cohnii* oil, respectively. These nutrients are promoted as essential building blocks for brain and eyesight development.

▶ **Indications**

Infant formulas are sources of nutrients to be used in place of or as a supplement to breastfeeding.

▶ **Warnings**

In conditions where the infant is losing abnormal quantities of one or more electrolytes, it may be necessary to supply electrolytes from sources other than formula. With premature infants weighing less than 1500 g at birth, it may be necessary to supply an additional source of sodium, calcium, and phosphorus during the period of very rapid growth.

Parents should be cautious of signs of cow's milk allergy, which include vomiting, diarrhea, excessive fussiness, irritability, and spitting up, loose stools, runny nose, and the eruption of a rash. In case of suspected milk allergy, it is recommended that the child be evaluated by a pediatrician.

FOOD PRODUCTS FOR TERM INFANTS

▶ **Actions**

The energy density of most formulas for term infants is 20 kcal/oz (670 kcal/L). Formulas with greater energy density (24 kcal/oz) have higher levels of macronutrients, but micronutrients are provided at the same concentrations per 100 kcal as in the 20 kcal/oz formulas.

Milk-based infant formulas: Various cow milk-derived products (eg, nonfat milk, casein, combinations of casein and whey proteins, or partially hydrolyzed whey protein concentrate) provide protein for these formulas. Lactose, corn syrup solids, sucrose, or corn maltodextrin provide carbohydrates, and vegetable oil blends provide fat.

Soy protein-based formulas: The soy protein is a specific protein isolate fortified with L-methionine; combinations of corn maltodextrin, sucrose, or corn syrup solids provide carbohydrate; and vegetable oil blends provide fat.

Protein hydrolysate-based formulas: For infants with milk allergy or intolerance to intact protein (eg, alimentum). Enzymatically hydrolyzed casein, fortified with selected amino acids, provides nitrogen; combinations of corn syrup solids, maltodextrin, or sucrose provide carbohydrate; and vegetable oil blends provide fat. One protein hydrolysate-based product also includes medium chain triglyceride (MCT) oils as a fat source.

▶ **Administration and Dosage**

93 to 120 kcal/kg/24 hr. Do not exceed 30 mL/kg/feeding. If formula intake exceeds 1000 mL/24 hr, supplement the diet with solid food. Feed healthy term infants iron-supplemented formula. Dilute formula as needed (see product instructions). After opening, refrigerate and use within 48 hours. Do not microwave; warm formula in hot water or a bottle warmer.

See individual product listings for specific labeling information and additional ingredients.

FOOD PRODUCTS FOR TERM INFANTS	
Trade name	**Doseform**
Bright Beginnings with Iron[1-3]	**Concentrated liquid and powder**: 2.2 g protein, 10.6 g carbohydrate, 5.3 g fat, 1.2 mg iron/100 calories
Enfamil with Iron[1,2]	**Liquid, concentrated liquid, and powder**: 2.1 g protein, 10.9 g carbohydrate, 5.3 g fat, 1.8 mg iron/100 calories
Enfamil LIPIL with Iron[1-3]	**Liquid (in bottles) and powder**: 2.1 g protein, 10.9 g carbohydrate, 5.3 g fat, 1.8 mg iron/100 calories
Enfamil Low Iron[1,2]	**Liquid, concentrated liquid, and powder**: 2.1 g protein, 10.9 g carbohydrate, 5.3 g fat, 0.7 mg iron/100 calories
Good Start Essentials[1,2]	**Powder**: 2.2 g protein, 11.2 g carbohydrate, 5.1 g fat, 1.5 mg iron/100 calories

FOOD PRODUCTS FOR TERM INFANTS	
Trade name	Doseform
Similac Advance[1-3]	**Liquid, concentrated liquid, and powder**: 2.07 g protein, 10.8 g carbohydrate, 5.4 g fat, 1.8 mg iron/100 calories
Similac with Iron[1,2]	**Liquid, concentrated liquid, and powder**: 2.07 g protein, 10.8 g carbohydrate, 5.4 g fat, 1.8 mg iron/100 calories
Similac Low Iron[1,2]	**Liquid, concentrated liquid, and powder**: 2.07 g protein, 10.8 g carbohydrate, 5.4 g fat, 0.7 mg iron/100 calories
Lactose-Free Products	
Bright Beginnings Soy with Iron	**Powder**: 2.7 g protein, 10.2 g carbohydrate, 5.3 g fat, 1.8 mg iron/100 calories
Good Start Essentials Soy	**Liquid, concentrated liquid, and powder**: 2.8 g protein, 11.1 g carbohydrate, 5.1 g fat, 1.8 mg iron/100 calories
Similac Lactose Free[4]	**Liquid, concentrated liquid, and powder**: 2.14 g protein, 10.7 g carbohydrate, 5.4 g fat, 1.8 mg iron/100 calories
Similac Lactose Free Advance[3,4]	**Liquid and powder**: 2.14 g protein, 10.7 g carbohydrate, 5.4 g fat, 1.8 mg iron/100 calories
Enfamil LactoFree LIPIL[3,4]	**Liquid, concentrated liquid, and powder**: 2.1 g protein, 10.9 g carbohydrate, 5.3 g fat, 1.8 mg iron/100 calories. Sucrose free.

Products listed are representative of currently available and widely distributed brands. Similar products, including regional and private label brands, may also exist.

[1] Contains milk.
[2] Contains lactose.
[3] Contains DHA and ARA.
[4] Contains milk protein.

FOOD PRODUCTS FOR PRETERM OR LOW BIRTH-WEIGHT INFANTS

▶ **Actions**

Premature infant formulas: Energy concentrations of these formulas are 24 kcal/oz and 20 kcal/oz. They also contain higher concentrations of protein and certain micronutrients to meet the needs of preterm infants. These formulas contain nonfat milk, whey protein concentrate, corn syrup solids, lactose, vegetable oil blends, or MCT as sources of macronutrients.

Transitional formulas: These formulas are consumed by many preterm infants as they approach hospital discharge and after discharge. The energy concentration of these formulas is 22 kcal/oz and they contain higher concentrations of certain nutrients than formulas for term infants. These formulas contain nonfat milk, whey protein concentrate, maltodextrin, lactose, or vegetable oil blends as sources of macronutrients.

Human milk fortifiers: Human milk fortifiers are nutritional supplement products that may be added to breast milk to supplement its nutrient content. These products contain corn syrup solids and milk proteins with or without MCT as energy sources. Addition of these powdered human milk fortifiers result in minimal volume increment to the fluid volume consumed by the preterm infant.

▶ **Administration and Dosage**

See individual product listings for specific labeling information and additional ingredients.

FOOD PRODUCTS FOR PRETERM OR LOW BIRTH-WEIGHT INFANTS	
Trade name	Doseform
Enfamil Human Milk Fortifier[1]	**Powder:** 1.1 g protein, < 0.4 g carbohydrate, 1 g fat, 1.44 mg iron/0.71 g
Enfamil Premature LIPIL[1-3]	**Liquid (in bottles):** 3 g protein, 11 g carbohydrate, 5.1 g fat, 0.5 mg iron/100 calories
Enfamil Premature LIPIL with Iron[1-3]	**Liquid (in bottles):** 3 g protein, 11 g carbohydrate, 5.1 g fat, 1.8 mg iron/100 calories
Similac Human Milk Fortifier[1]	**Powder:** 1 g protein, 1.8 g carbohydrate, 0.36 g fat, 0.4 mg iron/3.6 g
Similac Natural Care Advance[1-3]	**Liquid:** 2.71 g protein, 10.6 g carbohydrate, 5.43 g fat, 0.4 mg iron/100 calories
Similac NeoSure Advance[1-3]	**Liquid and powder:** 2.6 g protein, 10.3 g carbohydrate, 5.5 g fat, 1.8 mg iron/100 calories
Similac Special Care Advance 20[1-3]	**Liquid:** 2.71 g protein, 10.6 g carbohydrate, 5.43 g fat, 0.4 mg iron/100 calories
Similac Special Care Advance with Iron 24[1-3]	**Liquid:** 2.71 g protein, 10.6 g carbohydrate, 5.43 g fat, 1.8 mg iron/100 calories

Products listed are representative of currently available and widely distributed brands. Similar products, including regional and private label brands, may also exist.

[1] Contains milk.
[2] Contains lactose.
[3] Contains DHA and ARA.

FOOD PRODUCTS FOR OLDER INFANTS

▶ Actions

Follow-up or follow-on formulas: Follow-up or follow-on formulas are iron-fortified, cow milk-based, or isolated soy protein-based products intended for use by older infants (older than 6 months of age) and toddlers consuming solid foods. These formulas are marketed in powder, liquid concentrate, and liquid ready-to-feed forms. The nutrient concentrations of formulas for older infants must meet the nutrient requirements for formulas fed to younger infants. They typically contain higher levels of calcium and phosphorus than formulas for younger infants.

▶ Administration and Dosage

See individual product listings for specific labeling information and additional ingredients.

FOOD PRODUCTS FOR OLDER INFANTS	
Trade name	Doseform
Enfamil Next Step LIPIL[1-3]	**Powder:** 2.6 g protein, 10.5 g carbohydrate, 5.3 g fat, 2 mg iron/100 calories
Enfamil Next Step ProSobee LIPIL[3]	**Powder:** 3.3 g protein, 11.8 g carbohydrate, 4.4 g fat, 2 mg iron/100 calories
Good Start 2 Essentials[1]	**Liquid, concentrated liquid, and powder:** 2.6 g protein, 13.2 g carbohydrate, 4.1 g fat, 1.8 mg iron/100 calories
PediaSure	**Liquid:** 3 g protein, 11 g carbohydrate, 4.98 g fat, 1.4 mg iron/100 calories. Vanilla, banana cream, strawberry, and chocolate flavors.
Similac Isomil 2	**Powder:** 2.45 g protein, 10.3 g carbohydrate, 5.46 g fat, 1.8 mg iron/100 calories

Products listed are representative of currently available and widely distributed brands. Similar products, including regional and private label brands, may also exist.

[1] Contains milk.
[2] Contains lactose.
[3] Contains DHA and ARA.

SPECIALIZED INFANT FOODS

▶ **Actions**

Metabolic infant formulas: Metabolic infant formulas are formulated for use by infants with disorders of amino acid metabolism, such as phenylketonuria, maple syrup urine disease, tyrosinemia, or other inherited metabolic disorders. Metabolic infant formulas and other products for infants with special nutritional needs are available only in powder form. These formulas contain corn syrup solids, blends of vegetable oils, and selected balance of amino acids. Each is formulated without the primary offending amino acid(s) for the specific disorders. Unlike other formulas, these products are not intended to be fed as the sole source of nutrition to infants with metabolic disorders.

▶ **Administration and Dosage**

See individual product listings for specific labeling information and additional ingredients.

SPECIALIZED INFANT FOOD PRODUCTS	
Trade name	**Doseform**
Cyclinex-1	**Powder:** 7.5 g protein, 52 g carbohydrate, 27 g fat, 10 mg iron/100 g
Enfamil A.R. LIPIL[1-3]	**Liquid:** 2.5 g protein, 11 g carbohydrate, 5.1 g fat, 1.8 mg iron/100 calories
Enfamil Nutramigen LIPIL[1,4]	**Powder:** 2.8 g protein, 10.3 g carbohydrate, 5.3 g fat, 1.8 mg iron/100 calories
Enfamil Pregestimil[4]	**Liquid (in bottles) and powder:** 2.8 g protein, 10.2 g carbohydrate, 5.6 g fat, 1.8 mg iron/100 calories
Glutarex-1	**Powder:** 15 g protein, 46 g carbohydrate, 23.9 g fat, 9 mg iron/100 g
Hominex-1	**Powder:** 15 g protein, 46.3 g carbohydrate, 23.9 g fat, 9 mg iron/100 g
I-Valex-1	**Powder:** 15 g protein, 46.3 g carbohydrate, 23.9 g fat, 9 mg iron/100 g
Ketonex-1	**Powder:** 15 g protein, 46.3 g carbohydrate, 23.9 g fat, 9 mg iron/100 g
PediaSure with Fiber	**Liquid:** 3 g protein, 11.4 g carbohydrate, 4.98 g fat, 1.4 mg iron, 0.5 g dietary fiber/100 calories
Phenex-1	**Powder:** 15 g protein, 46.3 g carbohydrate, 23.9 g fat, 9 mg iron/100 g
Phenyl-Free 1	**Powder:** 16.2 g protein, 51 g carbohydrate, 26 g fat, 9.6 mg iron, 500 calories/100 g
Pro-Phree	**Powder:** 60 g carbohydrate, 31 g fat, 11.9 mg iron/100 g
Propimex-1	**Powder:** 15 g protein, 46.3 g carbohydrate, 23.9 g fat, 9 mg iron/100 g
RCF	**Liquid, concentrated:** 4 g protein, 0 g carbohydrate, 7.2 g fat, 2.4 mg iron, 81 calories/100 mL concentrated liquid
Similac Alimentum[4]	**Liquid and powder:** 2.75 g protein, 10.2 g carbohydrate, 5.54 g fat, 1.8 mg iron/100 calories
Similac Alimentum Advance[1,4]	**Liquid and powder:** 2.75 g protein, 10.2 g carbohydrate, 5.54 g fat, 1.8 mg iron/100 calories
Similac Isomil	**Liquid, concentrated liquid, and powder:** 2.45 g protein, 10.3 g carbohydrate, 5.46 g fat, 1.8 mg iron/100 calories

SPECIALIZED INFANT FOOD PRODUCTS

Trade name	Doseform
Similac Isomil Advance[1]	**Liquid, concentrated liquid, and powder**: 2.45 g protein, 10.3 g carbohydrate, 5.46 g fat, 1.8 mg iron/100 calories
Similac Isomil DF	**Liquid**: 2.66 g protein, 10.1 g carbohydrate, 5.46 g fat, 1.8 mg iron, 0.9 g dietary fiber/100 calories
Similac PM 60/40[2]	**Powder**: 2.22 g protein, 10.2 g carbohydrate, 5.59 g fat, 0.7 mg iron/100 calories

Products listed are representative of currently available and widely distributed brands. Similar products, including regional and private label brands, may also exist.

[1] Contains DHA and ARA.
[2] Contains lactose.
[3] Contains milk.
[4] Hypoallergenic formula.

PATIENT INFORMATION

Infant Foods

- Instructions accompany each product. Have the parent carefully read these instructions before use, preferably before leaving the pharmacy, in case they have any questions.
- Nursing mothers should not use medications while breastfeeding without consulting their physician or other health care providers.
- Caution parents about unsubstantiated advertising claims about dietary supplements.
- Assist parents in the selection of infant formulas that best meet their needs.
- Instruct parents in the proper technique when using products that require preparation and sterilization.
- In conditions where the infant is losing abnormal quantities of one or more electrolytes, it may be necessary to supply electrolytes from sources other than the formula. With premature infants weighing less than 1500 g at birth, it may be necessary to supply an additional source of sodium, calcium, and phosphorous during the period of very rapid growth.
- Do not use the microwave to prepare or warm formula; serious burns may occur. Warm formula in hot water or a bottle warmer.

OPHTHALMIC CONDITIONS

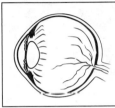

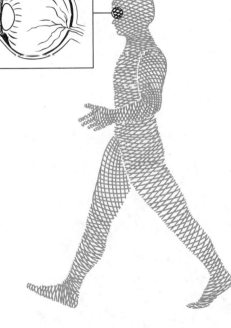

NONPRESCRIPTION DRUG THERAPY
TABLE OF CONTENTS

■ ■ ■

OPHTHALMIC CONDITIONS

INTRODUCTION

Ophthalmic conditions or complaints are not uncommon, especially considering the prevalence of contact lens wear. From dry eye to conjunctivitis to complaints of minor eye irritation or redness, it is not unusual for patients to present with ophthalmic conditions that pose a challenge when trying to determine the appropriate course of therapy. Because of the complexity of ocular surface problems, chronic cases can exacerbate if improperly diagnosed or treated, which in some cases can lead to permanent vision problems. It is therefore important to note that any patient who complains of an ophthalmic condition and is looking for self-treatment options must be handled with the utmost care, and proper referral cannot be overemphasized. Misdiagnosis of ocular surface insults, based solely on symptoms, can be avoided by appropriate clinical care.

The ocular surface, which consists of the cornea and conjunctiva, is protected from environmental exposure as well as microbial and other insult by the orbit, lids, lashes, and tear film. The glands of the lids and conjunctiva secrete this tri-layered matrix and nourish the exposed ocular surface as well. The tear film is composed of mucous, aqueous, and lipid layers. The most common tear film abnormality is aqueous deficiency. Its prevalence increases with age. If anomalies of the lid, specifically blepharitis are included, lipid-layer abnormalities become the most prevalent condition. Mucus-layer deficiencies are generally secondary to chemical insult or chronic disorders. Any of these may be exacerbated by or preclude contact lens wear. Nonspecific symptoms of ocular irritation (itching, burning, increased tearing, foreign-body sensation) may lead to self-treatment or a request for advice from the pharmacist.

Although pathways to infection and allergic response are well known, causes and treatment of the dry eye remain largely enigmatic. Dry eye may result from tear-layer deficiencies or other traumatic events, including contact lens wear. Intermittently symptomatic dry eye may become intransigent. Allergic conjunctivitis may develop more significant symptoms or tissue changes. Styes can become chronic, leading to lid tissue alterations. Inappropriate contact lens care or lens-care systems may lead to infection, perhaps serious enough in the case of corneal ulceration, to require hospitalization and result in vision loss. Because the ocular surface response to a spectrum of insults is nonspecific, delay in diagnosis or treatment may lead to these complications.

Perhaps the greatest cause of persistent dry eye symptoms is the preservatives in OTC ophthalmic preparations. When patients self-treat, they may not realize that application of preserved solutions more frequently than 4 times per day can do more harm than good. The only alternative until recently was nonpreserved unit-dose preparations. Fortunately, tear supplements are now available in transiently preserved versions. For mild symptoms of short duration, these represent a safe alternative for most patients without an eye care visit. Tear-supplement preparations also offer a cost advantage over unit-dose formulations.

Once a course of treatment is recommended or prescribed, adherence to the dosage schedule is critical. Patients should understand that both acute and chronic ophthalmic conditions might be alleviated quickly following appropriate treatment. Strict adherence to any dosing schedule, however protracted, should be integral with all patient information. A good rule of thumb is that when resolution extends beyond 2 days, an alternate diagnosis should be sought. This would be true when patients are self-medicating or if the initial recommendation fails to provide the intended relief.

Considering the large number of patients who use contact lenses and the resultant plethora of contact lens care products, it is essential that the health care professional be familiar with these products so that they can play an important role in the patient's self-care regimen. For contact lens products, separation of those products intended for rigid lenses from those used in the care of soft lenses is imperative. Products for heat disinfection (although now less common) versus chemical disinfection are also important distinctions. In addition, OTC ophthalmic products containing benzalkonium chloride (BAK) are contraindicated for use in the eyes of soft contact lens wearers. An easy mnemonic to share with these patients is that anything containing BAK means, "buy another kind." Benzalkonium chloride is concentrated in the soft lens and later creates a chronic allergic response. Patient confusion can easily be alleviated by appropriate counseling.

Ophthalmic conditions pose an interesting challenge for the health care professional. Many conditions can be treated with non-drug or OTC drug therapy, but it is essential that patients are immediately referred to an optometrist or ophthalmologist for conditions that are difficult to identify, conditions that clearly need an eye care professional's diagnosis or care, or conditions that do not resolve after 2 days of treatment with either prescription or nonprescription therapy. When it comes to a patient's vision, one can never be too cautious.

ALLERGIC CONJUNCTIVITIS

DEFINITION

Allergic conjunctivitis is an inflammatory reaction of the conjunctiva, which is the thin mucous membrane that lines the inner surface of the eyelids and the anterior surface of the white portion (sclera) of the eyeball. The reaction can occur acutely or chronically. The major symptoms are ocular itching, watering, and redness. The reaction includes conjunctival chemosis (swelling), engorgement of conjuctival vessels, and a conjunctival papillary response.

ETIOLOGY

Allergic conjunctivitis is an immunological response that is incited by a specific allergen. Common conjuctival allergens include airborne pollens, smoke, dust, environmental contaminants, vegetable substances, yeast, animal hair, and danders. Other provoking allergens include cosmetics, perfumes, soaps, detergents, aftershave lotions, hair dressings, contact lens solutions, and ophthalmic drugs. Ophthalmic drugs that more commonly trigger allergic responses are neomycin, sulfonamide preparations, proparacaine, cyclopentolate, atropine, timolol, and thimerosal.

Patients with mild and chronic allergic symptoms may have dry eyes as the primary problem. Inadequate tear production allows for allergens and allergic mediators to have longer contact time with the ocular surface before becoming washed away.

INCIDENCE

Allergic conjunctivitis is common in patients with a personal history or a family history of atopy, asthma, eczema, hay fever, or other allergies. In one study, the prevalence of allergies in a surveyed population was 9.4%. The prevalence of allergic conditions in other epidemiological estimates indicates that over 18% of the population (over 50 million people) has allergic conjunctivitis or allergic rhinitis. Often, allergic conjunctivitis is the only manifestation of allergic disease.

PATHOPHYSIOLOGY

Hypersensitivity reactions are humoral or cell-mediated immunologic interactions resulting in release of vasoactive amines and lymphokines. Type I, or immediate, Ig-mediated reactions occur within minutes of the re-exposure of a specific antigen. This response is mediated by serum immunoglobins (antibodies) and produces an eosinophilic cellular response. Seasonal allergies are examples of type I reactions. Type IV, or delayed, reactions are cell-mediated (lymphocytes) responses to an antigen and produce a primarily mononuclear cellular response. The reaction occurs within hours to days. Type IV reactions have signs and symptoms similar to type I reactions, along with possible mild follicular responses and basophils identified on conjunctival scrapings.

Hypersensitivity reactions involve a cascade of events initiated by mast cell degranulation (rupture). The conjunctiva has a mast cell density averaging 5000 cell/mm^3; the densest area is the limbus. Each mast cell contains granules filled with inflammatory chemical mediators, including histamines and precursors of prostaglandins, thromboxanes, and leukotrienes. IgE receptors on the mast cell membrane surface react with antigen-specific IgE antibodies synthesized from mature plasma cells. The ensuing degranulation of the mast cell causes release of large quantities of the chemical mediators. These mediators trigger vascular dilation and serous exudation, causing the conjuctival hyperemia and chemosis. The degranulation is also characterized by the annoying itching and tearing symptoms of allergic conjunctivitis.

SIGNS/SYMPTOMS

The distinguishing symptom of allergic conjunctivitis is itching. Often this itching is unrelenting. Other symptoms include a watery discharge, stringy whitish mucus, redness and swelling of the conjunctiva, and possibly the eyelids. A history of a specific allergen may be reported. Visual acuity is not reduced, but may fluctuate.

DIAGNOSTIC PARAMETERS/PHYSICAL ASSESSMENT

Clinical Observation: Allergic conjunctivitis may present unilaterally or bilaterally. The bulbar conjunctiva appears pink to red because of vascular engorgement. The chemotic mucous membranes have a shiny luster. A stringy mucus may be present. The eyelids may be red and edematous. Conjunctival papillary reaction is present. Mild superior punctate keratitis may be present. Preauricular nodes are not palpable, as they are with viral conjunctivitis.

Interview: It may be beneficial to ask the patient about the following:

- Recent redness, swelling, or itching of the eyelid(s).
- Discharge from the eye.
- History of atopy, asthma, eczema, hay fever, or other allergies.
- Recent changes in use of cosmetics, perfumes, soaps, detergents, aftershave lotions, haircare products, contact lens solutions, or ophthalmic drugs.
- Past occurrences of allergic conjunctivitis and success of past treatments.

TREATMENT

Approaches to therapy: If the cause of conjunctivitis (allergic, viral, bacterial) is uncertain, or if is nonresponsive to therapy, see an optometrist or ophthalmologist to rule out early bacterial and early viral conjunctivitis.

The best approach to treatment of allergic conjunctivitis is removal of the allergen. Because this is not always possible, other treatments are employed. Cold compresses, saline rinses, artificial tears, and drug therapy utilizing OTC topical vasoconstrictors and antihistamines are often successful in relieving signs and symptoms. Avoid rubbing eyes, which causes additional tissue irritation.

Patients with a history of atopy, hay fever, eczema, or other systemic allergy respond well to mast cell stabilizers. These are not OTC medications and require a prescription from an optometrist or ophthalmologist.

Desensitization is reserved for more severe cases in which an airborne or specific allergen can be unequivocally identified.

Nondrug therapy: Removal or avoidance of the inciting agent, if possible, is the best cure. Frequent cool compresses (to decrease the circulation and immunological cascade), and frequent eye rinsing with saline solutions or artificial tears (to dilute and irrigate the allergen) will provide relief of symptoms.

Pharmacotherapy: Ophthalmic decongestants (vasoconstrictors) or antihistamines are indicated for acute symptoms. Combinations of vasoconstrictors and antihistamines are slightly more effective because of synergism. OTC topical and oral combinations are available.

Decongestants, including naphazoline, phenylephrine, and oxymetazoline, cause vasoconstriction (alpha-adrenergic) that reduces conjunctival hyperemia, congestion, and edema, and greatly relieve symptoms. Topical preparations can be used 4 to 6 times daily. However, rebound hyperemia occurs in long-term use or with frequent use of phenylephrine. The dosage can be reduced to "as needed" as symptoms subside.

Histamine inhibitors relieve the symptoms of hyperemia, tearing, and itching due to immediate (type I) response of histamine release. Antazoline and pheniramine are antihistamines used in OTC topical combinations with decongestants (eg, *Vasocon-A, Naphcon-A, Opcon-A*). These preparations are quite effective in relieving allergy symptoms when used every 3 to 4 hours.

Oral antihistamines may be utilized in moderate to severe cases. Both OTC and prescription antihistamines are available. Dosage recommendations vary; use the smallest dose to relieve the symptoms. Refer to the package insert for instructions.

Allergic conjunctivitis treatment may require prescription medications (eg, levocabastine [*Livostin*], cromolyn sodium [*Crolom*], lodozamide [*Alomide*], olopatadine [*Patanol*], ketorolac [*Acular*], corticosteroids). If symptoms are not relieved through the OTC therapies, refer patients to an optometrist or ophthalmologist for further evaluation and treatment.

OPHTHALMIC DECONGESTANTS

▶ **Actions**

The effects of sympathomimetic agents on the eye are concentration-dependent and include: Pupil dilation, increase in outflow of aqueous humor, and vasoconstriction (alpha-adrenergic effects).

Higher drug concentrations (ie, phenylephrine 2.5% and 10%) cause vasoconstriction and pupillary dilation for diagnostic eye exams, during surgery, and to prevent synechiae formation in uveitis. Weak concentrations of phenylephrine (0.12%) and other alpha-adrenergic agonists (naphazoline, tetrahydrozoline) are used as ophthalmic decongestants (vasoconstriction of conjunctival blood vessels) and for symptomatic relief of minor eye irritations.

Nonprescription Ophthalmic Vasoconstrictors		
Vasoconstrictor	Duration of action (hrs)	Available concentrations
Naphazoline	3 to 4	0.012%, 0.02%, 0.03%
Oxymetazoline	4 to 6	0.025%
Phenylephrine	0.5 to 1.5	0.12%
Tetrahydrozoline	1 to 4	0.05%

▶ Indications

Itching, tearing, and redness of allergic conjunctivitis. Refer to individual product listings for specific indications.

▶ Contraindications

Hypersensitivity to any of these agents; narrow-angle glaucoma or anatomically narrow-angle (occludable) and no glaucoma; prior to peripheral iridectomy in eyes capable of angle closure because mydriatic action may precipitate angle closure. Certain health conditions and age restrictions are also contraindications. See package inserts for specific listings.

▶ Warnings

Ophthalmic solutions may sting or burn upon contact with the eye.

Anesthetics: Discontinue prior to use of anesthetics that sensitize the myocardium to sympathomimetics (eg, cyclopropane, halothane).

Local anesthetics can increase absorption of topical drugs; exercise caution when applying prior to use of phenylephrine. However, use of a local anesthetic prior to phenylephrine 2.5% or 10% may prevent stinging and enhance ocular drug penetration.

Overuse: Overuse may cause rebound vasodilation and increased redness of the eye.

Special risk patients: Use with caution in children of low body weight, the elderly, and in the presence of hypertension, diabetes, hyperthyroidism, cardiovascular abnormalities, and arteriosclerosis.

Narrow-angle glaucoma: Ordinarily, any mydriatic is contraindicated in patients with angle-closure glaucoma. However, when temporary pupil dilation may free adhesions, these advantages may temporarily outweigh danger from coincident pupil dilation.

Rebound congestion: Rebound congestion may occur with frequent or extended use of ophthalmic vasoconstrictors. Rebound miosis has occurred in older persons 1 day after receiving phenylephrine; reinstillation produced a reduction in mydriasis.

Systemic absorption: Exceeding recommended dosages of these agents or applying phenylephrine 2.5% to 10% solutions to the instrumented, traumatized, diseased, or postsurgical eye or adnexa, or to patients with suppressed lacrimation as during anesthesia, may result in the absorption of sufficient quantities to produce a systemic vasopressor response.

Pigment floaters: Older individuals may develop transient pigment floaters in the aqueous humor 30 to 45 minutes after instillation of phenylephrine. The appearance may be similar to anterior uveitis or to a microscopic hyphema.

Soft contact lenses: Any solution preserved with benzalkonium chloride (BAK) should not be used with soft contact lenses. When treatment ceases, lens wear may be resumed within a few hours after discontinuation of the drug.

Pregnancy: Category C. Safety for use in pregnancy is not established. Use only if clearly needed and if the potential benefits outweigh potential hazards to the fetus.

Lactation: Safety for use during breastfeeding has not been established. Use caution when administering to a nursing woman.

Children: Safety and efficacy have not been established. Phenylephrine 10% is contraindicated in infants.

Hazardous tasks: Phenylephrine and the other ophthalmic decongestants may cause temporary blurred or unstable vision; observe caution while driving or performing other hazardous tasks.

Sulfite sensitivity: Some of these products contain sulfites that may cause allergic-type reactions (eg, hives, itching, wheezing, anaphylaxis) in certain susceptible people. Although the overall prevalence of sulfite sensitivity in the general population is low, it is seen more frequently in asthmatics or in atopic nonasthmatic people.

▶ Drug Interactions

Ophthalmic Sympathomimetic Drug Interactions			
Precipitant drug	Object drug*		Description
Anesthetics	Ophthalmic sympathomimetics	↑	Cautiously use anesthetics that sensitize the myocardium to sympathomimetics (eg, cyclopropane, halothane). Local anesthetics can increase absorption of topical drugs; exercise caution when applying prior to use of phenylephrine.
Beta blockers	Ophthalmic sympathomimetics	↑	Systemic side effects may occur more readily in patients taking these drugs.
MAOIs	Ophthalmic sympathomimetics	↑	When given with, or up to 21 days after MAOIs, exaggerated adrenergic effects may result. Supervise and adjust dosage carefully.

* ↑ = Object drug increased.

Also consider drug interactions that may occur with systemic use of the sympathomimetics.

▶ Adverse Reactions

Ophthalmic: Overtreatment of acute or chronic conjunctivitis can cause conjunctival hyperemia and irritation. These symptoms are relieved after medication is withdrawn.

Transitory stinging on initial instillation; blurred vision; mydriasis; increased redness; irritation; discomfort; punctate keratitis; lacrimation; increased IOP. See individual package inserts.

Phenylephrine: Phenylephrine may cause rebound miosis and decreased mydriatic response to therapy in older persons.

Cardiovascular: Palpitation; tachycardia; cardiac arrhythmia; hypertension; collapse; extrasystoles; ventricular arrhythmias (ie, premature ventricular contractions); reflex bradycardia; coronary occlusion; subarachnoid hemorrhage; MI; stroke; death associated with cardiac reactions. Headache or browache may occur.

Miscellaneous: Blanching; sweating; dizziness; nausea; nervousness; drowsiness; weakness; hyperglycemia.

PHENYLEPHRINE HCL

▶ **Indications**

0.12%: A decongestant to provide relief of minor eye irritations.

▶ **Administration and Dosage**

Minor eye irritations: Instill 1 or 2 drops of the 0.12% solution in the affected eye(s) up to 4 times daily as needed.

Stability: Prolonged exposure to air or strong light may cause oxidation and discoloration. Do not use if solution changes color, becomes cloudy, or contains a precipitate.

PHENYLEPHRINE HCL PRODUCTS	
Trade name	Doseform
AK-Nefrin	**Solution**: 0.12%. 0.005% benzalkonium Cl, 1.4% polyvinyl alcohol, EDTA.
Prefrin Liquifilm	**Solution**: 0.12%. 1.4% polyvinyl alcohol, 0.004% benzalkonium Cl, EDTA.
Relief, Zincfrin	**Solution**: 0.12%. 0.01% benzalkonium Cl, polysorbate 80, 0.25% zinc sulfate.

Products listed are representative of currently available and widely distributed brands. Similar products, including regional and private label brands, may also exist.

PATIENT INFORMATION

Phenylephrine HCl

- Phenylephrine may cause temporary blurred or unstable vision; observe caution while driving or performing other hazardous tasks.
- Do not use beyond 48 to 72 hours without consulting a physician.
- If irritation, blurring, or redness persists, or if severe eye pain, headache, vision changes, floating spots, dizziness, decrease in body temperature, drowsiness, acute eye redness, or pain with light exposure occurs, discontinue use and consult a physician.
- Do not use if you have glaucoma except under the advice of a physician.
- If ocular stinging occurs, refrigeration of the solution prior to use may decrease this sensation. Artificial tears application prior to allergy drop may also reduce stinging.
- Discard any solution that becomes cloudy or discolored.
- Avoid consuming alcohol and other sedatives during use.
- May produce excitability in children.
- Discontinue use several days prior to allergy skin testing.
- Avoid contamination of tips of containers and recap immediately after use.
- Soft contact lens wear may need to be avoided during treatment.

NAPHAZOLINE HCL

▶ **Indications**

Redness: To soothe, refresh, and remove redness due to minor eye irritation such as smoke, smog, sun glare, allergies, or swimming.

▶ **Warnings**

Soft contact lenses: Any solution preserved with benzalkonium chloride (BAK) should not be used with soft contact lenses. When treatment ceases, lens wear may be resumed within a few hours after discontinuation of the drug.

▶ **Administration and Dosage**

Instill 1 or 2 drops into the conjunctival sac of the affected eye(s) every 3 to 4 hours, up to 4 times daily as needed.

Storage/Stability: Do not use if solution changes color or becomes cloudy.

NAPHAZOLINE HCL PRODUCTS	
Trade name	**Doseform**
Allerest Eye Drops	**Solution**: 0.012%. Benzalkonium Cl, EDTA.
Clear Eyes	**Solution**: 0.012%. Benzalkonium Cl, EDTA, 0.2% glycerin, boric acid.
Clear Eyes ACR	**Solution**: 0.012%. Benzalkonium Cl, EDTA, 0.25% zinc sulfate, 0.2% glycerin.
Degest 2	**Solution**: 0.012%. 0.0067% benzalkonium Cl, 0.02% EDTA, hydroxyethylcellulose, povidone.
Naphcon	**Solution**: 0.012%. 0.01% benzalkonium Cl, EDTA.
Allergy Drops	**Solution**: 0.012%. 0.2% PEG-300, 0.01% benzalkonium Cl.
Vaso Clear	**Solution**: 0.02%. 0.01% benzalkonium Cl, 0.25% polyvinyl alcohol, 1% PEG-400, EDTA.
Vaso Clear A	**Solution**: 0.02%. 0.005% benzalkonium Cl, EDTA, 0.25% zinc sulfate, 0.25% polyvinyl alcohol, 1% PEG-400.
Comfort Eye Drops	**Solution**: 0.03%. 0.005% benzalkonium Cl, 0.02% EDTA.
Maximum Strength Allergy Drops	**Solution**: 0.03%. 0.01% benzalkonium Cl, 0.5% hydroxypropyl methylcellulose, EDTA.

Products listed are representative of currently available and widely distributed brands. Similar products, including regional and private label brands, may also exist.

PATIENT INFORMATION

Naphazoline HCl

- Do not use beyond 48 to 72 hours without consulting a physician.
- If irritation, blurring, or redness persists, or if severe eye pain, headache, vision changes, floating spots, dizziness, decrease in body temperature, drowsiness, acute eye redness, or pain with light exposure occurs, discontinue use and consult a physician.
- Do not use if you have glaucoma except under the advice of a physician.
- If ocular stinging occurs, refrigeration of the solution prior to use may decrease this sensation. Artificial tears application prior to allergy drop may also reduce stinging.
- Discard any solution that becomes cloudy or discolored.
- Avoid consuming alcohol and other sedatives during use.
- May produce excitability in children.
- Discontinue use several days prior to allergy skin testing.
- Avoid contamination of tips of containers and recap immediately after use.
- Soft contact lens wear may need to be avoided during treatment.

TETRAHYDROZOLINE HCL

▶ **Indications**

Redness: For relief of redness of the eye due to minor irritations.

Burning/Irritation: For temporary relief of burning and irritation due to dryness of the eye, discomfort due to minor irritations, or to exposure to wind or sun.

▶ **Warnings**

Soft contact lenses: Any solution preserved with benzalkonium chloride (BAK) should not be used with soft contact lenses. When treatment ceases, lens wear may be resumed within a few hours after discontinuation of the drug.

▶ **Administration and Dosage**

Instill 1 or 2 drops into the affected eye(s) up to 4 times a day as needed.

Stability: Do not use if solution changes color or becomes cloudy.

TETRAHYDROZOLINE HCL PRODUCTS	
Trade name	Doseform
AR Eye Drops-Astringent Redness Reliever	**Solution**: 0.05%. 0.25% zinc sulfate.
Collyrium Fresh	**Solution**: 0.05%. 0.01% benzalkonium Cl, 0.1% EDTA, 1% glycerin.
Eye Drops, Eyesine, Mallazine Eye Drops	**Solution**: 0.05%. 0.01% benzalkonium Cl, EDTA.
Eye Drops Extra	**Solution**: 0.05%. 1% polyethylene glycol 400.
Geneye, Optigene 3, Visine	**Solution**: 0.05%. 0.01% benzalkonium Cl, 0.1% EDTA.
Geneye Extra, Tetrasine Extra	**Solution**: 0.05%. 1% polyethylene glycol 400, benzalkonium Cl, EDTA.
Murine Plus	**Solution**: 0.05%. Benzalkonium Cl, EDTA, 1.4% polyvinyl alcohol, 0.6% povidone.
Tetrasine	**Solution**: 0.05%. Benzalkonium Cl, EDTA.
Visine Allergy Relief	**Solution**: 0.05%. 0.01% benzalkonium Cl, 0.1% EDTA, 0.25% zinc sulfate.
Visine Moisturizing	**Solution**: 0.05%. 0.013% benzalkonium Cl, 0.1% EDTA, 1% PEG-400.

Products listed are representative of currently available and widely distributed brands. Similar products, including regional and private label brands, may also exist.

PATIENT INFORMATION
Tetrahydrozoline HCl
- Do not use beyond 48 to 72 hours without consulting a physician.
- If irritation, blurring, or redness persists, or if severe eye pain, headache, vision changes, floating spots, dizziness, decrease in body temperature, drowsiness, acute eye redness, or pain with light exposure occurs, discontinue use and consult a physician.
- Do not use if you have glaucoma except under the advice of a physician.
- If ocular stinging occurs, refrigeration of the solution prior to use may decrease this sensation. Artificial tears application prior to allergy drop may also reduce stinging.
- Discard any solution that becomes cloudy or discolored.
- Avoid consuming alcohol and other sedatives during use.
- May produce excitability in children.
- Discontinue use several days prior to allergy skin testing.
- Avoid contamination of tips of containers and recap immediately after use.
- Soft contact lens wear may need to be avoided during treatment.

OXYMETAZOLINE HCL

▶ Indications
Redness: For the relief of redness of the eye due to minor eye irritations.

▶ Warnings
Soft contact lenses: Any solution preserved with benzalkonium chloride (BAK) should not be used with soft contact lenses. When treatment ceases, lens wear may be resumed within a few hours after discontinuation of the drug.

▶ Administration and Dosage
Adults and children 6 years of age and older: Instill 1 or 2 drops in the affected eye(s) every 6 hours as needed.

Stability: Do not use if solution changes color or becomes cloudy as needed.

OXYMETAZOLINE HCL PRODUCTS	
Trade name	**Doseform**
OcuClear, Visine L.R.	**Solution:** 0.025%. 0.01% benzalkonium Cl, 0.1% EDTA.

Products listed are representative of currently available and widely distributed brands. Similar products, including regional and private label brands, may also exist.

PATIENT INFORMATION
Oxymetazoline HCl
- Do not use beyond 48 to 72 hours without consulting a physician.
- If irritation, blurring, or redness persists, or if severe eye pain, headache, vision changes, floating spots, dizziness, decrease in body temperature, drowsiness, acute eye redness, or pain with light exposure occurs, discontinue use and consult a physician.
- Do not use if you have glaucoma except under the advice of a physician.
- If ocular stinging occurs, refrigeration of the solution prior to use may decrease this sensation. Artificial tears application prior to allergy drop may also reduce stinging.
- Discard any solution that becomes cloudy or discolored.
- Avoid consuming alcohol and other sedatives during use.
- May produce excitability in children.
- Discontinue use several days prior to allergy skin testing.
- Avoid contamination of tips of containers and recap immediately after use.
- Soft contact lens wear may need to be avoided during treatment.

OPHTHALMIC ANTIHISTAMINES

▶ Actions
Topical antihistamines can be used alone or in combination with ophthalmic decongestants to provide relief of ocular irritation or congestion for the treatment of allergic or inflammatory ocular conditions. Antihistamines counteract the effects of histamine, a chemical released in the body in response to an antigen-antibody reaction that causes redness, itching, and irritation of tissues, and can cause watery eyes, runny nose, and sneezing.

▶ Indications
To provide relief of symptoms of allergic conjunctivitis (watering, itching eyes).

▶ Contraindications
Hypersensitivity to any component of the formulation; with monoamine oxidase (MAO) inhibitor use; patients with known risk of angle-closure glaucoma.

▶ Warnings
Topical antihistamines may produce a local sensitivity reaction.

Use with caution in the presence of asthma, coronary artery disease, digestive tract obstruction, enlarged prostate, glaucoma (narrow-angle), heart disease, hypertension, hyperthyroidism, irregular heartbeat, liver disease, peptic ulcer, pregnancy, urinary bladder obstruction.

Soft contact lenses: Any solution preserved with benzalkonium chloride (BAK) should not be used with soft contact lenses. When treatment ceases, lens wear may be resumed within a few hours after discontinuation of the drug.

Glaucoma: Because the formulation may produce angle closure, use with caution in people with a narrow-angle or a history of glaucoma.

Topical antihistamines: Topical antihistamines are potential sensitizers and may produce a local sensitivity reaction.

Pregnancy: Category C. Safety for use has not been established. Use only if clearly needed and if the potential benefits outweigh the potential hazards to the fetus.

Lactation: Antihistamines appear in breast milk. Breastfeeding should be discouraged while using these medications.

Children: Antihistamine overdosage in children may cause hallucinations, convulsions, and death. Antihistamines may decrease mental alertness and may produce hyperactivity in children. Use caution when given to children younger than 12 years of age.

Elderly: The elderly may require lower doses. Antihistamines are more likely to cause dizziness, sedation, confusion, and decreased blood pressure in the elderly.

▶ **Drug Interactions**

Because preparations are topical and instilled directly into the eye, no clinically significant drug/drug or drug/food interactions are expected if used appropriately. Excessive dosing increases the risk of drug interactions and systemic adverse effects.

Alcohol, sedatives (sleeping pills), antianxiety medications, and narcotic pain relievers are all known to interact adversely with antihistamines. The following drugs and drug classes also interact with antihistamines: Anticoagulants, epinephrine, fluconazole, isocarboxazid, itraconazole, ketoconazole, macrolides, metronidazole, miconazole, phenelzine, procarbazine, selegiline, tranylcypromine.

▶ **Adverse Reactions**

Ophthalmic: Blurred or double vision; eye pain; dryness; sensitivity to light.

Systemic: Stomachache; constipation; appetite changes; nausea; vomiting; diarrhea; drowsiness; dizziness; mental confusion; decreased coordination; fatigue; headache; sleeplessness; sleepiness; sore throat; pharyngitis; cough; dry nose, throat and mouth; thickening of mucus in respiratory tract; wheezing; stuffiness.

Cardiovascular: Irregular heartbeat; palpitations; hypotension.

Miscellaneous: Difficult urination; urine retention; ringing in the ears; rash; hives; excessive perspiration; chills.

PATIENT INFORMATION

Ophthalmic Antihistamines

- May cause drowsiness or dizziness. Use caution while driving or performing tasks requiring mental alertness. Avoid alcohol and other CNS depressants (eg, sedatives, hypnotics, tranquilizers).
- Elderly patients are more likely to experience dizziness, sedation, decreased coordination, mental confusion, and fainting when they take antihistamines.
- May produce unexpected excitation, restlessness, irritability, and insomnia in rare instances. This is most likely in children and elderly patients.
- Do not use for several days before allergy skin testing.
- To avoid contamination, do not touch tip of the container to any surface. Replace cap after use.

OPHTHALMIC DECONGESTANT/ANTIHISTAMINE COMBINATIONS

▶ **Actions**

Naphazoline HCl has decongestant action. See individual product listings for further information.

Hydroxypropyl methylcellulose and **polyvinyl alcohol** increase the viscosity of the solution, thereby increasing contact time.

Pheniramine maleate and **antazoline** are antihistamines.

▶ **Indications**

Temporary relief of the minor eye symptoms of itching and redness caused by allergens (eg, pollen, animal dander).

▶ **Warnings**

Soft contact lenses: Any solution preserved with benzalkonium chloride (BAK) should not be used with soft contact lenses. When treatment ceases, lens wear may be resumed within a few hours after discontinuation of the drug.

Antihistamines: Topical antihistamines are potential sensitizers and may produce a local sensitivity reaction. Because they may produce angle closure, use with caution in people with a narrow angle or a history of glaucoma.

▶ **Administration and Dosage**

Recommendations vary. Refer to manufacturer package insert for instructions.

DECONGESTANT/ANTIHISTAMINE COMBINATIONS	
Trade name	**Doseform**
Naphazoline HCl & Pheniramine Maleate	**Solution:** 0.025% naphazoline HCl, 0.3% pheniramine maleate
Naphazoline Plus, Naphcon-A	**Solution:** 0.025% naphazoline HCl, 0.3% pheniramine maleate, 0.01% benzalkonium Cl, EDTA
Opcon-A	**Solution:** 0.027% naphazoline HCl, 0.315% pheniramine maleate, 0.5% hydroxypropyl methylcellulose, 0.01% benzalkonium Cl, 0.1% EDTA, boric acid
Naphazoline HCl & Antazoline Phosphate	**Solution:** 0.05% naphazoline HCl, 0.5% antazoline phosphate
Vasocon-A	**Solution:** 0.05% naphazoline HCl, 0.5% antazoline phosphate, 0.01% benzalkonium Cl, PEG-8000, polyvinyl alcohol, EDTA

Products listed are representative of currently available and widely distributed brands. Similar products, including regional and private label brands, may also exist.

PATIENT INFORMATION

Decongestant/Antihistamine Combinations

- Shake well before using.
- To prevent contaminating the dropper tip and suspension, do not touch the eyelid or surrounding area with the dropper tip of the bottle. Recap immediately after use.
- Keep bottle tightly closed when not in use. Do not use if the suspension is discolored or cloudy. Store at controlled room temperature. Protect from freezing.
- Antihistamines may cause drowsiness or dizziness. Use caution while driving.
- If ocular stinging occurs, refrigeration of the solution prior to use may decrease this sensation. Artificial tears application prior to allergy drop may also reduce stinging.
- Discard any solution that becomes cloudy or discolored.
- Avoid taking alcohol and other sedatives during use.
- May produce excitability in children.
- Discontinue use several days prior to allergy skin testing.
- Soft contact lens wear may need to be avoided during treatment.

NonAllergic Conjunctivitis

DEFINITION

Conjunctivitis is an inflammation of the conjunctiva, the mucous membrane lining the inner surface the eyelids and the outer surface of the sclera (white portion of the eyeball). Symptoms include redness (vascular dilation), swelling (cellular infiltration), and discharge (exudation).

ETIOLOGY

Nonallergic causative agents include bacteria, viruses, chlamydia, and toxins. Differential diagnosis and classification of the conjunctivitis usually requires a thorough investigation of the onset, symptoms and signs (including biomicroscopic examination of the ocular and adnexal surfaces), and, if necessary, cultures.

Chronic conjunctivitis can also be associated with dermatologic conditions (acne rosacea and psoriasis), mucous membrane disorders (Stevens-Johnson syndrome and pemphigoid), collagen disorders (systemic lupus erythematosus, Reiters syndrome) and other conjunctival disorders (pinguccula, pterygium, lacerations, and abrasions).

Bacterial conjunctivitis: Staphylococcus aureus is the most common cause of bacterial conjunctivitis. *S. aureus, Streptococcus pneumoniae*, and *Haemophilus* species account for the great majority of bacterial infections. *S. pneumoniae* is a common cause of epidemic conjunctivitis among schoolchildren and is often associated with a respiratory tract infection. Rare causes of bacterial conjunctivitis are bacterial agents *Neisseria gonorrhoeae, Moraxella, Serratia marcescens, Proteus mirabilis*, and *Pseudomonas aeruginosa*. (Neonatal conjunctivitis has specific pathogens and medical treatment and is beyond the scope of this monograph.) Transmission occurs predominantly by hand-to-eye contact. Other modes of transmission include nasopharynx, oculogenital, contaminated eye drops, insect vectors, nosocomial outbreaks, and iatrogenic means. Unlike the hyperacute forms, acute bacterial conjunctivitis tends to be self-limiting. Important exceptions to this include the conversion of acute staphylococcal infection to a chronic blepharoconjunctivitis and an acute *Haemophilus* infection progressing to orbital cellulitis in infants. If improperly treated, conjunctivitis can become chronic and lead to substantial conjunctival and corneal disease.

Viral conjunctivitis: Several viruses are known to affect the eye. The more common ocular DNA viruses are adenovirus, herpes simplex, molluscum contagiosum (viral warts), papilloma (verrucae), and varicella (herpes zoster). The most common RNA virus is influenza. Adenovirus is the most common viral infection of the ocular surface and several different serotypes exist. Adenovirus is a spherical DNA virus that typically causes diseases of the respiratory tract. Pharyngoconjunctival fever (PCF) and epidemic keratoconjunctivitis

(EKC) are common manifestations of adenoviral ocular infections. Less common viral ocular pathogens include cytomegalovirus, Epstein-Barr (mononucleosis), vaccinia, variola (smallpox), varicella, HIV, coxsackie, enterovirus 70 (*Haemophilus*), measles (rubeola), mumps, Newcastle disease, poliovirus, rabies, rhinovirus, and rubella (German measles). Transmission principally occurs from direct contact with the virus in ocular secretions or on shared fomites (eg, towels, pillows, soaps, sunglasses). Although the condition is usually self-limiting, viral conjunctivitis causes significant morbidity. High absenteeism from work or school during contagious stages causes tremendous socioeconomic losses.

Chlamydial conjunctivitis: Chlamydia species produce several oculogenital diseases and commonly induce a chronic follicular conjunctivitis. *Chlamydia trachomatis* (TRIC) causes 2 distinct clinical diseases: Trachoma and inclusion conjunctivitis. Trachoma is endemic in many underdeveloped areas in the world, and is found among Native Americans in the Southwester US. In the US, chlamydia is the most common infective agent causing neonatal conjunctivitis. It affects 2% to 6% of all neonates through exposure to the maternal cervix. Chlamydial disease spreads by direct contact (eg, hands, sexual contact, cervical) and is associated with mild or asymptomatic genitourinary involvement. Chlamydia commonly causes an acute follicular conjunctivitis that becomes chronic.

Toxic conjunctivitis: Toxic conjunctivitis results from chronic exposure to injurious agents such as eye medications, eye makeup, bacterial or viral toxins, and contact lens solutions. Other causes include dry conditions, airborne irritants, allergens, radiation, soaps, and perfumes. The ocular immunologic response to these irritants is chronic inflammation.

INCIDENCE

Conjunctivitis is recognized as being very common. The precise incidence in the national general population is unknown. (National government health statistics indicate prevalence rates for chronic diseases, and acute conditions such as conjunctivitis are not gathered on extensive surveys.) Generally, bacterial conjunctivitis is more common among children and young adults than among older adults. Viral conjunctivitis has a higher incidence in people between the ages of 20 and 40 years and has no sexual, racial, socioeconomic, or nutritional status preference. Bacterial conjunctivitis occurs more commonly in the winter and spring, while viral conjunctivitis has a higher relative incidence in the summer. Incidence may become epidemic at schools, offices, work sites, or eye doctor offices because of contagious nature and ease of transmission.

PATHOPHYSIOLOGY

The conjunctiva is well protected from infection. Tears irrigate and dilute the infectious agents while tear lysozymes or antibodies destroy the organisms. Pathogens must have sufficient innoculum size and virulence to establish infection. The stages of infection are pathogen attachment, adhesion, invasion, multiplication, toxin production, protease release, and evasion of host defenses. The severity of the infection is determined by the hosts immunologic abilities, by the conjunctival structural integrity, and by the pathogen's ability to cause disease. Infection occurs when the ocular surface pathogen is able to overcome the mucosal defenses, penetrate the epithelial surface, multiply greatly, and evoke a host inflammatory response. This response is apparent through signs of epithelial toxicity and necrosis, vascular hyperemia, and exudative discharge.

Bacterial conjunctivitis: The more common bacterial pathogens are *Staphylococcus* and *streptococcus.* Staphylococci are gram-positive extracellular pyogenic organisms. They produce numerous toxins and enzymes that enhance their disease-causing ability. *Streptococcus pneumoniae* are gram-positive diplococci. These organisms are invasive and able to encapsulate themselves to retard or prevent phagocytosis by leukocytes. *Haemophilus aegyptius* is a gram-negative bacillus that can be pleomorphic, occurs more commonly in young children, and can be more severe and lengthy than the *Staphylococcus* or *Streptococcus* conjunctivitis.

Viral conjunctivitis: Viruses are single-cell organisms made up of a single DNA or RNA strand and cannot replicate without an external source of proteins. Some viruses tend to live in dormancy in ganglion cells or infected cells and become active when the host becomes stressed or immunocompromised. Adenoviral infection (the most common viral conjunctivitis) has an incubation period of 4 to 10 days before the onset of clinical symptoms, and length of viral replication varies (with pathogen virulence and host immunity) from less than 14 days to 21 days.

Chlamydial conjunctivitis: Inclusion conjunctivitis is caused by *Chlamydia trachomatis* organisms. Chlamydia are intracellular parasites that depend on the host cell for high-energy compounds to perform biosynthetic processes but are not true viruses. They have enzyme systems similar to bacteria. Chlamydia replicate within infected cells and form intracellular inclusion bodies. The host's immune system response is monocytic and neutrophilic. A distinctive characteristic of inclusion conjunctivitis is an approximately equal number of polymorphonuclear leukocytes and lymphocytes found on conjunctival scrapings.

Toxic conjunctivitis: A hypersensitivity response to a chronic foreign agent results in a follicular conjunctivitis. This condition is noncontagious, and the course duration is dependent upon presence of the causative offender.

SIGNS/SYMPTOMS

Bacterial: Bacterial conjunctivitis occurs in all age groups. The onset is unilateral, but frequently spreads to the other eye 2 to 3 days later. Initial complaints are tearing and irritation or foreign body sensation. Subsequently, the eye becomes red. There is no frank pain and no visual reduction. A history of a recent upper respiratory tract or ear infection is possible. Hyperemia and a mucopurulent discharge worsen for 2 to 3 days. The eyelashes are matted with the discharge and may be matted shut upon wakening.

Viral: Adenoviral conjunctivitis is frequently mild and has a short acute phase. The condition is unilateral or bilateral, the second eye becoming involved 3 to 7 days later. A recent upper respiratory tract infection or low-grade fever may precede the ocular symptoms (pharyngoconjunctival fever). Other symptoms include watery discharge, foreign-body sensation, mild visual fluctuations, and mild-to-moderate burning.

Chlamydial: Inclusion conjunctivitis presents with a variable degree of involvement. The mild follicular conjunctivitis form is less sight-threatening than severe forms that involve the cornea. Risk factors include sexual activity and a new sexual partner in the past few months. The onset is insidious and sudden after incubation of 5 to 12 days. The acute stage becomes chronic, lasting weeks to months. It can be unilateral or bilateral. Mucopurulent discharge, mild lid edema, and conjunctival chemosis may result. The patient notices conjuctival redness and a foreign body sensation, or is often asymptomatic. A concomitant vaginitis, cervicitis, or urethritis is common. No history of recent upper respiratory tract infection or fever exists.

Toxic: Toxic conjunctivitis patients experience chronic nonspecific irritation and inflammation. This condition can often be associated with other anterior segment diseases (eg, dry eyes, blepharitis), or injurious agents listed above. Symptom severity ranges from absent to moderate and may involve one or both eyes. The condition is aggravated by wind, rubbing, and contact lens wear.

DIAGNOSTIC PARAMETERS/PHYSICAL ASSESSMENT

Practitioners should rule out other causes of red eyes (eg, dry eyes, blepharitis, subconjunctival hemorrhage, iritis, episcleritis), determine if condition is primary or secondary to other conditions (eg, mucous membrane disorders, blepharitis, acne rosacea), and determine the causative type of conjunctivitis.

Clinical Observation:

Bacterial – Different bacterial etiologic agents may have slightly different signs. Inflammation is greatest toward the fornices, and occurs in a nonradiating pattern. The vessels are movable and blanche with a mild vasoconstrictor. The cornea is usually clear, but superficial punctate keratitis may result from exotoxins. The lower palpebral conjunctiva reveal a velvety-appearing papillary reaction. Papillae are small, round elevations of conjunctival epithelium and stroma with a vessel centered in the projection. A greenish yellow mucopurulent discharge is present.

Viral – The injection begins at the inner canthus and spreads laterally to involve the entire bulbar conjunctiva. Other signs include a rapid tear break-up time, superficial punctate keratitis, and serous (tearing, watery) discharge. Follicles (round, translucent elevations) present on the lower palpebral conjunctiva. Occasionally, an ipsilateral preauricular lymphadenopathy (node enlargement) is present. Epidemic keratoconjunctivitis

(EKC) has other distinctive findings: Petechiae and edema of caruncle and semilunar fold, pseudomembrane formation in severe cases, corneal involvement for approximately 4 weeks, and subepithelial opacities that disappear in 3 to 4 months. Secondary bacterial infections are common in EKC.

Chlamydial – Upper tarsal follicles, papillary hypertrophy, superior palpebral inflammation, and infiltration of conjunctiva is present. Older cases involve scarring.

Toxic – No discharge and an occasional phlyctenule (conjunctival nodule representing nonspecific delayed hypersensitivity to foreign protein).

Interview: It may be beneficial to ask the patient about the following:

- Symptoms such as tearing, irritation, redness, watery discharge, mild visual fluctuations, mild-to-moderate burning, swelling, foreign body sensation, or matting of eyelashes.
- Duration of condition.
- History of recent upper respiratory tract infection, ear infection, or low-grade fever.
- Sexual history.
- Prior occurrences of eye problems, infections, blepharitis, dry eye, etc.

TREATMENT

Approaches to therapy: The type of conjunctivitis must first be determined. If it is toxic, removal of the offending agent is curative. Toxic conjunctivitis is noninfectious; therefore supportive treatment (versus antibiotic) is used in relieving symptoms. If the conjunctivitis is bacterial, the use of a topical broad-spectrum antibiotic, prescribed by an optometrist or physician, hastens resolution. If it is a hyperacute form of bacterial conjunctivitis (rapidly advancing bacterial signs and symptoms and copious mucopurulent discharge), a laboratory work-up is indicated before initiation of antibiotic treatment. Another time to consider laboratory culturing is when the condition is nonresponsive to accepted treatment. If adenoviral, treatment is supportive because there is no drug cure for adenoviruses, and antibacterial agents are of no therapeutic value against conjunctival viral infection. Adult inclusion conjunctivitis (chlamydia) requires oral antibiotic treatment for resolution.

Nondrug therapy: Supportive therapy for viral and toxic conjunctivitis includes:

1.) Reassurance that the condition is usually self-limiting and will not cause permanent damage;
2.) sunglasses to reduce discomfort in bright light;
3.) use of artificial tears (1 drop in affected eye 4 to 8 times daily);
4.) saline rinses; and
5.) frequent cool compresses (every 3 to 4 hours) for 1 to 2 weeks.

Artificial tears supplement the natural tears by irrigating and diluting the pathogens and protecting the conjunctival surface from drying. A nonviscous formulation may be preferred for ocular clarity and nonpreserved preparations should be used if they need to be applied more frequently than 4 times daily. Saline rinses would also serve to dilute the infecting agent and increase comfort. Cool compresses cause vasoconstriction and reduce redness and congestion, thereby increasing comfort. Some practitioners recommend alternating warm and cold compresses. Warm compresses increase the immune response in the area and may hasten resolution, but also increase congestion and discomfort. Cold compresses will decrease vasodilation and help to increase patient comfort.

Pharmacotherapy: Limited usage (3 to 6 times daily) of topical OTC vasoconstrictors (eg, naphazoline, phenylephrine) will improve redness and may reduce symptoms and inflammation. Topical preparations with heavy metals such as zinc and mercuric oxides (eg, *Zincfrin, Visine A.C.*) may be of questionable value in reducing discharge. Aspirin or ibuprofen may be taken for discomfort if there are no contraindications for their use in the patient. (See the Aches and Pains monograph in the Musculoskeletal Conditions chapter for more information on these agents).

If corneal involvement exists in a viral or toxic conjunctivitis, or if a secondary reaction occurs (anterior uveitis, bacterial infection), an eyecare practitioner will prescribe appropriate therapy.

Bacterial conjunctivitis treatment includes ophthalmic antibiotic therapy, which requires a prescription from an optometrist or ophthalmologist. Topical antibiotic therapy manages most cases of acute bacterial conjunctivitis. Antibiotics differ in their mechanisms of action on bacteria. Antibiotics can affect bacterial cell wall synthesis, cell membrane osmotic integrity, protein synthesis, intermediary metabolism, or DNA synthesis. Chlamydial infection requires oral prescription antibiotic treatment. Topical tetracycline ointment, also requiring a prescription, may be used along with the oral antibiotic. Intimate associates should also be evaluated and treated, if necessary, with oral antibiotics.

OPHTHALMIC DECONGESTANTS

▶ Actions

The effects of sympathomimetic agents on the eye are concentration-dependent and include: Pupil dilation, increase in outflow of aqueous humor, and vasoconstriction (alpha-adrenergic effects).

Higher drug concentrations (ie, phenylephrine 2.5% and 10%) cause vasoconstriction and pupillary dilation for diagnostic eye exams, during surgery, and to prevent synechiae formation in uveitis. Weak concentrations of phenylephrine (0.12%) and other alpha-adrenergic agonists (naphazoline, tetrahydrozoline) are used as ophthalmic decongestants (vasoconstriction of conjunctival blood vessels) and for symptomatic relief of minor eye irritations.

Nonprescription Ophthalmic Vasoconstrictors		
Vasoconstrictor	Duration of action (hrs)	Available concentration
Naphazoline	3 to 4	0.012%, 0.02%, 0.03%
Oxymetazoline	4 to 6	0.025%
Phenylephrine	0.5 to 1.5	0.12%
Tetrahydrozoline	1 to 4	0.05%

▶ **Indications**

Red, swollen conjunctival membranes sometimes are accompanied by a mucopuru-
lant discharge. Refer to individual product listings for specific indications.

▶ **Contraindications**

Hypersensitivity to any of these agents; narrow-angle glaucoma or anatomically narrow (occludable) angle and no glaucoma; prior to peripheral iridectomy in eyes
capable of angle closure because mydriatic action may precipitate angle closure. Contact lenses should not be worn while the conjunctiva is infected.

▶ **Warnings**

If condition is painful, severe, or does not resolve, see an eyecare specialist (eg, ophthalmologist, optometrist).

If wearing disposable contact lenses, discard the lens that was on the infected eye.
Thoroughly clean and disinfect the contact lens case before using for new contact
lenses. If contact lenses are not disposable, thoroughly clean, and disinfect before
inserting in the eye.

Anesthetics: Local anesthetics can increase absorption of topical drugs; exercise caution when applying prior to use of phenylephrine.

Overuse: Overuse may produce rebound vasodilation and increased redness of the eye.

Special risk patients: Use with caution in children of low body weight, the elderly, and
in the presence of hypertension, diabetes, hyperthyroidism, cardiovascular abnormalities, and arteriosclerosis.

Rebound congestion: Rebound congestion may occur with frequent or extended use of
ophthalmic vasoconstrictors. Rebound miosis has occurred in older persons 1 day
after receiving phenylephrine; reinstillation produced a reduction in mydriasis.

Systemic absorption: Exceeding recommended dosages of these agents may result in
the absorption of sufficient quantities to produce a systemic vasopressor response.

Pigment floaters: Older individuals may develop transient pigment floaters in the aqueous humor 30 to 45 minutes after instillation of phenylephrine. The appearance may
be similar to anterior uveitis or to a microscopic hyphema.

Pregnancy: Category C. Safety for use in pregnancy has not been established. Use only
if clearly needed and if the potential benefits outweigh potential hazards to the fetus.

Lactation: Safety for use during breastfeeding has not been established. Use caution when administering to a nursing woman.

Children: Safety and efficacy have not been established.

Hazardous tasks: Phenylephrine may cause temporary blurred or unstable vision;
observe caution while driving or performing other hazardous tasks.

Sulfite sensitivity: Some of these products contain sulfites that may cause allergic-type
reactions (eg, hives, itching, wheezing, anaphylaxis) in certain susceptible persons.
Although the overall prevalence of sulfite sensitivity in the general population is low,
it is seen more frequently in asthmatics or in atopic nonasthmatic persons.

▶ **Drug Interactions**

Because preparations are topical, no drug/drug or drug/food interactions are expected
if used as prescribed. Temporary punctal occlusion (fingertip pressure just below the
inner corner of the eye) will decrease systemic absorption through the lacrimal
system.

Ophthalmic Sympathomimetic Drug Interactions			
Precipitant drug	Object drug*		Description
Anesthetics	Ophthalmic sympathomimetics	↑	Cautiously use anesthetics that sensitize the myocardium to sympathomimetics (eg, cyclopropane, halothane). Local anesthetics can increase absorption of topical drugs; exercise caution when applying prior to use of phenylephrine.
Beta blockers	Ophthalmic sympathomimetics	↑	Systemic side effects may occur more readily in patients taking these drugs.
MAOIs	Ophthalmic sympathomimetics	↑	When given with, or up to 21 days after MAOIs, exaggerated adrenergic effects may result. Supervise and adjust dosage carefully.

* ↑ = Object drug increased.

Also consider drug interactions that may occur with systemic use of the sympathomimetics.

▶ **Adverse Reactions**

Overtreatment of acute or chronic conjunctivitis can cause conjunctival hyperemia and irritation. These symptoms are relieved after medication is withdrawn.

Ophthalmic: Transitory stinging on initial instillation; blurring of vision; mydriasis; increased redness; irritation; discomfort; punctate keratitis; lacrimation; increased IOP. See individual package inserts.

Phenylephrine: Phenylephrine may cause rebound miosis and decreased mydriatic response to therapy in older persons.

Cardiovascular: Palpitation; tachycardia; cardiac arrhythmia; hypertension; collapse; extrasystoles; ventricular arrhythmias (ie, premature ventricular contractions); reflex bradycardia; coronary occlusion; subarachnoid hemorrhage; myocardial infarction; stroke; death associated with cardiac reactions. Headache or browache may occur.

Miscellaneous: Blanching; sweating; dizziness; nausea; nervousness; drowsiness; weakness; hyperglycemia.

PHENYLEPHRINE HCL

▶ **Indications**

0.12%: A decongestant to provide relief of minor eye irritations.

▶ **Administration and Dosage**

Minor eye irritations: Instill 1 or 2 drops of the 0.12% solution in the affected eye(s) up to 4 times daily as needed.

Stability: Prolonged exposure to air or strong light may cause oxidation and discoloration. Do not use if solution changes color, becomes cloudy, or contains a precipitate.

PHENYLEPHRINE HCL PRODUCTS	
Trade name	Doseform
AK-Nefrin	**Solution:** 0.12%. 0.005% benzalkonium Cl, 1.4% polyvinyl alcohol, EDTA.
Prefrin Liquifilm	**Solution:** 0.12%. 1.4% polyvinyl alcohol, 0.004% benzalkonium Cl, EDTA.
Relief, Zincfrin	**Solution:** 0.12%. 0.01% benzalkonium Cl, polysorbate 80, 0.25% zinc sulfate.

Products listed are representative of currently available and widely distributed brands. Similar products, including regional and private label brands, may also exist.

> # PATIENT INFORMATION
> ## Phenylephrine HCl
> - Phenylephrine may cause temporary blurred or unstable vision; observe caution while driving or performing other hazardous tasks.
> - Do not use beyond 48 to 72 hours without consulting a physician.
> - If irritation, blurring, or redness persists, or if severe eye pain, headache, vision changes, floating spots, dizziness, decrease in body temperature, drowsiness, acute eye redness, or pain with light exposure occurs, discontinue use and consult a physician.
> - Do not use if you have glaucoma except under the advice of a physician.
> - Viral conjunctivitis often becomes worse (first 4 to 7 days) before it begins to improve.
> - Viral treatment is palliative because there are no cures for viruses.
> - Due to the contagious nature of some types of conjunctivitis (bacterial, viral) especially during early mild stages, good hygiene and limited contact with others is critical. Children with nonallergic conjunctivitis should not attend school or camp as long as the eyes are red and weeping. Epidemic keratoconjunctivitis patients continue to shed virus in the tears and nasopharynx for 2 weeks, and should limit contact with others during this period. Frequent hand washing, avoiding hand contact with the eye(s), eliminating hand shaking, and use of separate towels, sheets, and pillowcases reduce the spread of the infectious disease. After resolution of the acute condition, some ocular viruses remain dormant in ganglion tissues or infected cells, so the potential exists for mild or moderate exacerbations with increasing stress.
> - Discontinue usage of contact lenses during acute conjunctivitis episodes.
> - Avoid contamination of tips of containers and recap immediately after use.
> - Soft contact lens wear may need to be discontinued during treatment.

NAPHAZOLINE HCL

▶ Indications
Redness: To soothe, refresh, and remove redness due to minor eye irritation such as smoke, smog, sun glare, allergies, or swimming.

▶ Warnings
Soft contact lenses: Any solution preserved with benzalkonium chloride (BAK) should not be used with soft contact lenses. When treatment ceases, lens wear may be resumed within a few hours after discontinuation of the drug.

▶ Administration and Dosage
Instill 1 or 2 drops into the conjunctival sac of affected eye(s) every 3 to 4 hours, up to 4 times daily as needed.

Storage/Stability: Do not use if solution changes color or becomes cloudy.

NAPHAZOLINE HCL PRODUCTS	
Trade name	**Doseform**
Allerest Eye Drops	**Solution:** 0.012%. Benzalkonium Cl, EDTA.
Clear Eyes	**Solution:** 0.012%. Benzalkonium Cl, EDTA, 0.2% glycerin, boric acid.

NAPHAZOLINE HCL PRODUCTS	
Trade name	Doseform
Clear Eyes ACR	**Solution**: 0.012%. Benzalkonium Cl, EDTA, 0.25% zinc sulfate, 0.2% glycerin.
Degest 2	**Solution**: 0.012%. 0.0067% benzalkonium Cl, 0.02% EDTA, hydroxyethylcellulose, povidone.
Naphcon	**Solution**: 0.012%. 0.01% benzalkonium Cl, EDTA.
Allergy Drops	**Solution**: 0.012%. 0.2% PEG-300, 0.01% benzalkonium Cl.
Vaso Clear	**Solution**: 0.02%. 0.01% benzalkonium Cl, 0.25% polyvinyl alcohol, 1% PEG-400, EDTA.
Vaso Clear A	**Solution**: 0.02%. 0.005% benzalkonium Cl, EDTA, 0.25% zinc sulfate, 0.25% polyvinyl alcohol, 1% PEG-400.
Comfort Eye Drops	**Solution**: 0.03%. 0.005% benzalkonium Cl, 0.02% EDTA.
Maximum Strength Allergy Drops	**Solution**: 0.03%. 0.01% benzalkonium Cl, 0.5% hydroxypropyl methylcellulose, EDTA.

Products listed are representative of currently available and widely distributed brands. Similar products, including regional and private label brands, may also exist.

PATIENT INFORMATION
Naphazoline HCl

- Do not use beyond 48 to 72 hours without consulting a physician.
- If irritation, blurring, or redness persists, or if severe eye pain, headache, vision changes, floating spots, dizziness, decrease in body temperature, drowsiness, acute eye redness, or pain with light exposure occurs, discontinue use and consult a physician.
- Do not use if you have glaucoma except under the advice of a physician.
- Viral conjunctivitis often becomes worse (first 4 to 7 days) before it begins to improve.
- Viral treatment is palliative because there are no cures for viruses.
- Due to the contagious nature of some types of conjunctivitis (bacterial, viral) especially during early mild stages, good hygiene and limited contact with others is critical. Children with nonallergic conjunctivitis should not attend school or camp as long as the eyes are red and weeping. Epidemic keratoconjunctivitis patients continue to shed virus in the tears and nasopharynx for 2 weeks, and should limit contact with others during this period. Frequent hand washing, avoiding hand contact with the eye(s), eliminating hand shaking, and use of separate towels, sheets, and pillowcases reduce the spread of the infectious disease. After resolution of the acute condition, some ocular viruses remain dormant in ganglion tissues or infected cells, so the potential exists for mild or moderate exacerbations with increasing stress.
- Discontinue usage of contact lenses during acute conjunctivitis episodes.
- Avoid contamination of tips of containers and recap immediately after use.
- Soft contact lens wear may need to be discontinued during treatment.

TETRAHYDROZOLINE HCL

▶ **Indications**

Redness: For relief of redness of the eye due to minor irritations.

Burning/Irritation: For temporary relief of burning and irritation due to dryness of the eye or discomfort due to minor irritations or to exposure to wind or sun.

▶ **Warnings**

Soft contact lenses: Any solution preserved with benzalkonium chloride (BAK) should not be used with soft contact lenses. When treatment ceases, lens wear may be resumed within a few hours after discontinuation of the drug.

▶ **Administration and Dosage**

Instill 1 or 2 drops into the affected eye(s) up to 4 times a day as needed.

Stability: Do not use if solution changes color or becomes cloudy.

TETRAHYDROZOLINE HCL PRODUCTS	
Trade name	Doseform
AR Eye Drops-Astringent Redness Reliever	**Solution:** 0.05%. 0.25% zinc sulfate.
Collyrium Fresh	**Solution:** 0.05%. 0.01% benzalkonium 0.1% EDTA, 1% glycerin.
Eye Drops, Eyesine, Mallazine Eye Drops	**Solution:** 0.05%. 0.01% benzalkonium Cl, EDTA.
Eye Drops Extra	**Solution:** 0.05%. 1% polyethylene glycol 400.
Geneye, Optigene 3, Visine	**Solution:** 0.05%. 0.01% benzalkonium Cl, 0.1% EDTA.
Geneye Extra, Tetrasine Extra	**Solution:** 0.05%. 1% polyethylene glycol 400, benzalkonium Cl, EDTA.
Murine Plus	**Solution:** 0.05%. Benzalkonium Cl, EDTA, 1.4% polyvinyl alcohol, 0.6% povidone.
Tetrasine	**Solution:** 0.05%. Benzalkonium Cl, EDTA.
Visine Allergy Relief	**Solution:** 0.05%. 0.01% benzalkonium Cl, 0.1% EDTA, 0.25% zinc sulfate.
Visine Moisturizing	**Solution:** 0.05%. 0.013% benzalkonium Cl, 0.1% EDTA, 1% PEG-400.

Products listed are representative of currently available and widely distributed brands. Similar products, including regional and private label brands, may also exist.

PATIENT INFORMATION
Tetrahydrozoline HCl

- Do not use beyond 48 to 72 hours without consulting a physician.
- If irritation, blurring, or redness persists, or if severe eye pain, headache, vision changes, floating spots, dizziness, decrease in body temperature, drowsiness, acute eye redness, or pain with light exposure occurs, discontinue use and consult a physician.
- Do not use if you have glaucoma except under the advice of a physician.
- Viral conjunctivitis often becomes worse (first 4 to 7 days) before it begins to improve.
- Viral treatment is palliative because there are no cures for viruses.
- Due to the contagious nature of some types of conjunctivitis (bacterial, viral) especially during early mild stages, good hygiene and limited contact with others is critical. Children with nonallergic conjunctivitis should not attend school or camp as long as the eyes are red and weeping. Epidemic keratoconjunctivitis patients continue to shed virus in the tears and nasopharynx for 2 weeks, and should limit contact with others during this period. Frequent hand washing, avoiding hand contact with the eye(s), eliminating hand shaking, and use of separate towels, sheets, and pillowcases reduce the spread of the infectious disease. After resolution of the acute condition, some ocular viruses remain dormant in ganglion tissues or infected cells, so the potential exists for mild or moderate exacerbations with increasing stress.
- Discontinue usage of contact lenses during acute conjunctivitis episodes.
- Avoid contamination of tips of containers and recap immediately after use.
- Soft contact lens wear may need to be discontinued during treatment.

OXYMETAZOLINE HCL

▶ **Indications**

Redness: For the relief of redness of the eye due to minor eye irritations.

▶ **Warnings**

Soft contact lenses: Any solution preserved with benzalkonium chloride (BAK) should not be used with soft contact lenses. When treatment ceases, lens wear may be resumed within a few hours after discontinuation of the drug.

▶ **Administration and Dosage**

Adults and children 6 years of age and older: Instill 1 or 2 drops in the affected eye(s) every 6 hours as needed.

Stability: Do not use if solution changes color or becomes cloudy.

OXYMETAZOLINE HCL PRODUCTS	
Trade name	**Doseform**
OcuClear, Visine L.R.	**Solution**: 0.025%. 0.01% benzalkonium Cl, 0.1% EDTA.

Products listed are representative of currently available and widely distributed brands. Similar products, including regional and private label brands, may also exist.

PATIENT INFORMATION
Oxymetazoline HCl
- Do not use beyond 48 to 72 hours without consulting a physician.
- If irritation, blurring, or redness persists, or if severe eye pain, headache, vision changes, floating spots, dizziness, decrease in body temperature, drowsiness, acute eye redness, or pain with light exposure occurs, discontinue use and consult a physician.
- Do not use if you have glaucoma except under the advice of a physician.
- Viral conjunctivitis often becomes worse (first 4 to 7 days) before it begins to improve.
- Viral treatment is palliative because there are no cures for viruses.
- Due to the contagious nature of some types of conjunctivitis (bacterial, viral) especially during early mild stages, good hygiene and limited contact with others is critical. Children with nonallergic conjunctivitis should not attend school or camp as long as the eyes are red and weeping. Epidemic keratoconjunctivitis patients continue to shed virus in the tears and nasopharynx for 2 weeks, and should limit contact with others during this period. Frequent hand washing, avoiding hand contact with the eye(s), eliminating hand shaking, and use of separate towels, sheets, and pillowcases reduce the spread of the infectious disease. After resolution of the acute condition, some ocular viruses remain dormant in ganglion tissues or infected cells, so the potential exists for mild or moderate exacerbations with increasing stress.
- Discontinue usage of contact lenses during acute conjunctivitis episodes.
- Avoid contamination of tips of containers and recap immediately after use.
- Soft contact lens wear may need to be discontinued during treatment.

DEFINITION

Blepharitis is a common low-grade inflammation of the eyelid margins that causes mild ocular itching, tearing, and burning. The eyelid margins are the lid edges where the lashes emerge (approximately 2 mm thick and approximately 30 mm long). Blepharitis is characterized by thickened, erythematous lid margins, telangiectatic blood vessels on the margins, and crusting on the lids or eye lashes, possibly with a mild discharge. Blepharitis is frequently associated with conjunctivitis, dry eyes, inferior superficial keratitis, corneal marginal infiltrates, and acne rosacea. It is usually a chronic condition. Severe cases may produce a mucopurulent discharge and permanent structural changes to the eyelids, such as loss of eyelashes (madarosis), misdirection of lashes (trichiasis), and thickened eyelid margins (tylosis ciliaris).

ETIOLOGY

Blepharitis has either an infectious cause or is a hypersensitivity reaction to the normal eyelid flora. Treatment is aimed at conservatively decreasing the normal population of these agents.

Classifications of chronic blepharitis are staphylococcal, seborrheic, primary meibomitis, and a combined etiology.

Infectious agents: Staphylococcus is the most common bacteria in and around the eye and is present on the lid margin 100% of the time. *Staphylococcus aureus* (most commonly) and *S. epidermidis* almost exclusively cause bacterial infection of the eyelid margin.

Propionibacterium acnes, Corynebacterium sp., and yeast *Pityrosporum* are less-common causative agents in blepharoconjunctivitis.

Streptococcus and gram-negative bacteria usually produce a unilateral hyper-acute form of blepharitis characterized by rapid onset, greater pain, a heavy mucopurulent discharge, and possibly preseptal cellulitis. This is treated differently than the chronic, low-grade lid inflammation of the staphylococcal infection; in most cases, systemic medications, as well as a topical agent, are prescribed by an ophthalmologist.

Other causes: Seborrheic blepharitis is typified by scaling and greasy deposits around the lids and lashes. The margins are typically less inflamed than with the staphylococcal variety. This blepharitis seems to be a localized form of a more generalized seborrheic dermatitis accompanied by scalp dandruff and chronic dry dermatitis. Young adults frequently have a blepharitis of combined seborrheic and staphylococcal origin.

Meibomitis is characterized by biomicroscopic changes in the meibomian glands and ducts of the eyelids. Meibomian glands are holocrine glands that supply essential lipids to the external tear layer. Meibomian seborrhea is excessive secretion of the glands in the absence of inflammation. Primary mei-bomitis is stagnation and inspissation of meibomian secretions. Secondary meibomitis is a localized glandular inflammatory response resulting from the anterior blepharitis.

Acne rosacea, a disease of the sebaceous glands of the skin, is a frequent cause of blepharitis. This blepharitis presents as a nonulcerative, bilateral plugging and inspissation of meibomian gland secretion. A staphylococcal super-infection may co-exist and become a contributing component.

Nonbacterial immunological etiologies include contaminated make-up, pollutants, soaps, and preservatives.

INCIDENCE

Data from the National Disease and Therapeutics Index indicates that blepharitis accounted for approximately 590,000 patient visits in 1982. This common condition is chronic; therefore, a high prevalence exists. Staphylococcal blepharitis has a gender predilection; 80% of patients are female. Systemic associations of blepharitis include acne rosacea and atopy. Atopic patients were found to have greater than normal skin colonization rates for *S. aureus*. Another possible explanation for blepharitis in atopic patients is a defect in cell-mediated immunity, possibly in local IgA antibody response.

Meibomian gland dysfunction was present in 39% of patients in a random series of patients presenting to a general eye clinic. The prevalence increases with advancing age and is associated with acne rosacea. One-third of patients with meibomian gland dysfunction have seborrheic dermatitis, and two-thirds have acne rosacea.

PATHOPHYSIOLOGY

Three possible mechanisms exist for staphylococcal blepharitis. The first is direct infection by the staphylococci. The second mechanism is a reaction to the staphylococcal dermonecrotic toxin (alpha-lysin). Third, patients may have an allergic response to the staphylococcal exotoxin.

The production of the staphylococcal sterile exotoxins probably accounts for the clinical manifestations of blepharitis. This toxin is believed to be the trigger that causes the stimulation of the immune inflammatory response. The result (inflammation, redness, discomfort, mild discharge) is a noninfectious reaction of the host's antibodies to staphylococcal antigens (40% of patients with chronic blepharitis demonstrated enhanced cell-mediated immunity to *S. aureus* in the absence of antibodies to teichoic acid).

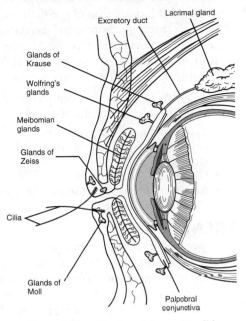

Figure 1. Cross-Section of Eye and Eyelid

Meibomian gland dysfunction is caused either by a hyperkeratinization of the meibomian gland ductal epithelium that results in ductal and acinar obstruction or by an alteration of meibomian secretions. There is an increase in the free fatty acid component of meibum and a shift toward lipids with higher melting points. A higher percentage of esterified cholesterol is also present in the altered secretions. Most investigators maintain that there is no pathogenic evidence that *Demodex folliculorum* or *brevis* (mites) play a role in blepharitis.

SIGNS/SYMPTOMS

Symptoms include bilateral ocular itching, burning, tearing, mild pain, foreign-body sensation, and mattering (crusting) around the eyes upon wakening. In the ulcerative form, which is less common, bleeding occurs when the hard crusts surrounding individual lashes are removed. Seborrheic blepharitis has greasy as opposed to flaky or scaly crusting.

DIAGNOSTIC PARAMETERS/PHYSICAL ASSESSMENT

Clinical Observation: Signs include crusting flakes or collarettes at the base of the lashes and red thickened eyelid margins and prominent blood vessels at the margins. Associated findings may include loss of eyelashes, misdirected lashes, chronic papillary conjunctivitis, superficial punctate epithelial keratitis (SPK) in the inferior third of the cornea, marginal infiltrates, swollen

eyelids, and mild mucus discharge. A secondary meibomitis (spotty congestion and inflammation of the meibomian glands) may manifest as a stagnation
or thickening of meibomian secretions. Chronic, dry dermatitis and dandruff or acne rosacea may also be present. A history of months to years duration and history of recurrences of styes (hordeolum or chalazia) are common
complaints with this chronic condition.

Interview: To aid in the diagnosis and proper treatment of blepharitis, it may
be helpful to ask patients about the following:

- Type and duration of symptoms.
- Concurrent signs of dermatitis, dandruff, or acne rosacea. (See related mono-
  graphs.)
- History of recurrent styes.
- Any recent changes in cosmetics or soap products.
- Use of contact lenses.

TREATMENT

Approaches to therapy: Because the causative agent is normal eyelid flora, treatment is meant to control the condition and relieve the symptoms rather than
to cure the condition. Blepharitis can become chronic and thus more difficult to treat; therefore, it should be treated early and aggressively. Attentive lid
hygiene is the mainstay of treatment. This is easily accomplished at home by
the patient.

Nondrug therapy: Prior to performance of lid hygiene treatments, wash hands
and face with soap and water. Remove contact lenses.

Initial therapy:

1.) Application of warm compresses (as hot as possible without burning or dis-
    comfort) to lid margins for 15 minutes (rewarming washcloth every 2 to
    3 minutes) 4 times a day. This will reduce the discomfort and increase blood
    flow to the region.
2.) Lid massage. Warm compresses can be followed by gentle lid massage, push-
    ing inward of the lower lid just below the lid margin. This will help to expel
    the now warmer and more liquefied glandular secretions from the possibly
    plugged or stagnant meibomian glands.
3.) With closed eyes, scrub the eyelid margins with a diluted mild shampoo (baby
    shampoo) on a *Q-tip*, washcloth, or gauze pad. Commercial lid cleaners are
    available and are reported to be as effective as baby shampoo, but may cause
    less ocular stinging and toxicity. Rinse thoroughly with water. Lid scrub-
    bing can be performed twice daily.
4.) If the patient also has dry eyes, artificial tears can be used at least 4 times daily.
    (See the Dry Eye monograph for more information on artificial tear prod-
    ucts.)
5.) If a seborrheic component is present, in addition to the scrupulous lid hygiene
    described above, shampooing of the scalp and eyebrows (not the eyelashes)
    with a selenium sulfide product is helpful. Reduction of fatty foods in the diet
    is also beneficial.
6.) Discontinue use of contaminated cosmetics. Use of water-based cosmetics
    instead of oil-based cosmetics on the lids and lashes is recommended.

If the acute symptoms are relieved after 2 to 8 weeks of the initial therapy, the frequency of lid hygiene may be reduced to the minimum amount of therapy required to maintain control. Because of the chronicity of the condition, this lid hygiene may need to be maintained indefinitely, especially if there is an underlying condition such as acne rosacea or seborrheic dermatitis.

If the condition does not respond or becomes worse, patients should contact an optometrist or ophthalmologist for further treatment.

Pharmacotherapy: If the condition is moderately severe or is not responsive to lid hygiene alone, an optometrist or ophthalmologist may prescribe a prescription ophthalmic antibiotic medication (eg, bacitracin or erythromycin ointment or oral antibiotics such as tetracycline, doxycycline, or erythromycin).

LID SCRUBS

▶ Indications

Eyelid cleansing: To aid in the removal of oils, debris, or desquamated skin.

▶ Contraindications

Contraindications include allergies or sensitivities to lid hygiene preparations or components of preparations and allergies to any antibiotic used in treatment.

▶ Warnings

For external use only. Do not instill directly into eye.

▶ Drug Interactions

Because lid hygiene involves topical preparations, no drug/drug or drug/food interactions are expected.

▶ Adverse Reactions

Ocular stinging or burning may occur with cleansing products.

▶ Administration and Dosage

Follow instructions for individual products. In general, for most lid scrubs, close eye(s) and gently scrub on eyelid(s) and lashes using lateral side-to-side strokes; rinse thoroughly.

Baby shampoo may also be used as a lid scrub. Dilute 3 drops of shampoo in 1 cup of warm water. Gently scrub on eyelids with a washcloth, *Q-tip*, or gauze pad.

LID SCRUB PRODUCTS	
Trade name	Doseform
Eye-Scrub	**Solution:** PEG-200 glyceryl tallowate, disodium laureth sulfosuccinate, cocoamido-propylamine oxide, PEG-78 glyceryl cocoate, benzyl alcohol, EDTA
Lid Wipes-SPF	**Solution:** PEG-200 glyceryl tallowate, PEG-80 glyceryl cocoate, laureth-23, cocoamido-propylamine oxide, NaCl, glycerin, sodium phosphate, sodium hydroxide
OCuSOFT	**Solution:** PEG-80 sorbitan laurate, sodium trideceth sulfate, PEG-150 distearate, cocoamido-propyl hydroxysultaine, lauroamphocarboxy-glycinate, sodium laureth-13 carboxylate, PEG-15 tallow polyamine, quaternium-15

Products listed are representative of currently available and widely distributed brands. Similar products, including regional and private label brands, may also exist.

PATIENT INFORMATION
Lid Scrubs

- Remove contact lenses before initiating lid hygiene.
- If using commercial lid scrubs, follow package directions on usage.
- If the condition does not respond to therapy or worsens, contact an optometrist or ophthalmologist for further treatment.
- Baby shampoo also may be used as a lid scrub. If using baby shampoo, dilute 3 drops of shampoo in 1 cup of warm water. Use this solution on a washcloth, *Q-tip*, or gauze pad.

DRY EYE
(Keratitis Sicca)

DEFINITION

Dry eye is a chronic, usually bilateral condition which is caused by a deficiency in the tear film. The symptoms include ocular burning, grittiness or foreign-body sensation and scratchiness. Excessive tearing may also result. There may be mattering (dried mucus) at the nasal corner or the eyelids. This irritation increases through the course of the day.

ETIOLOGY

Tear abnormalities can be classified by the specific layer of the tear film that is deficient, the mechanical (lid resurfacing) cause of poor tear coverage, or corneal epithelial irregularities. The tear film has 3 layers. The most superficial layer, the lipid or oily layer, is 0.9 to 0.2 mcm thick, and is secreted by the meibomian eyelid glands. The function of this layer is to inhibit evaporation of the underlying aqueous layer. The aqueous layer is the thickest potion of the tear film, measuring 6.5 to 7.5 mcm in thickness. The lacrimal glands and the accessory lacrimal glands of the eyelids secrete this water layer that also contains lysozymes and immunoglobin A and B lysin. The functions of this layer are to keep the epithelium of the cornea moist, to preserve the smooth light-refracting surface and to lubricate the front of the eyeball so that it moves freely underneath the lids. The mucin layer is the thin (0.5 mcm thick), deepest layer, and is secreted by the goblet cells in the conjunctiva. This mucus layer lowers the surface tension between the water layer and corneal surface and wets microvilli of the corneal epithelium.

1.) A deficiency in the oily layer results in rapid tear evaporation. This layer is secreted by the meibomian glands; therefore, any disease or condition that affects these glands (blepharitis or meibomianitis) could result in dry eyes.

2.) A decrease in aqueous production by the basic secretors is known to occur with advancing age, and can occur with no associated disease or drugs that decrease production. A variety of diseases can also diminish the basal (and reflex) lacrimal secretion. Collagen-vascular diseases such as Sjögren syndrome, systemic lupus erythematosus, rheumatoid arthritis, and Wegener's granulomatosis reduce tear production. Infiltration of the lacrimal grand, by a tumor, lymphocytes, or sarcoidosis, or postradiation of the lacrimal gland can cause a decrease in tear production. Cancers (especially lymphoma) and kidney disease may also influence tear secretion. Drugs that reduce aqueous tear secretion include: Antihistamines, beta blockers, oral contraceptives, phenothiazines, atropine and other anticholinergics, decongestants, diuretics, oral steroids, and alcohol.

3.) An instability of the tear film can result from a mucin layer deficiency. Causes of this mucus tear film deficiency include: Vitamin A deficiency (usually from malnutrition or malabsorption), Stevens-Johnson syndrome (erythema multiforme), conjunctival diseases such as ocular cicatricial pemphigoid and benign mucosal pemphigoid, goblet cell dysfunction secondary to conjunctival destruction or toxic etiologies (chemical burns, irradiation, or drug-induced pseudopemphigoid). Another cause of mucin layer deficiency is increased age. The number of goblet cells that secrete the mucin layer is greatest in children and young adults and decreases with age.

4.) The eyelids function with each blink to restore the tear film. A renewed tear film ensures complete tear coverage of the corneal surface. Lid-resurfacing disorders do not allow for tear film renewal, and result in dry eyes. Conditions causing lid surface abnormalities include conjunctival scarring, trauma, and burns. Bell's palsy, thyroid disorders, coloboma, ectropion, nocturnal lagophthalmos, and incomplete blinking can result in lack of tear film over certain corneal areas. The resulting drying causes corneal damage known as exposure keratopathy.

5.) Epithelial abnormalities that include ocular surface abnormalities decrease tear film adherence and contact time, and result in dryness. Epithelial basement membrane disorders (EBMD) can present as negative tear staining patterns and morning dryness symptoms that are worse than evening symptoms. Both EBMD and decreased tear production can be present.

INCIDENCE

Lacrimal insufficiency, or a decrease in basal tear production, is one of the most common causes of chronic low-grade irritations of the eyes, particularly in the elderly population. Dry eye due to an aqueous tear layer deficiency is common in adults during the fifth and sixth decades of life, especially post-menopausal women. In a population of elderly women, 24% had lacrimal aqueous insufficiency, while only 2% were classified with the diagnosis of Sjögren syndrome. Approximately 10 million Americans suffer from dry eye syndrome. The reported female to male ratio of diagnosis of dry eye ranges from 9 females per male to 3 females per 2 males.

SIGNS/SYMPTOMS

Dry eye usually has a gradual onset, with periods of exacerbation. Although not always symmetrical, it is usually bilateral and chronic. However, sometimes patients present with acute onset in one eye.

Ocular symptoms include burning, foreign body sensation, scratchiness, sandy or gritty irritation, excess tearing, nonspecific surface dryness, and discomfort. This irritation becomes more prevalent in mid to late day.

These symptoms are aggravated by dehumidified conditions, wind, dust, smoke, fumes, fine particles, and heating. Bright lights, extended reading, computer or other near work (prolonged use of eyes, which decrease blink rate), and chlorinated swimming pool water often exacerbate symptoms.

With these commonly mild-to-moderate symptoms, patients usually feel more discomfort than observable signs would indicate.

DIAGNOSTIC PARAMETERS/PHYSICAL ASSESSMENT

Clinical Observation: Clinical signs of keratitis sicca include a minimal height of tear meniscus seen at the inferior eyelid margin (less than 0.3 mm), and a decreased tear break-up time (less than 10 seconds). A consistently diminished Schirmer strip test is of diagnostic importance, indicating low aqueous tear secretion. The presence of punctate corneal or conjunctival fluorescein or rose bengal staining, particularly of inner palpebral conjunctiva and inferior cornea, are signs of dry eyes. Low-grade angular bulbar hyperemia and nonspecific papillary palpebral conjunctivitis can also be observed. Excess mucus or debris in tear film debris, which form filaments (helixes of mucin and dead epithelial cells), are also signs of dry eye.

Interview: It may be beneficial to ask the patient the following:

- Symptoms such as burning, irritation, gritty/rough feeling, dryness, excessive tearing, sensitivity to light, itching, or redness in one or both eyes.
- Duration of condition.
- Patient's age.
- Patient's medical history, including prior eye problems.
- Contact lens wearer.
- Patient's OTC and prescription drug history.
- Lifestyle and working conditions on job (eg, reading, working on computers).
- Effect of climate conditions on patient.

TREATMENT

Approaches to therapy: Treatment goals are to relieve symptoms, protect the cornea, and prevent complications. Treatment of contributing disorders such as blepharitis or exposure keratopathy is needed. If history suggests the presence of previously undiagnosed collagen-vascular disease, refer to an internist or rheumatologist.

Altering medications that reduce tear secretion should be considered.

Nondrug therapy: Alteration of the home and work environment to increase humidity increases patient comfort.

Mild cases of dry eye respond well to tear replacement with artificial tear drops applied 4 times per day.

Moderate cases will require more frequent use of (preservative-free) artificial tears, as often as every 1 to 2 hours during the day. Application of a lubricating ointment at bedtime will increase comfort and decrease drying.

Severe cases of dry eye require use of more viscous types of artificial tears that provide longer contact times, but may temporarily blur vision. Lubricating ointment may be needed 2 to 3 times per day, with preservative-free artificial tears applied every 1 to 2 hours.

Additional methods may need to be provided or prescribed by an optometrist or ophthalmologist. These strategies include punctal occlusion by plugs or cautery to decrease tear drainage, patching with lubrication at night, removal of corneal mucus filaments with forceps and use of acetylcysteine drops, artificial tear inserts (patient tolerance is variable), use of a low- to mid-water soft contact lenses along with certain replacement tears (risk of contact lens intolerance and superinfection requires careful monitoring), lateral tarsorrhaphy, moisture chambers, parotid duct transplants, and mechanized pumps with implanted tubes into the conjunctival pouch.

Pharmacotherapy: Artificial tear solutions should be compatible with the eye and provide all three of the major tear components: Mucin, aqueous, and lipids. Solutions usually contain inorganic electrolytes, preservatives, and water-soluble polymeric systems. Salts and buffers help to maintain tonicity and pH. Preservatives in the multidose tears prevent bacterial contamination. Preservative-free tears (frequently packaged in single-dose vials) are more expensive, but will not contribute to the corneal "preservative toxicity" found in long-term or frequent use of preparations containing preservatives. Thicker preparations contain vehicles such as methylcellulose or polyvinyl alcohol, which enhance viscosity, promote stability, and increase contact time, but may temporarily blur vision. Some artificial tears contain vitamins that may aid in the dry eye therapy.

ARTIFICIAL TEARS

▶ Actions

These products contain the following: Balanced amounts of salts to maintain ocular tonicity (0.9% NaCl equivalent); buffers to adjust pH; viscosity agents to prolong eye contact time; preservatives for sterility.

▶ Indications

To relieve ocular burning, dryness, scratchiness, gritty or sandy sensation.

Ophthalmic lubricants: These products offer tear-like lubrication for the relief of dry eyes and eye irritation associated with deficient tear production. Also used as ocular lubricants for artificial eyes.

▶ Contraindications

Allergies to any component in the preparations. Some artificial tears should not be used with soft contact lenses (eg, those containing the preservative benzalkonium chloride). Contact lenses are optional, and are usually discontinued when the patient becomes intolerant.

▶ Adverse Reactions

Solutions may cause mild stinging or temporary blurred vision. The preservative benzalkonium chloride can reduce tear break-up time and aggravate symptoms. Irritation may occur if using preserved solutions more often than 4 times daily. If eye condition worsens or persists for longer than 72 hours, discontinue use and contact an optometrist or ophthalmologist.

▶ Administration and Dosage

Artificial tears are used as needed for an occasional irritation, or are usually applied 3 to 4 times daily for chronic irritation. One drop is applied to each eye.

ARTIFICIAL TEAR SOLUTION PRODUCTS	
Trade name	Doseform
Akwa Tears	**Solution:** 0.01% benzalkonium Cl, 1.4% polyvinyl alcohol, sodium phosphate, EDTA, NaCl
AquaSite	**Solution:** 0.2% PEG-400, 0.1% dextran 70, polycarbophil, NaCl, EDTA, sodium hydroxide
Artificial Tears	**Solution:** 0.01% benzalkonium Cl. May also contain EDTA, NaCl, polyvinyl alcohol, hydroxypropyl methylcellulose.

ARTIFICIAL TEAR SOLUTION PRODUCTS

Trade name	Doseform
Artificial Tears Plus	Solution: 1.4% polyvinyl alcohol, 0.6% povidone, 0.5% chlorobutanol, NaCl
Bion Tears	Solution: 0.1% dextran 70, 0.3% hydroxypropyl methylcellulose 2910, NaCl, KCl, sodium bicarbonate
Celluvisc	Solution: 1% carboxymethylcellulose, NaCl, KCl, sodium lactate
Comfort Tears	Solution: Hydroxyethylcellulose, 0.005% benzalkonium chloride, 0.02% EDTA
Dakrina	Solution: Povidone, polyvinyl alcohol, antioxidant retinyl palmitate, boric acid, 0.09% EDTA, 0.001% WSCP, NaCl, KCl
Dry Eyes	Solution: 1.4% polyvinyl alcohol, 0.01% benzalkonium Cl, sodium phosphate, EDTA, NaCl
Dry Eye Therapy	Solution: 0.3% glycerin, NaCl, KCl, sodium citrate, sodium phosphate
Dwelle	Solution: 0.09% EDTA, NaCl, KCl, boric acid, povidone, 0.001% NPX
Eye-Lube-A	Solution: 0.25% glycerin, EDTA, sodium chloride, benzalkonium Cl
Gen Teal	Solution: Hydroxypropyl methylcellulose, boric acid, NaCl, KCl, phosphoric acid. Preservative: Sodium perborate
HypoTears	Solution: 1% polyvinyl alcohol, PEG-400, 1% dextrose, 0.01% benzalkonium Cl, EDTA
HypoTears PF	Solution: 1% polyvinyl alcohol, PEG-400, 1% dextrose, EDTA
Isopto Plain, Isopto Tears	Solution: 0.5% hydroxypropyl methylcellulose 2910, 0.01% benzalkonium Cl, NaCl, sodium phosphate, sodium citrate
Just Tears	Solution: Benzalkonium Cl, EDTA, 1.4% polyvinyl alcohol, NaCl, KCl
Liquifilm Tears	Solution: 1.4% polyvinyl alcohol, 0.5% chlorobutanol, NaCl
LubriTears	Solution: 0.3% hydroxypropyl methylcellulose 2906, 0.1% dextran 70, EDTA, KCl, NaCl, 0.01% benzalkonium Cl
Moisture Drops	Solution: 0.5% hydroxypropyl methylcellulose, 0.1% povidone, 0.2% glycerin, 0.01% benzalkonium Cl, EDTA, NaCl, boric acid, KCl, sodium borate
Murine	Solution: 0.5% polyvinyl alcohol, 0.6% povidone, benzalkonium Cl, dextrose, EDTA, NaCl, sodium bicarbonate, sodium phosphate
Murocel	Solution: 1% methylcellulose, propylene glycol, NaCl, 0.046% methylparaben, 0.02% propylparaben, boric acid, sodium borate
Nature's Tears	Solution: 0.4% hydroxypropyl methylcellulose 2910, KCl, NaCl, sodium phosphate, 0.01% benzalkonium Cl, EDTA
Nu-Tears	Solution: 1.4% polyvinyl alcohol, EDTA, sodium chloride, benzalkonium Cl, KCl
Nu-Tears II	Solution: 1% polyvinyl alcohol, 1% PEG-400, EDTA, benzalkonium Cl

ARTIFICIAL TEAR SOLUTION PRODUCTS

Trade name	Doseform
OcuCoat	Solution: 0.1% dextran 70, 0.8% hydroxypropyl methylcellulose, sodium phosphate, KCl, NaCl, 0.01% benzalkonium Cl, dextrose
OcuCoat PF	Solution: 0.1% dextran 70, 0.8% hydroxypropyl methylcellulose, sodium phosphate, KCl, NaCl, dextrose
Puralube Tears	Solution: 1% polyvinyl alcohol, 1% PEG 400, EDTA, benzalkonium Cl
Refresh	Solution: 1.4% polyvinyl alcohol, 0.6% povidone, NaCl
Refresh Plus	Solution: 0.5% carboxymethylcellulose sodium, KCl, NaCl
Refresh Tears	Solution: 0.5% carboxymethylcellulose sodium, boric acid, calcium chloride, magnesium chloride, potassium chloride, sodium chloride
Tear Drop	Solution: Polyvinyl alcohol, NaCl, EDTA, 0.01% benzalkonium chloride
TearGard	Solution: 0.25% sorbic acid, 0.1% EDTA, hydroxymethylcellulose
Teargen	Solution: 0.01% benzalkonium Cl, EDTA, NaCl, polyvinyl alcohol
Tearisol	Solution: 0.5% hydroxypropyl methylcellulose 0.01% benzalkonium Cl, EDTA, boric acid, KCl
Tears Naturale	Solution: 0.1% dextran 70, 0.01% benzalkonium Cl, 0.3% hydroxypropyl methylcellulose, NaCl, EDTA, hydrochloric acid, sodium hydroxide, KCl
Tears Naturale Forte	Solution: Boric acid, calcium chloride, glycine, hydrochloric acid, sodium hydroxide, magnesium chloride, polyquaternium-1 0.001%, polysorbate 80, potassium chloride, sodium chloride, zinc chloride
Tears Naturale Free	Solution: 0.3% hydroxypropyl methylcellulose 2910, 0.1% dextran 70, NaCl, KCl, sodium borate
Tears Naturale II	Solution: 0.1% dextran 70, 0.3% hydroxypropyl methylcellulose 2910, 0.001% polyquaternium-1, NaCl, KCl, sodium borate
Tears Plus	Solution: 1.4% polyvinyl alcohol, NaCl, 0.6% povidone, 0.5% chlorobutanol
Tears Renewed	Solution: 0.01% benzalkonium Cl, EDTA, 0.1% dextran 70, NaCl, 0.3% hydroxypropyl methylcellulose 2906
Thera Tears	Solution: 0.25%, sodium carboxymethylcellulose, NaCl, KCl, sodium phosphate
Ultra Tears	Solution: 1% hydroxypropyl methylcellulose 2910, 0.01% benzalkonium Cl, NaCl
Viva-Drops	Solution: Polysorbate 80, sodium chloride, EDTA, retinyl palmitate, mannitol, sodium citrate, pyruvate

Products listed are representative of currently available and widely distributed brands. Similar products, including regional and private label brands, may also exist.

PATIENT INFORMATION

Artificial Tear Solutions

- The condition of dry eye is usually chronic in nature. Treatment goals are aimed at protection of the cornea and prevention of complications; they are not curative. Decreased tear formation interferes with the normal lubrication and the cleansing function of the tears. It also is associated with decreased lysozyme content in tears, and therefore, places the patient at risk for chronic low-grade infections. Infections should be treated when necessary with appropriate antibiotics.
- Take care not to contaminate the tip or cap of the artificial tear containers. Recap the containers promptly.
- Transient blurring of vision with use of "increased viscosity" tear solutions and ointments is a concession for subjective benefits. Use caution when operating hazardous equipment/machinery or driving.
- Use a preservative-free artificial tear to prevent preservative toxicity if using more frequently than every 3 hours.
- Contact lenses may be worn as long as they are tolerated by the patient.

STYE
(Hordeolum)

DEFINITION

Hordeolii are focal acute eyelid infections arising from within the glands of the eyelids. A stye, or external hordeolum, is an eyelid lump or swelling that is mildly painful, tender, and red. An internal hordeolum is an inflammation that lies deeper in the eyelid and is usually more painful, with moderate-to-severe edema and erythema.

ETIOLOGY

The eyelids are composed of a superficial layer of skin that contains sebaceous glands of Zeiss and ciliary glands of Moll. Deeper lid structures are thin subcutaneous tissue, striated muscle, the tarsal plate, smooth muscle, and, internally, the conjunctiva. The tarsal plate is fibrous tissue that gives the lid shape and houses a row of 30 to 40 meibomian glands in the upper lid and 20 to 30 in the lower lid. The duct orifices are located in the lid margins.

A hordeolum is an acute infection, often staphylococcal, arising within the eyelid glands. Staphylococcus, the most common bacteria in and around the eye, is present continuously on the eyelid margin. An internal hordeolum infection usually results from blockage of the meibomian gland and is found more often in the upper lid. An external hordeolum is an acute staphylococcal infection of the glands of Zeiss or Moll. These styes are also frequently associated with fatigue, poor diet, and stress.

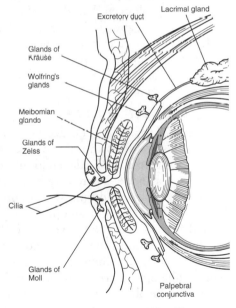

Figure 1. Eyelid Anatomy

INCIDENCE

A stye is one of the most common eyelid disorders that prompts patients into an eye doctor's office. Conditions such as chronic staphylococcal blepharitis or acne rosacea will increase the risk of hordeolii, although it is usually a localized area of inflammation.

PATHOPHYSIOLOGY

Acute staphylococcal infections may produce hordeolii from acute purulent occlusion of the glands of Zeiss or from acute inflammation of the meibomian glands. Dermatological/cutaneous disorders that cause hyperkeratinization of the meibomian gland epithelium result in ductal obstruction. Trapped secretions and cell debris provide a rich substrate for the normal bacterial flora. The bacteria are capable of producing extracellular lipolytic enzymes (triglyceride lipase, cholesterol lipase, and fatty wax esterase), which alter the biochemical composition of the secretions. Resulting free fatty acids are irritating to the skin. The infection of the gland results in the clinical presentation of the tender, swollen, and erythematous eyelid mass.

SIGNS/SYMPTOMS

External hordeolum: The primary symptom is usually localized eyelid pain of recent onset. A focal area of mild-to-moderate redness, tenderness, and swelling evolves near the lid margin. This area develops a yellow point within a few days of the onset of redness. This exudate points in a direction outward from the skin surface. It may suppurate through the gland orifice or break through the skin surface. In most cases, the abscess will spontaneously drain within 3 to 4 days after pointing.

Internal hordeolum: The onset and course of the internal hordeolum is usually more prolonged than those of the external hordeolum. Symptoms include increased pain and clinical signs: A deeper lid response, moderate-to-severe edema, and more erythema and tenderness. The lump may point inward toward the palpebral conjunctiva or upward through the meibomian orifice. A diffuse edema and redness can evolve, hiding the swollen gland and causing a preseptal cellulitis.

DIAGNOSTIC PARAMETERS/PHYSICAL ASSESSMENT

Clinical Observation: A hordeolum is a visible or palpable, well-defined subcutaneous nodule within the eyelid. Other signs are plugged meibomian orifices, eyelid erythema, edema, localized tenderness, and possibly a palpable preauricular node. There may be an associated blepharitis or acne rosacea. Nodules, lumps, and bumps that appear on or in eyelids and do not resolve should be examined by an optometrist or ophthalmologist to determine whether the lesion should be treated. Differential diagnoses for hordeolum include chalazion (nonpainful, noninfectious inflammation of a meibomian gland), preseptal cellulitis, sebaceous cell carcinoma, and pyogenic granuloma. The optometrist or ophthalmologist can also differentiate the clinical degree of involvement to determine an appropriate therapeutic approach.

Interview: To confirm the diagnosis of a hordeolum and to determine whether it is an external or internal hordeolum, it may be beneficial to ask the following questions:

- Duration and severity of eyelid pain.
- Symptoms of redness, tenderness, or swelling near the eyelid.
- Severity of redness, tenderness, or swelling.
- Presence of a lump.
- Fluid draining from the lump.
- Development of a yellow point.

TREATMENT

Approaches to therapy: External and mild internal hordeolii are usually responsive to conservative therapy (hot, moist compresses). If significant pointing occurs, refer the patient to an optometrist or ophthalmologist who may make a sterile puncture to allow drainage. Under these circumstances, a topical antibiotic ointment will be prescribed by the optometrist or ophthalmologist to prevent further infection.

Moderate-to-severe hordeolii may require systemic therapy in addition to conservative topical therapy. An optometrist or ophthalmologist may prescribe a prescription antibiotic. Some sources advocate the use of a topical antibiotic to aid in the resolution of infection and inflammation. Others advise oral antibiotic use because the external entry into the infected gland is obstructed. In cases resistant to conservative topical and oral systemic antibiotic therapy, sterile puncture and drainage by an eyecare provider may be necessary.

Nondrug therapy: Application of a warm, moist compress (washcloth) for 10 to 15 minutes 4 times a day usually resolves external and mild internal hordeolii. Remove contact lenses before applying compresses to the eyelids. Reheat the compress every 3 to 5 minutes. The heat and moisture increase vascular circulation and hasten pointing and drainage. Generally, this is all that is necessary for resolution. To hasten drainage, one or two of the involved eyelashes may be epilated. If not too tender, lightly massaging the involved region several times a day may help.

If the hordeolum is unresponsive to conservative therapy, seek an optometrist or ophthalmologist for additional treatment.

Pharmacotherapy: There are no effective OTC agents for treatment of stye. Because bacitracin and erythromycin are effective against both *Staphylococcus aureus* and *S. epidermidis*, these ophthalmic grade antibiotics are often prescribed by an optometrist or ophthalmologist for the treatment of hordeolii. Nonprescription antibiotic ointments should not be used in or near the eye.

Treatment for moderate-to-severe hordeolii includes prescription of oral antibiotics by an eyecare practitioner. Tetracycline 250 mg 4 times a day, doxycyline 100 mg/day, or erythromycin 250 mg 4 times a day will usually resolve the infection and inflammation in 1 to 2 weeks. The antibacterial action of the tetracycline does not appear to be the primary mechanism that produces effective treatment. The inhibition of the lipolytic enzymes produced by the ocular bacteria may be the therapeutic mechanism of the tetracycline in hordeolii treatment.

If the nodule is resistant to oral therapy, sterile puncture by an optometrist or an ophthalmologist into the area of pointing will allow drainage. Application of topical prescription ophthalmic antibiotic ointment after the puncture procedure will prevent further infection.

CONTACT LENS CARE

DEFINITION

Successful contact lens wear includes good vision, lens comfort, normal ocular health, and is dependent upon patient compliance in caring for contact lenses. The FDA defines compliance as the use of an approved contact lens care regimen in a manner consistent with good general hygiene and the manufacturer's instructions for any given contact lens care product. Contact lens care systems are FDA-approved product sets that are used for cleaning, disinfecting, rinsing, soaking/storing, and rewetting, which help to ensure healthy and comfortable contact lens wear.

INCIDENCE

More than 25 million Americans wear contact lenses, which offer patients a natural appearance, increased visual performance, and convenience. Contact lenses can successfully correct most refractive errors (eg, myopia, hyperopia, astigmatism). Research and development have produced a variety of new lens materials and designs. With new contact lens products and patient education, contact lens use should continue to grow. The number of contact lens care products has also increased dramatically. There are over 125 different products sold for contact lens care. With knowledge of contact lens care systems, health care professionals can educate patients, increase compliance, and therefore decrease lens-related complications.

Studies indicate that between 40% and 74% of soft contact lens patients do not adhere to the care regimen prescribed by their doctor. Another study found that 50% of patients harbor potentially pathogenic microorganisms in their care systems.

PATHOPHYSIOLOGY

When a soft or rigid contact lens is removed from the eye, it may be covered with lipids, proteins, eye makeup, and other debris. Inadequate cleaning can lead to lens discoloration and lens surface buildup of these and other environmental contaminants. Lens buildup can contribute to giant papillary conjunctivitis (GPC), an inflammation that is thought to be a response to eyelid trauma as it moves across a dirty lens, and a hypersensitivity response to antigens accumulated in the lens. Lens buildup can also damage the corneal epithelium, resulting in superficial punctate keratitis and corneal abrasion. Irregular or improper contact lens disinfection may lead to microbial contamination on the lens, and microbes can penetrate corneal lesions to cause severe ocular infections.

SIGNS/SYMPTOMS

Eye dryness is a common complaint, which may be associated with patient factors (eg, older patients have less tearing) and the differences in lens composition and hydration (eg, hard and rigid gas permeable [RGP] lenses tend to be hydrophobic and more drying than soft lenses, which are hydrophilic).

Patients may develop symptoms due to sensitivity to preservative-containing products, excessive duration of wear, and most commonly, improper care of lenses. Redness, lacrimation, and a sensation of foreign body in the eye are symptoms of preservative hypersensitivity. Prolonged duration of lens wear usually causes discomfort. Lacrimation, blepharospasm (eyelid tic), and photophobia may occur due to keratitis; worsening symptoms with pain may suggest corneal abrasion. Corneal abrasions are an invitation for infection, evidenced by ocular hyperemia, edema, and pain. A patient who experiences symptoms of corneal abrasions should consult an eyecare practitioner.

Early symptoms of improper lens care are eye discomfort, and blurred or distorted vision due to accumulated debris. GPC is characterized by itchy eyes, especially when lenses are removed, and reddened conjunctiva. Lowered tolerance to the lenses is evident by patients decreasing their periods of wear. Mucus may be seen in the inner eye corners. Later symptoms include increased pain and discomfort, with a sensation of a foreign body in the eye, and excess mucus, which may have a "glued eye" effect after sleeping; these symptoms require referral to an eyecare practitioner. Increased accumulation of mucus and other substances on the lens may lead to keratitis, abrasion, and infection; these symptoms were described earlier.

DIAGNOSTIC PARAMETERS/PHYSICAL ASSESSMENT

Interview: The following questions may assist in determining the cause of a patient's lens problems, recommending care systems, or deciding if the patient needs to be referred to an eyecare practitioner:

- Type of lenses (hard, soft, RGP).
- Recent change to new type of lens.
- Age of current set of lenses.
- Description of lens care regimen.
- List of lens care products used and any recent change in lens care products.
- Duration of daily wear (has duration decreased due to discomfort?).
- History of other eye problems (eg, conjunctivitis due to seasonal allergies).
- Current medication profile.

TREATMENT

LENS CARE SYSTEMS

▶ **Actions**

Management/Preventive Care: Patients should comply with a contact lens care regimen that is in agreement with their ophthalmologist's/optometrist's recommendations and the manufacturer's instructions. The care regimen should also be consistent with good general hygiene. Compliance is defined as meeting 4 criteria: 1) Patients should always wash hands before lens manipulation. 2) Patients should use an FDA-approved care system in an appropriate manner. 3) Lenses should be worn on a daily wear schedule unless they are FDA-approved for extended wear. 4) All solutions should be free of bacterial contamination.

The most common types of contact lenses are soft lenses and RGP lenses, which make up approximately 80% and 20% of contact lens wearers in the US, respectively. Hard contact lens wearers account for less than 1% of lens wearers. Although all contact lenses serve similar functions in correcting visual defects, each distinct type of lens material requires a unique lens care program. The typical lens care regimen includes appropriate products for cleaning, disinfecting, rinsing, wetting or rewetting, and enzymatic cleaning.

In selecting appropriate lens care solutions, it is essential to correctly identify the type of lens the patient is using (the patient may not always know). Products and care regimens for each lens type are outlined in the following sections.

▶ **Drug Interactions**

Some systemic medications may affect the physiology of the cornea, lids, and tear system. In addition, some drugs may discolor soft contact lenses. Pharmacists and eye-care practitioners should be aware of the interaction potential of systemic medications and contact lenses.

Drug Interference with Contact Lens Use		
Drug	**Lens type**	**Action**
Anticholinergics	RGP, hard, soft	Decrease tear volume
Antihistamines, Sympathomimetics	RGP, hard, soft	Decrease tear volume and blink rate
Chlorthalidone	RGP, hard, soft	Causes lid or corneal edema
Clomiphene	RGP, hard, soft	Causes lid or corneal edema
Diuretics, Thiazides	RGP, hard, soft	Decreased tear volume
Dopamine	RGP, hard, soft	Discolors lenses
Epinephrine, topical	RGP, hard, soft	Discolors lenses
Fluorescein, topical	RGP, hard, soft	Lens absorbs yellow dye
Hypnotics, Sedatives, Muscle Relaxants	RGP, hard, soft	Decreased blink rate
Iodine Groups	RGP, hard, soft	Discolors lenses
Nitrofurantoin	RGP, hard, soft	Discolors lenses
Oral Contraceptives	RGP, hard, soft	Increase mucus stickiness; fluid retention properties of estrogens cause corneal lid edema
Phenazopyridine	Soft	Discolors lenses
Phenolphthalein	Soft	Discolors lenses
Phenylephrine	Soft	Discolors lenses
Primidone	RGP, hard, soft	Causes lid or corneal edema
Rifampin	Soft	Lens absorbs drug, causing orange discoloration
Sulfasalazine	Soft	Stains lenses yellow
Tricyclic Antidepressants	RGP, hard, soft	Decrease tear volume

► **Adverse Reactions**

Dryness after several hours of wear (see Warnings); *Acanthamoeba keratitis* infection (see Warnings).

Sensitivity to preservative-containing agents may occur.

SOFT LENS CARE SYSTEMS

► **Actions**

Soft (hydrogel) contact lenses are manufactured from hydrophilic polymers containing 38% to 79% water. There are several types of soft contact lenses.

Hydrogel lenses must be maintained in a hydrated state in physiological saline to prevent them from becoming brittle. Hydrogel lenses will absorb many substances; therefore, use only solutions specifically formulated for hydrogel lenses. In addition, these lenses must be disinfected by heating in saline solution or by soaking in a chemical solution. Heating a lens in solutions designed only for chemical disinfection may cause the lens to become opaque.

Soft lens solutions are specially formulated to be compatible with, and to meet the particular needs of, soft contact lenses. Thorough cleaning to remove deposits that coat and potentially discolor the lens is especially important for soft lenses subjected to asepticizing by heating.

Types of soft lenses: **Daily wear soft lenses** may be worn 12 to 14 hours per day, but must be removed nightly for cleaning and disinfection. It is recommended that conventional soft lenses be discarded after 12 months of wear. Planned replacement lenses may be scheduled every 1, 3, or 6 months. Lens longevity is quite variable and patient-dependent. Factors influencing lens life include cleaning regimen and tear composition. Some lens wearers are "heavy depositors" (ie, produce a greater amount of lipids and proteins). A replacement schedule may be recommended by the eyecare practitioner.

Extended wear soft lenses may be worn for 24 hours or more. The FDA and most eyecare practitioners recommend a maximum wearing period of 7 days. The lenses must then be removed overnight for cleaning and disinfection. Extended lens use has decreased because of reported risk of infection.

Disposable soft lenses allow for frequent replacement of lenses and help to eliminate complications of lens deposits. They also offer the convenience of reduced lens care. Disposable lenses may be daily wear or extended wear (usually replaced every 1 to 2 weeks). If a disposable lens is not discarded immediately after lens removal, clean it with a surfactant cleaner and store in a disinfecting solution.

Single-use lenses: One-day, single-use lenses are designed to be worn one time and then discarded; a new, clean, sterile lens is used each day. Contact lens care products (lens case, cleaning solution, and disinfection solution) are not needed because a new sterile lens is being used each time.

► **Warnings**

Soft (hydrogel) contact lenses will absorb many substances; use only solutions specifically formulated for hydrogel lenses. Do not use rigid gas permeable or hard lens solutions on soft contact lenses.

In addition, these lenses must be disinfected by heating in saline solution or by soaking in a chemical solution. Heating a lens in solutions intended for chemical disinfection may cause the lens to become opaque; do not disinfect lenses by heating lenses in chemical disinfecting solutions.

Dryness: It is not uncommon for contact lens wearers to experience dryness after several hours of wear. Rewetting drops can provide temporary relief by rinsing debris off the lens surface and rewetting the eye and the lens.

Acanthamoeba keratitis: Contact lens wearers who use homemade saline solution are at risk of developing *Acanthamoeba* keratitis, a serious and painful corneal infection that may cause blindness or impaired vision. Homemade saline solutions are not recommended by the FDA; they may be used during the thermal disinfection phase but not after disinfecting. Do not use homemade saline solutions directly in the eye.

▶ **Administration and Dosage**

Cleaning: Cleaning solutions facilitate removal of oleaginous, proteinaceous, and other types of debris from the lens surface. Follow instructions on package labeling or directions given by an eyecare practitioner. Clean soft lenses thoroughly with a surfactant cleaner each time a lens is removed. Place lens in the palm of the hand, apply a few drops of cleaner, and use the fingertip to rub the lens for approximately 30 seconds to remove most contaminants. This process removes lipids, proteins, eye makeup, and other debris. After cleaning the lens, thoroughly rinse. All rinsing solutions contain 0.9% saline. Discourage use of saline made with salt tablets because of the risk of contamination and infection (see Warnings).

Enzymatic cleaners, which contain proteolytic enzymes (papain, pancreatin, or subtilisin) remove protein deposits from lenses and should be used once weekly or as needed. Inorganic deposits (eg, jelly bumps) become part of the soft lens matrix and are not removed by surfactant and enzymatic cleaners, and require lens replacement.

Disinfection: Disinfection is the most important step. It is achieved by using a thermal or chemical system.

Thermal Disinfection – Lenses are placed in saline and heated (above 80°C) in an electric unit for a minimum of 10 minutes. This method kills most microorganisms (including *Pseudomonas* species and HIV) and is quick and inexpensive. No preservatives are involved. Patients may find that this process shortens lens life (eg, lenses may stiffen and yellow), is inconvenient, and tends to "bake on" unremoved protein deposits.

Thermally disinfected lenses are then rinsed and stored in sterile saline solution.

Thermal disinfection is contraindicated with higher water lenses (approximately 55% and over) and tinted lenses.

Salt tablets for normal saline are available for use in conjunction with heat disinfection regimens, but are not recommended by the FDA. Use resulting saline solution only as a rinse prior to thermal disinfection and for storage during thermal disinfection (see *Acanthamoeba* keratitis in Warnings). Do not use these solutions to rinse and store after thermal disinfection.

Chemical Disinfection – Lenses are soaked in solutions containing one or more preservatives, which act as disinfecting agents, usually for 4 to 6 hours overnight. While typically more expensive than thermal disinfection, this method is simple and convenient and is associated with less detrimental effects on lens longevity. Patients may develop sensitivities to preservatives in chemical disinfecting solutions.

Multi-Purpose Solutions: These all-in-one solutions contain a weak cleaner and disinfectant. Such solutions are recommended for disposable lenses that are discarded before they become heavily deposited.

Rewetting: Solutions for rewetting lenses are instilled into the eyes as needed to improve comfort and wearing time by rehydrating the lens, which may become dry during wear. These solutions may also provide increased viscosity and added cushioning between the lens and cornea.

SURFACTANT CLEANING SOLUTIONS, SOFT CONTACT LENSES

▶ **Indications**

Cleaning solutions are used for daily cleaning to remove debris and to prevent the accumulation of proteinaceous (mucus) deposits.

SURFACTANT CLEANING SOLUTIONS FOR SOFT CONTACT LENSES	
Trade name	**Doseform**
Daily Cleaner for Sensitive Eyes	**Solution**: 0.2% EDTA, 0.1% sorbic acid. Cocamphocarboxyglycinate, sodium lauryl sulfate, hexylene glycol.
LC-65 Daily Contact Lens Cleaner	**Solution**: Surface-active, buffered. Cocoamphocarboxyglycinate, sodium lauryl sulfate, hexylene glycol, NaCl, sodium phosphate, EDTA.
Lens Plus Daily Cleaner[1]	**Solution**: Surface-active, buffered. Cocoamphocarboxyglycinate, sodium lauryl sulfate, hexylene glycol, NaCl, sodium phosphate.
MiraFlow Extra Strength Daily Cleaner[1,2]	**Solution**: 15.7% isopropyl alcohol, poloxamer 407, amphoteric 10.
Opti-Clean II Daily Cleaner Especially for Sensitive Eyes[2]	**Solution**: Buffered, isotonic. 0.1% EDTA, 0.001% polyquad. Polysorbate 21, polymeric cleaners.
Opti-Free Daily Cleaner	**Solution**: Buffered, isotonic. 0.01% EDTA, 0.001% polyquad. Polysorbate 21, polymeric cleaning agents.
Opti-Free Supra Clens Daily Protein Remover[1]	**Solution**: Propylene glycol, sodium borate, highly purified porcine pancreatin enzymes.
Pliagel[2]	**Solution**: 0.5% EDTA, 0.25% sorbic acid. Poloxamer 407, potassium chloride, NaCl.
Sensitive Eyes Daily Cleaner	**Solution**: Buffered, isotonic. 0.5% EDTA, sorbic acid. Hydroxypropyl methylcellulose, poloxamine, sodium borate, NaCl.
Sensitive Eyes Saline/Cleaning[2]	**Solution**: Buffered, isotonic. 0.15% sorbic acid, 0.1% EDTA. Boric acid, poloxamine, sodium borate, NaCl.
Sterile Daily Cleaner	**Solution**: Buffered, isotonic. 0.2% EDTA, 0.004% thimerosal. Sodium phosphates, NaCl, tyloxapol, hydroxymethylcellulose, polyvinyl alcohol.

Products listed are representative of currently available and widely distributed brands. Similar products, including regional and private label brands, may also exist.

[1] Preservative free.
[2] Thimerosal free.

RINSING/STORAGE SALINE SOLUTIONS, SOFT CONTACT LENSES

▶ **Indications**

Use these solutions for rinsing in many lens care systems, and for rinsing and storage in conjunction with heat disinfection. Prepared saline solutions may contain chelating agents (EDTA), which prevent calcium deposits from forming. Thimerosal-free preserved saline solutions may be used by patients sensitive to thimerosal or mercury-containing compounds. Preservative-free solutions are for patients intolerant to preservatives.

PRESERVED SALINE SOLUTIONS, SOFT CONTACT LENSES

PRESERVED SALINE SOLUTIONS FOR SOFT CONTACT LENSES	
Trade name	**Doseform**
Alcon Saline Especially for Sensitive Eyes[1]	**Solution**: Buffered, isotonic. Sorbic acid, EDTA. NaCl, borate buffer system.
ReNu Saline Solution[1]	**Solution**: Buffered, isotonic. 0.00003% poly-aminopropyl biguanide, EDTA. Boric acid, NaCl.
Sensitive Eyes Plus Saline	**Solution**: Buffered isotonic. 0.025% EDTA, 0.00003% polyaminopropyl biguanide. Boric acid, sodium borate, potassium chloride, NaCl.
Sensitive Eyes Saline[1]	**Solution**: Buffered, isotonic. 0.1% sorbic acid, 0.025% EDTA. Boric acid, sodium borate, NaCl.
SoftWear Saline for Sensitive Eyes[1]	**Solution**: Isotonic. NaCl, boric acid, sodium borate, sodium perborate (generating up to 0.006% hydrogen peroxide stabilized with phosphonic acid).
Sterile Preserved Saline Solution	**Solution**: Buffered, isotonic. 0.1% EDTA, 0.001% thimerosal. Boric acid, NaCl.

Products listed are representative of currently available and widely distributed brands. Similar products, including regional and private label brands, may also exist.

[1] Thimerosal free.

PRESERVATIVE-FREE SALINE SOLUTIONS, SOFT CONTACT LENSES

PRESERVATIVE-FREE SALINE SOLUTIONS FOR SOFT CONTACT LENSES	
Trade name	**Doseform**
Blairex Sterile Saline	**Solution**: Buffered, isotonic. NaCl, boric acid, sodium borate.
Clear Conscience Saline Solution[1]	**Solution**: Buffered, isotonic. NaCl, boric acid, sodium borate.
Lens Plus Sterile Saline	**Solution**: Buffered, isotonic. NaCl, boric acid, nitrogen.
Saline	**Solution**: Buffered, isotonic. NaCl, boric acid.
Sensitive Eyes Preservative Free Sterile Saline Spray	**Solution**: Buffered, isotonic. 0.4% NaCl, boric acid, sodium borate.
Unisol 4[1]	**Solution**: Buffered, isotonic. NaCl, boric acid, sodium borate.
Unisol Plus	**Solution**: Buffered, isotonic. NaCl, boric acid, sodium borate.

Products listed are representative of currently available and widely distributed brands. Similar products, including regional and private label brands, may also exist.

[1] Thimerosal free.

ENZYMATIC CLEANERS, SOFT CONTACT LENSES

▶ Indications

Enzymatic cleaning, by soaking in a solution prepared from enzyme tablets; it is recommended once weekly to remove protein and other lens deposits.

ENZYMATIC CLEANERS FOR SOFT CONTACT LENSES	
Trade name	Doseform
Allergan Enzymatic	**Tablets**: Papain, NaCl, sodium carbonate, sodium borate, EDTA.
Complete Weekly Enzymatic Cleaner	**Tablets**: Subtilisin A. Effervescing, buffering, and tableting agents.
Opti-Free Supra Clens Daily Protein Remover[1][2]	**Tablets**: Propylene glycol, sodium borate, highly purified pork pancreatin enzymes.
Opti-Zyme Enzymatic Cleaner Especially for Sensitive Eyes[1]	**Tablets**: Highly purified pork pancreatin.
ReNu 1 Step Enzymatic Cleaner	**Tablets**: Subtilisin, sodium carbonate, NaCl, boric acid.
ReNu Effervescent Enzymatic Cleaner	**Tablets**: Subtilisin, polyethylene glycol, sodium carbonate, NaCl, tartaric acid.
Sensitive Eyes Enzymatic Cleaner	**Tablets**: Subtilisin, polyethylene glycol, sodium carbonate, NaCl, tartaric acid.
Ultrazyme Enzymatic Cleaner	**Tablets**: Subtilisin A. Effervescing, buffering, and tableting agents.
Unizyme Enzymatic Cleaner	**Tablets**: Subtilisin A.

Products listed are representative of currently available and widely distributed brands. Similar products, including regional and private label brands, may also exist.

[1] Preservative free.
[2] Developed for use with *Opti-Free Rinsing, Disinfecting, and Storage Solution* and *Opti-Free Express Multi-Purpose Solution*. Effectiveness has not been demonstrated when used with other products.

CHEMICAL DISINFECTION SYSTEMS, SOFT CONTACT LENSES

▶ Indications

After cleaning lenses, use these solutions to disinfect and store lenses until next use.

CHEMICAL DISINFECTION SYSTEMS FOR SOFT LENSES	
Trade name	Doseform
Hydrogen Peroxide-Containing Systems	
AOSEPT[1]	**Disinfecting Solution**: Buffered. 3% hydrogen peroxide, 0.85% NaCl, phosphoric acid, phosphates.
	AODISC Neutralizer: Platinum-coated tablet.
Pure Eyes[1]	**Disinfectant/Soaking Solution**: Buffered. 3% hydrogen peroxide, 0.85% NaCl, phosphonic acid, phosphates.
	Cleaner/Rinse Solution: Buffered, isotonic. NaCl, boric acid, sodium borate, sodium perborate (generating up to 0.006% hydrogen peroxide stabilized with phosphonic acid), surfactant.
Ultra-Care	**Disinfecting Solution**: Buffered. 3% hydrogen peroxide, sodium stannate, sodium nitrate, phosphates.
	Neutralizing Tablets: Catalase, hydroxypropyl methylcellulose, cyanocobalamin, buffering and tableting agents.

CHEMICAL DISINFECTION SYSTEMS FOR SOFT LENSES

Trade name	Doseform
Non-Hydrogen Peroxide-Containing Systems	
Clear Conscience Multi-Purpose Solution[1]	**Solution:** Buffered, isotonic. 0.0001% poly-hexamethylene biguanide, EDTA. Polyoxyethylene polyoxypropylene block copolymer, phosphate salt, NaCl.
ContaClair	**Solution:** Buffered, isotonic. 0.0031% biguanide copolymer. EDTA.
Flex-Care Rinsing, Disinfecting and Storage Solution Especially for Sensitive Eyes[1]	**Solution:** Buffered, isotonic. 0.1% EDTA, 0.005% chlorhexidine gluconate. NaCl, sodium borate, boric acid.
Opti-Free Express Multi-Purpose Disinfecting Solution	**Solution:** Buffered, isotonic. 0.05% EDTA, 0.001% polyquad, 0.0005% myristamidopropyl dimethylamine. Sodium citrate, NaCl, boric acid, sorbitol, AMP-95, tetronic 1304.
Opti-Free Rinsing, Disinfecting and Storage Solution	**Solution:** Buffered, isotonic. 0.05% EDTA, 0.001% polyquad. Citrates, NaCl.
Opti-One Multi-Purpose Solution	**Solution:** Buffered, isotonic. 0.05% EDTA, 0.0011% polyquad. Borates, citrates, mannitol, NaCl, surfactants.
Purilens UV Disinfection System	**Solution:** Cleaning unit with UV-C radiation.
Quick CARE[1]	**Disinfecting Solution:** NaCl, disodium lauroamphodiacetate.
	Rinse and Neutralizer. Isotonic. Sodium borate, boric acid, sodium perborate (generating up to 0.006% hydrogen peroxide), phosphonic acid.
ReNu Multi-Purpose Solution	**Solution:** Isotonic. 0.00005% polyaminopropyl biguanide. Boric acid, EDTA, poloxamine, sodium borate, NaCl.
SOLO-care Multi-Purpose Solution[1]	**Solution:** Isotonic. 0.025% EDTA, 0.0001% polyhexanide. NaCl, polyoxyethylene polyoxypropylene block copolymer, sodium phosphate dibasic, sodium phosphate monobasic.

Products listed are representative of currently available and widely distributed brands. Similar products, including regional and private label brands, may also exist.

[1] Thimerosal free.

REWETTING SOLUTIONS, SOFT CONTACT LENSES

▶ **Indications**

These solutions are instilled into the eyes to relieve dryness and lens discomfort.

REWETTING SOLUTIONS FOR SOFT CONTACT LENSES

Trade name	Doseform
Clerz 2 Lubricating & Rewetting Drops[1]	**Solution:** Isotonic. NaCl, potassium chloride, sodium borate, EDTA, hydroxy ethylcellulose, boric acid, sorbic acid, poloxamer 407.
Complete Lubricating and Rewetting Drops[1]	**Solution:** Buffered, isotonic. 0.0001% poly-hexamethylene biguanide. NaCl, tromethamine, hydroxymethylcellulose, tyloxapol, EDTA.
Focus Lens Drops[1]	**Solution:** Buffered, isotonic. 0.2% EDTA, 0.15% sorbic acid. NaCl, borate buffer, *Oxy-Gentle*, polyoxyethylene polyoxypropylene block copolymer.

REWETTING SOLUTIONS FOR SOFT CONTACT LENSES	
Trade name	Doseform
Just Tears Lubricant Eye Drops	**Solution**: Isotonic. 1.4% polyvinyl alcohol, EDTA, benzalkonium chloride. NaCl, potassium chloride.
Lens Drops[1]	**Solution**: Buffered, isotonic. 0.2% EDTA, 0.15% sorbic acid. NaCl, borate buffer, carbamide, poloxamer 407.
Lens Plus Rewetting Drops[1,2]	**Solution**: Buffered, isotonic. NaCl, boric acid.
Opti-Free Rewetting Drops	**Solution**: Buffered, isotonic. 0.5% EDTA, 0.001% polyquad. Citrate buffer, NaCl.
Opti-One Rewetting Drops	**Solution**: Buffered, isotonic. 0.05% EDTA, 0.001% polyquad. Citrate buffer, NaCl.
Opti-Tears Soothing Drops[1]	**Solution**: Isotonic. 0.1% EDTA, 0.001% polyquad. Dextran, NaCl, potassium chloride, hydroxypropyl methylcellulose.
ReNu Lubricating & Rewetting Drops[1]	**Solution**: Isotonic. 0.15% sorbic acid, 0.1% EDTA. Boric acid, poloxamine, sodium borate, NaCl.
ReNu MultiPlus Lubricating & Rewetting Drops	**Solution**: 0.1% EDTA, 0.1% sorbic acid. Povidone, boric acid, potassium chloride, sodium borate, NaCl.
Sensitive Eyes Drops[1]	**Solution**: Buffered. 0.1% sorbic acid, 0.025% EDTA. Boric acid, sodium borate, NaCl.

Products listed are representative of currently available and widely distributed brands. Similar products, including regional and private label brands, may also exist.

[1] Thimerosal free.
[2] Preservative free.

RIGID GAS PERMEABLE (RGP) LENSES

▶ Actions

Approximately 20% of contact lens patients wear RGP lenses. These lenses are oxygen-permeable; therefore, the RGP lens patient does not have the severe physiological complications of the hard lens patient. Several lens polymers with a high degree of oxygen permeability have been approved by the FDA for extended wear. RGP lenses provide the patient with good vision, durability, and easy care.

▶ Warnings

Dryness: It is not uncommon for contact lens wearers to experience dryness after several hours of wear. This is especially true with RGP lens patients because of the hydrophobic nature of some lens materials. Rewetting drops can provide temporary relief by rinsing debris off the lens surface and providing moisture to the eye and the lens.

Acanthamoeba keratitis: Contact lens wearers who use homemade saline solution are at risk of developing *Acanthamoeba keratitis*, a serious and painful corneal infection that may cause blindness or impaired vision. Do not use homemade saline solutions directly in the eye.

Gas permeable lens materials: Some newer rigid gas permeable lens materials are made of softer plastics. Abrasive cleaners may scratch rigid gas permeable lens surfaces. RGP lenses also differ in materials and composition; use only the cleaning and soaking system prescribed by the contact lens product or eyecare practitioner.

▶ **Adverse Reactions**

Dryness after several hours of wear (see Warnings); *Acanthamoeba keratitis* infection (see Warnings); preservative sensitivity.

▶ **Administration and Dosage**

For optimum comfort, these lenses require care with separate wetting, cleaning, and soaking solutions. Lens care systems for RGP lenses contain more highly concentrated preservatives than soft lens care systems, due to the decreased lens adherence found with rigid lenses.

Cleaning: Cleaning solutions facilitate removal of oleaginous, proteinaceous, and other types of debris from the lens surface. These cleaners remove lipids, mucoprotein haze, and film, as well as increase lens surface wettability.

Surfactant cleaning solutions are used for daily prophylactic cleaning to prevent accumulation of proteinaceous (mucus) deposits and to remove other debris.

Some cleaners may contain abrasives to clean specific lens products, but can scratch or damage others. Lenses must be cleaned with solutions designed for them.

Follow package instructions or guidelines from an eyecare practitioner, place the lens in the palm of the clean hand immediately after removal. Apply a few drops of cleaner and use the fingertip to gently rub the lens surface for approximately 20 seconds, then rinse with sterile saline solution. This process removes most debris. If an abrasive cleaner is used, do not clean the lens forcefully between the fingers, because increases in minus power and warpage have been reported over time.

Many clinicians routinely recommend the weekly use of an enzymatic (papain) cleaner with RGP lenses. The weekly cleaning process is very effective in removing protein deposits from the lens surface.

Disinfecting/Soaking/Wetting: Solutions for disinfecting and soaking enhance lens surface wettability so that tears will spread evenly over the lens surface, hydration is maintained, and lens cushioning and viscosity are increased.

Chemical Disinfection: Lenses are usually soaked for 4 to 6 hours (or overnight). Patients may develop sensitivities to preservatives in soaking solutions. Soaking solution should not be reused; this could lead to bacterial growth.

Rewetting: Solutions for rewetting lenses are instilled into the eyes as needed to improve comfort and wearing time by rehydrating the lens. These solutions may also provide increased viscosity and added cushioning between the lens and cornea.

SURFACTANT CLEANING SOLUTIONS, RGP LENSES

▶ **Indications**

Surfactant cleaning solutions are used for daily prophylactic cleaning to prevent accumulation of proteinaceous (mucus) deposits and to remove other debris.

▶ **Warnings**

Solutions used strictly for cleaning should never be used for wetting/rewetting RGP lenses or chemical keratitis may result.

SURFACTANT CLEANING SOLUTIONS FOR RGP LENSES	
Trade name	Doseform
Boston Advance Cleaner	**Solution**: Concentrated homogenous surfactant. Alkyl ether sulfate, ethoxylated alkyl phenol, tri-quaternary cocoa-based phospholipid, titanium dioxide, silica gel.
Boston Original Formula Cleaner	**Solution**: Concentrated homogenous surfactant. Alkyl ether sulfate, silica gel, titanium dioxide.
Claris Cleaning and Soaking	**Solution**: 0.5% trisodium EDTA, 0.3% benzyl alcohol. Lauryl sulfate salt of imidazoline, octylphenoxypolyethoxyethanol.
Concentrated Cleaner	**Solution**: Concentrated homogenous surfactant. Alkyl ether sulfate, ethoxylated alkyl phenol, tri-quaternary cocoa-based phospholipid, silica gel.
LC-65 Daily Contact Lens Cleaner	**Solution**: Buffered surface-active. Cocoamphocarboxyglycinate, sodium lauryl sulfate, hexylene glycol, NaCl, sodium phosphate, EDTA.
Opti-Clean II Daily Cleaner Especially for Sensitive Eyes[1]	**Solution**: Buffered, isotonic. 0.1% EDTA, 0.001% polyquad. Polysorbate 21, polymeric cleaning agents.
Opti-Soak Daily Cleaner Especially for Sensitive Eyes[1]	**Solution**: Buffered, isotonic. 0.1% EDTA, 0.001% polyquad. Polysorbate, polymeric cleaning agents.
Resolve/GP Daily Cleaner[2]	**Solution**: Buffered. Cocoamphocarboxyglycinate, sodium lauryl sulfate, hexylene glycol, alkyl ether sulfate, fatty acid amide surfactants.

Products listed are representative of currently available and widely distributed brands. Similar products, including regional and private label brands, may also exist.

[1] Thimerosal free.
[2] Preservative free.

DISINFECTING/WETTING/SOAKING SOLUTIONS, RGP LENSES

▶ Indications

Solutions for disinfecting and soaking enhance lens surface wettability, maintain lens hydration similar to that achieved during contact lens wear, disinfect the lens, and act as a mechanical buffer between the lens and the cornea.

DISINFECTING/WETTING/SOAKING SOLUTIONS FOR RGP LENSES	
Trade name	Doseform
Boston Advance Comfort Formula Conditioning Solution	**Solution**: Buffered, slightly hypertonic. 0.05% EDTA, 0.003% chlorhexidine gluconate, 0.0005% polyaminopropyl biguanide. Cationic cellulose derivative polymer, PEG, cellulosic viscosifier, polyvinyl alcohol.
Boston Original Formula Conditioning	**Solution**: Buffered, slightly hypertonic, low viscosity. 0.05% EDTA, 0.006% chlorhexidine gluconate. Cationic cellulose derivative polymer, polyvinyl alcohol, hydroxyethyl cellulose.
Boston Simplicity Multi-Action Solution	**Solution**: Buffered, slightly hypertonic. 0.05% EDTA, 0.003% chlorhexidine gluconate, 0.0005% polyaminopropyl biguanide. PEO sorbitan monolaurate, betaine surfactant, silicone glycol copolymer, PEG, cellulosic viscosities.

DISINFECTING/WETTING/SOAKING SOLUTIONS FOR RGP LENSES

Trade name	Doseform
ComfortCare GP Wetting & Soaking	**Solution**: Buffered, isotonic. 0.02% EDTA, 0.005% chlorhexidine gluconate. Oxyethylene, povidone, polyvinyl alcohol, propylene glycol, NaCl, hydroxyethylcellulose, phosphates.
Flex-Care Rinsing, Disinfecting and Storage Solution Especially for Sensitive Eyes[1]	**Solution**: Buffered, isotonic. 0.1% EDTA, 0.005% chlorhexidine gluconate. NaCl, sodium borate, boric acid.
Opti-Soak Daily Cleaner Especially for Sensitive Eyes[1]	**Solution**: Buffered, isotonic. 0.1% EDTA, 0.001% polyquad. Polysorbate 21, polymeric cleaning agents.
Optimum C/D/S Solution	**Solution**: 0.1% EDTA, 0.1% benzyl alcohol, 0.05% sorbic acid, 0.02% sodium bisulfite. NaCl, potassium chloride, PVA, PVP, hydroxyethylcellulose.
Wet-N-Soak Plus Wetting and Soaking Solution	**Solution**: Buffered, isotonic. 0.003% benzalkonium chloride, polyvinyl alcohol, EDTA.
Wetting and Soaking Solution	**Solution**: Buffered, slightly hypertonic, low viscosity. 0.05% EDTA, 0.006% chlorhexidine gluconate. Cationic cellulose derivative polymer.

Products listed are representative of currently available and widely distributed brands. Similar products, including regional and private label brands, may also exist.

[1] Thimerosal free.

ENZYMATIC CLEANERS, RGP LENSES

▶ **Indications**

Enzyme cleaners are used as an adjunct to surfactant cleaning for the removal of adherent deposits. They are especially beneficial in dry eye patients who are more prone to deposit formation and for individuals who are not compliant with regular surfactant cleaning.

ENZYMATIC CLEANERS FOR RGP LENSES

Trade name	Doseform
Boston One-Step Liquid Enzymatic Cleaner[1]	**Solution**: Subtilisin A. Glycerol.
Opti-Free Supra Clens Daily Protein Remover[1]	**Solution**: Propylene glycol, sodium borate, highly purified porcine pancreatin enzymes.
Opti-Zyme Enzymatic Cleaner Especially for Sensitive Eyes[1]	**Tablets**: Highly purified pork pancreatin.
ProFree/GP Weekly Enzymatic Cleaner	**Tablets**: Papain, NaCl, sodium carbonate, sodium borate, EDTA.

Products listed are representative of currently available and widely distributed brands. Similar products, including regional and private label brands, may also exist.

[1] Preservative free.

REWETTING SOLUTIONS, RGP LENSES

▶ **Indications**

Rewetting solutions are needed when patients experience dryness or redness. They rewet the lens surface, rinse away trapped debris, and break up loosely-adherent deposits.

REWETTING SOLUTIONS FOR RGP LENSES	
Trade name	**Doseform**
Boston Rewetting Drops	**Solution**: Buffered, slightly hypertonic. 0.05% EDTA, 0.006% chlorhexidine gluconate. Cationic cellulose derivative polymer, polyvinyl alcohol, hydroxyethyl cellulose.
Claris Rewetting Drops	**Solution**: Buffered, isotonic. 0.006% polixetonium chloride, hydroxyethyl cellulose, borate buffer.
Lens Drops[1]	**Solution**: Buffered, isotonic. 0.2% EDTA, 0.15% sorbic acid. NaCl, borate buffer, carbamide, poloxamer 407.
Opti-Tears Soothing Drops[1]	**Solution**: Isotonic. 0.1% EDTA, 0.001% polyquad. Dextran, NaCl, potassium chloride, hydroxypropyl methylcellulose.
Optimum C/D/S Solution	**Solution**: 0.1% EDTA, 0.1% benzyl alcohol, 0.05% sorbic acid, 0.02% sodium bisulfite. NaCl, potassium chloride, PVA, PVP, hydroxyethylcellulose.
Sterile Sereine Wetting Solution	**Solution**: Buffered. 0.1% EDTA, 0.01% benzalkonium chloride.

Products listed are representative of currently available and widely distributed brands. Similar products, including regional and private label brands, may also exist.

[1] Thimerosal free.

HARD CONTACT LENS CARE SYSTEMS

▶ **Actions**

Conventional hard lenses are made of a rigid hydrophobic polymer, polymethylmethacrylate (PMMA). Their rigidness causes temporary alteration of the cornea, resulting in vision blurring "spectacle blur" that lasts approximately 30 minutes. PMMA does not transmit the oxygen needed for normal corneal integrity. Hard contact lenses have caused chronic corneal distortion, edematous corneal formations, polymegathism, and corneal abrasions. Because of these ocular complications, hard lenses are seldom the lens of choice for a new contact lens patient. Less than 1% of the contact lens population wear hard contact lenses.

▶ **Warnings**

Dryness: It is not uncommon for contact lens wearers to experience dryness after several hours of wear. Rewetting drops can provide temporary relief by rinsing debris off the lens surface and rewetting the eye and the lens.

Acanthamoeba keratitis: Contact lens wearers who use homemade saline solution are at risk of developing *Acanthamoeba keratitis*, a serious and painful corneal infection that may cause blindness or impaired vision. Do not use homemade saline solutions directly in the eye.

▶ **Adverse Reactions**

Dryness after several hours of wear (see Warnings); *Acanthamoeba keratitis* infection (see Warnings); hypersensitivity to preservatives.

▶ **Administration and Dosage**

For optimum comfort, hard contact lenses require care to achieve proper wetting, cleaning, and soaking. Lens care systems for these lenses contain more highly concentrated preservatives than soft lens care systems, due to the decreased lens adherence.

Cleaning: Cleaning solutions facilitate removal of oleaginous, proteinaceous, and other types of debris from the lens surface. These cleaners remove lipids, mucoprotein haze, and film, as well as increase lens surface wettability.

Surfactant cleaning solutions are used for daily prophylactic cleaning to prevent accumulation of proteinaceous (mucus) deposits and to remove other debris.

Solutions may contain abrasives to maintain lens smoothness to float freely over the eye.

Follow package instructions or guidelines from an eyecare practitioner; place lens in palm of clean hand immediately after removal. Apply a few drops of cleaner and use fingertip to gently rub lens surface for approximately 20 seconds, then rinse with sterile saline solution. This process removes most debris.

Soaking: Solutions for soaking lenses and enhancing lens surface wettability so that tears will spread evenly over the lens surface, maintaining a hydrated state and increasing lens cushioning and viscosity. Lenses are soaked in one or more preservatives, which act as disinfecting agents, usually for 4 to 6 hours (or overnight). Patients may develop sensitivities to preservatives in chemical disinfecting solutions. Soaking solution should not be reused; this could lead to bacterial growth.

Multipurpose solutions: These solutions fulfill the role of cleaning, wetting, and soaking, which are a convenience to some patients. However, they are not as effective as using separate solutions for each function.

Rewetting: Solutions for rewetting lenses are instilled into the eyes as needed to improve comfort and wearing time by rehydrating the lens, which may become dry and contaminated during wear. These solutions may also provide increased viscosity and added cushioning between the lens and cornea. In many cases, more benefit is obtained by actually removing and rewetting the lens.

CLEANING/SOAKING/WETTING SOLUTIONS FOR HARD LENSES	
Trade name	Doseform
LC-65	**Solution:** Buffered. 0.001% thimerosal, EDTA.
MiraFlow Extra Strength	**Solution:** 15.7% isopropyl alcohol, poloxamer 407, amphoteric 10. Preservative free.
Opti-Clean	**Solution:** Buffered, isotonic. Tween 21, hydroxyethylcellulose, polymeric cleaners, 0.004% thimerosal, 0.1% EDTA.
Opti-Clean II	**Solution:** Buffered, isotonic. Tween 21, polymeric cleaners, 0.1% EDTA, 0.001% polyquaternium-1.
Resolve/GP	**Solution:** Buffered. Cocoamphocarboxyglycinate, sodium lauryl sulfate, hexylene glycol, alkyl ether sulfate, fatty acid amide surfactants. Preservative free.
Sereine	**Solution:** Cocoamphodiacetate and glycols, 0.1% EDTA, 0.01% benzalkonium chloride.

Products listed are representative of currently available and widely distributed brands. Similar products, including regional and private label brands, may also exist.

WETTING SOLUTIONS FOR HARD LENSES

Trade name	Doseform
Liquifilm Wetting	**Solution**: 0.004% benzalkonium chloride, EDTA, hydroxypropyl methylcellulose, NaCl, KCl, polyvinyl alcohol.
Sereine	**Solution**: Buffered. 0.1% EDTA, 0.01% benzalkonium chloride.

Products listed are representative of currently available and widely distributed brands. Similar products, including regional and private label brands, may also exist.

WETTING/SOAKING SOLUTIONS FOR HARD LENSES

Trade name	Doseform
Sereine	**Solution**: Buffered, isotonic. 0.1% EDTA, 0.01% benzalkonium chloride.
Soac-Lens	**Solution**: Buffered. 0.004% thimerosal, 0.1% EDTA, wetting agents.
Wet-N-Soak Plus	**Solution**: Buffered, isotonic. 0.003% benzalkonium chloride, polyvinyl alcohol, EDTA.

Products listed are representative of currently available and widely distributed brands. Similar products, including regional and private label brands, may also exist.

MULTIPURPOSE CLEANING/SOAKING/WETTING SOLUTIONS FOR HARD LENSES

Trade name	Doseform
Clean-N-Soak	**Solution**: Buffered. Surfactant cleaning agent with 0.004% phenylmercuric nitrate.
Total	**Solution**: Buffered, isotonic. Polyvinyl alcohol, benzalkonium chloride, EDTA.

Products listed are representative of currently available and widely distributed brands. Similar products, including regional and private label brands, may also exist.

REWETTING SOLUTIONS FOR HARD LENSES

Trade name	Doseform
Adapettes	**Solution**: Buffered, isotonic. Povidone and other water-soluble polymers, sorbic acid, EDTA. Thimerosal free.
Clerz 2	**Solution**: Isotonic. Hydroxyethylcellulose, poloxamer 407, NaCl, KCl, sodium borate, boric acid, sorbic acid, EDTA. Thimerosal free.
Lens Lubricant	**Solution**: Buffered, isotonic. 0.004% thimerosal, 0.1% EDTA, povidone, polyoxyethylene.
Opti-Tears	**Solution**: Isotonic. 0.1% EDTA, 0.001% polyquaternium-1, dextran, NaCl, KCl, hydroxymethylcellulose. Thimerosal and sorbic acid free.
Lens Drops	**Solution**: Buffered, isotonic. NaCl, carbamide, poloxamer 407, 0.2% EDTA, 0.15% sorbic acid. Thimerosal free.

Products listed are representative of currently available and widely distributed brands. Similar products, including regional and private label brands, may also exist.

PATIENT INFORMATION
Contact Lens Care

- Proper contact lens care will increase lens wearing success and decrease complications.
- Always wash hands with a bar soap or liquid soap approved for use with contact lenses before lens manipulation. Do not use soft soaps or soaps containing lanolin, lotions, creams or oils, as these could leave a smeary film on the lens surface.
- Always rinse lenses after disinfection (eg, before lens placement in the eye).
- Use an FDA-approved care system in the appropriate manner.
- Wear lenses only on a daily wear schedule unless the lenses are approved by the FDA for extended wear.
- All solutions should be free of bacterial contamination. Cap bottles immediately after use. Discard expired solutions.
- Cleaning does not disinfect lenses; disinfecting does not clean lenses.
- Discard disinfecting/soaking solutions after each use. Do not "top off" previously used solutions.
- Clean, rinse, and air dry contact lens case daily.
- Enzymatic cleaning is not a substitute for disinfection.
- Do not insert contact lenses if eyes are red or irritated. If eyes become painful or vision worsens while wearing lenses, remove lenses, and consult an eyecare practitioner immediately.
- Do not wear contact lenses while sleeping unless they have been prescribed for extended wear.
- For soft lens care, use only products designed for soft lenses; for rigid lens care, use only products designed for rigid lenses.
- Do not change or substitute products from a different manufacturer without consulting a doctor.
- Always follow label directions or doctor's recommendations.
- Do not store lenses in tap water; do not use tap water for rinsing lenses.
- Never use saliva to wet contact lenses.
- Keep lens care products out of the reach of children.
- Do not instill topical medications in the eye while contact lenses are being worn unless directed by a doctor.
- Do not get cosmetic lotions, creams, or sprays in your eye or on lenses. It is best to insert lenses before putting on makeup and remove them before removing makeup. Water-based cosmetics are less likely to damage lenses than oil-based products.
- Schedule and keep follow-up appointments with your eyecare practitioner (every 6 to 12 months or as recommended).
- Contact lenses wear out with time; replace lenses regularly. Throw away disposable lenses after the recommended wearing period.
- Cases should be replaced every 3 to 6 months.

ORAL CAVITY
CONDITIONS

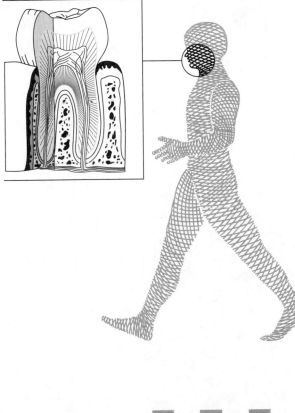

NONPRESCRIPTION DRUG THERAPY
TABLE OF CONTENTS

■ ■ ■

ORAL CAVITY CONDITIONS

INTRODUCTION

Conditions of the oral cavity can range from mild (halitosis) to severe (periodontitis), but all of the conditions are treatable, and in most cases, preventable. The goal is to increase patient awareness and self-care, mainly through education and encouragement of daily oral hygiene. Effective oral hygiene is a must, and cannot be overemphasized.

Ask most patients about oral hygiene, dental care, conditions of the oral cavity, etc., and the response will usually include the mention of a dentist. However, proper care of the teeth and gums must reach beyond the usual recommended care of a dentist. There is no question that a dentist must be the primary health care professional involved in the care of the oral cavity, but the role of the pharmacist can be key as well. Encourage patients to visit their dentist at least once a year (preferably every 6 months). However, in the interim, the pharmacist is in a position to further advocate proper oral hygiene and help patients choose the appropriate products and materials (eg, toothbrush, floss, toothpaste).

Patients must be made aware of the fact that standard daily care of their teeth and gums will help prevent severe, painful, and costly conditions such as cavities, gingivitis, and periodontitis. Treatment of these conditions costs billions of dollars annually in the US. Proper care can prevent these conditions and reduce the large health care expenditures associated with these conditions. Even halitosis, which is sometimes nothing more than a societal problem, can involve a more deep-seated problem that can be addressed and treated if recognized.

Proper flossing and brushing at least twice daily will go a long way toward preventing the build-up of plaque (the bacterial mass that adheres to and builds up on a tooth surface) that can eventually lead to gingivitis and potentially periodontitis, resulting in tooth loss. Patients need to understand that the proper mechanical process of brushing and flossing is as important, if not more so, than the specific products being used. There are many different types of toothbrushes available to consumers, manual and electric, that can be recommended to fit the specific needs of the patient. In addition, there are various types of floss that can be recommended, as well as devices that patients can use to make flossing more effective. Remember to stress proper mechanics and frequency of use.

Toothpaste type is an important aspect, especially with the multitude of brands available with a myriad of ingredients. Many available toothpaste products prevent cavities, reduce tarter and plaque, decrease sensitivity, whiten teeth, and reduce occurrence of canker sores. Help patients determine which product is best for them and their family members. Often a dentist will recommend a specific type or brand. There are also numerous mouthwashes that freshen breath, provide fluoride, and fight plaque. Again, determine what is best for the patient.

Great advances have been made over the years in the prevention and treatment of oral cavity conditions. The addition of fluoride to drinking water sources has significantly reduced the incidence of cavities, and dental care in general has made great strides in preventing and treating the various conditions. However, not all areas have fluoridated water, and some patients do not or cannot visit a dentist. Therefore, stressing the importance of self-care is essential. Be prepared to answer questions about toothbrush type, floss, toothpaste, mouthwash, and various other oral hygiene products. Patients that are pleased with their decisions will be more likely to use the products on a regular basis.

The goal is simple: Help educate patients on the importance of proper daily oral hygiene. Compliance will increase when patients understand the proper technique, use products that are satisfying to them, and understand the conditions that may result from improper or absent oral hygiene. The pharmacist is in a position to stress the importance of oral hygiene to patients and help identify the existence of various conditions of the oral cavity if referral to a dentist is appropriate.

DENTAL HYGIENE/PREVENTIVE ORAL CARE

DEFINITION

Dental hygiene and preventive oral care involve a certain knowledge of the oral environment, daily brushing and flossing, and regular dental check-ups that often include dental prophylaxis and examination of the teeth and gums.

ETIOLOGY

Plaque, the primary cause of dental disease, is a constantly present, thin bioactive film composed of bacteria and salivary by-products that adheres to the teeth and gingiva (ie, gums). The bacteria consume carbohydrates and cause a drop in pH that alters the normal ion exchange process between tooth and saliva. Rapid dissolution of calcium and phosphate ions ensues. Secondary colonization of the minutely dissolved tooth enamel by bacteria leads to caries. Plaque, coupled with a variety of genetic, medical, and iatrogenic factors, contributes to the destruction of the teeth and supporting periodontium.

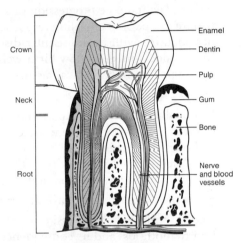

Figure 1. The Tooth

Calculus (tartar) is calcified plaque plus normal salivary constituents. This mass of concrescence forms around the base of teeth and often extends under the gingiva if left untreated. Unlike plaque, calculus cannot be removed by brushing alone; dental intervention is required to remove it. The presence of calculus is not always indicative of periodontitis.

Periodontal disease results from certain indigenous bacteria and bacterial toxins that cause a breakdown of connective tissues and bone around the roots of teeth. A resulting immune and inflammatory response compounds the problem by causing localized gingival tissue destruction, degradation of the deeper periodontal components, and, finally, resorption of alveolar bone.

The latest findings associate the host response with the severity and magnitude of periodontal disease. An overproduction of inflammatory agents, including collagenase and various prostaglandins, leads to excessive destruction of collagen, which is the primary organic component of the entire periodontium. It is still unclear why certain individuals are more susceptible to periodontal disease than others; genetics, diet, lifestyle, and oral hygiene may all play a role.

Recently, studies have shown that lack of a periodontal enzyme called Cathepsin S has been implicated in the progression of periodontal disease. Patients who lack this enzyme may benefit from future gene therapy. However, for now, increased vigilance and scrupulous periodontal maintenance by the dentist and patient are required. Periodontal disease may still progress despite these various dental modalities.

A compromised immune system, underlying medical conditions, and smoking can facilitate the progression of a diseased periodontium and also contribute to a poor oral healing response. Some other recent findings have linked periodontitis with cardiovascular disease, diabetes mellitus, stroke, infectious endocarditis, and low birth weight or premature babies. Age and oral cleanliness are rarely critical factors in the prediction of periodontal disease.

INCIDENCE

Dental disease (caries and periodontitis) has long been called the greatest ill of society. It has been present since ancient times and has not been eradicated. Although great strides have been made by developed nations to control dental ailments, the vast majority of the world's population continues to suffer from caries and periodontal disease.

Periodontitis remains the primary cause of adult tooth loss in the US.

Though seemingly harmless, if untreated, tooth decay and periodontitis often lead to tooth loss and its consequences, as well as severe morbidity and even mortality. The proportion of adults aged 35 to 44 years and 55 to 64 years with periodontal disease is estimated to exceed 70% and 90%, respectively. Increased longevity will probably increase the prevalence and severity of caries and periodontal disease in Americans.

SIGNS/SYMPTOMS

Besides regular dental appointments, proper home care is necessary to keep the teeth and gingiva clean. Some signs and symptoms of improper/inadequate oral hygiene include:

- Frequently bleeding gums when brushing and flossing.
- Spontaneously bleeding gums or gums that bleed while eating.
- Bleeding gingiva upon probing by dental professional.
- Pain when brushing or flossing.
- Toothaches or aches from the gingival region.
- Halitosis.
- Stained teeth.
- Receding gumline.
- Episodic gingival swellings or abscesses.

TREATMENT

Approaches to therapy: Proper home care for oral hygiene consists of a daily regimen of brushing, flossing, and rinsing. Because plaque is the major cause of caries and periodontal disease, proper home care is based on the need to remove as much of the bacteria as possible, thereby reducing the insult on the teeth and periodontium. Regular visits to the dentist for prophylactic cleaning are also necessary.

TOOTHBRUSHES

▶ Actions

Toothbrushes come in a variety of forms, styles, head angles, and bristle placement designs. No ADA-approved toothbrush is superior to any other. A soft, nylon, polished-bristle brush is recommended, although a new line of "periodontal" toothbrushes featuring very soft, feathered tufts at the ends of the bristles is now available. They are designed to improve subgingival cleaning. The thoroughness and degree of brushing supercede the particular brushes, bristle arrangement, and other design features. Ideally, one should brush at least twice daily. Discard toothbrushes when the bristles start to appear worn and splayed out, roughly every 3 months. Do not share toothbrushes because of the possible passage of infectious agents. A multitude of pediatric toothbrushes are available. Most resemble miniature adult brushes, but other types include combination teething ring/brushes to multiple-headed brushes for maximum efficacy. The act of brushing/flossing is considered more important than the particular dentifrice used.

TOOTHBRUSH PRODUCTS	
Trade name	**Description**
3800 Concept Series	**Toothbrush**: 38 tuft compact head, 0.007 Dupont Tynex bristles
3810 Concept Perio X-Soft	**Toothbrush**: 0.005 bristles
3815 Concept Perio	**Toothbrush**: Comes with cap
3820 Classic Colors Concept, 3830 Concept Colors, 3840 Concept Colors	**Toothbrush**: Available in various colors
3850 Concept Colors X-Soft	**Toothbrush**: Extra soft 0.006 bright white bristles
4200 Signature Series	**Toothbrush**: 42 tuft tapered head, 0.007 Dupont Tynex bristles
4210 Signature Adult X-Soft	**Toothbrush**: Interior 0.007 bristles and perimeter 0.006 bristles
4220 Signature Classic Adult, 4250 Signature Winter Series	**Toothbrush**: Available in various colors
Alert	**Toothbrush**: Built-in sensor
Angled Toothbrushes	**Toothbrush**: Soft bristle
Biotene Supersoft	**Toothbrush**: 0.003 bristles
Butler G•U•M Multi-Level Trim Toothbrush with Super-Tip	**Toothbrush**: Tapered and rounded head, tapered and texturized bristles
Butler G•U•M Pulse Plaque Remover	**Toothbrush**: 0.006 bristles
Butler G•U•M Super Tip	**Toothbrush**: Soft (0.009 to 0.007) and sensitive (0.008 to 0.006) bristles
Butler G•U•M	**Toothbrush**: Denture, Dr. Bass Right Kind, End Tuft, Orthodontic, Orthodontic Travel, Regular Travel, Soft and Sensitive, Stimulator, Sulcular, Bridge & Clasp

TOOTHBRUSH PRODUCTS

Trade name	Description
Colgate Navigator	**Toothbrush:** Full and compact flexible heads; soft and medium bristles
Colgate Plus	**Toothbrush:** Full and compact heads; soft and ultrasoft bristles; adult, youth, and child styles
Colgate Precision	**Toothbrush:** Full and compact, soft and ultrasoft
Colgate Star Wars	**Toothbrush:** Soft compact head; angled outer bristles, long inner bristles; extra soft diamond-shaped head
Crest Complete, Crest Deepsweep	**Toothbrush:** Rippled bristles
Dentax Adult	**Toothbrush:** 45° right angle brush
Dentec Super 40	**Toothbrush:** Diamond-shaped head, long handle
Dex-T-Brush	**Toothbrush:** Bulb-shaped handle, stabilizer bar
Diatech Deluxe Series, Diatech Economy Series	**Toothbrush:** 0.007 soft bristle
Dyna Flex	**Toothbrush:** Nylon bristles
E-Z	**Toothbrush:** Polished-end bristles
Echo, Flox 39, Flox 47	**Toothbrush:** 4 row
Improve "Deep V-Groove"	**Toothbrush:** 5 row, 45° angle
Mentadent Oral Care	**Toothbrush:** Flared side bristles, contoured inner bristles; compact and full heads; soft and medium bristles
Mentadent Procare	**Toothbrush:** Flexible handle, flared side bristles, contoured inner bristles; adult and youth sizes; extra soft, soft, or medium bristles
Oral-B Advantage and Advantage Control Grip with Micro-Textured Bristles	**Toothbrush:** Micro-textured bristles
Oral-B Indicator	**Toothbrush:** End-rounded bristles
Oral-B Specialty	**Toothbrush:** Denture brush, End-tufted, Ortho Travel, Orthodontic, Sensitive, Stimulator, Sulcus, Travel Brush
Pepsodent	**Toothbrush:** End-rounded, polished bristles
Pepsodent Professional	**Toothbrush:** Soft and medium
PHB	**Toothbrush:** 41 Tuft Bronze, Silver and Gold; All-American; Brush; Double-Header; Flexi-Brush; Flosser; Insidental Toothbrush; Large Denture Brush; Ortho; Rx Ultra Suave and Ultra Suave Petit; Small Denture Brush; V-Brush
Plax	**Toothbrush:** Adult soft and medium
Reach	**Toothbrush:** Adult & Kids, Advanced Design, Interdental, Plaque Sweeper, Tooth & Gum Care
Sensodyne	**Toothbrush:** Gentle, Pycopay, Search
Wernet Denture	**Toothbrush:** Double-brush
Wisdom	**Toothbrush:** Angle, Denture Fresh, Denture Fresh Deluxe Bath, Plaque Control, Spacemaster, Straight, Travel, Ultra-Soft

Products listed are representative of currently available and widely distributed brands. Similar products, including regional and private label brands, may also exist.

PATIENT INFORMATION

Toothbrushes
- Brush your teeth at least twice daily.
- Discard toothbrushes when the bristles start to appear worn and splayed out, approximately every 3 months.
- Do not share toothbrushes. Infectious agents can be passed by sharing toothbrushes.

FLOSS

▶ **Actions**

Flossing cleans adhered plaque and food debris from the spaces between teeth. Uncleaned interproximal tooth surfaces can readily develop caries, which can be difficult to detect and treat.

▶ **Product Selection**

Floss comes in a large variety of thickness, waxiness, roughness, and flavors. Newer flosses incorporate fluoride and pyrophosphates (tartar inhibitors). Many different types of floss aids are available to successfully clean around bridgework and other hard-to-clean areas. Personal preference and ease of use usually dictate floss selection. There is also a wide selection of OTC picks, miniature bristle-brushes, and other devices to help clean difficult areas.

DENTAL FLOSS PRODUCTS	
Trade name	Description
Butler G•U•M Dental, Wisdom Dental	**Floss:** Unwaxed, waxed, mint waxed
Colgate Total, Oral B New Improved Dental	**Floss:** Waxed, mint waxed
Dentax Dental	**Floss:** Waxed
E-Z	**Floss:** Unwaxed, mint waxed, cinnamon waxed
Glide	**Floss:** Polytetrafluorethylene
Johnson & Johnson Reach Dental Mint Waxed with Fluoride	**Floss:** Mint waxed, cinnamon waxed, waxed, unwaxed, mint unwaxed, baking soda, mint waxed with fluoride
Johnson & Johnson Reach Dentotape Ribbon, Johnson & Johnson Reach Easy Slide Dental	**Floss:** Regular and mint
Johnson & Johnson Reach Gentle Gum Care Dental	**Floss:** Mint, tartar control with tetrasodium pyrophosphate, mint with fluoride, grape floss for kids
Oral-B Mint Superfloss	**Floss:** Mint flavored, unwaxed
Oral-B Ultra	**Floss:** Regular, mint, mint ultra
Oral-B Unit-Dose	**Floss:** Aseptic with fluoride
PHB	**Floss:** Flat-waxed in mint or unflavored
PHB E-Z	**Floss:** Toothbrush and floss handle in 1 unit
PHB Perio	**Floss:** Acrylic yarn floss
Plaque Fighting Dental	**Floss:** Contains patented plaque-fighting ingredient
Quick	**Floss:** Y-design, contains flexible pick
Oral-B with Fluoride	**Floss:** Fluoride
	Tape: Fluoride

DENTAL FLOSS PRODUCTS	
Trade name	Description
Wisdom Dental	**Tape**: Waxed
Butler G•U•M Dental Tape	**Tape**: Waxed, mint waxed

Products listed are representative of currently available and widely distributed brands. Similar products, including regional and private label brands, may also exist.

PATIENT INFORMATION

Floss

• Floss at least twice daily.
• Consult your dentist on proper flossing technique.

TOOTHPASTE

▶ Actions

Fluoride helps prevent caries. Topically, the fluoride ion incorporates itself into the enamel, making the tooth less susceptible to acidic dissolution. It also has a direct topical antibacterial effect. Systemic fluoride supplementation in children markedly increases the resistance of adult tooth enamel to caries.

In particular, topical stannous fluoride is effective as a caries and gingivitis fighter.

▶ Product Selection

Dentifrices have developed from cleansing and polishing agents to caries-fighting fluoride carriers to the present genre of chemotherapeutic specialty pastes.

Toothpastes appear in a great assortment of flavors and colors. Although the primary active ingredient, fluoride, is now the industry standard, various other substances are frequently added to bolster the therapeutic efficacy of a particular dentifrice. Children's toothpastes contain less fluoride per dose than adult toothpaste and also come in various styles and flavors.

The following sections discuss the various toothpaste ingredients:

Pyrophosphates are compounds that chemically inhibit the formation of tartar (calculus) around the teeth. Most antitartar toothpastes contain pyrophosphates in various amounts; their overall in vivo efficacy in reducing tartar build-up has been open to debate.

Desensitizing toothpastes are marketed specifically for people with sensitive teeth. Strontium chloride (which occludes the tiny pores on the exposed tooth root surfaces) and potassium nitrate (which acts as an anesthetic at the tooth root-pore interface) have been effective in some individuals. To obtain maximum benefits, these toothpastes must be used for an extended period of time. These products are not intended for patients with a long duration of hypersensitive teeth; such patients should consult a dentist.

Baking soda and peroxide combinations have been added to some popular dentifrices. Baking soda is touted as a pH-raising, cleansing, antibacterial substance. Research has also confirmed that it has a mild lightening effect on teeth. It is not known whether this is due to an external cleansing effect or an internal mechanism. However, the amounts of baking soda/peroxide found in most toothpastes may not have profound bleaching results. Also, the therapeutic effects on the periodontium may not be significant.

Some toothpastes are dispensed in a dual chamber pump, and combine peroxide and baking soda, which releases oxygen. This bubbling oxygen helps kill odor-causing bacteria, cleanses the mouth, and acts as a topical tooth cleanser. This oxygenation mechanism, combined with peroxide (a known tooth whitener), is also being touted as a tooth lightener.

Carbamide peroxide in varying OTC percentages is used in some toothpastes. Vital bleaching (using carbamide peroxide) through OTC products, mail order products, or performed by a dentist, has become very much in vogue. Carbamide peroxide penetrates the enamel and bleaches the underlying tooth substance to a lighter color. So far, this has been deemed safe and effective by the ADA. While bleaching works in most individuals to a certain degree, the low percentage found in toothpastes is probably not high enough to produce a profound effect. A patient desiring bleaching should consult a dentist first. Many toothpastes containing "whiteners" such as titanium dioxide and various "cleansers," are being touted as "whitening toothpastes," but their overall effectiveness compared with true bleaching is questionable.

There has been a blurring between whitening and true bleaching toothpastes. Because baking soda and peroxide have inherent bleaching activity, their inclusion in many name-brand toothpastes, albeit in low concentrations, has created a new genre of dentifrices. Other "whitening" toothpastes contain only cleansers, surfactants, and various white colorants to externally affect the tooth. It is difficult to determine which of these 2 types of OTC toothpastes is more efficacious. In-office dental bleaching still has the most profound and long-lasting effects.

Sanguinaria root extract is a component of *Viadent Original* toothpaste and *Viadent* mouth rinse. This substance has been touted to clinically inhibit plaque formation on teeth and is recommended by some dentists. Some newer toothpastes are promoting a eutectic combination of **menthol/thymol/eucalyptol-type agents** (eg, *Listerine*), in addition to fluoride, as an aid to fighting caries and gingivitis.

Chlorhexidine, the active therapeutic antibacterial found in prescription mouthrinses *Peridex* and *Perioguard*, may soon be marketed in toothpaste form.

Another available dentifrice contains the antibacterial agent **triclosan**. Coupled with fluoride as an active ingredient, this toothpaste may indeed help prevent caries and gingivitis.

A new toothpaste (*Viadent Advanced Care*) containing the extra ingredient **zinc citrate** also shows promise in the control of plaque, gingivitis, and supragingival calculus.

The latest developments in toothpastes are the inclusion of specific chemicals that may someday supersede fluoride as the primary active ingredient. The first of these "new generation" dentifrices contains calcium sulfate and monoammonium phosphate in addition to fluoride. The current theory is that recalcification of early demineralized carious lesions is possible. Other toothpastes currently being developed include salivary enzymatic activity. This type of dentifrice seeks to mimic the protective nature of certain salivary proteins and thus help ward off tooth decay and gum disease.

Many toothpastes are being marketed as "natural." These dentifrices can be just as effective as their mainstream counterparts as long as they contain an acceptable percentage of fluoride.

The current bottom line for toothpaste selection remains the inclusion of fluoride. In addition, many dentifrices now contain a large variety of "therapeutic" substances that may or may not offer any advantages over fluoride alone. Further study is needed.

TOOTHPASTE PRODUCTS

Trade name	Doseform
Viadent Advanced Care Fluoride	**Toothpaste:** 2% zinc citrate trihydrate, 0.8% sodium monofluorophosphate. Sorbitol, saccharin.
Viadent Original Fluoride Formula Wintermint	**Toothpaste:** 0.8% sodium monofluorophosphate. Sorbitol, sanguinaria extract, saccharin.
Aim with Baking Soda Gel	**Toothpaste:** 0.14% sodium monofluorophosphate. Sorbitol, SD alcohol 38-B, sodium bicarbonate, saccharin.
Aim Regular Strength Gel, Close-Up with Baking Soda, Close-Up Classic Red Gel	**Toothpaste:** 0.14% sodium monofluorophosphate. Sorbitol, SD alcohol 38-B, saccharin.
Aim Tartar Control, Close-Up Tartar Control Mint Gel	**Toothpaste:** 0.14% sodium monofluorophosphate. Sorbitol, zinc citrate trihydrate, SD alcohol 38-B, saccharin.
Colgate Baking Soda and Peroxide Clean Mint, Colgate Baking Soda and Peroxide Fresh Mint	**Toothpaste:** 0.145% sodium monofluorophosphate. Sodium bicarbonate, calcium peroxide, saccharin.
Aquafresh Baking Soda	**Toothpaste:** 0.15% sodium monofluorophosphate. Sodium bicarbonate, sorbitol, saccharin.
Aquafresh Extra Fresh, Aquafresh Triple Protection	**Toothpaste:** 0.15% sodium monofluorophosphate. Saccharin, sorbitol.
Colgate Great Regular Flavor, Colgate Winter Fresh Gel	**Toothpaste:** 0.15% sodium monofluorophosphate. Glycerin/sorbitol, saccharin.
Aim Extra Strength Gel	**Toothpaste:** 0.21% sodium monofluorophosphate. Sorbitol, SD alcohol 38-B, saccharin.
Biotene Dry Mouth	**Toothpaste:** Lactoperoxidase, glucose oxidase, lysozyme, sodium monofluorophosphate. Sorbitol, xylitol, beta-d-glucose.
Caffree Anti-Stain Fluoride	**Toothpaste:** Sodium monofluorophosphate. Saccharin, parabens.
Cool Mint Listerine Tartar Control, Cool Mint Listerine Toothpaste and Gel	**Toothpaste:** Sodium monofluorophosphate. Sorbitol, saccharin.
Tom's of Maine Baking Soda Gingermint	**Toothpaste:** Sodium monofluorophosphate. Sodium bicarbonate, xylitol, ginger and peppermint oils.
Tom's of Maine Cinnamint Fluoride	**Toothpaste:** Sodium monofluorophosphate. Cinnamon and peppermint oils.
Tom's of Maine Fennel Fluoride	**Toothpaste:** Sodium monofluorophosphate. Fennel oil.
Tom's of Maine Orange Fluoride Toothpaste for Children, Tom's of Maine Silly Strawberry Fluoride Toothpaste for Children	**Toothpaste:** Sodium monofluorophosphate.
Tom's of Maine Peppermint Fluoride	**Toothpaste:** Sodium monofluorophosphate. Sodium bicarbonate, xylitol, peppermint oil.
Tom's of Maine Spearmint Fluoride	**Toothpaste:** Sodium monofluorophosphate. Xylitol, spearmint and peppermint oils.
Tom's of Maine Wintermint Fluoride	**Toothpaste:** Sodium monofluorophosphate. Xylitol, wintergreen oil.
Enamelon Anticavity Fluoride	**Toothpaste:** 0.14% sodium fluoride. Parabens, castor oil, saccharin, sorbitol.

TOOTHPASTE PRODUCTS

Trade name	Doseform
Aquafresh Tartar Control, Crest Cavity Protection Cool Mint Gel, Crest Cavity Protection Icy Mint Paste, Crest Cavity Protection Regular Flavor, Crest Tartar Control Original Flavor, Crest Tartar Protection Fresh Mint Gel, Colgate Junior, Interplak	**Toothpaste**: 0.15% sodium fluoride. Sorbitol, saccharin.
Colgate Tartar Control Gel and Paste	**Toothpaste**: 0.15% sodium fluoride. Glycerin/sorbitol, saccharin.
Crest Cavity Protection Mint Gel with Baking Soda, Crest Cavity Protection Mint Paste with Baking Soda, Crest Tartar Protection Mint Gel with Baking Soda, Crest Tartar Protection Mint Paste with Baking Soda	**Toothpaste**: 0.15% sodium fluoride. Sorbitol, sodium bicarbonate, saccharin.
Crest Multicare	**Toothpaste**: 0.15% sodium fluoride. Xylitol, sodium bicarbonate, saccharin, tartrazine (Cool Mint only).
Crest Tartar Protection Smooth Mint Gel	**Toothpaste**: 0.15% sodium fluoride. Sorbitol, saccharin, tartrazine.
Gleem Sodium Fluoride Anticavity	**Toothpaste**: 0.15% sodium fluoride. Saccharin.
Mentadent Baking Soda and Peroxide Cool Mint, Mentadent Baking Soda and Peroxide Fresh Mint, Mentadent Baking Soda and Peroxide Tartar Control	**Toothpaste**: 0.15% sodium fluoride. Sorbitol, sodium bicarbonate, SD alcohol 38-B, hydrogen peroxide, saccharin.
Mentadent Baking Soda Crystal Ice	**Toothpaste**: 0.15% sodium fluoride, menthol. Sorbitol, sodium bicarbonate, SD alcohol 38-B, hydrogen peroxide, saccharin.
Mentadent Tartar Control	**Toothpaste**: 0.15% sodium fluoride. Sorbitol, sodium bicarbonate, zinc citrate trihydrate, SD alcohol 38-B, hydrogen peroxide, saccharin.
Oral-B Children's Sesame Street Fruity and Bubblegum flavors, Oral-B Children's Nickelodeon Ice Mint Splash, Oral-B Children's Rugrats Blue Fruit Burst	**Toothpaste**: 0.15% sodium fluoride. Sorbitol.
Colgate Baking Soda Tartar Control Gel and Paste	**Toothpaste**: 0.156% sodium fluoride. Sodium bicarbonate, glycerin/sorbitol, saccharin.
Colgate Total, Colgate Total Fresh Stripe	**Toothpaste**: 0.24% sodium fluoride, 0.3% triclosan. Sorbitol, saccharin.
Arm & Hammer Dental Care Smooth Spearmint, Arm & Hammer Dental Care Tartar Control Toothgel	**Toothpaste**: 0.243% sodium fluoride. Sodium bicarbonate, saccharin, sorbitol.
Arm & Hammer Dental Care Tartar Control	**Toothpaste**: 0.243% sodium fluoride. Sodium bicarbonate, saccharin.
Arm & Hammer Dental Care Toothgel	**Toothpaste**: 0.243% sodium fluoride. Sodium bicarbonate, sorbitol/glycerin, saccharin.
Arm & Hammer Peroxicare Tartar Control	**Toothpaste**: 0.243% sodium fluoride. Sodium bicarbonate, sodium carbonate peroxide, saccharin.
Canker Cure Tooth Gel, Colgate Star Wars, Colgate Barbie	**Toothpaste**: Sodium fluoride. Sorbitol, saccharin.
Close-Up Cool Mint Gel	**Toothpaste**: Sodium fluoride. Sorbitol, SD alcohol 38-B, saccharin.
Crest Gum Care Thera Mint Gel and Paste	**Toothpaste**: 0.15% stannous fluoride. Sorbitol, saccharin.
AP-24 Anti-Plaque	**Toothpaste**: AP-24 (a patented melt-emulsion of medical grade dimethicone and the surfactants, poloxamer 407 and poloxamer 338). Sorbitol, saccharin.

TOOTHPASTE PRODUCTS

Trade name	Doseform
Pepsodent Anticavity	**Toothpaste**: Sorbitol, SD alcohol 38-B, saccharin
Pepsodent Baking Soda	**Toothpaste**: Sodium bicarbonate, SD alcohol 38-B, saccharin, sorbitol
Tom's of Maine Cinnamint Non-Fluoride	**Toothpaste**: Cinnamon and peppermint oils
Tom's of Maine Fennel Non-Fluoride	**Toothpaste**: Fennel oil
Tom's of Maine Peppermint Non-Fluoride	**Toothpaste**: Sodium bicarbonate, peppermint oil
Tom's of Maine Spearmint Non-Fluoride	**Toothpaste**: Spearmint and peppermint oils
Arm & Hammer Dental Care Tooth Powder	**Powder**: Sodium fluoride. Sodium bicarbonate, saccharin.
Products for Sensitive Teeth	
Crest Sensitivity Protection Mild Mint Paste	**Toothpaste**: Potassium nitrate, 0.15% sodium fluoride. Saccharin.
Sensodyne Cool Gel	**Toothpaste**: 5% potassium nitrate, 0.13% sodium fluoride. Saccharin, sorbitol.
Sensodyne Fresh Mint	**Toothpaste**: 5% potassium nitrate, 0.16% sodium monofluorophosphate. Parabens, sorbitol, saccharin.
Tom's of Maine Fennel for Sensitive Teeth	**Toothpaste**: Potassium nitrate. Sodium bicarbonate, xylitol, fennel oil.
Tom's of Maine Wintermint for Sensitive Teeth	**Toothpaste**: Potassium nitrate. Sodium bicarbonate, xylitol, wintergreen and peppermint oils.
Sensodyne-SC	**Toothpaste**: 10% strontium Cl hexahydrate. Parabens, saccharin, sorbitol.
Whitening Toothpastes	
Aquafresh Whitening	**Toothpaste**: 0.15% sodium monofluorophosphate. Saccharin, sorbitol.
Colgate Baking Soda and Peroxide Whitening, Ultra brite Baking Soda and Peroxide Whitening	**Toothpaste**: 0.15% sodium monofluorophosphate. Glycerin/sorbitol, sodium bicarbonate, calcium peroxide, saccharin.
Rembrandt Naturals Whitening Fluoride Toothpaste, Papaya & Ginseng, Aloe Vera & Echinacea, and Raspberry Leaf & Mint	**Toothpaste**: 0.15% sodium monofluorophosphate. Xylitol, natural products.
Colgate Platinum Whitening	**Toothpaste**: 0.76% sodium monofluorophosphate. Sorbitol, saccharin.
Plus+White	**Toothpaste**: 0.88% sodium monofluorophosphate
Close-Up Whitening Anticavity	**Toothpaste**: Sodium monofluorophosphate. Sorbitol, SD alcohol 38-B, saccharin.
Pearl Drops Extra Strength Whitening	**Toothpaste**: Sodium monofluorophosphate. Sorbitol, saccharin.
Enamelon Whitening Anticavity Fluoride	**Toothpaste**: 0.14% sodium fluoride. Parabens, castor oil, saccharin, sorbitol.
Crest Extra Whitening	**Toothpaste**: 0.15% sodium fluoride. Sorbitol, sodium bicarbonate, saccharin, tartrazine.
Mentadent Fluoride with Baking Soda and Peroxide: Advanced Whitening	**Toothpaste**: 0.15% sodium fluoride. Sorbitol, sodium bicarbonate, hydrogen peroxide, zinc citrate trihydrate, SD alcohol 38-B, hydrogen peroxide, saccharin.
Ultra brite All in One	**Toothpaste**: 0.15% sodium fluoride. Glycerin/sorbitol, saccharin.
Arm & Hammer Dental Care Extra Whitening	**Toothpaste**: 0.243% sodium fluoride. Sodium bicarbonate, saccharin.

TOOTHPASTE PRODUCTS	
Trade name	Doseform
Whitening Toothpastes	
Arm & Hammer Dental Care Advance White	**Toothpaste**: Sodium fluoride. Sodium bicarbonate, sodium carbonate peroxide, saccharin.
Pearl Drops Whitening Gel Toothpaste, Icy Cool Mint	**Gel**: Sodium fluoride. Sorbitol, saccharin.

Products listed are representative of currently available and widely distributed brands. Similar products, including regional and private label brands, may also exist.

PATIENT INFORMATION

Toothpaste

- Brush your teeth at least twice daily.
- Do not swallow toothpaste.

MOUTHWASHES/MOUTHRINSES

▶ Actions

Today's mouthwashes and rinses are slowly becoming more than cover-ups for halitosis. Most are still a combination of alcohol, anesthetics, astringents, and flavoring agents. All have some germ-fighting ability; most mask odors somewhat.

▶ Indications

As an adjunct to help freshen the mouth, remove debris, fight bad breath, or bathe the teeth in a weak fluoride solution; or as a therapeutic agent in the management of periodontal disease.

▶ Product Selection

Mouthrinses containing fluoride (0.05%) have proven beneficial in helping prevent caries in susceptible individuals. Prescription fluoride mouthrinses that are dispensed by the dentist have been found to be significantly effective in the diminution of new caries formation in susceptible patients. Use of such rinses twice yearly dramatically decreases the risk of caries.

Listerine, with its menthol/thymol/eucalyptol/methyl salicylate ingredients, has been approved by the ADA as a legitimate adjunct to periodontal therapy. However, it also contains a significant amount of alcohol.

Viadent mouth rinse contains the same extract as the *Viadent Original Fluoride Formula* toothpaste, but its low pH makes its therapeutic effectiveness a paradox.

Peridex and *Perioguard* (prescription only) mouthrinses contain chlorhexidine gluconate 0.12% as the active ingredient. These products prevent plaque from adhering to tooth structures and gingiva; they have a lingering topical germicidal effect as well. They are useful in combination with other dental therapies in the treatment of periodontal disease. Staining of the teeth, tongue, and a slightly disagreeable taste are some of the drawbacks of this particular rinse.

Oral-B Anti-Plaque, a new mouthrinse containing 0.05% cetylpyridinium chloride (an antibacterial already found in various OTC sore throat products), shows promise in reducing plaque and gingivitis.

Halitosis can now successfully be treated with new mouthwashes containing chlorine dioxide (a potent algaccide) and zinc chloride. The chlorine dioxide readily attacks the volatile sulfur compounds produced by bacteria and certain foods and neutralizes them. Not to be mistaken as a cure for an underlying dental or medical disorder, these particular mouthwashes work as promised. Certain prebrushing rinses are also available. They claim to loosen plaque prior to brushing. Although studies by the individual companies have shown efficacy, it remains a controversial subject within the dental community.

MOUTHWASH/MOUTHRINSE PRODUCTS	
Trade name	Doseform
Advanced Formula Plax New Mint Sensation Flavor, Advanced Formula Plax Original, Advanced Formula Plax Soft Mint Flavor	**Solution:** Glycerin, alcohol, benzoic acid, xanthan gum
AP-24 Anti-Plaque	**Mouthwash:** AP-24, sorbitol, glycerin, EDTA, citric acid
Betadine	**Mouthwash:** 0.5% povidone-iodine, 8% alcohol, glycerin, saccharin
Biotene Alcohol-Free	**Mouthwash:** Lysozyme, lactoferrin, glucose oxidase, lactoperoxidase
Cēpacol Mint Antiseptic	**Mouthwash:** Cetylpyridinium chloride, 0.05% alcohol, EDTA, tartrazine, saccharin, glycerin
Lavoris Crystal Fresh, Lavoris Original, Lavoris Peppermint	**Mouthwash:** SD alcohol 38-B, glycerin, citric acid, zinc oxide, saccharin
Lavoris Mint, Lavoris Original Cinnamon	**Mouthwash:** Low alcohol base, zinc chloride or zinc oxide, glycerin
Listerine Antiseptic	**Mouthrinse:** 0.064% thymol, 0.092% eucalyptol, 0.06% methyl salicylate, 0.042% menthol, 26.9% alcohol, benzoic acid
Listerine Cool Mint Antiseptic, Listerine Freshburst Antiseptic	**Mouthrinse:** 0.064% thymol, 0.092% eucalyptol, 0.06% methyl salicylate, 0.042% menthol, 21.6% alcohol, benzoic acid, saccharin
Listermint	**Mouthwash:** Glycerin, saccharin, benzoic acid, zinc chloride
Orajel Perioseptic Super Cleaning	**Mouthrinse:** 1.5% hydrogen peroxide, EDTA, 4% ethyl alcohol, parabens, sorbitol, saccharin
Oxyfresh Mint	**Mouthrinse:** Oxygene, mint oils
Oxyfresh Natural	**Mouthrinse:** Oxygene
Peroxyl Antiseptic Dental	**Mouthrinse:** 1.5% hydrogen peroxide, 6% alcohol
Prevention Regular Strength, Prevention Periodontal	**Mouthrinse:** Glycerin, 2.6% SD alcohol 38-B, 1.5% hydrogen peroxide, EDTA, zinc chloride, citric acid
Prevention Orthodontic	**Mouthrinse:** Glycerin, 2.6% SD alcohol 38-B, 1% hydrogen peroxide, EDTA, zinc chloride, citric acid
Reach ACT Anti-Cavity Fluoride Treatment	**Mouthrinse:** 0.05% sodium fluoride, EDTA, glycerin, saccharin. Available in bubble gum, cinnamon, or mint flavors.
Rembrandt Dazzling Fresh	**Mouthrinse:** Citric acid, sodium benzoate, parabens, saccharin
CloSYSII Oral Rinse	**Mouthrinse:** Trisodium phosphate, chlorine dioxide
Scope	**Mouthrinse:** 18.9% SD alcohol 38-B, glycerin, saccharin, benzoic acid
Signal	**Mouthwash:** 14.5% SD alcohol 38-B, sorbitol, saccharin
Targon Smokers'	**Mouthwash:** 15.6% alcohol, glycerin, saccharin, tartrazine

MOUTHWASH/MOUTHRINSE PRODUCTS	
Trade name	Doseform
Therasol	**Mouthwash**: 0.3% aqueous solution of C31G, 8% SD alcohol 38-B, 6% glycerin, saccharin
Tom's of Maine Natural Mouthwash with Aloe & Vitamin C	**Mouthwash**: Glycerin, witch hazel (non-alcoholic), menthol, ascorbic acid, aloe vera juice
Tom's of Maine Spearmint Mouthwash	**Mouthwash**: Glycerin, spearmint oil, menthol, natural products
Tom's of Maine Cinnamint Mouthwash	**Mouthwash**: Glycerin, cinnamon and peppermint oils, natural products
Vademecum	**Mouthwash**: Ethyl alcohol, menthol
Viadent	**Mouthrinse**: Sanguinaria extract, 10% SD-alcohol 38-F, glycerin, saccharin, citric acid
Gly-Oxide Liquid	**Liquid**: Carbamide peroxide, citric acid, glycerin

Products listed are representative of currently available and widely distributed brands. Similar products, including regional and private label brands, may also exist.

PATIENT INFORMATION
Mouthwash/Mouthrinse Products
- Do not swallow mouthwash.
- For severe halitosis, consult your dentist.

SPECIALTY AIDS

▶ Actions

Specialty flosses are made of different components and materials to aid in cleaning of difficult areas such as around implants and bridgework (eg, *Superfloss*).

Floss aids consist of floss threaders/holders to help facilitate flossing. There are also a variety of interdental cleaners (eg, *Flossbrush*, *Stimudents*, *Proxabrush*) that can be useful in plaque/debris removal.

Gingival irrigation products, such as the *Water Pik*, can greatly aid in the removal of large food particles from between teeth and help massage the gums. Antibacterial solutions can be substituted for water, making the oral irrigators suitable for fighting gum disease and for controlling plaque. However, their usefulness in plaque removal and as a substitute for brushing and flossing is questionable. The *Hydrofloss* magnetic oral irrigator claims to inhibit bacterial colonization on tooth and gum surfaces by altering the polarity of ions at the molecular level. It also functions as an irrigator.

Electric toothbrushes feature excellent brushing capabilities. They are especially well suited for individuals that possess minimal dexterity.

Electric flossing machines are also available. A thin monofilament is inserted between the teeth and oscillated. Tight tooth contacts may be difficult to clean.

Tongue scrapers come in a multitude of forms and materials. Proper tongue brushing and scraping with available OTC products help reduce halitosis and promote a healthier tongue. The scraping action removes debris and dead skin cells. The tongue surface can be altered by many medications and oral solutions, making proper tongue hygiene important.

For years, *Dentine* and *Trident* "dental" chewing gums advertised the benefits of after-meals chewing. Besides acquiring "fresher" breath, product advertisements also claimed that the gums helped promote better oral hygiene. Today, chewing gums specifically marketed as dental adjuncts are claimed to reduce plaque and tartar, promote gingival health, and help prevent caries. However, chewing any substance (with the exception of tobacco) after a meal increases saliva flow, raises the oral pH above the critical dissolution threshold (pH 5), and contributes to decreased caries formation. These newer gums are sugarless; they all contain various amounts of baking soda, pyrophosphate (tartar control) cleansers, mild abrasives, surfactants, antihalitosis ingredients (eg, chlorophyll), specialized polymers (eg, polydimethylsiloxane, plaque), and flavorings, etc. *Trident* and *Dentine* are still available, although in new and improved formulations. Like toothpastes, these new dental chewing gums contain many bioactive therapeutic agents; their usefulness may be warranted, although they cannot yet replace brushing and flossing.

There are also many OTC dental kits available containing a mirror, forceps, cotton, etc., that may aid the patient in home care oral hygiene.

A number of prescription items that specifically combat oral bacteria and the host inflammatory response are available. A caries vaccine, as well as new caries detecting agents, are available. Future dentistry will incorporate more pharmaceutical intervention in addition to a normal oral hygiene maintenance schedule to help combat caries and periodontitis.

TOOTH DISCOLORATION

DEFINITION

Coloration of tooth enamel/dentin other than the white or yellowish-white of healthy, normal teeth.

ETIOLOGY

Tooth discoloration can be caused by either discoloration of or damage to the formation of tooth enamel/dentin. Normal yellowing of teeth occurs with aging, due to the porosity of enamel allowing stains to accumulate in the underlying dentin layer. Excessive coffee or tea usage, smoking and tobacco products, certain fruits (eg, blueberries), and some medications (eg, antibiotics in infancy) can cause staining of teeth. Xerostomia and excessive soda usage can externally damage the enamel, causing staining.

INCIDENCE

It is difficult to determine how many people have this condition.

PATHOPHYSIOLOGY

The external (enamel) and internal (dentin) parts of the tooth are both affected. Obvious external stains exert a topical staining effect on the enamel. These same stains can then penetrate the enamel and stain the underlying dentin.

SIGNS/SYMPTOMS

Tooth discoloration presents fairly obviously: The teeth appear to be a color other than the white or yellowish-white of healthy teeth. Discoloration can be yellow, brown, black, grey, blue-grey, or pink.

Types of Tooth Discoloration	
Color of Stain	**Etiology**
White	Fluorosis
Blue-gray	Dentinogenesis imperfecta, erythroblastosis fetalis, tetracycline
Gray	Silver oxide from root canal sealers
Yellow	Fluorosis, physiological changes due to aging, obliteration of the pulp chamber
Brown	Fluorosis, caries, porphyria, tetracycline, dentinogenesis imperfecta
Black	Mercury stain (amalgam), caries, fluorosis
Pink	Internal resorption

DIAGNOSTIC PARAMETERS/PHYSICAL ASSESSMENT

Clinical Observation: The pharmacist must be careful in any diagnosis of tooth discoloration. There is considerable span in natural coloration of teeth. The teeth may be newly crowned at their current color, which may be an improvement over a previous shade. The teeth may be full of composite fillings; these teeth cannot be bleached as is. The teeth may have been bleached already and the results are the best that can be obtained.

Interview: Bleaching is most effective on teeth without fillings that are yellowed with age. Multiple white fillings, antibiotic staining, and caries are conditions that need to be evaluated by a dentist prior to the recommendation of a bleaching product or procedure. Patients with fractured teeth, severe erosion/abrasion areas, known hypersensitivity, or bad oral hygiene are not good candidates for a bleaching procedure. To aid in diagnosis and proper treatment, it may be beneficial to ask patients about the following, questioning the patient carefully to avoid embarrassment.

- Presence of fillings
- Recent dental procedures
- Age at onset of discoloration
- Presence of dentures
- Response of discoloration to good oral hygiene
- Precipitating factors, especially diet (eg, coffee, tea, milk, dairy products)
- Patient's medical history (eg, general health, medications being taken or taken in the past, family history of tooth discoloration, jaundice in infancy)
- Amount of fluoride exposure (eg, fluoridated water, fluoride supplements)
- Dental problem frequency (eg, cavities, gingivitis)
- Oral hygiene habits (eg, toothbrushing, flossing, brands used)

TREATMENT

Approaches to therapy: Evaluate patients using the previous diagnostic parameters. Depending on various factors (eg, extent of discoloration, existence of fillings, fractures) health care providers may recommend (1) a nondrug approach, (2) appropriate pharmacotherapy, or (3) immediate referral to a dentist for medical evaluation.

Nondrug therapy: Good oral hygiene with the use of toothpastes containing polymeric phosphates (eg, *Colgate Total*) and/or baking soda peroxide (eg, *Mentadent*) and the cessation of stain-inducing foods and tobacco products can be a first step to whitening teeth. Obviously, a dental evaluation is also important. Several whitening toothpastes available OTC have received the ADA Seal of Acceptance (eg, *Rembrandt*). These toothpastes contain polishing or chemical agents that remove surface stains through gentle polishing, chemical chelation, or other nonbleaching actions but may not achieve significant whitening due to the short duration of product-to-tooth contact.

Pharmacotherapy: Whitening is any process that makes the teeth appear whiter. This can be achieved in two ways: actually changing the natural tooth color or removing surface stains. Bleaching products contain peroxides, which whiten teeth by both methods. Nonbleaching products work by physical or chemical action to remove surface stains only. Whitening products may be administered or dispensed by dentists or puchased OTC.

The exact mechanism of action is not completely understood but it is thought that peroxide, a potent oxidizing agent, diffuses through the enamel and into the underlying dentin layer, where it releases free radicals. These free radicals oxidize any organic stains into lighter colored matter. The continual breaking of double bonds of stain material by the peroxide reaches a saturation point; no more increase in lightening of the tooth.

Bleaching agents are available OTC. Due to the importance of professional consultation to the procedure's safety and effectiveness only those dispensed through a dental office bear the ADA Seal of Acceptance. Since 1989, numerous studies have been conducted to establish the safety of oral bleaching products. Hydrogen peroxide as a chemical has been associated with the following major concerns: carcinogenicity, genotoxicity, pulpal effects, gingival irritations, and hard dental tissue alterations.

The least costly, most nonintrusive and time-efficient method to begin to whiten teeth is an external bleaching procedure. This type of bleaching can be done either in a dental office or at home under the dentist's supervision. OTC whitening products and procedures that bypass the dentist attempt to mimic the same results, but the outcomes can be variable. Whitening agents, although often mentioned interchangeably with bleaching materials, are actually different chemically and do not achieve the same degree of whiteness.

Yellowed teeth without fillings are the most amendable to bleaching, often surpassing the usual two-shade whitening. Tetracycline staining, characterized by a gray/brown intrinsic staining of the teeth, is a difficult situation to overcome. However, prolonged bleaching, regardless of the method used, can often successfully lighten the teeth to an acceptable shade. Heavy external staining such as from tobacco, tea, and coffee can be overcome but the patient has to drop the habits or the teeth will quickly return to baseline.

In vitro and clinical evidence has shown enamel is not significantly affected by the bleaching agents, even if overused.

WHITENING AGENTS

► **Actions**

Surfactant cleansing action coupled with a residue of white color pigment, which is deposited on the enamel surface.

OTC whitening toothpastes containing polymeric phosphates (eg, *Colgate Total*) and/or baking soda/peroxide (eg, *Mentadent*) have an extrinsic cleansing effect at best. Added white colorants can add to the "whitening" efforts. OTC bleaching toothpastes (eg, *Rembrandt*) contain peroxide.

STRIPS

► **Actions**

Hydrogen peroxide bleaches extrinsic and intrinsic enamel stains.

► **Indications**

To whiten teeth.

► **Contraindications**

Do not use whitening strips on caps, crowns, veneers, fillings, or braces.

► **Adverse Reactions**

Tooth sensitivity: Whitening strips may cause teeth to become temporarily sensitive.

Gum discomfort: Temporary gum discomfort may occur while using whitening strips due to vigorous brushing, using a medium- to hard-bristled toothbrush, or using a strong toothpaste.

► **Administration and Dosage**

Wear one strip for 30 minutes, twice daily, for 14 days.

WHITENING STRIP PRODUCTS	
Trade name	**Description**
Crest Whitestrips	**Strip**: 6% hydrogen peroxide, glycerin, sodium hydroxide

Products listed are representative of currently available and widely distributed brands. Similar products, including regional and private label brands, may also exist.

PATIENT INFORMATION
Whitening Strips

- Eating, drinking, smoking, or sleeping during use is not recommended.
- Begin treatment with upper teeth. After completing 14 days of treatment, proceed to treat lower teeth.
- Avoid brushing your teeth within 30 minutes of use.
- All types of bleaching should be done under the direct supervision of a dentist, complete with periodic check-ups.
- Store any unused portions of take-home bleaching systems away from children in a cool dry place.

GEL

► **Actions**

Carbamide peroxide bleaches extrinsic and intrinsic enamel stains. Polymers adhere gel to teeth.

► **Indications**

To whiten teeth.

► **Adverse Reactions**

If tooth sensitivity or gum irritation occur, discontinue use and consult a dentist.

► **Administration and Dosage**

Apply a thin layer to all teeth twice daily.

GEL PRODUCTS	
Trade name	**Description**
Colgate Simply White	**Gel**: Carbamide peroxide
Rembrandt 3 in 1	**Gel**: Peroxide
Rembrandt Quick White	**Gel**: Hydrogen peroxide

Products listed are representative of currently available and widely distributed brands. Similar products, including regional and private label brands, may also exist.

PATIENT INFORMATION
Gel

- Store in a cool place.
- Do not eat or drink within 30 minutes of use.
- Dry teeth completely before use.
- All types of bleaching should be done under the direct supervision of a dentist, complete with periodic check-ups.
- Store any unused portions of take-home bleaching systems away from children in a cool dry place.

EDENTULISM, DENTURES, AND DENTURE CARE

DEFINITION

Edentulism is the partial or complete absence of teeth. Complete or partial removable dentures are often the prescribed treatment for the restoration of masticatory function and pleasing dental aesthetics to the patient.

ETIOLOGY

Tooth loss resulting in edentulism is usually the terminal outcome of untreated dental disease (eg, caries and periodontitis). Many factors, including dental plaque, diet, oral hygiene, medical conditions, saliva constitution, genetics, and lifestyle, contribute to oral health problems. In addition, certain medications with anticholinergic properties (eg, antiparkinsonian agents, antianxiety agents, antihistamines) can cause xerostomia (dry mouth), which contributes to tooth loss. A compromised immune system or smoking also can lead to the early loss of teeth.

INCIDENCE

Although edentulism is on the decline in the US, an estimated 32 million Americans wear full or partial dentures. If current population and longevity forecasts are accurate, the number of denture wearers will continue to rise. This translates into more interaction between patient, dentist, and pharmacist.

Theoretically, proper dental care, nutrition, and periodic dental surveillance should maintain teeth for life; however, this is not always the case. And, although aging is not directly linked to tooth loss, most partially or totally edentulous patients are elderly.

TREATMENT

Approaches to therapy:

Full Dentures – A series of dental visits is required for the fabrication of a complete set of dentures. Impressions, bite records, and a try-in appointment followed by the insertion visit are the usual steps. The denture base is usually pink denture acrylic; the teeth, which can be porcelain or acrylic, come in a wide variety of shades and sizes. Acrylic denture teeth are used more frequently than the more aesthetically pleasing porcelain dentures because of better bonding to the denture base, ease of adjustment, and less potential for damage to the underlying bony ridge. In addition, acrylic teeth are less abrasive than porcelain teeth when opposing natural dentition. Over time, porcelain wears down and abrades natural teeth considerably; such wear may result in increased sensitivity and may require crowns to prevent further wear. Today's high-end acrylic teeth are durable, aesthetically pleasing, and a good substitute for porcelain teeth. Different grades, shades, and finishes of denture acrylic are available for the denture base itself. Retention of a complete denture is achieved by suction against the bony ridges, correct extensions of the denture borders, saliva, and proper occlusion. The technical mastery of the dentist and dental laboratory technician is paramount in producing a denture of pleasing appearance and proper form and function. However, patients should have realistic expectations; a denture is not an exact replacement of natural dentition. The biting force is greatly decreased, the retention may be less than ideal, speaking and eating may be difficult, etc. Unrealistic patient expectations can doom an otherwise successful denture.

Partial Dentures – As with the complete denture, much the same dental fabrication procedures are followed. The base is usually made of a thin, highly polished, cast base metal. The edentulous areas are filled in by pink denture base acrylic and denture teeth. Retention is achieved by frictional fit against the natural teeth and by finger-like metal projections called clasps; these encircle key natural teeth. These clasps are easily broken, necessitating dental consultation. A partial denture is much preferred over a complete denture; better retention, stability, and chewing power are the advantages. Mobile teeth, and even a few remaining teeth, can sometimes be successfully clasped with a retentive partial denture. Of course, as key teeth are lost, the partial situation may eventually evolve into a complete denture case. As with complete dentures, there are a variety of materials and techniques used to fabricate attractive and functional partial dentures.

Other Types of Dentures – Although the 2 most common types of dentures have been described, there are a multitude of "specialty" and "interim" dentures as well. Below are just a few examples of such dentures:

- *Immediate Denture:* An immediate denture is a complete denture made from a dentate-toothed patient and subsequently inserted immediately upon the extraction of all remaining teeth and roots. This is an excellent service for some patients because they avoid going toothless. Also, it quickly trains the patient to become used to the denture. On the other hand, this type of denture offers no try-in stage for the patient, and also no opportunity for the patient to see the denture in wax before the final production process (as such, no modifications can be made to the denture). With such dentures, the final product is an "estimation" by the dentist and lab technicians in terms of final aesthetics and function; therefore, it is possible that patient expectations may not be met. The immediate denture is often considered an interim treatment modality because healing-induced resorption of the alveolar ridge causes the denture to loosen. Successive temporary or permanent relines performed in the office or dental laboratory are often necessary for approximately 6 months until sufficient retention and stability are established. A new "final" denture is often fabricated, leaving the immediate denture as a back-up.

- *Cu-Sil or Gasket Denture:* This type of denture is basically a complete denture with holes for the few remaining natural teeth to fit through. The holes in the denture are lined by a softer, elastomeric material, allowing a tight fit over the remaining teeth. Often, these liners must be replaced every 3 to 6 months. This denture allows the patient increased stability and retention. If the natural teeth fail, this denture can easily be converted to a complete one by filling in the holes with denture acrylic and denture teeth.

- *Overdenture:* Usually a complete denture, the overdenture rests over a ridge with remaining roots, prepared teeth, or implants. The remaining dentition, though usually submerged, affords the patient increased retention of the denture and some proprioception.

- *Transitional or "Flipper" Dentures:* These are various temporary dentures made to replace 1 or 2 teeth until a more permanent denture or bridgework can be done. Such dentures are generally placed in the anterior areas of the mouth and are intended for aesthetic purposes only (eg, they are not to be used for mastication). Unfortunately, these emergency dentures too often become the final treatment because of the inability of the dentist to convince the patient of the temporary nature of these dentures or inadequate patient finances. They are usually claspless, offering poor retention.

- *Specialty Dentures:* Specialty dentures such as "precision" and "semi-precision" types with sophisticated interlocking pieces that fit into special bridgework along with implant-supported dentures are just 2 examples of additional dentures that can be made. They offer high retention but cost more. It should be stressed that if dentally, medically, and financially feasible, other treatment may be available to the patient seeking closure of edentulous spaces. Fixed bridgework and implants are such alternative therapies. Removable prostheses are often the easiest to fabricate and involve little tooth reduction. They are also the most economical for the patient.

Denture Care and Adjunctive Services – Good denture care begins with proper **cleaning** of the prosthesis. A "scrub and soak" method is advocated. Using a regular or specially designed denture toothbrush and toothpaste, the denture is first gently scrubbed to remove any food particles, debris, or plaque. Any available denture toothpaste or regular paste may be used. Mild soap is an alternative cleanser. Avoid bleach and other harsh chemicals because they can damage the denture. Cleaning the denture over a sink of water is highly recommended to help guard against falling and breakage. Using the specially designed effervescent soaking tablets after scrubbing increases plaque removal and bacterial destruction, and adds "freshness" to the denture. Using this method daily is highly recommended to achieve a clean denture. An annual professional cleaning of the prosthesis is also advised to remove any hard tartar deposits that may accumulate.

Proper **storage** is also important. Most denture acrylic must stay wet; thus, storing the prosthesis in a water-filled container when not in use is prudent. A dried-out denture may warp or crack. Hot water may also distort the denture acrylic, compromising the fit. An *otc* denture bath or equivalent may be used.

Constant wearing of the prosthesis is contraindicated. Constant use of dentures can cause a wide range of problems in the underlying mucosa. Although patients who have been wearing dentures for many years feel "unnatural" without them, it is actually natural not to wear them. The tissue lying underneath the dentures must have time to aerate and rest. A lack of proper aeration can lead to fungal growth (eg, *Candida*) in the underlying tissue, requiring medication to alleviate the problem.

In addition, failure to remove the denture to provide rest for tissues and to clean the soft tissue of the palate may produce palatal inflammatory hyperplasia. In this condition, the tissue appears red with a pebbly surface and is typically asymptomatic. Treatment generally involves removal of the denture to allow the edema to subside. More aggressive attempts to treat this condition involve surgery.

Wearing a dental prosthesis 24 hours a day may also cause negative effects to the bony ridges. For example, increased bone resorption may occur, which can result in an ill-fitting denture, loss of retention, and shortened life of the prosthesis. Multiple relines may be required to correct these problems. As the patient ages, bone resorption can eventually become so severe that achieving retention is nearly impossible because the ridges are given no chance to rest.

It is therefore recommended that patients remove their prostheses nightly to allow soft tissue and bony ridges to rest. Even short periods of rest are better than nothing; however, some patients do insist on wearing their dentures all the time.

Ill-fitting Dentures – Ill-fitting dentures may have many causes, including improper construction, patient weight loss, etc. By far, the most common cause is normal bone resorption of the bony ridges because of the aging process. The pharmacist may be asked to recommend a certain denture adhesive or cushion. Denture adhesives are available as creams or powders; either type is effective. Both dissolve in saliva after a few hours and should be reapplied for continued use. New dentures, immediate dentures, and mouths with very little bony ridge support stand to benefit most from the judicious application of adhesive. This is not the same as the chronic overuse of adhesives in old, ill-fitting prostheses; the result is often an accelerated destruction of supportive bone.

Nonprescription reliners and cushions are materials that, unlike adhesives, do not dissolve away intra-orally. They are similar to the soft temporary relines placed by the dentists. If the OTC device or material is not placed properly, the propensity for ridge destruction is great. Use of such products should be discouraged.

In some rare cases, bone resorption, especially on the lower ridge, is so extreme that a conventional denture may be too harsh on the thin underlying mucosa. When this occurs, it is more feasible to perform a laboratory soft reline to provide a cushion to the soft tissue and elevate chronic sore spots. Such relines last 1 to 2 years.

Patients often perceive dentures as definitive treatment and fail to realize that periodic check-ups are important. No denture, regardless of how precisely made, produces an ideal fit for life. If dentures become so loose as to require constant adhesive or cushion/reliner use, then a professional dental reline or new denture should be made.

Denture sores are small, painful, indurated lesions that appear on the ridges or in the fold of the cheeks. They can appear anywhere a denture rests and result from normal minute denture base discrepancies and bite problems. The rubbing of the denture base against the mucosa causes chafing and ultimately, the sore. Nonprescription denture anesthetics made especially for combatting denture sores have limited usefulness. A dentist must be seen; the dentist will shave off the particular high spot on the denture and adjust the bite, relieving the sore spot. Rapid healing occurs after the denture is adjusted; however, many adjustment visits may be required until proper fit and comfort is achieved. Remedies consisting of warm salt water rinses (2 to 3 times per day), milk, magnesium hydroxide (eg, *Milk of Magnesia*), and diphenhydramine (eg, *Benadryl*) may also be used to provide a soothing effect on the denture sores until a dentist is seen. Denture adhesives may also be temporarily effective. Avoid use of peroxides or mouthwashes (eg, *Listerine*, *Scope*) because these products will further irritate the affected areas.

In some cases, an ill-fitting denture may result in a condition called epulis fissuratum. This develops in association with the flange of an ill-fitting partial or complete denture. The epulis typically presents as multiple folds of tissue between the cheek and gum. Treatment involves surgical removal of the epulis and remaking or relining the ill-fitting denture.

Denture stomatitis is a candidal/bacterial infection and inflammation that usually occurs underneath an ill-fitting denture or in patients who wear dentures all day and night. Redness, burning, sloughing of mucosa, and odor are characteristic manifestations. After an underlying medical cause has been ruled out, the usual treatment consists of the application of a topical antifungal, such as nystatin (eg, *Mycostatin*) cream, directly to the underside of the denture. The patient is instructed to apply the antifungal and wear the prosthesis; a 7- to 10-day healing period is usually the norm. Antibiotic/antifungal drugs, systemic and topical, also may be used in refractory cases.

Use of dental repair kits should be discouraged. Avulsed (torn away) denture teeth and fractured dentures are common problems, resulting from trauma, falls, or blows. Many patients do not realize the importance of precision when it comes to dentures. An incorrect repair can have severe consequences, including gum irritation, bite problems, and ridge resorption. Repair with *Crazy Glue* or other household adhesives should be discouraged. A dentist is most qualified to properly repair the many types of broken dentures. If the dentist cannot repair the prosthesis in the office, it may have to be sent out to a dental laboratory for repair. This may take a few hours or a few days.

DENTURE CLEANSERS

▶ Actions

Cleansers added to overnight denture bath solutions include chelating agents, surfactants, and oxidizing bubbling agents such as peroxides, perborates, and hypochlorites. Several ultrasonic denture bath devices are available to aid in the cleaning of dentures.

▶ Warnings

Children: These alkaline products should be kept away from children.

▶ Guidelines for Use

See instructions that accompany individual products for appropriate directions for use. As previously mentioned, chemical cleansing alone is inadequate; mechanical scrubbing and professional cleaning are also required.

DENTURE CLEANSERS	
Trade name	**Doseform[1]**
Polident for Partials	**Crystals**
Fresh N' Brite Two Layer	**Gel**
Ban-A-Stain	**Liquid**
Dentu-Creme Denture Cleansing Toothpaste	**Paste**
Dentu-Gel Denture Cleansing Toothpaste	**Paste**
Kleenite Denture Cleanser	**Powder**
Polident Powder Denture Cleanser	**Powder**
Stain-Away "For Partials"	**Powder**
Stain-Away "Plus" Denture Cleanser	**Powder**
Efferdent 2-Layered Anti-Bacterial Denture Cleanser	**Tablets**
Efferdent Denture Cleanser	**Tablets**
Efferdent Plus Denture Cleanser	**Tablets**
Polident Double Action	**Tablets**
Polident Overnight	**Tablets**
Smokers' Polident Denture Cleanser	**Tablets**

Products listed are representative of currently available and widely distributed brands. Similar products, including regional and private label brands, may also exist.

[1] Many denture cleansers, adhesives, reliners, and cushions do not list active ingredients or composition in the package labeling.

PATIENT INFORMATION
Denture Cleansers

- Keep out of reach of children.
- These products are only for use on artificial teeth, outside the mouth. Do not ingest products or place them inside the mouth.
- Avoid contact with eyes, eyelids, and mucous membranes.
- Clean dentures over a sink half-filled with water to prevent damage if dropped.
- Rinse dentures thoroughly with tap water after cleaning.

DENTURE ADHESIVES, RELINERS, AND CUSHIONS

► Actions

Although very useful in certain situations and in certain individuals, adhesives usually should be used on a temporary basis only. Dental supervision is required. The consequences of chronic overuse in ill-fitting dentures include destruction of the bony alveolar ridges and overlying mucosa. Denture adhesive products contain inert, gummy, and adherent agents such as methylcellulose, ethylene oxide, karaya, and petroleum jelly. Some of these products are soluble in saliva; repeat application depends on the fit of the denture to start with. Denture adhesives come in powders, creams, strips, liquids, wafers, and cushions. Many patients prefer the creams, especially the newer creams with longer holding power.

DENTURE ADHESIVES, RELINERS, AND CUSHIONS	
Trade name	Doseform[1]
Confident Denture Adhesive	Cream
Effergrip Extra Strength Denture Adhesive	Cream
Fixodent	Cream
Rigident Denture Adhesive	Cream
Super Poli-Grip Free Denture Adhesive	Cream
Ezo Denture Cushions	Cushions
Snug Denture Adhesives	Cushions
Dentrol	Liquid
Endslip	Plate
Denture-Fit Adhesive	Powder
Denturite	Powder/Liquid
Fixodent	Powder
Klutch	Powder
Super Wernet's Denture Adhesive	Powder
Polident Dentu-Grip	Powder
Brimms Plasti-Liner	Strips
Sea Bond Denture Adhesive	Wafers

Products listed are representative of currently available and widely distributed brands. Similar products, including regional and private label brands, may also exist.

[1] Many denture cleansers, adhesives, reliners, and cushions do not list active ingredients or composition in the package labeling.

PATIENT INFORMATION

Denture Adhesives, Reliners, and Cushions

- Ill-fitting dentures may impair health. Consult your dentist regularly.
- If irritation occurs, discontinue use.
- Long-term use of denture adhesives, reliners, and cushions may lead to faster bone loss, continuing irritation, sores, and tumors. These products are for use only until a dentist can be seen.
- Some products should not be used on dentures with soft linings. Consult your dentist.

CANKER SORES

DEFINITION

Canker sores are painful mouth ulcerations that generally appear on the moveable oral mucosa (eg, tongue, inside lip, cheek). The ulcers are usually rounded, shallow, and painful, and rarely occur on the hard palate, soft palate, or gingiva. Canker sores are also known as aphthous ulcers or aphthous stomatitis.

ETIOLOGY

The cause of canker sores is poorly defined. The etiology may be multifactorial as a variety of etiological factors have been implicated. Local trauma precedes 50% to 70% of lesions. Physical or psychological stress may be a significant precipitating factor in some cases. Approximately 20% of canker sore sufferers have iron, B_{12}, or folic acid deficiencies. An autoimmune disorder or systemic disease may decrease host resistance and predispose to the development of canker sores. Viruses, streptococci, hormonal shifts, smoking, and gluten sensitivity may be precipitating or confounding factors. In addition, toothpastes containing sodium lauryl sulfate and acidic/citrus foods may induce aphthous ulcers.

INCIDENCE

Canker sores are common oral lesions, usually first experienced in individuals between 10 and 20 years of age. Approximately 20% of the population has experienced at least 1 episode of canker sores. Recurrent attacks are common, especially in patients with compromised immune systems. Multiple lesions (2 to 15 ulcers) per episode scattered over different areas of the mouth may occur, but lesions usually appear singly in one area and most are from 3 to 15 mm in diameter. An unexplained gender predisposition toward women exists. Canker sores also are seen more often in nonsmokers than in smokers or users of snuff or chewing tobacco. While canker sores occur most often in healthy individuals, lesions may be particularly severe and frequent in patients with systemic diseases such as celiac sprue, Behcet syndrome, Crohn disease, Reiter syndrome, HIV infection, AIDS, inflammatory bowel disease, and nutritional deficiencies (eg, iron, vitamin B_{12}, folic acid).

PATHOPHYSIOLOGY

Canker sores begin as shallow, elevated, solid, circumscribed, round or oval macules surrounded by red, edematous, inflamed margins. The lesions progress to shallow ulcerations over the next 4 to 7 days, with the ulcer crater coated by a gray-white pseudomembrane composed of coagulated tissue, fluids, bacteria, leucocytes, and cellular debris. The lesions heal spontaneously. Lesions less than 1 cm in diameter typically heal without scarring in 7 to 14 days. Lesions larger than 1 cm in diameter may not heal completely for weeks or months, and scarring is likely.

SIGNS/SYMPTOMS

The physical appearance of the canker sore is described above. Lesions invariably are painful, and the acutely painful phase lasts 3 to 5 days or more. Pain then begins to diminish in intensity as healing occurs. Friction of any type compounds the pain. Pain and discomfort caused by friction may inhibit eating, drinking, talking, or swallowing. Malaise, fever, and lymphadenopathy may accompany more severe attacks. Pain may mimic toothache if the lesion is near a tooth.

DIAGNOSTIC PARAMETERS/PHYSICAL ASSESSMENT

Clinical Observation: In assessing the oral lesion by history and observation, it is appropriate to determine the following:

• If lesions are not distinctive enough to differentiate canker sores from oral candidiasis (thrush), leukoplakia, primary or recurrent intraoral herpetic ulcers, or mucosal pemphigoid, refer the patient to a physician or dentist for further evaluation.

• Smokers and users of smokeless tobacco who develop white, thickened patches on the mucosa of the cheeks, gums, or tongue should be referred to a physician or dentist for further evaluation. Such lesions could be leukoplakia, a precancerous lesion associated with the use of tobacco products, particularly smokeless tobacco.

Interview: To help the patient determine if physician referral or self-treatment is warranted, it may be beneficial to ask about the following:

• Location of lesion(s).
• Number of lesions.
• Size and physical appearance of lesion(s).
• Length of time lesions have been present.
• Frequency of oral lesions.
• Presence of any potentially precipitating or confounding comorbidity or lifestyle factors (eg, systemic infection, autoimmune disease, local trauma, presence of unusual physical or psychological stress, nutritional status, smoking status).
• Pain intensity and level of physical discomfort.

TREATMENT

Approaches to therapy: There is no cure for canker sores. These lesions are self-limiting; thus the goals of pharmacotherapy should be directed at (1) controlling pain and discomfort and (2) promoting healing. Treatment is based on the severity of symptoms, duration of lesions, and concurrent underlying systemic disease. Nondrug therapy, as well as topical and systemic drug therapy, may be used.

Nondrug therapy:

Saline rinses – A warm saline rinse held in the oral cavity for 30 to 60 seconds, and repeated as necessary, can produce transient but therapeutic relief. Consider saline rinses adjunctive to oral protectant/lubricants and other analgesic therapies. One to three teaspoonfuls of table salt (sodium chloride) added to 4 to 8 ounces of warm tap water is a simple but useful mixture.

Avoidance of acidic foods – Patients should avoid acidic or citrus foods, which may aggravate aphthous ulcers.

Pharmacotherapy: Patients frequently attempt treatment of canker sores with OTC products. Generally, these products do more to control symptoms than to actually cure the lesions. Patients who experience recurrent aphthous ulcers should be referred to a physician for thorough evaluation.

Iron, vitamin B$_{12}$, or folic acid – These agents given alone or in combination with one another, or in a multivitamin formulation, may be employed as prophylactic, empirical therapy if canker sores recur and there is legitimate concern regarding dietary neglect (eg, confirmed or suspected nutritional deficiency).

Local anesthetics and oral protectants/lubricants – Most of the pain and discomfort associated with canker sores is caused by friction of the tongue, teeth, food, and oral tissue rubbing against the lesion. Products such as *Orabase* and *Zilactin* in their various formulations are bioadhesive to varying degrees and reduce friction because of their lubricant properties. Additionally, some formulations contain an astringent (eg, tannic acid), which promotes drying and healing. The duration of action of the oral protectants/lubricants ranges from 2 to 6 hours. Before applying an oral protectant/lubricant, dry the canker sore with a tissue. Hold the area of canker sore involvement away from other oral tissue for to 30 to 60 seconds after application to allow tissue healing. The oral protectant/lubricant can be administered 3 to 6 times daily as needed.

Local anesthetics (eg, benzocaine [5% to 20%], butacaine, lidocaine [0.5% to 4%], dyclonine [0.5% to 1%], dibucaine [0.25% to 1%], tetracaine [2%]) may be applied directly to the canker sore lesion alone or via an oral protectant/lubricant. The duration of action of topical anesthetics is relatively short (20 to 30 minutes), so they serve only as an adjunct to oral protectants/lubricants and systemic oral analgesics. As some patients are hypersensitive to local anesthetics, discontinue use if symptoms worsen.

Miscellaneous ingredients– –

Cetylpyridinium chloride, benzalkonium chloride, and povidone-iodine: Have mild antiseptic activity.

Menthol, camphor, and phenol: Counterirritants used for their antipruritic and very mild local anesthetic activities.

Allantoin (0.5% to 2%) and dimethicone (1% to 30%): Skin protectants/ moisturizers that prevent cracking and fissuring of lesions.

Tannic acid, benzoin compound tincture, zinc acetate, benzyl alcohol, and alcohol: Have astringent (drying) properties.

Systemic oral analgesics – Systemic oral analgesics are considered a mainstay of symptom management. Oral protectants/lubricants plus oral systemic analgesic therapy presents a dual opportunity to relieve discomfort. Use of therapeutic doses of aspirin, acetaminophen, and OTC doses of ibuprofen, naproxen, or ketoprofen is encouraged if there are no contraindications. For a complete discussion of OTC systemic analgesics, see the Aches and Pains monograph in the Musculoskeletal Conditions chapter.

Prescription products can be used to treat canker sores that do not respond to OTC therapy or when the patient has pre-existing conditions.

Antibiotic rinses – Antibiotic rinses are of little or no value in treating aphthous ulcers.

Chlorhexidine gluconate – Chlorhexidine gluconate oral rinse (eg, *Peridex*) has been reported to speed up healing of canker sores, but in one study, it did not offer any improvement over a placebo alcoholic mouthwash.

Triamcinolone acetonide – Triamcinolone acetonide dental paste (*Kenalog in Orabase*) is a synthetic corticosteroid preparation with anti-inflammatory properties. It has been used as adjunctive therapy and for relief of symptoms associated with inflammatory or ulcerative mouth lesions. Topical steroids, while anti-inflammatory, do not promote healing, and if used regularly, may interfere with the healing process.

Kenalog (triamcinolone) 20 to 40 mg also has been used with success as a local injection in AIDS patients with major aphthous ulcers to control profound inflammation (not to promote healing).

Amlexanox – Amlexanox (*Aphthasol*) paste is a prescription agent indicated for use in the treatment of aphthous ulcers in immunocompetent patients.

Miscellaneous prescription agents – Several other agents have been employed in the management of canker sores, but their value is either equivocal or highly inappropiate. Antibiotic rinses are of no documented value. Topical steroids, either alone or in oral protectant/lubricant vehicles, should not be employed routinely. The steroid may interfere with the healing process. Products containing counterirritants (eg, menthol, phenol, camphor, eugenol) may produce further inflammation. Silver nitrate should not be employed to "cauterize" canker sores as it produces a local inflammation and may stain teeth and surrounding tissue. The zinc in astringent mouthwashes has no proven value in promoting healing of canker sores. Antiseptics that release oxygen (eg, debriding/cleansing agents containing carbamide peroxide, hydrogen peroxide, perborates) are of no apparent value. Aspirin should never be applied directly to any oral lesion or toothache because of the risk of local trauma and of irreversible nerve damage in the case of a toothache.

Additional agents available by prescription that have been used in treating aphthous ulcers are topical and systemic corticosteroids (eg, dexamethasone, prednisone), cyclosporine, diclofenac, sucralfate, tetracyclines, colchicine, dapsone, pentoxifylline, and, for extremely debilitating aphthous ulcers, thalidomide. Use of these agents lacks significant evidence of efficacy; their use is largely experimental and should be directed and monitored by a physician.

BENZOCAINE

▶ Actions
The duration of action of benzocaine, a topical anesthetic, is relatively short (20 to 30 minutes), so it serves only as an adjunct to oral protectants/lubricants and systemic oral analgesics.

▶ Indications
Benzocaine may be applied directly to the canker sore lesion either alone or via an oral protectant/lubricant.

▶ Contraindications
Hypersensitivity to any component of these products.

▶ Warnings
For external or mucous membrane use only. Do not use in the eyes.

Systemic effects: Use the lowest effective dose to avoid adverse effects.

Methemoglobinemia. Benzocaine should not be used in those rare patients with congenital or idiopathic methemoglobinemia and in infants younger than 12 months of age who are receiving treatment with methemoglobin-inducing agents. Very young patients or patients with glucose-6-phosphate deficiencies are more susceptible to methemoglobinemia.

Traumatized mucosa: Use cautiously in patients with known drug sensitivities or in patients with severly traumatized mucosa and sepsis in the region of the application. If irritation or rash occurs, discontinue treatment and institute appropriate therapy.

Oral use: Topical anesthetics may impair swallowing and enhance danger of aspiration. Do not ingest food for 1 hour after anesthetic use in mouth or throat. This is particularly important in children because of their frequency of eating.

Pregnancy: Category C. Safety for use during pregnancy has not been established. Use in women of childbearing potential, and particularly in early pregnancy, only when the potential benefits outweigh the potential hazards to the fetus.

Lactation: Exercise caution when administering this drug to a nursing woman.

Children: Do not use benzocaine in infants younger than 1 year of age. Reduce dosages in children commensurate with age, body weight, and physical condition.

Tartrazine sensitivity: Some of these products may contain tartrazine, which may cause allergic-type reactions (including bronchial asthma) in susceptible individuals. Although the incidence of tartrazine sensitivity in the general population is low, it is frequently seen in patients who also have aspirin hypersensitivity.

Sulfite sensitivity: Some of these products may contain sulfites that may cause allergic-type reactions including anaphylactic symptoms and life-threatening or less severe asthmatic episodes in certain susceptible people. The overall prevalence of sulfite sensitivity in the general population is unknown and probably low. Sulfite sensitivity is seen more frequently in asthmatic or atopic nonasthmatic people.

▶ **Drug Interactions**

Class I antiarrhythmic agents: Use with caution in patients receiving class I antiarrhythmic drugs (eg, tocainide, mexiletine) because the toxic effects are additive and potentially synergistic.

▶ **Adverse Reactions**

Adverse reactions are, in general, dose-related and may result from high plasma levels caused by excessive dosage or rapid absorption, hypersensitivity, idiosyncrasy, or diminished tolerance. (See Overdosage.)

Hypersensitivity: Cutaneous lesions; urticaria; edema; contact dermatitis; bronchospasm; shock; anaphylactoid reactions. The detection of sensitivity by skin testing is of doubtful value.

Miscellaneous: Urethritis with and without bleeding. In a few case reports, methemoglobinemia characterized by cyanosis has followed topical application of benzocaine.

Local: Burning; stinging; tenderness; sloughing.

▶ **Overdosage**

Symptoms: Reactions caused by overdosage (high plasma levels) are systemic and involve the CNS (convulsions) or the cardiovascular system (hypotension).

CNS reactions are excitatory or depressant and may be characterized by the following: nervousness; apprehension; euphoria; confusion; dizziness; lightheadedness; tinnitus; blurred vision; vomiting; sensations of heat, cold, or numbness; twitching; tremors; drowsiness; convulsions; unconsciousness; respiratory depression or arrest. Excitatory reactions may be very brief or not occur at all. In this case, the first sign of toxicity may be drowsiness, merging into unconsciousness, and respiratory arrest.

Cardiovascular reactions are depressant and may be characterized by the following: hypotension; myocardial depression; bradycardia; cardiac arrest; cardiovascular collapse.

Treatment: Maintain airway and support ventilation. Cardiovascular support consists of vasopressors, preferably those that stimulate the myocardium, IV fluids, and blood transfusions. Control convulsions by slow IV administration of 0.1 mg/kg diazepam or 10 to 50 mg succinylcholine, with continued use of oxygen. Refer to General Management of Acute Overdosage.

Methemoglobinemia may be treated with 1% methylene blue, 0.1 mL/kg IV over 10 minutes.

▶ **Administration and Dosage**

Apply to affected areas using the proper technique (refer to specific package labeling).

BENZOCAINE-CONTAINING ORAL PROTECTANTS/LUBRICANTS	
Trade name	Doseform
Anbesol, Maximum Strength	**Liquid**: 20% benzocaine. Methylparaben, saccharin.
Hurricane	**Liquid**: 20% benzocaine.
Kank-A	**Liquid/Film**: 20% benzocaine. With benzoin compound tincture. SD alcohol 38B, benzyl alcohol, castor oil, saccharin.
Orajel Mouth Sore Medicine	**Liquid**: 20% benzocaine. 44.2% ethyl alcohol, tartrazine, sodium saccharin.

BENZOCAINE-CONTAINING ORAL PROTECTANTS/LUBRICANTS	
Trade name	Doseform
Tanac	**Liquid**: 10% benzocaine. 0.12% benzalkonium chloride, sodium saccharin.
Miradyne-3	**Liquid**: 9% benzocaine. SD alcohol 38B.
Orasol	**Liquid**: 6.3% benzocaine. 0.5% phenol, 70% alcohol, povidone-iodine.
Hurricane	**Spray**: 20% benzocaine
Anbesol, Maximum Strength	**Gel**: 20% benzocaine. Methylparaben.
Hurricane	**Gel**: 20% benzocaine
Orajel Cold and Canker Sore Relief	**Gel**: 20% benzocaine. 0.2% benzalkonium chloride, 0.1% zinc chloride, EDTA, sodium saccharide, alcohol.
Orajel, Maximum Strength	**Gel**: 20% benzocaine. Sodium saccharin.
Orajel Oral Pain Reliever	**Gel**: 10% benzocaine. Sodium saccharin.
Zilactin-B	**Gel**: 10% benzocaine. 70% alcohol.
Miradyne-3	**Gel**: 9% benzocaine. SD alcohol 38B.
Anbesol, Baby	**Gel**: 7.5% benzocaine. EDTA, parabens, saccharin.
Orabase B	**Paste**: 20% benzocaine
Anbesol	**Liquid**: 6.3% benzocaine. 0.5% phenol, 0.5% povidone-iodine, 70% alcohol.
	Gel: 6.3% benzocaine. 0.5% phenol, 70% alcohol.
Rembrandt Low Abrasion Whitening Toothpaste	**Toothpaste**: 0.15% fluoride ion (from sodium monofluorophosphate). Saccharin.
Rembrandt Canker Pain Relief Kit	**Gel**: 5% benzocaine
	Mouth rinse: Benzocaine, sodium benzoate. Methylparaben, saccharin.
	Toothpaste: 0.15% fluoride ion (from sodium monoflurophosphate). Saccharin.

Products listed are representative of currently available and widely distributed brands. Similar products, including regional and private label brands, may also exist.

PATIENT INFORMATION

Benzocaine

- Dry the canker sore lesion before applying an oral protectant/lubricant.
- Once applied, hold the affected area away from surface contact with other oral tissue for 30 to 60 seconds or longer. This ensures optimal binding to the lesion.
- Products can be administered 3 to 6 times/day for several days, then as needed.

NONBENZOCAINE-CONTAINING ORAL LUBRICANTS/PROTECTANTS

▶ **Actions**

Lidocaine (0.5% to 4%) and tetracaine (2%) are local anesthetics.

▶ **Warnings**

Do not use in or around the eyes. If contact occurs, flush immediately and continuously with water for 10 minutes. Consult physician immediately if pain or irritation persists.

Stinging sensation: A slight, temporary stinging sensation may occur when drugs are applied to an open sore or blister.

Infection: If lesions persist beyond 10 to 14 days or evidence of a secondary bacterial infection exists, discontinue use and consult a physician.

▶ **Administration and Dosage**

For dosage guidelines, refer to the specific package labeling.

NONBENZOCAINE-CONTAINING ORAL LUBRICANTS/PROTECTANTS	
Trade name	**Doseform**
Banadyne-3	**Solution**: 4% lidocaine, 1% menthol, 45% alcohol.
Colgate Orabase Soothe-N-Seal	**Liquid**: Formulated 2-octyl cyanoacrylate.
Zilactin-L	**Liquid**: 2.5% lidocaine HCl. 80% alcohol.
Amosan	**Powder**: Sodium perborate monohydrate, sodium bitartrate, sodium saccharin.
Tanac Medicated Gel	**Gel**: 1% dyclonine HCl, 0.5% allantoin.
Zilactin	**Gel**: 10% benzyl alcohol.
Cēpacol Viractin	**Cream**: 2% tetracaine. Methylparaben.
	Gel: 2% tetracaine. Parabens.

Products listed are representative of currently available and widely distributed brands. Similar products, including regional and private label brands, may also exist.

PATIENT INFORMATION

Nonbenzocaine-Containing Oral Lubricant/Protectants

- Dosing, method of administration, and duration of action of these products vary. Carefully read the instructions on the packaging before using these medications. Do not exceed the recommended dosage or dosing frequency.
- Do not swallow these products.
- Do not use benzocaine-containing products if you have a history of allergy to local anesthetics, such as procaine or other "-caine" anesthetics, or to any other ingredients.
- If lesions persist beyond 10 days, if irritation, pain, and redness persists or worsens, or if swelling, rash, or fever develops, consult a physician or dentist.
- Do not use longer than 5 to 10 days unless directed a physician or dentist. (Do not use *Tanac* longer than 5 consecutive days.)
- Mild burning may occur at application site.
- Allergic reactions at the site of application may occur after prolonged or repeated use; discontinue use and contact a physician if this occurs.
- Do not use in young children (refer to ages specified on packaging). Benzocaine products may make swallowing difficult or inhibit gag reflexes in infants and children.
- Avoid contact with eyes.
- Do not apply over large areas or cover with a bandage.

MISCELLANEOUS ANTISEPTICS FOR THE MOUTH

▶ **Indications**

These preparations contain various agents to provide relief and treatment of canker sores and other minor mouth or gum wounds and inflammation.

▶ **Warnings**

Not for prolonged use. If condition persists or rash or infection develops, discontinue use and consult a physician or dentist.

Children: Do not use products containing antiseptics in infants younger than 1 year of age. Consult a dentist or physician for use of these products in children younger than 6 years of age.

▶ **Administration and Dosage**

Varies by product; follow guidelines provided with individual products.

MISCELLANEOUS MOUTH ANTISEPTIC PRODUCTS	
Trade name	**Doseform**
Debacterol	**Liquid:** 22% sulphonated phenolics, 30% sulfuric acid.
Orasept	**Liquid:** 14.4 mg methylbenzethonium HCl, 14.4 benzocaine. Ethyl alcohol 38B, camphor, menthol, benzyl alcohol.
Peroxyl	**Liquid:** 1.5% hydrogen peroxide, 6% ethyl alcohol, 70% sorbitol solution, menthol, sodium saccharin.
Orasept Mouthwash/Gargle	**Liquid:** 1% methylbenzethonium chloride
Peroxyl	**Gel:** 1.5% hydrogen peroxide

Products listed are representative of currently available and widely distributed brands. Similar products, including regional and private label brands, may also exist.

PATIENT INFORMATION
Miscellaneous Mouth Antiseptics

- Do not swallow these products.
- Avoid contact with eyes and eyelids.
- Do not use longer than 7 days; if condition persists or worsens or if swelling, rash, or fever develops, discontinue use and consult a physician or dentist.
- For best results, do not consume food or liquids for 20 minutes after use of these products.

COLD SORES
(Fever Blisters; Recurrent Herpes Labialis [RHL])

DEFINITION

Cold sores, also known as fever blisters, are painful, recurrent lesions that can occur anywhere but most often are on the lip or areas that border the lips. The common name is derived from the fact that many patients develop the lesions during a cold or fever, with the initial lesion being a cluster of blisters (vesicles) on a red base.

ETIOLOGY

Of the 50 different herpes viruses, 5 affect humans. These are herpes simplex, varicella zoster (chicken pox), herpes zoster (shingles), Epstein-Barr virus (mononucleosis, possibly chronic fatigue syndrome), and cytomegalovirus (hepatitis, mononucleosis). Herpes simplex virus type 1 (HSV-1) typically causes cold sores and herpes simplex virus type 2 (HSV-2) typically causes genital herpes. Thus, as a general rule one can say that HSV-1 occurs "above the waist" and HSV-2 occurs "below the waist." Exceptions to this general rule exist, however, because of oral sex. HSV-2 lesions can occur on the lip or area bordering the lip, but the incidence of oral HSV-2 lesions is not high.

Cold sores are typically caused by the reactivation of the herpes simplex virus type 1 (HSV-1). The herpes virus enters the body after the patient is exposed to the virus and, after an initial appearance called "primary herpes infection," lies dormant until later when it reappears as a cold sore, called "recurrent herpes infection." Reactivation of HSV-1 oral lesions often occurs secondary to a "trigger" event such as sun exposure, wind, local trauma, stress, or fatigue.

Whether water contaminated with the herpes simplex virus can cause a recurrence of herpes labialis is not well defined; however, it is noteworthy that HSV-1 and HSV-2 can survive in nonchlorinated tap water and distilled water for up to 4.5 hours. For a variety of health reasons, users of swimming pools and hot tubs should seek assurances that the water is chlorinated.

INCIDENCE

Almost everyone gets a primary HSV infection by age 5. The majority of primary infections are subclinical. Approximately 80% of the population carries the herpes simplex virus. An estimated 15% of adults will have overt symptoms with primary infection; after the primary infection heals, effective immunity develops in some, although 20% to 45% of US adults are seropositive for HSV-1 and have recurrent lesions. It is estimated that 7% of the general population in North America has 2 or more bouts of recurrent herpes labialis (RHL) each year. More than 100 million episodes of herpes labialis occur every year in the US.

PATHOPHYSIOLOGY

Because of the extremely contagious nature of the herpes simplex virus, it is thought that primary infection with HSV-1 generally occurs after mucocutaneous contact with an infected individual. The virus may be spread via kissing, coughing, sneezing, or via contaminated objects (eg, drinking glasses, straws, eating utensils). After onset of the infection, viral excretion persists for 15 to 42 days. Predisposing factors ("triggers") that may result in recurrences of cold sores include fever, physical or emotional stress, physical trauma, ultraviolet radiation, wind burn, allergic reactions, systemic infections, and menses. Do not break cold sore blisters, as the blister fluid contains high concentrations of HSV. Most cold sores are self-limiting and heal within 10 to 14 days without scarring.

SIGNS/SYMPTOMS

In patients who are susceptible to cold sores, a prodrome often (in up to 60% of patients) precedes the onset of a visible lesion by 1 to 2 days and consists of symptoms such as low grade fever, headache, muscle aches, and malaise. Patients may experience tingling, itching, numbness, or burning in the area where the lesion generally appears (generally around the lips, usually the bottom lip). The first clinical finding is generally local pain, edema, swelling, and erythema; 4 to 8 hours later, a cluster of small fluid-filled vesicles of 1 to 3 mm in diameter appears, then ruptures and crusts over to form the typical cold sore, a yellowish-white lesion surrounded by a red halo. Sometimes many of the lesions will coalesce, resulting in a larger area of involvement. The lesions are very sensitive to friction and chemical irritation. The base of the lesion is usually red and edematous. Blisters will spontaneously rupture, producing a gelatinous, mucoid material. Within 24 hours, an adherent clot or "crust" forms, and the healing process begins. The presence of pus signals the existance of a secondary bacterial infection and requires immediate medical referral and antibiotic treatment. Healing of recurrent, uncomplicated cold sores is usually complete in 10 to 14 days with no scarring.

DIAGNOSTIC PARAMETERS/PHYSICAL ASSESSMENT

Clinical Observation: The classic cold sore is very easy to identify based on appearance and locale (see Signs/Symptoms above).

Interview: To help the patient determine if physician referral or self-treatment is warranted, it may be beneficial to ask about the following:

• Frequency of cold sore occurrence
• Occurrence of prodrome
• Sunlight or wind exposure
• Recent cold, fever, or other illness
• Recent stressful periods (physical or emotional)
• Recent local trauma to the lip

TREATMENT

Approaches to therapy: Evaluate patients using the previous diagnostic parameters. Depending on various factors (eg, symptoms, duration, recurrence), health care providers may recommend: (1) a nondrug approach, (2) appropriate pharmacotherapy, or (3) immediate referral to a physician for medical evaluation.

Goals of therapy – There is no cure for an active cold sore, so the treatment objective is to treat the symptoms. This is best done by the following:

• Controlling patient discomfort
• Promoting healing
• Preventing complications

Nondrug therapy: There is no known nondrug therapy to prevent the recurrence of cold sores except to avoid known exacerbating or precipitating factors (eg, sunburn, wind burn, stress, fatigue). Further, it is appropriate to recommend avoidance of acidic foods such as citrus fruits, tomatoes, pickles, or other foods high in salt, as they irritate active lesions. Mouthwashes and saline rinses may help soothe cold sores and reduce irritation. Do not squeeze or pinch cold sores. Wash contaminated washcloths and towels as soon as possible after use. Little that has been proven to shorten the healing time, anecdotal reports suggest that ice applied within 24 hours of the onset of the prodrome for 45 to 60 continuous minutes will either prevent a cold sore, or if the lesion appears, it will accelerate healing. The ice treatment must be started as soon as possible after the initial prodromal signs.

Lip balm with a high SPF (30) may help reduce photoactivation of the virus in patients exposed to sunlight or tanning beds for prolonged periods. Keep lesions clean and moist and keep hands clean to prevent autoinoculation of the lesion with bacteria.

Pharmacotherapy: As with nondrug therapy, there are no proven, effective OTC treatments to prevent cold sores. Most topical treatments are nonprescription drugs and are meant to relieve the pain, itching, and discomfort of the lesion, promote healing, or prevent complications. These include topical skin protectants and analgesic/anesthetic products containing benzocaine (5% to 20%), lidocaine (0.5% to 4%), dibucaine (0.25% to 1%), or dyclonine (0.5% to 1%); benzyl alcohol (10% to 33%); camphor (0.1% to 3%); menthol (0.1% to 1%); topical antibiotics; and others. Cool compresses with tap water or Burow solution also can be used.

Higher concentrations of ingredients such as menthol and camphor, as well as topical corticosteroids, are contraindicated. Highly astringent products (eg, tannic acid, zinc sulfate) are of limited value; avoid caustic agents (eg, phenol, silver nitrate).

Consumers should realize that local anesthetics (eg, benzocaine, lidocaine, dibucaine, tetracaine) have a relatively short duration of pain-relieving action (20 to 30 minutes), so frequent applications consistent with the instructions on the package may be necessary.

Systemic oral analgesics (eg, acetaminophen, aspirin, ibuprofen, naproxen, ketoprofen) may provide longer-acting pain relief and can be used along with the topical local anesthetics.

Other treatments that have not been clearly proven useful but are used by patients to self-medicate include the following:

Topical treatments
- Ethyl ether: It has been suggested (but not proven) that the use of topical ether (which can be obtained from a service station as "car starter") as soon as the prodrome begins will shorten the outbreak or even abort it.
- Chloroform
- Zinc
- Alcohol
- Silver sulfadiazine
- Povidone iodine

Oral treatments
- *Lactobacillus acidophilus* and *L. bulgaricus*
- L-lysine (an essential amino acid)
- Citrus bioflavanoids
- Red marine algae
- Vitamins B_6, B_{12}, C, and E

In truth, most of the OTC products used to treat this condition relieve symptoms but do not abort the condition. Soaking the area with cool compresses appears to be the most effective way to relieve swelling and keep the area clean.

DOCOSANOL

▶ **Actions**

Docosanol is unique among cold sore treatments as it has antiviral properties. It enters cells and prevents viral replication by blocking movement of the virus within the cell. Docosanol is most effective when used early in the course of an outbreak. Viral resistance to docosanol has not been reported to date.

▶ **Indications**

Docosanol cream treats cold sores or fever blisters on the face or lips and significantly shortens healing time and duration of tingling, pain, burning, or itching symptoms.

▶ **Contraindications**

Hypersensitivity to docosanol or any component of the product.

▶ **Warnings**

Children: Use in children younger than 12 years of age is not recommended; consult a physician.

Pregnancy: There are no adequate and well-controlled studies; use during pregnancy only if clearly needed.

Lactation: There are no adequate and well-controlled studies; use only if clearly needed.

For external use only: When using this product, apply only to the affected areas. Do not use in or near the eyes. Avoid applying directly inside the mouth.

► **Administration and Dosage**

Do not share this product with anyone; this may spread infection.

Stop using and consult a physician if cold sore worsens (eg, pain, redness, itching, oozing of pus) or is not healed within 10 days.

Wash hands before and after applying cream. Apply only to infected areas. Remove all cosmetics from the affected area and apply the cream to the affected area on face or lips at the first sign of a cold sore or fever blister (eg, tingle sensation). Cosmetics can be reapplied over this medication. Early treatment ensures the best results. Rub a thin layer in gently but completely. Use 5 times/day until healed.

DOCOSANOL PRODUCTS	
Trade name	Doseform
Abreva	**Cream**: 10% docosanol. Benzyl alcohol, light mineral oil, sucrose distearate, sucrose stearate.

Products listed are representative of currently available and widely distributed brands. Similar products, including regional and private label brands, may also exist.

PATIENT INFORMATION

Docosanol

- For external use only. Use as directed. Avoid contact with eyes, nose, mouth, or other mucous membranes.
- Apply as soon as you notice the first symptom (tingling, redness, bump, or itch).
- Do not apply over large areas or cover with a bandage.
- Cleanse and dry the area to be treated before application; wash hands thoroughly with soap and water before and after application.
- Use the medication for the recommended treatment time. Strict adherence to the dosage schedule is essential for optimal clinical response.
- If you miss a dose, take the next dose as soon as you remember, and then reapply the next dose as scheduled.
- Do not use longer than 10 days unless directed by a physician or dentist. If lesions persist beyond 10 days, if irritation, pain, and redness persist or worsen, or if swelling, rash, or fever develops, consult a physician or dentist.
- Allergic reactions at the application site may occur after prolonged or repeated use; discontinue use and contact a physician if this occurs.
- Do not use in children younger than 12 years of age.
- Do not share this product with anyone; this may spread infection.

MISCELLANEOUS COLD SORE PRODUCTS

► **Actions**

Benzocaine (5% to 20%), lidocaine (0.5% to 4%), dyclonine (0.5% to 1%), dibucaine (0.25% to 1%), and tetracaine (2%) are local anesthetics.

Cetylpyridinium chloride and benzalkonium chloride have mild antiseptic activity.

Menthol, camphor, and phenol are counterirritants used for their antipruritic and very mild local anesthetic activities.

Allantoin (0.5% to 2%) and dimethicone (1% to 30%) are skin protectants/moisturizers that prevent cracking and fissuring of lesions.

Tannic acid, benzoin compound tincture, zinc acetate, zinc sulfate, benzyl alcohol, and alcohol have astringent (drying) properties. Scientific evidence supporting the use of astringents in managing cold sores is lacking. Drying properties may lead to cracking and fissuring of a lesion and predispose to secondary bacterial infections. Tannic acid precipitates a protein-taimate layer over cold sores that may encourage the colonization of bacteria underneath.

▶ Indications

These products are indicated for cold sore management.

▶ Warnings

Do not use in or around the eyes. If contact occurs, flush immediately and continuously with water for 10 minutes. Consult physician immediately if pain or irritation persists.

Stinging sensation: A slight, temporary stinging sensation may occur when drugs are applied to an open sore or blister.

Infection: If lesions persist beyond 10 to 14 days or evidence of a secondary bacterial infection exists, discontinue use and consult a physician.

▶ Administration and Dosage

For dosage guidelines, refer to the specific package labeling.

MISCELLANEOUS COLD SORE PRODUCTS	
Trade name	Doseform
Anbesol Cold Sore Therapy	**Ointment**: 1% allantoin, 20% benzocaine, 3% camphor, 64.9% white petrolatum. Aloe extract, benzyl alcohol, glyceryl stearate, menthol, sodium lauryl sulfate, white wax, parabens.
Blistex	**Ointment**: 1% allantoin, 0.5% camphor, 0.5% phenol, 0.6% menthol. Beeswax, cetyl alcohol, glycerin, lanolin, mineral oil, petrolatum, polyglyceryl-3, SD alcohol 36, stearyl alcohol.
Blistex Lip Medex	**Ointment**: 59.14% petrolatum, 1% camphor, 1% menthol, 0.54% phenol. Lanolin, mixed waxes, oil of cloves, beeswax, benzyl alcohol, saccharin.
Viractin	**Cream**: 2% tetracaine. Eucalyptus oil, methylparaben.
Pfieffer's Cold Sore	**Lotion**: 3% camphor, 0.75% menthol. 85% alcohol, thymol, eucalyptol, gum benzoin.
Banadyne-3	**Solution**: 5% benzocaine, 1% menthol, 45% alcohol. Propylene glycol, dimethicone.
Campho-Phenique	**Liquid**: 4.7% phenol, 10.8% camphor. Eucalyptus oil, light mineral oil.
Kank-A	**Liquid/Film**: 20% benzocaine, benzoin compound tincture
Orasept	**Liquid**: 114.9 mg/mL tannic acid, 14.4 mg/mL methylbenzethonium HCl, 14.4 mg/mL benzocaine, 61% ethyl alcohol
Tanac	**Liquid**: 10% benzocaine, 0.12% benzalkonium chloride. Sodium saccharin.
Zilactin-L	**Liquid**: 2.5% lidocaine. Alcohol.
Campho-Phenique Cold Sore	**Gel**: 4.7% phenol, 10.8% camphor. Eucalyptus oil, glycerin, light mineral oil.
Orajel Mouth-Aid	**Gel**: 20% benzocaine, 0.2% benzalkonium chloride, 0.1% zinc chloride. Peppermint oil, stearyl alcohol, allentoin, sodium saccharin, EDTA.
Orajel Multi-Action	**Gel**: 0.5% allantoin, 20% benzocaine, 3% camphor, 2% dimethicone, 65% white petrolatum. Menthol.

MISCELLANEOUS COLD SORE PRODUCTS	
Trade name	Doseform
Tanac	**Gel**: 1% dyclonine HCl, 0.5% allantoin. Hydroxylated lanolin, petrolatum.
Viractin	**Gel**: 2% tetracaine HCl. Eucalyptus oil, maleated soybean oil, parabens.
Zilactin	**Gel**: 10% benzyl alcohol
Orabase B	**Paste**: 20% benzocaine
Carmex	**Lip balm**: Menthol, camphor, salicylic acid, phenol. Petrolatum, lanolin, fragrance, wax base.
ChapStick Medicated	**Lip balm**: 41% petrolatum, 1% camphor, 0.6% menthol, 0.5% phenol. Paraffin wax, mineral oil, white wax, oleyl alcohol, lanolin, cetyl alcohol, parabens.
Herpecin-L (SPF 30)	**Lip balm**: 7.5% octyl methoxycinnamate, 6% oxybenzone, 5% octyl salicylate, 1% dimethicone. Beeswax, hybrid sunflower oil, mineral oil, petrolatum, titanium dioxide, zinc oxide.
Pure Lip Prevention	**Lip balm**: 85% white petrolatum, 0.5% zinc oxide. Zinc glycerolate glycerin.
Pure Lip Remedy	**Lip balm**: 57% white petrolatum, 0.5% allantoin, 0.25% zinc oxide. Meadowfoam seed oil, green tea extract, grapeseed extract.
Zilactin-Lip (SPF 24)	**Lip balm**: 7% octyl methoxycinnamate, 4% homosalate, 3% oxybenzone, 1.5% dimethicone, 0.5% menthol

Products listed are representative of currently available and widely distributed brands. Similar products, including regional and private label brands, may also exist.

PATIENT INFORMATION
Cold Sore Products

- Dosing, method of administration, and duration of action of these products varies. Carefully read the instructions on the packaging before using these medications. Do not exceed the recommended dosage or dosing frequency.
- Do not swallow these products.
- Do not use benzocaine-containing products if you have a history of allergy to local anesthetics, such as procaine or other "-caine" anesthetics, or to any other ingredients.
- If lesions persist beyond 14 days, if irritation, pain, and redness persist or worsen, or if swelling, rash, or fever develops, consult a physician or dentist.
- Do not use longer than 14 days unless directed by a physician or dentist. Do not use *Tanac* for longer than 5 consecutive days.
- Mild burning may occur at application site.
- Allergic reactions at the application site may occur after prolonged or repeated use; discontinue use and contact a physician if this occurs.
- Do not use in young children (refer to ages specified on packaging). Benzocaine products may make swallowing difficult or inhibit gag reflexes in infants and children.
- Avoid contact with eyes.
- Do not apply over large areas or cover with a bandage.

HALITOSIS
(Bad Breath)

DEFINITION

Halitosis, also referred to as bad breath, malodor, breath odor, bromopnea, or *fetor ex ore*, is an offensive odor emanating from the mouth, nose, sinuses, or pharynx, although the mouth, tongue, and teeth are most often implicated in the majority of cases. Halitosis is nothing more than a significant social disability unless it results from an underlying medical condition.

ETIOLOGY

As with other body odors, halitosis is generally caused by bacteria in the oral cavity, mainly from the tongue coating and plaque. Putrefaction of food or debris may occur under anaerobic conditions, involving a wide range of gram-negative organisms such as *Fusobacterium* sp, *Haemophilus* sp, *Veillonella* sp, *Treponema denticola*, *Porphyromonas gingivalis*, and *Bacteroides forsythus*. It recently has been suggested that *Stomatococcus mucilaginus*, a gram-positive organism, may also contribute to malodor.

Oral cavity disorders cause up to 85% of all halitosis cases. Rarely is the GI tract involved. It is most frequently associated with dental plaque or caries, poor oral hygiene, gingivitis, stomatitis, periodontitis, oral carcinoma, and salivary dysfunction. Other potential causes of halitosis include: Respiratory conditions (eg, sinusitis, tonsillitis, rhinitis, tuberculosis, bronchiectasis), GI disorders, smoking, hepatic failure, azotemia, and diabetic ketoacidosis.

INCIDENCE

The incidence of halitosis is difficult to objectively assess. An estimated 25 million Americans have chronic halitosis, and approximately 25% of adults 60 years of age or older may have this condition. It is likely that the majority of adults have bad breath at least occasionally. Most people are unaware of their bad breath.

PATHOPHYSIOLOGY

Retention of large quantities of food and debris on the tongue and papillary structure may generate volatile sulfur compounds (eg, hydrogen sulfide, methylmercaptan), contributing to the malodor. These compounds can also be produced by the organisms mentioned above (see Etiology). Volatile non-sulfur compounds may also play a role.

Even in people with a healthy mouth, there is frequently a malodor upon waking ("morning breath") because of decreased saliva flow during sleep, resulting in putrefaction of food and debris that is not cleared by the low saliva level. Mouth-breathers during sleep especially experience bad breath in the morning.

Foods such as garlic and onions and alcoholic beverages can cause a very distinct odor that can last up to 72 hours after ingestion because of salivary excretion of the compounds or excretion through the lungs.

Some patients may have halitophobia, the belief that they have chronic halitosis that cannot be detected by an observer. In severe cases, delusional halitosis may be a sign of a more severe condition such as depression or obsessive-compulsive disorder, and these olfactory hallucinations may also occur in patients with schizophrenia, temporal lobe epilepsy, or organic brain disease.

SIGNS/SYMPTOMS

Halitosis is detected by the presence of a foul odor emanating from a person's mouth. However, in the absence of common identifiable causes (ingestion of garlic or onions, smoking, poor oral hygiene), signs and symptoms are more unique, for example halitosis because of systemic causes. These are identified as follows:

- Hepatic failure - Fishy or mousy odor.
- Uremia - Urinous smell.
- Lung abscess or bronchiectasis - Putrid odor.
- Diabetic ketosis - Presence of acetone smell.

Patients with halitophobia avoid social situations and are continually preoccupied with concealing the supposed odor with constant brushing of teeth, continuous gum chewing or use of candy, keeping a safe distance, and talking sideways.

DIAGNOSTIC PARAMETERS/PHYSICAL ASSESSMENT

Clinical Observation: In most cases, clinical observation is unnecessary. The patient's self-assessment of halitosis generally will suffice; however, it may be necessary to smell the person's breath, especially if the complaint is of a chronic nature. The initial challenge is to determine if the complaints are well founded or are exaggerated. Personal and medical history can provide important information, but self-reports of halitosis are extremely subjective. Take all complaints of bad breath seriously, regardless of whether they appear justified.

Interview: To help the patient determine if referral to a physician or dentist or self-treatment is warranted, it may be beneficial to ask the patient about the following:

- Duration of bad breath condition.
- Smoking and alcohol consumption.
- Recent or regular consumption of garlic (including garlic capsules), onions, or spicy foods.
- Recent oral cavity conditions (eg, gingivitis, caries), periodontitis, old leaking fillings, pericoronitis, many other dental causes.
- Description of odor (noted by self or others).
- Origin of odor (mouth or nose).
- Detection of odor by others.
- Current medications.
- Current medical conditions.

TREATMENT

Approaches to therapy: Evaluate patients using the previous diagnostic parameters. Depending on various factors (eg, symptoms, duration, recurrence), health care providers may recommend (1.) a non-drug approach, (2.) appropriate pharmacotherapy, or (3.) immediate referral to a physician or dentist for medical evaluation.

Nondrug therapy: The importance of good dental hygiene cannot be overemphasized. Because most cases of halitosis originate from the oral cavity, this will be the most effective form of therapy. This includes regular flossing, use of interdental cleaners, deep tongue cleaning, and proper toothbrushing. Other helpful measures include drinking ample amounts of water and chewing gum (sugarless, and only for a short period of time).

Pharmacotherapy: A pharmacotherapeutic approach to halitosis treatment is the use of mouthwashes (or mouthrinses). Today's mouthwashes/rinses are slowly becoming more than cover-ups for halitosis. Most are still a combination of alcohol, anesthetics, astringents, and flavoring agents. All have some germ-fighting ability; most mask odors somewhat. Most of these products may be subclassified into 2 categories: Cosmetic and therapeutic. The cosmetic products are those that are intended to eliminate or suppress mouth odor of local origin in healthy people with healthy mouths, and do not contain antimicrobial or other therapeutic agents. The therapeutic products are generally used to combat/prevent plaque and gingivitis, which, if left untreated, can result in halitosis.

Some newer mouthwash products contain chlorine dioxide (a potent algaecide) or zinc chloride. The chlorine dioxide readily attacks the volatile sulfur compounds produced by bacteria and certain foods and neutralizes them. However, these products should not be mistaken for curative agents for underlying dental or medical disorders.

For more severe cases of halitosis, stronger mouthwash formulations may be available only from the dentist. Examples of such products include *Tri-Oral Anti-Halitosis Treatment Rinse, Oxygene Mouthrinse with Zinc,* and the *BreathRx ProActive Care Prophy Pak* (includes antibacterial mouthrinse, breath spray, toothpaste, sugar-free gum, breathmints, and tongue cleaning gel/scraper).

MOUTHWASHES (MOUTHRINSES)

▶ **Indications**

Cosmetic mouthwashes are used to eliminate or suppress mouth odor of local origin. Therapeutic mouthwashes are intended to treat or prevent plaque and gingivitis, which in turn may help eliminate halitosis. These products may contain antibacterial ingredients such as cetylpyridinium chloride, chlorhexidine and triclosan, alcohol, fluoride, surfactants (to remove debris), aromatic oils (eg, menthol, eucalyptol, thymol, methyl salicylate), and phenol.

▶ **Contraindications**

Use of products high in alcohol content by children.

▶ **Warnings**

Oral cancer: There may be a potential association between alcohol-containing mouthwashes and oral cancer. Further studies are needed.

Masking of underlying problems: If marked breath odor persists after proper oral hygiene, the use of a cosmetic mouthwash may mask an underlying condition. Consider a dental examination.

Children: Children may be attracted to the bright colors and pleasant flavors of mouthwashes, resulting in the potential ingestion of mouthwashes high in alcohol content. Keep out of reach of children. Child-resistant packaging is required for mouthwashes containing 3 g or more of absolute ethanol per package.

▶ **Drug Interactions**

None known. However, if a significant amount of an alcohol-containing mouthwash is ingested, usual effects of alcohol can be expected to occur, including potential drug interactions (eg, with CNS agents).

▶ **Adverse Reactions**

None known, other than usual effects of alcohol if a significant amount of an alcohol-containing mouthwash is ingested, especially in children.

▶ **Administration and Dosage**

Follow labeled directions. Generally, use twice daily after brushing. Vigorously swish 1 to 2 tablespoons of mouthwash in mouth for approximately 30 seconds and expectorate. Do NOT swallow.

MOUTHWASH/MOUTHRINSE PRODUCTS	
Trade name	**Doseform**
Advanced Formula Plax New Mint Sensation Flavor, Advanced Formula Plax Original, Advanced Formula Plax Soft Mint Flavor	**Solution:** Glycerin, alcohol, benzoic acid, xanthan gum
AP-24 Anti-Plaque	**Mouthwash:** AP-24, sorbitol, glycerin, EDTA, citric acid
Betadine	**Mouthwash:** 0.5% povidone-iodine, 8% alcohol, glycerin, saccharin sodium
Biotene Alcohol-Free	**Mouthwash:** Lysozyme, lactoferrin, glucose oxidase, lactoperoxidase
Cēpacol Mint Antiseptic	**Mouthwash:** Cetylpyridinium chloride, 0.05% alcohol, EDTA, tartrazine, saccharin, glycerin
Lavoris Crystal Fresh, Lavoris Original, Lavoris Peppermint	**Mouthwash:** SD alcohol 38-B, glycerin, citric acid, zinc oxide, saccharin
Lavoris Mint, Lavoris Original Cinnamon	**Mouthwash:** Low alcohol base, zinc chloride or zinc oxide, glycerin
Listerine Antiseptic	**Mouthrinse:** 0.064% thymol, 0.092% eucalyptol, 0.06% methyl salicylate, 0.042% menthol, 26.9% alcohol, benzoic acid
Listerine Cool Mint Antiseptic, Listerine Freshburst Antiseptic	**Mouthrinse:** 0.064% thymol, 0.092% eucalyptol, 0.06% methyl salicylate, 0.042% menthol, 21.6% alcohol, benzoic acid, sodium saccharin
Listermint	**Mouthwash:** Glycerin, sodium saccharin, benzoic acid, zinc chloride
Listermint with Fluoride	**Mouthwash:** 0.02% sodium fluoride, 6.65% SD alcohol 38-B, glycerin, sodium saccharin, zinc chloride, citric acid

MOUTHWASH/MOUTHRINSE PRODUCTS

Trade name	Doseform
Mentadent Dual Action with Baking Soda & Peroxide	**Mouthwash**: 12% alcohol, sorbitol, sodium saccharin
Natural Mouthwash with Aloe & Vitamin C	**Mouthwash**: Glycerin, witch hazel (non-alcoholic), menthol, ascorbic acid, aloe vera juice
Orajel Perioseptic Super Cleaning	**Mouthrinse**: 1.5% hydrogen peroxide, EDTA, 4% ethyl alcohol, parabens, sorbitol, sodium saccharin
Oral-B Anti-Cavity Dental	**Mouthrinse**: 0.05% sodium fluoride
Oral-B Anti-Plaque	**Mouthrinse**: 0.05% cetylpyridinium chloride
Oral-B Fluorinse	**Mouthrinse**: 0.2% sodium fluoride
Oxyfresh Mint	**Mouthrinse**: Oxygene, mint oils
Oxyfresh Natural	**Mouthrinse**: Oxygene
Perimax Hygienic Perio	**Mouthrinse**: 1.5% hydrogen peroxide
Peroxyl Antiseptic Dental	**Mouthrinse**: 1.5% hydrogen peroxide, 6% alcohol
Prevention Regular Strength, Prevention Periodontal	**Mouthrinse**: Glycerin, 2.6% SD alcohol 38-B, 1.5% hydrogen peroxide, EDTA, zinc chloride, citric acid
Prevention Orthodontic	**Mouthrinse**: Glycerin, 2.6% SD alcohol 38-B, 1% hydrogen peroxide, EDTA, zinc chloride, citric acid
Reach ACT Anti-Cavity Fluoride Treatment	**Mouthrinse**: Available in bubble gum, cinnamon, or mint. 0.05% sodium fluoride, EDTA, glycerin, sodium saccharin.
Rembrandt Mouth Refreshing Rinse	**Mouthrinse**: Citric acid, sodium benzoate, parabens, sodium saccharin
Retardex Oral Rinse	**Mouthrinse**: Trisodium phosphate, chlorine dioxide
Scope	**Mouthrinse**: 18.9% SD alcohol 38-B, glycerin, sodium saccharin, benzoic acid
Signal	**Mouthwash**: 14.5% SD alcohol 38-B, sorbitol, sodium saccharin
Targon Smokers'	**Mouthwash**: 15.6% alcohol, glycerin, sodium saccharin, tartrazine
Therasol, Therasol Sub-Gingival Irrigant	**Mouthwash**: 0.3% aqueous solution of C31G, 8% SD alcohol 38-B, 6% glycerin, saccharin
Vademecum	**Mouthwash**: Ethyl alcohol, menthol
Viadent	**Mouthrinse**: Sanguinaria extract, 10% SD-alcohol 38-F, glycerin, sodium saccharin, citric acid
Gly-Oxide Liquid	**Liquid**: Carbamide peroxide, citric acid, glycerin
Cavity Guard Home Fluoride Treatment	**Gel**: Glycerin, ascorbic acid, citric acid
Lactona Vince Gum and Mouth Care Oral Rinse and Dentrifice	**Powder**: Sodium alum, calcium carbonate, sodium perborate monohydrate, sodium carbonate, magnesium trisilicate, tricalcium phosphate, sodium saccharin

Products listed are representative of currently available and widely distributed brands. Similar products, including regional and private label brands, may also exist.

PATIENT INFORMATION

Mouthwashes

- Use these products as directed.
- Keep alcohol-containing products out of the reach of children.
- To prevent bad breath, the importance of good dental hygiene cannot be over-emphasized. Because most cases of halitosis originate from the oral cavity, this will be the most effective form of therapy. This includes regular flossing, use of interdental cleaners, deep tongue cleaning, and proper toothbrushing.
- If marked breath odor persists after proper dental hygiene, the use of a cosmetic mouthwash may mask an underlying condition. Consider a dental examination.

TEETHING

DEFINITION

Teething, or deciduous dentition, is defined as the eruption of the primary teeth in infancy. The term is not used for the eruption of permanent teeth.

PATHOPHYSIOLOGY

The eruption of deciduous (baby) teeth typically begins around 6 months of age and is complete by 30 months of age. Teething may cause pain or discomfort, but the mechanism is not known. Possible causes include irritation of the trigeminal nerve, infection of the dental sac, decreased local resistance to infection, or release of toxins during the eruption process. Before the teeth erupt, the gums often swell and are tender. Molars are usually the most troublesome teeth. The eruption of permanent teeth is relatively asymptomatic.

SIGNS/SYMPTOMS

While the signs and symptoms of teething are controversial, teething has been touted as the cause of irritability, increased salivation, fever, increased mucus secretions, change in bowel habits, anorexia, pain on chewing, wakefulness, increased mouthing and biting, rash or flushing of cheeks, ear pulling, inflammation of gums, colic, cough, and otitis media. There is no support to the claims that teething causes bronchitis, fever, diarrhea, or convulsions.

DIAGNOSTIC PARAMETERS/PHYSICAL ASSESSMENT

When a child of teething age presents signs of an illness (ie, fever, excessive irritability), it is important that a thorough evaluation rules out an organic cause (eg, otitis, upper respiratory tract infection, meningitis). Parents need to be educated about the need for prompt medical attention if the child experiences significant lethargy, drowsiness, or irritability.

Interview: To aid parents in the proper treatment or relief of teething and its symptoms, it may be beneficial to ask about the following:

- Age of the child.
- Signs of tooth eruption.
- Additional signs and symptoms the child has been experiencing.
- Duration of symptoms (especially fever, rash, ear pulling, cough, or bowel changes, if present).
- Symptoms of lethargy, drowsiness, or irritability.
- Any attempted non-drug therapy (eg, teething rings or biscuits) for relief of symptoms.
- Child's current medication profile.
- Any known drug hypersensitivities.

TREATMENT

Approaches to therapy: Reassuring parents of a child experiencing teething pain is essential. Teething discomfort can often be relieved for short periods with topical anesthetic agents that soothe the gums or with oral systemic analgesic agents.

Nondrug therapy: Often the discomfort a child experiences with teething can be minimized or relieved through the use of teething rings or biscuits, which satisfy the child's need to chew. Items that are cold may provide more relief and help relieve inflammation. Some children find frozen bagels helpful.

Pharmacotherapy: Drugs that are effective for relieving teething pain include topical local anesthetics or oral systemic analgesics. The use of aspirin in children has been associated with Reye syndrome; therefore, use of aspirin for relieving teething pain is not recommended.

ACETAMINOPHEN

▶ Actions

The mechanism of the analgesic effect of acetaminophen is uncertain. It acts directly on the hypothalamic heat-regulating centers, which increases dissipation of body heat (via vasodilatation and sweating). It is almost as potent as aspirin on a mg for mg basis for inhibiting prostaglandin synthetase in the CNS, but its peripheral inhibition of prostaglandin synthesis is minimal, which may account for its lack of clinically significant antirheumatic or anti-inflammatory effects.

Acetaminophen does not inhibit platelet aggregation, affect prothrombin response, or produce GI ulceration.

▶ Indications

For the treatment of mild-to-moderate pain, such as pain associated with teething. This agent has other labeled indications as well.

▶ Contraindications

Hypersensitivity to acetaminophen.

▶ Warnings

Do not exceed recommended dosage.

If a sensitivity reaction occurs, discontinue use.

Severe or recurrent pain or high or continued fever may indicate serious illness. If pain persists for longer than 5 days, consult a physician immediately.

Concurrent medications: Many other medications, specifically multi-ingredient cough and cold products, also contain aspirin or acetaminophen. It is important to advise patients of this possibility and to inquire about other medications they might be taking before recommending an analgesic.

Children: Consult a physician before using in children younger than 3 years old or for use for longer than 3 days (adults and children) for fever reduction.

▶ Drug Interactions

Acetaminophen Drug Interactions			
Precipitant drug	**Object drug***		**Description**
Anticholinergics	APAP	⟷	The onset of acetaminophen effect may be delayed or decreased slightly, but the ultimate pharmacological effect is not significantly affected by anticholinergics.
Beta blockers, propranolol	APAP	↑	Propranolol appears to inhibit the enzyme systems responsible for glucuronidation and oxidation of APAP. Therefore, the pharmacologic effects of acetaminophen may be increased.
Charcoal, activated	APAP	↓	Reduces acetaminophen absorption when administered as soon as possible after overdose.
Probenecid	APAP	↑	Probenecid may increase the therapeutic effectiveness of acetaminophen slightly.
APAP	Loop diuretics	↓	The effects of the loop diuretic may be decreased because APAP may decrease renal prostaglandin excretion and decrease plasma renin activity.
APAP	Zidovudine	↓	The pharmacologic effects of zidovudine may be decreased because of enhanced nonhepatic or renal clearance of zidovudine.

* ↑ = Object drug increased. ↓ = Object drug decreased. ⟷ = Undetermined clinical effect.

The potential hepatotoxicity of acetaminophen may be increased by large doses or long term administration of barbiturates, carbamazepine, hydantoins, rifampin, and sulfinpyrazone. The therapeutic effects of acetaminophen may also be decreased.

▶ Adverse Reactions

When used as directed, acetaminophen rarely causes severe toxicity or side effects. However, the following adverse reactions have been reported:

Hematologic: Hemolytic anemia; neutropenia; leukopenia; pancytopenia; thrombocytopenia.

Hepatic: Jaundice.

Metabolic: Hypoglycemia.

Hypersensitivity: Skin rash; fever.

▶ Overdosage

Symptoms: Acute poisoning may be manifested by nausea, vomiting, drowsiness, confusion, liver tenderness, low blood pressure, cardiac arrhythmias, jaundice, and acute hepatic and renal failure. These occur within the first 24 hours and may persist for 1 week or longer. Death has occurred because of liver necrosis. Acute renal failure may also occur. However, there are often no specific early symptoms or signs. The course of acetaminophen poisoning is divided into 4 stages (postingestion time):

Stage 1 (12 to 24 hours) – Nausea; vomiting; diaphoresis; anorexia.

Stage 2 (24 to 48 hours) – Clinically improved; AST, bilirubin, and prothrombin levels begin to rise.

Stage 3 (72 to 96 hours) – Peak hepatotoxicity; AST of 20,000 not unusual.

Stage 4 (7 to 8 days) – Recovery.

Hepatotoxicity may result. The minimal toxic dose is 10 g (140 mg/kg), but liver damage has occurred with a single 5.85 g dose; doses 20 to 25 g or larger are potentially fatal. Children appear less susceptible to toxicity than adults because children have less capacity for glucuronidation metabolism. Initial signs of toxicity may include nausea, vomiting, anorexia, malaise, diaphoresis, abdominal pain, and diarrhea. Hepatotoxicity is usually not apparent for 48 to 72 hours. Hepatic failure may lead to encephalopathy, coma, and death.

Plasma acetaminophen levels more than 300 mcg/mL at 4 hours postingestion were associated with hepatic damage in 90% of patients; minimal hepatic damage is anticipated if plasma levels at 4 hours are less than 120 mcg/mL or less than 30 mcg/mL at 12 hours after ingestion.

Chronic excessive use (over 4 g/day) may lead to transient hepatotoxicity. The kidney(s) may undergo tubular necrosis; the myocardium may be damaged.

Treatment: Perform gastric lavage in all cases, preferably within 4 hours of ingestion. Refer also to General Management of Acute Overdosage. It is important to contact a local poison control center or emergency room if overdosage is suspected.

▶ **Administration and Dosage**

Children: The usual dose is 10 mg/kg/dose, which may be repeated 4 to 5 times daily. Do not exceed 5 doses in 24 hours.

Adult and junior strength products should not be used for relief of teething.

Acetaminophen Dosages for Children			
Weight	Dosage (mg)	Weight	Dosage (mg)
6-11 lbs	40	48-59 lbs	320
12-17 lbs	80	60-71 lbs	400
18-23 lbs	120	72-95 lbs	480
24-35 lbs	160	> 95 lbs	640
36-47 lbs	240		

Suppositories:

Children – (3 to 11 months of age): 80 mg every 6 hours.

(1 to 3 years of age): 80 mg every 4 hours.

Storage – Store suppositories below 27°C (80°F) or refrigerate. Store tablets and oral solutions at 15° to 30°C (59° to 86°F).

ACETAMINOPHEN PRODUCTS	
Trade name	Doseform
Children's Genapap, Children's Panadol, Children's Tylenol	**Tablets, chewable**: 80 mg
Children's Silapap	**Elixir**: 80 mg/2.5 mL
Children's Genapap, Children's Mapap, Children's Tylenol	**Elixir**: 160 mg/5 mL
Children's Panadol	**Liquid**: 160 mg/5 mL
Liquiprin Drops for Children	**Solution**: 80 mg/1.66 mL
Genapap Infants' Drops, Mapap Infant Drops, Infants' Panadol Drops, Infants' Silapap	**Solution**: 100 mg/mL
Infants' Tylenol Drops	**Suspension**: 80 mg/0.8 mL
Children's Tylenol	**Suspension**: 160 mg/5 mL
Infants FeverAll	**Suppositories**: 80 mg

Products listed are representative of currently available and widely distributed brands. Similar products, including regional and private label brands, may also exist.

■ ■ ■

PATIENT INFORMATION

Acetaminophen

- For liquid preparations, only use the measuring device included in the packaging or a measuring device specifically for medication. Do **not** use household measuring spoons or standard teaspoons.
- Keep out of reach of children.
- In case of accidental overdose, contact your local poison control center immediately.
- Do not use with other products containing acetaminophen (eg, cough and cold products).
- Severe or recurrent pain may indicate a serious illness. Consult a physician.
- Do not exceed the recommended dosage.
- Fever and nasal congestion are not symptoms of teething and may indicate an infection.
- Consult a physician for use in children younger than 3 years old.
- Do not give acetaminophen to children for longer than 5 days. If symptoms persist, worsen, or if new symptoms develop, contact a physician.

IBUPROFEN

▶ Actions

Ibuprofen and other nonsteroidal anti-inflammatory drugs (NSAIDs) have analgesic and antipyretic activities. The major mechanism of action of ibuprofen is believed to be inhibition of cyclooxygenase activity and prostaglandin synthesis. While naproxen and ketoprofen are also available without a prescription, these agents are not appropriate for use in children, unless directed by a physician.

▶ Indications

For the treatment of mild to moderate pain, such as pain associated with teething. This agent has other labeled indications as well.

▶ Contraindications

NSAID hypersensitivity: Because of potential cross-sensitivity to other NSAIDs, do not give this agent to patients in whom aspirin, iodides, or other NSAIDs have induced symptoms of asthma, rhinitis, urticaria, nasal polyps, angioedema, bronchospasm, and other symptoms of allergic or anaphylactoid reactions.

▶ Warnings

Acute renal insufficiency: Patients with preexisting renal disease or compromised renal perfusion are at greatest risk. A form of renal toxicity seen in patients with prerenal conditions leads to reduced renal blood flow or blood volume. NSAID use may cause a dose-dependent reduction in prostaglandin formation and precipitate renal decompensation. Patients at greatest risk are the elderly, premature infants, those with heart failure, those with renal or hepatic dysfunction, systemic lupus erythematosus (SLE), chronic glomerulonephritis, and those receiving diuretics. Recovery usually follows discontinuation.

Hypersensitivity: Severe hypersensitivity reactions with fever, rash, abdominal pain, headache, nausea, vomiting, signs of liver damage, and meningitis have occurred in patients receiving ibuprofen, especially those with SLE or other collagen diseases. Anaphylactoid reactions have occurred in patients with aspirin hypersensitivity.

Renal function impairment: NSAID metabolites are eliminated primarily by the kidneys; use with caution with impaired renal function. Reduce dosage to avoid excessive accumulation.

Platelet aggregation: NSAIDs can inhibit platelet aggregation; the effect is quantitatively less and of shorter duration than that seen with aspirin. These agents prolong bleeding time (within normal range) in healthy subjects. This may be exaggerated in patients with underlying hemostatic defects; use with caution in people with intrinsic coagulation defects and in those on anticoagulant therapy.

Cardiovascular effects: May cause fluid retention and peripheral edema. Use caution in compromised cardiac function, hypertension, or other conditions predisposing to fluid retention. Agents may be associated with significant deterioration of circulatory hemodynamics in severe heart failure and hyponatremia, presumably because of inhibition of prostaglandin-dependent compensatory mechanisms.

Infection: NSAIDs may mask the usual signs of infection (eg, fever, muscle aches). Use with extra care in the presence of existing controlled infection.

Photosensitivity: Photosensitivity may occur; caution patients to take protective measures (ie, sunscreens, protective clothing) against UV or sunlight until tolerance is determined.

GI effects: GI toxicity (including NSAID-induced ulcers and GI bleeding disorders) can occur with or without warning with chronic use of NSAIDs. High-dose NSAIDs probably carry a greater risk of causing GI adverse effects. Have patients with a history of GI lesions consult a physician before using these products. GI adverse effects are more likely to occur in elderly patients.

Duration of therapy: Do not take for longer than 10 days for pain. If symptoms persist, worsen, or if new symptoms develop, contact a physician.

▶ **Drug Interactions**

NSAID Drug Interactions			
Precipitant drug	**Object drug***		**Description**
NSAIDs	Anticoagulants	↑	Coadministration may prolong prothrombin time (PT). Also consider the effects NSAIDs have on platelet function and gastric mucosa. Monitor PT and patients closely, and instruct patients to watch for signs and symptoms of bleeding.
NSAIDs	Beta blockers	↓	The antihypertensive effect of beta blockers may be impaired. Naproxen did not affect atenolol.
NSAIDs	Cyclosporine	↑	Nephrotoxicity of both agents may be increased.
NSAIDs	Digoxin	↑	Ibuprofen may increase digoxin serum levels.
NSAIDs	Hydantoins	↑	Serum phenytoin levels may be increased, resulting in an increase in pharmacologic and toxic effects of phenytoin.
NSAIDs	Lithium	↑	Serum lithium levels may be increased.
NSAIDs	Loop diuretics	↓	Effects of loop diuretics may be decreased.
NSAIDs	Methotrexate	↑	The risks of methotrexate toxicity (eg, stomatitis, bone marrow suppression, nephrotoxicity) may be increased.
NSAIDs	Thiazide diuretics	↓	Decreased antihypertensive and diuretic action of thiazides may occur with concurrent naproxen.
Cimetidine	NSAIDs	↔	NSAID plasma concentrations may be increased or decreased by cimetidine; some studies report no effect.

NSAID Drug Interactions			
Precipitant drug	Object drug*		Description
Probenecid	NSAIDs	↑	Probenecid may increase the concentrations and possibly the toxicity of NSAIDs.
Salicylates	NSAIDs	↓	Plasma concentrations of NSAIDs may be decreased by salicylates. Avoid concurrent use because it offers no therapeutic advantage and may significantly increase the incidence of GI effects.

* ↑ = Object drug increased.   ↓ = Object drug decreased.   ↔ = Undetermined clinical effect.

▶ **Adverse Reactions**

Cardiovascular: Edema; congestive heart failure.

CNS: Dizziness; drowsiness; headache; lightheadedness; vertigo.

Dermatologic: Erythema; pruritus; rash.

GI: Bleeding; diarrhea; dyspepsia; heartburn; nausea; vomiting.

Miscellaneous: Muscle cramps; thirst.

▶ **Administration and Dosage**

Children (6 months to 12 years of age): 5 to 10 mg/kg/dose repeated 3 to 4 times daily as needed. Maximum daily dose is 40 mg/kg.

IBUPROFEN PRODUCTS	
Trade name	Doseform
Children's Advil, Children's Motrin	**Suspension**: 100 mg/5 mL
Pediatric Advil Drops	**Suspension**: 50 mg/5 mL

Products listed are representative of currently available and widely distributed brands. Similar products, including regional and private label brands, may also exist.

PATIENT INFORMATION

Ibuprofen

- For liquid preparations, only use the measuring device included in the packaging or a measuring device specifically for medication. Do **not** use household measuring spoons or standard teaspoons.
- Keep out of reach of children.
- In case of accidental overdose, contact your local poison control center immediately.
- Severe or recurrent pain may indicate a serious illness. Consult a physician.
- May cause GI upset; take with food or after meals.
- Fever and nasal congestion are not symptoms of teething and may indicate an infection.
- Do not take OTC ibuprofen for longer than 10 days for pain. If symptoms persist, worsen, or if new symptoms develop, contact a physician.

TOPICAL AGENTS

▶ **Actions**

Benzocaine is a local anesthetic agent.

Eucalyptus oil is an antiseptic agent.

Menthol and camphor have local anesthetic and counterirritant activity.

▶ **Indications**

These products are indicated for minor irritations of the mouth.

▶ **Warnings**

For external or mucous membrane use only. Do not use in the eyes.

Methemoglobinemia: Benzocaine should not be used in those rare patients with congenital or idiopathic methemoglobinemia and in infants younger than 12 months of age who are receiving treatment with methemoglobin-inducing agents (eg, TMP-SMZ, phenazopyridine). Very young patients or patients with glucose-6-phosphate deficiencies are more susceptible to methemoglobinemia.

Traumatized mucosa: Use cautiously in patients with known drug sensitivities or in patients with severly traumatized mucosa and sepsis in the region of the application. If irritation or rash occurs, discontinue treatment and institute appropriate therapy.

Oral use: Topical anesthetics may impair swallowing and enhance danger of aspiration. Do not ingest food for 1 hour after anesthetic use in mouth or throat. This is particularly important in children because of their frequency of eating.

Children: Do not use benzocaine in infants younger than 1 year of age. Reduce dosages in children commensurate with age, body weight, and physical condition.

Tartrazine sensitivity: Some of these products contain tartrazine, which may cause allergic-type reactions (including bronchial asthma) in susceptible individuals. Specific products containing sulfites are identified in the product listings.

Sulfite sensitivity: Some of these products contain sulfites that may cause allergic-type reactions, including anaphylactic symptoms and life-threatening or less severe asthmatic episodes in certain susceptible people. The overall prevalence of sulfite sensitivity in the general population is unknown and probably low. Sulfite sensitivity is seen more frequently in asthmatic or atopic nonasthmatic people. Specific products containing sulfites are identified in the product listings.

▶ **Administration and Dosage**

For specific dosing information refer to package labeling of individual products.

TOPICAL TEETHING PRODUCTS	
Trade name	**Doseform**
Baby Numzit	**Gel**: 7.5% benzocaine, clove and peppermint oil. Saccharin.
Baby Anbesol	**Gel**: 7.5% benzocaine. EDTA, parabens, saccharin.
Baby Orajel	**Gel**: 7.5% benzocaine. Saccharin, sorbitol.
Baby Orajel Nighttime	**Gel**: 10% benzocaine. Saccharin, sorbitol.
Orabase Baby	**Gel**: 7.5% benzocaine
Baby Orajel	**Liquid**: 7.5% benzocaine. Parabens, saccharin, sorbitol.
Babee Teething (sf)	**Lotion**: 2.5% benzocaine, 0.02% cetalkonium chloride, camphor, eucolyptol, menthol. Alcohol.
Zilactin Baby	**Lotion**: 10% benzocaine. Parabens.

Products listed are representative of currently available and widely distributed brands. Similar products, including regional and private label brands, may also exist.

sf = Sugar free.

PATIENT INFORMATION

Topical Teething Products

- Dosing and uses for specific products may vary. Read instructions for individual products carefully before using these medications.
- Do not exceed the recommended dosage.
- Do not swallow these products.
- Do not use benzocaine-containing products if your child has a history of allergy to local anesthetics, such as procaine, butacaine, benzocaine, or other "-caine" anesthetics. Do not use if the child has an allergy to any other ingredient in these products.
- If sore mouth conditions last for longer than 7 days; if irritation, pain, and redness persists or worsens; or if swelling, rash, or fever develops, see a physician.
- Do not use for longer than 5 to 7 days unless directed by a physician.
- Fever and nasal congeston are not symptoms of teething and may indicate an infection.
- Mild burning may occur at application site.
- Allergic reactions at site of application may occur after prolonged or repeated use; discontinue use and contact a physician if this occurs.
- Benzocaine products may make swallowing difficult or inhibit gag reflexes in infants and children.
- Avoid contact with eyes. If contact occurs, flush with water and contact a physician.
- Use only in children of ages specified on packaging of individual products.

TOOTHACHE

DEFINITION

Toothache is usually the result of a localized dental insult to the integrity of a particular tooth. The surrounding periodontium may also be involved. A majority of toothaches are caused by dental caries and periodontal disease. Both of these causes are multifactorial, are initiated by certain bacteria, and culminate in pain, tooth mobility, and possible tooth loss.

ETIOLOGY

Dental plaque, the ever-present bacterial/bioactive film covering the teeth and gums, is considered the precursor of caries and periodontitis. A combination of factors, including oral hygiene, bacteria, diet, host-immune response, saliva quantity/quality, time, and genetics determine the individual's susceptibility to dental disease. As a carious or periodontal lesion progresses in and around a tooth, the nerves in the tooth pulp and periodontium become stimulated. Different dental insults will elicit various pains. This variation is often useful for the dentist in determining the cause of the toothache. Besides caries and periodontal disease, there are a multitude of other sources of toothaches and conditions whose symptoms mimic those of toothache.

INCIDENCE

Although recent studies indicate a worldwide decline in dental diseases, caries and periodontal disease are still considered to be 2 of the most common international health problems. Industrialized nations that have access to fluoride, improved patient education, diet awareness, dental care, and dental products typically manage dental disease better than Third World countries.

SIGNS/SYMPTOMS

The pulp/root canal of a tooth is composed of a network of nerves and blood vessels. The surrounding periodontium is highly vascular and innervated. Microscopic odontoblastic processes, which radiate outward from the center of the tooth into the dentin, function as conduits of sensation to the pulp. A hydrodynamic theory has been proposed to explain how the odontoblastic processes conduct sensation. Insult to the dentin causes a water pressure change in the processes that is relayed to the pulp. Minute nerve endings also extend partially outward from the pulp. An injury to the tooth or temperature changes stimulate the nerve endings/odontoblastic processes, causing various types of dental pain or sensation, ranging from distinct throbbing to hypersensitivity to cold. Periodontal structures do not translate pain to the extent that a tooth would. Therefore, periodontal disease is sometimes called "silent killer dental disease."

TREATMENT

Approaches to therapy: All dental pain, intra-oral swellings, fractured teeth, lost fillings, lesions, or lacerations should be evaluated by a dentist. However, many types of toothache may be successfully triaged and, until the patient can see a dentist, may be treated by a pharmacist with OTC dental products or proper advice.

Caries – Lancinating, intermittent, or constant pain is often exacerbated by food, sweets, and hot or cold liquids. It is important to remember that a carious lesion is not always visible intra-orally and may remain asymptomatic for years. In such cases, it will only be discovered on a dental x-ray. An untreated carious lesion will usually progress, eventually causing painful pulpitis, nerve death, and other sequelae. Dental care should be sought if caries is suspected.

Interim OTC treatment:

• Topical analgesics/anesthetics or OTC oral analgesics (eg, acetaminophen, NSAIDs) may provide some pain relief.
• Limit aggravating food/drinks.
• Eugenol-containing products applied to the tooth and gums may help. (Eugenol acts as an obtundant and anesthetic).
• Protectants, including OTC products and home remedies such as paraffin and cotton, may help.
• Zinc oxide/eugenol products (available OTC) are good sealants/protectants.
• Petroleum jelly and cream denture adhesives are also good protectants.

Chipped/Fractured Teeth – Such conditions may or may not be painful, depending on the proximity of the underlying nerve to the loss of tooth structure. The tooth may be relatively painless if only enamel is lost; it may be sensitive if dentin or the nerve is exposed. "Cracked tooth syndrome" is a unique and sometimes baffling dental condition, whereby biting pressure causes intense pain in a tooth upon release. The actual fracture may or may not be visible to the eye or detected on an x-ray but should be suspected based on the specific symptoms. Posterior molars with large amounts of filling are most likely to be fracture candidates.

Interim OTC treatment:

• Protect the tooth from further insults such as cold, heat, and pressure.
• Nonprescription oral analgesics may provide some pain relief.
• Nonprescription protectants or petroleum jelly may help.
• Directly applied eugenol-containing products may either help or irritate.

See a dentist for any broken tooth. The dentist will either rebuild or crown the tooth, or begin endodontics, depending on the condition of the nerve. If rebuilt, the tooth may still require eventual endodontic therapy because of traumatic nerve death.

Gingival/Periodontal Abscess – The origin of this type of painful abscess is bacterial, coupled with the body's own host-immune response. It usually presents as a purulent, fluctuant swelling of the gingiva, most often adjacent to a periodontally involved tooth. This condition must be differentiated from a true periapical abscess of the tooth.

A dentist must be seen. The dentist will drain the abscess, debride the area, prescribe an antibiotic/analgesic, and evaluate the gingiva involved. The offending tooth or area may need periodontal therapy and endodontics, hemisection, or extraction.

Interim OTC treatment:

- Nonprescription oral analgesics/topical anesthetics may provide some pain relief.
- Hot/cold packs applied to the face may provide some pain relief.
- Saline rinses may help.
- Proper, regular oral hygiene performed by the patient helps keep the area clean and facilitates healing.

Leaking or Lost Filling – A leaking or lost filling usually causes an intermittent sharp pain after consuming certain foods, hot or cold beverages, or sweet, sour, or spicy items, without necessarily progressing to a constant toothache. A lost filling may not be painful; it depends on the depth of the exposed cavity and patient sensitivity. A leaking filling is one that has gradually deteriorated or fractured, allowing oral fluids to penetrate into the relatively porous and sensitive dentin section of the tooth.

Interim OTC treatment:

- Avoid offending food substances and hot or cold beverages.
- Eugenol-containing products, such as *Den Temp, Den Temp O.S.*, or *Dent's Extra-Strength Toothache Gum* may be used as temporary filling material. (The patient must be quick, dexterous, and have cotton and tweezers available.)
- Topical eugenol-containing products may ease the pain.
- Paraffin/beeswax/denture adhesive cream may be inserted into the cavity. Cotton pellets also work.
- Brushing with desensitizing toothpaste (containing potassium nitrate) may help.
- Topical protectants with or without benzocaine may help.
- Nonprescription oral analgesics may provide some pain relief.

Periapical Abscess – One of the most painful and debilitating types of toothache, periapical abscess is also potentially threatening to tooth life, especially if the lower jaw is involved. The abscess occurs at the apex of the affected tooth's root. It can occur because of untreated caries, iatrogenic causes, periodontal disease, fractured cusps, failed endodontic therapy, or other dental injuries. The tissues in the root canal become bacterially infected and undergo necrosis. At this point, the root canal contents become composed of bacteria, leukocytes, and suppuration. Edema, cellulitis, and fluctuant swelling occur around the affected tooth. Pain increases as pus formation continues and periapical pressure builds. The patient will often appear sick, with a swollen face and an elevated temperature. The offending tooth will often be tender to percussion and palpation. Advise the patient of the seriousness of this dental condition, especially when it occurs in the lower jaw. Fulminant cases have been known to close off the airway, cause septic shock, and possibly cause death. The patient should seek emergency dental or medical care immediately. The abscess will usually be drained through the fluctuant mass, and an antibiotic/analgesic will be prescribed. Draining the abscess usually causes immediate diminution of pain but may be accompanied by shivering and syncope on the part of the patient. The dentist may also begin endodontics on the tooth or advise the patient to have it extracted once the infection subsides. If left untreated, a periapical abscess can lead to chronic infection and form a fistula draining into the mouth. This sets up a long-standing oral infection that requires treatment.

Traumatic Injury – Trauma to a tooth usually occurs because of a blow or a fall. The tooth's position may become altered during the accident.

Interim OTC treatment:

- A dentist should be seen promptly. In the meantime, the tooth should be repositioned as much as possible.
- Apply cold compresses to the affected oral areas to decrease swelling and help alleviate pain.
- Nonprescription eugenol-containing products and topical anesthetics may help relieve pain.
- Nonprescription oral analgesics may provide some pain relief.
- Avoidance of chewing stress on the tooth is prudent.

A dentist must be seen, especially if the pain continues after a short period of time. The dentist will x-ray the tooth to rule out an obvious fracture and the possibility of a root abscess. The tooth may require repositioning in its socket; it may require endodontics if the pain is intractable. An antibiotic may be prescribed, especially if the trauma extensively involves surrounding soft tissues. Ultimately, the tooth may die, turn dark, become painful, and need root canal therapy or become exfoliated. Any of these reactions can happen immediately after the accident or many years later.

Trauma from Occlusion – This condition, also called "primary occlusal traumatism," can be a painful condition originating from one of the following causes: Periodontal disease, a filling placed too high, orthodontic tooth movement, natural malocclusion of the jaws, or tooth loss that subjects the remaining teeth to increased biting pressure. Possible sequelae include the following: Pain subsides but the tooth becomes mobile, resembling periodontal disease; the pain increases, sometimes causing tooth fracture; or gradual wear of the tooth, with formation of abfraction areas along the gumline. A dentist should be seen. The dentist will perform an overall bite evaluation. Possible dental solutions may include selective grinding of tooth surfaces to even out the bite, fabrication of fixed/removable prostheses to stabilize the teeth and occlusion, or orthodontic intervention.

Teething Pain in Children – Teething begins at 6 months of age. Besides the obvious pain associated with the eruption of primary teeth, other signs and symptoms may include elevated temperature, salivation, irritability, sleeplessness, and diarrhea. For more information, refer to the Teething monograph in this chapter.

Interim OTC treatment:

- Cold teething toys/food may work best to alleviate the discomfort (supervision required).
- Nonprescription oral analgesics may provide pain relief.
- Nonprescription topical anesthetics (be aware of benzocaine allergies) may be useful.
- Alcohol is contraindicated as a topical anesthetic in children.

Hypersensitive Dentin/Root Areas – The area of a tooth at the junction of the gingiva can be extremely painful, especially if some gum recession exists. This area is not covered by enamel; it is root surface of a porous nature. According to the hydrodynamic pain theory, these microscopic pore openings convey sensitivity to the tooth nerve. However, cold is usually the only sensation felt. The hypersensitive, exposed root areas are a result of abfraction because of occlusal problems, caries, abrasion, chemical insult, gum disease, or gradual gingival recession. Sensitivity varies in individuals and does not always correlate to the degree of root exposure.

Interim OTC treatment:

- Desensitizing dentifrices containing the obtundant potassium nitrate are effective.
- Fluoride rinses and high-fluoride OTC toothpastes help alleviate the sensitivity.
- Petroleum jelly and other protectants applied directly to the area may help.
- Avoid offending food and drink.

Ultimately, a dentist must be seen. The hypersensitive area may be a carious lesion, a lost filling, etc. Dental treatments include selective grinding of the occlusion to alleviate abfraction stresses coupled with bonding agents applied directly to the affected area. High-fluoride dentifrices (eg, *Prevident, Gel Kam*) and oral rinses, all of which are available by prescription, can also be used as desensitizers. If the lesions are deep and refractory to simple desensitizing procedures, a composite restoration may have to be placed. Dentinal hypersensitivity can be a chronic and annoying problem; patients may need periodic OTC/dental management.

Toothache Due to Occlusal Attrition/High Filling – Severe bruxism (tooth grinding), malocclusion, diet, or a combination of these factors may cause the occlusal surfaces of teeth to become unevenly worn, often resulting in painful toothaches exacerbated by temperature extremes and certain foods. This is frequently a problem of long-standing duration; proper dental care is the only solution.

A new filling inadvertently placed even slightly high in occlusion often results in sensitivity to cold. In the absence of other symptoms, a cold-sensitive, newly filled tooth should be promptly treated by a dentist to relieve the occlusion and pain.

Impacted Wisdom Tooth Pain – Usually occurring in young adults, pain from impacted wisdom teeth is episodic in nature; the pressure/pain is due to the movement of the wisdom tooth in a tight, closed area of the jaw. Cystic formation is possible along with trismus of the surrounding musculature. Temporomandibular joint (TMJ) syndrome-type symptoms can sometimes be related to an impacted wisdom tooth.

Interim OTC treatment:

- Nonprescription oral analgesics may provide pain relief.
- Extraction is the only long-term solution if symptoms persist and are substantiated by a panoramic x-ray.

Pericoronitis – The tissue around a partially erupted wisdom tooth can become episodically infected in susceptible individuals. The partial eruption, coupled with an often hard-to-reach, difficult-to-clean area, can lead to a localized but very painful infection. The infection can cause difficulty in mastication and swallowing and may also cause TMJ-type symptoms. The gingiva around the affected molar is usually red, swollen, and exudative. An offensive odor may be present.

Interim OTC treatment:

- Nonprescription oral analgesics may provide pain relief.
- Nonprescription oral rinses and saline rinses may help.
- Thorough brushing is necessary to prevent/minimize the symptoms of pericoronitis.

Patients with pericoronitis must see a dentist. Antibiotics and analgesics will usually be prescribed along with localized debridement of the area. The offending wisdom tooth should be flushed out regularly and ultimately extracted if the condition recurs.

Maxillary Sinus Pain Mimicking Toothache – The maxillary sinuses occupy the spaces between the maxillary premolars, molars, and eyes, roughly just below the cheekbones. Any infection, inflammation, or congestion of these spaces can cause the premolars and molars to ache. The ache can be unilateral or bilateral, can be severe, and frequently involves more than one tooth. Mastication and bending forward usually cause pain. Patients should see a dentist. X-rays and a differential diagnosis will be used to determine if the sinus is the cause of toothache. An antibiotic and a decongestant will usually be prescribed. Symptoms gradually resolve as the sinus starts clearing.

Failing Endodontics Toothache – Root canal therapy is often perceived as definitive dental treatment. However, recurrent infection due to missed canals, post fractures, root fractures, and iatrogenic factors can all cause endodontic failure. The offending tooth may become abscessed, develop a fistula, and have swollen surrounding tissue. This condition may be painful and confusing to a patient who assumed nothing further could go wrong with the affected tooth.

Interim OTC treatment:

• Nonprescription oral analgesics may provide pain relief.

A dentist must be seen. The tooth may need to be endodontically retreated, undergo surgery, or be extracted.

Deep Filling/Composite Filling Toothache – It is normal to have pain and sensitivity for a short duration after a new filling is placed. Nerve proximity to the restoration often determines the severity of pain. Although most of this type of pain is short-lived, a dental visit is prudent if symptoms escalate. Though infrequent, an unusual phenomenon has been observed with composite restorations. Sometimes, even a shallow-placed composite will cause postoperative pain. Recent studies have shown that shrinkage of the filling next to the bottom of the cavity induces a hydrodynamic effect on the dentinal tubules, causing the pain.

Interim OTC treatment:

• Nonprescription oral analgesics may provide pain relief.

If any pain continues or escalates over time, consult a dentist. The dentist will check the occlusion, replace the filling with a temporary sedative filling (containing zinc oxide and eugenol), check the status of the nerve on an x-ray, and determine the best course of action.

Referred Aphthous Ulcer Pain – Close proximity of an aphthous ulcer to a tooth can be readily mistaken for a toothache. The intense pain is in fact generated by the small aphthous lesion.

Interim OTC treatment:

• Topical anesthetics and protectants work well.
• Nonprescription oral analgesics may provide pain relief.
• Antibacterial, peroxide, and saline rinses may help.

A dentist should be seen to rule out a genuine toothache if the pain persists. For severe or chronic aphthous ulcers, amlexanox (*Aphthasol*) or triamcinolone acetonide (*Kenalog in Orabase*) may be prescribed. For more information, see the Canker Sores monograph in this chapter.

Neuropathies Arising from Tooth Extraction – Although rare, if nerves such as the inferior alveolar nerve (the third branch of the trigeminal nerve found in the lower jaw) are accidentally abraded, punctured, or bruised by an injection, paresthesia and other neuropathies may develop. Most of these resolve in time with no lingering sequelae. Patients must be told that there is always risk involved in some difficult dental procedures, such as implant placement. If numbness, tingling, loss of taste, or other symptoms continue after any dental treatment, consult a dentist.

Dry Socket Toothache – This is one of the most painful dental problems. It results from an avulsed blood clot or poor initial healing of a recent extraction site. The exposed jaw bone can become secondarily infected, causing this very painful condition. Smoking and improper wound care greatly contribute to dry socket formation.

Interim OTC treatment:

• Nonprescription oral analgesics may provide pain relief.

A dentist will usually debride the infected socket, prescribe an antibiotic/analgesic, and sometimes pack the affected area with a special antibacterial poultice. This condition, when properly treated, resolves rapidly.

Nontraditional Toothaches – A large number of factors causing tooth pain are not of the "normal" variety. Any oral medicine textbook is replete with a multitude of rare, and unlikely, but legitimate, causes of toothache. Systemic diseases, genetic malformations, viral/bacterial infections, a compromised immune system, etc., all may contribute to a specific toothache situation. It is beyond the scope of this monograph to list the eccentric toothaches not commonly found in the population.

Iatrogenic Toothache – A toothache caused by the dentist. This can be more commonplace than might be expected, especially in high-risk dental procedures.

Braces Pain/Partial Denture Pain – Any immediate stress placed upon a tooth may elicit pain. Initial irritation of the lips, tongue, and cheeks is normal. Clasping, binding, and forced tooth movement can cause a throbbing pain until the tooth adjusts to the new pressure and stressors.

Braces Pain/Broken or Loose Parts – A patient should consult his or her orthodontist or dentist if any brackets or wires come loose or if pain continues.

Interim OTC treatment:

• There are OTC products available (eg, ortho wax) to cover offending wires and brackets.
• Nonprescription oral analgesics may provide pain relief.
• Paraffin or beeswax may be used.

Partial denture pain – A dentist must be seen to relieve the tight clasping, alter the occlusion, adjust the partial denture, or to reassure the patient that some pressure is normal in an initially placed removable partial denture.

TMJ Pain Mimicking Toothache – True temporomandibular disc derangement, myofacial pain dysfunction symptoms, and other TMJ-type syndromes can mimic a toothache in the posterior regions of the mouth, and vice versa. This particular type of posterior "tooth" pain can be challenging for dentists to correctly diagnose.

Toothache of Unknown Origin – A toothache without an obvious cause can be frustrating and painful, and sometimes baffling to the dentist. Early nerve death, a torqued tooth (from biting something very hard), temperature extremes, viral infection, and a host of other traditional but not-so-easily spotted causes may be the source of pain. X-rays and typical diagnostic criteria may not show anything unusual during the dental visit. However, in time, the cause of the toothache will become evident, or conversely, the pain will disappear. Patience can sometimes be the best approach to treating diagnostically difficult toothaches.

Toothache from a Lost, Temporary, or Permanent Crown/Bridge – Provisional (temporary) crowns and bridgework are usually cemented by the dentist using a "temporary" cement while waiting for the permanent prostheses to be fabricated by a dental laboratory. They can loosen and fall out or be swallowed. Permanent crowns and bridges should remain in place after permanent cementation but may occasionally suffer the same fate as the temporaries. An uncovered "live" tooth will become extremely sensitive to multiple oral insults including certain foods, beverages, and temperature extremes. Bacterial invasion and infection are also possible.

Interim OTC treatment:

- It is important to keep the tooth covered.
- If the prosthesis is available, it should be put back on using dental cream adhesive, petroleum jelly, *Den Temp* cement, or as is.

A dentist should be seen as quickly as possible, even if the tooth has had endodontics and is not painful. Uncovered teeth may not only become sensitive, but the bite may change quite rapidly as well, to the detriment of a well-fitting crown and proper occlusion. The dentist will either recement the existing prosthesis back on or fabricate a provisional one until a new crown or bridge can be made.

Toothache from Uncleaned Teeth/Early Gingivitis – Tartar build-up around the necks of teeth may be responsible for gingival bleeding, foul mouth odor, pain on mastication, various painful gingival abcesses, "itchy gums," and toothaches that are actually related to the gingiva and surrounding periodontium. The patient should be advised to have a dental cleaning/prophylaxis/examination, even though the initial visit may be somewhat uncomfortable because of gingival pain and inflammation. In the absence of frank periodontal disease, the gums will usually heal and toughen up; subsequent cleanings will not be as painful. After proper dental care has been initiated, various specialty toothpastes (eg, *Colgate Total*, *Viadent Advance Care*), toothbrushes, and oral rinses can be recommended to the patient.

ORAL TOPICAL OBTUNDENT/ANALGESIC PRODUCTS

▶ **Indications**

For the temporary relief of throbbing, persistent toothache pain caused by a cavity until a dentist can be seen.

EUGENOL

▶ **Contraindications**

Allergy to eugenol.

▶ **Administration and Dosage**

Rinse the affected tooth with water to remove any food particles from the cavity. Use tweezers (provided) to moisten cotton pellet, shake off excess water, and place in cavity.

EUGENOL PRODUCTS	
Trade name	Doseform
Red Cross Toothache Medication	**Cotton pellets:** Eugenol 85%, sesame oil.

Products listed are representative of currently available and widely distributed brands. Similar products, including regional and private label brands, may also exist.

PATIENT INFORMATION
Eugenol Products

• Do not swallow.
• Do not exceed recommended dosage.
• Do not use for longer than 7 days.
• Do not use in children younger than 2 years of age.
• Closely supervise children younger than 12 years of age in the use of this product.
• If irritation persists, or if inflammation, infection, or fever develop, discontinue use and consult a dentist or physician promptly.
• In case of accidental ingestion, seek professional assistance or contact a poison control center.
• Avoid touching tissues other than the affected tooth cavity when applying the product.
• Do not apply more than 4 times daily or more frequently than directed by a dentist or physician.

ORAL TOPICAL ANESTHETIC/ANALGESIC PRODUCTS

BENZOCAINE

▶ **Indications**

For the temporary relief of pain associated with toothache.

▶ **Contraindications**

History of allergy to local anesthetics such as procaine, butacaine, benzocaine, or other "-caine" anesthetics.

▶ **Administration and Dosage**

Adults and children 2 years of age and older: Apply to the affected area up to 4 times daily or as directed by a dentist or doctor.

Gum: Cleanse tooth cavity by rinsing with warm water. Use scissors to cut a piece of the gum product and press it into the cavity.

BENZOCAINE PRODUCTS	
Trade name	Doseform
Dent's Extra Strength Toothache Gum	**Gum:** Benzocaine 20%. Beeswax, petrolatum, cotton.
Zilactin Maximum Strength Toothache Swabs	**Medicated swabs:** Benzocaine 20%

BENZOCAINE PRODUCTS

Trade name	Doseform
Anbesol Cool Mint	**Gel**: Benzocaine 10%. Glycerin, methylparaben, saccharin.
Maximum Strength Anbesol	**Gel**: Benzocaine 20%. Glycerin, methylparaben, saccharin.
Orajel Regular Strength	**Gel**: Benzocaine 10%. Polyethylene glycols, saccharin, sorbic acid.
Orajel Maximum Strength	**Gel**: Benzocaine 20% in special base. Clove oil, polyethylene glycols, saccharin, sorbic acid.
Orajel Mouth-Aid	**Gel**: Benzocaine 20%, benzalkonium chloride 0.02%, zinc chloride 0.1%. Allantoin, carbomer, EDTA, peppermint oil, polyethylene glycol, polysorbate 60, propyl gallate, propylene glycol, povidone, saccharin, sorbic acid, stearyl alcohol.
hda Toothache	**Gel**: Benzocaine 6.5%. Benzyl alcohol, clove oil, glycerin, propylene glycol.
Liquid Anbesol	**Liquid**: Alcohol 70% w/v, benzocaine 6.4% w/v, phenol 0.5% w/v. Camphor, glycerin, menthol, povidone iodine.
Maximum Strength Anbesol	**Liquid**: Benzocaine 20%. Methylparaben, phenylcarbinol, polyethylene glycol, propylene glycol, saccharin.
Orajel Maximum Strength	**Liquid**. Benzocaine 20%. Ethyl alcohol 44.2% by weight, tartrazine, polythylene glycol, sodium saccharin.
Miradyne-3	**Liquid**: Benzocaine 9%. Glycerin USP, SD alcohol 388, myrrh extract, goldenseal extract.

Products listed are representative of currently available and widely distributed brands. Similar products, including regional and private label brands, may also exist.

PATIENT INFORMATION

Benzocaine Products

- Do not use any benzocaine product for longer than 7 days unless directed by a dentist or physician.
- If symptoms do not improve within 7 days, if irritation, pain, or redness persists or worsens, or if swelling, rash, or fever develops, discontinue use, and consult a dentist or physician promptly.
- Do not exceed recommended dosage.
- Consult a dentist or physician before using in children younger than 2 years of age.
- Supervise children younger than 12 years of age in the use of these products.
- Avoid contact with the eyes.
- In the event of overdose, seek professional assistance or contact a poison control center.

COMBINATION TOPICAL TOOTHACHE PRODUCTS

EUGENOL AND BENZOCAINE

▶ **Indications**

For the temporary relief of throbbing, persistent toothache pain until a dentist can be seen.

▶ **Contraindications**

History of allergy to eugenol or local anesthetics such as procaine, butacaine, benzocaine, or other "-caine" anesthetics.

▶ **Administration and Dosage**

Apply as needed and according to package directions to control symptoms.

COMBINATION TOOTHACHE PRODUCTS	
Trade name	Doseform
Dent's Double-Action Toothache Kit	**Tablets**: *Maranox Aspirin-Free Analgesic* tablets (acetaminophen 325 mg)
	Drops: *Dent's Maxi-Strength Toothache Drops* (see below)
Dent's Maxi-Strength Toothache Drops Treatment	**Drops**: Benzocaine 20%. Alcohol 74%, chlorobutanol anhydrous 0.09%, eugenol.

Products listed are representative of currently available and widely distributed brands. Similar products, including regional and private label brands, may also exist.

PATIENT INFORMATION

Combination Toothache Products

- If pain persists for longer than 10 days or redness is present, consult a dentist or physician.
- Consult a physician before using acetaminophen-containing products in children younger than 12 years of age.
- Apply drops to tooth only; avoid using product on gums.
- Do not exceed recommended dose.
- Avoid contact with eyes.

XEROSTOMIA
(Dry Mouth)

DEFINITION

Xerostomia is a condition that is referred to as dry mouth, generally caused by limited or absent salivary flow.

ETIOLOGY

The most frequent causes of xerostomia are drugs, autoimmune diseases (eg, Sjogren syndrome), and irradiation of the salivary glands. However, there are many potential causes of xerostomia:

1.) Factors affecting salivary gland function - Sjogren syndrome, obstruction/infection, salivary tumors, irradiation, cerebrovascular accident, Alzheimer disease, excision, mouth breathing, smoking.
2.) Factors affecting fluid/electrolyte balance - Vomiting, diarrhea, edema, dehydration, cardiac failure, sweating, hemorrhage.
3.) Factors affecting the salivary center - Depression, emotions (eg, fear, excitement, stress), brain tumors, Parkinson disease, drugs (morphine, levodopa).
4.) Factors affecting autonomic nervous system - Encephalitis, cerebrovascular accidents, brain tumors, neurosurgery, drugs (eg, antidepressants, antiparkinson agents, diuretics, antihistamines, antipsychotics, antihypertensives, anticholinergics, antineoplastics).

Although salivary gland function theoretically remains constant throughout life, some atrophic changes occur because of aging.

INCIDENCE

The incidence of xerostomia is more common in elderly patients. The exact incidence in this population varies, but has been reported to occur in 13% to 49% of people older than 55 years of age and in up to 60% of patients in long-term care facilities. There appears to be no significant difference in incidence between males and females.

PATHOPHYSIOLOGY

The amount of saliva produced on a daily basis is approximately 1.5 L, 99% of which is water. The submandibular glands are responsible for approximately 50%, the parotid glands for 40%, the sublingual glands for 5%, and the minor salivary glands (eg, lips, tongue, palate) for 5%. Normal functions of saliva include digestive enzymes, lubricant, antibacterial activity, buffer capacity, taste, water balance, and oral mucosa protection. Therefore, any change in saliva flow can dramatically affect these important functions and result in caries; periodontal diseases; difficulty with denture wearing, eating, and talking; altered taste sensation; and increased risk of candidiasis and mucositis. Although structure and function of salivary glands change with age, resulting in reduced salivary flow, xerostomia, more common in the elderly, is not caused by the aging process alone and is unlikely to occur unless the patient's health is compromised by one of the factors listed above (see Etiology). Therefore, the older the patient, the more likely he or she is to have one of these conditions or to be taking a medication that affects salivary flow.

SIGNS/SYMPTOMS

The complaint of dry mouth is subjective and highly individualized. Symptoms vary depending on whether or not the patient is eating. Common symptoms of xerostomia when not eating include: Dryness (often localized to tongue), increased need of water (especially during the night), rapidly developing and severe dental caries or atypical caries, gingivitis, candidiasis, speech difficulties, cracks/fissures at corners of mouth, bad breath, and sore throat. Common symptoms of xerostomia when eating include: Difficulty chewing dry food, sipping water at nearly every mouthful, difficulty swallowing, intense burning sensation after salty or spicy food, and pain localized to major, sometimes swollen, salivary glands (occurs in 30% to 60% of cases, most often unilateral).

DIAGNOSTIC PARAMETERS/PHYSICAL ASSESSMENT

Clinical Observation: Because xerostomia is caused by some underlying condition or drug therapy, observation of the condition itself is difficult. Patients must describe the symptoms they are experiencing to aid the health care professional in his or her assessment. It is likely that the patient will have been experiencing some or most of the symptoms described above. In addition, some of the physical, outward signs can often be detected (eg, cracks/fissures on corner of mouth, signs of gingivitis/caries, halitosis, speech changes).

Interview: To help the patient determine if physician referral or self-treatment is warranted, it may be beneficial to ask about the following:

- Duration and frequency of dry mouth.
- Difficulties in swallowing/sore throat.
- Difficulties in speech.
- Increased need for water, especially at night or with each mouthful of food.
- Recent teeth or gum changes.
- Bad breath.
- Intense burning sensation after salty/spicy foods.

TREATMENT

Approaches to therapy: Evaluate patients using the previous diagnostic parameters. Depending on various factors (eg, symptoms, duration, recurrence), health care providers may recommend (1.) a non-drug approach, (2.) appropriate pharmacotherapy, or (3.) immediate referral to a physician for medical evaluation. Because xerostomia is caused by some underlying condition or drug therapy, physician referral is appropriate in almost every case of suspected xerostomia.

Nondrug therapy: Most non-drug therapies are temporary in nature. These include: Avoidance of dry, spicy, or acidic foods, alcohol, and tobacco; sipping water throughout the day; sucking on ice chips or hard candy (preferably sugarless); chewing dill pickles; chewing gum (preferably sugarless); maintenance of humidified air in the home.

Pharmacotherapy: Saliva substitutes are the most common OTC agents for this condition, and usually contain some combination of carboxymethyl-cellulose and glycerin (for viscosity) and xylitol and sorbitol (for flavoring). There is some belief that evening primrose oil increases parotid and sub-mandibular flow in some patients and may be beneficial for dry mouth treatment. Consider modifying or changing the dosing schedule of drug therapy that may be causing dry mouth. Pilocarpine tablets (*Salagen*) are used for treatment of xerostomia, but are available by prescription only and have a variety of systemic adverse effects.

SALIVA SUBSTITUTES

▶ Indications
These products are used as saliva substitutes for relief of dry mouth and throat in xerostomia and hyposalivation. These products contain some combination of carboxy-methylcellulose and glycerin (for viscosity) and xylitol and sorbitol (for flavoring).

▶ Contraindications
None known.

▶ Warnings
None known.

▶ Drug Interactions
Systemic effects of these agents should be minimal.

▶ Adverse Reactions
None known.

▶ Administration and Dosage
Check individual products for specific instructions.

Solutions: Squirt or spray a small quantity into mouth as often as needed to moisten and lubricate mouth. Close container between uses.

Tablets: Allow to move around and slowly dissolve in mouth. Repeat 1 tablet per hour as necessary.

Lozenges: Allow 1 lozenge to move around and slowly dissolve in mouth. Repeat as necessary. In severe dry mouth cases, 1 lozenge per hour is recommended.

Gel: Use twice a day and at bedtime.

Entertainer's Secret: Spray into each nostril while inhaling to apply drug to upper throat.

SALIVA SUBSTITUTE PRODUCTS	
Trade name	**Doseform**
Saliva Substitute	**Solution:** Sorbitol, sodium carboxymethycellulose
Optimoist Oral Moisturizer	**Solution:** Xylitol, citric acid, hydroxyethyl cellulose, fluoride, deionized water, calcium phosphate monobasic, sodium hydroxide, sodium benzoate, aceculfame potassium, polysorbate 20, sodium monofluorophosphate
Moi-Stir, Moi-Stir Swabsticks	**Solution:** Sorbitol, sodium carboxymethylcellulose, methylparaben, propylparaben, potassium chloride, dibasic sodium phosphate, calcium chloride, magnesium chloride, sodium chloride
Entertainer's Secret	**Solution:** Carboxymethylcellulose, glycerin
Salivart Synthetic Saliva Spray	**Solution:** Sodium carboxymethylcellulose, sorbitol, sodium chloride, potassium chloride, calcium chloride dihydrate, magnesium chloride hexahydrate
Mouthkote Oral Moisturizer	**Solution:** Xylitol, sorbitol, yerba santa, citric acid, ascorbic acid, sodium benzoate, sodium saccharin
Glandosane Mouth Moisturizer	**Solution:** Sodium carboxymethylcellulose, sorbitol, sodium chloride, potassium chloride, calcium chloride dihydrate, magnesium chloride hexahydrate, dipotassium hydrogen phosphate
Salix	**Lozenges:** Sorbitol, hydroxypropyl methylcellulose, carboxymethycellulose, citric acid
Oral Balance Moisturizing	**Gel:** Glucose oxidase, lactoperoxidase, lysozyme, lactoferrin, xylitol, hydroxymethyl cellulose

Products listed are representative of currently available and widely distributed brands. Similar products, including regional and private label brands, may also exist.

PATIENT INFORMATION
Saliva Substitutes

- Use these products as directed.
- These products are not meant to cure or treat the underlying disease or condition. See a physician if the dry mouth symptoms do not subside with standard use of these products.
- Avoid dry, spicy, or acidic foods, alcohol, and tobacco.
- Sipping water throughout the day, sucking on ice chips or hard candy (preferably sugarless), chewing dill pickles, chewing gum (preferably sugarless), and maintaining humidified air in the home may be helpful in relieving dry mouth symptoms.
- Although changing the dose or frequency of medications that may cause dry mouth may be beneficial, this should not be undertaken without the guidance of a physician.
- Store at room temperature.
- Solution may be swallowed or expectorated.
- Do not drink water immediately after use.

OTIC
CONDITIONS

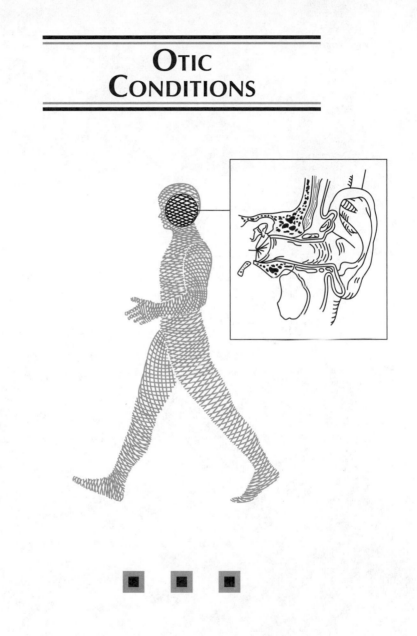

NONPRESCRIPTION DRUG THERAPY
TABLE OF CONTENTS

■ ■ ■

OTIC CONDITIONS

INTRODUCTION

The ear is composed of three major sections: The external, middle, and inner ear. The external ear includes the auricle (pinna) and the ear canal, which conveys sound into the tympanic membrane and the middle ear. The tympanic membrane, or eardrum, is a thin membrane that separates the external ear from the middle ear and is considered functionally as part of the middle ear. The middle ear also consists of the ossicles, malleus, incus, and stapes. When these bony structures are moved by the eardrum, sound waves are amplified and transmitted into the inner ear. The middle ear is connected by the eustachian tube to the nasopharynx. The eustachian tubes aid in pressure equilibrium on both sides of the eardrum. The inner ear is composed of the cochlea, a tube essential for hearing, and the vestibular apparatus, a structure that maintains balance and equilibrium. Infections can occur in each section of the ear and can occur in 3% to 10% of the population.

Afflictions of the outer ear, often causing discomfort and pain, are very common. Most otic conditions are minor and easily treatable. If left untreated, however, serious complications may arise. It is very important that patients realize that safe and effective nonprescription treatments for the ear are available; however, these treatments are restricted to those conditions relating to the external ear. In such cases, OTC products can be used effectively to help the body's normal defenses and improve/restore the external ear canal environment. With the rapid rise in the cost of health care and a more informed public, many patients now self-medicate. Patients often question when an OTC product is appropriate and which one to select for their particular condition.

Earwax buildup or cerumen impaction is the most common disorder affecting the outer ear. Patients often try to manage excessive earwax accumulation on their own; however, patients need to be educated about not putting any object, including matches, bobby pins, or cotton applicators, into the ear canal. Many external otitis conditions are caused by objects such as cotton applicators that push the wax further into the ear, resulting in impaction, or that scratch and puncture the epithelial lining of the ear canal. If cerumen impaction occurs, proper earwax removal systems are advised and are available for OTC use.

If symptoms such as itching, ear pain, and feeling of fullness in the ear develop, suspect an external ear infection (otitis externa), such as swimmer's ear. If the pain is sharp and knife-like or intolerable, consult a physician. As long as the symptoms have started within the last day or so and are limited to itching, a feeling of fullness, and mild discomfort, OTC products can be used to irrigate the ear and to acidify and dry the ear. Instruct patients on how to properly irrigate the ear and on how to instill ear preparations (drops and ointments).

Educate patients on preventive measures. Use of drying agents, such as alcohol- or glyerin-containing products after swimming, bathing, or showering will help remove excess moisture in the ears that can lead to an infection. Earplugs can be used to prevent water from entering the ear canal during swimming. Good management of seborrhea or dandruff can also aid in preventing the onset of an infection. Warn children with tympanostomy tubes to avoid diving, deep underwater swimming, and swimming in unchlorinated pools or ponds.

Pharmacists can provide a valuable service by identifying and recommending treatments that are for a wide variety of ear afflictions such as earaches, impacted earwax, and otic itching and irritation secondary to an infection. Before recommending an OTC product, pharmacists should be able to recognize potentially serious otic problems requiring physician referral and patient-specific conditions such as diabetes or immunosuppression that would also necessitate a physician referral. The pharmacist can also be key in advising on prevention of recurring problems and in instructing the patient on how to administer the otic products.

CERUMEN IMPACTION

DEFINITION

The outer ear canal has self-cleansing properties. The squamous epithelium from the eardrum migrates to the external area of the ear naturally, but this process is sensitive to various physical and environmental factors. Movement of the jaw by chewing aids in the migratory process.

Cerumen, or earwax, is a secretory product formed by glands in the external ear canal. Cerumen protects the ear canal by trapping dust, insects, and miscellaneous particles that can lead to infection. Cerumen is acidic and oily; these factors aid in keeping the ear canal water-resistant. It also contains various anti-infective substances.

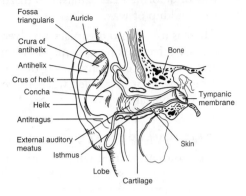

Figure 1. Anatomy of the Ear

Excessive accumulation of earwax can cause discomfort, pruritus, temporary hearing loss, and vertigo. Water and bacteria or fungi trapped behind excessive accumulations of cerumen can cause an ear infection. The cerumen needs to be removed if any of these symptoms occur.

ETIOLOGY

There are several causes of cerumen impaction, including the following:
1.) An overactive ceruminous gland may produce excessive cerumen.
2.) The ear canal may be abnormally narrow, interfering with the normal outward migration of epithelial tissue and cerumen.
3.) Abnormal cerumen may be either drier or softer than normal cerumen and may interfere with normal migration of epithelial cells.

When water enters the ears from swimming or bathing, it can sometimes cause sudden hearing loss. This may be caused by water trapped behind the earwax.

Cerumen can be pushed deeper into the ear canal when attempts are made to remove the earwax with devices such as cotton swabs, bobby pins, or matchsticks. At times, hair located in the ear canal will mix with the earwax and form a matted material that occludes the canal. This blocks the normal, natural migration and elimination process.

INCIDENCE

Cerumen impaction is a common disorder of the external auditory canal. Cerumen impaction occurs in approximately 2% to 6% of healthy adults.

PATHOPHYSIOLOGY

A variety of factors, such as improper attempts to remove the earwax, or narrow or deformed ear canals, can disrupt the self-cleansing process and lead to a buildup of wax.

There is usually no organism involved in cerumen impaction. However, a secondary infectious process may develop, and is usually accompanied by pain and fever if the epithelial lining of the ear is damaged by poking or prodding to remove wax, or if trapped water macerates the skin and fissures form, leading to a portal for infection. (See Swimmer's Ear and Otitis Externa monographs.)

SIGNS/SYMPTOMS

Symptoms associated with cerumen impaction are mild-to-severe discomfort, pruritus, pain, tinnitus, and hearing loss. Dizziness or motion sickness may occur. These symptoms can be present in one or both ears.

DIAGNOSTIC PARAMETERS/PHYSICAL ASSESSMENT

Clinical Observation: The diagnosis of cerumen impaction is usually based on specific complaints by the patient, including hearing loss, tinnitus, discomfort, and dizziness or motion sickness. Previous experience with this condition may help aid the proper diagnosis as well.

Interview: To ensure the proper diagnosis and treatment, it may be beneficial to ask the patient about the following:

- Description of symptoms, especially hearing loss, pain, or tinnitus.
- Nature of ear discharge (if any)—does it have a bad odor or unusual appearance?
- Duration of condition.
- Attempts to treat the condition.
- Previous experience with cerumen impaction.
- Presence of fever.
- Any recent ear injuries.
- Recent use of a cotton swab or other device (eg, bobby pin) in the ear.
- Recent exposure to water (eg, bathing or swimming).

TREATMENT

Approaches to therapy: An ideal approach is to help the patient avoid cerumen impaction in the future.

For general prevention of cerumen impaction, patients may be instructed to follow these guidelines:

1.) Do not put any foreign objects in the ear (eg, bobby pins, matches, toothpicks, pencils) that are not specifically designed for insertion into the ear.
2.) Remove earwax only when it is in the outer part of the external ear canal, using a warm, soapy washcloth that has been wrung out.
3.) Apply 2 to 3 drops of alcohol, glycerin, or alcohol-acetic acid solution in the proper concentration to ears after swimming, bathing, or showering to help remove excess moisture in the ears. (See Swimmer's Ear monograph.)

For current conditions, it may be best to recommend a pharmacotherapeutic approach; however, a physician referral may be appropriate if the condition is severe or if OTC therapy is ineffective.

Nondrug therapy: Prevention of cerumen impaction is the best approach. (See Approaches to Therapy.)

Pharmacotherapy: Earwax softening agents help soften and loosen the earwax; however, these agents do not remove the earwax. After using the earwax softening agents for 3 to 4 days, the earwax can be removed by rinsing the ear with an ear syringe using warm water or an irrigation solution for the ear. If pain or dizziness is present or if the earwax is not readily removed, consult a physician. Instruct patients to follow the directions for applying ear drops.

EARWAX SOFTENING AGENTS

CARBAMIDE PEROXIDE

▶ Actions

Mechanically removes debris and softens earwax through effervescence caused by nascent oxygen release.

These agents aid in softening, lubricating, and facilitating the elimination of earwax and other debris.

▶ Indications

Earwax softener and cleansing agent.

▶ Contraindications

Do not use if ear drainage, dizziness, or pain is present; do not use if the eardrum is injured or perforated, or if ear surgery was performed within the past 6 weeks. Do not use if a hypersensitivity reaction occurs with carbamide peroxide use.

▶ Warnings

Discontinue use if rash or irritation develops.

▶ Administration and Dosage

Warm the carbamide peroxide to body temperature by holding the bottle in the hands for several minutes. Place 5 to 10 drops (or enough to fill the ear canal) into affected ear twice daily. Allow the ear drops to remain in the ear for 15 minutes or more. See directions for instilling ear drops in Appendix D, Administration Techniques. Maximum use: 4 consecutive days. If there is no relief within 3 to 4 days, contact a physician. When the head is repositioned, have a tissue available to catch drainage from the ear.

OLIVE OIL ("SWEET OIL")

▶ Actions

Softens earwax.

▶ Contraindications

Hypersensitivity reaction to olive oil.

▶ Warnings

Discontinue use if rash or irritation develops.

▶ **Administration and Dosage**

Warm the olive oil to body temperature by holding the bottle in the hands for several minutes. Place 5 drops (or enough to fill the ear canal) into affected ear twice daily and allow drops to remain in the affected ear for several minutes. See directions for instilling ear drops in Appendix D, Administration Techniques. When the head is repositioned, have a tissue available to catch drainage from the ear.

LIGHT MINERAL OIL (BABY OIL)

▶ **Actions**

Emollient properties; softens earwax.

▶ **Indications**

Earwax softener.

▶ **Contraindications**

Hypersensitivity reaction to mineral oil.

▶ **Warnings**

Discontinue use if rash or irritation develops.

▶ **Drug Interactions**

None with otic use.

▶ **Administration and Dosage**

After filling an ear dropper with mineral oil, warm the ear dropper by holding the dropper in dry, clean hands for several minutes. Place 5 to 10 drops (or enough to fill the ear canal) into affected ear twice daily. Allow ear drops to remain in the ear for several minutes. See directions for instilling ear drops in Appendix D, Administration Techniques. When the head is repositioned, have a tissue available to catch drainage from the ear.

ANHYDROUS GLYCERIN

▶ **Actions**

Its hygroscopic properties aid in softening, lubricating, and facilitating the elimination of earwax. It also helps reduce moisture in the ear.

▶ **Indications**

Earwax softener.

▶ **Contraindications**

Hypersensitivity reaction to glycerin.

▶ **Warnings**

Discontinue use if rash or irritation develops.

▶ **Administration and Dosage**

Never use alone. Use with other products such as alcohol, carbamide peroxide, or other OTC otic preparations, as directed. Do not rinse ear dropper with water because water dilutes glycerin, making it less effective.

IRRIGATION SOLUTIONS FOR THE EAR

3% HYDROGEN PEROXIDE

▶ **Actions**

Aids in softening earwax and facilitates its removal from the ear.

Irrigation solutions are used after an earwax softening agent has been used for 3 to 4 days and if further earwax removal is necessary. These solutions aid in softening the earwax and facilitate its removal from the ear. Irrigation solutions may simply be warm water or a hydrogen peroxide solution at body temperature.

▶ **Indications**

Earwax softener; cleansing agent.

▶ **Contraindications**

Hypersensitivity reaction to hydrogen peroxide.

▶ **Warnings**

Discontinue use if rash or irritation develops. Do not use solutions if there is moderate-to-severe pain or if dizziness is present. If the earwax is not readily removed, consult a physician. Do not use these solutions on a chronic basis because this can lead to maceration of the epithelial tissue and a portal for infection.

▶ **Administration and Dosage**

Dilute 3% hydrogen peroxide with an equal amount of warm water (½ pint of each ingredient). Mix well. Follow directions for using an ear syringe in Appendix D, Administration Techniques.

2.5% ACETIC ACID SOLUTION (VINEGAR & WATER)

▶ **Actions**

Aids in softening earwax and facilitates its removal from the ear.

▶ **Indications**

Cleansing agent; acidifying agent.

▶ **Contraindications**

Hypersensitivity reaction to acetic acid or vinegar.

▶ **Warnings**

Discontinue use if rash or irritation develops. Do not use acetic acid solution routinely because it can lead to maceration or softening of the epithelial tissue, which can lead to an infection.

▶ **Administration and Dosage**

Dilute household vinegar (5% acetic acid) with an equal amount of warm water (½ pint of each ingredient). Mix well. Make a fresh solution prior to each irrigation. Discard unused solution. Follow directions for using an ear syringe in Appendix D, Administration Techniques.

Note: May combine vinegar with 70% isopropyl alcohol (preferred), 70% ethyl alcohol, propylene glycol, or glycerin instead of water. Higher alcohol concentrations increase the drying effect but may cause a burning sensation; lower alcohol concentrations reduce the burning sensation.

NONPRESCRIPTION EARWAX REMOVAL PRODUCTS

▶ **Administration and Dosage**

These products come with instructions and an ear dropper. They offer a combination of products that aid in earwax removal. Any earwax remaining after use of these products can then be removed by gently flushing with warm water with a soft rubber bulb ear syringe. Follow directions for using an ear syringe in Appendix D, Administration Techniques.

Refer to labeling for guidelines on individual products.

EARWAX REMOVAL PRODUCTS	
Trade name	Doseform
Debrox	**Drops**: 6.5% carbamide peroxide, glycerin, propylene glycol, sodium stannate
	Dose: Instill 5 to 10 drops twice daily for up to 4 days.
Murine Ear	**Drops**: 6.5% carbamide peroxide, 6.3% alcohol, glycerin, polysorbate 20
	Dose: Instill 5 to 10 drops twice daily for up to 4 days.
Auro Ear Drops, Aurocaine Ear Wax Removal Aid	**Drops**: 6.5% carbamide peroxide in an anhydrous glycerin base
	Dose: Instill 5 to 10 drops twice daily for up to 4 days.
E•R•O Ear Drops, Mollifene Ear Wax Removal Aid, Bausch & Lomb Earwax Removal System	**Drops**: 6.5% carbamide peroxide, anhydrous glycerin. *Mollifene* also contains propylene glycol and sodium stannate.
	Dose: Instill 5 to 10 drops twice daily for up to 4 days.

Products listed are representative of currently available and widely distributed brands. Similar products, including regional and private label brands, may also exist.

PATIENT INFORMATION

Earwax Removal Preparations

• Patient instructions accompany each product. Read these instructions carefully before use, preferably before leaving the pharmacy, in case of any questions.
• If burning or itching occurs or persists after use, contact a physician.
• Do not use if ear drainage, dizziness, or pain is present, or if you have injured your eardrum or undergone ear surgery within the past 6 weeks.
• Discontinue use if rash or irritation develops.
• If earwax is not readily removed with these preparations, consult a physician.

OTITIS EXTERNA

DEFINITION

Otitis externa refers to inflammation in the external ear canal. Otitis externa can be categorized into several different types: Inflammatory otitis externa, fungal otitis externa, eczematoid otitis externa, and seborrheic otitis externa. Inflammatory otitis externa can be further subdivided into swimmer's ear and acute localized external otitis. Swimmer's ear is a common type of otitis externa (see Swimmer's Ear monograph). Another type of otitis externa is necrotizing external otitis. It occurs primarily in diabetic and immunocompromised patients. Because of the potential for serious complications, refer a suspected ear infection in a diabetic or immunocompromised patient to a doctor immediately.

ETIOLOGY

Inflammatory otitis externa/Acute localized external otitis: An infection associated with a furuncle formation over a hair follicle. No OTC treatment is appropriate; therefore, this infection will be presented as an overview so that it can be differentiated from the other types of otitis externa and the patient referred to a physician. (See Swimmer's Ear monograph.)

Necrotizing otitis externa: Consult a physician. Usually associated with diabetic or immunocompromised patients. No OTC treatment is appropriate; therefore, this infection will not be discussed. Refer all diabetic or immunosuppressed patients with ear inflammation to a physician for diagnosis and treatment.

Fungal otitis externa: A fungal infection of the external ear canal.

Eczematoid otitis externa: Hypersensitivity of the external ear canal skin resulting in lesions.

Seborrheic otitis externa: Ear inflammation associated with the presence of seborrheic dermatitis.

INCIDENCE

Otitis externa occurs in 3% to 10% of the patient population.

PATHOPHYSIOLOGY

Inflammatory otitis externa: Acute localized external otitis is an infection of the hair follicles that forms furuncles. Furuncles are usually caused by a staphylococcal infection. Occasionally, a furuncle can form in a sebaceous gland. This gland can become blocked, leading to swelling, possible occlusion of the ear canal, and possible inoculation of bacteria into the ear canal.

Fungal otitis externa: Chronic diffuse external otitis resulting from a fungal infection. The fungi most commonly involved are *Aspergillus niger, Actinomyces,* or yeast. This infection often occurs secondary to an underlying bacterial infection, and may also occur as a result of prolonged topical antibiotic use. Susceptible patients include those whose ear canals are chronically exposed to moisture, those who wear hearing aids, the immunocompromised, those who have had mastoidectomies, and those receiving topical antibiotics. These situations provide an environment promoting fungal growth via chronic exposure to moisture that can lead to maceration of the epithelium lining the ear canal. This can lead to the development of fissures, especially in patients who use foreign objects (eg, bobby pins) to scratch the inside of the external ear canal secondary to pruritus. Fissures provide a portal of entry for fungi that are the normal flora of the ear. The fungi then enter into a fertile environment where they can proliferate. The infection may perforate the eardrum and spread into the middle ear.

Eczematoid otitis externa: Inflammation of the external ear canal resulting from a hypersensitivity reaction can result from many dermatologic conditions, such as atopic dermatitis, contact dermatitis, psoriasis, and lupus. These dermatologic conditions can cause fissures, vesicles, oozing, and urticaria in the external ear canal. Note that any nonprescription otic product, if used for longer than 10 days, may produce an eczematoid external otitis. The condition can lead to inflammatory otitis externa caused by breaks in the skin, thus providing portals of entry for pathogenic organisms.

Seborrheic otitis externa: An external ear canal inflammation resulting from seborrheic areas near the ear, such as the scalp. Seborrheic lesions are found in and on the ear and result in pruritus. Etiology is unknown for seborrhea. Seborrheic otitis externa is primarily recurrent rather than continually present. The condition may lead to inflammatory otitis externa because breaks in the skin provide portals of entry for pathogenic organisms.

SIGNS/SYMPTOMS

Inflammatory otitis externa/Acute localized external otitis: Inflamed, erythematous, raised lesion(s) or pustule(s) present in the ear canal. Pain is usually severe and without discharge, unless an abscess ruptures. (See Swimmer's Ear monograph.)

Fungal otitis externa: Pruritus is the most common early symptom, followed in a day or two by otorrhea. Systemic symptoms are only seen in severe cases. Pain, if any, occurs when chewing or manipulating the ear. Physical exam reveals mild erythema and edema in the ear canal. Fungal growth presents as white, black, gray, bluish green, or yellow exudate.

Eczematoid external otitis: Eczema-like skin conditions, such as erythema, edema, and crusting are present in and around the ear canal. Vesicles, fissures, and otorrhea may also be present. Pruritus is present, whereas pain is usually not a problem.

Seborrheic external otitis: Areas of yellowish, greasy scales can be found on the skin lining the external ear and ear canal. The ear canal is generally not erythematous. Pruritus is present. The surrounding scalp area often reveals seborrheic lesions and flaking. Patients often correlate the pruritus with dry skin rather than secondary to seborrhea.

DIAGNOSTIC PARAMETERS/PHYSICAL ASSESSMENT

Interview: To aid in the diagnosis and proper treatment of otitis externa, it may be beneficial to ask about the following:

- Patient's medical history. If patient is diabetic or immunosuppressed, refer to a physician.
- Any contraindications to the use of an NSAID (eg, history/presence of ulcer, GI bleeding, uncontrolled or severe hypertension, renal dysfunction, taking an ACE inhibitor, taking an anticoagulant such as warfarin, fluid-restricted).
- Current medication profile (ask specifically about antibiotics).
- OTC products (if any) used for otitis externa in the past (including medication for the pain). Also, duration and success of therapy.
- The patient's drug allergies.
- Signs and symptoms that the patient is experiencing. Consider OTC treatment in the case of pruritus, mild-to-moderate pain, or recent onset of symptoms. Refer the patient to a physician in the following cases: Knife-like pain; steady pain; systemic symptoms (eg, chills, fever, sore throat); hearing loss.
- What led to this ear infection (eg, patient put a foreign object in the affected ear[s] recently, used a wax removal kit, had recurring exposure to moisture/water activity, has a history of furuncles, or has the observed presence of dandruff or eczema).

Once the above issues have been addressed, decide whether the patient can be treated with a nonprescription product or if the patient should be referred to a physician. Always advise patients to seek medical attention immediately if symptoms worsen or if hearing loss, systemic symptoms, or severe knife-like pain occurs.

With mild cases of otitis externa, topical nonprescription medications can be used as alternatives to antibiotics and antifungals.

TREATMENT

Approaches to therapy: For general prevention of otitis externa, patients may be instructed to follow these general guidelines:

- Do not put any foreign objects into the ear (eg, bobby pins, matches, toothpicks, pencils) that are not specifically designed for insertion into the ear.
- Remove earwax only when it is in the outer part of the ear canal, using a warm, soapy wash cloth that has been wrung out.
- Applying 2 to 3 drops of alcohol, glycerin, or alcohol-acetic acid solutions to ears after swimming, bathing, or showering will help remove excess moisture in the ears and may help prevent swimmer's ear.
- Keep the ear as dry as possible for 6 weeks or longer after the ear infection has subsided.
- Whenever any medication is obtained, it should be completely understood how the medication should be given (ie, taken orally or put in the ear). Many patients think that during an ear infection all medications should be applied directly into the ear, which in many cases is not true. If there is any question as to how the medication should be taken, consult a pharmacist or physician.

- As with all medications, keep these agents out of children's reach. Only adults should administer these agents or treatments.
- Earplugs: Water-tight or molded earplugs or even swim caps may help prevent water from entering the ear canal. This can be very helpful when the ear is to be kept dry for 6 weeks or longer after the ear infection has subsided. Avoid diving and deep underwater swimming.
- Prophylactic advice for children with tympanostomy tubes: Patients with tympanostomy tubes (tubes in the ears) should avoid diving and deep underwater swimming, swimming in ponds (swimming holes), and submerging the head into bath water to rinse off shampoos. It is highly recommended that scuba diving be prohibited.

Nondrug therapy: Warming the ear canal with a blow dryer on a low setting can aid in drying of the ear canal and can be soothing to the patient. Use caution by touching the ear frequently to avoid overheating the area and hurting the patient if someone else is applying the blow dryer to the patient's ear(s). Application of heat locally using a hot pack, hot water bottle, or heating pad is often helpful in reducing discomfort.

Pharmacotherapy: Treat otitis externa as soon as possible to prevent development and spread of infection. Before any treatment is recommended, it is advised that the interview questions above be addressed.

Each of the various types of otitis externa requires a specific treatment regimen. In most variations of this condition, hydrogen peroxide, acidifying agents, drying agents, and medicated shampoos (not appropriate for fungal external otitis) are the initial nonprescription treatment agents. See nonprescription treatment recommendations for the various types of otitis externa below.

In certain cases (eg, acute localized external otitis, persistent pruritus, or initial treatment failure), physician referral is warranted.

Note – Instructions for using an ear syringe and instilling ear drops are in Appendix D, Administration Techniques.

Inflammatory Otitis Externa –
- *Acute localized external otitis:* Refer patient to a physician.
- *Swimmer's ear:* See Swimmer's Ear monograph.

Fungal Otitis Externa – Irrigate the affected ear with hydrogen peroxide, then use an otic acidifying agent or antifungal topical ear drops (eg, gentian violet, thimerosal). Once inflammation in the ear has diminished, a drying agent can be used. If a drying agent causes burning or pain upon application, the inflammation has not subsided enough to use these agents. It is important to remove the offending agent (if applicable). If severe pruritus is present and does not improve after initial treatment, use an antipruritic agent that contains hydrocortisone.

Eczematoid Otitis Externa – Irrigate the affected ear with hydrogen peroxide, then use an otic acidifying agent. Use a warm washcloth containing a medicated shampoo (refer to the Dandruff and Seborrheic Dermatitis monographs in the Dermatological Conditions chapter for complete information on these products) to remove any scaling skin around the ear. Once the inflammation in the ear has diminished, a drying agent can be used. If a drying agent causes burning or pain upon application, the inflammation has not subsided enough to use these agents. It is important to remove any offending agent, if known and possible, and to manage the underlying dermatologic condition. If necessary to relieve pruritus, use hydrocortisone otic drops for inflammation in the ear canal and hydrocortisone cream for external ear lesions. Oral antihistamines may also be effective.

> *Prevention:* Patients should avoid any irritants that cause or aggravate the eczema such as soaps, shampoos, and cosmetics. Patients may use the drying agents as needed to avoid inflammation.

Seborrheic Otitis Externa – Irrigate the affected ear with hydrogen peroxide, and follow with an otic acidifying agent. Once the inflammation in the ear has diminished, a drying agent can be used. If a drying agent causes burning or pain upon application, the inflammation has not subsided enough to use these agents. Controlling seborrhea is important, not only in the treatment phase, but also in the prevention of recurrent seborrheic external otitis. Various medicated shampoos are available for seborrhea, such as shampoos containing selenium sulfide, pyrithione zinc, sulfur with salicylic acid, and coal tar. These products may be used directly on the lesions. Patients should shampoo with one of these products daily during the flare-up, and then use 2 to 3 times per week as a preventive measure. Allow the shampoo to enter the ear canal using a warm wash cloth and try to gently remove any debris. Patients should avoid oily hair rinses or tonics. Gentian violet can be used in the ear canal as an astringent. If severe pruritus is present and does not improve after initial treatment, a topical antipruritic agent may be used that contains hydrocortisone.

> *Prevention:* Control the seborrheic dermatitis with medicated shampoos, applied directly to all seborrheic areas 2 to 3 times weekly after the inflammation has subsided. (See the Seborrheic Dermatitis monograph in the Dermatological Conditions chapter for detailed information on this condition.)

THIMEROSAL SOLUTION/TINCTURE (49% MERCURY)

▶ **Actions**

An antiseptic with sustained fungistatic and bacteriostatic activity against common pathogens.

▶ **Indications**

Topical antifungal agent.

▶ **Contraindications**

Hypersensitivity to thimerosal or mercury.

▶ **Warnings**

Avoid contact with eyes.

Prolonged/Repeated use: Frequent or prolonged use may cause serious mercury poisoning.

Incompatibilities: Thimerosal is incompatible with strong acids, salts of heavy metals, potassium permanganate, and iodine; do not use in combination with or immediately following their application.

Discontinue use and consult physician if redness, swelling, pain, infection, rash, or irritation persists or increases.

▶ Drug Interactions

Do not use in combination with strong acids, salts of heavy metals, potassium permanganate, and iodine.

▶ Overdosage

In case of ingestion of the tincture, consider alcohol and acetone content. Treatment includes supportive therapy; refer to General Management of Acute Overdosage.

▶ Administration and Dosage

Apply enough solution to fill the ear canal 2 to 3 times daily for 1 week. Follow directions for irrigating the external ear canal in Appendix D, Administration Techniques. After applying the drops, hold a tissue to the ear to catch run-off when head position is changed. Allow the solution to dry and remain in the ear canal. If symptoms worsen or do not improve, consult a physician. Avoid contact with clothing, because thimerosal may stain some fabrics.

THIMEROSAL PRODUCTS	
Trade name	**Doseform**
Mersol	**Tincture:** 1:1000. 50% alcohol. Red or colorless.
Aeroaid	**Antiseptic spray:** 1:1000. 72% alcohol.

Products listed are representative of currently available and widely distributed brands. Similar products, including regional and private label brands, may also exist.

PATIENT INFORMATION

Thimerosal

- Patient instructions accompany each product. Read these instructions carefully before use, preferably before leaving the pharmacy, in case of any questions.
- Not for prolonged use.
- Discontinue use and consult physician if rash or irritation persists or worsens.

IRRIGATION SOLUTIONS FOR THE EAR

▶ Actions

Gentle rinsing of the ear will help rid the ear of bacteria, fungi, and debris, as well as assist in reestablishing an environment that does not promote bacterial/fungal growth.

3% HYDROGEN PEROXIDE SOLUTION

▶ Actions

Aids in the softening of earwax and facilitates its removal from the ear.

▶ Indications

Earwax softener; cleansing agent.

► **Contraindications**

Hypersensitivity reaction to hydrogen peroxide.

► **Warnings**

Discontinue use if a rash or irritation develops. Do not use hydrogen peroxide routinely because it can lead to maceration or softening of the epithelial tissue, which can lead to an infection.

► **Drug Interactions**

None with otic use.

► **Administration and Dosage**

Dilute 3% hydrogen peroxide with an equal amount of warm water (½ pint of each ingredient). Mix well. Follow directions for irrigating the external ear canal in Appendix D, Administration Techniques.

2.5% ACETIC ACID SOLUTION (VINEGAR & WATER)

► **Actions**

Aids in the softening of earwax and facilitates its removal from the ear.

► **Indications**

Cleansing agent; acidifying agent.

► **Contraindications**

Hypersensitivity reaction to acetic acid or vinegar.

► **Warnings**

Discontinue use if a rash or irritation develops. Do not use acetic acid solution routinely because it can lead to maceration or softening of the epithelial tissue, which can lead to an infection.

► **Drug Interactions**

None with otic use.

► **Administration and Dosage**

Dilute household vinegar (5% acetic acid) with an equal amount of warm water (½ pint of each ingredient). Mix well. Follow directions for irrigating the ear in Appendix D, Administration Techniques. Make a fresh solution prior to each irrigation. Discard unused solution.

Note: May substitute 70% isopropyl alcohol (preferred), 70% ethyl alcohol, propylene glycol, or glycerin instead of water to be combined with the vinegar. Higher alcohol concentrations increase the drying effect but may cause a burning sensation; lower alcohol concentrations reduce the burning sensation.

ASTRINGENT AGENTS

ALUMINUM ACETATE SOLUTION ("BUROW'S SOLUTION")

► **Actions**

Acts as an astringent (drying agent) that creates an environment hostile to bacterial and fungal growth.

► **Indications**

To help alleviate the pain, inflammation, and pruritus associated with otitis externa.

In mild cases of otitis externa, these agents can be used as alternatives to antibiotics.

► **Contraindications**

Hypersensitivity reaction to aluminum acetate.

► **Warnings**

Discontinue use if rash or irritation develops. Do not use to treat otitis externa on a chronic basis. If itching, inflammation, or pain persists after 3 to 4 days or worsens, contact a physician.

► **Administration and Dosage**

For most products, place 2 to 3 drops (or enough drops to fill the ear canal) into the affected ear(s) every 2 to 3 hours while awake, keeping head tilted to the side. Follow directions for irrigating the external ear canal in Appendix D, Administration Techniques. Allow the drops to remain in the ear canal and allow the solution to contact as much of the surface area of the ear as possible before straightening the head. Use until the pain and inflammation subsides, then as needed for itching. May use as a prophylactic agent: 2 drops into each ear after exposure to water.

ALUMINUM ACETATE SOLUTION PRODUCTS	
Trade name	Doseform
Buro-Sol	**Powder**: 0.23% aluminum acetate. One packet placed in a pint of water produces a modified Burow's Solution.
Bluboro Powder, Boropak Powder, Domeboro Powder and Tablets	**Powder, tablets**: Aluminum sulfate and calcium acetate. One packet or tablet placed in a pint of water produces a modified 1:40 Burow's Solution.
Star-Otic	**Solution**: Nonaqueous acetic acid, Burow's Solution, boric acid, propylene glycol

Products listed are representative of currently available and widely distributed brands. Similar products, including regional and private label brands, may also exist.

PATIENT INFORMATION

Aluminum Acetate Solution

- Patient instructions accompany each product. Read these instructions carefully before use, preferably before leaving the pharmacy, in case of any questions.
- If condition worsens or symptoms persist after 3 to 4 days, discontinue use of the product and consult a physician.
- For external use only. Avoid contact with the eyes.

ACIDIFYING/DRYING AGENTS

► **Indications**

Treatment of otitis externa also should include agents that aid in removing excess moisture from the ear. Keeping the ear dry will provide a less desirable environment for bacteria, preventing reinfection. Once the inflammation in the ear has diminished, a drying agent can be used. If a drying agent causes burning or pain upon application, the inflammation has not subsided enough to use these agents. These agents can also be used as prophylactic therapy. Usually 1 to 2 drops in each ear after water exposure (eg, swimming, showering) is sufficient.

2.5% ACETIC ACID IN 70% ALCOHOL

► Actions

Equal parts of household vinegar (5% acetic acid) and 70% isopropyl or ethyl alcohol provides an acidic environment that restores the ear canal to its normal pH, which is antibacterial and antifungal. It also acts as an astringent and drying agent.

► Indications

To help alleviate the pain and inflammation associated with swimmer's ear. May also be used prophylactically against otitis externa after swimming.

► Contraindications

Hypersensitivity reaction to acetic acid or alcohol.

► Warnings

Discontinue use if rash or irritation develops. Do not use to treat otitis externa on a chronic basis. If itching, inflammation, or pain persists after 3 to 4 days or worsens, contact a physician.

► Administration and Dosage

Place 2 to 3 drops (or enough drops to fill the ear canal) into the affected ear(s) every 2 to 3 hours, keeping head tilted to the side. Follow directions for irrigating the external ear canal in Appendix D, Administration Techniques. Allow the drops to remain in the ear canal and allow the solution to contact as much of the surface area of the ear as possible before straightening the head. Use until the pain and inflammation subsides, then as needed for itching. May use as a prophylactic agent: 2 drops into each ear after exposure to water.

BORIC ACID 2.75% IN ISOPROPYL ALCOHOL

► Actions

Provides an acidic environment that restores the ear canal to its normal pH, which is antibacterial and antifungal. It also acts as an astringent and drying agent.

► Indications

Helps alleviate the pain and inflammation associated with otitis externa.

► Contraindications

Hypersensitivity reaction to boric acid or isopropyl alcohol.

► Warnings

Discontinue use if rash or irritation develops. Do not use to treat otitis externa on a chronic basis. If itching, inflammation, or pain persists after 3 to 4 days or worsens, contact a physician.

► Drug Interactions

None with otic use.

► Administration and Dosage

Place 2 to 3 drops (or enough drops to fill the ear canal) into the affected ear(s) every 2 to 3 hours, keeping head tilted to the side. Follow directions for irrigating the external ear canal in Appendix D, Administration Techniques. Allow the drops to remain in the ear canal and allow the solution to contact as much of the surface area of the ear as possible before straightening the head. Use until the pain and inflammation subsides, then as needed for itching. May use as a prophylactic agent: 2 to 3 drops (or enough drops to fill the ear canal) into each ear after exposure to water.

BORIC ACID PRODUCTS	
Trade name	Doseform
Aurocaine2	**Liquid**: 97.25% isopropyl alcohol and boric acid

Products listed are representative of currently available and widely distributed brands. Similar products, including regional and private label brands, may also exist.

PROPYLENE GLYCOL/ANHYDROUS GLYCERIN/ISOPROPYL ALCOHOL

▶ **Actions**

These agents extract moisture from the ear canal.

▶ **Indications**

Drying agent.

▶ **Contraindications**

Hypersensitivity reaction to propylene glycol, anhydrous glycerin, or isopropyl alcohol.

▶ **Warnings**

Discontinue use if rash or irritation develops. Do not use if burning occurs upon application.

▶ **Administration and Dosage**

Follow instructions for individual products. For most products, instill 4 to 6 drops (or enough drops to fill the ear canal) in affected ear twice daily for 4 to 6 days. Refer to the directions for irrigating the external ear canal in Appendix D, Administration Techniques. May use 2 drops in each ear after exposure to water on a chronic basis to aid in preventing the onset of swimmer's ear.

EAR DRYING PRODUCTS	
Trade name	Doseform
Ear-Dry, Swim-Ear	**Liquid**: 95% isopropyl alcohol, 5% anhydrous glycerin
Dri/Ear	**Liquid**: 95% isopropyl alcohol, 5% glycerin
Auro-Dri	**Liquid**: 95% isopropyl alcohol in anhydrous glycerin

Products listed are representative of currently available and widely distributed brands. Similar products, including regional and private label brands, may also exist.

PATIENT INFORMATION

Ear Acidifying/Drying Products

- Patient instructions accompany each product. Read these instructions carefully before use, preferably before leaving the pharmacy, in case of any questions.
- For external use only; avoid contact with eyes.
- Do not use on mucous membranes or broken skin.
- Do not use these products if you have a history of hypersensitivity reactions to alcohol.
- Do not use if ear drainage, dizziness, or pain is present, or if you have injured your eardrum.
- Discontinue use and consult a physician if irritation persists or worsens.

ANTIPRURITIC THERAPY

OTIC HYDROCORTISONE PREPARATIONS

► Actions

Reduces inflammation associated with an ear infection and helps dry the ear.

Ear drops containing hydrocortisone will help alleviate the pruritus associated with otitis externa.

► Indications

To relieve itching associated with ear inflammation.

► Contraindications

Hypersensitivity reaction to hydrocortisone or other topical steroids, alcohol, or propylene glycol.

► Warnings

Do not use in children younger than 2 years of age.

For external use only. Avoid contact with eyes.

Discontinue use if a rash or irritation develops. Do not use on a chronic basis. If itching persists after 3 to 4 days, contact a physician.

► Drug Interactions

None with otic use.

► Administration and Dosage

Place 4 to 6 drops (or enough drops to fill the ear canal) into affected ear(s) not more than 3 to 4 times daily. See individual product labeling for guidelines. Follow directions for irrigating the external ear canal in Appendix D, Administration Techniques.

OTIC HYDROCORTISONE PRODUCTS	
Trade name	Doseform
EarSol-HC	Solution: 1% hydrocortisone. 44% alcohol, propylene glycol.

Products listed are representative of currently available and widely distributed brands. Similar products, including regional and private label brands, may also exist.

PATIENT INFORMATION

Otic Hydrocortisone

- Patient instructions accompany each product. Read these instructions carefully before use, preferably before leaving the pharmacy, in case of any questions.
- Do not use in children younger than 2 years of age.
- For external use only. Avoid contact with eyes.
- If condition worsens or if symptoms persist after 4 days, discontinue use and consult a physician.

SWIMMER'S EAR

DEFINITION

Swimmer's ear, or acute diffuse otitis externa, refers to an infection in the external auditory canal. This infection can be caused by bacteria or fungi. Swimmer's ear is a very common infection that occurs in people of all ages and both sexes. It occurs more frequently in the summer months.

ETIOLOGY

Moisture, heat, and humidity can lead to swelling of the stratum corneum, which blocks the follicular canals. The introduction of excessive moisture or water into the ear during swimming or bathing can cause extreme softening or maceration of the skin lining the ear canal. This may lead to a fissure or break in the skin and allow the bacteria to enter. Water containing chlorine or salt can also cause irritation and damage to this lining and lead to infection.

INCIDENCE

Swimmer's ear is the most common cause of otitis externa. Otitis externa occurs in 3% to 10% of the patient population. (See also Otitis Externa monograph)

PATHOPHYSIOLOGY

The ear canal is a dark, warm, skin-lined area that readily collects moisture. Prolonged accumulation of moisture can cause maceration with the development of fissures, which provide a portal of entry for bacteria that make up the normal flora of the ear. The bacteria then enter a fertile environment where they can proliferate, leading to a bacterial infection with inflammation. The infection has the potential to perforate the eardrum and spread into the middle ear but only in extremely severe cases.

The most common bacteria associated with swimmer's ear are *Pseudomonas*, *Staphylococcus*, *Bacillus*, and *Proteus*; however, other less common bacteria can lead to swimmer's ear. Bacterial growth is promoted when the pH of the external auditory canal changes from mildly acidic at a pH of 4 to 5 (which discourages antimicrobial growth) to a more alkaline pH, allowing for the growth or spread of bacteria. This change in pH is caused by a retention of water from swimming or some other recreational water activity. Accumulation of water can promote tissue maceration, making the ear canal susceptible to infection. Heat, humidity, and moisture can cause edema and occlusion of the follicular glands, promoting infection. Cerumen also absorbs water and expands, thereby trapping water and providing a favorable environment for bacterial growth.

SIGNS/SYMPTOMS

The first symptoms are itching, a feeling of fullness or wetness in the ear canal, and ear discomfort. These symptoms occur within a few hours to 1 day following exposure to excessive moisture. Later, pain develops with increased itching. With mild swimmer's ear, mild erythema and swelling are evident when the ear is examined. Minor scaling or shedding of the ear epithelium may occur, along with a small amount of clear or cloudy secretions. Moderate swimmer's ear is present if pain and itching extend and include the outer ear (auricle) along with ear canal pain. Ear secretions become more profuse. With severe swimmer's ear, the pain extends to the area around the ear. The ear is constantly producing a purulent discharge. The inner part of the ear canal may become occluded secondary to swelling, leading to temporary hearing loss. As described above, itching and pain are the main symptoms of swimmer's ear. The pain may increase when chewing gum or eating. However, if the pain becomes sharp or knife-like and intolerable, or if external redness and swelling develop, then the infection has progressed and a physician should be consulted.

DIAGNOSTIC PARAMETERS/PHYSICAL ASSESSMENT

Physical examination of the ear demonstrates erythema and edema of the external auditory canal. Weeping secretions, purulent otorrhea, and exfoliation of the skin are often present. Pain may occur secondary to manipulation of the ear. Partial or complete closure of the ear canal may be present with hearing loss. With advanced disease, erythema, edema, or lymphadenopathy may be present in the preauricular, postauricular, and anterior cervical regions. The eardrum is normal or erythematous but is not perforated or bulging.

Interview:

1.) Patient's medical history. If the patient is diabetic or immunosuppressed, refer to a physician. Any contraindications to the use of an NSAID (history/presence of ulcer, GI bleeding, uncontrolled or severe hypertension, renal dysfunction, taking an ACE inhibitor, taking an anticoagulant such as warfarin, fluid-restricted).
2.) Current medication profile.
3.) Current treatment of swimmer's ear, including duration and success.
4.) Drug allergies.
5.) Signs and symptoms. Consider OTC treatment in the case of pruritus, mild-to-moderate pain or recent onset of symptoms. The patient should be referred to a physician in the following cases: Knife-like pain; steady pain; severe pain; systemic symptoms (eg, chills, fever, sore throat); hearing loss.
6.) What led to this ear infection (eg, the patient has put some foreign object in the affected ear[s] lately, used a wax-removal kit, participated in a recreational water activity, been in a warm, humid area, or around a lot of moisture).
7.) Past occurences and treatments of swimmer's ear.

TREATMENT

Approaches to therapy: Treat swimmer's ear as soon as possible before the infection is allowed to spread. Once the above questions have been addressed, decide whether the patient can be treated with an OTC product or if the patient should be referred to a physician. Always advise patients to seek medical attention immediately if symptoms worsen or if hearing loss, systemic symptoms, or severe knife-like pain occurs.

Nondrug therapy:

Heat – Warming the ear canal with a blow dryer on a low setting can aid in drying the ear canal and can be soothing to the patient. Use caution by touching the ear frequently to avoid overheating the area and hurting the patient, particularly if someone else is applying the blow dryer to the patient's ear(s). Applying heat locally using a hot pack, hot water bottle, or heating pad is often very helpful in reducing discomfort.

Pharmacotherapy: In mild cases of swimmer's ear, topical nonprescription medications can be used as alternatives to systemic antibiotics.

Analgesics – Swimmer's ear often involves pain and discomfort. At times a fever will also develop. These symptoms can often be alleviated by nonprescription analgesics such as acetaminophen and NSAIDs. For complete information, please refer to the Aches and Pains and Fever monographs in Musuloskeletal Conditions and CNS Conditions chapters.

Prevention – For prevention of swimmer's ear, provide patients with the following guidelines:

- Do not insert objects or devices in the ear (eg, bobby pins, matches, toothpicks, pencils) unless the device is specifically designed for insertion into the ear.
- Remove earwax only when it is in the outer part of the external ear canal, using a warm, soapy wash cloth that has been wrung out.
- Applying 2 to 3 drops of alcohol, glycerin, or alcohol-acetic acid solutions to ears after swimming, bathing, or showering will help remove excess moisture from the ears and may help prevent swimmer's ear.
- Keep the ear dry as much as possible for 6 weeks or more after the ear infection has subsided.
- Whenever any medication is obtained, it should be completely understood how the medication should be given (ie, taken orally or put into the ear). Many patients assume that during an ear infection all medications should be applied directly into the ear, which in many cases is not true. If there is any question as to how the medication should be taken, consult a pharmacist or physician.
- As with all medications, keep these agents out of children's reach. Only adults should administer these agents or treatments.
- *Earplugs:* Water-tight or molded earplugs or even swim caps can be helpful in preventing water from entering the ear canal. This can be very helpful

when the ear is to be kept dry for at least 6 weeks after the ear infection has subsided. Avoid diving and deep underwater swimming.

- *Children with tympanostomy tubes:* Patients with tympanostomy tubes (tubes in the ears) should avoid diving and deep underwater swimming, swimming in ponds (swimming holes), and submerging the head into bath water to rinse off shampoo. It is highly recommended that scuba diving be prohibited.

IRRIGATION SOLUTIONS FOR THE EAR

▶ **Actions**

Gentle rinsing of the ear will help rid the ear of bacteria, fungi, and debris, as well as assist in reestablishing an environment that does not promote bacterial/fungal growth.

3% HYDROGEN PEROXIDE SOLUTION

▶ **Actions**

Aids in softening earwax and facilitates its removal from the ear.

▶ **Indications**

Earwax softener; cleansing agent.

▶ **Contraindications**

Hypersensitivity reaction to hydrogen peroxide.

▶ **Warnings**

Discontinue use if rash or irritation develops. Do not use hydrogen peroxide routinely because it can lead to maceration or softening of the epithelial tissue, which can lead to an infection.

▶ **Drug Interactions**

None with otic use.

▶ **Administration and Dosage**

Dilute 3% hydrogen peroxide with an equal amount of warm water (½ pint of each ingredient). Mix well. Follow directions for irrigating the external ear canal in Appendix D, Administration Techniques.

2.5% ACETIC ACID SOLUTION (VINEGAR & WATER)

▶ **Actions**

Aids in softening earwax and facilitates its removal from the ear.

▶ **Indications**

Cleansing agent; acidifying agent

▶ **Contraindications**

Hypersensitivity reaction to acetic acid or vinegar.

▶ **Warnings**

Discontinue use if rash or irritation develops. Do not use acetic acid solution routinely because it can lead to maceration and irritation of the epithelial tissue, which can lead to an infection.

▶ **Drug Interactions**

None with otic use.

▶ **Administration and Dosage**

Dilute household vinegar (5% acetic acid) with an equal amount of warm water (½ pint of each ingredient). Mix well. Follow directions for irrigating the ear in Appendix D, Administration Techniques. Make a fresh solution prior to each irrigation. Discard unused solution.

Note: May substitute 70% isopropyl alcohol (preferred), 70% ethyl alcohol, propylene glycol, or glycerin instead of water to be combined with the vinegar. Higher alcohol concentrations increase the drying effect but may cause a burning sensation; lower alcohol concentrations reduce the burning sensation.

ASTRINGENT AGENTS

ALUMINUM ACETATE SOLUTION ("BUROW'S SOLUTION")

▶ **Actions**

Acts as an astringent that creates an environment that is antibacterial and antifungal.

▶ **Indications**

To help alleviate the pain and inflammation associated with swimmer's ear.

In mild cases of swimmer's ear, these agents can be used as alternatives to antibiotics.

▶ **Contraindications**

Hypersensitivity reaction to aluminum acetate.

▶ **Warnings**

Discontinue use if a rash or irritation develops. Do not use to treat swimmer's ear on a chronic basis. If itching, inflammation, or pain persists after 3 to 4 days or worsens, contact a physician.

▶ **Administration and Dosage**

For most products, place 2 to 3 drops (or enough drops to fill the ear canal) into the affected ear(s) every 2 to 3 hours while awake, keeping head tilted to the side. Follow directions for irrigating the external ear canal in Appendix D, Administration Techniques. Allow the drops to remain in the ear canal and to allow the solution to contact as much of the surface area of the external ear canal before straightening the head. Use until the pain and inflammation subsides, then as needed for itching. May use as a prophylactic agent: 2 drops into each ear after exposure to water.

ALUMINIUM ACETATE SOLUTION PRODUCTS	
Trade name	**Doseform**
Buro-Sol	**Powder**: 0.23% aluminum acetate. One packet placed in a pint of water produces a modified Burow's Solution.
Bluboro Powder, Boropak Powder, Domeboro Powder and Tablets	**Powder, tablets**: Aluminum sulfate and calcium acetate. One packet or tablet placed in a pint of water produces a modified 1:40 Burow's Solution.
Star-Otic	**Solution**: Nonaqeous acetic acid, Burow's Solution, boric acid, propylene glycol

Products listed are representative of currently available and widely distributed brands. Similar products, including regional and private label brands, may also exist.

PATIENT INFORMATION
Aluminum Acetate Solution
- Patient instructions accompany each product. Read these instructions carefully before use, preferably before leaving the pharmacy, in case of any questions.
- If condition worsens or symptoms persist after 3 to 4 days, discontinue use of the product and consult a physician.
- For external use only. Avoid contact with the eyes.

ACIDIFYING/DRYING AGENTS

▶ **Indications**

Treatment of swimmer's ear should also include agents that aid in removing excess moisture from the ear. Keeping the ear dry will provide a less desirable environment for bacteria, preventing reinfection. Once the inflammation in the ear has diminished, a drying agent can be used. If a drying agent causes burning or pain upon application, the inflammation has not subsided enough to use these agents. These agents can also be used as prophylactic therapy. Usually 1 to 2 drops in each ear after water exposure (eg, swimming, showering) is sufficient.

2.5% ACETIC ACID IN 70% ALCOHOL

▶ **Actions**

Equal parts of household vinegar (5% acetic acid) and 70% isopropyl or ethyl alcohol provide an acidic environment that restores the ear canal to its normal pH, which is antibacterial and antifungal. It also acts as an astringent and drying agent.

▶ **Indications**

To help alleviate the pain and inflammation associated with swimmer's ear.

▶ **Contraindications**

Hypersensitivity reaction to acetic acid or alcohol.

▶ **Adverse Reactions**

Discontinue use if a rash or irritation develops. Do not use to treat swimmer's ear on a chronic basis. If itching, inflammation, or pain persists after 3 to 4 days or worsens, contact a physician.

▶ **Administration and Dosage**

Place 2 to 3 drops (or enough drops to fill the ear canal) into the affected ear(s) every 2 to 3 hours, keeping the head tilted to the side. Follow directions for irrigating the external ear canal in Appendix D, Administration Techniques. Allow the drops to remain in the ear canal and allow the solution to contact as much of the surface area of the ear as possible before straightening the head. Use until the pain and inflammation subsides, then as needed for itching. May use as a prophylactic agent: 2 drops into each ear after swimming, bathing, or showering.

BORIC ACID 2.75% IN ISOPROPYL ALCOHOL

▶ **Actions**

Provides an acidic environment that restores the ear canal to its normal pH, which is antibacterial and antifungal. It also acts as an astringent and drying agent.

▶ **Indications**

To help alleviate pain and inflammation associated with swimmer's ear.

▶ **Contraindications**

Hypersensitivity reaction to boric acid or isopropyl alcohol.

▶ **Warnings**

Discontinue use if a rash or irritation develops. Do not use to treat swimmer's ear on a chronic basis. If itching, inflammation, or pain persists after 3 to 4 days or worsens, contact a physician.

▶ **Drug Interactions**

None with otic use.

▶ **Administration and Dosage**

Place 2 to 3 drops (or enough drops to fill the ear canal) into the affected ear(s) every 2 to 3 hours while awake, keeping head tilted to the side. Follow directions for irrigating the external ear canal in Appendix D, Administration Techniques. Allow the drops to remain in the ear canal and allow the solution to contact as much of the surface area of the ear as possible before straightening the head. Use until the pain and inflammation subside, then as needed for itching. May use as a prophylactic agent: 2 to 3 drops (or enough drops to fill the ear canal) into each ear after swimming, bathing, or showering.

BORIC ACID PRODUCTS	
Trade name	Doseform
Aurocaine2	**Liquid**: 97.25% isopropyl alcohol and boric acid

Products listed are representative of currently available and widely distributed brands. Similar products, including regional and private label brands, may also exist.

PROPYLENE GLYCOL/ANHYDROUS GLYCERIN/ISOPROPYL ALCOHOL

▶ **Actions**

These agents extract moisture from the auditory canal.

▶ **Indications**

Drying agent.

▶ **Contraindications**

Hypersensitivity reaction to propylene glycol, anhydrous glycerin, or isopropyl alcohol.

▶ **Adverse Reactions**

Discontinue use if rash or irritation develops. Do not use if burning occurs upon application.

▶ **Administration and Dosage**

Follow instructions for individual products. For most products, instill 4 to 6 drops (or enough drops to fill the ear canal) in affected ear twice daily for 4 to 6 days. Refer to the directions for irrigating the external ear canal in Appendix D, Administration Techniques. May use 2 drops in each ear after swimming, bathing, or showering on a chronic basis to aid in preventing the onset of swimmer's ear.

EAR DRYING PRODUCTS	
Trade name	**Doseform**
Ear-Dry, Swim-Ear	**Liquid**: 95% isopropyl alcohol, 5% anhydrous glycerin
Dri/Ear	**Liquid**: 95% isopropyl alcohol, 5% glycerin
Auro-Dri	**Liquid**: 95% isopropyl alcohol in anhydrous glycerin

Products listed are representative of currently available and widely distributed brands. Similar products, including regional and private label brands, may also exist.

PATIENT INFORMATION
Ear Acidifying/Drying Products

- Patient instructions accompany each product. Read these instructions carefully before use, preferably before leaving the pharmacy, in case of any questions.
- For external use only; avoid contact with eyes.
- Do not use on mucous membranes or broken skin.
- Do not use these products if you have a history of hypersensitivity reactions to alcohol.
- Do not use if ear drainage, dizziness, or pain is present, or if you have injured your eardrum.
- Discontinue use and consult a physician if irritation persists or worsens.

ANTIPRURITIC THERAPY

OTIC HYDROCORTISONE PREPARATIONS

▶ Actions

Reduces inflammation associated with an ear infection and helps dry the ear.

Ear drops containing hydrocortisone will help alleviate the pruritus associated with swimmer's ear.

▶ Indications

Relieves itching associated with ear inflammation secondary to an infectious process.

▶ Contraindications

Hypersensitivity to hydrocortisone or other topical steroids, alcohol, or propylene glycol.

▶ Warnings

Do not use in children younger than 2 years of age.

For external use only. Avoid contact with eyes.

Discontinue use if rash or irritation develops. Do not use on a chronic basis. If itching persists after 3 to 4 days, contact a physician.

▶ Drug Interactions

None with otic use.

▶ Administration and Dosage

Place 4 to 6 drops (or enough drops to fill the ear canal) into affected ear(s) not more than 3 to 4 times daily. See individual product labeling for guidelines. Follow directions for irrigating the external ear canal in Appendix D, Administration Techniques.

OTIC HYDROCORTISONE PRODUCTS	
Trade name	Doseform
EarSol-HC	Solution: 1% hydrocortisone. 44% alcohol, propylene glycol.

Products listed are representative of currently available and widely distributed brands. Similar products, including regional and private label brands, may also exist.

PATIENT INFORMATION

Otic Hydrocortisone

- Patient instructions accompany each product. Read these instructions carefully before use, preferably before leaving the pharmacy, in case of any questions.
- Do not use in children younger than 2 years of age.
- For external use only. Avoid contact with eyes.
- If condition worsens or if symptoms persist after 4 days, discontinue use and consult a physician.

PODIATRIC CONDITIONS

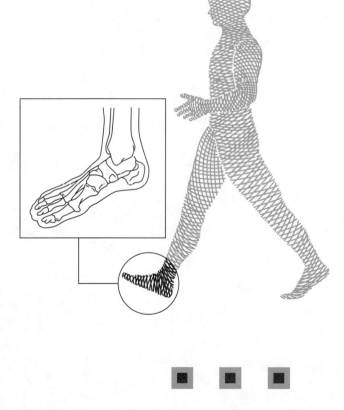

NONPRESCRIPTION DRUG THERAPY
TABLE OF CONTENTS
■ ■ ■

PODIATRIC CONDITIONS

INTRODUCTION

The American Podiatric Medical Association estimates that approximately 75% of Americans will experience foot health problems at some time in their lives. Women have approximately 4 times as many foot problems as men, their shoes often causing most complaints. Only a small percentage of the US population is born with foot problems. Most podiatry related visits occur from worn-out shoes, ill-fitting shoes, and general neglect from a lack of awareness of proper foot care. Podiatrists receive more than 55 million visits a year from people with a variety of foot ailments.

Each foot contains 26 bones, 33 joints, 107 ligaments, 19 muscles, and tendons that allow for the tri-planar movement of walking and running. The average person takes 8000 to 10,000 steps in a day, approximately 115,000 miles in a lifetime. Coupled with an increase in health-related sport activity, sports-related foot injuries and fatigue are on the increase. Running increases pressure on the feet by 3 to 4 times body weight. Without adequate training and pre-activity stretching, more frequent complaints of heel and arch pain as well as tendinitis and stress fracture occur.

Increased sports activity also leads to the condition of tinea pedis. Tinea pedis is caused by a fungal infection of the skin that can be mild and asymptomatic or acutely painful. Tinea is exacerbated by increased moisture and perspiration. Left untreated, tinea pedis can cause a secondary bacterial infection or onychomycosis. Athlete's foot is the most common fungal infection in the United States.

A corn or an ingrown toenail is the chief complaint of more than 40% of all patients who visit a podiatrist. Corns are caused by the underlying bones of the foot rubbing abnormally on the skin, secondary to shoe pressure or going barefoot. Treating the external symptoms of the corn will not prevent the recurrence of a corn. Ingrown toenails are a common hereditary condition that can be irritated by tight shoes or improper trimming. Some ingrown toenails can cause infection, which in the diabetic or vascular compromised patient is a medical emergency. Unfortunately, many patients feel that painful corns and ingrown toenails are normal and do not seek treatment.

Wart lesions or "verrucae" are a common viral infection of the foot. Unlike a bacterial infection, it is purely a nuisance and poses no medical problems except in the immunocompromised patient. It is necessary to treat warts to prevent spread, pain in the foot when walking, and transfer to other patients.

General care of the feet will keep the average patient walking pain-free from infancy through adulthood. Purchase of shoe gear in the afternoon will allow for better fit, as feet tend to swell later in the day. To ensure a better fit, measure the feet each time shoes are purchased. When purchasing shoes it is important to note where the shoes were manufactured, because shoes made outside of the

United States tend to be smaller in size and do not always correspond to the US sizing system. To help prevent shoe-related pain, rotate shoes and regularly replace shoes.

Toenail problems can be avoided by trimming the nails straight across with an appropriate clipper. Trimming in the corners and the use of OTC ingrown toenail preparations are the most common cause of toenail infection. Toenail preparations should never be used in the diabetic or vascular compromised patient.

Self-treatment of foot conditions is on the rise due to more restrictive medical insurance and the advent of managed care. However, delaying foot care or self-treatment of a foot ailment can lead to increased costs, disability, and hospitalization. Therefore, it is important for the pharmacist to be aware of these various conditions to help patients make proper decisions regarding their treatment options. It is also essential to remind patients of preventive measures, such as proper shoe fit and toenail trimming. When foot products are used, direct careful attention to the instructions as well as the contraindications for each product. Used judiciously, many OTC preparations can provide relief and keep a patient walking. Consult a podiatrist if certain medical conditions exist (eg, diabetes, peripheral vascular disease) or if OTC remedies fail to provide relief.

ACHILLES TENDINITIS

DEFINITION

Achilles tendinitis is inflammation and swelling of the Achilles tendon (see Figure 1). The Achilles tendon is one of the strongest tendons of the lower extremity. It is subject to much stress in normal everyday activity. Achilles tendinitis can occur with changes in daily activity, change of footwear, the abrupt onset of physical activity, or an exercise program without adequate training of the muscle-tendon group.

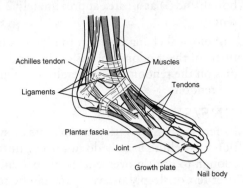

Figure 1. Foot Muscles, Tendons, and Ligaments

ETIOLOGY

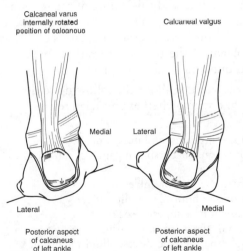

Figure 2. Calcaneal Varus and Calcaneal Valgus, Posterior View of Left Ankle

Achilles tendinitis may be caused by injury or abnormal biomechanical forces. Injury may be caused by a trauma to the tendon complex, such as a direct blow to the back of the leg or a severe ankle sprain. In the athlete, overuse and strain of the tendon will cause moderate-to-severe swelling and discomfort and mild loss of muscle/tendon power. A severe injury to the Achilles tendon can cause weakening of the tendon that may lead to partial or complete tendon rupture. Biomechanical causes of Achilles tendinitis may include an unstable ankle and calcaneal varus or valgus (internal or external rotation of the calcaneous [heel]; see Figure 2.) associated with the high arched or flexible flat foot. A Haglund's deformity (inflammation and projection of the posterior aspect of the heel bone, which is often associated with wearing high-heeled shoes) of the calcaneus is another common cause of Achilles tendinitis.

PATHOPHYSIOLOGY

Pathology of the Achilles tendon may occur at 3 areas: 1) At the insertion of the tendon into the middle one-third of the posterior aspect of the calcaneus (heel bone); 2) at the myotendinous junction (eg, the point at which muscle tissue changes to fibrous tendon tissue, which attaches the muscle to bone); and 3) at an area approximately 2 to 6 cm above the insertion of the tendon.

Pathological changes within the tendon include microscopic changes of the fibers of the tendon, fibrosis of the tendon, thickening and formation of nodules on the tendon, and generalized inflammation along the entire course of the tendon.

SIGNS/SYMPTOMS

Patients may have varied complaints or symptoms. Symptoms of inflammation or swelling usually do not occur until after activity and may be severe enough to limit movement. Some patients have no complaints of discomfort after rest or sleep; however, pain can be severe.

DIAGNOSTIC PARAMETERS/PHYSICAL ASSESSMENT

Clinical Observation: Although a patient's general complaints may lead one to consider the potential of Achilles tendinitis, physical assessment and diagnosis must be done by a physician. Swelling and thickening of the tendon just above the posterior aspect of the calcaneus, mild loss of plantarflexion power against resistance because of discomfort, specific complaints of discomfort on side-to-side pressure, and exam of the tendon are various parameters that should be evaluated by trained medical personnel.

Interview: It may be beneficial to ask patients about the following to determine whether Achilles tendinitis is likely, and whether physician referral is necessary:

• Location of problem, including signs, symptoms, and duration.
• Description of pain, type of pain, situations that result in pain (eg, standing, walking).
• Recent sprain, strain, or other injury to the foot or ankle.
• Recent changes in activity level or working hours or conditions.
• Recent changes of footwear (or the use of new shoes or socks).
• If patient exercises, obtain description of the warm-up routine.
• History of GI ulceration or bleeding, renal/hepatic disease, fluid retention, hypertension, or heart disease. Current medical treatment (including medication profile) for any other medical conditions.
• Pregnancy or breastfeeding.
• Description and success of self-treatment.

Refer the patient to a physician for further evaluation if Achilles tendinitis is suspected.

TREATMENT

Nondrug therapy: As with any tendon injury, rest, application of ice, compression, and elevation are the standard elements of non-drug therapy for acute tendinitis. Discontinuation of the activity associated with tendinitis allows the tendon to rest and should be continued for at least 2 weeks. Application of ice at 20-minute intervals 2 to 3 times daily for a minimum of 3 days should help reduce inflammation. Medical evaluation is necessary if minor swelling does not subside. Use an ace wrap or similar elastic bandage for compression and immobilization of the tendon and elevate the affected extremity.

In the chronic Achilles tendon injury, warm, moist heat is recommended instead of ice. An elastic bandage may also be used in conjunction with a heel cup for immobilization and reduction of tendon tension. Although these products are available without a prescription, self-treatment is generally not recommended.

Pharmacotherapy: Numerous OTC nonsteroidal anti-inflammatory agents, (NSAIDs), as well as aspirin, are available for the treatment of tendinitis. Combined with non-drug therapy, these agents provide optimum relief of symptoms. For further information about aspirin and NSAIDs, refer to the Aches and Pains monograph in the Musculoskeletal Conditions chapter. Acetaminophen may provide pain relief, but this agent has no anti-inflammatory properties.

In the chronic tendinitis patient, topical deep-heating analgesic creams or lotions may also be considered. Such agents may reduce inflammation in chronic tendinitis and provide some relief of symptoms.

RUBS AND LINIMENTS

▶ Indications
These products are used for relief of pain of muscular aches, neuralgia, rheumatism, arthritis, sprains, and like conditions, when skin is intact.

Individual components include:

Counterirritants: Camphor, capsicum preparations (capsicum oleoresin, capsaicin), eucalyptus oil, menthol, methyl nicotinate, methyl salicylate, mustard oil, wormwood oil.

Antiseptics: Thymol.

Analgesics: Trolamine salicylate, methyl salicylate.

▶ Contraindications
Allergy to components of any formulation or to salicylates.

▶ Warnings
For external use only: Avoid contact with eyes, eyelids, and mucous membranes.

Apply to affected parts only: Do not apply to irritated skin; discontinue use if excessive irritation develops. Consult a physician if pain persists for longer than 7 to 10 days, or if redness is present, or in conditions affecting children younger than 10 years of age.

Heat therapy: Do not use an external source of high heat (eg, heating pad) with these agents because irritation and burning of the skin may occur.

Protective covering: Applying a tight bandage or wrap over these agents is not recommended because increased absorption may occur.

▶ Drug Interactions
Anticoagulants: An enhanced anticoagulant effect (eg, increased prothrombin time) occurred in several patients receiving an anticoagulant and using topical methyl salicylate concurrently.

▶ **Adverse Reactions**

If applied to large skin areas and used over a prolonged period of time, salicylate side effects (eg, tinnitus, nausea, vomiting) may occur.

Products may be toxic if ingested.

Counterirritants may cause local irritation, especially in patients with sensitive skin.

▶ **Administration and Dosage**

Apply to affected areas as needed.

RUBS AND LINIMENTS	
Trade name	**Doseform**
Icy Hot	**Balm**: 29% methyl salicylate, 7.6% menthol, white petrolatum
Epiderm	**Balm**: Isopropyl alcohol, parabens, ureas, menthol, EDTA
JointFlex	**Cream**: 3.1% camphor, lanolin, aloe, urea, EDTA, glycerin, peppermint oil
Capzasin-P	**Cream**: 0.025% capsaicin
ArthriCare for Women Silky Dry	**Cream**: 0.025% capsaicin, parabens, mineral oil
ArthriCare for Women Extra Moisturizing	**Cream**: 0.025% capsaicin, aloe vera gel, cetyl and stearyl alcohol, parabens
ArthriCare for Women Multi-Action	**Cream**: 0.025% capsaicin, 1.25% menthol, 0.25% methyl nicotinate, aloe vera gel, cetyl alcohol, parabens
Capzasin-HP	**Cream**: 0.075% capsaicin
ArthriCare for Women Ultra Strength	**Cream**: 0.075% capsaicin, 2% menthol, aloe vera gel, cetyl and stearyl alcohol, parabens
Vicks VapoRub	**Cream**: 2.8% menthol, 5.2% camphor, 1.2% eucalyptus oil, cedarleaf oil, cetyl and stearyl alcohol, EDTA, glycerin, urea, parabens, turpentine oil
BenGay S.P.A.	**Cream**: 10% menthol, cetyl alcohol, urea, EDTA, glycerin
Arthritic Hot	**Cream**: Methyl salicylate, menthol
Ziks	**Cream**: 12% methyl salicylate, 1% menthol, 0.025% capsaicin, cetyl alcohol, urea
Thera-Gesic	**Cream**: 15% methyl salicylate, 1% menthol, glycerin, parabens
BenGay Greaseless	**Cream**: 15% methyl salicylate, 10% menthol, cetyl alcohol, glycerin
Pain Bust-R II	**Cream**: 17% methyl salicylate, 12% menthol, cetyl and stearyl alcohol
ArthriCare for Women Nighttime	**Cream**: 30% methyl salicylate, 1.25% menthol, 0.25% methyl nicotinate, glycerin, isopropyl alcohol
Arthritis Formula BenGay	**Cream**: 30% methyl salicylate, 8% menthol, lanolin
Icy Hot	**Cream**: 30% methyl salicylate, 10% menthol
Ultra Strength BenGay	**Cream**: 30% methyl salicylate, 10% menthol, 4% camphor, EDTA, lanolin
Panalgesic Gold	**Cream**: 35% methyl salicylate, 4% menthol, lanolin, cetyl and stearyl alcohol, mineral oil
Myoflex	**Cream**: 10% triethanolamine salicylate, cetyl and stearyl alcohol, EDTA

RUBS AND LINIMENTS

Trade name	Doseform
Myoflex Extra, Myoflex Arthritic	**Cream**: 15% triethanolamine salicylate
Sportscreme	**Cream**: 10% trolamine salicylate, cetyl alcohol, glycerin, parabens, mineral oil
Aspercreme	**Cream**: 10% trolamine salicylate, aloe vera gel, cetyl alcohol, glycerin, parabens, mineral oil
Mobisyl	**Cream**: 10% trolamine salicylate, aloe vera gel, cetyl alcohol, urea, glycerin, parabens, mineral oil, sweet almond oil, EDTA
Icy Hot Arthritis Therapy	**Gel**: 0.025% capsaicin, aloe vera gel, benzyl alcohol, urea, maleated soybean oil, parabens
Flexall Quik Gel	**Gel**: Menthol, methyl salicylate
Vanishing Scent BenGay	**Gel**: 2.5% menthol, urea, isopropyl alcohol
Vicks VapoRub	**Gel**: 2.6% menthol, 4.8% camphor, 1.2% eucalyptus oil, cedarleaf oil, nutmeg oil, petrolatum, turpentine oil
Flexall 454	**Gel**: 7% menthol, aloe vera gel, eucalyptus oil, glycerin, peppermint oil, thyme oil
Maximum Strength Flexall 454	**Gel**: 16% menthol, aloe vera gel, eucalyptus oil, glycerin, peppermint oil, thyme oil
Flexall Ultra Plus	**Gel**: 16% menthol, 10% methyl salicylate, 3.1% camphor, aloe vera gel, eucalyptus oil, glycerin, peppermint oil, thyme oil
Icy Hot Chill Stick	**Gel**: 30% methyl salicylate, 10% menthol, hydrogenated castor oil, stearyl alcohol
Myoflex Ice Cold Plus	**Gel**: 15% triethanolamine salicylate
Absorbine Jr Arthritis Strength	**Liquid**: Capsaicin, echinacea, calendula, and wormwood extracts
Absorbine Jr	**Liquid**: 1.27% menthol, echinacea, calendula, and wormwood extracts, wormwood oil
Extra Strength Absorbine Jr	**Liquid**: 4% menthol, echinacea, calendula, and wormwood extracts, wormwood oil
Yager's	**Liniment**: Camphor, turpentine oil, clove oil
Panalgesic Gold	**Liniment**: 55.01% methyl salicylate, 1.25% menthol, 3.1% camphor, emollient oils, alcohol
Banalg	**Lotion**: 4.9% methyl salicylate, 1% menthol, 2% camphor, parabens, eucalyptus oil
Banalg Hospital Strength	**Lotion**: 14% methyl salicylate, 3% menthol, parabens
Aspercreme	**Lotion**: Trolamine salicylate
Eucalyptamint	**Ointment**: 16% menthol, eucalyptus oil, lanolin, mineral oil
Original Formula BenGay	**Ointment**: 18.3% methyl salicylate, 16% menthol, lanolin
Absorbine Jr	**Patch**: Menthol, camphor, eucalyptus
Absorbine Jr Deep Pain Relief	**Patch**: Menthol, glucosamine, MSM
Icy Hot	**Patch**: Methyl salicylate, menthol

Products listed are representative of currently available and widely distributed brands. Similar products, including regional and private label brands, may also exist.

PATIENT INFORMATION
Rubs and Liniments
- For external use only. Avoid contact with eyes, eyelids, and mucous membranes.
- Apply to affected areas only. Do not apply to irritated skin; discontinue use if excessive irritation develops.
- Consult a physician if pain persists for longer than 7 to 10 days, if redness is present, or in conditions affecting children younger than 10 years of age.
- Do not use an external source of high heat (eg, heating pad) with these agents because irritation and burning of the skin may occur.
- Do not apply tight bandages or wraps over these agents.
- Do not apply to broken skin.

CORNS

DEFINITION

Corns are noncontagious hyperkeratotic tissue that forms in response to bony friction, rubbing, and pressure on the skin. Typically, corns are described as lesions that occur on the top of or between the toes. Heloma durum is a hard corn that occurs on the dorsal aspect of a digit with or without a central "core." This central core is sometimes described as a "seed corn." Heloma molle is a soft, interdigital corn that may appear white or macerated and is caused by absorption of moisture. A distal clavus is a hard corn that occurs at the tip of the toe.

ETIOLOGY

The most common cause of a corn lesion is the formation of a hammertoe. A corn is a symptom of an underlying bony condition such as contracture (hammertoe) or bone spur of a toe. Hammertoes involving corn lesions may be an inherited trait associated with orthopedic and biomechanical causes. Another cause of corn lesions in a noncontracted toe is wearing ill-fitting or tight-fitting shoes that form a blister, which progresses into a corn lesion.

INCIDENCE

Approximately 40% of all patient visits to podiatrists are initially due to corn problems. Patients spend millions of dollars each year on various OTC products to relieve symptoms. In the United States, countless visits are made to the podiatrist and orthopedist for surgical and nonsurgical treatment of painful corn conditions.

PATHOPHYSIOLOGY

The hammertoe digital deformity that can cause corn lesions has its pathology in the improper function of the long flexor tendon. The improper function causes dorsiflexion of the proximal interphalangeal joint, and plantarflexion of the middle and distal interphalangeal joint causing the contracted digit. Secondary to the contraction of the digit, the head of the proximal phalanx becomes more prominent and is exposed to friction and rubbing of the bone on other digits or shoes. A corn lesion forms in response to this friction and reacts by building a layer of hyperkeratotic skin. This layer is protective of the joint; however, as the corn lesion increases in size and thickness, the patient experiences varying degrees of discomfort and irritation. With continued increase in thickness of the corn, a breakdown of the skin can occur and an infection may ensue. An infection in this area is of great concern in diabetic and vascular compromised patients.

A corn lesion can also occur when a bone spur is present. Bone spurs are a result of degenerative or arthritic changes in the joint. This irregular growth of bone may be seen at the digits or metatarsal joint areas in a bunion or Taylor's bunion.

SIGNS/SYMPTOMS

Corns usually become cone-shaped lesions of thickened, calloused skin. Symptoms include pain in the corn area with shoe wear. Use of ill-fitting or tight-fitting shoes may initially cause a blister, which progresses into a corn lesion. Corns may exist as a single lesion or may occur on several different areas of the foot. Corns are generally not painful without shoes; however, the pressure of socks or bed sheets may cause sensitivity. A corn that is infected shows redness, swelling, and purulent drainage. Systemic symptoms of fever and chills may also be present. Interdigital corns may appear white or macerated because of absorption of interdigital moisture.

DIAGNOSTIC PARAMETERS/PHYSICAL ASSESSMENT

Clinical Observation: Patients with corns may display a contracted digit with prominence of 1 or more joints, heavy build-up of hyperkeratotic tissue with or without redness or swelling, and deformation of the shoe corresponding to the corn area of the foot.

Weight-bearing x-rays in the AP, lateral, and oblique positions may be warranted. Perform culture and sensitivity tests and CBC if clinical signs of infection are present.

Interview: It may be beneficial to ask about the following to assist patients in the diagnosis and proper treatment of corns:

- Description, location, and duration of corn lesion.
- Presence of pain (while walking, with shoes), bleeding, or discharge.
- History of injury or trauma to the toes or feet.
- Previous occurrence of corns.
- Concurrent medical conditions, such as arthritis (or other degenerative joint disease), diabetes, infection, peripheral vascular disease, Raynaud disease, asthma, chronic obstructive pulmonary disease, a history of smoking, cyanosis of the digits, frostbite or other thermal injury. Physician referral would be appropriate in these cases.
- Recent use of tight or ill-fitting shoes.
- Past self-treatment of corns, including success of treatment.

TREATMENT

Approaches to therapy: Direct treatment of corn lesions at eliminating the cause of the lesion; however, treatment of the symptomatic corn will provide temporary relief for the patient. Physician referral is appropriate with presence of bleeding or discharge, if concurrent medical conditions exist (see Interview section), or if the patient is refractory to non-drug or OTC therapy.

Nondrug therapy: The following may provide relief from corn lesions: Change of shoes to provide more room in the toe box area, eliminating friction and rubbing of the toe on the shoes; foot soaks in warm, soapy water to soften the corn lesion followed by filing with an emery board or pumice stone; use of accommodative padding such as nonmedicated mole skin, tube foam, toe caps, lamb's wool or silicone pads; reduction of the lesion by a podiatrist.

Pharmacotherapy: When the patient is unresponsive to nondrug therapy, the use of medicated (salicylic acid) corn plasters or liquids may be indicated. Salicylic acid is the only OTC medicine considered safe and effective for treatment of corns. Pad- or disc-type products, as well as flexible collodions, are usually preferable because they allow the salicylic acid to act longer and penetrate deeper into the corn lesion.

SALICYLIC ACID

▶ **Actions**

Salicylic acid is the only OTC product considered safe and effective by the FDA for use as a keratolytic for corns. Medicated corn plasters or liquids, which contain salicylic acid, cause keratolysis and attempt chemical debridement or exfoliation of the corn lesion. This is applied directly to the corn lesion area.

▶ **Indications**

A topical aid in the removal of excessive keratin in hyperkeratotic skin disorders, including corns.

▶ **Contraindications**

Sensitivity to salicylic acid; prolonged use (especially in infants); use on moles, birthmarks, warts with hair growing from them, genital or facial warts, warts on mucous membranes irritated skin, or any infected or reddened area.

Do not use when diabetes, infection, peripheral vascular disease, Raynaud disease, asthma, chronic obstructive pulmonary disease, history of smoking, cyanosis of the digits, frostbite or other thermal injury, bleeding or purulent discharge from lesion, or pain severe enough to interfere with daily activities exist.

▶ **Warnings**

Salicylate toxicity: Prolonged use over large areas, especially in young children and those patients with significant renal or hepatic impairment could result in salicylism. Limit the area to be treated and be aware of signs of salicylate toxicity (eg, nausea, vomiting, dizziness, loss of hearing, tinnitus, lethargy, hyperpnea, diarrhea, psychic disturbances). In the event of salicylic acid toxicity, discontinue use.

Infection: Not to be used in the presence of infection. Topical OTC agents containing salicylic acid may mask pain associated with infection and trap bacteria within the lesion, thus increasing severity of the infection.

For external use only: Avoid contact with eyes, mucous membranes, and normal skin surrounding warts. If contact with eyes or mucous membranes occurs, immediately flush with water for 15 minutes. Avoid inhaling vapors.

Flammable: Liquid salicylic acid products are extremely flammable; do not use near open flames.

Pregnancy: Category C. There are no adequate and well-controlled studies in pregnant women. Use during pregnancy only if the potential benefit justifies the potential risk to the fetus.

Lactation: Topical salicylic acid may be excreted in breast milk. Use with caution in nursing mothers.

▶ **Drug Interactions**

Prolonged use of topical salicylates could result in systemic absorption. Interactions have been reported with both topical and oral salicylates. Consider this possibility when using in patients receiving other medications.

▶ **Adverse Reactions**

Irritation or allergic reaction to the components of the product or bandages supplied may occur. Local irritation may occur from contact with normal skin surrounding the affected area.

Nonresolution of the painful corn lesion or quick return of symptoms may occur after discontinuation, especially if tight shoes continue to be worn. Worsening of symptoms is often seen if the hyperkeratosis does not resolve following use.

▶ **Administration and Dosage**

Carefully follow instructions supplied with individual products. Some general tips for getting favorable results with salicylic acid treatment are as follows:

• To accelerate destruction of the corn, use a nail file or pumice stone to remove dead skin every 2 days.
• If skin surrounding the corn becomes inflamed or injured, apply a thin layer of petrolatum to this area (not on the corn itself) before applying salicylic acid.
• Doughnut-shaped adhesive foot pads may be helpful for relief of pressure and pain to the corn. After wearing such pads, corns tend to protrude through the open hole in the pad, making application of medication easier.

SALICYLIC ACID PRODUCTS	
Trade name	**Doseform**
Maximum Strength Freezone	**Liquid**: 17.6% with 33% alcohol and 65.5% ether
Mosco	**Liquid**: 17.6% in a flexible collodion with 33% alcohol and 65% ether
Dr. Scholl's Corn/Callus Remover	**Liquid**: 12.6% in flexible collodion with 18% alcohol, 55% ether, acetone, hydrogenated vegetable oil. With cushions.
Dr. Scholl's Corn Removers	**Disk**: 40% in rubber-based vehicle. With cushions.
Dr. Scholl's Extra-Thick Corn Removers	**Disk**: 40% in rubber-based vehicle. With cushions.
Dr. Scholl's Moisturizing Corn Remover Kit	**Disk**: 40% in rubber-based vehicle. With moisturizing cream, cushions, and disks.
Dr. Scholl's One Step Corn Removers	**Strips**: 40% in rubber-based vehicle
Dr. Scholl's Cushlin Gel Corn Removers	**Disk**: 40% in rubber-based vehicle. With cushions.
Dr. Scholl's Ultra-Thin Corn Removers	**Disk**: 40% in rubber-based vehicle. With cushions.
Dr. Scholl's Waterproof Corn Removers	**Disk**: 40% in rubber-based vehicle. With cushions.
Maximum Strength Freezone One Step Corn Remover	**Medicated pads**: 40% in a plaster vehicle
Mediplast	**Plaster**: 40%

Products listed are representative of currently available and widely distributed brands. Similar products, including regional and private label brands, may also exist.

PATIENT INFORMATION

Salicylic Acid Products

- The patient must understand that severe consequences may ensue if corn removal products are used in the presence of certain medical conditions (eg, diabetes); see Contraindications.
- If corn symptoms are not relieved by OTC products, consult the podiatrist or orthopedist to determine the underlying cause and appropriate treatment.
- Follow product instructions carefully. Misuse can result in complications. Following proper administration technique and length of therapy is of great importance.
- If bleeding or discharge of the lesion occurs, discontinue treatment and see a physician.
- Use of daily warm water soaks for 5 minutes may help facilitate removal of corn. Use of an abrasive stick or pumice stone for tissue removal may be beneficial.
- Properly fitted footwear/hosiery is essential. Avoid high heels (which apply increased pressure on the toes and ball of the foot) and shoes that narrow sharply at the toes. Use shoes with cushioned soles and soft upper liners. Athletic socks or double layers of socks help pad uncomfortable shoes, but may make them tighter.
- With presence of soft corns, use of foot powder during treatment is recommended.
- Corn pads or similar products may help relieve pressure.

INGROWN TOENAILS

DEFINITION

Onychocryptosis, or ingrown toe-nail, is the most common nail condition. It is characterized by an abnormal curvature of the nail plate. The ingrown nail may be present with or without paronychia (inflammation of the skin of the nail fold). Symptoms may include pain, tenderness, and swelling of the nail borders. More advanced cases may demonstrate drainage, malodor, erythema, abscess, paronychia, and pyogenic granuloma. A nonhealing, chronic, infected ingrown toenail may lead to osteomyelitis in some cases,

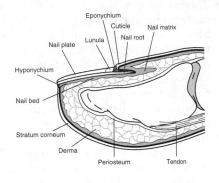

Figure 1. Nail Anatomy

ETIOLOGY

Improper cutting of the toenail is the most common cause of ingrown toenails. Secondary causes may include poorly fitting shoes, tight hosiery, obesity, trauma, sport injury, hyperhidrosis, subungual exostosis, and heredity. When an infection is present, the most common organisms involved are *Staphylococcus* and *Streptococcus*. The hallux, or great toe, is the most common location of an ingrown toenail.

INCIDENCE

Paronychia, an acute or chronic infection of marginal tissues around the nail, is most common in the diabetic patient, and can be found in 3% of nondiabetic female patients. Early paronychia is associated with an incurvated nail or a normal nail that is cut too short or torn into the nail fold. Improper trimming or tearing of the nail may cause an irritation of the periungual skin with redness and swelling.

PATHOPHYSIOLOGY

Ingrown toenails may result from the following various causes:

- *Improper nail trimming* - When an ingrown toenail is cut too short or torn into the nail fold, a small portion of the remaining nail may puncture the periungual skin. This can cause a reaction leading to inflammation or the introduction of bacteria into the skin to cause infection. Tapering nail edges or leaving sharp, jagged edges on the nails can also lead to ingrown toenails.
- *Poorly fitting shoes* - Ingrown toenails are often associated with dress shoes or tight or improperly fitting shoes and hosiery, which may exert pressure on the nail or nail fold, causing paronychia or pushing the nail corners into the skin.

- *Obesity* - Weight gain or fluid retention associated with congestive heart failure (CHF), pregnancy, or other medical conditions may lead to pain and swelling of the nail fold that may progress to infection.
- *Trauma and sport injuries* - Trauma to the nail matrix or root of the nail may cause permanent damage to the nail cells. This is most common with a direct blow to the nail plate or, in the athlete, with repetitive injury and pressure to the nail plate. Injury can cause changes in the cells of the matrix, making the external appearance of the nail thicker or ingrown. Athletes commonly experience subungual hematoma or black toenail syndrome, which ultimately causes thickening and ingrowing of the nail.
- *Hyperhidrosis* - Hyperhidrosis of the nail causes maceration of the skin of the nail fold, accumulation of perspiration, and bacteria leading to paronychia.
- *Subungual exostosis* - A bone spur at the distal phalanx of the toe may cause dorsal (upward) pressure on the nail plate. The bone spur causes deformation of the nail bed and incurvation of the nail plate.
- *Heredity* - Familial inheritance of ingrown toenails is common. Inherited ingrown toenails may not be painful but similar nail shape, size, thickness, and incurvation may be seen in many family members.

SIGNS/SYMPTOMS

Redness, swelling, and sensitivity of the toenail are the first symptoms. Symptoms may present as tenderness when wearing shoes or socks, or when touched by bed clothes. Clear or purulent drainage may occur with redness and abscess formation at the distal aspect of the toenail. In the chronic ingrown toenail, formation of pyogenic granuloma (inflamed, pus-producing) tissue is seen.

DIAGNOSTIC PARAMETERS/PHYSICAL ASSESSMENT

Clinical Observation: Observable signs include redness and swelling with or without drainage, as well as increased sensitivity to touch. Discoloration of the toe may also occur. The toe may appear bright pink-to-red or dark red-to-purple in color. Malodor and calor may be present. Maceration of the toe is common when the patient attempts to wear an adhesive bandage for protection.

Interview: To aid patients in the diagnosis and proper treatment of an ingrown nail, it may be beneficial to ask about the following:

- Location of problem
- Duration of signs and symptoms
- Description of condition
- Recent use of ill-fitting shoes, or new shoes/socks
- Recent trauma to the affected toe or nail (eg, via a blow or repetitive pressure to the nail)
- Recent change in activity level (eg, walking, standing, jogging)
- Description of pain, type of pain, situations that result in pain (eg, standing, walking)
- Familial occurrence of ingrown nails
- Concurrent medical conditions such as diabetes, vascular disease, asthma, COPD, or other medical conditions
- Current medication profile (including prescription and nonprescription drugs)
- Self-treatment and efficacy of self-treatment
- Excessive sweating of feet

TREATMENT

Approaches to therapy: The ingrown toenail is a local irritation that can affect every walking step. It is important to initiate early treatment to relieve symptoms and prevent infection. Treatment of the ingrown toenail is directed toward resolution of symptoms and elimination of the cause(s).

Nondrug therapy: If the condition is treated early or the symptoms are minor, twice-daily warm foot soaks with antibacterial soap or Epsom salts is indicated. Advise the patient of proper nail trimming techniques to prevent recurrence and discuss properly fitted, well-ventilated footwear and absorbent hosiery.

Pharmacotherapy: Topical OTC preparations are indicated when nondrug therapy has not resolved symptoms. Topical OTC products are indicated for local treatment of the symptoms of paronychia and inflammation with minor drainage and symptoms. Local anesthetic agents may help relieve pain for short periods of time. None of these agents correct the underlying problem of ingrown toenails. Any recommendation for use of these agents as a treatment for ingrown toenails should come from a pharmacist or physician. Topical creams and ointments may be applied to the nail groove twice daily following a warm foot soak in soapy water or Epsom salts. Reapply the topical medication following bathing. Repeat twice daily for 7 to 10 days. If OTC preparations do not provide relief and symptoms do not resolve, a simple trimming of the offending nail by a podiatrist or other medical professional may be indicated. Refer patients to a physician if an infection is present. If purulent drainage occurs, a culture and sensitivity test may be warranted, especially in the diabetic or vascular-compromised patient. Toenail infections may not resolve without a podiatrist or other medical professional's removal of the ingrown nail spicule or abscess. Seek the advice of a physician if symptoms have not resolved within 2 weeks with OTC medications.

ANTISEPTIC PREPARATIONS

▶ **Indications**

The goal of wound cleansing or antisepsis is to remove necrotic tissue, excess wound exudate, dressing residue, and metabolic waste from the wound surface with as little chemical and mechanical trauma as possible. In general, normal saline is considered to be the "gold standard" for wound cleansing. Antiseptic agents may not be necessary in most superficial, clean wounds and should not be used on healthy granulating tissue because of their toxicity.

Active Ingredient	Actions	Indications
Benzalkonium chloride (BAC)	Cationic surfactant and rapidly-acting anti-infective agent with antimicrobial effects on gram-positive and gram-negative bacteria, and some viruses, fungi, and protozoa, but not on spores. The antimicrobial activity may involve the disruption of cell membranes and denaturation of lipoprotein of microbes. Solutions are bacteriostatic or bactericidal depending on concentration. Solutions also have deodorant, wetting, detergent, keratolytic, and emulsifying activities.	First-aid antiseptic

Active Ingredient	Actions	Indications
Camphorated compounds	Antibacterial agent.	First-aid antiseptic
Chlorhexidine gluconate	Antimicrobial effects against a wide range of organisms, including gram-positive and gram-negative bacteria, such as *Pseudomonas aeruginosa*.	Skin wound cleanser
Hydrogen peroxide	Antimicrobial oxidizing agent. When hydrogen peroxide comes in contact with blood and tissue fluids, oxygen is enzymatically released, which has a physical cleansing effect on a wound. The duration of action is only as long as the period of active oxygen release (fizzing).	First-aid antiseptic and wound cleanser
Iodine	Broad antimicrobial spectrum against bacteria, fungi, virus, spores, protozoa, and yeast.	First-aid antiseptic pre-op skin preparation. 2% iodine and 2.5% sodium iodide are used as antiseptics for superficial wounds. Do not use strong iodine solution as an antiseptic.
Isopropyl alcohol	Stronger bactericidal activity and lower surface tension than ethanol.	First-aid antiseptic
Phenolic compounds	Bacteriostatic at low concentration and bactericidal and fungicidal at higher concentrations.	First-aid antiseptic
Povidone-iodine	Water-soluble complex of iodine with povidone. Povidone-iodine contains 9% to 12% available iodine. It retains the bactericidal activity of iodine but is less potent, and therefore causes less irritation to skin and mucous membranes.	First-aid antiseptic and skin cleanser
Sodium hypochlorite	Has germicidal, deodorizing, and bleaching properties. It is effective against vegetative bacteria and viruses and, to some degree, against spores and fungi.	Skin antiseptic
Triclosan	Bacteriostatic agent with activity against a wide range of gram-positive and gram-negative bacteria.	Skin disinfectant

► Contraindications

In general, hypersensitivity to the active antiseptic ingredient listed. Avoid use of benzalkonium chloride in occlusive dressings because of the risk of irritation and chemical burning. Avoid triclosan application on burned or denuded skin, mucous membranes, or for prophylactic total body bathing.

► Warnings

In general, antiseptic agents are to be applied to intact skin surrounding the wound because direct application of antiseptics to the wound bed can cause tissue irritation.

BENZALKONIUM CHLORIDE

► Indications

Aqueous solutions in appropriate dilutions: Antisepsis of skin, mucous membranes, and wounds; treatment of wounds.

Tinctures and sprays: Treatment of minor skin wounds and abrasions.

► Contraindications

Use in occlusive dressings, casts, and anal or vaginal packs because irritation or chemical burns may result.

▶ Warnings

Diluents: Use Sterile Water for Injection as a diluent for aqueous solutions intended for deep wounds. Otherwise, use freshly distilled water. Tap water containing metallic ions and organic matter may reduce antibacterial potency. Do not use resin deionized water because it may contain pathogenic bacteria.

Storage: Organic, inorganic, and synthetic materials and surfaces may adsorb sufficient quantities to significantly reduce the antibacterial potency in solutions, resulting in serious contamination of solutions with viable pathogenic bacteria. Do not use corks to stopper bottles containing BAC solution. Do not store cotton, wool, rayon, or other materials in solutions. Use sterile gauze sponges and fiber pledgets to apply solutions to the skin, and store in separate containers; immerse in BAC solutions immediately prior to application.

Soaps: BAC solutions are inactivated by soaps and anionic detergents; therefore, rinse thoroughly if these agents are employed prior to BAC use.

Sterilization: Do not rely on antiseptic solutions to achieve complete sterilization; they do not destroy bacterial spores and certain viruses, including the etiologic agent of infectious hepatitis, and may not destroy *Mycobacterium tuberculosis* and other bacteria. In addition, when applied to the skin, BAC may form a film under which bacteria remain viable.

Flammable solvents: The tinted tincture and spray contain flammable organic solvents; do not use near an open flame or cautery.

Eyes/Mucous membranes: If solutions stronger than 1:3,000 enter the eyes, irrigate immediately and repeatedly with water; obtain medical attention promptly. Do not use concentrations over 1:5,000 on mucous membranes, except the vaginal mucosa (see recommended dilutions). Keep the tinted tincture and spray, which contain irritating organic solvents, away from the eyes or other mucous membranes.

Inflamed/Irritated tissues: Solutions used must be more dilute than those used on normal tissues (see recommended dilutions).

▶ Adverse Reactions

Solutions in normal concentrations have low systemic and local toxicity and are generally well tolerated, although a rare individual may exhibit hypersensitivity.

▶ Overdosage

(Systemic—via accidental ingestion/poisoning):

Symptoms – Marked local GI tract irritation (eg, nausea, vomiting) may occur after ingestion. Signs of systemic toxicity include restlessness, apprehension, weakness, confusion, dyspnea, cyanosis, collapse, convulsions, and coma. Death occurs as a result of respiratory muscle paralysis.

Treatment – Immediately administer several glasses of mild soap solution, milk, or egg whites beaten in water. This may be followed by gastric lavage with a mild soap solution. Avoid alcohol as it promotes absorption. Contact the Poison Control Center immediately (800-222-1222).

To support respiration, clear airway and administer oxygen; employ artificial respiration if necessary. If convulsions occur, a short-acting parenteral barbiturate may be given with caution.

► **Administration and Dosage**

Thoroughly rinse anionic detergents and soaps from the skin or other areas prior to use of solutions because they reduce the antibacterial activity of BAC.

Incompatibilities: The following are incompatible with BAC solutions: iodine, silver nitrate, fluorescein, nitrates, peroxide, lanolin, potassium permanganate, aluminum, kaolin, pine oil, zinc sulfate, zinc oxide, yellow oxide of mercury.

Recommended dilutions for specific applications of BAC solutions:

Deeply infected wounds – 1:3,000 to 1:20,000 aqueous solution.

Denuded skin and mucous membranes – 1:5,000 to 1:10,000 aqueous solution.

Minor wounds/lacerations – 1:750 tincture or spray.

Oozing and open infections – 1:2,000 to 1:5,000 aqueous solution.

Wet dressings – Less than 1:5,000 aqueous solution.

Clean the affected area and apply a thin layer 1 to 3 times daily. Cover with sterile bandage if desired. Do not use for longer than 1 week.

BENZALKONIUM CHLORIDE PRODUCTS	
Trade name	Doseform
Benzalkonium Chloride	**Concentrate**: 17% (requires dilution before use)
Bactine	**Liquid**: 0.13%. 2.5% lidocaine HCl, EDTA, octoxynol 9.
	Spray: 0.13%. 2.5% lidocaine HCl, EDTA, octoxynol 9.
	Wipes: 0.13%. 1% pramoxine HCl, EDTA, octoxynol 9.
Benza	**Solution**: 0.13%
Ony-Clear	**Solution**: Benzalkonium chloride, urea, tea tree oil
Zephiran	**Solution, aqueous**: 1:750. Alcohol.
Unguentine Plus	**Cream**: Benzalkonium chloride, benzocaine.

Products listed are representative of currently available and widely distributed brands. Similar products, including regional and private label brands, may also exist.

PATIENT INFORMATION
Benzalkonium Chloride

- Doses and frequency of use depend on the condition, the area to be treated, individual tolerance, and doseform. Individual products should be reviewed for their use and dosage guidelines. Consult your doctor or pharmacist for product-specific information.
- For external use only. Avoid contact with eyes. If contact occurs, immediately flush with water.
- Do not apply over large areas of the body or in large quantities.
- Thoroughly rinse anionic detergents and soaps from the skin or other areas prior to use of solutions because they reduce the antibacterial activity of benzalkonium chloride.
- Do not apply over raw surfaces or blistered areas.
- Consult your doctor before use if you have deep or puncture wounds, animal bites, or serious burns.
- Do not use for longer than 1 week, unless directed by your doctor.
- Stop use and consult your doctor if conditions worsen or if symptoms persist for more than 7 days or clear up and occur again within a few days.
- Discontinue use and consult your doctor if redness, irritation, swelling, or pain increases.
- Benzalkonium chloride's effects are deactivated by soap
- Clean the affected area and apply a thin layer 1 to 3 times daily. Cover with sterile bandage if desired.

CAMPHORATED COMPOUNDS

▶ **Warnings**

Apply to dry skin only; may have caustic effects if applied to moist areas.

▶ **Administration and Dosage**

Clean the affected area before applying. Apply with cotton 1 to 3 times daily.

CAMPHORATED COMPOUND PRODUCTS	
Trade name	**Doseform**
Campho-phenique	**Liquid**: 10.8% camphor, 4.7% phenol, eucalyptus oil, light mineral oil
	Gel: 10.8% camphor, 4.7% phenol, eucalyptus oil, glycerin, light mineral oil

Products listed are representative of currently available and widely distributed brands. Similar products, including regional and private label brands, may also exist.

PATIENT INFORMATION
Camphorated Compounds

- Doses and frequency of use depend on the condition, the area to be treated, individual tolerance, and doseform. Individual products should be reviewed for their use and dosage guidelines. Consult your doctor or pharmacist for product-specific information.
- For external use only. Avoid contact with eyes. If contact occurs, immediately flush with water.
- Do not apply over large areas of the body or in large quantities.
- Consult your doctor before use if you have deep or puncture wounds, animal bites, or serious burns.
- Do not use for longer than 1 week, unless directed by your doctor.
- Stop use and consult your doctor if conditions worsen or if symptoms persist for more than 7 days or clear up and occur again within a few days.
- Discontinue use and consult your doctor if redness, irritation, swelling, or pain increases.
- Clean the affected area and apply liquid with cotton 1 to 3 times daily.
- Do not bandage.
- In case of accidental ingestion, contact your doctor or the Poison Control Center immediately (800-222-1222).

CHLORHEXIDINE GLUCONATE

▶ Indications
Skin wound cleanser.

▶ Contraindications
Hypersensitivity to chlorhexidine gluconate or any component of the product.

▶ Warnings
There have been several case reports of anaphylaxis following disinfection with 0.05% to 1% chlorhexidine. Symptoms included generalized urticaria, bronchospasm, cough, dyspnea, wheezing, and malaise. Symptoms resolved following therapy with various agents including oxygen, aminophylline, epinephrine, corticosteroids, or antihistamines. Refer to Management of Acute Hypersensitivity Reactions.

For external use only: Keep out of eyes, ears, and mouth; if contact accidentally occurs, rinse out promptly and thoroughly with water. Do not use as a preoperative skin preparation of the face or head (except *Hibiclens* liquid).

Excessive heat: Avoid exposing the drug to excessive heat (higher than 40°C [104°F]).

Routine use: Do not use routinely on wounds involving more than superficial layers of skin or for repeated general skin cleansing of large body areas, except in those patients whose underlying condition makes it necessary to reduce the bacterial population of the skin.

Deafness: May cause deafness when instilled in the middle ear. Take particular care in the presence of a perforated eardrum to prevent exposure of inner ear tissues.

Lactation: In one case report, a mother sprayed chlorhexidine gluconate on her breasts to prevent mastitis. Her 2-day-old infant developed bradycardia episodes after breastfeeding; symptoms resolved when the topical chlorhexidine was discontinued by the mother.

▶ **Adverse Reactions**

Irritation; dermatitis; photosensitivity (rare); deafness (see Warnings). Sensitization and generalized allergic reactions have occurred, especially in the genital areas. If adverse reactions occur, discontinue use immediately. If severe, contact a physician.

▶ **Administration and Dosage**

Skin wound and general skin cleanser: Rinse affected area thoroughly with water. Apply a sufficient amount to cover skin or wound area and wash gently. Rinse thoroughly again.

CHLORHEXIDINE GLUCONATE PRODUCTS	
Trade name	Doseform
Hibistat	**Liquid**: 0.5% 70% isopropyl alcohol.
Dyna-Hex, Operand	**Liquid**: 2%. 4% isopropyl alcohol.
Betasept, Dyna-Hex, Hibiclens, Operand	**Liquid**: 4%. 4% isopropyl alcohol.
Hibistat	**Wipes**: 0.5%. 70% isopropyl alcohol.

Products listed are representative of currently available and widely distributed brands. Similar products, including regional and private label brands, may also exist.

PATIENT INFORMATION

Chlorhexidine Gluconate

- Doses and frequency of use depend on the condition, the area to be treated, individual tolerance, and doseform. Individual products should be reviewed for their use and dosage guidelines. Consult your doctor or pharmacist for product-specific information.
- For external use only. Avoid contact with eyes, ears, and mouth, or mucous membranes. If contact occurs, immediately flush with water.
- Consult your doctor before use if you have deep or puncture wounds, animal bites, or serious burns.
- Discontinue use and consult your doctor if redness, irritation, swelling, or pain increases.
- In case of accidental ingestion, contact your doctor or the Poison Control Center immediately (800-222-1222).

HYDROGEN PEROXIDE

▶ **Warnings**

Do not use in abscesses, and do not apply bandages before the compound dries.

▶ **Adverse Reactions**

Generally safe, nonirritating, and noncorrosive.

▶ **Administration and Dosage**

Use on intact skin is of minimal value because the release of nascent oxygen is too slow. Do not use in abscesses. Do not apply bandages before the compound dries. Avoid contact with eyes and mucous membranes.

HYDROGEN PEROXIDE PRODUCTS	
Trade name	Doseform
Hydrogen Peroxide	**Liquid**: 3%

Products listed are representative of currently available and widely distributed brands. Similar products, including regional and private label brands, may also exist.

PATIENT INFORMATION
Hydrogen Peroxide

- Doses and frequency of use depend on the condition, the area to be treated, individual tolerance, and doseform. Individual products should be reviewed for their use and dosage guidelines. Consult your doctor or pharmacist for product-specific information.
- For external use only. Avoid contact with eyes. If contact occurs, immediately flush with water.
- Do not apply over large areas of the body or in large quantities.
- Consult your doctor before use if you have deep or puncture wounds, animal bites, or serious burns.
- Do not use for longer than 1 week, unless directed by your doctor.
- Stop use and consult your doctor if conditions worsen or if symptoms persist for more than 7 days or clear up and occur again within a few days.
- Discontinue use and consult your doctor if redness, irritation, swelling, fever, or pain develop.
- In case of accidental ingestion, contact your doctor or the Poison Control Center immediately (800-222-1222).
- Clean the affected area and apply a thin layer 1 to 3 times daily. Cover with sterile bandage if desired.

IODINE

▶ Indications

Iodine preparations are used externally for their broad microbicidal spectrum against bacteria, fungi, viruses, spores, protozoa, and yeasts. Iodine may be used to disinfect intact skin preoperatively. Potassium iodide is added to increase the solubility of the iodine. Sodium iodide is present to stabilize the tincture and make it miscible with water in all proportions.

▶ Contraindications

Hypersensitivity to iodine.

▶ Warnings

For external use only: Avoid contact with the eyes and mucous membranes.

Highly toxic: Highly toxic if ingested. Sodium thiosulfate is the most effective chemical antidote.

Staining: Iodine preparations stain skin and clothing.

▶ Adverse Reactions

Iodine tincture may be irritating to the tissue.

▶ Administration and Dosage

Do not use with occlusive dressing or bandages.

IODINE PRODUCTS	
Trade name	**Doseform**
Iodine Topical	**Solution**: 2%. 2.4% sodium iodide.
Iodine Tincture Mild	**Solution**: 2%. 2.4% sodium iodide, 47% alcohol.
	Solution, swabsticks: 2%

IODINE PRODUCTS	
Trade name	Doseform
Strong Iodine Tincture	**Solution**: 7%. 5% potassium iodide, 85% alcohol.
Iodex	**Ointment**: 4.7%. Petrolatum.

Products listed are representative of currently available and widely distributed brands. Similar products, including regional and private label brands, may also exist.

PATIENT INFORMATION

Iodine

- Doses and frequency of use depend on the condition, the area to be treated, individual tolerance, and doseform. Individual products should be reviewed for their use and dosage guidelines. Consult your doctor or pharmacist for product-specific information.
- For external use only. Avoid contact with eyes or mucous membranes. If contact occurs, immediately flush with water.
- Do not apply over large areas of the body or in large quantities.
- Consult your doctor before use if you have deep or puncture wounds, animal bites, or serious burns.
- Do not use for longer than 1 week, unless directed by your doctor.
- Stop use and consult your doctor if conditions worsen or if symptoms persist for more than 7 days or clear up and occur again within a few days.
- Discontinue use and consult your doctor if redness, irritation, swelling, or pain develop.
- In case of accidental ingestion, contact your doctor or the Poison Control Center immediately (800-222-1222).
- Highly toxic if ingested.
- May stain skin and clothing or fabrics.
- Use only in well-ventilated areas. Fumes may be harmful.
- Clean the affected area and apply a thin layer 1 to 3 times daily. Do not use with tight-fitting dressings.

ISOPROPYL ALCOHOL

▶ **Warnings**

Flammable; keep away from fire or flame.

▶ **Adverse Reactions**

Tissue irritation with direct application to wound bed. Will dehydrate the skin when applied topically at high concentration. Greater potential for drying the skin than alcohol.

▶ **Administration and Dosage**

May apply on intact skin 1 to 3 times daily. Avoid contact with eyes and mucous membranes.

ISOPROPYL ALCOHOL PRODUCTS	
Trade name	Doseform
Isopropyl Alcohol	**Liquid**: 70% (typically)

Products listed are representative of currently available and widely distributed brands. Similar products, including regional and private label brands, may also exist.

PATIENT INFORMATION
Isopropyl Alcohol

- Doses and frequency of use depend on the condition, the area to be treated, individual tolerance, and doseform. Individual products should be reviewed for their use and dosage guidelines. Consult your doctor or pharmacist for product-specific information.
- For external use only. Avoid contact with eyes or mucous membranes. If contact occurs, immediately flush with water.
- Do not apply over large areas of the body or in large quantities.
- Consult your doctor before use if you have deep or puncture wounds, animal bites, or serious burns.
- Do not use for longer than 1 week, unless directed by your doctor.
- Stop use and consult your doctor if conditions worsen or if symptoms persist for more than 7 days or clear up and occur again within a few days.
- Discontinue use and consult your doctor if redness, irritation, swelling, or pain develop.
- In case of accidental ingestion, contact your doctor or the Poison Control Center immediately (800-222-1222).
- Use only in well-ventilated areas. Fumes may be harmful.
- Clean the affected area and apply a thin layer 1 to 3 times daily. Cover with sterile bandage if desired.

PHENOLIC COMPOUNDS

▶ Warnings

May only be used on the skin as a keratolytic or chemical peel because, in aqueous solutions of more than 1%, it is a primary irritant.

▶ Adverse Reactions

In aqueous solutions of more than 1%, it is a primary irritant and should not be used on the skin except as a keratolytic or peeling agent.

▶ Administration and Dosage

Clean the affected area. Apply with cotton 1 to 3 times daily.

PHENOLIC COMPOUNDS PRODUCTS	
Trade name	Doseform
Campho-phenique	**Liquid**: 10.8% camphor, 4.7% phenol, eucalyptus oil, light mineral oil
	Gel: 10.8% camphor, 4.7% phenol, eucalyptus oil, glycerin, light mineral oil
Castellani Paint Modified	**Liquid**: 1.5% phenol, 13% alcohol
Unguentine	**Ointment**: 1% phenol

Products listed are representative of currently available and widely distributed brands. Similar products, including regional and private label brands, may also exist.

PATIENT INFORMATION
Phenolic Compounds

- Doses and frequency of use depend on the condition, the area to be treated, individual tolerance, and doseform. Individual products should be reviewed for their use and dosage guidelines. Consult your doctor or pharmacist for product-specific information.
- For external use only. Avoid contact with eyes. If contact occurs, immediately flush with water.
- Do not apply over large areas of the body or in large quantities.
- Consult your doctor before use if you have deep or puncture wounds, animal bites, or serious burns.
- Do not use for longer than 1 week, unless directed by your doctor.
- Stop use and consult your doctor if conditions worsen or if symptoms persist for more than 7 days or clear up and occur again within a few days.
- Discontinue use and consult your doctor if redness, irritation, swelling, or pain develop.
- In case of accidental ingestion, contact your doctor or the Poison Control Center immediately (800-222-1222).
- Cleanse affected area as directed. Check individual package labels for directions.
- May stain skin and clothing or fabrics.
- Clean the affected area and apply a thin layer 1 to 3 times daily. Do not bandage.

POVIDONE-IODINE

▶ Warnings

Hypothyroidism: A 6-week-old infant developed low serum total thyroxine concentration and high thyroid stimulating hormone concentration following maternal use of topical povidone-iodine during pregnancy and lactation. In 1 study, the use of povidone-iodine solution on very low birth weight infants resulted in neonatal hypothyroidism. In contrast, women who used povidone-iodine douche daily for 14 days did not develop overt hypothyroidism; however, there was a significant increase in serum total iodine concentration and urine iodine excretion. Use with caution during pregnancy and lactation and in infants.

Open wounds: Avoid solutions containing a detergent if treating open wounds with povidone-iodine. The value of povidone-iodine on open wounds has not been established.

▶ Adverse Reactions

Hypothyroidism may develop when used to treat large wounds in patients with abnormal renal function. May cause a hypersensitivity reaction.

▶ Administration and Dosage

Unlike iodine tincture, treated areas may be bandaged.

POVIDONE-IODINE PRODUCTS	
Trade name	Doseform
Betadine	**Aerosol**: 5%. Glycerin, dibasic sodium phosphate.
	Ointment: 10%. Polyethylene glycols.
	Skin cleanser: 7.5%. Ammonium nonoxynol-4-sulfate, lauramide DEA.
	Solution: 10%. Glycerin, nonoxynol-9.
	Solution, swab aid: 10%. Glycerin, nonoxynol-9.
	Solution, swabsticks: 10%. Glycerin, nonoxynol-9.
Minidyne	**Solution**: 10%. Citric acid and sodium phosphate dibasic.
Operand	**Gel**: 10%. 1% iodine
	Solution: 10%. 1% iodine
	Scrub: 7.5%. 0.75% iodine
	Solution, pads: 10%. 1% iodine
	Solution, swabsticks: 10%. 1% iodine

Products listed are representative of currently available and widely distributed brands. Similar products, including regional and private label brands, may also exist.

PATIENT INFORMATION
Povidone-Iodine

- Doses and frequency of use depend on the condition, the area to be treated, individual tolerance, and doseform. Individual products should be reviewed for their use and dosage guidelines. Consult your doctor or pharmacist for product-specific information.
- For external use only. Avoid contact with eyes or mucous membranes. If contact occurs, immediately flush with water.
- Do not apply over large areas of the body or in large quantities.
- Consult your doctor before use if you have deep or puncture wounds, animal bites, or serious burns.
- Do not use for longer than 1 week, unless directed by your doctor.
- Stop use and consult your doctor if conditions worsen or if symptoms persist for more than 7 days or clear up and occur again within a few days.
- Discontinue use and consult your doctor if redness, irritation, swelling, or pain increases.
- In case of accidental ingestion, contact your doctor or the Poison Control Center immediately (800-222-1222).
- Clean the affected area and apply a thin layer 1 to 3 times daily. Cover with sterile bandage if desired.

SODIUM HYPOCHLORITE

▶ Indications

Applied topically to the skin as an antiseptic.

▶ Warnings

Avoid eye contact with this solution. Use with caution as chemical burns may be produced.

Chemical burns: Chemical burns may be produced; avoid eye contact with this solution.

▶ **Administration and Dosage**

Administer as lavage solution for wounds.

SODIUM HYPOCHLORITE PRODUCTS	
Trade name	**Doseform**
Di-Dak-Sol (Diluted Dakin's Solution)	**Solution**: 0.0125%
Dakin's Half Strength	**Solution**: 0.25%
Dakin's Full Strength	**Solution**: 0.5%

Products listed are representative of currently available and widely distributed brands. Similar products, including regional and private label brands, may also exist.

PATIENT INFORMATION

Sodium Hypochlorite

- Doses and frequency of use depend on the condition, the area to be treated, individual tolerance, and doseform. Individual products should be reviewed for their use and dosage guidelines. Consult your doctor or pharmacist for product-specific information.
- For external use only. Avoid contact with eyes or mucous membranes. Chemical burns may be produced. If contact occurs, immediately flush with water.
- Do not apply over large areas of the body or in large quantities.
- Consult your doctor before use if you have deep or puncture wounds, animal bites, or serious burns.
- Do not use for longer than 1 week, unless directed by your doctor.
- Stop use and consult your doctor if conditions worsen or if symptoms persist for more than 7 days or clear up and occur again within a few days.
- Discontinue use and consult your doctor if redness, irritation, swelling, or pain increases.
- In case of accidental ingestion, contact your doctor or the Poison Control Center immediately (800-222-1222).

TRICLOSAN

▶ **Indications**

Skin cleanser. May use as hand/body wash, shampoo, or bed or towel bath.

▶ **Contraindications**

Use on burned or denuded skin or mucous membranes; routine prophylactic total body bathing.

Not a surgical scrub; do not use in preparation for surgery.

▶ **Warnings**

Septi-Soft is not a surgical scrub and should not be used in preparation for surgery. Avoid contact with the eyes.

For external use only: Avoid contact with the eyes.

▶ **Administration and Dosage**

Dispense a small amount (5 mL) on hands, rub thoroughly for 30 seconds, rinse thoroughly, and dry.

TRICLOSAN PRODUCTS	
Trade name	Doseform
Septi-Soft	**Body wash and shampoo**: 0.25%

Products listed are representative of currently available and widely distributed brands. Similar products, including regional and private label brands, may also exist.

PATIENT INFORMATION

Triclosan

- Doses and frequency of use depend on the condition, the area to be treated, individual tolerance, and doseform. Individual products should be reviewed for their use and dosage guidelines. Consult your doctor or pharmacist for product-specific information.
- For external use only. Avoid contact with eyes or mucous membranes. Chemical burns may be produced. If contact occurs, immediately flush with water.
- Do not apply over large areas of the body or in large quantities.
- Consult your doctor before use if you have deep or puncture wounds, animal bites, or serious burns.
- Do not use for longer than 1 week, unless directed by your doctor.
- Stop use and consult your doctor if conditions worsen or if symptoms persist for more than 7 days or clear up and occur again within a few days.
- Discontinue use and consult your doctor if redness, irritation, swelling, or pain increases.
- In case of accidental ingestion, contact your doctor or the Poison Control Center immediately (800-222-1222).

FIRST-AID ANTIBIOTICS

▶ Indications

Infection in minor cuts, burns, wounds, and scrapes may be alleviated by topical OTC antibiotics (eg, tetracycline, bacitracin/neomycin/polymyxin B sulfate combination). The pharmacist should assess the wound and possible infection before recommending any topical product. Consider referral to a physician in the following situations:

- Uncertainty over cause of infection.
- Top layer of skin is missing from a large area.
- Wound continues to drain a large amount of exudate. Draining and pain are aided by lancing.
- Infection is widespread.
- Deep lesions cover a wide area of skin.
- Underlying illness (eg, diabetes, systemic infection, immune deficiency), which may predispose patients to serious abrasions.
- Unsuccessful initial attempt at treatment or worsened condition.

Active Ingredient	Actions	Indications
Bacitracin	Polypeptide bactericidal antibiotic that inhibits cell wall synthesis in several gram-positive organisms.	Help prevent infection in minor cuts, burns, wounds, and scrapes.
Neomycin	Aminoglycoside antibiotic that exerts its bacterial activity by inhibiting protein synthesis in gram-negative organisms and some species of *Staphylococcus*.	Help prevent infection in minor cuts, burns, wounds, and scrapes.
Polymyxin B Sulfate	Polypeptide antibiotic effective against several gram-negative organisms by altering cell wall permeability.	Help prevent infection in minor cuts, burns, wounds, and scrapes.

▶ **Contraindications**

Hypersensitivity to any of the listed ingredients. Do not use in eyes or in external ear canal if the eardrum is perforated.

▶ **Warnings**

For topical use only. Deeper cutaneous infections may require systemic antibiotic therapy in addition to local treatment. Because of the potential nephrotoxicity and ototoxicity of neomycin, use with care in treating extensive burns, trophic ulceration, or other extensive conditions in which absorption is possible. Do not apply more than once daily in burn cases involving more than 20% of body surface, especially if the patient has impaired renal function or is receiving other aminoglycoside antibiotics concurrently. Chronic application of neomycin to inflamed skin of individuals with allergic contact dermatitis increases the possibility of sensitization.

Neomycin: Low-grade reddening with swelling, dry scaling, and itching, or a failure to heal are usually manifestations of this hypersensitivity. During long-term use of neomycin-containing products, perform periodic examinations and discontinue use if symptoms appear. These symptoms regress upon withdrawal of medication, but avoid neomycin-containing products thereafter.

Cross-sensitization: Sensitization is frequent, and patients may experience cross-reaction to gentamicin.

▶ **Drug Interactions**

None significant.

▶ **Adverse Reactions**

Bacitracin: Allergic contact dermatitis has been reported. Case reports of anaphylaxis.

Neomycin: Ototoxicity and nephrotoxicity have been reported with its use.

Polymyxin B sulfate: Rare sensitizer.

BACITRACIN

▶ **Administration and Dosage**

Clean the affected area and apply a thin layer 1 to 3 times daily. Cover with sterile bandage if desired. Do not use for longer than 1 week.

BACITRACIN PRODUCTS	
Trade name	**Doseform**
Bacitracin	**Ointment**: 500 units/g

Products listed are representative of currently available and widely distributed brands. Similar products, including regional and private label brands, may also exist.

NEOMYCIN

▶ Administration and Dosage

Clean the affected area and apply a thin layer 1 to 3 times daily. Cover with sterile bandage if desired. Do not use for longer than 1 week.

NEOMYCIN PRODUCTS	
Trade name	Doseform
Neomycin	**Ointment**: 3.5 mg (as sulfate)/g

Products listed are representative of currently available and widely distributed brands. Similar products, including regional and private label brands, may also exist.

POLYMYXIN B SULFATE AND NEOMYCIN

▶ Administration and Dosage

Clean the affected area and apply a thin layer 1 to 3 times daily. Cover with sterile bandage if desired. Do not use for longer than 1 week.

POLYMYXIN B SULFATE/NEOMYCIN PRODUCTS	
Trade name	Doseform
Neosporin Plus	**Cream**: 10,000 units polymyxin B, 3.5 mg neomycin, 10 mg pramoxine HCl/g. Methylparaben, mineral oil, white petrolatum.

Products listed are representative of currently available and widely distributed brands. Similar products, including regional and private label brands, may also exist.

POLYMYXIN B SULFATE AND BACITRACIN

▶ Administration and Dosage

Clean the affected area and apply a thin layer 1 to 3 times daily. Cover with sterile bandage if desired. Do not use for longer than 1 week.

POLYMYXIN B SULFATE/BACITRACIN PRODUCTS	
Trade name	Doseform
Betadine, Polysporin[1]	**Ointment**: 10,000 units polymyxin B sulfate, 500 units bacitracin zinc/g
Betadine Plus	**Ointment**: 10,000 units polymyxin B sulfate, 500 units bacitracin zinc, 1% pramoxine HCl/g

Products listed are representative of currently available and widely distributed brands. Similar products, including regional and private label brands, may also exist.

[1] Contains white petrolatum.

POLYMYXIN B SULFATE, NEOMYCIN, AND BACITRACIN

▶ **Administration and Dosage**

Clean the affected area and apply a thin layer 1 to 3 times daily. Cover with sterile bandage if desired. Do not use for longer than 1 week.

POLYMYXIN B SULFATE/NEOMYCIN/BACITRACIN PRODUCTS	
Trade name	Doseform
Lanabiotic	**Ointment**: 10,000 units polymyxin B sulfate, 5 mg neomycin, 500 units bacitracin, 40 mg lidocaine, aloe, lanolin, mineral oil, petrolatum
Bactine, Neosporin Plus, Spectrocin Plus	**Ointment**: 10,000 units polymyxin B sulfate, 3.5 mg neomycin, 500 units bacitracin, 10 mg pramoxine HCl/g. White petrolatum.
Triple Antibiotic[1], Neosporin[2,3]	**Ointment**: 5000 units polymyxin B sulfate, 3.5 mg neomycin, 400 units bacitracin zinc/g

Products listed are representative of currently available and widely distributed brands. Similar products, including regional and private label brands, may also exist.

[1] Contains white petrolatum, light mineral oil.
[2] Contains cottonseed oil, olive oil, white petrolatum.
[3] Available in portable pocket-sized packets.

PATIENT INFORMATION
First-Aid Antibiotics

- Doses and frequency of use depend on the condition, the area to be treated, individual tolerance, and doseform. Individual products should be reviewed for their use and dosage guidelines. Consult your doctor or pharmacist for product-specific information.
- For external use only. Avoid contact with eyes or mucous membranes. If contact occurs, immediately flush with water.
- Do not apply over large areas of the body or in large quantities.
- Do not apply over raw surfaces or blistered areas.
- Consult your doctor before use if you have deep or puncture wounds, animal bites, or serious burns.
- Do not use for longer than 1 week, unless directed by your doctor.
- Stop use and consult your doctor if conditions worsen or if symptoms persist for more than 7 days or clear up and occur again within a few days.
- Discontinue use and consult your doctor if redness, irritation, swelling, or pain increases.
- In case of accidental ingestion, contact your doctor or the Poison Control Center immediately (800-222-1222).
- Clean the affected area and apply a thin layer 1 to 3 times daily. Cover with sterile bandage if desired.

PLANTAR WARTS

DEFINITION

Verrucae plantaris, or plantar warts, are caused by the human papillomavirus (HPV). The virus invades the outer layers of skin and does not grow below the dermis. The term "plantar" refers to the plantar aspect of the foot. Verrucae tend to recur frequently and are difficult to cure.

ETIOLOGY

HPV is the cause of wart lesions. A wart lesion forms when excessive perspiration or a break in the integrity of the skin such as a scratch, blister, or puncture wound allows the virus to enter the superficial skin layer. The virus invades individual cells, takes over the function of the nucleus and begins to replicate. The virus is most commonly transmitted in warm moist places such as shoes, indoor pools, and locker rooms.

INCIDENCE

Verrucae plantaris is the most common viral disease of the foot. It is most often found in children and young adults and is associated with excessive perspiration and high levels of activity in sports, which predisposes one to HPV. Verrucae plantaris infection can occur in the immunocompromised patient during treatment of cancer, HIV/AIDS, and other medical conditions requiring immunosuppressant therapy.

PATHOPHYSIOLOGY

The abnormal growth of the HPV occurs in the outer skin layers. The infection begins in the epidermis but never grows below the dermis. Warts on the plantar aspect or bottom of the foot appear deep but do not "grow down to the bone" as patients may insist. This perception exists because the wart lesion presses on deep nerves, causing pain that feels as if it is originating from a deep lesion. As the virus replicates, epithelial hyperplasia occurs, causing an irregular appearance of the skin. On the foot, the wart may appear on the toes, between the toes, or on the dorsal aspect of the foot. However, the plantar aspect of the foot is the most common location. Pressure from standing causes the lesions to be painful, because it causes further pressure on the deep nerves.

SIGNS/SYMPTOMS

The patient may relate rapid growth of what was originally thought to be a callous on the bottom of the foot. The lesion begins as a small, smooth-surfaced, skin-colored lesion that enlarges after a period of time. Initially, these lesions are not painful, but as they enlarge, can cause discomfort with and without shoe wear.

DIAGNOSTIC PARAMETERS/PHYSICAL ASSESSMENT

Clinical Observation: At the plantar aspect of the foot, the lesion appears white or skin-colored with a rough epithelial surface. This surface is described as papillary in nature, similar in appearance to a head of broccoli or cauli-flower. Additionally, there is interruption of the skin lines; normal skin lines do not transverse the lesion. Dark capillary endings are also seen and are often described as the "seeds" of the wart. These dark capillary endings appear to be caused by friction and rubbing of the lesion and show pinpoint bleeding on debridement. The final clinical observation is discomfort with side-to-side pressure of the lesion. Verrucae may occur singularly or occur in multiple patches called mosaic verrucae. On the plantar aspect of the foot, the lesions are flat and circular in shape, whereas on the top of the foot or toes, the lesions are dome-shaped above the skin.

Interview: To aid patients in the diagnosis and proper treatment of plantar warts, it may be beneficial to ask about the following:

- Signs and symptoms, duration, and frequency of occurrence.
- The location and the shape of the lesions.
- Description of pain, if any, including pain while walking, standing, or at rest.
- Infection or broken skin on the feet, bleeding, discharge, hair growing from the area.
- Concurrent medical conditions, such as diabetes, COPD, asthma, or cardiovascular disease, and medication profile (prescription and nonprescription).
- Pregnancy or breastfeeding.
- Family history of warts.
- Self-treatment.

The patient will describe a long-standing or recent occurrence of the lesion with or without discomfort. Multiple recurrences of the lesions are common and are associated with heavy perspiration or hyperhidrosis.

TREATMENT

Approaches to therapy: Treatment is focused on resolution of symptoms and destruction of the wart lesion, by desiccation, keratolysis, or surgical removal.

Nondrug therapy: Although most patients do not seek treatment until warts have reached advanced stages, the wart, if caught early, can be destroyed by desiccation because the virus cannot live without moisture. Following use of a drying foot soak, change socks and shoes twice daily with the use of a talc or cornstarch powder to absorb moisture. Cotton socks are recommended for their ability to absorb moisture.

Pharmacotherapy: Pharmacotherapy is aimed at drying of the lesion, or complete destruction of the wart lesion. Nonprescription therapy is intended to dry the lesion via foot soaks in Epsom salts or a vinegar/water solution. Other astringent products include *Domeboro* or *Pedi-Boro* soaking agents. Prescription drying agents are also available but should be used in conjunction with a topical wart preparation. Topical agents (eg, plasters, collodions) contain salicylic acid as the main component to cause keratolysis and destruction of the skin cells that contain the HPV.

When drying agents are unsuccessful, other treatments by a physician may include the following: Hyfrecation, laser ablation, surgical excision, or the use of bleomycin or liquid nitrogen. Each of these treatment methods have equal successes and failures caused by the viral nature of these lesions. Recurrence of wart lesions may occur no matter which method is selected.

SALICYLIC ACID

► Actions
The topical products contain salicylic acid in a 17% to 40% concentration and cause keratolysis of the lesion and destruction of the HPV.

► Indications
Topical products are indicated for the treatment of common plantar verrucae that have not resolved with non-drug therapy.

► Contraindications
Nonprescription products should not be used in the presence of infection, broken skin, diabetes, COPD, asthma, or peripheral vascular disease. The products should not be used on genital warts, facial lesions, or lesions on mucosal surfaces, moles, or lesions with hair growing from them or on the face.

► Warnings
These products are for external use only and should be kept away from fire, flame, or heat. Consult obstetrician/gynecologist prior to use during pregnancy or when breastfeeding. Discontinue treatment if excessive irritation occurs. Avoid inhaling vapors. Avoid contact with healthy skin, eyes, eyelids, or mucous membranes.

► Drug Interactions
There are no known drug/drug or drug/food interactions associated with these topical agents.

► Adverse Reactions
Local irritation of the non-involved healthy skin may occur if application of the topical medication is beyond the borders of the wart lesion. The adverse reactions may involve blistering of the skin, redness and irritation of the normal skin surrounding the wart, or irritation of the skin secondary to the adhesive on bandages or patches supplied to secure the medication. On rare occasions, formation of a sterile abscess has occurred with the overzealous application of medication. Adverse reactions can be reversed by temporarily discontinuing the product, soaking foot in warm water, and resuming medication only when symptoms are completely resolved. Consult a physician.

► Administration and Dosage
Prior to the application of the wart medications, most products recommend a warm foot soak followed by filing of the lesion with an emory board, brush, or wash cloth to remove any loose skin. The area is dried thoroughly, and the medication is applied according to package instructions. The usual dose is applied twice daily for a minimum of 4 to 6 weeks.

SALICYLIC ACID PRODUCTS	
Trade name	**Doseform**
Dr. Scholl's Wart Remover Kit, Maximum Strength Wart Remover, Wart-Off	**Liquid**: 17%
DuoPlant	**Gel**: 17%
Mediplast	**Transdermal Patch**: 40%
Dr. Scholl's Clear Away Plantar	**Disk**: 40% in rubber-based vehicle.
Sal-Acid	**Plaster**: 40%

Products listed are representative of currently available and widely distributed brands. Similar products, including regional and private label brands, may also exist.

PATIENT INFORMATION
Salicylic Acid Products

- Wart lesions are a benign medical condition. Treatment is initiated to relieve painful symptoms involved in the location of the wart and to prevent spread in the patient or to other family members.
- The most common problem in treating warts is discontinuing treatment with topical medication before the lesion is completely destroyed. Although most products list 4 to 6 weeks as an appropriate treatment time, larger or more resistant lesions may require up to 12 or more weeks of treatment.
- Once a wart lesion is completely resolved, steps must be taken to prevent recurrence of this viral lesion. Topical foot antiperspirants, foot powders, and frequent changing of socks and shoes will help prevent recurrent infections. The use of water shoes and thongs in public showers is also recommended to prevent reinnoculation.
- If warts do not resolve with topical products following diligent use for 12 weeks, the patient should seek the advice of a podiatrist, dermatologist, or physician.
- Wart removal products are for external use only.
- Avoid contact with healthy skin, eyes, eyelids, or mucous membranes.
- Do not use on other dermatological lesions (eg, genital warts, moles, facial lesions, or skin growths on other areas of the body).
- Keep liquid products away from fire, flame, or heat.
- If excessive irritation occurs with the use of these products, discontinue use and contact a health care professional.
- Avoid inhaling vapors of liquid wart removal products.
- If you are pregnant or breastfeeding, consult a physician before using wart removal products.
- If you suffer from diabetes, cardiovascular disease, COPD, asthma, or peripheral vascular disease, consult a physician before using wart removal products.
- Do not use in the presence of an infection or broken skin.

ALUMINUM ACETATE SOLUTION

▶ **Indications**

Aluminum acetate solution provides an astringent wet dressing for relief of inflammatory conditions of the skin.

▶ **Warnings**

Discontinue use if intolerance, irritation, or extension of the inflammatory condition being treated occurs. If symptoms persist longer than 7 days, discontinue use and consult a physician.

Do not use plastic or other impervious material to prevent evaporation.

For external use only. Avoid contact with the eyes.

▶ **Drug Interactions**

Collagenase: The enzyme activity of topical collagenase may be inhibited by aluminum acetate solution because of the metal ion and low pH. Cleanse the site of the solution with repeated washings of normal saline before applying the enzyme ointment.

▶ **Administration and Dosage**

One packet or tablet in a pint of water produces a modified 1:40 Burow's solution. Apply for 15 to 30 minutes for 4 to 6 times daily. Wetting gauze with the solution is a suggested method for application to smaller, defined areas (eg, hand, arm, face, foot).

ALUMINUM ACETATE SOLUTION PRODUCTS	
Trade name	Doseform
Domeboro Astringent Solution, Pedi-Boro Soak Paks	**Powder, tablets**: Aluminum sulfate and calcium acetate.

Products listed are representative of currently available and widely distributed brands. Similar products, including regional and private label brands, may also exist.

PATIENT INFORMATION

Aluminum Acetate Solution

- For external use only. Do not use in eyes or allow to come in contact with the eye(s) or eyelid(s).
- Do not use if you are allergic to any ingredient of the products.
- Do not use on irritated or broken skin without consulting a physician or pharmacist.
- If the condition persists or worsens, or if irritation develops, discontinue use and consult a physician.
- Apply to affected skin with gentle massage as instructed by a physician

TINEA PEDIS
(Athlete's Foot)

DEFINITION
Also known as athlete's foot, tinea pedis is a common, superficial fungal infection of the skin of the foot. Other terms used to describe tinea pedis are foot fungus, ringworm of the foot, and jungle rot.

ETIOLOGY
The most common organisms associated with tinea pedis are *Trichophyton rubrum*, *T. mentagrophytes*, and *Epidermophyton floccosum*. These fungi flourish in the warm moist environment of enclosed shoes and excessive perspiration. The fungal infection, spread by contact with contaminated surfaces, begins as dermatophytes grow on dead keratin cells of the skin. Many of the fungi are normal flora of the skin.

INCIDENCE
Tinea pedis is the most common fungal infection in humans, with approximately 70% of all fungal infections occurring on the feet. The incidence is approximately 38.7 per 1000 people, with most people developing some type of mild infection at least once in their lifetime. The highest incidence of fungal infection is noted in teenagers, athletes, and those who work long hours wearing tight-fitting, poorly ventilated shoes and nonabsorbent socks.

PATHOPHYSIOLOGY
Stages of tinea pedis infection include the following: incubation, enlargement, refractory period, and involution. When the infection becomes established, the rate of organism growth and epidermal cell turnover will determine the duration and size of the lesions. The infection does not spread beyond the foot and remains within the stratum corneum. The signs and symptoms of tinea pedis depend on the infecting fungus: *T. rubrum* causes a dry hyperkeratotic pattern; *T. mentagrophytes* causes a vesicular pattern; *E. floccosum* presents a mixed pattern. However, because the specific organism does not dictate the type of therapy, isolation of the specific fungus is not essential.

SIGNS/SYMPTOMS
Unilateral or bilateral itching, peeling, and maceration of the foot are likely to be present. In the acute stages of infection, a red, pruritic vesicular reaction is seen. This is characterized by small blisters filled with a clear or straw-colored fluid. Surrounding the vesicles, redness, weeping of the vesicular lesions, mild swelling, and evidence of excoriation are seen. Fissuring of the skin at the interdigital spaces, especially at the fourth digital interspace and fifth toe, is common. The patient may describe pruritus and a burning sensation of the foot. Conversely, the chronic fungal infection manifests as dry, scaling skin with a mild underlying redness. This is commonly misinterpreted as dry skin and is usually otherwise asymptomatic.

DIAGNOSTIC PARAMETERS/PHYSICAL ASSESSMENT

Clinical Observation: Heavy moisture may appear on the skin and socks. In the acute presentation, a red, vesicular rash forms with weeping of the skin and foot odor (which may indicate a concurrent bacterial infection). A severe, acute bacterial infection may form bullae and pustules. In chronic tinea pedis, there is dry scaling of the skin with an underlying margin of redness. In refractory cases, physician referral is recommended to confirm the condition: A potassium hydroxide slide preparation or dermatophyte test media (DTM) will confirm the presence of fungal elements; a gram stain will rule out secondary bacterial infection. Differential diagnoses include contact dermatitis, atopic eczema, psoriasis, and hyperhidrosis of the feet.

Interview: To aid the patient in the diagnosis and proper treatment of tinea pedis, it may be beneficial to ask about the following:

- Description, location, and duration of signs and symptoms of the condition
- Presence of pain, swelling, or whitish discharge from lesions
- History of tinea pedis (either in adolescence or adulthood)
- Toenail involvement
- Family members with the same condition
- Description of any past self-treatment, including success of treatment and recurrence of the condition
- History of excessive sweating of the feet
- Recent changes in footwear (eg, different shoes, new type of socks [eg, wool, nylon] or nylon stockings, no socks), laundry detergent, fabric softener, or soap
- Recent increase in physical activity
- Exposure to contaminated surfaces (eg, public shower facilities)
- Presence of foot odor
- Overall nutritional status
- Coexisting diseases (eg, diabetes, cancer)
- Presence of immunosuppressant drugs in the regimen

TREATMENT

Approaches to therapy: Therapy is dependent on duration and severity of symptoms and can include nondrug therapy with pharmacotherapy or treatment by a physician. A severe case of tinea pedis involves sloughing and blistering of the skin or secondary bacterial infection and requires a prescription medication for treatment.

Nondrug therapy: Nondrug therapy is appropriate in patients with mild symptoms or early onset as adjunctive therapy only. Such therapy consists of keeping the foot dry via astringent foot soaks in epsom salt solution or vinegar and water solution (for wet forms of the condition only). The goal of such therapy is to convert the condition to a dry form. Essential nondrug adjuncts to pharmacotherapy include the following: daily foot hygiene, light cotton socks (changed daily), well-ventilated footwear, medicated or nonmedicated foot powder, rubber sandals in public or family shower facilities.

Pharmacotherapy: If nondrug therapy has failed or symptoms are more severe, numerous OTC agents are available. Most products contain agents that are fungicidal against the most common dermatophytes, including yeast. The initial treatment is aimed at relieving symptoms; however, to produce complete resolution, treatment must continue for at least 2 weeks following resolution of symptoms.

UNDECYLENIC ACID AND DERIVATIVES

▶ Actions

Antifungal agents impair the synthesis of ergosterol, a component of the fungus cell membrane, ultimately causing the destruction of the fungus cell membrane and rendering the fungus nonviable.

Undecylenic acid and its derivatives are antifungal and antibacterial agents for tinea pedis, exclusive of the nails and hairy areas. These agents have additional indications (eg, for the relief and prevention of diaper rash, itching, burning and chafing, prickly heat, tinea cruris [jock itch], excessive perspiration and irritation in the groin area, bromhidrosis [foul-smelling perspiration]).

▶ Indications

For the relief of the signs and symptoms of tinea pedis (athlete's foot) associated with fungus or yeast infection. These agents have additional indications (eg, prickly heat, eczema, tinea cruris [jock itch], tinea corporis [ringworm]).

▶ Contraindications

Allergy or sensitivity to the preparation or its components; patients with diabetes or peripheral vascular disease.

Self-care is contraindicated in the following situations: toenail involvement; purulent discharge; whitish, soggy, foul-smelling toe webs; inflammation or swelling of a major portion of the foot.

▶ Warnings

External use: For external use only. Avoid inhaling. Do not use in mouth, eyes, or vagina.

Pregnancy: Consult an obstetrician/gynecologist prior to use in pregnancy.

Lactation: Topical preparations are known to be excreted in breast milk. Use with caution.

Children: Do not use in children younger than 2 years of age unless directed by a physician.

▶ Drug Interactions

There are no known drug/drug or drug/food interactions with topical undecylenic acid.

▶ Adverse Reactions

Adverse reactions are usually limited to the local application sites. Erythema, stinging, pruritus, and general irritation of the skin may occur. Local allergic reactions have been seen on the skin from the components of the topical spray products.

▶ Administration and Dosage

Follow dosing guidelines for individual products. Twice-daily application is recommended. Cleanse and dry area well before application; smooth on. Wash hands with soap and water after use to avoid spreading infection. The condition generally resolves within 2 weeks, although treatment should continue for at least 2 weeks following resolution of symptoms (maximum recommended duration of treatment is 4 weeks for most patients).

The choice of vehicle is important for these products. Solutions are used as primary therapy. In general, powders are used as adjunctive therapy, but they may be acceptable as primary therapy in very mild conditions.

UNDECYLENIC ACID AND DERIVATIVES PRODUCTS	
Trade name	Doseform
Blis-To-Sol	**Powder**: 12% zinc undecylenate
Fungi Nail	**Solution**: 25% undecylenic acid
Elon Dual Defense Anti-Fungal Formula	**Solution**: 25% undecylenic acid. Ethyl alcohol, lime oil, tea tree oil.
Blis-To-Sol	**Liquid**: 1% undecylenic acid

Products listed are representative of currently available and widely distributed brands. Similar products, including regional and private label brands, may also exist.

PATIENT INFORMATION
Undecylenic Acid and Derivatives

- The most important factor in treating tinea pedis (athlete's foot) is the duration and consistency in treatment. It is common for the patient to discontinue use of a product after a few days when relief of symptoms is experienced. However, it is very important to continue treatment for at least 2 weeks after symptoms have been relieved to prevent recurrence or infection of the toenails.
- For external use only. Avoid contact with eyes, nose, mouth, or other mucous membranes.
- Cleanse skin with soap and water and dry thoroughly before applying product. Wash hands after applying the medication to the affected areas.
- Do not apply to blistered, oozing, or raw skin.
- Notify your pharmacist or physician if there is no improvement after 4 weeks of treatment.
- Avoid the use of occlusive dressings unless directed by your physician.
- Patients with decreased circulation, including diabetic patients, should consult their physician before using these products.
- Frequency of application and duration of therapy is dependent on the location of the condition, the drug, the strength of the drug, and the doseform used. For assistance in drug selection and dosage guidelines, consult your pharmacist or physician.
- If condition persists or worsens, or if irritation (burning, itching, stinging, redness) occurs, discontinue use and notify your pharmacist or physician.
- Inform your pharmacist or physician if the area of application shows signs of increased irritation (eg, redness, itching, burning, blistering, swelling, oozing) indicative of possible sensitization.
- Do not use on children younger than 2 years of age unless directed by a physician.
- Essential adjuncts to antifungal therapy that should be undertaken by the patient include the following: daily foot hygiene, light cotton socks (changed daily), well-ventilated footwear, medicated or nonmedicated foot powder, and rubber sandals in public or family shower facilities.
- Wear well-fitting, ventilated shoes. Change shoes and socks at least once daily.

TOLNAFTATE

▶ Actions

Effective in the treatment of superficial fungal infections of the skin.

▶ Indications

For the treatment of tinea pedis (athlete's foot), tinea cruris (jock itch), or tinea corporis (ringworm) caused by *Trichophyton rubrum*, *T. mentagrophytes*, *T. tonsurans*, *Microsporum canis*, *M. audouini*, *Epidermophyton floccosum*, and *Malassezia furfur*, the active organism in tinea versicolor.

Powder and powder aerosol: Effective prophylactically against athlete's foot.

▶ Contraindications

Allergy or sensitivity to the preparation or its components; patients with diabetes or peripheral vascular disease.

Self-care is contraindicated in the following situations: toenail involvement; purulent discharge; whitish, soggy, foul-smelling toe webs; inflammation or swelling of a major portion of the foot.

▶ Warnings

If symptoms do not improve after 10 days of use as recommended by the labeling, discontinue use unless otherwise directed.

External use: For external use only. Avoid inhaling. Do not use in mouth, eyes, or vagina.

Sensitivity: If sensitization or irritation occurs, discontinue use and contact your pharmacist or physician.

Pregnancy: Consult an obstetrician/gynecologist prior to use in pregnancy.

Lactation: Topical preparations are known to be excreted in breast milk. Use with caution.

▶ Adverse Reactions

A few cases of sensitization have been confirmed; mild irritation has occurred.

▶ Administration and Dosage

Follow dosing guidelines for individual products. Twice-daily application for 2 or 3 weeks is usually adequate, although 4 to 6 weeks may be required if the skin has thickened. Cleanse and dry area well before application. Creams, sprays, solutions, and gels should be applied generously to all involved areas and between toes. Wash hands with soap and water after use to avoid spreading infection. The condition generally resolves within 2 weeks, although treatment should continue for at least 2 weeks following resolution of symptoms.

The choice of vehicle is important for these products. Creams, gels, and liquids are used as primary therapy. In general, powders are used as adjunctive therapy, but they may be acceptable as primary therapy in very mild conditions.

TOLNAFTATE PRODUCTS	
Trade name	Doseform
Tinactin	**Cream**: 1%. Cetearyl alcohol, mineral oil, petrolatum.
Ting	**Cream**: 1%. White petrolatum.
Quinsana Plus, Tinactin	**Powder**: 1%
Blis-To-Sol Antifungal, Tinactin	**Solution**: 1%

TOLNAFTATE PRODUCTS	
Trade name	Doseform
Absorbine Jr Antifungal	**Liquid**: 1%. Wormwood oil.
Absorbine Jr Antifungal	**Gel**: 1%. SD alcohol, tea tree oil.
Aftate for Athlete's Foot, Tinactin	**Spray Powder**: 1%. 14% alcohol SD-40-2, talc.
Aftate for Athlete's Foot	**Spray Liquid**: 1%. 36% alcohol SD-40-2.
Tinactin	**Spray Liquid**: 1%. 36% alcohol SD-40-2.
Ting	**Spray Liquid**: 1%. 41% alcohol SD-40-8.
Tinactin	**Pump Spray**: 1%. 70% alcohol SD-40.

Products listed are representative of currently available and widely distributed brands. Similar products, including regional and private label brands, may also exist.

PATIENT INFORMATION
Tolnaftate

- The most important factor in treating tinea pedis (athlete's foot) is the duration and consistency in treatment. It is common for the patient to discontinue use of a product after a few days when relief of symptoms is experienced. However, it is very important to continue treatment for at least 2 weeks after symptoms have been relieved to prevent recurrence or infection of the toenails.
- For external use only. Avoid contact with eyes, nose, mouth, or other mucous membranes.
- Cleanse skin with soap and water and dry thoroughly before applying product. Wash hands after applying the medication to the affected areas.
- Do not apply to blistered, oozing, or raw skin.
- Notify your pharmacist or physician if there is no improvement after 4 weeks of treatment.
- Avoid the use of occlusive dressings unless directed by your physician.
- Patients with decreased circulation, including diabetic patients, should consult their physician before using these products.
- Frequency of application and duration of therapy is dependent on the location of the condition, the drug, the strength of the drug, and the doseform used. For assistance in drug selection and dosage guidelines, consult your pharmacist or physician.
- If condition persists or worsens, or if irritation (burning, itching, stinging, redness) occurs, discontinue use and notify your pharmacist or physician.
- Inform your pharmacist or physician if the area of application shows signs of increased irritation (eg, redness, itching, burning, blistering, swelling, oozing) indicative of possible sensitization.
- Essential adjuncts to antifungal therapy that should be undertaken by the patient include the following: daily foot hygiene, light cotton socks (changed daily), well-ventilated footwear, medicated or nonmedicated foot powder, and rubber sandals in public or family shower facilities.
- Wear well-fitting, ventilated shoes. Change shoes and socks at least once daily.

MICONAZOLE

▶ Actions

Miconazole alters cellular membrane permeability and interferes with mitochondrial and peroxisomal enzymes, resulting in intracellular necrosis. It inhibits growth of the common dermatophytes, *Trichophyton rubrum*, *T. mentagrophytes*, *Epidermophyton floccosum*, *Candida albicans*, and *Malassezia furfur*, the active organism in tinea versicolor.

▶ Indications

For the treatment of tinea pedis (athlete's foot), tinea cruris (jock itch), and tinea corporis (ringworm) caused by *T. rubrum*, *T. mentagrophytes*, and *E. floccosum*.

▶ Contraindications

Allergy or sensitivity to the preparation or its components; patients with diabetes or peripheral vascular disease.

Self-care is contraindicated in the following situations: toenail involvement; purulent discharge; whitish, soggy, foul-smelling toe webs; inflammation or swelling of a major portion of the foot.

▶ Warnings

External use: For external use only. Avoid inhaling. Do not use in mouth, eyes, or vagina.

Sensitivity: If sensitization or irritation occurs, discontinue use and contact your pharmacist or physician.

Pregnancy: Consult an obstetrician/gynecologist prior to use in pregnancy.

Lactation: Topical preparations are known to be excreted in breast milk. Use with caution.

▶ Adverse Reactions

Infrequent reports of irritation, burning, maceration (softening of the skin due to excessive moisture), and allergic contact dermatitis have occurred.

▶ Administration and Dosage

Follow dosing guidelines for individual products. Twice-daily application of most topical creams or solutions is recommended. Cleanse and dry area well before application. Creams, solutions, and sprays should be applied generously to all involved areas and between toes. Wash hands with soap and water after use to avoid spreading infection. The condition generally resolves within 2 weeks, although treatment should continue for at least 2 weeks following resolution of symptoms (maximum recommended duration of treatment is 4 weeks for most patients).

Cream and solution: Cover affected areas twice daily, morning and evening. Solution is preferred in intertriginous areas; if cream is used, apply sparingly to avoid maceration effects.

Powder: Spray or sprinkle liberally over affected area morning and evening. Early relief of symptoms occurs in most patients; clinical improvement may be seen within 2 to 3 days after beginning treatment. However, treat tinea pedis daily for at least 4 weeks, to reduce chance of recurrence. If no clinical improvement is observed after 4 weeks, reevaluate the diagnosis.

MICONAZOLE PRODUCTS	
Trade name	Doseform
Micatin Athlete's Foot, Micatin Jock Itch	**Cream**: 2%. Mineral oil.
Desenex	**Powder**: 2%. Talc.
Lotrimin AF	**Powder**: 2%
Zeasorb-AF	**Powder**: 2%. 36% alcohol, EDTA.
Desenex, Ting	**Spray Powder**: 2%. 10% alcohol SD-40-8.
Lotrimin AF, Micatin Athlete's Foot, Micatin Jock Itch	**Spray Powder**: 2%. 10% alcohol SD 40, talc.
Lotrimin AF	**Spray Liquid**: 2%. 17% alcohol SD 40.
Micatin Athlete's Foot	**Spray Liquid**: 2%. Benzyl alcohol, 16.8% alcohol SD-40.
Neosporin AF Athlete's Foot	**Spray Liquid**: 2%

Products listed are representative of currently available and widely distributed brands. Similar products, including regional and private label brands, may also exist.

PATIENT INFORMATION
Miconazole

- The most important factor in treating tinea pedis (athlete's foot) is the duration and consistency in treatment. It is common for the patient to discontinue use of a product after a few days when relief of symptoms is experienced. However, it is very important to continue treatment for at least 2 weeks after symptoms have been relieved to prevent recurrence or infection of the toenails.
- For external use only. Avoid contact with eyes, nose, mouth, or other mucous membranes.
- Cleanse skin with soap and water and dry thoroughly before applying product. Wash hands after applying the medication to the affected areas.
- Do not apply to blistered, oozing, or raw skin.
- Notify your pharmacist or physician if there is no improvement after 4 weeks of treatment.
- Avoid the use of occlusive dressings unless directed by your physician.
- Patients with decreased circulation, including diabetic patients, should consult their physician before using these products.
- Frequency of application and duration of therapy is dependent on the location of the condition, the drug, the strength of the drug, and the doseform used. For assistance in drug selection and dosage guidelines, consult your pharmacist or physician.
- If condition persists or worsens, or if irritation (burning, itching, stinging, redness) occurs, discontinue use and notify your pharmacist or physician.
- Inform your pharmacist or physician if the area of application shows signs of increased irritation (eg, redness, itching, burning, blistering, swelling, oozing) indicative of possible sensitization.
- Essential adjuncts to antifungal therapy that should be undertaken by the patient include the following: daily foot hygiene, light cotton socks (changed daily), well-ventilated footwear, medicated or nonmedicated foot powder, and rubber sandals in public or family shower facilities.
- Wear well-fitting, ventilated shoes. Change shoes and socks at least once daily.

CLOTRIMAZOLE

▶ **Actions**

Antifungal agent that impairs the synthesis of ergosterol, a component of the fungus cell membrane, ultimately causing the destruction of the fungus cell membrane and rendering the fungus nonviable.

Clotrimazole, a broad-spectrum antifungal agent, inhibits growth of pathogenic dermatophytes, yeasts, and *Malassezia furfur*. It exhibits fungistatic and fungicidal activity in vitro against isolates of *Trichophyton rubrum*, *T. mentagrophytes*, *Epidermophyton floccosum*, *Microsporum canis*, and *Candida* species, including *C. albicans*. No single-step or multiple-step resistance to clotrimazole has developed during successive passages of *C. albicans* and *T. mentagrophytes*.

▶ **Indications**

Topical treatment of tinea pedis (athlete's foot), tinea cruris (jock itch), and tinea corporis (ringworm) caused by *T. rubrum*, *T. mentagrophytes*, *E. floccosum*, and *M. canis*.

▶ **Contraindications**

Allergy or sensitivity to the preparation or its components; patients with diabetes or peripheral vascular disease.

Self-care is contraindicated in the following situations: toenail involvement; purulent discharge; whitish, soggy, foul-smelling toe webs; inflammation or swelling of a major portion of the foot.

▶ **Warnings**

External use: For external use only. Do not use in mouth, eyes, or vagina.

Sensitivity: If sensitization or irritation occurs, discontinue use and contact your pharmacist or physician.

Pregnancy: Category B. Consult an obstetrician/gynecologist prior to use in pregnancy.

There are no adequate and well-controlled studies in pregnant women during the first trimester of pregnancy. Use only if clearly indicated during the first trimester.

Lactation: Topical preparations are known to be excreted in breast milk. Use with caution.

▶ **Adverse Reactions**

Adverse reactions are usually limited to the local application sites. Erythema, stinging, pruritus, and general irritation of the skin may occur.

▶ **Administration and Dosage**

Follow dosing guidelines for individual products. Twice-daily application of most topical creams or solutions is recommended. Cleanse and dry area well before application. Creams and solutions should be applied generously to all involved areas and between toes. Wash hands with soap and water after use to avoid spreading infection. The condition generally resolves within 2 weeks, although treatment should continue for at least 2 weeks following resolution of symptoms (maximum recommended duration of treatment is 4 weeks for most patients).

Gently massage into affected and surrounding skin areas. Clinical improvement, with relief of pruritus, usually occurs within the first week of treatment. If patient shows no clinical improvement after 4 weeks, reevaluate the diagnosis.

CLOTRIMAZOLE PRODUCTS	
Trade name	**Doseform**
Lotrimin AF	**Cream**: 1%. Cetearyl alcohol, benzyl alcohol.
Lotrimin AF	**Lotion**: 1%
Lotrimin AF	**Solution**: 1%

Products listed are representative of currently available and widely distributed brands. Similar products, including regional and private label brands, may also exist.

PATIENT INFORMATION
Clotrimazole

- The most important factor in treating tinea pedis (athlete's foot) is the duration and consistency in treatment. It is common for the patient to discontinue use of a product after a few days when relief of symptoms is experienced. However, it is very important to continue treatment for at least 2 weeks after symptoms have been relieved to prevent recurrence or infection of the toenails.
- For external use only. Avoid contact with eyes, nose, mouth, or other mucous membranes.
- Cleanse skin with soap and water and dry thoroughly before applying product. Wash hands after applying the medication to the affected areas.
- Do not apply to blistered, oozing, or raw skin.
- Notify your pharmacist or physician if there is no improvement after 4 weeks of treatment.
- Avoid the use of occlusive dressings unless directed by your physician.
- Patients with decreased circulation, including diabetic patients, should consult their physician before using these products.
- Frequency of application and duration of therapy is dependent on the location of the condition, the drug, the strength of the drug, and the doseform used. For assistance in drug selection and dosage guidelines, consult your pharmacist or physician.
- If condition persists or worsens, or if irritation (burning, itching, stinging, redness) occurs, discontinue use and notify a pharmacist or physician.
- Inform your pharmacist or physician if the area of application shows signs of increased irritation (eg, redness, itching, burning, blistering, swelling, oozing) indicative of possible sensitization.
- Essential adjuncts to antifungal therapy that should be undertaken by the patient include the following: daily foot hygiene, light cotton socks (changed daily), well-ventilated footwear, medicated or nonmedicated foot powder, and rubber sandals in public or family shower facilities.
- Wear well-fitting, ventilated shoes. Change shoes and socks at least once daily.

TERBINAFINE

▶ **Actions**

Terbinafine exerts its antifungal effect by inhibiting squalene epoxidase, a key enzyme in sterol biosynthesis in fungi. This action results in a deficiency in ergosterol and a corresponding accumulation of squalene within the fungal cell and causes fungal cell death.

Terbinafine is active against most strains of the following organisms, both in vitro and in clinical infections: *Trichophyton rubrum*; *T. mentagrophytes*; *Epidermophyton floccosum*.

▶ **Indications**

For the relief of the signs and symptoms of interdigital tinea pedis (athlete's foot), tinea cruris (jock itch), or tinea corporis (ringworm of the body) caused by *T. rubrum*, *T. mentagrophytes*, or *E. floccosum*.

▶ **Contraindications**

Allergy or sensitivity to the preparation or its components.

▶ **Warnings**

External use: For external use only. Do not use in mouth, eyes, or vagina.

Sensitivity: If sensitization or irritation occurs, discontinue use and contact your pharmacist or physician.

Pregnancy: Category B. There are no adequate and well-controlled studies in pregnant women. Use during pregnancy only if clearly needed.

Lactation: It is not known if terbinafine is excreted in breast milk. Exercise caution when administering to a breastfeeding woman. Breastfeeding mothers should avoid application of terbinafine cream to the breast.

Children: Safety and efficacy in children younger than 12 years of age have not been established.

▶ **Adverse Reactions**

In clinical trials, 0.2% of patients discontinued therapy because of adverse events and 2.3% reported adverse reactions. These reactions included the following: irritation (1%); burning (0.8%); itching, dryness (0.2%).

▶ **Administration and Dosage**

Spray, cream, solution: Follow dosing guidelines for individual products. Cleanse and dry area well before application. Wash hands with soap and water after use to avoid spreading infection. Do not cover the treated skin with any bandages.

For athlete's foot between the toes, spray or apply cream or solution twice a day (morning and night) for 1 week or as directed by a physician. Duration of therapy should be for a minimum of 1 week (if only interdigital tinea pedis is present) or 2 weeks (for tinea pedis present on the bottom or sides of the feet), or as directed. Wear well-fitting, ventilated shoes. Change shoes and socks at least once daily.

Many people get relief from their symptoms after the completion of 1 week of treatment, although treatment should continue for at least 2 weeks following resolution of symptoms. Skin may continue to show some of the signs of infection until the outer layer of the treated skin naturally replaces itself. Skin replacement takes longer on some parts of the body than others. If no improvement is seen within 4 weeks, consult a physician.

TERBINAFINE PRODUCTS	
Trade name	Doseform
DesenexMax, Lamisil AT	**Cream**: 1%. Benzyl, cetyl, and stearyl alcohols.
Lamisil AT	**Solution, dropper**: 1%. Ethanol.
Lamisil AT	**Spray**: 1%. Ethanol.

Products listed are representative of currently available and widely distributed brands. Similar products, including regional and private label brands, may also exist.

PATIENT INFORMATION
Terbinafine

- For external use only. Avoid contact with eyes, nose, mouth, or other mucous membranes.
- Cleanse skin with soap and water and dry thoroughly before applying product. Wash hands after applying the medication to the affected areas.
- Do not apply to blistered, oozing, or raw skin.
- Notify your pharmacist or physician if there is no improvement after 4 weeks of treatment.
- Avoid the use of occlusive dressings unless directed by your physician.
- If condition persists or worsens, or if irritation (burning, itching, stinging, redness) occurs, discontinue use and notify a pharmacist or physician.
- Inform your pharmacist or physician if the area of application shows signs of increased irritation (redness, itching, burning, blistering, swelling, oozing) indicative of possible sensitization.
- Do not use on children younger than 12 years of age unless directed by a physician.
- Essential adjuncts to antifungal therapy that should be undertaken by the patient include the following: daily foot hygiene, light cotton socks (changed daily), well-ventilated footwear, medicated or nonmedicated foot powder, and rubber sandals in public of family shower facilities.
- Wear well-fitting, ventilated shoes. Change shoes and socks at least once daily.

BUTENAFINE

▶ Actions

Antifungal agent that impairs the synthesis of ergosterol, a component of the fungus cell membrane, ultimately causing the destruction of the fungus cell membrane and rendering the fungus nonviable.

Butenafine is active against most strains of the following microorganisms, both in vitro and in clinical infections: *Trichophyton rubrum, T. mentagrophytes, T. tonsurans, Epidermophyton floccosum,* and *Malassezia furfur.*

▶ Indications

For the relief of the signs and symptoms of interdigital tinea pedis (athlete's foot), tinea cruris (jock itch), or tinea corporis (ringworm of the body) caused by *T. rubrum, T. mentagrophytes, T. tonsurans,* or *E. floccosum.*

▶ Contraindications

Allergy or sensitivity to the preparation or its components.

▶ **Warnings**

External use: For external use only. Do not use in mouth, eyes, or vagina.

Sensitivity: If sensitization or irritation occurs, discontinue use and contact your pharmacist or physician. Patients known to be sensitive to allylamine antifungals should use butenafine with caution; it is possible that these drugs may be cross-reactive.

Pregnancy: Category B. There are no adequate and well-controlled studies in pregnant women. Use during pregnancy only if clearly needed.

Lactation: It is not known if butenafine is excreted in breast milk. Exercise caution when administering to a breastfeeding woman. Breastfeeding mothers should avoid application of butenafine cream to the breast.

Children: Do not use on children younger than 12 years of age unless directed by a physician.

▶ **Adverse Reactions**

Burning, stinging, itching, and worsening of the condition (approximately 1%); contact dermatitis; erythema, irritation, and itching (less than 2%).

In provocative testing in over 200 subjects, there was no evidence of allergic contact sensitization for either cream or vehicle base.

▶ **Administration and Dosage**

Cleanse and dry area well before application. Apply sufficient butenafine to cover the affected area and immediately surrounding skin. Wash hands with soap and water after use to avoid spreading infection.

Apply butenafine once daily for 2 weeks. The condition generally resolves within 2 weeks, although treatment should continue for at least 2 weeks following resolution of symptoms (maximum recommended duration of treatment is 4 weeks for most patients). If a patient shows no clinical improvement after the treatment period, consult a physician.

BUTENAFINE PRODUCTS	
Trade name	**Doseform**
Lotrimin Ultra	**Cream**: 1%. Benzyl and cetyl alcohol, glycerin, white petrolatum.

Products listed are representative of currently available and widely distributed brands. Similar products, including regional and private label brands, may also exist.

PATIENT INFORMATION
Butenafine

- The most important factor in treating tinea pedis (athlete's foot) is the duration and consistency in treatment. It is common for the patient to discontinue use of a product after a few days when relief of symptoms is experienced. However, it is very important to continue therapy for at least 2 weeks after symptoms have been relieved to prevent recurrence or infection of the toenails.
- For external use only. Use as directed. Avoid contact with eyes, nose, mouth, or other mucous membranes.
- Cleanse skin with soap and water and dry thoroughly before applying product. Wash hands after applying the medication to the affected areas.
- Do not apply to blistered, oozing, or raw skin.
- Notify your pharmacist or physician if there is no improvement after 4 weeks of treatment.
- Avoid the use of occlusive dressings unless directed by your pharmacist or physician.
- Frequency of application and duration of therapy is dependent on the location of the condition, the drug, the strength of the drug, and the doseform used. For assistance in drug selection and dosage guidelines, consult your pharmacist or physician.
- If condition persists or worsens, or if irritation (burning, itching, stinging, redness) occurs, discontinue use, and notify a pharmacist or physician.
- Inform your pharmacist or physician if the area of application shows signs of increased irritation (redness, itching, burning, blistering, swelling, oozing) indicative of possible sensitization.
- Do not use on children younger than 12 years of age unless directed by a physician.
- Essential adjuncts to antifungal therapy that should be undertaken by the patient include the following: daily foot hygiene, light cotton socks (changed daily), well-ventilated footwear, medicated or nonmedicated foot powder, and rubber sandals in public or family shower facilities.
- Wear well-fitting, ventilated shoes. Change shoes and socks at least once daily.

RESPIRATORY CONDITIONS

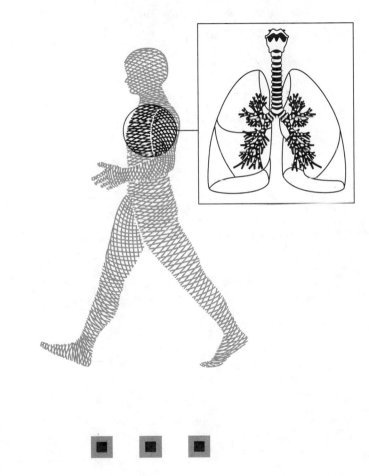

NONPRESCRIPTION DRUG THERAPY
TABLE OF CONTENTS
■ ■ ■

RESPIRATORY CONDITIONS

INTRODUCTION

The respiratory tract, including the sinuses, is a common site of infection and irritation in the general population. Viral infections account for the majority of complaints associated with the respiratory tract; however, allergic rhinitis and bacterial infections (sinusitis, bronchitis) cause or contribute to chronic conditions that are persistent problems for many patients. Symptoms associated with seasonal allergic rhinitis, colds, nasal congestion, cough, and viral sinusitis are usually amenable to nonprescription self-medication. These conditions tend to be mild in severity and are often self-limiting. The primary purpose of self-medication is to relieve the patient's symptoms of nasal congestion (the most frequent complaint), cough, sneezing, chest congestion, and ocular irritation. However, incomplete treatment of viral upper respiratory tract infections and allergic rhinitis may lead to secondary bacterial infections of the middle ear or sinuses caused by transmission of infected mucus via the eustachian tubes. Prolonged presence of these symptoms increases the likelihood of secondary infection caused by diminished immune resistance. Any suspicion of bacterial infection of these areas should be referred to a physician for evaluation and possible antibiotic therapy. However, empiric treatment of these infections with antibiotics, many of which are viral in nature, may induce the development of resistance. Therefore, it is important for the pharmacist to be able to educate the patient about the warning signs of a bacterial infection, such as fever, chills, purulent sputum, and rash. Any evidence of a lower respiratory tract infection, such as bronchitis or pneumonia, requires immediate referral to a physician.

Nonprescription medications generally are effective for the relief of many symptoms of upper respiratory tract conditions. Many of these medications necessitate caution when used in certain populations. For example, oral decongestants are to be used cautiously in patients with hypertension because of the potential for increased blood pressure through systemic vasoconstriction. Also, most oral cold preparations (including antihistamines, decongestants, and cough suppressants) should be avoided by pregnant women because of the lack of information about the teratogenic potential of the drugs. Use of topical decongestant sprays are limited to short courses (less than 4 consecutive days) because of the potential for irritation of the nasal mucosa and resultant rebound congestion. Because of the dynamics (economic, social, and political) of the health care delivery system in the US, patients are more inclined than in previous years to self-medicate for conditions that may require direct medical attention. The pharmacist is well positioned to provide immediate advice and to screen for potential inappropriate selection and use of nonprescription medications. Topics the pharmacist may ask about to access the most useful information from the patient include the following:

1.) Description of symptoms.
2.) Duration of symptoms.
3.) Medications (prescription and OTC) that have been used to treat symptoms.
4.) Any conditions (eg, high blood pressure, diabetes, pregnancy) or drugs that may interact with a nonprescription medication.

The answers elicited from such questioning not only provide an avenue to improve patient care, but also forge a bond between patient and pharmacist that is unique among health care professionals. After the proper selection of medication has been made, the pharmacist may then reinforce correct administration techniques (as for a nasal spray), proper dosage, administration to children, if applicable, and monitoring for common adverse effects.

Most mild upper respiratory tract conditions are minor nuisances that are managed sufficiently with self-medication. In assisting with the selection of these medications, the pharmacist is a partner in improving patient health outcomes and quality of life. The ability to recognize and teach patients how to recognize warning signs of medical conditions and complications requiring prescription treatment will allow the pharmacist to become an even more vital link in providing patient care to the community.

COMMON COLD

DEFINITION

The common cold is an acute, usually afebrile, viral infection of the upper respiratory tract with inflammation of all or part of the airways (eg, nose, paranasal sinuses, throat, larynx, trachea, bronchi).

ETIOLOGY

The common cold is caused by viruses and some atypical bacteria. Rhinoviruses (more than 100 subtypes) cause approximately 60% of all colds; coronaviruses cause about 10% to 20% of all colds. Less common pathogens include influenza viruses (1% to 10%), parainfluenza viruses (1% to 10%), respiratory syncytial virus (1% to 10%), adenoviruses (1% to 10%), enteroviruses (1% to 10%), *Mycoplasma pneumoniae* (1% to 10%), and *Chlamydia pneumoniae* (1% to 10%).

Rhinoviruses, which are hardy viruses that remain infectious for several hours after drying on hard surfaces, cause colds year-round with peaks in the fall and spring. Coronaviruses and parainfluenza viruses also cause colds year round but are associated with winter peaks. The respiratory syncytial virus is associated with discrete yearly winter epidemics; the remainder of the viruses cause sporadic illnesses. *Mycoplasma pneumoniae* is associated with 5-year epidemic cycles. The true incidence and pattern of illness associated with *Chlamydia pneumoniae* is unknown.

INCIDENCE

The common cold is the most frequent acute illness in the US with an incidence of 25.4 episodes per 100 people per year or approximately 66 million colds per year. Costs associated with the common cold include direct treatment costs of approximately $15 billion/year and indirect costs of approximately $9 billion/year. Preschoolers have the highest number of colds (6 to 10 colds per year); adults may experience 2 to 4 colds per year.

Risk factors for the common cold include decreased individual immunity, smoking, psychological stress, poor nutrition, increased population density, and family structures that include preschool and school-age children. The common cold is not caused by drafts, wet weather, or exposure to cold temperatures; an infectious organism must be present. A recent report suggests that aspirin and acetaminophen suppress seroneutralizing antibodies and are associated with increased nasal signs and symptoms and a trend toward longer viral shedding. These findings are not conclusive and require further validation.

PATHOPHYSIOLOGY

The most common route of transmission is direct hand-to-hand contact with an infected individual. Less common routes of transmission include contact with large or small aerosolized particles, kissing, and contact with inanimate objects. Viruses can survive on the hands for several hours. The typical sequence of transmission is from donor's nose to donor's hand, donor's hand to recipient's hand, then recipient's hand to recipient's nose or eye. Scrupulous handwashing, particularly in day care centers, schools, and the workplace can decrease transmission of infecting viruses.

Viruses deposited in the nose or eye are transported to the nasopharynx (see Figure 1). The adenoids, rich in viral receptors, usually are the initial sites of infection. Viral infection activates inflammatory mediators such as kinins, prostaglandins, leukotrienes, cytokines, interferons, chemokines, and tumor necrosis factor, resulting in vasodilation, increased vascular permeability with serum transudation, and increased mucus production. Stimulation of pain, sneeze, and cough fibers and receptors results in the symptoms of myalgia, sneezing, and coughing. Viral shedding starts approximately 24 hours after the initial infection, peaks at approximately 48 hours, and persists for approximately 3 weeks.

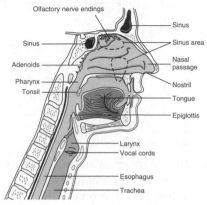

Figure 1. Upper Respiratory System

SIGNS/SYMPTOMS

All colds, regardless of the infectious etiology, cause the same symptoms in the same sequence. However, the incubation period, frequency, and severity vary with the infectious agent. The sore throat usually appears first, followed by malaise, nasal symptoms (eg, stuffiness, rhinorrhea, postnasal drip), watery eyes, sneezing, and then coughing.

One-third to 50% of patients have sore throat and hoarseness. Nasal symptoms are most common, occurring in 45% to 75% of patients; less than 20% have cough. Constitutional symptoms, including headache, low-grade fever, and myalgia are less frequent. Many patients are afebrile, but have a feverish feeling. Performance may be impaired during the incubation period, while the patient is symptomatic, and after the symptoms have resolved. Symptoms peak on day 2 or 3. Most symptoms resolve in approximately 1 week (mean duration 7 to 13 days), except for cough, which may last longer.

Complications include sinusitis, otitis media, bronchitis, and exacerbations of asthma and chronic lung disease. Sinus abnormalities are relatively common but usually are self-limited. Epistaxis is relatively common, with nosebleed occurring in 6.8% to 11% of patients and blood in mucosal tissues in 9% to 15.4% of patients. Pneumonia may follow upper respiratory tract infections with influenza viruses but is unusual with other viruses; however, secondary bacterial infections may occur.

DIAGNOSTIC PARAMETERS/PHYSICAL ASSESSMENT

Clinical Observation: The specific etiologic diagnosis can only be made by isolation of the virus from nasal secretions but is rarely necessary. Other laboratory tests, including a white blood cell count and differential, are not indicated for routine diagnosis of the common cold. Throat cultures may help to rule out streptococcal pharyngitis.

Patients with signs and symptoms suggestive of secondary bacterial infection (eg, discolored sputum, earache, facial pain) or secondary pneumonia (chest pain with breathing that is exacerbated by cough), wheezing, difficulty breathing, or with symptoms persisting longer than 2 weeks should be referred to a physician.

Interview: The common cold is relatively easy to recognize based on the specific signs and symptoms discussed above. It is sometimes difficult to differentiate between a common cold and acute or chronic rhinitis, sinusitis, or sore throats secondary to bacterial infection and influenza. Information that may help distinguish these conditions includes:

- Description and duration of symptoms.
- The sequence of symptoms, such as sore throat, which is often the initial symptom in colds, whereas nasal symptoms occur initially with allergic rhinitis. Sore throats caused by bacteria tend to develop more quickly, be more severe, and appear in conjunction with marked constitutional symptoms (eg, fever). Patients typically develop lymphadenopathy but do not report upper or lower respiratory tract symptoms.
- Presence and degree of fever, muscle or joint aches or pains, runny nose, nasal congestion, sneezing more frequently than usual, watery or scratchy eyes, and earache. The presence of paranasal pressure and eye symptoms are more likely to occur with sinusitis. Influenza tends to be associated with higher fevers (higher than 102°F to 104°F), more prominent headache, profound myalgia and arthralgia, fatigue, weakness, and less prominent rhinorrhea, nasal congestion, and sneezing.
- Description of cough (ie, productive vs nonproductive, appearance of sputum).
- Past and current treatment (prescription and nonprescription) for relief of symptoms.
- Smoking habits.
- Presence of other medical conditions (eg, asthma, chronic obstructive pulmonary disease, diabetes, coronary heart disease, glaucoma).

TREATMENT

Approaches to therapy: Treatment is symptomatic; antibiotics are not routinely indicated as they possess no antiviral activity. In general, single-entity products selected specifically to treat the most bothersome symptoms are recommended over combination products containing unneeded active ingredients that increase the risk of adverse effects and drug-drug interactions. Oral decongestants are preferred for nasal congestion or obstruction; limited use (no more than 3 to 5 consecutive days) of intranasal decongestant sprays or drops is an alternative to systemic decongestants. Dextromethorphan or codeine is preferred for cough suppression. Analgesics are preferred for headache and sore throat.

Lozenges (medicated and nonmedicated) or topical throat sprays or gargles may soothe sore throats. There is an epidemiological association between ingestion of salicylates during antecedent viral illness (eg, influenza, chickenpox) and the subsequent development of Reye syndrome in children. Therefore, children and teenagers should not be treated with salicylates for cold symptoms.

Nondrug therapy: Humidifiers (cool mist) and vaporizers raise environmental humidity and may provide symptomatic relief of upper respiratory tract symptoms. Warm salt water gargles (1 to 3 tsp of salt per 8 to 12 ounces of warm tap water) may soothe sore throats. Hot liquids such as chicken soup and sweetened milk or tea mobilize nasal secretions; chicken soup may improve mucociliary clearance. Regular hand washing may help to prevent the spread of infection.

Pharmacotherapy: Decongestants, expectorants, cough suppressants, and analgesics are the mainstays for symptomatic treatment of the common cold. Medicated lozenges containing local anesthetics (eg, benzocaine) and throat sprays may soothe sore throats. There are many multi-ingredient products marketed as agents to treat the multi-symptomatic cold; however, use of these products is controversial. A shotgun approach to treating a patient without all symptoms is generally not recommended and may be considered mismanagement of the condition. When possible, consider single-ingredient agents that target a specific symptom. It is important to counsel patients that dry, hacking nonproductive coughs are best treated with an antitussive, whereas productive or "loose" coughs are best treated with expectorants that will not suppress the helpful cough reflex. This is especially important when considering multi-ingredient products.

For complete information on OTC analgesics, refer to the Headache and Fever monographs in the CNS Conditions chapter.

> *Treatment controversies* – The pervasiveness of the common cold, along with the lack of curative treatment, has led to numerous treatment controversies:
>
> *Antihistamines* – No definitive data support the efficacy of antihistamines in the treatment of the common cold as the symptoms produced by the common cold are not histamine-mediated. Critical analyses of published controlled, clinical trials from 1947 to 1995 identified important study design and analytical flaws. For more information on antihistamines, see the Allergic Rhinitis monograph in this chapter. Neither the short-term nor long-term efficacy of antihistamine-decongestant combinations has been established in young children. Diphenhydramine has been shown to suppress the cough center. It may be helpful in decreasing cough caused by

minor irritations, but its anticholinergic drying effect would not be desirable for productive cough. See the Cough monograph in this chapter.

Zinc – Zinc, in the form of zinc gluconate or acetate lozenges, is said to reduce the severity and duration of the common cold. As with antihistamines, there are numerous study design problems. Zinc is not FDA-approved for treatment of the common cold. It is currently marketed as a homeopathic product.

Vitamin C supplementation – There is no evidence that vitamin C, even in doses of more than 1 g/day, decreases the incidence of the common cold in the general population. The few patients with vitamin C deficiency may benefit from vitamin C supplementation. There is some evidence that vitamin C, taken during a cold, may reduce the duration and severity of the cold approximately 23%.

Withholding milk and milk products – There is no evidence that milk or milk products stimulate mucus production or aggravate the common cold.

Nasal hyperthermia – It was hypothesized that the direct application of heated, moist air up the nasal passages would abort rhinovirus replication. However, there is no evidence that nasal hyperthermia is any better than placebo.

NASAL DECONGESTANTS

▶ **Actions**

The sympathomimetic agents constrict nasal and ocular blood vessels, reducing mucosal swelling and decreasing nasal airflow resistance and nasal and ocular congestion. Decongestants are applied directly to inflamed membranes or taken systemically. Oral agents are not as effective as topical products, especially when needed for immediate relief, but generally have a longer duration of action. However, oral agents cause less local irritation and are not associated with rebound congestion following prolonged use.

▶ **Indications**

Intranasal decongestants are indicated for the short-term relief of more severe nasal congestion and have a rapid onset of action (30 seconds to 10 minutes). Regular use for more than 3 to 5 consecutive days causes rebound congestion (rhinitis medicamentosa) and should be avoided. Oral decongestants are indicated for the symptomatic relief of nasal mucosal swelling and congestion and can be administered indefinitely without the risk of rebound congestion.

▶ **Contraindications**

Oral decongestants are contraindicated in patients with severe hypertension and coronary artery disease; monoamine oxidase inhibitor (MAOI) therapy; or hypersensitivity or idiosyncrasy to sympathomimetic amines or any component of the product (some nasal decongestant products contain sulfites). Ophthalmic naphazoline, oxymetazoline, and tetrahydrozoline are contraindicated in patients with glaucoma. Topical decongestants are associated with fewer systemic effects than oral decongestants, but use caution in the conditions listed for oral agents. Adverse reactions are more likely with excessive use, in the elderly, and in children.

▶ Warnings

Special risk patients: Administer with caution to patients with hyperthyroidism, diabetes mellitus, cardiovascular disease, coronary artery disease, ischemic heart disease, increased intraocular pressure, or prostatic hypertrophy. Sympathomimetics may cause CNS stimulation, convulsions, or cardiovascular collapse with hypotension. More serious effects generally occur at high doses and in very fragile patients.

Hypertension: Hypertensive patients should use these products with caution because they may elevate blood pressure. However, some studies report that these products do not significantly increase blood pressure in normotensive and hypertensive patients. Sustained-action preparations may affect the cardiovascular system less. Excessive use of decongestants or individual sensitivity may cause systemic effects (eg, nervousness, dizziness, sleeplessness), which are more likely to occur in infants and the elderly. Habituation and toxic psychosis have followed long-term high-dose therapy. Rebound congestion (rhinitis medicamentosa) may occur following prolonged intranasal application. Some patients increase the amount of the intranasal drug and the frequency of use, producing toxicity and perpetuating the rebound congestion. Use topical decongestants only in acute states and no longer than 3 to 5 consecutive days.

Stinging sensation: Some individuals may experience a mild, transient stinging sensation after topical application. This often disappears after a few applications.

Pregnancy: Give only when clearly needed. One study reported that topical oxymetazoline did not affect maternal blood pressure and pulse rates and, therefore, is safe to use in the third trimester of a normal pregnancy.

Lactation: Oral pseudoephedrine is contraindicated in the nursing mother. Consult a physician or pharmacist before using intranasal preparations.

Children: Use in children is product-specific. Naphazoline (topical) and pseudoephedrine (oral) are not recommended in children younger than 12 years of age. Nose drops, syrups, or elixirs are generally preferred to nasal sprays in children age 2 to 6 years because their reflexes are not generally developed adequately to ensure efficient use of a nasal spray. Refer to individual product information.

Elderly: Patients 60 years of age and older are more likely to experience adverse reactions to sympathomimetic decongestants. A lower dose may be sufficient and safe. Demonstrate safe use of a short-acting sympathomimetic before using a sustained-action formulation in elderly patients.

Sulfite sensitivity: Some of the oral nasal decongestant products contain sulfites that may cause allergic-type reactions, including anaphylactic symptoms and life-threatening or less severe asthmatic episodes in susceptible people. The overall prevalence of sulfite sensitivity in the general population is unknown but is probably low. Patients allergic to sulfites should check product ingredients.

▶ Drug Interactions

Most interactions listed apply to sympathomimetics when used as vasopressors; however, consider these interactions when using the nasal decongestants.

Nasal Decongestant Drug Interactions			
Precipitant drug	**Object drug***		**Description**
Furazolidone	Nasal decongestants	↑	The pressor sensitivity to mixed-acting agents (eg, ephedrine) may be increased. Direct-acting agents (eg, epinephrine) are not affected.
Guanethidine	Nasal decongestants Direct Mixed	↑ ↓	Guanethidine potentiates the effects of the direct-acting agents (eg, epinephrine) and inhibits the effects of the mixed-acting agents (eg, ephedrine).
Nasal decongestants	Guanethidine	↓	Guanethidine's hypotensive action may be reversed.
Methyldopa	Nasal decongestants	↑	Concurrent administration may result in an increased pressor response.
MAO inhibitors	Nasal decongestants	↑	Concurrent use of MAOIs and mixed-acting agents (eg, ephedrine) may result in severe headache, hypertension, and hyperpyrexia, possibly resulting in hypertensive crisis. Direct-acting agents (eg, epinephrine) interact minimally, if at all.
Phenothiazines	Nasal decongestants	↓	Phenothiazines may antagonize and, in some cases, reverse the action of the nasal decongestants.
Rauwolfia alkaloids	Nasal decongestants Direct Mixed	↑ ↓	Reserpine potentiates the pressor response of direct-acting agents (eg, epinephrine) which may result in hypotension. The pressor response of mixed-acting agents (eg, ephedrine) is decreased.
Tricyclic antidepressants (TCAs)	Nasal decongestants Direct Mixed	↑ ↓	TCAs potentiate the pressor response of direct acting agents (eg, epinephrine); dysrhythmia have occurred. The pressor response of mixed-acting agents (eg, ephedrine) is decreased.
Urinary acidifiers	Nasal decongestants	↓	Acidification of the urine may increase the elimination of the nasal decongestant; therapeutic effects may be decreased.
Urinary alkalinizers	Nasal decongestants	↑	Conversely, urinary alkalinization may decrease the elimination of these agents, possibly increasing therapeutic or toxic effects.
Nasal decongestants	Theophylline	↔	Enhanced toxicity, particularly cardiotoxicity, has occurred. Decreased theophylline levels may occur. Ephedrine may cause theophylline toxicity.

* ↑ = Object drug increased.   ↓ = Object drug decreased.   ↔ = Undetermined effect.

▶ **Adverse Reactions**

Oral decongestants may cause restlessness, nervousness, irritability, insomnia, dizziness, tremor, headache, tachycardia, and elevated blood pressure. Tachycardia and elevated blood pressure are dose-proportional. Locally applied nasal decongestants (eg, drops, sprays) may cause burning, stinging, and dryness; rebound congestion may occur after 3 to 5 days of continued use.

PSEUDOEPHEDRINE

▶ **Administration and Dosage**

Adults: 60 mg every 4 to 6 hours (120 mg sustained release every 12 hours) as needed. Do not exceed 240 mg in 24 hours.

Children (6 to 12 years): 30 mg every 4 to 6 hours as needed. Do not exceed 120 mg in 24 hours.

Children (2 to 5 years): 15 mg every 4 to 6 hours as needed. Do not exceed 60 mg in 24 hours.

Drops:

> *Children (2 to 3 years)* – 2 droppersful (1.6 mL) every 4 to 6 hours up to 4 doses/day.

> *Children (younger than 2 years)* – Consult a physician.

PSEUDOEPHEDRINE PRODUCTS	
Trade name	**Doseform**
Sudodrin	**Tablets**: 30 mg
Genaphed	**Tablets**: 30 mg. Parabens, sucrose.
Efidac 24 Hour, Sudafed 24 Hour	**Tablets, extended release**: 240 mg (60 mg immediate release/180 mg controlled release)
Children's Sudafed Nasal Decongestant Chewables (sf)	**Tablets, chewable**: 15 mg. Aspartame, phenylalanine.
Sinustop Pro	**Capsules**: 60 mg
Drixoral Non-Drowsy Nasal Decongestant, Sudafed 12 Hour Caplets	**Tablets, extended release**: 120 mg
Children's Sudafed Nasal Decongestant (sf)	**Liquid**: 15 mg/5 mL. EDTA, glycerin, saccharin, sorbitol. Alcohol free.
Triaminic Allergy Congestion	**Liquid**: 15 mg/5 mL. EDTA, saccharin, sorbitol.
Cenafed Decongestant Syrup	**Liquid**: 30 mg/5 mL
Children's Decofed	**Liquid**: 30 mg/5 mL. Glycerin, parabens, saccharin, sucrose.
PediaCare Infants' Drops	**Drops**: 7.5 mg/0.8 mL. Glycerin, sorbitol, sucrose. Alcohol free.

Products listed are representative of currently available and widely distributed brands. Similar products, including regional and private label brands, may also exist.

sf = Sugar free.

PROPYLHEXEDRINE

▶ **Administration and Dosage**

Adults and children (6 years and older): 2 inhalations in each nostril (while blocking the other nostril) not more than every 2 hours as needed. Do not exceed recommended dosage. Do not use for more than 3 days.

Abuse: Propylhexedrine has been extracted from inhalers and injected IV as an amphetamine substitute. It also has been ingested by soaking the fibrous interior in hot water. Chronic abuse has caused cardiomyopathy (severe left and right ventricular failure), pulmonary hypertension, foreign body granuloma (emboli), dyspnea, and sudden death.

PROPYLHEXEDRINE PRODUCTS	
Trade name	Doseform
Benzedrex	Inhaler: 250 mg. Lavender oil, menthol.

Products listed are representative of currently available and widely distributed brands. Similar products, including regional and private label brands, may also exist.

DESOXYEPHEDRINE

▶ **Administration and Dosage**

Adults and children (6 years and older): 1 to 2 inhalations in each nostril (while blocking the other nostril) not more than every 2 hours as needed. Do not exceed recommended dosage. Do not use for more than 7 days.

DESOXYEPHEDRINE PRODUCTS	
Trade name	Doseform
Vicks Vapor Inhaler	Inhaler: 50 mg l-desoxyephedrine. Bornyl acetate, camphor, lavender oil, menthol.

Products listed are representative of currently available and widely distributed brands. Similar products, including regional and private label brands, may also exist.

NAPHAZOLINE HCL

▶ **Administration and Dosage**

Adults and children (12 years and older): 1 or 2 drops or sprays in each nostril as needed, no more than every 6 hours (spray). Do not use for more than 3 to 5 consecutive days. Do not use in children younger than 12 years of age, unless directed by physician.

NAPHAZOLINE HCL PRODUCTS	
Trade name	Doseform
Privine Nasal Drops	Solution: 0.05%. Benzalkonium chloride, EDTA.
Privine Nasal Spray	Spray: 0.05%. Benzalkonium chloride, EDTA.

Products listed are representative of currently available and widely distributed brands. Similar products, including regional and private label brands, may also exist.

OXYMETAZOLINE HCL

▶ **Administration and Dosage**

Adults and children (6 years and older): 2 or 3 sprays or 2 or 3 drops of 0.05% solution in each nostril twice daily, morning and evening as needed. Do not use for more than 3 to 5 consecutive days.

OXYMETAZOLINE HCL PRODUCTS	
Trade name	Doseform
Afrin 12-Hour Original, Afrin Sinus, Afrin Extra Moisturizing 12 Hour[1], Dristan 12 Hour Nasal[1], 4-Way 12 Hour[2], Nōstrilla[2], Sinex Ultra Fine Mist 12-Hour[3], Neo-Synephrine 12 Hour[2], Neo-Synephrine 12-Hour Extra Moisturizing[2]	Spray: 0.05%

Products listed are representative of currently available and widely distributed brands. Similar products, including regional and private label brands, may also exist.

[1] Contains benzalkonium Cl, EDTA.
[2] Contains benzalkonium Cl.
[3] Contains benzalkonium Cl, camphor, EDTA.

XYLOMETAZOLINE HCL

▶ **Administration and Dosage**

Adults (12 years and older): 2 to 3 drops or 2 to 3 sprays (0.1%) in each nostril every 8 to 10 hours as needed. Do not use for more than 3 to 5 consecutive days.

Children (2 to 12 years): 2 to 3 drops or 1 spray (0.05%) in each nostril every 8 to 10 hours as needed. Do not use for more than 3 to 5 consecutive days.

XYLOMETAZOLINE HCL PRODUCTS	
Trade name	Doseform
Natru-vent	**Spray**: 0.05%

Products listed are representative of currently available and widely distributed brands. Similar products, including regional and private label brands, may also exist.

PATIENT INFORMATION

Nasal Decongestants

- Patient instructions accompany each product. Read these instructions carefully before use, preferably before leaving the pharmacy, in case of any questions.
- No single drug or combination of drugs completely eliminates all symptoms of the common cold.
- Patients with hypertension, coronary artery disease or other cardiovascular diseases, hyperthyroidism, diabetes mellitus, or prostatic hypertrophy should use these products with caution.
- Topical administration may cause stinging, burning, sneezing, increased nasal discharge, or drying of the nasal mucosa. Do not use for more than 3 to 5 consecutive days.
- Oral decongestants may cause nervousness, dizziness, or sleeplessness.
- Do not use any out-of-date product or exceed recommended dosages.
- Do not crush or chew sustained-release preparations.
- Do not use any solution that changes color or becomes cloudy.
- Do not share intranasal containers with other people.

SALINE NASAL PRODUCTS

▶ **Actions**

Saline solutions provide moisture to loosen and liquefy mucus secretions to allow drainage from nose and sinuses.

▶ **Indications**

To provide moisture to inflamed nasal passages and facilitate drainage of thickened nasal secretions.

▶ **Contraindications**

Hypersensitivity to any product component.

▶ **Administration and Dosage**

Refer to individual product labeling for dosing information.

SALINE NASAL PRODUCTS	
Trade name	Doseform
SalineX[1]	**Spray**: 0.4% sodium chloride
NaSal[2], Breathe Free[3], Ocean[3], Nasal Moist	**Spray**: 0.65% sodium chloride

SALINE NASAL PRODUCTS	
Trade name	**Doseform**
Simply Saline	**Solution**: 0.9% sodium chloride

Products listed are representative of currently available and widely distributed brands. Similar products, including regional and private label brands, may also exist.

[1] Contains benzalkonium chloride, EDTA.
[2] Contains thimerosal and benzalkonium chloride.
[3] Contains benzalkonium chloride, phenylcarbinol.

PATIENT INFORMATION
Saline Nasal Products

- Patient instructions accompany each product. Read these instructions carefully before use, preferably before leaving the pharmacy, in case of any questions.
- Do not share intranasal containers with other patients.
- Do not use out-of-date products or exceed recommended dosages.

ANTITUSSIVES

▶ **Actions**

Note: Many antitussives are available as combination products. For a complete listing of these products, see the Cough monograph.

DEXTROMETHORPHAN HBR

▶ **Actions**

Dextromethorphan is a preferred antitussive, equally potent to codeine as a cough suppressant on a mg-for-mg basis. It increases the cough threshold in the brainstem and is a narcotic analogue devoid of analgesic or habit-forming characteristics.

▶ **Indications**

For control of nonproductive cough and temporary relief of cough caused by minor throat and bronchial irritation as may occur with the common cold or inhaled irritants.

▶ **Contraindications**

Hypersensitivity to the drug or any of its components.

▶ **Warnings**

Do not use for persistent or chronic cough (eg, cough due to smoking, asthma, emphysema) or when cough is accompanied by excessive secretions. If cough persists for more than 1 week, tends to recur, or is accompanied by fever, rash, or persistent headache, consult a physician.

Drug abuse and dependence: Anecdotal reports of abuse of dextromethorphan-containing cough/cold products have increased, especially among teenagers. The FDA Drug Abuse Advisory Committee states that additional data are needed before determining the abuse and dependency potential of dextromethorphan.

▶ **Drug Interactions**

MAO inhibitors: Patients may develop hypotension, hyperpyrexia, nausea, myoclonic leg jerks, and coma following coadministration.

Quinidine: Coadministration may cause increased dextromethorphan plasma concentrations, increasing toxic effects (eg, nervousness, fatigue, unsteady gait, dizziness, confusion).

Sibutramine: A potentially fatal "serotonin syndrome", including CNS irritability, motor weakness, shivering, myoclonus, and altered consciousness, may occur. Coadministration is not recommended.

Terbinafine: Coadministration may cause increased dextromethorphan plasma concentrations, which increases toxic effects.

Drug-food interactions: Coadministration with grapefruit juice may cause increased dextromethorphan plasma concentrations, which increases toxic effects.

▶ Overdosage

Symptoms:

Adults – Altered sensory perception; ataxia; slurred speech; dysphoria.

Children – Ataxia; respiratory depression; convulsions.

▶ Administration and Dosage

Lozenges:

Adults and children (older than 12 years of age) – 10 mg every 4 hours as needed, not to exceed 60 mg in 24 hours.

Children (6 to 12 years of age) – 5 mg every 4 hours as needed, not to exceed 30 mg in 24 hours.

Children (younger than 6 years of age) – Do not give lozenges to children younger than 6 years of age.

Liquid:

Adults and children (older than 12 years of age) – 30 mg every 6 to 8 hours as needed, not to exceed 120 mg in 24 hours.

Children (6 to 12 years of age) – 15 mg every 6 to 8 hours as needed, not to exceed 60 mg in 24 hours.

Children (2 to 6 years of age) – 7.5 mg every 6 to 8 hours as needed, not to exceed 30 mg in 24 hours.

Children (younger than 2 years of age) – Use only as directed by a physician.

Syrup:

Adults and children (older than 12 years of age) – 30 mg every 6 to 8 hours as needed, not to exceed 120 mg in 24 hours.

Children (6 to 12 years of age) – 15 mg every 6 to 8 hours as needed, not to exceed 60 mg in 24 hours.

Children (younger than 6 years of age) – Use only as directed by a physician.

Extended-release suspension:

Adults and children (older than 12 years of age) – 60 mg every 12 hours as needed, not to exceed 120 mg in 24 hours.

Children (6 to 12 years of age) – 30 mg every 12 hours as needed, not to exceed 60 mg in 24 hours.

Children (2 to 6 years of age) – 15 mg every 12 hours as needed, not to exceed 30 mg in 24 hours.

Children (younger than 2 years of age) – Use only as directed by a physician.

DEXTROMETHORPHAN HBR PRODUCTS

Trade name	Doseform
DexAlone (sf)	**Gelcaps**: 30 mg. Alcohol free.
Hold DM	**Lozenges**: 5 mg. Corn syrup, sucrose, vegetable oil. Original, honey lemon, and cherry flavor.
Scot-Tussin DM Cough Chasers (sf)	**Lozenges**: 5 mg. Dye free. Peppermint oil, sorbitol.
Trocal	**Lozenges**: 7.5 mg. Cherry flavor.
Simply Cough	**Liquid**: 5 mg/mL. Alcohol free. Corn syrup, glycerin, sucralose. Cherry berry flavor.
Benylin Pediatric (sf)	**Liquid**: 7.5 mg/5 mL. Alcohol free. Glycerin, saccharin, sorbitol. Grape flavor.
ElixSure Cough	**Liquid**: 7.5 mg/5 mL. Glycerin, propylparaben, sorbitol. Cherry and bubble gum flavor.
Robitussin Pediatric Cough	**Liquid**: 7.5 mg/5 mL. Corn syrup, glycerin, saccharin.
Vicks 44 Cough Relief	**Liquid**: 10 mg/5 mL. Alcohol, corn syrup, saccharin.
Benylin Adult Formula (sf)	**Liquid**: 15 mg/5 mL. Alcohol free. Glycerin, menthol, saccharin, sorbitol.
Robitussin Honey Cough	**Syrup**: 10 mg/5 mL. Alcohol free. Glycerin, methylparaben.
Robitussin Maximum Strength Cough	**Syrup**: 15 mg/5 mL. Alcohol, corn syrup, glycerin, menthol, saccharin.
Delsym 12-Hour Cough Relief	**Suspension, extended release**: Dextromethorphan polistirex (equivalent to 30 mg dextromethorphan HBr/5 mL). Alcohol free. Corn syrup, parabens, sucrose, vegetable oil. Orange flavor.

Products listed are representative of currently available and widely distributed brands. Similar products, including regional and private label brands, may also exist.

sf = Sugar free.

PATIENT INFORMATION

Dextromethorphan HBr

- Patient instructions accompany each product. Read these instructions carefully before use, preferably before leaving the pharmacy, in case of any questions.
- Take as directed. Do not use any out-of-date products or exceed recommended dosages.
- Do not take for persistent or chronic cough (eg, cough due to smoking, asthma, emphysema) or when cough is accompanied by excessive secretions, except under supervision of a physician.
- A persistent cough may be a sign of a serious condition. Consult a physician if cough persists longer than 7 days, tends to recur, or is accompanied by fever, rash, or persistent headache.
- Do not take if you are now taking a prescription monoamine oxidase inhibitor (MAOI) or for 2 weeks after stopping the MAOI drug.
- Do not take this product if you have asthma or glaucoma, except under supervision of a physician.
- Do not use any solution that has changed color or become cloudy.

MOUTH AND THROAT PRODUCTS

▶ **Actions**

Benzocaine and dyclonine are local anesthetics and account for most of the symptomatic relief provided. Cetylpyridinium chloride, eucalyptus oil, and hexylresorcinol have minor antiseptic activity. Camphor, capsicum, dyclonine, menthol, and phenol are used for their antipruritic, local anesthetic, and counterirritant activities. Some throat products include dextromethorphan. Lozenges, not withstanding their active ingredients, have value because of the soothing action of their sialagogue (saliva-producing) and demulcent (lubricating) effect.

▶ **Indications**

These products are indicated for the symptomatic treatment of minor sore throat and minor irritation of the throat or mouth associated with conditions such as a viral upper respiratory tract infection (common cold), postnasal drip associated with a cold or allergic rhinitis, breathing through the mouth, smoking, or inhalation of smoke or irritating gas.

▶ **Contraindications**

Hypersensitivity to any component. Patients taking disulfiram should not take any alcohol-containing product.

▶ **Warnings**

Severe and persistent sore throat (lasting beyond 7 to 10 days) or sore throat accompanied by high fever, rash, severe headache, nausea, and vomiting may be serious. Consult a physician promptly.

▶ **Drug Interactions**

No known drug interactions.

▶ **Adverse Reactions**

Oral overdoses may cause systemic reactions. Seek professional advice (eg, physician, pharmacist) if overdose is suspected.

▶ **Administration and Dosage**

Do not use for more than 2 days or in children younger than 2 years of age unless directed by physician. For dosage guidelines, refer to the product-specific package labeling.

MOUTH AND THROAT PRODUCTS	
Trade name	**Doseform**
Chloraseptic Sore Throat	**Lozenges:** 6 mg benzocaine, 10 mg menthol. Corn syrup, sucrose.
Trocaine	**Lozenges:** 10 mg benzocaine
Sepasoothe	**Lozenges:** 10 mg benzocaine, 0.5 mg cetylpyridinium Cl
Cēpacol Regular Strength Cherry (sf)	**Lozenges:** 4.5 mg menthol. Cetylpyridinium Cl, sucrose.
Cēpacol Maximum Strength Cherry	**Lozenges:** 10 mg benzocaine, 3.6 mg menthol. Cetylpyridinium Cl, sucrose.
Cēpacol Maximum Strength Cherry (sf)	**Lozenges:** 10 mg benzocaine, 4.5 mg menthol. Cetylpyridinium Cl, sorbitol.
Cēpacol Maximum Strength Cool Mint (sf)	**Lozenges:** 10 mg benzocaine, 2.5 mg menthol. Cetylpyridinium Cl.
Cylex (sf)	**Lozenges:** 15 mg benzocaine, 5 mg cetylpyridinium Cl.

MOUTH AND THROAT PRODUCTS

Trade name	Doseform
Mycinettes (sf)	**Lozenges**: 15 mg benzocaine
Cēpacol Throat	**Lozenges**: 0.07% cetylpyridinium Cl, 0.3% benzyl alcohol
Sucrets Children's Formula	**Lozenges**: 1.2 mg dyclonine HCl. Sucrose.
Vapor Lemon Sucrets	**Lozenges**: 2 mg dyclonine HCl
Sucrets Maximum Strength	**Lozenges**: 3 mg dyclonine HCl
Sucrets Sore Throat	**Lozenges**: 2.4 mg hexylresorcinol
Cēpastat Extra Strength (sf)	**Lozenges**: 29 mg phenol, menthol, eucalyptus oil
Cēpastat Cherry (sf)	**Lozenges**: 14.5 mg phenol, menthol
Robitussin Liquid Center Cough Drops	**Lozenges**: 10 mg menthol
N'ice (sf)	**Lozenges**: 5 mg menthol
Medikoff (sf)	**Lozenges**: 6.1 mg menthol
Vicks Cherry Cough Drops	**Lozenges**: Menthol
Vicks Menthol Cough Drops	**Lozenges**: Menthol, thymol, eucalyptus oil, camphor, tolu balsam
Throat Discs	**Lozenges**: Capsicum, peppermint oil, mineral oil
Halls Plus Maximum Strength	**Lozenges**: 10 mg menthol. Eucalyptus oil, glucose, glycerin, sucrose.
Robitussin Cough Drops	**Lozenges**: 7.4 mg and 10 mg menthol
Cēpacol Anesthetic	**Troches**: 10 mg benzocaine, 0.07% cetylpyridinium Cl
Chloraseptic Sore Throat	**Liquid**: 1.4% phenol. Glycerin, saccharin.
Vicks Cough Drops	**Drops**: 1.7 mg menthol. Eucalyptus oil, sucrose.
Cēpacol Honey Lemon, Cēpacol Cherry	**Throat Spray**: 0.1% dyclonine HCl. Cetylpyridinium Cl, glycerin, sorbitol.
Cēpacol Cool Menthol	**Throat Spray**: 0.1% dyclonine HCl. Cetylpyridinium Cl, glycerin, saccharin, sorbitol.
Sucrets (sf)	**Throat Spray**: 0.1% dyclonine HCl, 10% alcohol
Kids Chloraseptic (sf)	**Throat Spray**: 0.5% phenol. Glycerin, saccharin, sorbitol. Alcohol free.
Chloraseptic Pocket Pump (sf), Cheracol Sore Throat (sf)	**Throat Spray**: 1.4% phenol. Glycerin, saccharin. Alcohol free.
Mycinettes (sf)	**Throat Spray**: 1.4% phenol, 0.3% alum (aluminum ammonium sulfate).
N'ice	**Throat Spray**: 0.12% menthol, 25% glycerin, 23% alcohol.
Children's Vicks Chloraseptic	**Throat Spray**: 0.5% phenol.

Products listed are representative of currently available and widely distributed brands. Similar products, including regional and private label brands, may also exist.

sf = Sugar free.

PATIENT INFORMATION
Lozenges and Throat Sprays

- Patient instructions accompany each product. Read these instructions carefully before use, preferably before leaving the pharmacy, in case of any questions.
- No single drug or combination of drugs completely eliminates all symptoms of the common cold.
- Local anesthetic effects linger for 20 to 30 minutes, but should not be administered more often than every 3 to 4 hours in most cases. Continuous relief of sore throat should not be a goal of therapy.
- Do not use any out-of-date product or exceed recommended dosages.
- Do not use for more than 2 days.
- Do not use in children younger than 2 years of age.
- Allow 1 lozenge to dissolve slowly in mouth.

TOPICAL RUB AND VAPOR AGENTS

▶ Actions

The active ingredients include the counterirritants camphor and menthol. Camphor and menthol aromatic vapors have modest local anesthetic activity.

▶ Indications

For temporary relief of nasal congestion and coughs associated with colds.

▶ Contraindications

Hypersensitivity to any component. Do not ingest orally.

▶ Warnings

For external use only. Avoid contact with eyes. Do not use unless directed by a physician or pharmacist if cough is associated with smoking, excess mucus, asthma, or emphysema, or if the cough is persistent or chronic. Do not take by mouth, place in nostrils, bandage tightly, or apply to damaged skin. Consult a physician if cough persists for more than 7 to 10 days, recurs, or is accompanied by a fever, rash, or persistent headache.

Precautions: Do not apply to irritated skin; if excessive irritation develops, discontinue use. If pain persists for more than 7 to 10 days, or if redness is present, or in conditions affecting children younger than 10 years of age, consult a physician.

▶ Drug Interactions

No known drug interactions.

▶ Adverse Reactions

Toxic if ingested. Oral ingestion may cause systemic reactions. Seek professional advice if oral ingestion is suspected. Counterirritants may cause local irritation, especially in patients with sensitive skin.

▶ Administration and Dosage

Rubs: Rub a thick layer on chest or throat. May cover with a soft, dry cloth, but keep clothing loose to allow vapors to reach nose and mouth.

Vaporizers: Add directly to the water in the warm- or hot-steam vaporizer. Do not direct steam too closely to face. Breathe in medicated vapors. May be repeated up to 3 times daily or as directed by a physician or pharmacist.

TOPICAL RUB AND VAPOR AGENTS	
Trade name	**Doseform**
Vicks VapoCream	**Cream**: 5.2% camphor, 2.8% menthol, 1.2% eucalyptus oil, cedarleaf oil, EDTA, nutmeg oil, parabens, thymol, turpentine oil, titanium dioxide.
Mentholatum	**Ointment**: 9% camphor, 1.3% natural menthol, petrolatum, titanium dioxide.
Mentholatum Cherry Chest Rub for Kids	**Ointment**: 4.7% camphor, 1.2% eucalyptus oil, 2.6 % natural menthol. Petrolatum, titanium dioxide.
Vicks VapoRub	**Ointment**: 4.8% camphor, 2.6% menthol, 1.2% eucalyptus oil, cedarleaf oil, nutmeg oil, special petrolatum, thymol, turpentine oil.
Vicks Vaposteam for Hot Steam Vaporizers	**Liquid**: 6.2% camphor, 78% alcohol, cedarleaf oil, eucalyptus oil, menthol, nutmeg oil.
Triaminic Vapor Patch	**Patch**: 4.7% camphor, 2.6% menthol, eucalyptus oil, glycerin, aloe vera gel, spirits of turpentine.

Products listed are representative of currently available and widely distributed brands. Similar products, including regional and private label brands, may also exist.

PATIENT INFORMATION
Rubs and Vaporizer Products

- Patient instructions accompany each product. Read these instructions carefully before use, preferably before leaving the pharmacy, in case of any questions.
- No single drug or combination of drugs completely eliminates all symptoms of the common cold.
- Do not use any out-of-date product or exceed recommended dosages.
- *Rubs:*
  For external use only.
  Avoid contact with eyes and mucous membranes.
  Rub a thick layer of the cream or ointment on the throat or chest.
  After application, the cream or ointment may be covered with a soft, dry cloth, but patient must keep clothing loose enough for the vapors to reach the nose and mouth.
  Do not apply to irritated skin. Discontinue use if excess irritation occurs. May cause local irritation in patients with sensitive skin.
- *Vaporizer products:*
  Add measured amount of vaporizer liquid medication directly to the water in the warm- or hot- steam vaporizer.
  Avoid directing the steam too closely to the face.
  Clean the vaporizer thoroughly after each use according to each specific manufacturer's directions.

EXPECTORANTS

GUAIFENESIN

▶ Actions

Although their clinical efficacy is not proven, expectorants may reduce the adherence, surface tension, and viscosity of mucus and other respiratory secretions, which facilitate clearance of the upper airway. These agents have not been shown to appreciably affect nasal clearance of secretions. Theoretically, improving airway clearance may reduce the urge to cough. Guaifenesin is the only OTC expectorant recognized as safe and effective by the FDA.

▶ Indications

For the symptomatic relief of respiratory conditions by facilitating removal of mucus from the respiratory tract.

▶ Contraindications

Hypersensitivity to guaifenesin.

▶ Warnings

Not for persistent, nonproductive cough, such as occurs with smoking, asthma, or emphysema, or where cough is accompanied by excessive secretions.

▶ Adverse Reactions

The following side effects occur infrequently: nausea, vomiting, dizziness, headache, rash (including urticaria).

▶ Administration and Dosage

Adults and children (12 years and older): 100 to 400 mg every 4 hours. Do not exceed 2.4 g/day.

Children (6 to 12 years): 100 to 200 mg every 4 hours. Do not exceed 1.2 g/day.

Children (2 to 6 years): 50 to 100 mg every 4 hours. Do not exceed 600 mg/day.

GUAIFENESIN PRODUCTS	
Trade name	**Doseform**
Hytuss (sf)	**Tablets**: 100 mg
Glytuss	**Tablets**: 200 mg
Breonesin[1], *Hytuss 2X*	**Capsules**: 200 mg
Guiatuss[2], *Robitussin*[3], *Diabetic Tussin*[4] (sf)	**Syrup**: 100 mg/5 mL
Scot-Tussin Expectorant (sf)	**Syrup**: 100 mg/5 mL. Glycerin, menthol, parabens. Alcohol free.
Naldecon Senior Ex	**Liquid**: 200 mg/5 mL. Saccharin, sorbitol.

Products listed are representative of currently available and widely distributed brands. Similar products, including regional and private label brands, may also exist.

sf = Sugar free.
[1] Sugar coated.
[2] Glycerin, corn syrup, saccharin.
[3] Contains 3.5% alcohol, saccharin, glucose, corn syrup.
[4] Contains aspartame, parabens, menthol. Alcohol free.

PATIENT INFORMATION

Expectorants

- Patient instructions accompany each product. Read these instructions carefully before use, preferably before leaving the pharmacy, in case of any questions.
- Do not take these products for persistent or chronic nonproductive cough such as occurs with smoking, asthma, chronic bronchitis, or emphysema, or when cough is accompanied by excessive phlegm, unless directed by a physician.
- A persistent cough may be a sign of a serious condition. If cough persists for more than 7 to 10 days, tends to recur, or is accompanied by fever, rash, or persistent headache, consult a physician.
- Guaifenesin is the only expectorant approved by the FDA as safe and effective.
- Drink a glass of water or other fluid with each dose of expectorant. Most medical professionals believe a well-hydrated body (due to fluid intake) is responsible for thinning respiratory tract mucus and may be as valuable or more so than the expectorant itself.

RESPIRATORY COMBINATION PRODUCTS

▶ **Indications**

Common nonprescription combination products for the common cold include decongestants and antihistamines; decongestants and analgesics; antihistamines and analgesics; decongestants, antihistamines, and analgesics; decongestants and expectorants; and decongestants, expectorants, and analgesics.

Note: Many of these combination products include antihistamines. For complete information on single-agent OTC antihistamines, see the Allergic Rhinitis monograph in this chapter.

Many multi-agent products also are available for the treatment of cough. For a complete listing of these products, see the Cough monograph in this chapter.

Synergistic activity with decongestant/antihistamine combinations and patient convenience are advantages of combination products.

Disadvantages include the inability to titrate the dose of individual ingredients, possible administration of a drug for which there are no symptoms, and unnecessary risk of side effects and drug interactions if more than one active ingredient is not needed to treat current symptoms. Locally administered drugs offer quick relief with fewer systemic side effects. However, topical antihistamines are potential sensitizers and may produce a local sensitivity reaction. Because of anticholinergic effects, use decongestants with caution in patients with narrow-angle or a history of glaucoma. Rebound nasal congestion and ocular hyperemia may occur with excessive use of topical products containing a decongestant.

ORAL DECONGESTANT/ANTIHISTAMINE COMBINATIONS

▶ **Administration and Dosage**

Dosages vary; refer to specific product information.

ORAL DECONGESTANT/ANTIHISTAMINE PRODUCTS	
Trade name	**Doseform**
Allerest Maximum Strength	**Tablets:** 30 mg pseudoephedrine HCl, 2 mg chlorpheniramine maleate
Advil Allergy Sinus Caplets	**Tablets:** 30 mg pseudoephedrine HCl, 2 mg chlorpheniramine maleate, 200 mg ibuprofen
Benadryl Allergy & Sinus Fastmelt	**Tablets, dissolving:** 30 mg pseudoephedrine HCl, 19 mg diphenhydramine citrate. Aspartame, phenylalanine.
Benadryl Allergy/Congestion	**Tablets:** 60 mg pseudoephedrine HCl, 25 mg diphenhydramine HCl
Genac	**Tablets:** 60 mg pseudoephedrine HCl, 2.5 mg triprolidine HCl. Lactose.
Cenafed Plus	**Tablets:** 60 mg pseudoephedrine HCl, 2.5 mg triprolidine HCl
Actifed Cold & Allergy	**Tablets:** 60 mg pseudoephedrine HCl, 2.5 mg triprolidine HCl. Lactose, sucrose.
Chlor-Trimeton Allergy-D 4 Hour	**Tablets:** 60 mg pseudoephedrine HCl, 4 mg chlorpheniramine maleate
Sudafed Cold & Allergy	**Tablets:** 60 mg pseudoephedrine HCl, 4 mg chlorpheniramine maleate. Lactose.
Chlor-Trimeton Allergy-D 12 Hour	**Tablets:** 120 mg pseudoephedrine sulfate, 8 mg chlorpheniramine maleate. Butylparaben, lactose, sugar.
Drixoral Cold & Allergy 12 Hour	**Tablets:** 120 mg pseudoephedrine sulfate, 6 mg dexbrompheniramine maleate. Butylparaben, lactose, sugar.
Histatab Plus	**Tablets:** 5 mg phenylephrine HCl, 2 mg chlorpheniramine maleate
A.R.M.	**Caplets:** 60 mg pseudoephedrine HCl, 4 mg chlorpheniramine maleate
PediCare (sf)	**Liquid:** 15 mg pseudoephedrine HCl, 1 mg chlorpheniramine maleate/5mL. Glycerin, sorbitol. Alcohol free.
Scot-Tussin Hayfebrol	**Liquid:** 30 mg pseudoephedrine HCl, 2 mg chlorpheniramine maleate/5 mL. Menthol, parabens. Alcohol free.
Ryna (sf)	**Liquid:** 30 mg pseudoephedrine HCl, 2 mg chlorpheniramine maleate/5 mL. Sorbitol. Alcohol free.
Triaminic Cold & Allergy	**Syrup:** 15 mg pseudoephedrine HCl, 1 mg chlorpheniramine maleate/5 mL. EDTA, sorbitol, sucrose.
Bromfed	**Syrup:** 30 mg pseudoephedrine HCl, 2 mg brompheniramine maleate/5 mL. Methylparaben, saccharin, sorbitol, sucrose.

Products listed are representative of currently available and widely distributed brands. Similar products, including regional and private label brands, may also exist.

ORAL DECONGESTANT/ANALGESIC COMBINATIONS

▶ Administration and Dosage

Differs among individual products. Follow instructions on package labeling. For contraindications and warnings, refer to Nasal Decongestants group monograph.

ORAL DECONGESTANT/ANALGESIC PRODUCTS	
Trade name	Doseform
Children's Tylenol Sinus Chewables	**Tablets:** 7.5 mg pseudoephedrine HCl, 80 mg acetaminophen. Aspartame, mannitol.
Triaminic Softchews Allergy Sinus & Headache	**Tablets:** 15 mg pseudoephedrine HCl, 160 mg acetaminophen. Aspartame, mannitol, sorbitol, sucrose.
Medi-Synal, Medi-First Sinus Pain & Pressure, Ornex Caplets	**Tablets:** 30 mg pseudoephedrine HCl, 325 mg acetaminophen
Dristan Maximum Strength Cold, Sinutab Sinus, Sudafed Non-Drowsy Sinus Headache, Tylenol Maximum Strength Sinus Non-Drowsy	**Tablets:** 30 mg pseudoephedrine HCl, 500 mg acetaminophen
Motrin Sinus/Headache	**Tablets:** 30 mg pseudoephedrine HCl, 200 mg ibuprofen
Advil Cold & Sinus, Dristan Sinus Caplets, Iprin Cold & Sinus	**Tablets:** 30 mg pseudoephedrine HCl, 200 mg ibuprofen. Paraben, sucrose.
Alka-Seltzer Plus Cold & Sinus Liqui-Gels, Sudafed Multi-Symptom Cold & Sinus Liquicaps	**Capsules:** 30 mg pseudoephedrine HCl, 325 mg acetaminophen. Sorbitol.
Tavist Maximum Strength Sinus	**Caplets:** 30 mg pseudoephedrine HCl, 500 mg acetaminophen. Lactose, methylparaben.
Tylenol Maximum Strength Sinus Non-Drowsy Geltabs and Gelcaps	**Capsules:** 30 mg pseudoephedrine HCl, 500 mg acetaminophen. Benzyl alcohol, EDTA, parabens.
Aleve Sinus & Headache, Aleve Cold & Sinus	**Caplets, extended-release:** 120 mg pseudoephedrine HCl, 220 mg naproxen sodium. Lactose.
Children's Tylenol Sinus Suspension	**Liquid:** 15 mg pseudoephedrine HCl, 160 mg acetaminophen/5 mL. Glycerin, parabens, sorbitol.
Children's Motrin Non-Staining Dye-Free Cold Suspension	**Liquid:** 15 mg pseudoephedrine HCl, 100 mg ibuprofen/5 mL. Glycerin, sucrose.
Cēpacol Sore Throat Formula Multi Symptom Relief, Cherry (sf)	**Liquid:** 30 mg pseudoephedrine HCl, 320 mg acetaminophen/15 mL. Cetylpyridinium Cl, glycerin, saccharin, sorbitol. Alcohol free.
Cēpacol Sore Throat Formula Multi Symptom Relief, Honey Lemon	**Liquid:** 30 mg pseudoephedrine HCl, 320 mg acetaminophen/15 mL. Cetylpyridinium Cl, glycerin, saccharin, sorbitol, tartrazine. Alcohol free.

Products listed are representative of currently available and widely distributed brands. Similar products, including regional and private label brands, may also exist.

ORAL ANTIHISTAMINE/ANALGESIC COMBINATIONS

▶ **Administration and Dosage**

Dosages vary; refer to specific product information.

ORAL ANTIHISTAMINE/ANALGESIC PRODUCTS	
Trade name	Doseform
Coricidin HBP Cold & Flu	**Tablets:** 2 mg chlorpheniramine maleate, 325 mg acetaminophen. Lactose, parabens, sugar.
Percogesic Extra Strength, Tylenol Severe Allergy	**Tablets:** 12.5 mg diphenhydramine HCl, 500 mg acetaminophen
Aceta-Gesic, Major-Gesic	**Tablets:** 30 mg phenyltoloxamine citrate, 325 mg acetaminophen
Percogesic	**Tablets:** 30 mg phenyltoloxamine citrate, 325 mg acetaminophen. Sucrose.

Products listed are representative of currently available and widely distributed brands. Similar products, including regional and private label brands, may also exist.

ORAL DECONGESTANT/ANTIHISTAMINE/ANALGESIC COMBINATIONS

▶ **Administration and Dosage**

Dosages vary; refer to specific product information/package labeling.

ORAL DECONGESTANT/ANTIHISTAMINE/ANALGESIC PRODUCTS	
Trade name	Doseform
Onset Forte	**Tablets:** 5 mg phenylephrine hydrochloride, 2 mg chlorpheniramine maleate, 162.5 mg acetaminophen
Dristan Cold Multi-Symptom	**Tablets:** 5 mg phenylephrine hydrochloride, 2 mg chlorpheniramine maleate, 325 mg acetaminophen
Medicidin-D	**Tablets:** 5 mg phenylephrine hydrochloride, 2 mg chlorpheniramine maleate, 325 mg acetaminophen. Sucrose, tartrazine.
Coricidin D Cold, Flu & Sinus	**Tablets:** 30 mg pseudoephedrine sulfate, 2 mg chlorpheniramine maleate, 325 mg acetaminophen. Lactose.
Children's Tylenol Cold	**Tablets, chewable:** 7.5 mg pseudoephedrine hydrochloride, 0.5 mg chlorpheniramine maleate, 80 mg acetaminophen. Aspartame, mannitol, 6 mg phenylalanine. Grape flavor.
Alka-Seltzer Plus Cold Orange Zest	**Tablets, effervescent:** 5 mg phenylephrine hydrochloride, 2 mg chlorpheniramine maleate, 250 mg acetaminophen. Aspartame, saccharin, sorbitol, 4.2 mg phenylalanine.
Drixoral Allergy Sinus	**Tablets, extended-release:** 60 mg pseudoephedrine sulfate, 3 mg dexbrompheniramine, 500 mg acetaminophen. Parabens.
Kolephrin	**Caplets:** 30 mg pseudoephedrine hydrochloride, 2 mg chlorpheniramine maleate, 325 mg acetaminophen
Tylenol Allergy Sinus Day Time, Sinutab Sinus Allergy	**Caplets:** 30 mg pseudoephedrine hydrochloride, 2 mg chlorpheniramine maleate, 500 mg acetaminophen
Tylenol Maximum Strength Sinus Night-Time	**Caplets:** 30 mg pseudoephedrine hydrochloride, 6.25 mg doxylamine succinate, 500 mg acetaminophen

ORAL DECONGESTANT/ANTIHISTAMINE/ANALGESIC PRODUCTS

Trade name	Doseform
Benadryl Allergy/Cold, Benadryl Allergy/Sinus Headache	**Caplets**: 30 mg pseudoephedrine hydrochloride, 12.5 mg diphenhydramine hydrochloride, 500 mg acetaminophen
Benadryl Severe Allergy & Sinus Headache, Tylenol Allergy Sinus Night Time	**Caplets**: 30 mg pseudoephedrine hydrochloride, 25 mg diphenhydramine hydrochloride, 500 mg acetaminophen
Tylenol Sinus Day/Night Convenience Pack*	**Caplets, day**: 30 mg pseudoephedrine hydrochloride, 500 mg acetaminophen
	Caplets, night: 30 mg pseudoephedrine hydrochloride, 6.25 mg doxylamine succinate, 500 mg acetaminophen
Comtrex Day & Night Maximum Strength Allergy-Sinus Treatment, Comtrex Day/Night Flu Therapy	**Caplets, day**: 30 mg pseudoephedrine hydrochloride, 500 mg acetaminophen. Mineral oil.
	Tablets, night: 30 mg pseudoephedrine hydrochloride, 2 mg chlorpheniramine maleate, 500 mg acetaminophen. Mineral oil, parabens.
Tylenol Allergy Sinus Day/Night Convenience Pack	**Caplets, day**: 30 mg pseudoephedrine hydrochloride, 2 mg chlorpheniramine maleate, 500 mg acetaminophen
	Caplets, night: 30 mg pseudoephedrine hydrochloride, 25 mg diphenhydramine hydrochloride, 500 mg acetaminophen
Contac Day & Night Cold/Flu	**Caplets, day**: 60 mg pseudoephedrine hydrochloride, 30 mg dextromethorphan HBr, 650 mg acetaminophen
	Caplets, night: 60 mg pseudoephedrine hydrochloride, 50 mg diphenhydramine hydrochloride, 650 mg acetaminophen
Contac Day & Night Allergy/Sinus*	**Caplets, day**: 60 mg pseudoephedrine hydrochloride, 650 mg acetaminophen
	Caplets, night: 60 mg pseudoephedrine hydrochloride, 50 mg diphenhydramine hydrochloride, 650 mg acetaminophen
Alka-Seltzer Plus Cold	**Softgels**: 30 mg pseudoephedrine hydrochloride, 2 mg chlorpheniramine maleate, 325 mg acetaminophen. Glycerin, sorbitol.
Tylenol Flu NightTime	**Gelcaps**: 30 mg pseudoephedrine hydrochloride, 25 mg diphenhydramine hydrochloride, 500 mg acetaminophen. Benzyl alcohol, castor oil, EDTA, parabens.
Tylenol Allergy Sinus Day Time	**Gelcaps/geltabs**: 30 mg pseudoephedrine hydrochloride, 2 mg chlorpheniramine maleate, 500 mg acetaminophen. Benzyl alcohol, castor oil, EDTA, parabens.
Tylenol Flu Day/Night Convenience Pack*	**Gelcaps, day**: 30 mg pseudoephedrine hydrochloride, 15 mg dextromethorphan HBr, 500 mg acetaminophen. Benzyl alcohol, castor oil, EDTA, parabens.
	Gelcaps, night: 30 mg pseudoephedrine hydrochloride, 25 mg diphenhydramine hydrochloride, 500 mg acetaminophen. Benzyl alcohol, castor oil, EDTA, parabens.
Children's Tylenol Cold	**Liquid**: 15 mg pseudoephedrine hydrochloride, 1 mg chlorpheniramine maleate, 160 mg acetaminophen/5 mL. Butylparaben, corn syrup, glycerin, sorbitol. Grape flavor.

ORAL DECONGESTANT/ANTIHISTAMINE/ANALGESIC PRODUCTS	
Trade name	Doseform
TheraFlu Flu & Sore Throat Maximum Strength Night Time	**Packets**: 60 mg pseudoephedrine hydrochloride, 4 mg chlorpheniramine maleate, 1,000 mg acetaminophen. Sucrose, aspartame, 22 mg phenylalanine. Alcohol free.

Products listed are representative of currently available and widely distributed brands. Similar products, including regional and private label brands, may also exist.

* Only night caplets/gelcaps contain an antihistamine.

DECONGESTANT/EXPECTORANT COMBINATIONS

▶ **Administration and Dosage**

Dosages vary; refer to specific product information/package labeling.

DECONGESTANT/EXPECTORANT PRODUCTS	
Trade name	Doseform
Congestac	**Caplets**: 60 mg pseudoephedrine hydrochloride, 400 mg guaifenesin
Robitussin Severe Congestion	**Softgels**: 30 mg pseudoephedrine hydrochloride, 200 mg guaifenesin. Glycerin, mannitol, sorbitol.
Sudafed Non-Drying Sinus	**Liquicaps**: 30 mg pseudoephedrine hydrochloride, 200 mg guaifenesin. Glycerin, sorbitol.
Rescon GG	**Liquid**: 5 mg phenylephrine hydrochloride, 100 mg guaifenesin/5 mL. Glycerin, parabens, sorbitol, sugar. Alcohol free. Wild cherry flavor.
Triaminic Chest & Nasal Congestion	**Liquid**: 15 mg pseudoephedrine hydrochloride, 50 mg guaifenesin/5 mL. EDTA, glycerin, sorbitol, sucrose. Alcohol free.
Robitussin PE	**Syrup**: 30 mg pseudoephedrine hydrochloride, 100 mg guaifenesin/5 mL. Corn syrup, glucose, glycerin, saccharin. Alcohol free.

Products listed are representative of currently available and widely distributed brands. Similar products, including regional and private label brands, may also exist.

DECONGESTANT/EXPECTORANT/ANALGESIC COMBINATIONS

▶ **Administration and Dosage**

Dosages vary; refer to specific product information/package labeling.

DECONGESTANT/EXPECTORANT/ANALGESIC PRODUCTS	
Trade name	Doseform
Decorel Forte	**Caplets**: 10 mg phenylephrine hydrochloride, 200 mg guaifenesin, 325 mg acetaminophen, 32.4 mg caffeine
Robitussin Cold, Sinus & Congestion	**Caplets**: 30 mg pseudoephedrine hydrochloride, 200 mg guaifenesin, 325 mg acetaminophen. Lactose.
Tylenol Sinus Severe Congestion	**Caplets**: 30 mg pseudoephedrine hydrochloride, 200 mg guaifenesin, 325 mg acetaminophen. Mannitol, polyvinyl alcohol.

Products listed are representative of currently available and widely distributed brands. Similar products, including regional and private label brands, may also exist.

PATIENT INFORMATION

Respiratory Combination Products

- Patient instructions accompany each product. Read these instructions carefully before use, preferably before leaving the pharmacy, in case of any questions.
- Take as directed. Do not use any out-of-date products or exceed recommended dosages.
- May cause GI upset; take with food.
- Do not crush or chew sustained-release preparations.
- Do not consume alcohol or other CNS depressants (eg, sedatives, hypnotics, narcotics, tranquilizers) concurrently with respiratory combination products without consulting a physician or pharmacist.
- May cause drowsiness or dizziness. Do not drive or perform other tasks requiring alertness, coordination, or physical dexterity while taking these products.
- Inform a physician of antihistamine use prior to diagnostic skin or blood allergy tests.
- Inform a physician if you have glaucoma, peptic ulcer, urinary retention, benign prostatic hypertrophy, or if you are pregnant before taking these products.
- May cause nervousness, dizziness, or sleeplessness.
- Inform a physician if a medication appears to lose its effectiveness over time.
- No single drug or combination of drugs completely eliminates all symptoms.
- Do not use any solution that has changed color or become cloudy.

ALLERGIC RHINITIS

DEFINITION

Allergic rhinitis, characterized by inflammation of the lining of the nasal passages, is caused by an adverse reaction to environmental stimuli. Typical symptoms include rhinorrhea, sneezing, conjunctivitis, and itching of the nose, eyes, and palate. Nasal congestion may occur. Sore throat may be associated with postnasal drip. Seasonal allergic rhinitis is characterized by episodic symptoms that occur during specific seasons. Perennial allergic rhinitis is characterized by symptoms that occur throughout the year. The two types of allergic rhinitis may coexist.

ETIOLOGY

Allergic rhinitis is caused by type I (immunoglobulin E; IgE) reactions to inhaled antigenic substances. Seasonal allergic rhinitis generally is caused by airborne plant pollens. Pollinating seasons vary geographically; however, tree pollens generally are present in the spring, grass pollens in May and June, and ragweed pollens in mid-August to the first killing frost. Perennial allergic rhinitis is caused by continual allergen exposure throughout the year. Typical antigens are house dust mites, mold spores, cosmetics, and animal dander.

INCIDENCE

Allergic rhinitis is the most commonly occurring atopic (allergy-mediated) medical condition. It is estimated that approximately 10% of the world's population and approximately 20 to 30 million Americans have symptoms of seasonal allergic rhinitis. Approximately 3% to 5% suffer from perennial allergic rhinitis. These conditions are most prevalent in children and young adults. The symptoms of allergic rhinitis generally become milder as one grows older but seldom disappear entirely. Asthma develops in approximately 20% of children with allergic rhinitis.

PATHOPHYSIOLOGY

In both seasonal and perennial allergic rhinitis, the pathophysiology is triggered by an inflammatory response to an allergen. Small quantities of antigenic protein deposited on the respiratory mucosa sensitize nasal mucosal inflammatory cells (mast cells, eosinophils, basophils). Subsequent exposure to the same protein results in the immediate release of pro-inflammatory mediators, including histamine, interleukins, tumor necrosis factor-alpha, and various enzymes that interact with neural and vascular sites within the nasal mucosa. Histamine is a primary mediator of the allergic response. Inflammatory cell activation also stimulates synthesis of additional pro-inflammatory mediators (leukotrienes, prostaglandins), which contribute to the inflammatory response and "prime" the nasal mucosa. Priming causes an exaggerated response to the same or smaller amounts of allergen. Histamine is primarily responsible for the symptoms of itching and sneezing. The inflammatory response of vasodilation and mucosal edema and secretion result in nasal obstruction and nasal discharge. Similar inflammatory response mechanisms in the eye produce the symptoms of edema and tearing.

SIGNS/SYMPTOMS

Symptoms include nasal obstruction, congestion, rhinorrhea, sneezing (multiple single episodes or paroxysms), pruritus (eyes, nose, and palate), impaired sense of smell, postnasal drip, chronic pharyngitis, hoarseness, eyelid edema, sensitivity to light and watering, irritated eyes. Marked conjunctival edema is seen rarely. Nasal congestion is the most prominent chronic symptom. Other symptoms may include malaise, fatigue, irritability, anorexia, and insomnia. In allergic rhinitis, the nasal mucosa usually appear pale blue but may appear red and inflamed or purple-gray, and nasal polyps may be present. Complications of allergic rhinitis include ear congestion, diminished hearing acuity, sinus headache and discomfort, recurrent sinus infections, otitis media, eustachian tube dysfunction, and acute asthma exacerbations.

DIAGNOSTIC PARAMETERS/PHYSICAL ASSESSMENT

Clinical Observation: Many symptoms of allergic rhinitis are similar to other upper respiratory tract diseases. The patient interview is helpful for the diagnosis.

Interview: To ensure the proper diagnosis and treatment of allergic rhinitis, it may be beneficial to ask about the following:

- Description of symptoms
- Onset of symptoms, and whether there is a seasonal pattern
- Factors that trigger the symptoms, such as outdoor activities that increase pollen exposure, or visits to a particular home with animal dander
- A family history of atopy or allergy
- Concomitant acute and chronic disorders to rule out the possibility of other disorders, such as sinusitis or a viral cold. If concurrent sinusitis (purulent nasal discharge with fever and parasinal pressure) or ear infection are present, secondary bacterial infection may be a complication, and the patient should see a physician
- Concurrent medications, especially topical decongestants, to rule out possible rebound congestion from overuse. Aspirin and other NSAIDs may cause a nonallergic rhinitis
- Nasal discharge, which tends to be clear and watery, in contrast to the purulent discharge of sinusitis and the mid-cycle of a common cold
- Hallmarks of allergic rhinitis, especially in children, include the linea nasalis, a crease across the nose caused by the "allergic salute" (pushing the palm upward against the nose to relieve itching) and "allergic shiners" (darkened eyelids secondary to chronic venous stasis)

Tests to determine the causative allergen include skin tests or radioallergosorbent tests (RAST) of the blood. Quantitative in vitro tests use enzymatic, fluorometric, and other markers of IgE reactivity. Fiberoptic nasopharyngoscopy, sinus transillumination, acoustic rhinometry, anterior rhinomanometry, and nasal cytology are sometimes used to determine the presence of nasal polyps or deformities, the extent of nasopharyngeal inflammation or response to therapy, or to rule out nonallergenic rhinitis.

TREATMENT

Approaches to therapy: The treatment of allergic rhinitis is directed at relief of symptoms, avoidance of allergens (if possible), and prevention of complications. It involves a combination of avoidance measures and pharmacotherapy; immunotherapy (desensitization) may be indicated if avoidance measures and pharmacotherapy do not control the symptoms.

Nondrug therapy: Avoidance of known allergens is essential; high-efficiency particulate (HEPA) filtration may decrease airborne antigens.

- *Pollens and other outdoor allergens*: Keep doors and windows closed whenever possible and avoid unnecessary outdoor activities, especially early in the morning when pollen counts are high. A nose and mouth mask may reduce exposure during outdoor activities such as lawn mowing.
- *House dust mites*: If possible, eliminate common sources of dust, such as rugs, upholstered furniture, and stuffed animals. Enclose bedding in plastic or other mite-impermeable material, wash bedding in hot water (at least 130°F), and change furnace filters regularly.
- *Mold spores*: Vent moisture-generating areas (eg, kitchens, bathrooms) to reduce household humidity. Repair wet basements, use a dehumidifier if necessary, and avoid raking piles of leaves.
- *Animal dander*: Remove the pet from the household or at least from the patient's bedroom; weekly bathing of pet cats may be helpful.

To relieve irritated nasal mucosa and relieve obstruction, saline solutions instilled or sprayed into the nostril may be helpful. Irrigation solutions can be prepared (7 oz of water with ¼ tsp salt) and instilled with a bulb syringe. Cool compresses applied to the eyes can soothe irritation.

Pharmacotherapy: Antihistamines, nasal decongestants, mast cell stabilizers, and corticosteroids provide symptomatic relief of seasonal and perennial allergic rhinitis. Several antihistamines and decongestants are available OTC.

Mild allergic rhinitis generally is treated with an oral antihistamine with or without a decongestant; intranasal cromolyn sodium may be effective as single-drug therapy. Moderate and severe allergic rhinitis are treated with antihistamines, decongestants, and intranasal corticosteroids. A short course (3 to 7 days) of oral corticosteroid therapy may be considered for patients with severe allergic rhinitis. Allergic conjunctivitis generally will improve with oral antihistamines but also may be treated with ocular antihistamines and decongestants. More severe ocular symptoms are treated with ocular NSAIDs and/or ocular steroids.

Immunotherapy: Specific immunotherapy is indicated if 1) avoidance measures and pharmacotherapy do not control symptoms; 2) the patient has undesirable and intolerable side effects from pharmacotherapy; 3) the patient has a history of allergic rhinitis for at least 2 seasons (seasonal) or 6 months (perennial); or 4) the patient has positive skin tests or serum-specific IgE that correlate with the symptoms. Because immunotherapy requires several months, is expensive, and may only partially reduce symptoms if multiple allergens are involved, it usually is recommended only in severe cases.

For administration techniques of nasal sprays, drops, inhalers, metered dose pumps, and eye drops, **see Appendix C: Administration Techniques.**

RESPIRATORY COMBINATION PRODUCTS

▶ **Indications**

Common nonprescription combination products for the common cold include decongestants and antihistamines; decongestants and analgesics; antihistamines and analgesics; decongestants, antihistamines, and analgesics; decongestants and expectorants; and decongestants, analgesics, and expectorants. Intranasal and ocular decongestant and antihistamine combination products are also available.

Advantages of combination products include synergistic activity with decongestant/ antihistamine combinations and patient convenience.

Disadvantages include the inability to titrate the dose of individual ingredients, possible administration of a drug for which there are no symptoms, and unnecessary risk of side effects and drug interactions if more than one active ingredient is not needed to treat current symptoms. Locally administered drugs offer quick relief with fewer systemic side effects. However, topical antihistamines are potential sensitizers and may produce a local sensitivity reaction. Because of anticholinergic effects, use decongestants with caution in persons with narrow-angle, or a history of, glaucoma. Rebound nasal congestion and ocular hyperemia may occur with excessive use of topical products containing a decongestant. **See Respiratory Combination Products in the Common Cold monograph.**

ANTIHISTAMINES

▶ **Actions**

Antihistamines are first-line agents for the symptomatic treatment of allergic rhinitis. They competitively antagonize histamine at the H_1 receptor, reducing sensory nerve stimulation, mucus production, and vascular permeability. Some antihistamines have been shown to inhibit mediator release from mast cells and basophils and decrease the synthesis of leukotrienes and kinins. Histamine release is the primary trigger event in allergic rhinitis; thus, antihistamines generally reduce overt symptoms of allergic rhinitis by 40% to 60%.

▶ **Indications**

Antihistamines are indicated for the symptomatic relief of itching, sneezing, rhinorrhea, post-nasal drip, and watery eyes associated with allergic rhinitis. They have little attenuating effect on nasal congestion.

▶ **Contraindications**

Hypersensitivity to antihistamines; newborn or premature infants; nursing mothers; narrow-angle glaucoma; stenosing peptic ulcer; symptomatic prostatic hypertrophy; bladder neck obstruction; pyloroduodenal obstruction; monoamine oxidase inhibitor (MAOI) therapy.

▶ **Warnings**

Respiratory disease: In general, antihistamines are not recommended to treat lower respiratory tract symptoms (eg, emphysema, chronic bronchitis, asthma) because their anticholinergic (drying) effects may thicken secretions and impair expectoration.

However, several reports indicate antihistamines can be used safely in asthmatic patients with severe perennial allergic rhinitis without exacerbating the asthma.

Hazardous tasks: Antihistamines have varying degrees of sedative effects; some may cause drowsiness and reduce mental alertness (especially first-generation antihistamines). Patients using such products should use caution when driving or performing other tasks requiring alertness, coordination, or physical dexterity. The nonsedating antihistamines (eg, loratadine) may produce mild sedation in some users, but this effect generally is less than that seen with other OTC antihistamines. Supervise children who are taking antihistamines when they engage in potentially hazardous activities (eg, bicycle riding).

Sleep apnea: Avoid sedatives and CNS depressants in patients with a history of sleep apnea.

Drug abuse: Nonmedical parenteral use of concurrent butorphanol and diphenhydramine has been reported.

Renal/hepatic function impairment: Use caution in patients with cirrhosis or other liver diseases. Use a lower dose of loratadine (10 mg every other day) in patients with renal or hepatic impairment.

Anticholinergic effects: Antihistamines have varying degrees of atropine-like actions; use with caution in patients with a predisposition to urinary retention, history of bronchial asthma, increased intraocular pressure, hyperthyroidism, cardiovascular disease, or hypertension. Antihistamines may thicken bronchial secretions caused by anticholinergic properties and may inhibit expectoration and sinus drainage.

Pregnancy:
- *Category B* — Chlorpheniramine, diphenhydramine, brompheniramine, clemastine, loratadine.
- *Category C* — Dexbrompheniramine.

Safe use during pregnancy has not been established. Use only when clearly needed and when the potential benefits outweigh the potential hazards to the fetus. Do not use during the third trimester; newborn and premature infants may have severe reactions (eg, convulsions) to some antihistamines.

Lactation: Because of the general higher risk of adverse effects for infants, and for newborns and prematures in particular, antihistamine therapy is contraindicated in nursing mothers.

Children: Safety and efficacy have not been established for all drugs in all age groups; refer to specific product information. Antihistamines may diminish mental alertness; conversely, they may occasionally produce excitation, particularly in young children.

Elderly: Antihistamines are more likely to cause dizziness, excessive sedation, syncope, confusional states, and hypotension in patients 60 years of age and older and also may cause paradoxical stimulation. Dosage reduction may be required.

Photosensitivity: Photosensitization may occur; caution patients to take protective measures (eg, sunscreens, protective clothing) against exposure to ultraviolet light or sunlight until tolerance is determined.

Sulfite sensitivity: Some products may contain sulfites, which may cause allergic-type reactions (eg, hives, itching, wheezing, anaphylaxis) in certain susceptible people.

► **Drug Interactions**

MAOIs: MAOIs may prolong and intensify the anticholinergic effects of some antihistamines.

Alcohol, CNS depressants: Sedating antihistamines have additive CNS depressant effects with alcohol and other CNS depressants (eg, tranquilizers, hypnotics, muscle relaxants, antidepressants).

Loratadine:

  Azole antifungal agents (eg, ketoconazole) – Ketoconazole administration may increase loratadine plasma concentrations.

  Cimetidine – Concomitant use resulted in substantially increased plasma levels of loratadine.

  Erythromycin – Plasma levels (including metabolites) may be increased. No clinically relevant changes were noted in the loratadine safety profile.

  Food – Food may increase absorption of loratadine.

Diphenhydramine: Do not use oral OTC diphenhydramine products concomitantly with other diphenhydramine products, including topical ones.

Drug-lab interactions: Discontinue antihistamines approximately 4 to 7 days prior to skin-testing; these drugs may prevent or diminish otherwise positive reactions to dermal reactivity indicators.

► **Adverse Reactions**

First-generation antihistamines are associated, to varying degrees, with CNS-depressant side effects manifested by drowsiness, dizziness, fatigue, weakness, decreased attention, slowed reaction time, impaired coordination, and impaired cognitive function. The ethanolamine antihistamines (eg, diphenhydramine, clemastine) are the most sedating OTC antihistamines and have the highest degree of anticholinergic activity. The alkylamine antihistamines (eg, brompheniramine maleate, chlorpheniramine maleate, triprolidine) are the least sedating OTC antihistamines and have relatively low anticholinergic activity (see table).

Second-generation antihistamines (of which loratadine is the only agent currently available OTC) are relatively free from anticholinergic activity, produce substantially less sedative activity, and are selective for the peripheral H_1 receptors. Penetration into the CNS is less, therefore producing a lower degree of side effects such as drowsiness, dizziness, fatigue, headache, and dry mouth.

Antihistamines: Effects			
Antihistamine	**Antihistaminic activity**	**Sedative activity**	**Anticholinergic activity**
Ethanolamines (OTC)			
Clemastine	low to moderate	moderate	high
Diphenhydramine	low to moderate	high	high
Alkylamines (OTC)			
Brompheniramine[1]	high	low	moderate
Chlorpheniramine	high	low	moderate
Dexbrompheniramine[1]	high	low	moderate
Triprolidine[1]	moderate to high	low	low
Piperidines (OTC)			
Phenindamine[1]	moderate	low to none	moderate
Loratadine	moderate to high	low to none	low

[1] Available OTC only in combination products.

A paradoxical stimulatory effect may occur in children and the elderly, with symptoms of appetite stimulation, seizures, insomnia, nervousness, irritability, tremor, anxiety, hallucinations, and psychosis. Anticholinergic effects occur to varying degrees with first-generation antihistamines and may be associated with dilated pupils, blurred vision, dry eyes, dry mouth, urinary retention, and constipation.

▶ Overdosage

Symptoms: Effects may vary from mild CNS depression (eg, sedation, apnea, diminished mental alertness) and cardiovascular collapse to stimulation (eg, insomnia, hallucinations, tremors, convulsions), especially in children and the elderly. Profound hypotension, respiratory depression, unconsciousness, coma, and death may occur, particularly in infants and children. Convulsions rarely occur and indicate a poor prognosis. The convulsant dose lies near the lethal dose.

Toxic effects are seen within 30 minutes to 2 hours after ingestion and result in drowsiness, dizziness, ataxia, tinnitus, blurred vision, and hypotension. Anticholinergic effects may result in fixed, dilated pupils, flushing, dry mouth, hyperthermia (especially in children), and fever. GI symptoms also may occur. Hyperpyrexia to 41.8°C (107°F) and acute oral and facial dystonic reactions have been reported.

Children often manifest CNS stimulation and may have hallucinations, toxic psychosis, delirium tremens, excitement, ataxia, incoordination, muscle twitching, athetosis, hyperthermia, cyanosis, convulsions, and hyperreflexia, followed by postictal depression and cardiorespiratory arrest. Seizures resistant to therapy may be preceded and followed by mild depression. CNS stimulation in adults usually manifests as seizures. Marked cerebral irritation, resulting jerking of muscles, and possible convulsions may be followed by deep stupor. Occasionally, respiratory depression, cardiovascular collapse, and death follow a latent period.

Treatment: Take adequate precautions to protect against aspiration, especially in infants and children. Administer activated charcoal as a slurry with water and a cathartic to minimize absorption. Correct acidosis and electrolyte imbalances. Do not induce emesis in unconscious patients. Gastric lavage is indicated within 3 hours after ingestion and even later if large amounts were taken. Isotonic or half isotonic saline is the lavage of choice, particularly for children. For adults, tap water can be used. Continue therapy directed at reversing the effects of timed-release medication and at supporting the patient. Hemoperfusion may be used in severe cases. Loratadine does not appear to be dialyzable. **Refer to General Management of Acute Overdosage.**

Hypotension is an early sign of impending cardiovascular collapse; treat vigorously using general supportive measures or specific vasopressor treatment (eg, norepinephrine, phenylephrine, dopamine). Avoid epinephrine; it may worsen hypotension. Propranolol may be used for refractory ventricular arrhythmias.

Administer 0.1 mg/kg IV diazepam slowly for convulsions; repeat as needed. IV physostigmine may reverse central anticholinergic effects. Use with caution. Avoid analeptics; they may cause convulsions.

Ice packs and cooling sponge baths with water, not alcohol, can help reduce a child's fever.

LORATADINE

▶ **Administration and Dosage**

Tablets:

Adults and children (6 years of age and older) – 10 mg once daily.

Children (2 to 6 years of age) – Use only as directed by a physician.

Extended-release tablets:

Claritin-D 12 Hour and Alavert D-12:

Adults and children (12 years of age and older) – 10 mg every 12 hours. Do not exceed 20 mg daily.

Children (younger than 12 years of age) – Use only as directed by a physician.

Claritin-D 24 Hour:

Adults and children (12 years of age and older) – 10 mg every 24 hours.

Children (younger than 12 years of age) – Use only as directed by a physician.

Orally disintegrating tablets: Place tablets on the tongue. Tablet disintegration occurs rapidly. Administer with or without water. Use within 6 months of opening laminated foil pouch and immediately upon opening individual tablet blister.

Adults and children (6 years of age and older) – 10 mg once daily.

Children (younger than 6 years of age) – Use only as directed by a physician.

Syrup:

Adults and children (older than 6 years of age) – 10 mg (10 mL) syrup once daily.

Children (2 to 6 years of age) – 5 mg (5 mL) syrup once daily.

Hepatic/renal function impairment:

Adults and children (6 years of age and older) – 10 mg every other day as starting dose.

Children (2 to 5 years of age) – 5 mg every other day as starting dose.

LORATADINE PRODUCTS	
Trade name	**Doseform**
Alavert, Claritin 24 Hour, Tavist ND	**Tablets**: 10 mg. Lactose.
Alavert D-12 Hour, Claritin-D 12 Hour	**Tablets, extended-release**: 5 mg loratadine, 120 mg pseudoephedrine sulfate. Lactose.
Claritin-D 24 Hour	**Tablets, extended-release**: 10 mg loratadine, 240 mg pseudoephedrine sulfate. Sugar.
Claritin Reditabs 24 Hour	**Tablets, orally disintegrating**: 10 mg. Mannitol. Mint flavor.
Alavert	**Tablets, orally disintegrating**: 10 mg. Aspartame, corn syrup, mannitol, 8.4 mg phenylalanine.
Children's Claritin	**Syrup**: 5 mg/5 mL. EDTA, glycerin, sugar. Fruit flavor.

Products listed are representative of currently available and widely distributed brands. Similar products, including regional and private label brands, may also exist.

BROMPHENIRAMINE MALEATE

▶ **Indications**

Brompheniramine is available OTC only as a combination product. **See Respiratory Combination Products in the Common Cold monograph.**

CHLORPHENIRAMINE MALEATE

▶ **Administration and Dosage**

Immediate-release tablets:

Adults and children (12 years of age and older) – 4 mg every 4 to 6 hours as needed. Do not exceed 24 mg in 24 hours.

Children (6 to 12 years of age) – 2 mg every 4 to 6 hours as needed. Do not exceed 12 mg in 24 hours.

Children (younger than 6 years of age) – Use only as directed by a physician.

Sustained-release release:

Adults and children (12 years of age and older) – 8 to 12 mg at bedtime or every 8 to 12 hours as needed during the day. Do not exceed 24 mg in 24 hours.

Children (younger than 12 years of age) – Use only as directed by a physician.

Liquid:

Adults and children (12 years of age and older) – 4 mg (10 mL) every 4 to 6 hours. Do not exceed 24 mg (60 mL) in 24 hours.

Children (6 to 12 years of age) – 2 mg (5 mL) every 4 to 6 hours. Do not exceed 12 mg (30 mL) in 24 hours.

CHLORPHENIRAMINE MALEATE PRODUCTS	
Trade name	**Doseform**
Chlorpheniramine Maleate	**Tablets**: 4 mg
Teldrin HBP	**Tablets**: 4 mg
Chlor-Trimeton Allergy 4 Hour	**Tablets, immediate-release**: 4 mg. Lactose, sugar, talc.
Chlor-Trimeton Allergy-D 4 Hour	**Tablets, immediate-release**: 4 mg chlorphenir-amine maleate, 60 mg pseudoephedrine sulfate. Lactose.
Chlor-Trimeton Allergy 12 Hour	**Tablets, sustained-release**: 12 mg. Lactose, sugar, talc.
Diabetic Tussin (sf)	**Liquid**: 2 mg/5 mL. Saccharin, methylparaben. Alcohol and dye free.
Tricodene (sf)	**Liquid**: 2 mg chlorpheniramine maleate, 10 mg dextromethorphan hydrobromide/5 mL. Saccharin, glycerin, sorbitol. Alcohol free.

Products listed are representative of currently available and widely distributed brands. Similar products, including regional and private label brands, may also exist.

CLEMASTINE FUMARATE

▶ **Administration and Dosage**

Adults and children (12 years of age and older): 1.34 mg (1 mg clemastine) twice daily as needed. Dosage may be increased as needed. Do not exceed 2.68 mg (2 mg clemastine) daily.

Children (younger than 12 years of age): Use only as directed by a physician.

CLEMASTINE FUMARATE PRODUCTS	
Trade name	Doseform
Tavist Allergy	**Tablets**: 1.34 mg (1 mg clemastine). Lactose, talc.

Products listed are representative of currently available and widely distributed brands. Similar products, including regional and private label brands, may also exist.

DEXBROMPHENIRAMINE MALEATE

▶ **Indications**

Dexbrompheniramine maleate is available OTC only as a combination product. **See Respiratory Combination Products in the Common Cold monograph.**

DIPHENHYDRAMINE HCL

▶ **Administration and Dosage**

Tablets, caplets, capsules, and softgels:

Adults and children (12 years of age and older) – 25 to 50 mg every 4 to 6 hours as needed. Do not exceed 300 mg in 24 hours.

Children (6 to 12 years of age) – 12.5 to 25 mg every 4 to 6 hours as needed. Do not exceed 150 mg in 24 hours.

Children (younger than 6 years of age) – Use only as directed by a physician.

Liquid and elixir:

Adults and children (12 years of age and older) – 25 to 50 mg (10 to 20 mL) every 4 to 6 hours as needed. Do not exceed 300 mg (120 mL) in 24 hours.

Children (6 to 12 years of age) – 12.5 to 25 mg (5 to 10 mL) every 4 to 6 hours as need. Do not exceed 150 mg (60 mL) in 24 hours.

Children (younger than 6 years of age) – Use only as directed by a physician.

DIPHENHYDRAMINE HCL PRODUCTS	
Trade name	Doseform
Benadryl Allergy Ultratabs, Diphenhist Captabs[1]	**Tablets**: 25 mg
Children's Benadryl Allergy	**Tablets, chewable**: 12.5 mg. Aspartame, 4.2 mg phenylalanine. Grape flavor.
Maximum Strength AllerMax	**Caplets**: 50 mg. Lactose.
Benadryl Allergy Kapseals	**Capsules**: 25 mg. Lactose.
Benadryl Dye-Free Allergy Liqui-Gels	**Softgels**: 25 mg. Sorbitol, glycerin.
AllerMax Allergy & Cough Formula[2], Children's Benadryl Allergy[3], Children's Benadryl Dye-Free Allergy[4], Genahist[4], Scot-Tussin[5], Siladryl Allergy[6]	**Liquid**: 12.5 mg/5 mL
Banophen	**Elixir**: 12.5 mg/5 mL

Products listed are representative of currently available and widely distributed brands. Similar products, including regional and private label brands, may also exist.

[1] Contains lactose.
[2] Contains 0.5% alcohol, saccharin, sugar, and sorbitol.
[3] Contains sugar and glycerin. Alcohol free.
[4] Contains saccharin, sorbitol, and glycerin. Alcohol and sugar free.
[5] Contains parabens, glycerin, and menthol. Alcohol and sugar free.
[6] Contains parabens, saccharin, and sorbitol.

PHENINDAMINE TARTRATE

▶ Administration and Dosage

Adults and children (12 years of age and older): 25 mg every 4 to 6 hours as needed. Do not exceed 150 mg in 24 hours.

Children (6 to 12 years of age): 12.5 mg every 4 to 6 hours as needed. Do not exceed 75 mg in 24 hours.

Children (younger than 6 years of age): Use only as directed by a physician.

PHENINDAMINE TARTRATE PRODUCTS	
Trade name	Doseform
Nolahist	**Tablets**: 25 mg. Sucrose.

Products listed are representative of currently available and widely distributed brands. Similar products, including regional and private label brands, may also exist.

TRIPROLIDINE HCL

▶ Indications

Triprolidine is available OTC only as a combination product. **See Respiratory Combination Products in the Common Cold monograph.**

PATIENT INFORMATION

Antihistamines

- Patient instructions accompany each product. Read these instructions carefully before use, preferably before leaving the pharmacy, in case of any questions.
- Start medication a few days prior to allergen exposure if possible, and continue for the duration of exposure.
- Sedation may be minimized by initiating therapy with a low dose and gradually increasing the dose when well tolerated.
- May cause drowsiness or dizziness. Use caution while driving or trying to perform tasks requiring alertness, coordination, or physical dexterity.
- Do not consume alcohol or use other CNS depressants (eg, sedatives, hypnotics, tranquilizers, antianxiety agents) concurrently.
- Inform a physician of antihistamine use prior to diagnostic skin or blood allergy tests.
- Inform a physician of presence of glaucoma, peptic ulcer, urinary retention, or pregnancy before starting antihistamine therapy.
- Antihistamines with moderate to high levels of anticholinergic activity may worsen dementia and cognition in the elderly and those with Alzheimer disease.
- Avoid prolonged exposure to sunlight; some agents may cause photosensitivity.
- Some antihistamines may cause nervousness, insomnia, and dry mouth.
- Take with food if the antihistamine causes GI upset.
- Do not crush or chew sustained-release preparations.
- Do not use any solution that changes color or becomes cloudy.
- Take as directed. Do not use any out-of-date products or exceed recommended dosages.

NASAL DECONGESTANTS

▶ **Actions**

The sympathomimetic vasoconstrictors constrict nasal and ocular blood vessels, reducing mucosal swelling, hyperemia, nasal airflow resistance, and congestion. Decongestants have no effect on sneezing or itching. Locally applied agents (nasal or ocular) have a fast onset of action and minimal systemic side effects, but regular use after 3 to 5 days causes rebound congestion (rhinitis medicamentosa) or ocular hyperemia and should be avoided.

▶ **Indications**

Oral decongestants: Oral decongestants are indicated for the symptomatic treatment of nasal and ocular congestion.

Intranasal decongestants: Intranasal decongestants are indicated for the short-term relief (3 to 5 days) of severe nasal congestion.

Ocular decongestants: Ocular decongestants are indicated for the temporary relief of conjunctival inflammation and hyperemia.

▶ **Contraindications**

Oral decongestants: Severe hypertension and coronary artery disease; MAOI therapy; hypersensitivity or idiosyncrasy to sympathomimetic amines. Naphazoline and sustained-release pseudoephedrine are contraindicated in children younger than 12 years of age.

Ocular decongestants: Ocular naphazoline is contraindicated in patients with glaucoma.

Topical decongestants: Topical decongestants are associated with fewer systemic adverse effects than oral decongestants, but use caution in the conditions listed for oral agents. Adverse reactions are more likely with excessive use in the elderly and in children.

▶ **Warnings**

Special-risk patients: Administer with caution to patients with hyperthyroidism, diabetes mellitus, cardiovascular disease, coronary artery disease, ischemic heart disease, increased intraocular pressure, or prostatic hypertrophy. Sympathomimetics may cause CNS stimulation and convulsions or cardiovascular collapse with hypotension.

Hypertension: Hypertensive patients should use these products only with medical advice, as these patients may experience increased blood pressure. However, some studies report that these products do not significantly increase blood pressure in normotensive and hypertensive patients. Sustained-release preparations may affect the cardiovascular system less.

Pregnancy: Give only when clearly needed. One study reported that oxymetazoline did not affect maternal blood pressure and pulse rates and is therefore safe in the third trimester of a healthy pregnancy.

Lactation: Oral pseudoephedrine is contraindicated in the nursing mother. Consult a physician before using other preparations. It is not known if topical decongestants are excreted in breast milk. Exercise caution when administering to a nursing woman.

Children: Use in children is product-specific. Refer to individual product information.

Elderly: Patients 60 years of age and older are more likely to experience adverse reactions to sympathomimetics. A lower dose may be safe and sufficient. Demonstrate safe use of a short-acting sympathomimetic before use of a sustained-action formulation in elderly patients.

▶ **Drug Interactions**

Most interactions listed apply to sympathomimetics when used as vasopressors; however, consider the interactions when using the nasal decongestants.

Nasal Decongestant Drug Interactions			
Precipitant drug	**Object drug***		**Description**
Beta blockers	Epinephrine	↑	An initial hypertensive episode followed by bradycardia may occur.
Furazolidone	Nasal decongestants	↑	The pressor sensitivity to mixed-acting agents may be increased. Direct-acting agents (eg, epinephrine) are not affected.
Guanethidine	Nasal decongestants Direct Mixed	 ↑ ↓	Guanethidine potentiates the effects of the direct-acting agents (eg, epinephrine) and inhibits the effects of the mixed-acting agents.
Nasal decongestants	Guanethidine	↓	Guanethidine's hypotensive action may be reversed.
Methyldopa	Nasal decongestants	↑	Concurrent administration may result in an increased pressor response.
MAO inhibitors	Nasal decongestants	↑	Concurrent use of MAOIs and mixed-acting agents may result in severe headache, hypertension, and hyperpyrexia, possibly resulting in hypertensive crisis. Direct-acting agents (eg, epinephrine) interact minimally, if at all.
Phenothiazines	Nasal decongestants	↓	Phenothiazines may antagonize and, in some cases, reverse the action of the nasal decongestants.
Rauwolfia alkaloids	Nasal decongestants Direct Mixed	 ↑ ↓	Reserpine potentiates the pressor response of direct-acting agents (eg, epinephrine) which may result in hypotension. The pressor response of mixed-acting agents is decreased.
Tricyclic anti-depressants (TCAs)	Nasal decongestants Direct Mixed	 ↑ ↓	TCAs potentiate the pressor response of direct-acting agents (eg, epinephrine); dysrhythmias have occurred. The pressor response of mixed-acting agents is decreased.
Urinary acidifiers	Nasal decongestants	↓	Acidification of the urine may increase the elimination of the oral nasal decongestant; therapeutic effects may be decreased.
Urinary alkalinizers	Nasal decongestants	↑	Urinary alkalinization may decrease the elimination of these agents, possibly increasing therapeutic or toxic effects.
Nasal decongestants	Theophylline	↔	Enhanced toxicity, particularly cardiotoxicity, has occurred. Decreased theophylline levels may occur.
Epinephrine	Insulin or oral hypoglycemic agents	↓	Diabetics may require an increased dose of the hypoglycemic agent.

* ↑ = Object drug increased.   ↓ = Object drug decreased.   ↔ = Undetermined effect.

► **Adverse Reactions**

Oral decongestants may cause restlessness, nervousness, irritability, insomnia, dizziness, tremor, headache, tachycardia, and elevated blood pressure. Tachycardia and elevated blood pressure are dose-proportional.

Locally applied nasal decongestants (drops, sprays) may cause burning, stinging, dryness, or rebound nasal congestion. Ocular hyperemia may occur after 3 to 5 days of continued use of an ophthalmic decongestant.

PSEUDOEPHEDRINE

► **Administration and Dosage**

Adults and children (at least 12 years of age): 60 mg every 4 to 6 hours (120 mg sustained release every 12 hours) as needed. Do not exceed 240 mg in 24 hours.

Children (6 to 12 years of age): 30 mg every 4 to 6 hours as needed. Do not exceed 120 mg in 24 hours.

Children (2 to 5 years of age): 15 mg every 4 to 6 hours as needed. Do not exceed 60 mg in 24 hours.

Children (1 to 2 years of age): 7 drops (0.2 mL)/kg body weight every 4 to 6 hours as needed, up to 4 doses/day.

Children (3 to 12 months of age): 3 drops/kg body weight every 4 to 6 hours as needed, up to 4 doses/day.

Abuse: Pseudoephedrine has been used in the production of illicit drugs.

PSEUDOEPHEDRINE PRODUCTS	
Trade name	Doseform
Good Sense	**Tablets:** 30 mg
Cenafed	**Tablets:** 60 mg
Children's Sudafed Nasal Decongestant Chewables[1]*, Triaminic Softchews Allergy Congestion*[2]	**Tablets, chewable:** 15 mg
Contac 12 Hour Cold Relief, Drixoral Non-Drowsy 12-Hour, Sudafed 12 Hour	**Tablets, extended-release:** 120 mg
Efidac 24 Pseudoephedrine, Sudafed 24 Hour	**Tablets, extended-release:** 240 mg (60 mg immediate release/180 mg controlled release)
Dimetapp Non-Drowsy Liqui-Gels[3]*, Nature's Way Cold Care Nighttime Rest, Nature's Way Hayfever Allergy Sinus*	**Capsules:** 30 mg
Sinustop Pro	**Capsules:** 60 mg
Children's Sudafed Nasal Decongestant[4]*, Triaminic Allergy Congestion*[5]	**Liquid:** 15 mg/5 mL
Cenafed	**Syrup:** 30 mg/5 mL
Infants' PediaCare Decongestant[5]*, Children's Dimetapp Decongestant*[5]	**Drops:** 7.5 mg/0.8 mL

Products listed are representative of currently available and widely distributed brands. Similar products, including regional and private label brands, may also exist.

[1] Contains aspartame.
[2] Contains aspartame, sorbitol, sucrose.
[3] Contains sorbitol.
[4] Contains saccharin, sorbitol.
[5] Contains sorbitol, sucrose.

PHENYLEPHRINE HCL

▶ **Administration and Dosage**

Tablets:

Adults and children (12 years of age and older) – 1 or 2 tablets every 4 hours.

Children 6 to 12 years of age – 1 tablet every 4 hours.

Sprays and drops:

Adults (12 years of age and older) – 2 to 3 sprays or drops in each nostril. Repeat every 3 to 4 hours (0.25% and 0.5%). The 1% solution should be repeated no more often than every 4 hours. The 0.25% solution is adequate in most cases. However, in resistant cases or if more powerful decongestion is desired, use the 0.5% or 1% solution.

Children (6 to 12 years of age) – 0.25%: 2 to 3 sprays or drops into each nostril every 3 to 4 hours.

Infants (older than 6 months of age) – 0.16%: 1 or 2 drops in each nostril every 3 hours.

PHENYLEPHRINE HCL PRODUCTS	
Trade name	**Doseform**
AH-chew D	**Tablets, chewable:** 10 mg
Tur-Bi-Kal Nasal Drops[1]	**Solution:** 0.17%
Afrin Children's Nasal Decongestant Spray[2], Neo-Synephrine Mild Strength Nasal Spray[3], Rhinall Nose Drops and Spray[4]	**Solution:** 0.25%
Neo-Synephrine Regular Strength Nasal Drops and Spray[3], Vicks Sinex Nasal Spray and Ultra Fine Mist[5]	**Solution:** 0.5%
4-Way Fast Acting Nasal Spray[1], Neo-Synephrine Extra Strength Nasal Drops and Spray[3]	**Solution:** 1%

Products listed are representative of currently available and widely distributed brands. Similar products, including regional and private label brands, may also exist.

[1] Contains benzalkonium chloride.
[2] Contains benzalkonium chloride, disodium EDTA.
[3] Contains benzalkonium chloride, thimerosal.
[4] Contains benzalkonium chloride, sodium bisulfite.
[5] Contains benzalkonium chloride, disodium EDTA, menthol.

PROPYLHEXEDRINE

▶ **Administration and Dosage**

Adults and children (at least 6 years of age): 1 to 2 inhalations in each nostril (while blocking the other nostril) not more than every 2 hours as needed. Do not exceed recommended dosage. Do not use for more than 3 days.

Abuse: Propylhexedrine has been extracted from inhalers and injected IV as an amphetamine substitute. It has also be made into an ingestable form by soaking the fibrous interior in hot water. Chronic abuse has caused cardiomyopathy (severe left and right ventricular failure), pulmonary hypertension, foreign body granuloma (emboli), dyspnea, and sudden death.

PROPYLHEXEDRINE PRODUCTS	
Trade name	Doseform
Benzedrex	**Inhaler:** 250 mg. Lavender oil, menthol.

Products listed are representative of currently available and widely distributed brands. Similar products, including regional and private label brands, may also exist.

DESOXYEPHEDRINE

▶ **Administration and Dosage**

Adults and children (6 years of age and older): 1 to 2 inhalations in each nostril (while blocking the other nostril) not more than every 2 hours as needed. Do not exceed recommended dosage. Do not use for more than 7 days.

DESOXYEPHEDRINE PRODUCTS	
Trade name	Doseform
Vicks Vapor Inhaler	**Inhaler:** 50 mg l-desoxyephedrine. Bornyl acetate, camphor, lavender oil, menthol.

Products listed are representative of currently available and widely distributed brands. Similar products, including regional and private label brands, may also exist.

NAPHAZOLINE HCL

▶ **Administration and Dosage**

Adults and children (at least 12 years of age): 1 or 2 drops or sprays in each nostril as needed, no more than every 6 hours (spray). Do not use in children younger than 12 years of age, unless directed by a physician.

NAPHAZOLINE HCL PRODUCTS	
Trade name	Doseform
Privine Nasal Spray	**Solution:** 0.05%. Benzalkonium chloride, EDTA, sodium chloride.

Products listed are representative of currently available and widely distributed brands. Similar products, including regional and private label brands, may also exist.

OXYMETAZOLINE HCL

▶ **Administration and Dosage**

Adults and children (at least 6 years of age): 2 or 3 sprays or 2 or 3 drops of 0.05% solution in each nostril twice daily, morning and evening, as needed.

OXYMETAZOLINE HCL PRODUCTS	
Trade name	Doseform
4-Way 12 Hour Fast Relief Nasal Spray[1], Afrin Extra Moisturizing Nasal Spray[2], Afrin No Drip Sinus Nasal Spray[3], Afrin Original Nasal Spray[2], Afrin Severe Congestion Nasal Spray[4], Dristan 12-hr Nasal Spray[5], Duramist Plus Nasal Spray[2], Long-Acting Nasal Relief[2], Neo-Synephrine 12-Hour Nasal Spray[5], Neo-Synephrine 12-Hour Extra Moisturizing Nasal Spray[5], Nōstrilla 12 Hour Nasal Decongestant Nasal Spray[1], Vicks Sinex 12 Hour Nasal Spray[2], Vicks Sinex 12 Hour Ultra Fine Mist[2]	**Solution:** 0.05%. Benzalkonium chloride.

Products listed are representative of currently available and widely distributed brands. Similar products, including regional and private label brands, may also exist.

[1] Contains sorbitol.
[2] Contains EDTA.
[4] Contains benzyl alcohol, EDTA, menthol.
[5] Contains thimerosal.

XYLOMETAZOLINE HCL

▶ **Administration and Dosage**

Adults and children (at least 12 years of age): 2 to 3 drops or 2 to 3 sprays (0.1%) in each nostril every 8 to 10 hours as needed.

Children (2 to 12 years of age): 2 to 3 drops (0.05%) in each nostril every 8 to 10 hours as needed.

XYLOMETAZOLINE HCL PRODUCTS	
Trade name	Doseform
Otrivin Pediatric Nasal Drops	**Solution**: 0.05%. Benzalkonium chloride, EDTA.
Natru-vent Nasal Spray[1], Otrivin Nasal Spray[2]	**Solution**: 0.1%

Products listed are representative of currently available and widely distributed brands. Similar products, including regional and private label brands, may also exist.

[1] Contains sorbitol.
[2] Contains benzalkonium acetate, EDTA.

PATIENT INFORMATION

Nasal Decongestants

- Patient instructions accompany each product. Read these instructions carefully before use, preferably before leaving the pharmacy, in case of any questions.
- Take as directed. Do not use any out-of-date products or exceed recommended dosage.
- Nasal obstruction complicated by nasal polyps or a deviated septum may reduce the effectiveness of these agents.
- Expect prompt relief (30 seconds to 10 minutes) from topical decongestants.
- The distribution of topical nasal decongestants over the largest surface area is better with sprays than drops.
- Contact a physician if you experience persistent abdominal pain or vomiting.
- Patients with hypertension, coronary artery disease, angina, irregular heartbeat, or other cardiovascular diseases, hyperthyroidism, diabetes mellitus, or prostatic hypertrophy should use these products only with medical advice.
- Do not crush or chew sustained-release preparations.
- Oral decongestants may cause nervousness, dizziness, or sleeplessness. If symptoms do not improve within 7 days of using an oral preparation or are accompanied by a high fever, consult a physician before continuing use.
- Do not use any solution that changes color or becomes cloudy.
- Topical agents may cause stinging, burning, sneezing, increased nasal discharge, or drying of the nasal mucosa. Notify a physician if insomnia, dizziness, weakness, tremor, or irregular heartbeat occurs while using topical agents. Do *not* use for more than 3 to 5 days.
- Do not share intranasal containers with other patients.

SALINE NASAL PRODUCTS

▶ **Actions**

Saline solutions provide moisture to help loosen and liquefy mucus secretions to allow drainage from the nose and sinuses.

▶ **Indications**

To provide moisture to inflamed nasal passages and facilitate drainage of thickened nasal secretions.

▶ **Contraindications**

Hypersensitivity to any product component.

▶ **Administration and Dosage**

Refer to individual product labeling for dosing information and administration technique.

SALINE NASAL PRODUCTS	
Trade name	**Doseform**
SalineX Nasal Mist[1]	**Solution:** 0.4% sodium chloride
Pretz Nasal Spray[2]	**Solution:** 0.6% sodium chloride
Afrin Non-Medicated Nasal Spray[1]	**Solution:** 0.64% sodium chloride
Ayr Nasal Mist[3], Baby Ayr Nasal Spray and Drops[1], Breathe Free Nasal Spray, Breathe Right Nasal Spray, Little Noses Nasal Spray and Drops[1], NaSal Nasal Spray and Drops[3], Nasal Moist Nasal Spray and Mist, Ocean Nasal Mist and Drops[4]	**Solution:** 0.65% sodium chloride
Pretz Irrigation Nasal Drops[2], Pretz Moisturizing Nasal Spray[2]	**Solution:** 0.75% sodium chloride
Blairex Broncho Saline Nasal Mist, Simply Saline Nasal Mist	**Solution:** 0.9%

Products listed are representative of currently available and widely distributed brands. Similar products, including regional and private label brands, may also exist.
[1] Contains benzalkonium chloride, EDTA.
[2] Contains *Mucoprotective Factor* yerba santa, phenylmercuric acetate.
[3] Contains benzalkonium chloride, thimerosal.
[4] Contains benzalkonium chloride, benzyl alcohol.

PATIENT INFORMATION
Saline Nasal Products

- Patient instructions accompany each product. Read these instructions carefully before use, preferably before leaving the pharmacy, in case of any questions.
- Do not share intranasal containers with other patients.
- Take as directed. Do not use any out-of-date products or exceed recommended dosages.

MAST CELL STABILIZERS

▶ **Actions**

Saline solutions provide moisture to help loosen and liquefy mucus secretions to allow drainage from the nose and sinuses.

▶ **Indications**

To prevent and treat the symptoms of seasonal and perennial allergic rhinitis, such as runny or itchy nose, sneezing, and allergic stuffy nose.

▶ **Contraindications**

Hypersensitivity to any product component.

▶ **Administration and Dosage**

Refer to individual product labeling for dosing information and administration technique.

MAST CELL STABILIZERS	
Trade name	Doseform
BenaMist Allergy Prevention Nasal Spray, Children's NasalCrom Nasal Spray, Nasal-Crom Nasal Spray	**Solution:** 4% cromolyn sodium. Benzalkonium chloride, EDTA.

Products listed are representative of currently available and widely distributed brands. Similar products, including regional and private label brands, may also exist.

PATIENT INFORMATION
Mast Cell Stabilizers

- Patient instructions accompany each product. Read these instructions carefully before use, preferably before leaving the pharmacy, in case of any questions.
- Do not share intranasal containers with other patients.
- Take as directed. Do not use any out-of-date products or exceed recommended dosages.

COUGH

DEFINITION

Cough, an important physiologic and protective respiratory tract defense mechanism, is a rapid, forceful expiration of air manifested by a sudden, noisy outburst from the upper airway. This response is usually caused by the presence of irritating substances or mechanical stimulation of the pharynx or upper airway. Two types of cough exist: nonproductive (dry) cough, which does not produce sputum and serves to clear the airway of particulate matter or herald underlying disease; and productive cough, which assists in the removal of mucus or other respiratory secretions through mobilization and expectoration.

ETIOLOGY

Although patients with common colds may develop a cough, other causes also are likely. The most common causes of dry cough include viral upper respiratory tract infections ("colds"), allergic rhinitis, sinusitis, and postnasal drip. These conditions tend to produce excessive nasal mucus and its retrograde migration into the upper airway. Inhalation of a foreign body, particulate matter, irritant gases, or smoke also can stimulate cough. A productive cough usually is induced by the presence of mucus congestion in the lower airway (chest congestion). Cough is a relatively common side effect of angiotensin-I-converting enzyme (ACE) inhibitors and is thought to be caused by the inhibition of bradykinin degradation by this drug class. Patients with asthma, chronic bronchitis, acute rhinitis, pneumonia, pulmonary embolism, or gastroesophageal reflux disease (GERD) also may present with complaints of cough. Other infectious sources of cough include pharyngitis, laryngitis, bronchiolitis, pertussis, and influenza. Noninfectious causes include allergic rhinitis, cystic fibrosis, immune deficiencies, bronchiectasis (chronic dilation of the bronchi secondary to disease or obstruction), some tumors, congestive heart failure, hypersensitivity pneumonitis, atelectasis (reduced breathing capacity), some drugs, smoking, and dry air. Cough also may be psychogenic.

INCIDENCE

Cough is a common presenting symptom in patients seeking medical attention. Chronic cough is estimated to be a persistent complaint in nearly 25% of nonsmoking adults in the United States.

PATHOPHYSIOLOGY

The complete pathophysiology of cough remains unclear. Cough appears to arise from either mechanical or chemical stimulation of the cough receptors in the upper airway, including the pharynx and larynx (see Figure 1). Activation of pulmonary stretch receptors and C fibers initiate a neural reflex response that involves transmission of the stimulatory signal through afferent neurons to the central cough center in the brain. The result is a sudden increase in intrathoracic and tracheal pressure followed by opening of the glottis, which expels a burst of air.

SIGNS/SYMPTOMS

Cough may be dry or productive. Isolated cough is uncommon and, depending upon the cause, accompanying symptoms may vary. Postnasal drip and nasal congestion generally accompany cough in upper respiratory tract infections, allergic rhinitis, or sinusitis. A hoarse cough with difficult breathing occurs in children with croup. A productive cough with discolored mucus and shortness of breath is seen with chronic bronchitis and pneumonia; whitish mucus plugs may be seen in productive coughs in patients with asthma. Patients with persistent cough (longer than 2 weeks in duration) or cough accompanied by bloody sputum (hemoptysis), wheezing, fainting, severe fatigue, fever, night sweats, or vomiting should be referred immediately to a physician for evaluation.

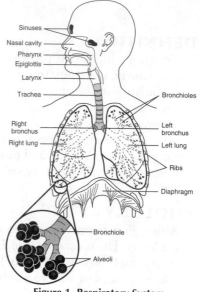

Figure 1. Respiratory System

DIAGNOSTIC PARAMETERS/PHYSICAL ASSESSMENT

Clinical Observation: While many patients have cough in association with mild airway irritation or upper respiratory tract infection, some patients may have bacterial infections or more serious pulmonary diseases. If physician referral is warranted, a complete physical assessment likely will be performed. Examination, gram stain, and culture of purulent sputum will assist in the identification of infectious causes. Chest radiography is necessary in patients in whom pneumonia, carcinoma, or other intrapulmonary processes are suspected. Perform pulmonary function tests in patients with cough and persistent obstruction or wheezing; bronchoscopy is reserved for the diagnosis of alveolar or parenchymal disease.

Interview: The diagnostic approach to cough is directed at isolating the cause. An accurate patient history is crucial in the initial assessment of the patient. The following information from the patient should be helpful:

- The time course of the cough (chronic vs acute, seasonal vs continuous)
- Duration of the cough
- Associated symptoms such as fever, nasal congestion, sore throat, or ear pain
- Production of sputum
- The color, viscosity, odor, and quantity of sputum, if produced
- Exposure to environmental or occupational irritants
- Smoking history
- Allergies

- Concurrent medications (especially ACE inhibitors or drugs that may cause pulmonary reactions where cough is a symptom)
- Pertinent medical problems, including cardiopulmonary and infectious disease history

TREATMENT

Approaches to therapy: Management of cough nearly always relies on treatment of its specific causes. This may involve treatment of an infection, pulmonary disease, cardiac disease, GERD, or nasal congestion. Cough is a natural reflex to help expectorate mucus. Symptomatic treatment is reserved for short-term use and when cough disturbs sleep or is a distraction (eg, in a meeting or a public place).

Nondrug therapy: Reduction of exposure to inhaled irritants is an effective method of cough reduction in many patients. Smoking cessation and avoidance of known allergens are common examples of this approach. Drinking copious amounts of water (more than 8 glasses per day) is beneficial in keeping the patient hydrated and may aid expectoration by thinning respiratory tract mucus. Moisturizing the throat with saliva-producing hard candy also may help reduce the frequency and intensity of cough.

Pharmacotherapy: Symptomatic relief of cough may be achieved by the use of nonprescription antitussives. Expectorants, in proper doses, loosen mucus to facilitate a productive cough and may decrease the urge to cough. Diphenhydramine is said to have antitussive activity. There are many multi-ingredient products marketed as agents to treat the multi-symptomatic cold; however, use of these products is controversial. A "shotgun" approach to treating a patient without all of the symptoms is generally not recommended and may be considered mismanagement of the condition. When possible, consider single-ingredient agents that target a specific symptom. It is important to counsel patients that dry, hacking coughs are best treated with an antitussive, whereas productive or "loose" coughs are best treated with the expectorant guaifenesin. This is especially important when considering multi-ingredient products.

ANTITUSSIVES

DEXTROMETHORPHAN HBR

▶ **Actions**

Dextromethorphan is a preferred antitussive, equally potent to codeine as a cough suppressant on a mg-for-mg basis. It increases the cough threshold in the brainstem and is a narcotic analogue devoid of analgesic or habit-forming characteristics.

▶ **Indications**

For control of nonproductive cough and temporary relief of cough caused by minor throat and bronchial irritation as may occur with the common cold or inhaled irritants.

▶ **Contraindications**

Hypersensitivity to the drug or any of its components.

▶ **Warnings**

Do not use for persistent or chronic cough (eg, cough due to smoking, asthma, emphysema) or when cough is accompanied by excessive secretions. If cough persists for more than 1 week, tends to recur, or is accompanied by fever, rash, or persistent headache, consult a physician.

Drug abuse and dependence: Anecdotal reports of abuse of dextromethorphan-containing cough/cold products have increased, especially among teenagers. The FDA Drug Abuse Advisory Committee states that additional data are needed before determining the abuse and dependency potential of dextromethorphan.

▶ **Drug Interactions**

MAO inhibitors: Patients may develop hypotension, hyperpyrexia, nausea, myoclonic leg jerks, and coma following coadministration.

Quinidine: Coadministration may cause increased dextromethorphan plasma concentrations, increasing toxic effects (eg, nervousness, fatigue, unsteady gait, dizziness, confusion).

Sibutramine: A potentially fatal "serotonin syndrome", including CNS irritability, motor weakness, shivering, myoclonus, and altered consciousness, may occur. Coadministration is not recommended.

Terbinafine: Coadministration may cause increased dextromethorphan plasma concentrations, which increases toxic effects.

Drug-food interactions: Coadministration with grapefruit juice may cause increased dextromethorphan plasma concentrations, which increases toxic effects.

▶ **Overdosage**

Symptoms:

   Adults – Altered sensory perception; ataxia; slurred speech; dysphoria.

   Children – Ataxia; respiratory depression; convulsions.

▶ **Administration and Dosage**

Lozenges:

   Adults and children (older than 12 years of age) – 10 mg every 4 hours as needed, not to exceed 60 mg in 24 hours.

   Children (6 to 12 years of age) – 5 mg every 4 hours as needed, not to exceed 30 mg in 24 hours.

   Children (younger than 6 years of age) – Do not give lozenges to children younger than 6 years of age.

Liquid:

   Adults and children (older than 12 years of age) – 30 mg every 6 to 8 hours as needed, not to exceed 120 mg in 24 hours.

   Children (6 to 12 years of age) – 15 mg every 6 to 8 hours as needed, not to exceed 60 mg in 24 hours.

   Children (2 to 6 years of age) – 7.5 mg every 6 to 8 hours as needed, not to exceed 30 mg in 24 hours.

   Children (younger than 2 years of age) – Use only as directed by a physician.

Syrup:

> *Adults and children (older than 12 years of age)* – 30 mg every 6 to 8 hours as needed, not to exceed 120 mg in 24 hours.

> *Children (6 to 12 years of age)* – 15 mg every 6 to 8 hours as needed, not to exceed 60 mg in 24 hours.

> *Children (younger than 6 years of age)* – Use only as directed by a physician.

Extended-release suspension:

> *Adults and children (older than 12 years of age)* – 60 mg every 12 hours as needed, not to exceed 120 mg in 24 hours.

> *Children (6 to 12 years of age)* – 30 mg every 12 hours as needed, not to exceed 60 mg in 24 hours.

> *Children (2 to 6 years of age)* – 15 mg every 12 hours as needed, not to exceed 30 mg in 24 hours.

> *Children (younger than 2 years of age)* – Use only as directed by a physician.

DEXTROMETHORPHAN HBR PRODUCTS	
Trade name	**Doseform**
DexAlone (sf)	**Gelcaps**: 30 mg. Alcohol free.
Hold DM	**Lozenges**: 5 mg. Corn syrup, sucrose, vegetable oil. Original, honey lemon, and cherry flavor.
Scot-Tussin DM Cough Chasers (sf)	**Lozenges**: 5 mg. Dye free. Peppermint oil, sorbitol.
Trocal	**Lozenges**: 7.5 mg. Cherry flavor.
Simply Cough	**Liquid**: 5 mg/mL. Alcohol free. Corn syrup, glycerin, sucralose. Cherry berry flavor.
Benylin Pediatric (sf)	**Liquid**: 7.5 mg/5 mL. Alcohol free. Glycerin, saccharin, sorbitol. Grape flavor.
ElixSure Cough	**Liquid**: 7.5 mg/5 mL. Glycerin, propylparaben, sorbitol. Cherry and bubble gum flavor.
Robitussin Pediatric Cough	**Liquid**: 7.5 mg/5 mL. Corn syrup, glycerin, saccharin.
Vicks 44 Cough Relief	**Liquid**: 10 mg/5 mL. Alcohol, corn syrup, saccharin.
Benylin Adult Formula (sf)	**Liquid**: 15 mg/5 mL. Alcohol free. Glycerin, menthol, saccharin, sorbitol.
Robitussin Honey Cough	**Syrup**: 10 mg/5 mL. Alcohol free. Glycerin, methylparaben.
Robitussin Maximum Strength Cough	**Syrup**: 15 mg/5 mL. Alcohol, corn syrup, glycerin, menthol, saccharin.
Delsym 12-Hour Cough Relief	**Suspension, extended release**: Dextromethorphan polistirex (equivalent to 30 mg dextromethorphan HBr/5 mL). Alcohol free. Corn syrup, parabens, sucrose, vegetable oil. Orange flavor.

Products listed are representative of currently available and widely distributed brands. Similar products, including regional and private label brands, may also exist.

sf = Sugar free.

PATIENT INFORMATION

Dextromethorphan HBr

- Patient instructions accompany each product. Read these instructions carefully before use, preferably before leaving the pharmacy, in case of any questions.
- Take as directed. Do not use any out-of-date products or exceed recommended dosages.
- Do not take for persistent or chronic cough (eg, cough due to smoking, asthma, emphysema) or when cough is accompanied by excessive secretions, except under supervision of a physician.
- A persistent cough may be a sign of a serious condition. Consult a physician if cough persists longer than 7 days, tends to recur, or is accompanied by fever, rash, or persistent headache.
- Do not take if you are now taking a prescription monoamine oxidase inhibitor (MAOI) or for 2 weeks after stopping the MAOI drug.
- Do not take this product if you have asthma or glaucoma, except under supervision of a physician.
- Do not use any solution that has changed color or become cloudy.

CODEINE

▶ **Actions**

Codeine is a narcotic possessing good antitussive activity; side effects are infrequent at the usual antitussive dose. The dose required to suppress coughing is lower than the dose required for analgesia.

▶ **Indications**

For suppression of a nonproductive cough and relief of mild to moderate pain.

▶ **Contraindications**

Hypersensitivity to the drug or any of its components; premature infants or during labor when delivery of a premature infant is anticipated (see Warnings).

▶ **Warnings**

Head injury and increased intracranial pressure: The respiratory depressant effects of the opiates and their capacity to elevate cerebrospinal fluid pressure may be markedly exaggerated in the presence of head injury, intracranial lesions, or a preexisting increase in intracranial pressure. Usual therapeutic oral doses of codeine produce little respiratory depression; however, exercise caution, particularly with larger doses. Furthermore, opiates may produce adverse reactions that may obscure the clinical course of patients with head injuries.

Respiratory disease: Use with extreme caution in patients having an acute asthmatic attack, patients with chronic obstructive pulmonary disease or cor pulmonale, patients having a substantially decreased respiratory reserve, and patients with preexisting respiratory depression, hypoxia, or hypercapnia. Usual therapeutic doses may decrease respiratory drive while simultaneously increasing airway resistance to the point of apnea. In asthma and pulmonary emphysema, codeine may, because of its drying action on the respiratory mucosa, precipitate insufficiency resulting from increased viscosity of the bronchial secretions and suppression of the cough reflex.

Acute abdominal conditions: Administration of codeine or other opiates may obscure the diagnosis or clinical course in patients with acute abdominal conditions.

Special-risk patients: Administer with caution and reduce the initial dose in patients with acute abdominal conditions, convulsive disorders, significant hepatic or renal impairment, fever, hypothyroidism, Addison disease, ulcerative colitis, prostatic hypertrophy, urethral stricture, recent GI or urinary tract surgery, and in very young, elderly, or debilitated patients.

Drug abuse and dependence:

Abuse – The abuse potential of codeine is less than that of heroin or morphine but significant nonetheless.

Most patients who receive opiates for medical indications do not develop drug-seeking behavior or compulsive drug use. However, give under close supervision to patients with a history of drug abuse or dependence.

Dependence – Psychological and physical dependence and tolerance may occur with regular, long-term use.

The severity of the abstinence syndrome is related to the degree of dependence, abruptness of withdrawal, and the drug used. If the syndrome is precipitated by a narcotic antagonist, symptoms appear in a few minutes and are maximal within 30 minutes.

While codeine can partially suppress the symptoms of morphine withdrawal, the codeine withdrawal syndrome (after 1.2 to 1.8 g codeine/day), though similar to that seen with morphine, is less intense. Withdrawal symptoms in patients dependent on codeine include yawning, sweating, lacrimation, rhinorrhea, restless sleep, dilated pupils, gooseflesh, irritability, tremor, nausea, vomiting, and diarrhea. Treatment is primarily symptomatic and supportive, including maintenance of proper fluid and electrolyte balance.

Pregnancy: Category C. Dependence has been reported in newborns whose mothers regularly took opiate narcotics during pregnancy. Withdrawal signs include irritability, excessive crying, tremors, hyperreflexia, fever, vomiting, and diarrhea. Signs usually appear during the first few days of life. Use during pregnancy only if the potential benefits outweigh the potential hazards to the fetus.

Labor and delivery – Opiates cross the placental barrier. The closer to delivery and the larger the dose used, the greater the possibility of respiratory depression in the newborn. Avoid use during labor if a premature infant is anticipated. If the mother has received opiates during labor, closely observe the newborn for signs of respiratory depression. Resuscitation may be required; in severe depression, naloxone also may be required. Codeine also may prolong labor.

Lactation: Exercise caution. Some studies have reported detectable amounts of codeine in breast milk. The levels are probably not clinically significant after usual therapeutic dosage. Clinically important amounts may be excreted in breast milk in individuals abusing codeine.

Children: Do not use opiates, including codeine, in premature infants. Opiates cross the immature blood-brain barrier to a greater extent, producing disproportionate respiratory depression. Give opiates to infants and small children only with great caution and carefully monitor dosage. Safety and efficacy in newborn infants have not been established.

▶ **Drug Interactions**

CNS depressants (eg, other opiates, general anesthetics, antihistamines, phenothiazines, hypnotics, tricyclic antidepressants, tranquilizers) and alcohol: Use codeine cautiously and in reduced dosage to avoid additive effects when given concomitantly.

Because opiates may increase biliary tract pressure with resultant increases in plasma amylase or lipase levels, determination of these enzyme levels may be unreliable for 24 hours after an opiate has been given.

▶ **Adverse Reactions**

Allergic reactions: Allergic reactions (eg, rash, itching) to opiates occur infrequently; pruritus, giant urticaria, angioneurotic edema, and laryngeal edema have occurred following IV administration.

Cardiovascular: Tachycardia; bradycardia; palpitation; faintness; syncope; orthostatic hypotension.

CNS: CNS depression, particularly respiratory depression, and, to a lesser extent, circulatory depression; respiratory arrest, shock, and cardiac arrest, particularly with overdosage or with rapid IV administration. Other effects include the following: lightheadedness; dizziness; sedation; euphoria; dysphoria; weakness; headache; hallucinations; disorientation; impaired coordination and dexterity; visual disturbances; convulsions. These effects are more common with larger oral or parenteral doses, in ambulatory patients, and in those patients who are not experiencing severe pain. Some reactions in ambulatory patients may be alleviated by lying down.

GI: Nausea; vomiting; constipation; biliary tract spasm. Patients with ulcerative colitis may experience increased colonic motility or toxic dilation.

GU: Oliguria; urinary retention; antidiuretic effect.

▶ **Overdosage**

The lethal oral dose of codeine in an adult is in the range of 0.5 to 1 g. Infants and children are relatively more sensitive to opiates on a body-weight basis. Elderly patients also are comparatively intolerant.

Refer to General Management of Acute Overdosage.

▶ **Administration and Dosage**

Adults and children (older than 12 years of age): 20 mg every 4 hours as needed, not to exceed 120 mg in 24 hours.

Children (6 to 12 years of age): 10 mg every 4 hours as needed, not to exceed 60 mg in 24 hours.

Children (younger than 6 years of age): Use only as directed by a physician.

Infants: Do not use in premature infants. Safety and efficacy in newborn infants have not been established.

Codeine, as a single agent, is not available without a prescription. It is available in many schedule *c-v* multi-ingredient respiratory preparations as an antitussive and may be purchased under limited circumstances without a prescription. Refer to individual state laws.

CODEINE PRODUCTS	
Trade name	**Doseform**
Tricodene Cough & Cold	**Liquid**: 8.2 mg codeine phosphate, 12.5 mg pyrilamine maleate/5 mL
Guiatuss AC (sf)	**Syrup**: 10 mg codeine phosphate, 100 mg guaifenesin/5 mL. 3.5% alcohol, glycerin, saccharin, sorbitol. Cherry flavor.
Mytussin AC Cough, Robafen AC (sf)	**Syrup**: 10 mg codeine phosphate, 100 mg guaifenesin/5 mL. Menthol, saccharin, sorbitol.

Products listed are representative of currently available and widely distributed brands. Similar products, including regional and private label brands, may also exist.

sf = Sugar free.

PATIENT INFORMATION

Codeine

- Patient instructions accompany each product. Read these instructions carefully before use, preferably before leaving the pharmacy, in case of any questions.
- May cause GI upset; take with food or milk.
- Do not take for persistent or chronic cough (eg, cough due to smoking, asthma, emphysema) or when cough is accompanied by excessive secretions, except under supervision of a physician.
- A persistent cough may be a sign of a serious condition. Consult a physician if cough persists longer than 7 days, tends to recur, or is accompanied by fever, rash, or persistent headache.
- The concomitant use of alcohol or other CNS depressants, including sedatives, hypnotics, tricyclic antidepressants, tranquilizers, phenothiazines, and antihistamines, may have an additive effect.
- Adults and children who have a chronic pulmonary disease or shortness or breath or children who are taking other drugs should not take this product unless instructed by a physician.
- May cause drowsiness or dizziness. Do not drive or perform other tasks requiring alertness, coordination, or physical dexterity while taking these products.
- May produce orthostatic hypotension (dizziness or light-headedness when rising quickly from a sitting or lying position) in some ambulatory patients.
- May cause dry mouth or constipation.

DIPHENHYDRAMINE HCL

▶ Actions

Diphenhydramine is an antihistamine that has been shown to suppress the cough center in the medulla of the brain. It also competitively antagonizes histamine at the H_1 receptor, reducing sensory nerve stimulation, mucus production, and vascular permeability.

▶ Indications

For control of coughs due to colds or allergy; considered a distant, secondary choice as a therapeutic cough suppressant. For dosing and product information, **see Diphenhydramine in the Allergic Rhinitis monograph.**

EXPECTORANTS

GUAIFENESIN

▶ Actions

Although the clinical efficacy is not proven, expectorants at proper doses may reduce the adherence, surface tension, and viscosity of mucus and other respiratory secretions that facilitate clearance of the upper airway. These agents have not been shown to appreciably affect nasal clearance of secretions. Theoretically, improving airway clearance may reduce the urge to cough. Guaifenesin is the only OTC expectorant recognized as safe and effective by the FDA. Guaifenesin works best when the patient is well hydrated by fluid intake.

▶ Indications

For temporary relief of coughs associated with respiratory tract infections and related conditions such as sinusitis, pharyngitis, bronchitis, and asthma when these conditions are complicated by tenacious mucus and/or mucus plugs and congestion. The drug is effective in productive as well as nonproductive cough, but is of particular value in dry, nonproductive cough that tends to injure the mucous membranes of the air passages.

▶ Contraindications

Hypersensitivity to the drug or any of its components.

▶ Warnings

Persistent cough: Not for persistent cough (eg, cough due to smoking, asthma, emphysema) or when cough is accompanied by excessive secretions.

Kidney stone formation: Reports have suggested consumption of large quantities of guaifenesin-containing products may be associated with an increased risk or drug-induced kidney stone formation.

Pregnancy: Category C.

▶ Adverse Reactions

The following side effects occur infrequently: nausea; vomiting; dizziness; headache; rash (including urticaria).

▶ Administration and Dosage

Adults and children (older than 12 years of age): 200 to 400 mg every 4 hours as needed, not to exceed 2.4 g in 24 hours. The minimum intake required to achieve any significant effect is 1200 mg/day.

Children (6 to 12 years of age): 100 to 200 mg every 4 hours as needed, not to exceed 1.2 g in 24 hours.

Children (2 to 6 years of age): 50 to 100 mg every 4 hours as needed, not to exceed 600 mg in 24 hours.

GUAIFENESIN PRODUCTS	
Trade name	Doseform
Hytuss	**Tablets**: 100 mg
Mucinex	**Tablets, extended release**: 600 mg
Hytuss 2X	**Capsules**: 200 mg. Benzyl alcohol, EDTA, parabens, talc.
Robitussin	**Liquid**: 100 mg/5 mL. Alcohol free. Corn syrup, glycerin, menthol, saccharin.

GUAIFENESIN PRODUCTS	
Trade name	Doseform
Scot-Tussin Expectorant (sf)	**Liquid**: 100 mg/5 mL. Alcohol free. Aspartame, glycerin, menthol, parabens, phenylalanine. Grape flavor.
Guiatuss	**Syrup**: 100 mg/5 mL. Corn syrup, glycerin, saccharin.

Products listed are representative of currently available and widely distributed brands. Similar products, including regional and private label brands, may also exist.

sf = Sugar free.

PATIENT INFORMATION

Expectorants

- Patient instructions accompany each product. Read these instructions carefully before use, preferably before leaving the pharmacy, in case of any questions.
- Do not take for persistent or chronic cough (eg, cough due to smoking, asthma, emphysema) or when cough is accompanied by excessive secretions, except under supervision of a physician.
- A persistent cough may be a sign of a serious condition. Consult a physician if cough persists for longer than 7 days, tends to recur, or is accompanied by fever, rash, or persistent headache.
- Guaifenesin is the only expectorant approved by the FDA as safe and effective.
- Drink a glass of water or other fluid with each dose of expectorant. Most authorities believe a well-hydrated body (because of fluid intake) is responsible for thinning respiratory tract mucus and may be as, or more, valuable than the expectorant itself.

TOPICAL RUBS, PATCHES, AND VAPOR AGENTS

▶ **Actions**

Products containing the aromatic agents camphor and menthol are FDA-approved for the relief of nasal and chest congestion and cough. Inhalation of camphor or menthol vapor theoretically produces an antitussive effect through their local anesthetic properties. Clinical value remains debatable.

▶ **Indications**

For relief of nasal and chest congestion and cough when applied topically to the chest or via inhalation of vapors.

▶ **Contraindications**

Hypersensitivity to the drug or any of its components.

▶ **Warnings**

For external use only: Do not ingest. Avoid contact with eyes. Do not take these products for persistent or chronic cough (eg, cough due to smoking, excess mucus, asthma, emphysema) unless directed by a physician. Do not take by mouth, place in nostrils, bandage tightly, or apply to damaged skin. Consult a physician if cough persists for longer than 7 to 10 days, recurs, or is accompanied by fever, rash, or persistent headache.

Heat therapy: Do not use an external source of heat (eg, heating pad) with these agents because irritation or burning of the skin may occur.

Never expose patches to flame, heat, microwave, or containers of heating water.

▶ **Drug Interactions**

There are no known drug interactions.

▶ **Adverse Reactions**

Toxic if ingested; oral ingestion may cause systemic reactions. Seek professional advice if ingestion is suspected. Counterirritants may cause local irritation, especially in patients with sensitive skin.

▶ **Administration and Dosage**

Rubs: Rub a thick layer on chest or throat. May cover with a soft, dry cloth but keep clothing loose to allow vapors to reach nose and mouth. Repeat up to 3 times/day.

Patches: Apply patch to throat or chest. Do not leave patch on for more than 12 hours. Applications may be repeated up to 3 times/day. If repeated application is desired, place patch on a new area of the skin. More than 1 patch may be used at a time.

Vaporizers: Add directly to the water in the warm or hot steam vaporizer. Do not direct steam too closely to face. Breathe in medicated vapors. May be repeated up to 3 times/day or as directed by a physician or pharmacist.

TOPICAL RUBS, PATCHES, AND VAPOR AGENTS	
Trade name	**Doseform**
Tom's of Maine Natural Cough & Cold Rub	**Ointment**: 4.8% camphor, 2.6% menthol. Canola oil, eucalyptus oil, white pine oil. Eucalyptus and lemon verbena fragrance.
Vicks VapoRub	**Ointment**: 4.8% camphor, 2.6% menthol, 1.2% eucalyptus oil. Cedarleaf oil, nutmeg oil, petrolatum, turpentine oil.
Mentholatum	**Ointment**: 9% camphor, 1.3% menthol. Petrolatum.
Vicks VapoCream	**Cream**: 5.2% camphor, 2.8% menthol, 1.2% eucalyptus oil. Cedarleaf oil, cetyl alcohol, EDTA, glycerin, imidazolidinyl urea, nutmeg oil, parabens, stearyl alcohol, turpentine oil.
Vicks VapoSteam for Hot Steam Vaporizers	**Liquid**: 6.2% camphor. 78% alcohol, cedarleaf oil, eucalyptus oil, menthol, nutmeg oil.
TheraPatch Vapor Chest	**Patch**: 4.7% camphor, 2.6% menthol. Aloe vera, eucalyptus oil, glycerin, turpentine spirits.
TheraPatch Vapor for Kids, Triaminic Vapor Patch	**Patch**: 4.7% camphor, 2.6% menthol. Aloe vera, eucalyptus oil, glycerin. Wild cherry fragrance.
Triaminic Vapor Patch	**Patch**: 4.7% camphor, 2.6% menthol. Aloe vera, eucalyptus oil, glycerin, turpentine spirits. Menthol fragrance.

Products listed are representative of currently available and widely distributed brands. Similar products, including regional and private label brands, may also exist.

PATIENT INFORMATION
Topical Rubs, Patches, and Vapor Products

- Patient instructions accompany each product. Read these instructions carefully before use, preferably before leaving the pharmacy, in case of any questions.
- Take as directed. Do not use any out-of-date products or exceed recommended dosages.
- For external use only. Avoid contact with eyes.
- Do not take for persistent or chronic cough (eg, cough due to smoking, asthma, emphysema,) or when cough is accompanied by excessive secretions, except under supervision of a physician.
- A persistent cough may be a sign of a serious condition. Consult a physician if cough persists for longer than 7 days, tends to recur, or is accompanied by fever, rash, or persistent headache.
- Never expose products to flame, heat, microwave, or containers of heating water.
- *Rubs:*
  Rub a thick layer of the cream or ointment on the throat or chest.
  After application, the cream or ointment may be covered with a soft, dry cloth, but keep clothing loose enough to allow vapors to reach the nose and mouth.
  Do not apply to irritated skin. Discontinue use if excess irritation occurs. May cause local irritation in patients with sensitive skin.
- *Patches:*
  Do not apply to wounds or irritated, sensitive, or damaged skin.
  Keep clothing loose around throat and chest to allow vapors to reach nose and mouth.
  In case of difficulty in removing the patch, moisten patch with water.
- *Vaporizer products:*
  Add measured amount of vaporizer liquid medication directly to the water in the warm or hot steam vaporizer.
  Avoid directing the steam too closely to the face.
  Clean the vaporizer thoroughly after each use according to specific manufacturer's directions.

COMBINATION PRODUCTS FOR COUGH

▶ **Indications**

Common nonprescription combination products for the common cold include: decongestants and antihistamines; decongestants and analgesics; antihistamines and analgesics; decongestants, antihistamines, and analgesics; and decongestants, antihistamines, analgesics, and expectorants. Intranasal and ocular combination products of decongestants and antihistamines are also available.

Advantages of combination products include complementary activity with decongestant/antihistamine combinations and patient convenience in those with histamine-mediated inflammation and nasal congestion.

Disadvantages of combination products include the inability to titrate the dose of individual ingredients, possible administration of a drug for which there are no symptoms, and an unnecessary risk of side effects and drug interactions if one or more active ingredient is not needed to treat specific current symptoms. Because of variable anticholinergic effects, use antihistamines with caution in patients with narrow-angle glaucoma or a history of glaucoma. Rebound nasal congestion and ocular hyperemia may occur with excessive use of topical nasal decongestants. **See Respiratory Combination Products in the Common Cold monograph.**

DECONGESTANT/ANTITUSSIVE COMBINATIONS

▶ Administration and Dosage

Dosages vary; refer to specific product information.

DECONGESTANT/ANTITUSSIVE COMBINATIONS	
Trade name	Doseform
Children's PediaCare Long-Acting Cough Plus Cold	**Tablets, chewable**: 15 mg pseudoephedrine HCl, 7.5 mg dextromethorphan HBr. Aspartame, mannitol, sucrose. 5 mg phenylalanine. Grape flavor.
Children's Sudafed Cold & Cough (sf)	**Liquid**: 15 mg pseudoephedrine HCl, 5 mg dextromethorphan HBr/5 mL. Alcohol free. EDTA, glycerin, saccharin, sorbitol. Cherryberry flavor.
Children's PediaCare Long-Acting Cough Plus Cold	**Liquid**: 15 mg pseudoephedrine HCl, 7.5 mg dextromethorphan HBr/5 mL. Alcohol free. Corn syrup, glycerin, sorbitol. Grape flavor.
Triaminic Cough & Congestion	**Liquid**: 15 mg pseudoephedrine HCl, 7.5 mg dextromethorphan HBr/5 mL. Alcohol free. EDTA, sorbitol, sucrose. Orange-strawberry flavor.
Vicks 44D Cough & Head Congestion Relief	**Liquid**: 20 mg pseudoephedrine HCl, 10 mg dextromethorphan HBr/5 mL. Alcohol, corn syrup, saccharin.
Robitussin Maximum Strength Cough & Cold	**Liquid**: 30 mg pseudoephedrine HCl, 15 mg dextromethorphan HBr/5 mL. Alcohol, corn syrup, glycerin, menthol, saccharin.
Infants' PediaCare Decongestant & Cough	**Liquid, drops**: 7.5 mg pseudoephedrine HCl, 2.5 mg dextromethorphan HBr/0.8 mL. Alcohol free. Glycerin, sorbitol. Cherry flavor.
Children's Dimetapp Long Acting Cough Plus Cold	**Syrup**: 15 mg pseudoephedrine HCl, 7.5 mg dextromethorphan HBr/5 mL. Corn syrup, glycerin, saccharin. Fruit punch flavor.
Robitussin Pediatric Cough & Cold	**Syrup**: 15 mg pseudoephedrine HCl, 7.5 mg dextromethorphan HBr/5 mL. Corn syrup, glycerin, saccharin.

Products listed are representative of currently available and widely distributed brands. Similar products, including regional and private label brands, may also exist.

sf = Sugar free.

ANTIHISTAMINE/ANTITUSSIVE COMBINATIONS

▶ Administration and Dosage

Dosages vary; refer to specific product information.

ANTIHISTAMINE/ANTITUSSIVE COMBINATIONS	
Trade name	Doseform
NyQuil Cough	**Liquid**: 6.25 mg doxylamine succinate, 15 mg dextromethorphan HBr/15 mL. Alcohol, corn syrup, saccharin.
Tricodene Cough and Cold Medication (sf)	**Liquid**: 2 mg chlorpheniramine maleate, 10 mg dextromethorphan HBr/5 mL. Mannitol, sorbitol.

Products listed are representative of currently available and widely distributed brands. Similar products, including regional and private label brands, may also exist.

sf = Sugar free.

ANTIHISTAMINE/ANTITUSSIVE/ANALGESIC COMBINATIONS

▶ **Administration and Dosage**

Dosages vary; refer to specific product information.

ANTIHISTAMINE/ANTITUSSIVE/ANALGESIC COMBINATIONS	
Trade name	Doseform
Alka-Seltzer Plus Flu Honey Orange	**Tablets, effervescent**: 2 mg chlorpheniramine maleate, 15 mg dextromethorphan HBr, 500 mg aspirin. Aspartame, mannitol, saccharin, 6.7 mg phenylalanine.

Products listed are representative of currently available and widely distributed brands. Similar products, including regional and private label brands, may also exist.

ANTITUSSIVE/EXPECTORANT COMBINATIONS

▶ **Warnings**

The combination of an expectorant with a cough suppressant, which retards expectoration, is considered illogical. Use of such combination products is generally discouraged.

▶ **Administration and Dosage**

Dosages vary; refer to specific product information.

ANTITUSSIVE/EXPECTORANT COMBINATIONS	
Trade name	Doseform
Robitussin DM Infant Drops	**Liquid**: 5 mg dextromethorphan HBr, 100 mg guaifenesin/2.5 mL. Alcohol free. Corn syrup, glycerin, saccharin.
Benylin Expectorant (sf)	**Liquid**: 5 mg dextromethorphan HBr, 100 mg guaifenesin/5 mL. Alcohol free. EDTA, saccharin, sorbitol.
Cheracol Plus, Cheracol D Cough	**Liquid**: 10 mg dextromethorphan HBr, 100 mg guaifenesin/5 mL. 4.75% alcohol, fructose, glycerin, sucrose.
Diabetic Tussin DM Regular Strength (sf)	**Liquid**: 10 mg dextromethorphan HBr, 100 mg guaifenesin/5 mL. Alcohol and dye free. Aspartame, menthol, methylparaben, 8.4 mg phenylalanine.
Kolephrin GG/DM	**Liquid**: 10 mg dextromethorphan HBr, 150 mg guaifenesin/5 mL
Diabetic Tussin DM Maximum Strength (sf)	**Liquid**: 10 mg dextromethorphan HBr, 200 mg guaifenesin/5 mL. Alcohol and dye free. Aspartame, menthol, methylparaben, 8.4 mg phenylalanine.
Vicks 44E Cough & Chest Congestion Relief	**Liquid**: 20 mg dextromethorphan HBr, 200 mg guaifenesin/15 mL. Alcohol, corn syrup, saccharin.
Guiatuss DM	**Syrup**: 10 mg dextromethorphan HBr, 100 mg guaifenesin/5 mL. Alcohol free. Cherry-mint flavor.
Robitussin DM Cough, Genatuss DM	**Syrup**: 10 mg dextromethorphan HBr, 100 mg guaifenesin/5 mL. Alcohol free. Corn syrup, glycerin, menthol, saccharin.

Products listed are representative of currently available and widely distributed brands. Similar products, including regional and private label brands, may also exist.

sf = Sugar free.

DECONGESTANT/ANTIHISTAMINE/ANTITUSSIVE COMBINATIONS

▶ Administration and Dosage

Dosages vary; refer to specific product information.

DECONGESTANT/ANTIHISTAMINE/ANTITUSSIVE COMBINATIONS	
Trade name	**Doseform**
Children's PediaCare Multi-Symptom Cold	**Tablets, chewable**: 15 mg pseudoephedrine HCl, 1 mg chlorpheniramine maleate, 5 mg dextromethorphan HBr. Aspartame, mannitol, sucrose. 8.4 mg phenylalanine. Cherry flavor.
Triaminic Softchews Cold & Cough	**Tablets, chewable**: 15 mg pseudoephedrine HCl, 1 mg chlorpheniramine maleate, 5 mg dextromethorphan HBr. Aspartame, mannitol, sucrose, 17.7 mg phenylalanine.
Alka-Seltzer Plus NightTime Cold	**Tablets, effervescent**: 5 mg phenylephrine HCl, 6.25 mg doxylamine succinate, 10 mg dextromethorphan HBr. Aspartame, sorbitol, 7.8 mg phenylalanine.
Father John's Medicine Plus	**Liquid**: 5 mg phenylephrine HCl, 2 mg chlorpheniramine maleate, 5 mg dextromethorphan HBr/15 mL. Alcohol free.
Children's PediaCare Multi-Symptom Cold	**Liquid**: 15 mg pseudoephedrine HCl, 1 mg chlorpheniramine maleate, 5 mg dextromethorphan HBr/5 mL. Alcohol free. Corn syrup, glycerin, sorbitol. Cherry flavor.
Triaminic Cold & Cough	**Liquid**: 15 mg pseudoephedrine HCl, 1 mg chlorpheniramine maleate, 5 mg dextromethorphan HBr/5 mL. Alcohol free. Sorbitol, sucrose. Cherry flavor.
Children's PediaCare NightRest Cough & Cold	**Liquid**: 15 mg pseudoephedrine HCl, 1 mg chlorpheniramine maleate, 7.5 mg dextromethorphan HBr/5 mL. Alcohol free. Corn syrup, glycerin, sorbitol. Cherry flavor.
Robitussin PM Cough & Cold	**Liquid**: 15 mg pseudoephedrine HCl, 1 mg chlorpheniramine maleate, 7.5 mg dextromethorphan HBr/5 mL. Corn syrup, glycerin, saccharin.
Triaminic Cold & NightTime Cough	**Liquid**: 15 mg pseudoephedrine HCl, 1 mg chlorpheniramine maleate, 7.5 mg dextromethorphan HBr/5 mL. Sorbitol, sucrose.
Children's Vicks NyQuil Cold/Cough Relief	**Liquid**: 30 mg pseudoephedrine HCl, 2 mg chlorpheniramine maleate, 15 mg dextromethorphan HBr/15 mL. Sucrose.
Pediatric Vicks 44m Cough & Cold Relief	**Liquid**: 30 mg pseudoephedrine HCl, 2 mg chlorpheniramine maleate, 15 mg dextromethorphan HBr/15 mL. Corn syrup, saccharin.
Robitussin Pediatric Night Relief	**Syrup**: 15 mg pseudoephedrine HCl, 1 mg chlorpheniramine maleate, 7.5 mg dextromethorphan HBr/5 mL. Corn syrup, glycerin, saccharin.
Children's Dimetapp DM Cold & Cough	**Elixir**: 15 mg pseudoephedrine HCl, 1 mg brompheniramine maleate, 5 mg dextromethorphan HBr/5 mL. Corn syrup, glycerin, saccharin, sorbitol.

Products listed are representative of currently available and widely distributed brands. Similar products, including regional and private label brands, may also exist.

sf = Sugar free.

DECONGESTANT/ANTITUSSIVE/ANALGESIC COMBINATIONS

▶ **Administration and Dosage**

Dosages vary; refer to specific product information.

DECONGESTANT/ANTITUSSIVE/ANALGESIC COMBINATIONS	
Trade name	**Doseform**
Sudafed Non-Drowsy Severe Cold Formula	**Tablets**: 30 mg pseudoephedrine HCl, 15 mg dextromethorphan HBr, 500 mg acetaminophen
Triaminic Soft Chews Cough & Sore Throat	**Tablets, chewable**: 15 mg pseudoephedrine HCl, 5 mg dextromethorphan HBr, 160 mg acetaminophen. Aspartame, mannitol, 28.1 mg phenylalanine.
Tylenol Cold Day Non-Drowsy	**Caplets**: 30 mg pseudoephedrine HCl, 15 mg dextromethorphan HBr, 325 mg acetaminophen
Tylenol Cold Day Non-Drowsy	**Gelcaps**: 30 mg pseudoephedrine HCl, 15 mg dextromethorphan HBr, 325 mg acetaminophen. Benzyl alcohol, castor oil, EDTA, parabens.
Tylenol Flu Day Non-Drowsy	**Gelcaps**: 30 mg pseudoephedrine HCl, 15 mg dextromethorphan HBr, 500 mg acetaminophen. Benzyl alcohol, castor oil, EDTA, parabens.
Vicks DayQuil Multi-Symptom Cold/Flu Relief	**Softgels**: 30 mg pseudoephedrine HCl, 10 mg dextromethorphan HBr, 250 mg acetaminophen. Glycerin, sorbitol.
Alka-Seltzer Plus Flu Non-Drowsy	**Softgels**: 30 mg pseudoephedrine HCl, 10 mg dextromethorphan HBr, 325 mg acetaminophen. Glycerin, sorbitol.
Infants' Tylenol Cold Plus Cough Concentrated Drops	**Liquid**: 15 mg pseudoephedrine HCl, 5 mg dextromethorphan HBr, 160 mg acetaminophen/1.6 mL. Corn syrup. Cherry flavor.
Vicks DayQuil Multi-Symptom Cold/Flu Relief	**Liquid**: 30 mg pseudoephedrine HCl, 15 mg dextromethorphan HBr, 325 mg acetaminophen/15 mL. Sucrose, saccharin.

Products listed are representative of currently available and widely distributed brands. Similar products, including regional and private label brands, may also exist.

DECONGESTANT/ANTITUSSIVE/EXPECTORANT COMBINATIONS

▶ **Warnings**

The combination of an expectorant with a cough suppressant, which retards expectoration, is considered illogical. Use of such combination products is generally discouraged.

▶ **Administration and Dosage**

Dosages vary; refer to specific product information/package labeling.

DECONGESTANT/ANTITUSSIVE/EXPECTORANT COMBINATIONS	
Trade name	**Doseform**
Robitussin Cold & Congestion	**Softgels**: 30 mg pseudoephedrine HCl, 10 mg dextromethorphan HBr, 200 mg guaifenesin. Glycerin, mannitol, sorbitol.
Robitussin CF	**Liquid**: 30 mg pseudoephedrine HCl, 10 mg dextromethorphan HBr, 100 mg guaifenesin/5 mL. Saccharin, sorbitol.

Products listed are representative of currently available and widely distributed brands. Similar products, including regional and private label brands, may also exist.

DECONGESTANT/ANTITUSSIVE/EXPECTORANT/ANALGESIC COMBINATIONS

▶ Warnings

The combination of an expectorant with a cough suppressant, which retards expectoration, is considered illogical. Use of such combination products is generally discouraged.

▶ Administration and Dosage

Dosages vary; refer to specific product information/package labeling.

DECONGESTANT/ANTITUSSIVE/EXPECTORANT/ANALGESIC PRODUCTS	
Trade name	Doseform
Robitussin Multi-Symptom Cold & Flu	**Caplets**: 30 mg pseudoephedrine hydrochloride, 10 mg dextromethorphan HBr, 200 mg guaifenesin, 325 mg acetaminophen
Tylenol Cold Severe Congestion Non-Drowsy	**Caplets**: 30 mg pseudoephedrine hydrochloride, 15 mg dextromethorphan HBr, 200 mg guaifenesin, 325 mg acetaminophen
Robitussin Multi-Symptom Cold & Flu	**Softgels**: 30 mg pseudoephedrine hydrochloride, 10 mg dextromethorphan HBr, 100 mg guaifenesin, 250 mg acetaminophen. Glycerin, mannitol, sorbitol.
Comtrex Multi-Symptom Deep Chest Cold & Congestion Relief	**Softgels**: 30 mg pseudoephedrine hydrochloride, 10 mg dextromethorphan HBr, 100 mg guaifenesin, 250 mg acetaminophen. Glycerin, sorbitol.
TheraFlu Maximum Strength Non-Drowsy Chest Congestion & Cough	**Packets for hot water**: 60 mg pseudoephedrine hydrochloride, 30 mg dextromethorphan HBr, 400 mg guaifenesin, 1,000 mg acetaminophen. Aspartame, sucrose, 25 mg phenylalanine. Honey lemon flavor.

Products listed are representative of currently available and widely distributed brands. Similar products, including regional and private label brands, may also exist.

DECONGESTANT/ANTIHISTAMINE/ANTITUSSIVE/ANALGESIC COMBINATIONS

▶ Administration and Dosage

Dosages vary; refer to specific product information/package labeling.

DECONGESTANT/ANTIHISTAMINE/ANTITUSSIVE/ANALGESIC PRODUCTS	
Trade name	Doseform
Tylenol Children's Cold Plus Cough	**Tablets, chewable**: 7.5 mg pseudoephedrine hydrochloride, 0.5 mg chlorpheniramine maleate, 2.5 mg dextromethorphan HBr, 80 mg acetaminophen. Aspartame, mannitol, 4 mg phenylalanine. Cherry flavor.
Alka-Seltzer Plus NightTime Cold	**Tablets, effervescent**: 5 mg phenylephrine hydrochloride, 6.25 mg doxylamine succinate, 10 mg dextromethorphan HBr, 250 mg acetaminophen. Aspartame, sorbitol, 5.6 mg phenylalanine.
Tylenol Cold NightTime Complete Formula	**Caplets**: 30 mg pseudoephedrine hydrochloride, 2 mg chlorpheniramine maleate, 15 mg dextromethorphan HBr, 325 mg acetaminophen

DECONGESTANT/ANTIHISTAMINE/ANTITUSSIVE/ANALGESIC PRODUCTS

Trade name	Doseform
TheraFlu Severe Cold & Congestion Maximum Strength NightTime	**Caplets**: 30 mg pseudoephedrine hydrochloride, 2 mg chlorpheniramine maleate, 15 mg dextromethorphan HBr, 500 mg acetaminophen. Methylparaben.
Tylenol Cold Day/Night Convenience Pack*	**Caplets, day**: 30 mg pseudoephedrine hydrochloride, 15 mg dextromethorphan HBr, 325 mg acetaminophen
	Caplets, night: 30 mg pseudoephedrine hydrochloride, 2 mg chlorpheniramine maleate, 15 mg dextromethorphan HBr, 325 mg acetaminophen
Contac Day & Night Cold and Flu Relief*†	**Caplets, day**: 60 mg pseudoephedrine hydrochloride, 30 mg dextromethorphan HBr, 650 mg acetaminophen
	Caplets, night: 60 mg pseudoephedrine hydrochloride, 50 mg diphenhydramine hydrochloride, 650 mg acetaminophen
Alka-Seltzer Plus Cold & Cough	**Softgels**: 30 mg pseudoephedrine hydrochloride, 2 mg chlorpheniramine maleate, 10 mg dextromethorphan HBr, 325 mg acetaminophen. Glycerin, sorbitol.
Alka Seltzer Plus NightTime Cold	**Softgels**: 30 mg pseudoephedrine hydrochloride, 6.25 mg doxylamine succinate, 10 mg dextromethorphan HBr, 325 mg acetaminophen. Glycerin, sorbitol. Alcohol free.
Tylenol Flu Day/Night Convenience Pack*†	**Gelcaps, day**: 30 mg pseudoephedrine hydrochloride, 15 mg dextromethorphan HBr, 500 mg acetaminophen. Benzyl alcohol, castor oil, EDTA, parabens.
	Gelcaps, night: 30 mg pseudoephedrine hydrochloride, 25 mg diphenhydramine hydrochloride, 500 mg acetaminophen. Benzyl alcohol, castor oil, EDTA, parabens.
Tylenol Children's Cold Plus Cough	**Liquid**: 15 mg pseudoephedrine hydrochloride, 1 mg chlorpheniramine maleate, 5 mg dextromethorphan HBr, 160 mg acetaminophen/5 mL. Butylparaben, corn syrup, glycerin, sorbitol. Cherry flavor.
Triaminic Flu, Cough & Fever	**Liquid**: 15 mg pseudoephedrine hydrochloride, 1 mg chlorpheniramine maleate, 7.5 mg dextromethorphan HBr, 160 mg acetaminophen/5 mL. EDTA, glycerin, sucrose. Alcohol free. Bubble gum flavor.
Tylenol NightTime Severe Cold & Flu	**Liquid**: 30 mg pseudoephedrine hydrochloride, 6.25 mg doxylamine succinate, 15 mg dextromethorphan HBr, 500 mg acetaminophen/15 mL. Corn syrup, saccharin, sorbitol.
NyQuil Multi-Symptom Cold/Flu Relief	**Liquid**: 30 mg pseudoephedrine hydrochloride, 6.25 mg doxylamine succinate, 15 mg dextromethorphan HBr, 500 mg acetaminophen/15 mL. Alcohol, corn syrup, saccharin. Original and cherry flavors.
TheraFlu Severe Cold & Congestion Maximum Strength NightTime	**Packets for hot water**: 60 mg pseudoephedrine hydrochloride, 4 mg chlorpheniramine maleate, 30 mg dextromethorphan HBr, 1,000 mg acetaminophen. Alcohol free. Natural lemon flavor.

■ ■ ■

DECONGESTANT/ANTIHISTAMINE/ANTITUSSIVE/ANALGESIC PRODUCTS	
Trade name	Doseform
TheraFlu Flu & Cough Maximum Strength NightTime	**Packets for hot water**: 60 mg pseudoephedrine hydrochloride, 4 mg chlorpheniramine maleate, 30 mg dextromethorphan HBr, 1,000 mg acetaminophen. Aspartame, sucrose, 26 mg phenylalanine. Alcohol free. Cherry flavor.

Products listed are representative of currently available and widely distributed brands. Similar products, including regional and private label brands, may also exist.

* Only night caplets/gelcaps contain an antihistamine.
† Only day caplets/gelcaps contain an antitussive.

ANTITUSSIVE/LOCAL ANESTHETIC COMBINATIONS

▶ Administration and Dosage

Dosages vary; refer to specific product information/package labeling.

ANTITUSSIVE/LOCAL ANESTHETIC PRODUCTS	
Trade name	Doseform
Halls	**Lozenges**: 3.1 mg menthol. Glucose, sucrose. Strawberry, tropical fruit flavors.
	Lozenges: 5.6 mg menthol. Glucose, sucrose. Spearmint flavor.
	Lozenges: 6.5 mg menthol. Glucose, sucrose. Mentho-lyptus flavor.
	Lozenges: 7 mg menthol. Glucose. Cherry flavor.
	Lozenges: 8 mg menthol. Glucose, sucrose. Honey-lemon flavor.
	Lozenges: 11.2 mg menthol. Glucose, sucrose. Ice-blue peppermint flavor.
Halls Sugar Free	**Lozenges**: 5 mg menthol. Aspartame, 2 mg phenylalanine. Black cherry flavor.
	Lozenges: 5 mg menthol. Aspartame, tartrazine, 2 mg phenylalanine. Citrus blend flavor.
	Lozenges: 5.8 mg menthol. Aspartame, 2 mg phenylalanine. Menthol flavor.
Halls Plus	**Lozenges**: 10 mg menthol. Glycerin, pectin, partially hydrogenated cottonseed oil, sucrose. Cherry, honey-lemon, and mentho-lyptus flavors.
Luden's Cough Drops with Vitamin C	**Lozenges**: 3 mg menthol, 60 mg vitamin C. Corn syrup, eucalyptus oil, soybean oil, sucrose. Black cherry flavor.
	Lozenges: 3 mg menthol, 60 mg vitamin C. Corn syrup, eucalyptus oil, soybean oil, sucrose, tartrazine. Honey citrus flavor.

ANTITUSSIVE/LOCAL ANESTHETIC PRODUCTS

Trade name	Doseform
Robitussin Cough Drops	**Lozenges**: 1 mg menthol. Corn syrup, glycerin, sucrose. Herbal berry flavor.
	Lozenges: 2.5 mg menthol. Corn syrup, glycerin, sorbitol, sucrose. Herbal almond flavor.
	Lozenges: 2.5 mg menthol. Corn syrup, sucrose. Herbal honey citrus flavor.
	Lozenges: 5 mg menthol. Corn syrup, glycerin, sorbitol, sucrose. Herbal with natural honey center flavor.
	Lozenges: 5 mg menthol. Corn syrup, lemon oil, parabens, sucrose. Honey lemon flavor.
	Lozenges: 5 mg menthol. Corn syrup, parabens, sucrose. Cherry flavor.
	Lozenges: 5 mg menthol. Corn syrup, sucrose. Honey lemon tea flavor.
Robitussin Sugar Free	**Lozenges**: 2.5 mg menthol. Aspartame, canola oil, 3.37 mg phenylalanine. Natural citrus, tropical fruit flavors.
Robitussin Extra Strength	**Lozenges**: 10 mg menthol. Corn syrup, eucalyptus oil, sucrose. Menthol eucalyptus flavor.
Fisherman's Friend	**Lozenges**: 10 mg menthol. Eucalyptus oil, sugar. Original flavor.
Vicks Cough Drops	**Lozenges**: 1.7 mg menthol. Corn syrup, eucalyptus oil, sucrose. Cherry flavor.
	Lozenges: 3.3 mg menthol. Corn syrup, eucalyptus oil, sucrose. Menthol flavor.

Products listed are representative of currently available and widely distributed brands. Similar products, including regional and private label brands, may also exist.

PATIENT INFORMATION
Combination Products for Cough

- Patient instructions accompany each product. Read these instructions carefully before use, preferably before leaving the pharmacy, in case of any questions.
- Take as directed. Do not use any out-of-date products or exceed recommended dosages.
- May cause GI upset; take with food.
- Do not crush or chew sustained-release preparations.
- Do not consume alcohol or other CNS depressants (eg, sedatives, hypnotics, narcotics, tranquilizers) concurrently with respiratory combination products without consulting a physician or pharmacist.
- May cause drowsiness or dizziness. Do not drive or perform other tasks requiring alertness, coordination, or physical dexterity while taking these products.
- Inform a physician of antihistamine use prior to diagnostic skin or blood allergy tests.
- Inform a physician if you have glaucoma, peptic ulcer, urinary retention, high blood pressure, or if you are pregnant before taking these products.
- May cause nervousness, dizziness, or sleeplessness.
- Inform a physician if a medication appears to lose its effectiveness over time.
- No single drug or combination of drugs completely eliminates all symptoms.
- Do not use any solution that has changed color or become cloudy.

SINUSITIS

DEFINITION

Sinusitis refers to inflammation of the paranasal sinus mucosa. The paranasal sinuses are located in the bony structure around the nose from the forehead to the upper jaw (see Figure 1). Infection may or may not be involved; if involved, it may be viral, bacterial, or fungal. Sinusitis conditions include acute, recurrent acute, chronic, and acute superimposed on chronic sinusitis. Acute sinusitis is defined as a symptomatic sinus infection lasting for 8 weeks or less. Recurrent acute sinusitis is defined as

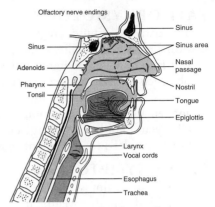

Figure 1. Upper Respiratory System

episodes of acute sinusitis separated by symptom-free intervals of at least 8 weeks. Chronic sinusitis is defined as persistent evidence of sinusitis despite continuous treatment for 2 months.

ETIOLOGY

Acute sinusitis is frequently a complication of upper respiratory tract viral infections. Sinusitis may also follow allergic rhinitis, presence of a nasal foreign body, air pressure changes which might occur when diving or swimming, or may be a complication of a tooth abscess. The swelling and impaired drainage that occur with sinusitis may result in secondary bacterial infection. The primary pathogens are *Streptococcus pneumoniae* and unencapsulated *Haemophilus influenzae*. Less frequent pathogens include *Streptococcus pyogenes*, *Staphylococcus aureus*, *Moraxella catarrhalis*, and gram-negative bacteria; mixed anaerobes are seen when a tooth abscess is involved. Predisposing conditions for recurrent and chronic sinusitis include anatomic abnormalities (nasal polyps, septal deformities, or nasal valvular collapse), immune suppression (AIDS, transplantation, or chemotherapy), humoral immunodeficiencies, immotile cilia syndrome, and cystic fibrosis. Anaerobes (*Peptostreptococcus*, *Corynebacterium*, and *Bacteroides* species), *Staphylococcus aureus*, and gram-negative bacteria (*Pseudomonas aeruginosa* and *Klebsiella pneumoniae*) predominate. Additionally, *Actinomyces*, *Nocardia*, and other fungi, such as mucormycosis in diabetic patients, are occasional causative agents.

INCIDENCE

Sinusitis is one of the most prevalent conditions in the United States. It affects almost 35 million people, and it is estimated that more than $2 billion a year

is spent on medical and surgical treatments. Because most cases are a complication of respiratory tract infections, acute sinusitis is prevalent during viral
cold seasons.

PATHOPHYSIOLOGY

The paranasal sinuses are maintained in a healthy state by adequate ventilation and by a mucociliary transport mechanism that keeps mucus flowing out-
wards to remove pollutants and accumulated debris. Any condition that
obstructs or restricts nasal air flow or mucociliary clearance can contribute to
mucosal stasis, inflammation, and microbial infection. As airflow and drainage remain blocked, secretions stagnate, obstruction becomes more severe, and
ciliary and epithelial damage become more pronounced. Recurrent acute
bouts may lead to permanent mucosal damage and result in chronic sinusitis.

SIGNS/SYMPTOMS

Facial pain is almost universal in acute
sinusitis due to the swelling in the paranasal sinuses (see Figure 2). Pain and
pressure may be present above or below
the eyes, around the cheekbone, and
in the upper jaw and teeth. Additional
symptoms include dysosmia (altered
sense of smell) or anosmia (loss of sense
of smell), nasal obstruction, and
purulent rhinorrhea. The secretions
may drain posteriorly into the throat,
causing sore throat and cough. Fever
and headache may also be present.
There may also be complaints of pop-
ping or clicking in the ears, muffled

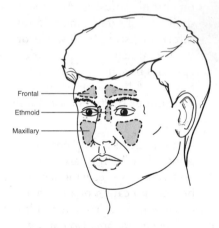

Figure 2. Paranasal sinus cavities

hearing, and halitosis. Facial pain without nasal symptoms is unlikely to be
sinusitis.

Any combination of the above symptoms may be present in chronic sinusitis,
but the primary complaint is nasal congestion or obstruction. The symptoms may be as subtle as fatigue; in other cases, nasal congestion, increased
postnasal drainage, or cough may be present. Complications of sinusitis
include orbital cellulitis, proptosis (protrusion of eyeballs), and subperiosteal
orbital abscess. CNS complications (brain abscess, subdural emphysema,
cavernous sinus thrombosis, and meningitis) may also occur, but are rare.

DIAGNOSTIC PARAMETERS/PHYSICAL ASSESSMENT

Clinical Observation: Symptoms of sinusitis are nonspecific and may be difficult to distinguish from other respiratory conditions. Because many cases are
self-limited, diagnostic tests such as detailed nasopharyngoscopy, x-rays,
ultrasonography, and computed tomography are usually not done for acute
cases, but only to evaluate chronic disease or cases with serious complications.

Interview: Patient interview is the main basis for diagnosis and questions might address the following information:

- Duration of symptoms: The classic presentation of acute sinusitis is the "cold that won't go away." Symptoms often evolve over 3 to 5 days following a cold. In chronic sinusitis, symptoms may be present continuously for weeks to months. Immunocompromised patients may mask the severity of symptoms and should be referred to their physicians.
- Nasal discharge: The discharge is purulent and often discolored, in contrast to the watery discharge of a viral "cold" or allergic rhinitis.
- Pain: Pain and discomfort tend to be localized in the area of the infected sinus, and are typically worsened when bending over, coughing, sneezing, or experiencing pressure changes in an airplane.
- Medical history: An upper respiratory tract infection is the most common preceding event, but trauma to the nasal area may also cause sinusitis. A recent or existing tooth infection may be a source for infection in sinusitis. Nasal polyps or tumors, deviated septum, or other nasal structure abnormalities are predisposing factors. Patients who are immunocompromised, such as those on chemotherapy or immunosuppressant drugs, or those having underlying immunodeficiencies such as AIDS, are more susceptible to sinusitis.

TREATMENT

Approaches to therapy: Because acute sinusitis often follows an upper respiratory tract infection, early use of decongestants may prevent its occurrence, although evidence is lacking. If purulent discharge with fever has been present for several days, bacterial infection is likely, and physician referral is warranted. Chronic sinusitis is managed symptomatically, with the addition of antibiotics for acute exacerbations.

Nondrug therapy: Steam inhalation, or humidification, with or without added astringents (eucalyptus, pine oil, or menthol), soothes irritated mucosa and moistens thickened secretions to facilitate drainage and decongestion. Steam inhalation can be accomplished by breathing through a warm, damp cloth over the face, inhaling from a basin of hot water, taking a hot shower, or using a commercially available humidifier. Topical nasal saline solutions also moisturize nasal mucous membranes and help mobilize secretions to provide a decongestant effect. Nasal saline is administered either as a topical spray or instilled with a bulb syringe (dropper) directly into the nasal passages. Nasal irrigation solutions (¼ teaspoon of table salt to 7 ounces of warm tap water) are administered with the head maintained parallel to the horizon and held over a sink. Chronic sinusitis with permanent mucosal damage may require surgery.

Pharmacotherapy: Antibiotic therapy is the mainstay of sinusitis therapy and is directed against the likely pathogens. Amoxicillin, sulfamethoxazole-trimethoprim, or an appropriate cephalosporin is commonly prescribed. Nonprescription agents to treat the symptoms of congestion, pain, and headache may be useful adjuncts. Early use of decongestants during an upper respiratory tract infection in patients with a history of acute sinusitis may prevent conditions for bacterial growth. Sympathomimetic agents are effective decongestants. Expectorants may facilitate mucus removal at high doses. Headache and local pain will resolve with improved sinus drainage but may be treated with mild analgesics (refer to the Aches and Pains monograph in the Musculoskeletal Conditions chapter for more information on these agents). Topical inhaled corticosteroids (available by prescription) are useful for chronic sinusitis.

RESPIRATORY COMBINATION PRODUCTS

▶ Indications

Common nonprescription combination products for the common cold include decongestants and antihistamines; decongestants and analgesics; antihistamines and analgesics; decongestants, anthistamines, and analgesics; and decongestants, antihistamines, analgesics, and expectorants. Intranasal and ocular combination products of decongestants and antihistamines are also available.

Advantages of combination products include synergistic activity with decongestant/antihistamine combinations and patient convenience.

Disadvantages include the inability to titrate the dose of individual ingredients, possible administration of a drug for which there are no symptoms, and unnecessary risk of side effects and drug interactions if more than one active ingredient is not needed to treat current symptoms. Locally administered drugs offer quick relief with fewer systemic side effects. However, topical antihistamines are potential sensitizers and may produce a local sensitivity reaction. Because of anticholinergic effects, use decongestants with caution in persons with narrow-angle or a history of glaucoma. Rebound nasal congestion and ocular hyperemia may occur with excessive use of topical products containing a decongestant. See Respiratory Combination Products in the Common Cold monograph.

NASAL DECONGESTANTS

▶ Actions

The sympathomimetic vasoconstrictors constrict blood vessels, reducing mucosal swelling and congestion and decreasing nasal airflow resistance. Decongestants have no effect on sneezing or itching. Decongestants are applied directly to inflamed membranes or taken systemically. Oral agents are not as effective as topical products, especially when needed for immediate relief, but generally have a longer duration of action. However, oral agents cause less local irritation and are not associated with rebound congestion following prolonged use.

▶ Indications

Decongestants are indicated for relief of nasal congestion. Regular use of intranasal products for more than 3 to 5 consecutive days may cause rebound congestion (rhinitis medicamentosa) and should be avoided. Oral agents may be used chronically.

▶ Contraindications

Oral decongestants are contraindicated in patients with severe hypertension and coronary artery disease, monoamine oxidase inhibitor (MAOI) therapy, and hypersensitivity or idiosyncrasy to sympathomimetic amines. Topical decongestants are associated with fewer systemic effects than oral decongestants, but should be used with caution in these conditions. Naphazoline and pseudoephedrine are contraindicated in children younger than 12 years of age.

► **Warnings**

Special risk patients: Administer with caution to patients with hyperthyroidism, diabetes mellitus, cardiovascular disease, coronary artery disease, ischemic heart disease, increased intraocular pressure, or prostatic hypertrophy. Sympathomimetics may cause CNS stimulation and convulsions or cardiovascular collapse with hypotension, but these severe adverse effects are rare. Hypertensive patients should use these products only with medical advice, as they may elevate blood pressure. However, some studies report that these products do not significantly increase blood pressure in normotensive and hypertensive patients. Sustained action preparations may affect the cardiovascular system less.

Rebound congestion (rhinitis medicamentosa): Use topical decongestants only in acute states and not longer than 3 to 5 consecutive days. Rebound congestion with chronic swelling of nasal mucosa may occur following prolonged use of nasal decongestants.

Pregnancy: Give only when clearly needed. One study reported that oxymetazoline did not affect maternal blood pressure and pulse rates and, therefore, is safe in the third trimester of a normal pregnancy.

Lactation: Oral pseudoephedrine is contraindicated in the breastfeeding mother. Nursing mothers should consult a physician before using other oral or topical decongestant preparations.

Children: Use in children is product-specific. Refer to individual product information.

Elderly: Patients 60 years of age or older are more likely to experience adverse reactions to sympathomimetic decongestants. A lower dose may be sufficient and safe. Use a short-acting sympathomimetic decongestant before using a sustained action formulation in elderly patients.

► **Drug Interactions**

Most interactions listed apply to sympathomimetics when used as vasopressors; however, consider the interactions when using the nasal decongestants.

Nasal Decongestant Drug Interactions			
Precipitant drug	**Object drug***		**Description**
Beta blockers	Epinephrine	↑	An initial hypertensive episode followed by bradycardia may occur.
Furazolidone	Nasal decongestants	↑	The pressor sensitivity to mixed-acting agents may be increased. Direct-acting agents (eg, epinephrine) are not affected.
Guanethidine	Nasal decongestants		Guanethidine potentiates the effects of the direct acting agents (eg, epinephrine) and inhibits the effects of the mixed-acting agents.
	Direct	↑	
	Mixed	↓	
Nasal decongestants	Guanethidine	↓	Guanethidine's hypotensive action may be reversed.
Methyldopa	Nasal decongestants	↑	Concurrent administration may result in an increased pressor response.
MAO inhibitors	Nasal decongestants	↑	Concurrent use of MAOIs and mixed-acting agents may result in severe headache, hypertension, and hyperpyrexia, possibly resulting in hypertensive crisis. Direct-acting agents (eg, epinephrine) interact minimally, if at all.

Nasal Decongestant Drug Interactions			
Precipitant drug	**Object drug***		**Description**
Phenothiazines	Nasal decongestants	↓	Phenothiazines may antagonize and, in some cases, reverse the action of the nasal decongestants.
Rauwolfia alkaloids	Nasal decongestants		Reserpine potentiates the pressor response of direct-acting agents (eg, epinephrine) which may result in hypotension. The pressor response of mixed-acting agents is decreased.
	Direct	↑	
	Mixed	↓	
Tricyclic antidepressants (TCAs)	Nasal decongestants		TCAs potentiate the pressor response of direct-acting agents (eg, epinephrine); dysrhythmias have occurred. The pressor response of mixed-acting agents is decreased.
	Direct	↑	
	Mixed	↓	
Urinary acidifiers	Nasal decongestants	↓	Acidification of the urine may increase the elimination of the nasal decongestant; therapeutic effects may be decreased.
Urinary alkalinizers	Nasal decongestants	↑	Urinary alkalinization may decrease the elimination of these agents, possibly increasing therapeutic or toxic effects.
Nasal decongestants	Theophylline	↔	Enhanced toxicity, particularly cardiotoxicity, has occurred. Decreased theophylline levels may occur.
Epinephrine	Insulin or oral hypoglycemic agents	↓	Diabetics may require an increased dose of the hypoglycemic agent.

* ↑ = Object drug increased.   ↓ = Object drug decreased.   ↔ = Undetermined effect.

▶ **Adverse Reactions**

Oral decongestants may cause restlessness, nervousness, irritability, insomnia, dizziness, tremor, headache, tachycardia, and elevated blood pressure. Tachycardia and elevated blood pressure are dose-proportional. Locally applied decongestants (drops, sprays) may cause burning, stinging, and dryness; rebound congestion may occur after 3 to 5 days of continued use. Adverse reactions are more likely with excessive use and in the elderly and children.

PSEUDOEPHEDRINE

▶ **Administration and Dosage**

Adults: 60 mg every 4 to 6 hours (120 mg sustained release every 12 hours) as needed. Do not exceed 240 mg in 24 hours.

Children (6 to 12 years): 30 mg every 4 to 6 hours as needed. Do not exceed 120 mg in 24 hours.

Children (2 to 5 years): 15 mg every 4 to 6 hours as needed. Do not exceed 60 mg in 24 hours.

Children (1 to 2 years): 7 drops (0.2 mL)/kg body weight every 4 to 6 hours as needed, up to 4 doses/day.

Children (3 to 12 months): 3 drops/kg body weight every 4 to 6 hours as needed, up to 4 doses/day.

PSEUDOEPHEDRINE PRODUCTS	
Trade name	**Doseform**
Sudafed	**Tablets:** 30 mg. Sucrose.
Cenafed	**Tablets:** 60 mg

PSEUDOEPHEDRINE PRODUCTS	
Trade name	Doseform
Drixoral Non-Drowsy Formula, Sudafed 12 Hour Caplets	Tablets, extended release: 120 mg
Efidac 24 Pseudoephedrine, Sudafed 24 Hour	Tablets, extended release: 240 mg (60 mg immediate release/180 mg controlled release)
Children's Sudafed Nasal Decongestant Chewables	Tablets, chewable: 15 mg. Aspartame, phenylalanine.
Allermed, Sinustop Pro	Capsules: 60 mg
Children's Sudafed Nasal Decongestant	Liquid: 15 mg/5 mL.
Triaminic AM Decongestant Formula	Liquid: 15 mg/5 mL. Alcohol and dye-free. Sorbitol, sucrose.
PediaCare Infants' Decongestant	Drops: 7.5 mg/0.8 mL. Alcohol free. Sorbitol, sucrose.

Products listed are representative of currently available and widely distributed brands. Similar products, including regional and private label brands, may also exist.

PHENYLEPHRINE HCL

▶ Administration and Dosage

Tablets:

> *Adults and children (12 years of age and older)* – 1 or 2 tablets every 4 hours.

> *Children 6 to 12 years of age* – 1 tablet every 4 hours.

Sprays and drops:

> *Adults (12 years of age and older)* – 2 to 3 sprays or drops in each nostril. Repeat every 3 to 4 hours (0.25% and 0.5%). The 1% solution should be repeated no more often than every 4 hours. The 0.25% solution is adequate in most cases. However, in resistant cases or if more powerful decongestion is desired, use the 0.5% or 1% solution.

> *Children (6 to 12 years of age)* – 0.25%: 2 to 3 sprays or drops into each nostril every 3 to 4 hours.

> *Infants (older than 6 months of age)* – 0.16%: 1 or 2 drops in each nostril every 3 hours.

PHENYLEPHRINE HCL PRODUCTS	
Trade name	Doseform
AH-chew D	Tablets, chewable: 10 mg
Tur-Bi-Kal Nasal Drops[1]	Solution: 0.17%
Afrin Children's Nasal Decongestant Spray[2], Neo-Synephrine Mild Strength Nasal Spray[3], Rhinall Nose Drops and Spray[4]	Solution: 0.25%
Neo-Synephrine Regular Strength Nasal Drops and Spray[3], Vicks Sinex Nasal Spray and Ultra Fine Mist[5]	Solution: 0.5%
4-Way Fast Acting Nasal Spray[1], Neo-Synephrine Extra Strength Nasal Drops and Spray[3]	Solution: 1%

Products listed are representative of currently available and widely distributed brands. Similar products, including regional and private label brands, may also exist.

[1] Contains benzalkonium chloride.
[2] Contains benzalkonium chloride, disodium EDTA.
[3] Contains benzalkonium chloride, thimerosal.
[4] Contains benzalkonium chloride, sodium bisulfite.
[5] Contains benzalkonium chloride, disodium EDTA, menthol.

EPINEPHRINE HCL

▶ **Administration and Dosage**

Adults and children (at least 6 years of age): Apply locally as drops or spray, or with a sterile swab as required. Do not use in children younger than 6 years of age, except on physician's advice.

EPINEPHRINE HCL PRODUCTS	
Trade name	Doseform
Adrenalin Chloride	**Solution:** 0.1%. Chlorobutanol, sodium sulfite.

Products listed are representative of currently available and widely distributed brands. Similar products, including regional and private label brands, may also exist.

PROPYLHEXEDRINE

▶ **Administration and Dosage**

Adults and children (at least 6 years of age): 1 to 2 inhalations in each nostril (while blocking the other nostril) not more than every 2 hours as needed. Do not exceed recommended dosage. Do not use for more than 3 days.

Abuse: Propylhexedrine has been extracted from inhalers and injected IV as an amphetamine substitute. It has also been ingested by soaking the fibrous interior in hot water. Chronic abuse has caused cardiomyopathy (severe left and right ventricular failure), pulmonary hypertension, foreign body granuloma (emboli), dyspnea, and sudden death.

PROPYLHEXEDRINE PRODUCTS	
Trade name	Doseform
Benzedrex	**Inhaler:** 250 mg. Menthol, lavender oil.

Products listed are representative of currently available and widely distributed brands. Similar products, including regional and private label brands, may also exist.

DESOXYEPHEDRINE

▶ **Administration and Dosage**

Adults and children (at least 6 years of age): 1 to 2 inhalations in each nostril (while blocking the other nostril) not more than every 2 hours as needed. Do not exceed recommended dosage. Do not use for more than 7 days.

DESOXYEPHEDRINE PRODUCTS	
Trade name	Doseform
Vicks Vapor Inhaler	**Inhaler:** 50 mg l-desoxyephedrine. Bornyl acetate, camphor, lavender oil, menthol.

Products listed are representative of currently available and widely distributed brands. Similar products, including regional and private label brands, may also exist.

NAPHAZOLINE HCL

▶ **Administration and Dosage**

Adults and children (at least 12 years of age): 1 or 2 drops or sprays in each nostril as needed, no more than every 6 hours (sprays). Do not use in children older than 12 years of age, unless directed by a physician.

NAPHAZOLINE HCL PRODUCTS

Trade name	Doseform
Privine	**Solution:** 0.05%. Benzalkonium chloride, EDTA.

Products listed are representative of currently available and widely distributed brands. Similar products, including regional and private label brands, may also exist.

OXYMETAZOLINE HCL

▶ Administration and Dosage

Adults and children (at least 6 years): 2 to 3 sprays or drops of 0.05% solution in each nostril twice daily, morning and evening, as needed.

Children (2 to 5 years): 2 or 3 drops or 0.025% solution in each nostril twice daily, morning and evening, as needed.

OXYMETAZOLINE HCL PRODUCTS

Trade name	Doseform
Afrin Children's Nose Drops[1]	**Solution:** 0.025%
Afrin Original[1], Afrin Sinus[2], Allerest 12 Hour Nasal[3], Dristan 12 Hour Nasal[4], Duramist Plus[5], Duration 12 Hour Nasal Spray[1], 4-Way 12 Hour[6], Neo-Synephrine 12 Hour, Nōstrilla[7], NTZ Long Acting Nasal[3], 12 Hour Sinarest[8], Sinex Long-Acting[6,8]	**Solution:** 0.05%

Products listed are representative of currently available and widely distributed brands. Similar products, including regional and private label brands, may also exist.

[1] Contains benzalkonium chloride, glycine, phenylmercuric acetate, sorbitol.
[2] Contains benzyl alcohol.
[3] Contains benzalkonium chloride, EDTA.
[4] Contains benzalkonium chloride, hydroxypropylmethylcellulose, thimerosal.
[5] Contains thimerosal.
[6] Contains benzalkonium chloride, glycerin, sorbitol, EDTA, phenylmercuric acetate.
[7] Contains benzalkonium chloride, glycine, sorbitol.
[8] Contains aromatics (ie, menthol, camphor, eucalyptol).

XYLOMETAZOLINE HCL

▶ Administration and Dosage

Adults (at least 12 years old): 2 to 3 drops or sprays (0.1%) in each nostril every 8 to 10 hours as needed.

Children (2 to 12 years): 2 to 3 drops (0.05%) in each nostril every 8 to 10 hours as needed.

XYLOMETAZOLINE HCL PRODUCTS

Trade name	Doseform
Otrivin Pediatric Nasal Drops	**Solution:** 0.05%. Benzalkonium chloride, EDTA.
Otrivin	**Solution:** 0.1%. Benzalkonium chloride, EDTA.

Products listed are representative of currently available and widely distributed brands. Similar products, including regional and private label brands, may also exist.

PATIENT INFORMATION
Nasal Decongestants

- Patient instructions accompany each product. Read these instructions carefully before use, preferably before leaving the pharmacy, in case of any questions.
- Patients with hypertension or other cardiovascular disease (eg, angina, cardiac rhythm disturbance), hyperthyroidism, diabetes mellitus, increased intraocular pressure, or prostatic hypertrophy should use these products only with medical advice.
- Topical products: Stinging, burning, sneezing, increased nasal discharge, or drying of the nasal mucosa may occur from use of drops or spray. Do not use for more than 3 to 5 consecutive days.
- Oral products: May cause nervousness, dizziness or sleeplessness.

SALINE NASAL PRODUCTS

► Actions

Saline solutions provide moisture to loosen and liquefy mucus secretions to allow drainage from nose and sinuses.

► Indications

To provide moisture to inflamed nasal passages and facilitate drainage of thickened nasal secretions.

► Contraindications

Hypersensitivity to any product component.

► Administration and Dosage

Refer to individual product labeling for dosing information.

SALINE NASAL PRODUCTS	
Trade name	**Doseform**
SalineX[1]	**Solution:** 0.4% sodium chloride
Pretz	**Solution:** 0.6% sodium chloride
Afrin Moisturizing Saline Mist[2]	**Solution:** 0.64% sodium chloride
Ayr Saline[3], Breathe Free[4], HuMist Nasal Mist[5], NaSal[3], Nasal Moist[6], Ocean[6], SeaMist[7]	**Solution:** 0.65% sodium chloride
Pretz Irrigation[8]	**Solution:** 0.75% sodium chloride
Pretz Moisturizing[8]	**Drops:** 0.75% sodium chloride

Products listed are representative of currently available and widely distributed brands. Similar products, including regional and private label brands, may also exist.

[1] Contains benzalkonium chloride, propylene glycol, polyethylene glycol.
[2] Contains benzalkonium chloride and 0.002% phenylmercuric acetate.
[3] Contains thimerosal and benzalkonium chloride.
[4] Contains benzalkonium chloride.
[5] Contains chlorobutanol.
[6] Contains benzyl alcohol.
[7] Contains benzyl alcohol and benzalkonium chloride.
[8] Contains 3% glycerin, Mucoprotective Factor yerba santa, phenylmercuric acetate.

PATIENT INFORMATION
Saline Nasal Products

- Patient instructions accompany each product. Read these instructions carefully before use, preferably before leaving the pharmacy, in case of any questions.
- Do not share intranasal containers with other patients.
- Do not use out-of-date products or exceed recommended dosages.

NASAL CONGESTION

DEFINITION

Nasal congestion is the subjective feeling of stuffiness due to swollen nasal turbinates. Associated nasal symptoms include increased discharge of nasal mucus (rhinorrhea), decreased nasal ventilation with resultant mouth breathing, reduced smell sensation, and altered voice tone.

ETIOLOGY

Causes of nasal congestion include viral upper respiratory infections (URIs) primarily due to rhinovirus (30% to 40% of reported cases), influenza virus (10% to 15% of cases), coronavirus, parainfluenza virus, and respiratory syncytial virus; allergic rhinitis; nonallergic rhinitis with eosinophilia (NARES); vasomotor rhinitis; pregnancy; hypothyroidism; and anatomic nasal obstruction. Allergic rhinitis and viral upper respiratory tract infections are the most commonly encountered causes; the others are diagnoses of exclusion.

INCIDENCE

As the most commonly reported complaint associated with the common cold, nasal congestion occurs an average of 2 to 4 times annually in adults and 6 to 8 times annually in children. It is also the most common manifestation of allergic rhinitis (seasonal and perennial), which has an estimated incidence of 15% to 20% in adults in the US.

PATHOPHYSIOLOGY

Upper respiratory tract infections are implicated in causing a local inflammatory response that produces mobization of extracellular fluid into the nasal mucosa via the nasal arterial supply. Increased production and secretion of nasal mucus results in swelling of nasal turbinates, culminating in symptoms of nasal fullness, nasal stuffiness, and rhinorrhea. In allergic rhinitis, these symptoms are evoked by histamine release upon exposure to an allergen to which the patient has previously been exposed. Sensitized nasal inflammatory cells (particularly mast cells and eosinophils) are thought to be responsible for the release of chemical mediators of inflammation in allergic rhinitis.

SIGNS/SYMPTOMS

Nasal congestion is itself a hallmark symptom of several disorders, including viral URIs and allergic rhinitis. The 2 disorders are distinguished by the presence of known triggers, such as pollen or other allergens, which would strongly suggest allergic rhinitis. In this disorder, sneezing, irritated and itchy eyes and nose, facial swelling, and headache are observed much more frequently than in viral URIs. The latter are usually self-limiting and resolve after 7 to 10 days. The former is either seasonal or perennial, depending on the persistency and cyclical nature of the symptoms. In either condition, the patient may report sinus pressure and headache, ear and nasal fullness due to the accumulation of nasal mucus and extracellular fluid in the nasal passages, eustachian tube, middle ear, and sinuses. Nocturnal drainage of nasal mucus into the oropharynx often produces throat pain and irritation and a foul taste in the mouth that interferes with taste sensation. Throat irritation is exacerbated by mouth breathing due to diminished nasal ventilation.

Nasal congestion also compromises olfactory sensation, sometimes rendering patients unable to taste ingested substances. Rhinorrhea is a universal symptom, and frequent forceful nose blowing increases the risk of transmission of nasal mucus into the sinuses and the middle ear via the eustachian tube, thus predisposing the patient to secondary bacterial infection of these spaces. The voice usually adopts a nasal tone when air is expelled through fluid-filled nasal passages during speaking.

DIAGNOSTIC PARAMETERS/PHYSICAL ASSESSMENT

Clinical Observation: Self-reporting by the patient is the most common method of assessment. Most affected individuals will not seek medical attention, but will attempt to self-medicate with nonprescription drugs.

Interview: Patient interview is the main basis for ascertaining the underlying cause of nasal congestion, and questions might address the following information:

- Duration of symptoms: If cessation of nasal congestion does not occur within 10 days or if fever is present, a bacterial infection must be considered.
- Nasal discharge: If the patient reports persistent clear, watery rhinorrhea not accompanied by other URI symptoms, vasomotor rhinitis may be suspected. Vasomotor rhinitis is a relatively rare condition that produces nasal congestion arising from an autonomic imbalance.
- Presence of other symptoms: If nasal congestion occurs with allergic symptoms (frequent sneezing, ocular irritation, nasal itching, facial puffiness, and headache), then allergic rhinitis is considered.

TREATMENT

Approaches to therapy: For nasal congestion associated with viral URIs, short-term self-medication is appropriate. If nasal congestion occurs with allergic rhinitis, nonprescription medication may provide relief. Referral to a physician may be necessary if severe allergic rhinitis, vasomotor rhinitis, nasal obstruction, or sinusitis is suspected.

Nondrug therapy: Symptomatic relief of nasal congestion may be achieved with inspiration of humidified air. The use of vaporizers or inhalers in the delivery of mentholated air into the nasal passages provides a feeling of warmth, which may produce weak vasoconstriction and temporary dilation of nasal passages. However, these treatments have not been shown to be significantly better than placebo in diminishing nasal congestion. Maintenance of adequate hydration is suggested; it may decrease the viscosity of nasal mucous secretions. At bedtime, the head should be raised to facilitate gravity-driven postnasal drainage of nasal secretions.

Pharmacotherapy: Drug treatment of nasal congestion may be achieved with short-term (3 or fewer consecutive days) use of topical decongestants, use of systemic decongestants, or a combination of the two.

RESPIRATORY COMBINATION PRODUCTS

▶ Indications

Common nonprescription combination products for the common cold include decongestants and antihistamines; decongestants and analgesics; antihistamines and analgesics; decongestants, antihistamines, and analgesics; and decongestants, antihistamines, analgesics, and expectorants. Intranasal and ocular combination products of decongestants and antihistamines are also available.

Advantages of combination products include synergistic activity with decongestant/antihistamine combinations and patient convenience.

Disadvantages include the inability to titrate the dose of individual ingredients, possible administration of a drug for which there are no symptoms, and unnecessary risk of side effects and drug interactions if more than one active ingredient is not needed to treat current symptoms. Locally administered decongestants offer quick relief with fewer systemic side effects. Topical antihistamines are potential sensitizers and may produce a local sensitivity reaction. Use decongestants with caution in persons with narrow-angle or a history of glaucoma. Rebound nasal congestion and ocular hyperemia may occur with excessive use of topical products containing a decongestant. **See Respiratory Combination Products in the Common Cold monograph.**

NASAL DECONGESTANTS

▶ Actions

Decongestants are sympathomimetic amines administered directly to swollen membranes (eg, via spray, drops) or systemically via the oral route. Sympathomimetic vasoconstrictors constrict blood vessels, reducing mucosal swelling and congestion and decreasing nasal airflow resistance. They are used in acute conditions such as hay fever, allergic rhinitis, vasomotor rhinitis, sinusitis, and the common cold to relieve mucous membrane congestion.

Oral systemic decongestants are indirect-acting sympathomimetics. These agents cause the release of norepinephrine in the nasal vasculature, which produces vasoconstriction, decreased edema of the nasal mucosa, and enlargement of the lumen of nasal passages. Sympathetic stimulation may also modestly decrease the production of nasal mucus; this contributes to drying of the nasal mucosa. Due to the systemic nature of these oral medications, they produce a slower and less intense relief of nasal congestion than the topical nasal decongestants. The nonprescription oral decongestants available are pseudoephedrine and phenylephrine, which have an onset and duration of effect of 3 to 6 hours.

Oral agents are not as effective as topical products, especially on an immediate basis, but generally have a longer duration of action, cause less local irritation, and are not associated with rebound congestion (rhinitis medicamentosa) following prolonged use.

▶ Indications

Oral: For temporary relief of nasal congestion due to the common cold, hay fever, or other upper respiratory allergies and nasal congestion associated with sinusitis; to promote nasal or sinus drainage; relief of eustachian tube congestion.

Topical: Symptomatic relief of nasal and nasopharyngeal mucosal congestion caused by the common cold, sinusitis, hay fever, or other upper respiratory allergies.

▶ Contraindications

Monoamine oxidase inhibitor (MAOI) therapy; hypersensitivity or idiosyncrasy to sympathomimetic amines manifested by insomnia, dizziness, weakness, tremor, or arrhythmias.

Oral: Severe hypertension and coronary artery disease. Sustained-release preparations are contraindicated in nursing mothers. Sustained-release pseudoephedrine should not be used in children younger than 12 years of age.

Topical: Systemic effects are less likely from topical use, but use caution in the conditions listed for oral agents. Adverse reactions are more likely with excessive use, in the elderly, and in children.

▶ Warnings

Special risk patients: Administer with caution to patients with hyperthyroidism, diabetes mellitus, cardiovascular disease, ischemic heart disease, mild to moderate hypertension, increased intraocular pressure, or prostatic hypertrophy. Sympathomimetics may cause CNS stimulation and convulsions or cardiovascular collapse with hypotension if overdosed.

Hypertension: Hypertensive patients should use these products only with caution, as they may produce an elevation in blood pressure because of the added vasoconstriction. Studies suggest pseudoephedrine is the drug of choice for treating nasal congestion in hypertensive patients.

Excessive use: Excessive use of decongestants may cause systemic effects (eg, nervousness, irritability, jitteriness, dizziness, sleeplessness) which are more likely to occur in infants and in the elderly. Habituation and toxic psychosis have followed long-term high-dose therapy.

Rebound congestion (rhinitis medicamentosa): Rebound congestion may occur following topical application after the vasoconstriction subsides. Patients who increase the amount of drug, length of use, and frequency of use increase the risk of toxicity and perpetuate rebound congestion.

A simple but uncomfortable treatment for rhinitis medicamentosa (RM) is to completely withdraw the topical medication. A more acceptable method is to gradually withdraw therapy by initially discontinuing the medication in one nostril, followed by total withdrawal. Substituting an oral decongestant for a topical one may also be useful. Use of a saline nasal spray is soothing. Prescription intranasal steroid preparations may also be used.

Pregnancy: It is not known whether these agents can cause fetal harm or affect reproduction capacity. Give only when clearly needed. One study reported that topical oxymetazoline did not affect maternal blood pressure and pulse rates, and therefore is safe for up to 3 consecutive days of use in the third trimester of a normal pregnancy.

Lactation: Oral pseudoephedrine is contraindicated in the nursing mother because of the higher than usual risks to infants from sympathomimetic agents. Nursing women should consult a physician before using other oral decongestant preparations.

It is not known if topical decongestant agents are excreted in breast milk. Exercise caution when administering to a nursing woman.

Children: Use in children is product-specific. Refer to individual product listings.

Sulfite sensitivity: Some nasal decongestant products contain sulfites that may cause allergic-type reactions including anaphylactic symptoms and life-threatening or less severe asthmatic episodes in certain susceptible people.

▶ Drug Interactions

Nasal Decongestant Drug Interactions			
Precipitant drug	**Object drug***		**Description**
Furazolidone	Nasal decongestants	↑	The pressor sensitivity to mixed-acting agents may be increased. Direct-acting agents (eg, epinephrine) are not affected.
Guanethidine	Nasal decongestants Direct Mixed	 ↑ ↓	Guanethidine potentiates the effects of the direct acting agents (eg, epinephrine) and inhibits the effects of the mixed-acting agents.
Nasal decongestants	Guanethidine	↓	Guanethidine's hypotensive action may be reversed.
Methyldopa	Nasal decongestants	↑	Concurrent administration may result in an increased pressor response.
MAO inhibitors	Nasal decongestants	↑	Concurrent use of MAOIs and mixed-acting agents may result in severe headache, hypertension, and hyperpyrexia, possibly resulting in hypertensive crisis. Direct-acting agents (eg, epinephrine) interact minimally, if at all.
Phenothiazines	Nasal decongestants	↓	Phenothiazines may antagonize and, in some cases, reverse the action of the nasal decongestants.
Rauwolfia alkaloids	Nasal decongestants Direct Mixed	 ↑ ↓	Reserpine potentiates the pressor response of direct-acting agents (eg, epinephrine) which may result in hypotension. The pressor response of mixed-acting agents is decreased.
Tricyclic anti-depressants (TCAs)	Nasal decongestants Direct Mixed	 ↑ ↓	TCAs potentiate the pressor response of direct-acting agents (eg, epinephrine); dysrhythmias have occurred. The pressor response of mixed-acting agents is decreased.
Urinary acidifiers	Nasal decongestants	↓	Acidification of the urine may increase the elimination of the nasal decongestant; therapeutic effects may be decreased.
Urinary alkalinizers	Nasal decongestants	↑	Urinary alkalinization may decrease the elimination of these agents, possibly increasing therapeutic or toxic effects.
Nasal decongestants	Theophylline	⟷	Enhanced toxicity, particularly cardiotoxicity, has occurred. Decreased theophylline levels may occur.

* ↑ = Object drug increased.   ↓ = Object drug decreased.   ⟷ = Undetermined effect.

▶ Adverse Reactions

Oral decongestants: Oral decongestants may cause restlessness, nervousness, irritability, insomnia, dizziness, tremor, headache, tachycardia, and elevated blood pressure. Tachycardia and elevated blood pressure are dose-proportional.

Topical decongestants: Locally applied decongestants (drops, sprays) may cause burning, stinging, and dryness; rebound congestion may occur after 3 to 5 days of continued use.

PSEUDOEPHEDRINE

▶ Administration and Dosage

Adults: 60 mg every 4 to 6 hours (120 mg extended-release every 12 hours, 240 mg extended-release every 24 hours) as needed. Do not exceed 240 mg in 24 hours.

Children (6 to 12 years of age): 30 mg every 4 to 6 hours as needed. Do not exceed 120 mg in 24 hours.

Children (2 to 5 years of age): 15 mg every 4 to 6 hours as needed. Do not exceed 60 mg in 24 hours.

Children younger than 2 years of age: Consult a physician.

PSEUDOEPHEDRINE PRODUCTS	
Trade name	**Doseform**
Genafed, Medi-First Sinus Decongestant, Ridafed, Sudafed, Sudodrin, SudoGest	**Tablets:** 30 mg (as HCl)
Children's Sudafed, Triaminic Allergy Congestion Softchews	**Tablets, chewable:** 15 mg (as HCl). Phenylalanine.
Dimetapp 12 Hour Non-Drowsy Extentabs, Sudafed 12 Hour Caplets, Suphedrine 12 Hour	**Tablets, extended release:** 120 mg (as HCl)
Drixoral Non-Drowsy 12 Hour Relief	**Tablets, extended release:** 120 mg (as sulfate)
Efidac 24 Pseudoephedrine, Sudafed 24 Hour	**Tablets, extended release:** 240 mg (60 mg immediate release/180 mg controlled release) (as HCl)
Dimetapp Decongestant Liqui-Gels	**Capsules:** 30 mg (as HCl)
Sinustop[1]	**Capsules:** 60 mg (as HCl)
Dimetapp Decongestant Infant Drops, PediaCare Infants' Drops	**Liquid:** 7.5 mg/0.8 mL (as HCl)
Children's Sudafed, Triaminic AM	**Liquid:** 15 mg/5 mL (as HCl)
Children's Decofed, Children's Silfedrine	**Liquid:** 30 mg/5 mL (as HCl)

Products listed are representative of currently available and widely distributed brands. Similar products, including regional and private label brands, may also exist.

[1] Contains echinacea, ginger, goldenseal root.

PHENYLEPHRINE HCL

▶ Administration and Dosage

Adults and children (12 years of age and older): 1 or 2 tablets every 4 hours.

Children 6 to 12 years of age: 1 tablet every 4 hours.

PHENYLEPHRINE HCL PRODUCTS	
Trade name	**Doseform**
AH-chew D	**Tablets, chewable:** 10 mg

Products listed are representative of currently available and widely distributed brands. Similar products, including regional and private label brands, may also exist.

PATIENT INFORMATION
Oral Decongestants

- Patient instructions accompany each product. Read these instructions carefully before use, preferable before leaving the pharmacy, in case of questions.
- Do not exceed recommended dosage; higher doses may cause nervousness, dizziness, or sleeplessness. If these effects occur, discontinue use and contact your physician or pharmacist.
- Patients with hypertension, coronary artery disease or other cardiovascular diseases, thyroid disease, glaucoma, diabetes mellitus, or enlarge prostate should use these products only under medical supervision.
- Do not crush or chew sustained-release preparations.
- Contact a physician if persistent abdominal pain or vomiting occur.
- If symptoms do not improve within 7 days or are accompanied by a high fever, consult a physician before continuing use.

TOPICAL DECONGESTANTS

▶ Actions

All nonprescription topical decongestants act through binding of alpha-adrenergic receptors in the nasal vasculature. Phenylephrine stimulates alpha$_1$ receptors while the imidazolines (oxymetazoline, tetrahydrozoline, and xylometazoline) selectively stimulate alpha$_1$- and alpha$_2$-adrenergic receptors. The resultant vasoconstriction reduces blood flow to the swollen nasal mucosa, hastens outflow of excess extracellular fluid from the site, and increases the diameter of the nasal passages. These actions provide quick relief (within 3 to 5 minutes) of nasal congestive symptoms.

▶ Warnings

Rhinitis medicamentosa: Continued use of topical decongestants for more than 3 consecutive days has been associated with the development of rhinitis medicamentosa (RM). RM is also described as rebound congestion, which occurs when topical decongestants are required in greater doses or with greater frequency to achieve adequate relief of nasal congestion. The etiology of RM is unclear, but may be due to direct irritation of the nasal mucosa by the vasoconstrictor drug or benzalkonium chloride, a preservative used in topical decongestant preparations.

Nasal irritation: If instillation of the topical decongestant produces local stinging, burning, or other irritation, the patient should cease the use of this agent and flush the nose with saline nasal spray.

Hypertension: Topical phenylephrine appears to be safe in patients with controlled hypertension if used properly.

Pregnancy: Topical oxymetazoline did not significantly affect maternal or fetal blood flow in 1 study of its use in pregnancy. Topical phenylephrine and oxymetazoline were not associated with a significantly increased risk of congenital malformations in 1 study. However, these agents should be used only when necessary.

Children: Topical decongestants are not recommended for use in children younger than 6 years of age. Administration of nasal drops may be easier than sprays in some children due to small nasal cavities.

▶ Adverse Reactions

Burning; stinging; sneezing; dryness of the nasal mucosa; rhinitis medicamentosa.

PHENYLEPHRINE HCL

▶ **Administration and Dosage**

Adults (12 years of age and older): 2 to 3 sprays or drops in each nostril. Repeat every 3 to 4 hours (0.25% and 0.5%). The 1% solution should be repeated no more often than every 4 hours. The 0.25% solution is adequate in most cases. However, in resistant cases or if more powerful decongestion is desired, use the 0.5% or 1% solution.

Children (6 to 12 years of age): 0.25%: 2 to 3 sprays or drops into each nostril every 3 to 4 hours.

Infants (older than 6 months of age): 0.16%: 1 or 2 drops in each nostril every 3 hours.

PHENYLEPHRINE HCL PRODUCTS	
Trade name	Doseform
Tur-Bi-Kal Nasal Drops	**Solution:** 0.17%. Benzalkonium chloride.
Afrin Children's Nasal Decongestant Spray[1], Neo-Synephrine Mild Strength Nasal Spray[2], Rhinall Nose Drops and Spray[3]	**Solution:** 0.25%
Neo-Synephrine Regular Strength Nasal Drops and Spray[2], Vicks Sinex Nasal Spray and Ultra Fine Mist[4]	**Solution:** 0.5%
4-Way Fast Acting Nasal Spray[5], Neo-Synephrine Extra Strength Nasal Drops and Spray[2]	**Solution:** 1%

Products listed are representative of currently available and widely distributed brands. Similar products, including regional and private label brands, may also exist.

[1] Contains benzalkonium chloride, disodium EDTA.
[2] Contains benzalkonium chloride, thimerosal.
[3] Contains benzalkonium chloride, sodium bisulfite.
[4] Contains benzalkonium chloride, disodium EDTA, menthol.
[5] Contains benzalkonium chloride.

PROPYLHEXEDRINE

▶ **Administration and Dosage**

Adults and children (6 years of age and older): 1 to 2 inhalations in each nostril (while blocking the other nostril) not more than every 2 hours as needed. Do not exceed recommended dosage. Do not use for more than 3 days.

Abuse: Propylhexedrine has been extracted from inhalers and injected IV as an amphetamine substitute. It has also been ingested by soaking the fibrous interior in hot water. Chronic abuse has caused cardiomyopathy (severe left and right ventricular failure), pulmonary hypertension, foreign body granuloma (emboli), dyspnea, and sudden death.

PROPYLHEXEDRINE PRODUCTS	
Trade name	Doseform
Benzedrex	**Inhaler:** 250 mg. Menthol.

Products listed are representative of currently available and widely distributed brands. Similar products, including regional and private label brands, may also exist.

LEVMETAMFETAMINE

▶ **Administration and Dosage**

Adults and children (6 years of age and older): 1 to 2 inhalations in each nostril (while blocking the other nostril) not more than every 2 hours as needed. Do not exceed recommended dosage. Do not use for more than 7 days.

LEVMETAMFETAMINE PRODUCTS	
Trade name	**Doseform**
Vicks Vapor Inhaler	**Inhaler**: 50 mg. Menthol.

Products listed are representative of currently available and widely distributed brands. Similar products, including regional and private label brands, may also exist.

OXYMETAZOLINE HCL

▶ **Administration and Dosage**

Adults and children (6 years of age and older): 2 or 3 sprays or 2 or 3 drops of 0.05% solution in each nostril twice daily, morning and evening, or every 10 to 12 hours.

Children (2 to 5 years): 2 or 3 drops of 0.025% solution in each nostril twice daily, morning and evening.

OXYMETAZOLINE HCL PRODUCTS	
Trade name	**Doseform**
4-Way 12 Hour Nasal Spray[1], Afrin Extra Moisturizing Nasal Spray[2], Afrin Original 12 Hour Decongestant Nasal Spray[3], Afrin Severe Congestion Nasal Spray with Menthol[3], Afrin Sinus 12 Hour Nasal Spray[4], Dristan 12-hr Nasal Spray[5], Duramist Plus Nasal Spray[3], Duration 12 Hour Nasal Spray[3], Genasal Nasal Spray[3], Long-Acting Nasal Relief Spray[3], Nasal Relief Spray[6], Neo-Synephrine 12-Hour Extra Moisturizing Nasal Spray[1], Neo-Synephrine 12-Hour Nasal Spray[1], Nōstrilla 12 Hour Nasal Spray[7], Twice-A-Day 12 Hour Nasal Spray[2], Vicks Sinex 12 Hour Nasal Spray[8], Vicks Sinex 12 Hour Ultra Fine Mist[8]	**Solution**: 0.05%

Products listed are representative of currently available and widely distributed brands. Similar products, including regional and private label brands, may also exist.

[1] Contains benzalkonium chloride, phenylmercuric acetate.
[2] Contains benzalkonium chloride, benzyl alcohol, disodium EDTA.
[3] Contains benzalkonium chloride, disodium EDTA.
[4] Contains benzalkonium chloride, benzyl alcohol, disodium EDTA, menthol.
[5] Contains benzalkonium chloride, dibasic sodium phosphate.
[6] Contains disodium EDTA, phenylmercuric acetate.
[7] Contains benzalkonium chloride.
[8] Contains benzalkonium chloride, disodium EDTA, menthol.

TETRAHYDROZOLINE HCL

▶ Administration and Dosage

Adults and children (6 years of age and older): 2 to 4 drops (or 3 or 4 sprays) in each nostril as needed, never more often than every 3 hours.

TETRAHYDROZOLINE HCL PRODUCTS	
Trade name	Doseform
Tyzine Pediatric Nasal Drops	**Solution**: 0.05%. Benzalkonium chloride, disodium EDTA.
Tyzine Nasal Drops and Spray	**Solution**: 0.1%. Benzalkonium chloride, disodium EDTA.

Products listed are representative of currently available and widely distributed brands. Similar products, including regional and private label brands, may also exist.

XYLOMETAZOLINE HCL

▶ Administration and Dosage

Adults (12 years of age and older): 2 to 3 drops or 2 to 3 sprays (0.1%) in each nostril every 8 to 10 hours.

Children (2 to 12 years): 2 to 3 drops (0.05%) in each nostril every 8 to 10 hours.

XYLOMETAZOLINE HCL PRODUCTS	
Trade name	Doseform
Otrivin Pediatric Nasal Drops	**Solution**: 0.05%. Benzalkonium chloride, disodium EDTA.
Natru-vent Nasal Spray, Otrivin Nasal Drops and Spray[1]	**Solution**: 0.1%

Products listed are representative of currently available and widely distributed brands. Similar products, including regional and private label brands, may also exist.

[1] Contains benzalkonium chloride, disodium EDTA.

TOPICAL DECONGESTANT COMBINATION PRODUCTS

TOPICAL DECONGESTANT COMBINATION PRODUCTS	
Trade name	Doseform
Dristan Fast Acting Formula Nasal Spray[1]	**Solution**: 0.5% phenylephrine HCl, 0.2% pheniramine maleate. Benzalkonium chloride, benzyl alcohol, disodium EDTA.

Products listed are representative of currently available and widely distributed brands. Similar products, including regional and private label brands, may also exist.

[1] In this combination, phenylephrine HCl is a decongestant. Pheniramine maleate is an antihistamine.

PATIENT INFORMATION

Topical Decongestants

- Patient instructions accompany each product. Read these instructions carefully before use, preferably before leaving the pharmacy, in case of questions.
- Patients with hypertension, coronary artery disease or other cardiovascular diseases, hyperthyroidism, diabetes mellitus, or prostatic hypertrophy should use these products only under medical supervision.
- Patients should notify a physician if they experience insomnia, dizziness, weakness, tremor, or irregular heartbeat while using topical decongestant preparations.
- Do not exceed the recommended dosage
- Do not use longer than 3 to 5 days.
- Stinging, burning, sneezing, increased nasal discharge, or drying of the nasal mucosa may occur.
- Do not share containers with other patients. Do not allow the tip of the container to touch the nasal passage. The container should be discarded after the medication is no longer required.
- If rebound congestion occurs from excessive doses and frequent use, withdraw the drug gradually. Stop using the medication in 1 nostril, then both nostrils. An oral decongestant may be used instead. Consult a physician or pharmacist if symptoms persist.

SALINE NASAL PRODUCTS

▶ Actions

Saline solutions provide moisture to loosen and liquefy mucus secretions to allow drainage from nose and sinuses.

▶ Indications

To provide moisture to inflamed nasal passages and facilitate drainage of thickened nasal secretions.

▶ Contraindications

Hypersensitivity to any product component.

▶ Administration and Dosage

Refer to individual product labeling for dosing information.

SALINE NASAL PRODUCTS	
Trade name	**Doseform**
Afrin Saline Nasal Spray[1], Pediamist Nasal Spray, Pretz Irrigation, Pretz Nasal Spray	**Solution:** Sodium chloride
SalineX Nasal Drops and Spray[1]	**Solution:** 0.4% sodium chloride
Ayr Saline Nasal Drops and Spray[1], Baby Ayr Nasal Drops and Spray[1], Breathe Free Nasal Spray, Breathe Right Saline Nasal Spray[2], HuMist Moisturizing Nasal Mist, Little Noses Saline Nasal Drops and Spray[2], Moisturizing Nasal Spray[3], Nasal Moist Nasal Spray, NaSal Nasal Drops and Spray[4], Ocean Nasal Drops and Spray[5]	**Solution:** 0.65% sodium chloride
Natru-vent Saline Nasal Spray, Simply Saline Nasal Spray	**Solution:** 0.9% sodium chloride

SALINE NASAL PRODUCTS	
Trade name	Doseform
Ayr Saline, Little Noses Moisturizing Saline, Nasal Moist	**Gel**: Sodium chloride

Products listed are representative of currently available and widely distributed brands. Similar products, including regional and private label brands, may also exist.

[1] Contains benzalkonium chloride, disodium EDTA.
[2] Contains benzalkonium chloride.
[3] Contains benzalkonium chloride, benzyl alcohol.
[4] Contains benzalkonium chloride, thimerosal.
[5] Contains benzalkonium chloride, phenylcarbinol.

PATIENT INFORMATION
Saline Nasal Products

- Patient instructions accompany each product. Read these instructions carefully before use, preferably before leaving the pharmacy, in case of questions.
- Do not share intranasal containers with other patients.
- Do not use out-of-date products or exceed recommended dosages.

NASAL STRIP PRODUCTS

▶ Actions

Opens nasal passages to ease breathing. Each nasal strip consists of two parallel plastic bands embedded in a special adhesive pad. When properly placed across the nose, the bands lift the sides of the nose, widening the intranasal space and making breathing easier.

▶ Indications

Used for snoring, nasal congestion due to cold or allergies, breathing difficulties caused by a deviated septum, and troubled sleep caused by minor breathing problems.

▶ Contraindications

Do not use over sores, sunburn, or irritated skin.

▶ Administration and Dosage

Wash and dry the nose. For sensitive skin, place a small drop of lotion under the center of the strip before applying. Remove liner and position as shown in the product literature. Gently rub to secure.

After use, remove slowly with warm water while washing your face or showering. Loosen the tabs at the ends, then gently lift both sides.

NASAL STRIP PRODUCTS	
Trade name	Doseform
Breathe Right Nasal Strips for Colds with Vicks Mentholated Vapors	**Nasal Strips**: Available in small/medium, large, and children's sizes
Breathe Right Nasal Strips	**Nasal Strips**: Available in small/medium and large sizes, in original tan and clear colors
Breathe Right Nasal Strips for Kids	**Nasal Strips**

Products listed are representative of currently available and widely distributed brands. Similar products, including regional and private label brands, may also exist.

PATIENT INFORMATION
Nasal Strip Products

- Patient instructions accompany each product. Read these instructions carefully before use, preferably before leaving the pharmacy, in case of questions.
- Always apply to a clean, dry nose.
- Avoid touching the adhesive at the ends of the strip.
- Use each strip only once, and discard after use.
- Apply at least 20 minutes before exercising.
- If rash or skin irritation occurs, discontinue use.

SORE THROAT
(Pharyngitis)

DEFINITION

Sore throat (pharyngitis) is a complaint that arises from swollen and irritated mucosal tissues of the oropharynx. Sore throat is usually self-limiting and responds to nonprescription symptomatic treatment, although the pharmacist should be aware that bacterial pharyngitis requires referral to a physician. Sore throat pain may occur only with swallowing, or it may be constant and associated with rhinorrhea, cough, fever, swollen cervical lymph nodes, tonsillar enlargement, or purulent discharge from the throat or tonsils.

ETIOLOGY

The most common causes of sore throat are infections, more than 90% of which are caused by viruses. The rhinovirus, coronavirus, influenza virus, and parainfluenza virus are responsible for the majority of acute pharyngitis. Such infections are usually short-lived (less than 7 days) and self-limiting (spontaneously resolve), requiring only symptomatic relief of sore throat pain. Infectious mononucleosis is a self-limiting, though often prolonged, viral disease occurring primarily in young adults and producing pharyngitis with lymphadenopathy. *Streptococcus pyogenes* (group A streptococcus, "strep throat") is the most common bacterial pathogen associated with the pathogenesis of acute pharyngitis; it accounts for 15% to 20% of acute pharyngitis in children between 5 and 15 years of age. *S. pyogenes* is highly communicable and is most common in populations housed in closed conditions, such as schools and dormitories. In children younger than 5 years of age, *Haemophilus influenza* type B may cause acute epiglottitis and severe throat pain. Diphtheria is an uncommon cause of pharyngitis in the United States because of the routine immunization of children against this pathogen; however, it remains a significant concern in developing countries.

Less common bacterial causes of acute pharyngitis include upper respiratory tract infections caused by *Mycoplasma pneumoniae* and *Chlamydia pneumoniae*. Painful oropharyngeal ulcers may indicate infection caused by herpes viruses (herpes simplex 1 or 2) or coxsackievirus A. Oral candidiasis with white, patchy lesions in the mouth and on the tongue may occur in patients on antibiotics or those receiving immunosuppressants. Finally, noninfectious causes such as the pres-

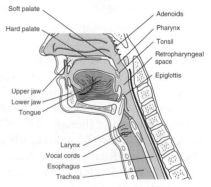

Figure 1. The Throat

ence of a tumor, a foreign body, or thyroiditis may produce sore throat. Sore throat may also follow excessive coughing caused by irritants or excessive yelling.

INCIDENCE

Sore throat from all causes is a complaint of approximately 100 million people per year in the United States.

PATHOPHYSIOLOGY

Viral infection of the pharynx has been shown to stimulate production of bradykinin in the nose, which travels in a retrograde fashion and potentiates local pain sensation. Streptococcal invasion of the pharyngeal and tonsillar tissue promotes the production and local infiltration of cellular mediators of inflammation, which cause mucosal inflammation, erythema, and pain, especially upon swallowing. Purulent secretions (exudate) may emanate from inflamed tissue; local hemorrhage and bloody sputum occur rarely.

SIGNS/SYMPTOMS

Recognition of key symptoms is important to distinguish self-limiting viral pharyngitis from more severe bacterial pharyngitis. Mild throat pain, irritation, scratchiness, or hoarseness not associated with fever or lymph node enlargement, especially in the presence of rhinorrhea, usually indicates a viral infection that should resolve within 4 to 7 days.

S. pyogenes should be suspected in any patient with pharyngitis, pharyngeal exudate, tender or enlarged lymph nodes, and high-grade fever (more than 38.3°C [101°F]). Because the consequences of delayed treatment of *S. pyogenes* include rheumatic fever and renal failure (post-streptococcal glomerulonephritis), suspected *S. pyogenes* pharyngitis should be referred for medical treatment. Any occurrence of rash with pharyngitis (scarlet fever) may also represent *S. pyogenes*; prompt referral is necessary for definitive diagnosis and antibiotic therapy.

Otalgia (ear pain) may accompany severe pharyngitis because of pain transmitted via the glossopharyngeal nerve after swallowing; referral to rule out bacterial otitis media is usually indicated in such situations. The presence of a creamy white exudate on the tonsils with lymph node tenderness and enlargement often signals mononucleosis. Rash and periorbital edema may occur occasionally. The course of the disease persists for several weeks and is not amenable to antibiotic therapy. Referral for diagnosis of mononucleosis is indicated with prolonged pharyngitis unresponsive to antibiotics; indeed, more than 90% of patients with mononucleosis who are treated with a penicillin antibiotic will develop a macular rash. Care of mononucleosis is symptomatic and supportive.

Creamy white patches in the oral mucosa are typically indicative of candidiasis. Painful superficial ulcers of the oral and pharyngeal mucosa usually are caused by viral pathogens. Coxsackieviruses cause fever without lymphadenopathy and ulcers limited to the soft palate in children approximately 4 to

12 years of age. This syndrome, herpangina, usually resolves within 3 to 5 days without therapy. Herpes viruses cause ulcers with an erythematous base in the gingiva, palate, and pharynx and respond well to symptomatic treatment with systemic analgesics and saline throat gargles. Referral for evaluation and antiviral therapy is indicated for immunocompromised patients with sore throat and oropharyngeal ulcers.

DIAGNOSTIC PARAMETERS/PHYSICAL ASSESSMENT

Clinical Observation: A patient's description of his symptoms, especially duration, will help determine the proper course of therapy. If the patient is willing, check inside his mouth for redness, ulcers, white patches, exudate, etc. If a physician referral is indicated, the patient likely will undergo a throat swab for bacterial culture. Physical assessment will likely include palpation of the lymph node chain, examination of the skin for rash, and examination of the oropharynx to elicit potential causes. Associated symptoms, phonation, and swallowing also will be observed. Given the level of suspicion for bacterial pharyngitis, empiric antibiotic therapy may be prescribed until the culture results are reported.

Interview: The focus of the patient interview is to ascertain the severity and duration of the sore throat and any associated findings that may determine the need for physician referral for specific antibacterial treatment vs symptomatic management. Obtaining the following information from the patient may assist the clinician:

- Time course of the sore throat (number of days since onset)
- Type of sore throat pain (eg, constant or only when swallowing)
- Presence of any of the following: swollen lymph nodes ("swollen glands"), fever symptoms, oral ulcers, common cold symptoms (eg, cough, rhinorrhea, sneezing, nasal congestion), rash, tonsillitis
- Similar symptoms known to be present in classmates or contacts
- Concurrent medications such as antibiotics or immunosuppressants
- History of similar complaints or episodes

TREATMENT

Approaches to therapy: Symptomatic treatment with topical or systemic agents may relieve mild sore throat pain associated with local irritation or a viral infection. Indiscriminate antibiotic use in patients with pharyngitis leads to increased bacterial resistance and, possibly, fungal superinfection. However, antibiotic treatment may be indicated for infectious pharyngitis. Therefore, careful evaluation by the pharmacist is necessary before referring the patient to a physician.

Nondrug therapy: Ingestion of cold liquids or solids produces a counterirritant effect and temporarily provides relief of mild sore throat pain. Salt water gargles (1 to 3 tsp of salt per 8 to 12 ounces of warm tap water) may soothe sore throats. Hard candies (preferably sugarless) increase the production of saliva, which bathes irritated pharyngeal mucosa, and may provide a brief soothing (demulcent) effect. Repetitive use of candy as a demulcent may predispose to dental caries; sugar-free products are useful substitutes.

Pharmacotherapy: Nonprescription drug therapy is limited to topical anesthetics, antiseptics, and systemic analgesics. The local anesthetic agent benzocaine is found in many nonprescription lozenges and sprays intended for use in treating sore throat pain. Benzocaine is safe at doses far greater than those found in marketed products; topical numbness and interference with the gag reflex are not significant concerns with benzocaine as with the more potent local anesthetics (eg, lidocaine). Benzocaine is minimally absorbed; ingestion of large quantities may cause GI upset. Dyclonine is a mild local anesthetic found in nonprescription lozenge and spray products. Both benzocaine and dyclonine alter the perception of pain at the nerves in the pharynx.

Aromatic oils and volatile compounds including menthol, eucalyptus oil, thymol, hexylresorcinol, and phenol induce the production of saliva and exert weak local anesthetic effects; they are also bacteriostatic agents. Additionally, menthol produces a counterirritant effect that results in a cold sensation. The pleasant sensation produced by these compounds accounts for a substantial placebo effect, which hampers the ability to demonstrate significant reduction in sore throat pain in controlled trials.

Cetylpyridinium chloride is a quarternary ammonium agent with minor antiseptic activity.

Nonsteroidal anti-inflammatory agents (NSAIDs) play an important role in the symptomatic treatment of sore throat pain. Aspirin, ibuprofen, and naproxen are effective for this indication. A placebo-controlled trial of acetaminophen and ibuprofen demonstrated that both drugs were superior to placebo and that ibuprofen was superior to acetaminophen in reducing the time to sore throat pain relief and the subjective sensation of swollen throat. Aspirin delivered in a chewing gum dosage form has not been shown to be any more effective than systemic aspirin tablets. However, the demulcent effect of aspirin-containing gum may account for some of the subjective relief it imparts. Do not use aspirin in children with sore throat if a viral etiology (eg, influenza, chicken pox) is suspected because its use has been associated with Reye syndrome. Do *not* encourage patients to utilize an aspirin "gargle," as this is ineffective and can be harmful in children. **For a complete discussion of NSAIDs, see the Aches and Pains monograph in the Musculoskeletal Conditions chapter.**

SORE THROAT PRODUCTS

▶ **Actions**

Sore throat products contain numerous active chemical ingredients. The following table lists the active chemicals and their actions:

Chemical Activity of Typical Sore Throat Products	
Ingredients	Actions
Benzocaine and phenol	Local anesthetic
Cetylpyridinium chloride, eucalyptus oil, thymol, hexylresorcinol, menthol, and alcohol	Antiseptic activity
Menthol and dyclonine	Antipruritic, local anesthetic, and counterirritant
Pectin	Protective colloid

▶ **Indications**

These products are indicated for the treatment of minor sore throat and minor irritation of the throat.

▶ **Warnings**

Severe and persistent sore throat or sore throat accompanied by high fever, headache, nausea, and vomiting may be serious. Consult a physician promptly.

Tartrazine sensitivity: Some of these products may contain tartrazine, which may cause allergic-type reactions (including bronchial asthma) in some susceptible individuals. Although the incidence of tartrazine sensitivity in the general population is low, it is frequently seen in patients who also have aspirin hypersensitivity.

▶ **Administration and Dosage**

Do not use for more than 2 days or in children younger than 2 years of age, unless directed by a physician. For dosage guidelines, refer to the specific package labeling.

SORE THROAT PRODUCTS	
Trade name	Doseform
Chloraseptic Sore Throat	**Lozenges:** 6 mg benzocaine, 10 mg menthol. Corn syrup, sucrose. Cherry flavor.
Cēpacol Maximum Strength	**Lozenges:** 10 mg benzocaine, 2 mg menthol. Cetylpyridinium chloride, sucrose. Mint flavor.
	Lozenges: 10 mg benzocaine, 2.6 mg menthol. Cetylpyridinium chloride, sucrose. Honey lemon flavor.
	Lozenges: 10 mg benzocaine, 3.6 mg menthol. Cetylpyridinium chloride, sucrose. Cherry flavor.
Cēpacol Sugar Free Maximum Strength	**Lozenges:** 10 mg benzocaine, 2.5 mg menthol. Cetylpyridinium chloride, sorbitol. Mint flavor.
	Lozenges: 10 mg benzocaine, 4.5 mg menthol. Cetylpyridinium chloride, sorbitol. Cherry flavor.
Cylex	**Lozenges:** 15 mg benzocaine, 5 mg cetylpyridinium chloride. Sorbitol. Cherry flavor.
Ricola Refreshers (sf)	**Lozenges:** 0.8 mg menthol. Assorted herb extracts. Lemon-mint flavor.

SORE THROAT PRODUCTS

Trade name	Doseform
Robitussin Cough Drops	**Lozenges**: 1 mg menthol. Corn syrup, sucrose, glycerin. Herbal berry flavor.
	Lozenges: 2.5 mg menthol. Corn syrup, sucrose, glycerin, sorbitol. Herbal almond flavor.
	Lozenges: 2.5 mg menthol. Corn syrup, sucrose. Herbal honey citrus flavor.
	Lozenges: 5 mg menthol. Corn syrup, sucrose. Honey lemon tea flavor.
	Lozenges: 5 mg menthol. Corn syrup, parabens, sucrose. Cherry and honey lemon[1] flavors.
	Lozenges: 5 mg menthol. Glycerin, corn syrup, sorbitol, sucrose. Herbal with natural honey center.
Ricola (sf)	**Lozenges:** 1.1 mg menthol. Assorted herb extracts. Natural lemon-mint.
Ricola	**Lozenges:** 1.5 mg menthol. Assorted herb extracts, sugar, peppermint oil, lemon oil. Natural lemon-mint flavor.
	Lozenges: 2 mg menthol. Assorted herb extracts, sugar, starch syrup. Natural cherry-honey and honey-herb[2] flavors.
Vicks Cough Drops	**Lozenges:** 1.7 mg menthol. Corn syrup, sucrose, eucalyptus oil. Cherry flavor.
	Lozenges: 3.3 mg menthol. Caramel corn syrup, sucrose, eucalyptus oil. Menthol flavor.
Cēpacol	**Lozenges:** 2 mg menthol. Cetylpyridinium chloride, sucrose. Original mint flavor.
	Lozenges: 3.6 mg menthol. Cetylpyridinium chloride, sucrose. Cherry flavor.
Robitussin Throat Drops (sf)	**Lozenges**: 2.5 mg menthol. Aspartame, canola oil, 3.37 mg phenylalanine. Natural citrus and tropical fruit flavors.
Luden's Cough Drops with Vitamin C	**Lozenges:** 3 mg menthol, 60 mg vitamin C. Corn syrup, eucalyptus oil, soybean oil, sucrose. Black cherry and honey citrus[3] flavors.
Halls	**Lozenges**: 3.1 mg menthol. Sucrose, glucose syrup. Strawberry flavor.
	Lozenges: 5.6 mg menthol. Sucrose, glucose syrup. Spearmint flavor.
	Lozenges: 6.5 mg menthol. Sucrose, glucose syrup. Mentholyptus flavor.
	Lozenges: 7 mg menthol. Glucose syrup. Cherry flavor.
	Lozenges: 8 mg menthol. Sucrose, glucose syrup. Honey lemon flavor.
	Lozenges: 11.2 mg menthol. Sucrose, glucose syrup. Ice blue peppermint flavor.
Halls Sugar Free (sf)	**Lozenges:** 5 mg menthol. Aspartame, 2 mg phenylalanine. Black cherry and citrus blend flavors.
	Lozenges: 5.8 mg menthol. Aspartame, 2 mg phenylalanine. Menthol flavor.

SORE THROAT PRODUCTS

Trade name	Doseform
N'ice (sf)	**Lozenges:** 5 mg menthol. 2.7 g sorbitol. Assorted, cherry, citrus, honey lemon, and menthol eucalyptus flavors.
	Lozenges: 10 mg menthol. Aspartame, sorbitol. Contains phenylalanine. Lemon ice[3], powerful peppermint, and cherry frost flavors.
Halls Plus Maximum Strength	**Lozenges:** 10 mg menthol, pectin. Eucalyptus oil, glycerin, sucrose, glucose syrup. Cherry, honey lemon, mentholyptus flavors
Robitussin Extra Strength Cough Drops	**Lozenges:** 10 mg menthol. Corn syrup, eucalyptus oil, sucrose. Menthol eucalyptus flavor.
Cēpastat (sf)	**Lozenges:** 14.5 mg phenol. Menthol, sorbitol, saccharin. Cherry flavor.
Cēpastat Extra Strength (sf)	**Lozenges:** 29 mg phenol. Eucalyptus oil, menthol, sorbitol. Menthol eucalyptus flavor.
Sucrets Children's	**Lozenges:** 1.2 mg dyclonine HCl. Corn syrup, sucrose. Cherry flavor.
Sucrets	**Lozenges:** 2 mg dyclonine HCl. Corn syrup, sucrose. Assorted, wild cherry, and vapor lemon flavors.
	Lozenges: 2.4 mg hexylresorcinol. Corn syrup, sucrose. Original mint flavor.
Sucrets Maximum Strength	**Lozenges:** 3 mg dyclonine HCl. Corn syrup, menthol, sucrose. Vapor black cherry flavor.
	Lozenges: 3 mg dyclonine HCl. Corn syrup, sucrose. Wintergreen flavor.
Luden's Sugar Free Throat Drops (sf)	**Lozenges:** Contains pectin. Soybean oil. Wild cherry flavor.
Luden's Throat Drops	**Lozenges:** Contains pectin. Corn syrup, soybean oil, sucrose. Honey lemon[3], berry assortment[4], citrus assortment[3,4] flavors.
	Lozenges: Contains menthol. Corn syrup, soybean oil, sucrose. Original menthol, honey licorice[5], wild cherry[4] flavors.
Halls Fruit Breezers	**Lozenges:** 7 mg pectin. Sucrose, partially hydrogenated cottonseed oil. Cool berry, cool citrus blend, and tropical chill[3] flavors.
Grape Zinkers (sf)	**Lozenges:** 5.5 mg zinc, 30 mg vitamin C. Grape flavor.
Dimetapp Get Better Bear Sore Throat Pops	**Lozenge on a stick:** 19 mg pectin. Corn syrup, parabens, sucrose. Grape and cherry flavors.
Cēpacol Sore Throat Multi Symptom Relief	**Liquid:** Acetaminophen 320 mg, pseudoephedrine HCl 30 mg/15 mL. Cetylpyridinium chloride, glycerin, saccharin, sorbitol. Alcohol free. Honey lemon[3] and cherry flavors.
Tylenol Sore Throat Maximum Strength	**Liquid:** Acetaminophen 1000 mg/30 mL. Saccharin, sorbitol, corn syrup. Honey lemon and cherry flavors.
Cēpacol	**Throat Spray:** 0.1% dyclonine HCl. Cetylpyridinium chloride, glycerin, sorbitol. Cherry, honey lemon, and cool menthol[6] flavors.
Chloraseptic Sore Throat Spray for Kids (sf)	**Throat Spray:** 0.5% phenol. Glycerin, saccharin, sorbitol. Grape flavor.
Cheracol Sore Throat (sf)	**Throat Spray:** 1.4% phenol. Alcohol 12.5%, glycerin, saccharin, sorbitol.

SORE THROAT PRODUCTS

Trade name	Doseform
Chloraseptic Sore Throat Spray (sf)	**Throat Spray:** 1.4% phenol. Glycerin, saccharin. Alcohol free. Cherry flavor.
Green Throat Spray AF (sf), Red Throat Spray AF (sf)	**Throat Spray:** 1.4% phenol. Glycerin, saccharin. Alcohol free.
Maximum Strength TheraFlu Flu and Cold	**Packets:** Acetaminophen 1000 mg, pseudoephedrine HCl 60 mg, chlorpheniramine maleate 4 mg. Aspartame, sucrose, 25 mg phenylalanine. Apple cinnamon flavor.

Products listed are representative of currently available and widely distributed brands. Similar products, including regional and private label brands, may also exist.

sf = Sugar free.
[1] Also contains lemon oil
[2] Also contains peppermint oil.
[3] Also contains tartrazine.
[4] Also contains mineral oil.
[5] Also contains glycerin.
[6] Also contains saccharin.

PATIENT INFORMATION

Sore Throat Products

- Patient instructions accompany each product. Read these instructions carefully before use, preferably before leaving the pharmacy, in case of any questions.
- Take as directed. Do not use any out-of-date products or exceed recommended dosage.
- *Lozenges:* Allow lozenge to dissolve slowly in the mouth.
- If sore throat is severe, persists for more than 2 days, and is accompanied by fever, headache, swelling, rash, nausea, or vomiting, contact a physician immediately.
- Do not use products containing benzocaine if you are allergic to procaine, lidocaine, butacaine, benzocaine, or other "-caine" anesthetics.

WOMEN'S HEALTH

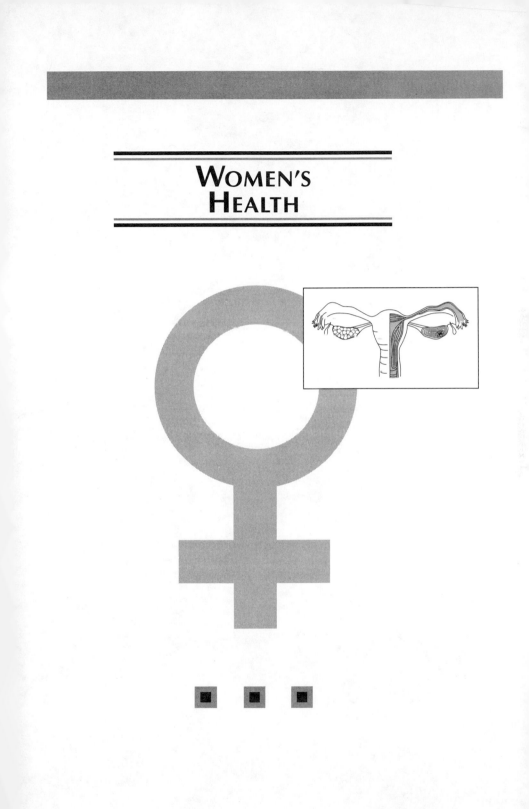

NONPRESCRIPTION DRUG THERAPY
TABLE OF CONTENTS
■ ■ ■

WOMEN'S HEALTH

INTRODUCTION

Conditions associated with women's health include problems pertaining to feminine hygiene, the menstrual or reproductive cycle, and menopause. Symptoms experienced by the female patient may be mild to severe, occur as a result of normal physiology, or be indicative of pathology. Educating the patient about appropriate feminine hygiene and proper use of feminine hygiene products, normal physiologic processes, the importance of annual gynecologic examinations, and a healthy lifestyle (eg, a balanced diet, exercise, not smoking) will empower the female patient to make informed decisions concerning her health.

The addition of vaginal antifungals and several NSAIDs (ie, ibuprofen, naproxen, ketoprofen) to the expanding OTC market has resulted in a significant benefit to women's health. In many instances, vaginal candidiasis, and symptoms experienced as a result of dysmenorrhea and premenstrual syndrome, may now be effectively treated with nonprescription medications. Increased access to effective therapy promotes self-medication practices for problems that are often recurrent. The need for fewer visits to the physician's office may potentially result in a decrease in health care expenditures associated with these conditions.

Agents used to treat conditions and symptoms associated with women's health encompass a myriad of product categories. Vaginal lubricants may be used to treat vaginal dryness associated with atrophic vaginitis. Vaginal antifungals effectively treat most cases of vaginal candidiasis when properly diagnosed. Nonprescription analgesics are often used successfully to relieve symptoms associated with dysmenorrhea and premenstrual syndrome. Other product categories include vaginal cleansers and deodorants, and sanitary protection products used during the menstrual cycle.

The vast assortment of available nonprescription products is certainly a benefit to the informed female consumer. However, improper assessment of the problem or inappropriate use of the product(s) may produce an exacerbation of the condition or result in cumulative complications. Thus, it is imperative that the pharmacist be familiar with these conditions as well as the ingredients contained in the recommended products.

Many symptoms may result from underlying pathology. Thus, it is important for the pharmacist to obtain detailed information in assessing signs and symptoms related to women's health. This may be accomplished by establishing good rapport with the patient by extending courtesy, being attentive to the patient's problems and concerns, and compiling information in an unhurried manner. Appropriate gestures and a nonjudgmental approach to questions will encourage the patient to feel at ease while discussing the conditions and use of products with the pharmacist. This approach enables the health care provider to determine what is most appropriate for the patient.

Discussing specific recommendations pertaining to product selection and use is important. Patients should be instructed to carefully follow product use guidelines. Information should be provided or reinforced concerning contraindications, warnings, and precautions associated with the use of nonprescription products. If symptoms are not alleviated or worsen within a given period of time, the patient should be referred to a physician for physical examination and further treatment.

Prevention and early detection of disease are key issues in promoting women's health. The use of nonprescription medications to provide symptomatic relief should not preclude advising the female patient to visit her physician regularly. These agents are best utilized as adjunctive measures to provide relief of symptoms after an appropriate diagnosis has been made. Thus, the importance of yearly gynecologic exams and a healthy lifestyle cannot be overemphasized.

FEMININE HYGIENE

DEFINITION

Feminine hygiene refers to the daily cleansing techniques and lifestyle practices employed by women, which promote the integrity of the normal vaginal flora and good urogenital health.

ETIOLOGY

There are two classifications of feminine hygiene products. One category of products encompasses the devices women use during menses (sanitary napkins, tampons, and maxipads/pantiliners) to absorb the menstrual blood flow and vaginal secretions. Vaginal douches and deodorants comprise the second category of products. These products make cosmetic claims; they are generally used to cleanse and deodorize the vaginal canal and to provide a soothing, refreshing effect. Efficacy testing is not required for products which limit their use to cosmetic purposes. However, douche products are considered to be drugs when the active ingredient(s) is present in a therapeutic concentration or when a physician prescribes the use of the product for a legitimate medical purpose.

Generally, good feminine hygiene may be accomplished through daily cleansing of the vulva with soap and water. However, many women use feminine hygiene products to "treat" the normal occurrence of vaginal secretions/discharge. When used inappropriately, douche products and feminine deodorants may disrupt the normal physiology of the external genitalia and vaginal tract. Preparations often contain chemicals which irritate the epithelial surface. The use of these products may result in irritation, burning, inflammation, or infection. Douching is also a risk factor for pelvic inflammatory disease (PID) and ectopic pregnancy.

INCIDENCE

Use of feminine hygiene products is widespread during the reproductive years. Surveys indicate that at least 1 person buys sanitary protection products (ie, sanitary pads, tampons, and pantiliners) at an average of 6.3 times each year in 61% of all households. Furthermore, approximately 22 million women use vaginal douches each month.

PATHOPHYSIOLOGY

The vaginal canal has self-cleansing properties. The position of the vagina, pH, microbial flora, and vaginal secretions are factors contributing to this property. The vagina has an acidic pH (3.8 to 4.2) that promotes the maintenance of protective bacteria that inhabit the birth canal. When the pH is altered and becomes more alkaline, pathogenic organisms are allowed to flourish, often leading to infection. Vaginal secretions are usually clear or milky white. Secretions are comprised of cervical and vaginal mucus, desquamated epithelial cells and bacteria. Gravity allows the secretions to travel downward; their function is to cleanse and wash the folds of the vaginal tract. Consistency and volume of secretions may change in periods of stress and normal monthly hormonal fluctuations. Vaginal odors may be present when residual secretions are left on the skin for long periods of time. Odors may also be caused by perspiration, the presence of semen or old blood, gynecological neoplasms, the presence of foreign bodies (eg, remnants of tampons), or infections.

SIGNS/SYMPTOMS

A malodorous discharge, burning, irritation, inflammation, recurrent infection, and dyspareunia (painful coitus) are symptoms of genitourinary problems (refer to the Vaginal Candidiasis monograph in this chapter); these symptoms may or may not be indicative of poor vaginal hygiene practices. Studies have shown the above problems are often correlated with the overuse or misuse of feminine hygiene products (eg, douches and vaginal deodorants).

DIAGNOSTIC PARAMETERS/PHYSICAL ASSESSMENT

Clinical Observation: Feminine hygiene is not a clinical condition. It consists of the cleansing techniques and lifestyle practices employed by women to control odor and deter complications associated with normal vaginal physiology. Factors associated with poor hygiene will usually be apparent only to the female.

Interview: Physician referral may be warranted if the patient is experiencing signs and symptoms correlating to infection or other disease processes. It may be helpful to inquire about the following:

- Pregnancy status.
- Medical conditions.
- Sexual history.
- Use of feminine deodorants and douches (eg, types of products, frequency of use).
- Nature and location of irritation.
- Pelvic pain.
- Association of symptoms with menses.
- Prescription and nonprescription medication use.

TREATMENT

Approaches to therapy:

> *Approach to hygiene* – The appropriate approach to feminine hygiene is to promote safe and adequate cleansing measures. Patients should be educated on the risks and benefits of using various products. This will allow the patient to make informed decisions about whether to purchase a particular product.

Nondrug therapy:

> *Daily cleansing technique* – The outside portion of the female genitalia should be thoroughly washed on a daily basis. Spreading the outer vaginal lips and using a soft cloth to clean the area will aid in washing away secretions. Warm, preferably unscented, soapy water should be used.

VAGINAL MENSTRUAL PRODUCTS

▶ **Actions**

Tampons, maxipads, and pantiliners contain no active ingredients and are simply used for their absorbent properties. These products are available in various shapes, sizes, and absorbency ranges to accommodate personal preferences and needs of the individual.

▶ **Indications**

These devices/products are used to absorb menstrual blood flow and vaginal secretions during menses. The "average" blood loss during menses is approximately 80 mL, but may be less or as much as 150 to 200 mL. Absorbency is an important consideration in product selection.

▶ **Warnings**

Toxic shock syndrome: Toxic shock syndrome (TSS) is a rare but potentially serious disease that has been associated with tampon use. Patients may avoid or reduce the risk of developing tampon-associated TSS by not using tampons, or by alternating tampon use with maxipads or other tampon alternatives.

It is estimated that TSS occurs in 1 to 17 menstruating females per 100,000 annually. Studies indicate that tampons with higher absorbency ranges increase the risk of developing TSS; thus, tampons with minimum absorbency ranges to control menstrual flow should be recommended. Patients who have experienced previous symptoms of TSS should be advised to avoid the use of tampons.

Early symptoms of TSS may be easily mistaken for other disease or illness. If patients experience the following symptoms while using tampons, they should contact a physician immediately: Sudden high fever (102°F or higher), sunburn-like rash, nausea, vomiting, diarrhea, muscle ache, sore throat, or confusion.

▶ **Guidelines for Use**

Consult product labeling for proper administration and use of all feminine hygiene products.

Tampon absorbency ranges: Tampons are available in several absorbencies to meet individual needs.

Tampon Absorbency	
Absorbency Range	**Absorbency Term**
≤ 6 g	Junior absorbency
6-9 g absorbed	Regular absorbency
9-12 g absorbed	Super absorbency
12-15 g absorbed	Super Plus absorbency

VAGINAL MENSTRUAL PRODUCTS

Trade name	Description
Maxipads, Minipads, and Pantiliners	
Stayfree	**Maxipads:** Deodorant, Super, Regular, Thin, Ultra Thin with Wings, Ultra Thin Overnight with Wings, Sure and Natural
Kotex New Freedom	**Maxipads:** Super, Thin, Regular
Kotex	**Maxipads:** Overnites, Regular, Long Super, Secure Hold Super, Secure Hold, Thin Super, Occasions, Ultra Thin Long, Thin Curved Overnites
Always	**Maxipads:** Ultra, Overnight, Regular, Long, Thin, Ultra
Kotex	**Minipads:** Lightdays Longs
Kotex New Freedom	**Pantiliners:** Lightdays Odor Absorbing Long, Light Days Odor Absorbing Regular
Always	**Pantiliners:** Freshweave Regular, Freshweave Wings, Alldays
Kotex Lightdays	**Pantiliners:** Regular (unscented and deodorant), Wraparound
Care Free	**Pantiliners:** Longs (original and lightly scented), Ultra Dry, Breathable To Go, To Go with Baking Soda, Ultra Dry Unscented
Tampons	
Tampax	**Flushable/Biodegradable Applicator Tampons:** Lites (junior absorbency), Slender Regular, Regular, Super, Super Plus, Multi-Pack (Super, Regular, and Lites), Satin Touch Regular, Satin Touch Super, Satin Touch Super Plus
Tampax Naturals (100% cotton)	**Flushable/Biodegradable Applicator Tampons:** Regular, Super
O.B.	**Flushable/Biodegradable Non-Applicator Tampons:** Regular, Super, Super Plus
	Flushable/Biodegradable Applicator Tampons: Regular, Super, Super Plus
Playtex Silk Glide	**Flushable/Biodegradable Applicator Tampons:** Regular, Super
Tampax	**Plastic Applicator Tampons:** Regular and Regular Unscented, Super
Kotex Security	**Plastic Applicator Tampons:** Slender Regular, Regular, Super, Super Plus
Playtex Gentle Glide Odor Absorbing Non-Deodorant	**Plastic Applicator Tampons:** Regular, Super, Super Plus
Playtex Non Deodorant	**Plastic Applicator Tampons:** Regular, Super, Super Plus
Playtex Deodorant	**Plastic Applicator Tampons:** Regular, Super, Super Plus
Playtex Soft Comfort	**Plastic Applicator Tampons:** Deodorant
Playtex Slimfits	**Plastic Applicator Tampons:** Deodorant, Non-Deodorant
Miscellaneous Vaginal Menstrual Products	
Instead	**Tampon Alternatives:** (disposable plastic reservoir; 12-hour wearing time)

Products listed are representative of currently available and widely distributed brands. Similar products, including regional and private label brands, may also exist.

■ ■ ■

PATIENT INFORMATION

Menstrual Products

- Consult manufacturer's recommendations for proper use of these products.
- If using tampons, select those with the minimum absorbency range needed to control menstrual flow.
- If you experience a sudden high fever (102°F or higher), sunburn-like rash, nausea, vomiting, diarrhea, muscle ache, sore throat, or confusion while using tampons, contact your physician immediately. Such symptoms may be indicative of toxic shock syndrome (TSS), a rare but potentially fatal illness that has been associated with tampon use.

VAGINAL DOUCHES

▶ Actions

Douche products contain numerous active chemical ingredients. The following table lists the activity and active chemicals contained in many products:

Chemical Activity of Typical Ingredients of Douche Products	
Ingredients	**Actions**
Lactic acid, sodium bicarbonate, sodium perborate	Alters pH to prevent infections.
Aloe vera (stabilized), ammonium alum	Astringents to reduce inflammation.
Benzethonium chloride, cetylpyridinium chloride, eucalyptol, menthol, oxyquinoline sulfate, phenol, povidone-iodide, sodium perborate, thymol	Antimicrobials and antiseptics to suppress bacterial growth.
Eucalyptol, menthol, methyl salicylate, phenol, thymol	Counterirritants and anesthetics to retard burning and itching.
Alkyl aryl sulfonate, octoxynol-9, sodium lauryl sulfate	Surfactants that lower surface tension to help remove vaginal secretions and facilitate spreading of product over the vaginal mucosa.

▶ Indications

Vaginal douches are used for general cleansing of the vaginal and perineal areas. These products are used for deodorizing; for relief of itching, burning, and edema; for removing vaginal secretions or discharge; or for altering vaginal pH.

▶ Contraindications

Hypersensitivity to any product component.

Douche products should not be used during pregnancy except under supervision of physician.

▶ Warnings

Povidone-iodine may be absorbed from the vagina. Advise patients with thyroid disorders, iodine allergies, and pregnant women to avoid iodine-containing feminine hygiene products.

▶ Guidelines for Use

Consult product labeling for proper administration and use of all feminine hygiene products.

VAGINAL DOUCHE PRODUCTS

Trade name	Doseform
Powders	
Triva	**Douche**: 2% oxyquinoline sulfate, 35% alkyl aryl sulfonate, 0.33% EDTA, 53% sodium sulfate, 9.67% lactose
Massengill	**Douche**: Ammonium alum, phenol, methyl salicylate, eucalyptus oil, menthol, thymol, PEG-8
Trichotine	**Douche**: Sodium lauryl sulfate, sodium perborate, monohydrate silica
Solutions	
Trichotine	**Douche**: Sodium lauryl sulfate, sodium borate, 8% SD alcohol 23-A, EDTA
Feminique Disposable	**Douche**: Sodium benzoate, sorbic acid, lactic acid, octoxynol-9
Massengill Baking Soda Freshness	**Douche**: Sodium bicarbonate
Betadine Medicated	**Douche**: 10% povidone-iodine (0.3% when diluted)
Yeast-Gard Medicated Disposable Premix	**Douche**: Octoxynol-9, lactic acid, sodium lactate, sodium benzoate, aloe vera
Betadine Medicated Disposable	**Douche**: 10% povidone-iodine (0.3% when diluted)
Betadine Premixed Medicated Disposable	**Douche**: 10% povidone-iodine (0.3% when diluted)
Massengill Medicated Disposable w/Cepticin	**Douche**: 10% povidone-iodine (0.3% when diluted)
Summer's Eve Medicated Disposable	**Douche**: 0.3% povidone-iodine when reconstituted
Yeast-Gard Medicated Disposable	**Douche**: 0.3% povidone-iodine when reconstituted.
Massengill Disposable	**Douche**: SD alcohol 40, lactic acid, sodium lactate, octoxynol-9, cetylpyridinum chloride, propylene glycol, diazolidinyl urea, parabens, EDTA
Summer's Eve Disposable	**Douche**: *Regular:* Citric acid, sodium benzoate. *Scented:* Citric acid, octoxynol-9, sodium benzoate, EDTA. In herbal, musk, and white flowers scents
Summer's Eve Post-Menstrual Disposable	**Douche**: Sodium lauryl sulfate, parabens, monosodium and disodium phosphates, EDTA
Feminique Disposable	**Douche**: Vinegar
Massengill Disposable	**Douche**: Vinegar
Massengill Vinegar & Water Extra Mild	**Douche**: Vinegar. Preservative free.
Summer's Eve Disposable	**Douche**: Vinegar
Summer's Eve Disposable Extra Cleansing	**Douche**: Vinegar, sodium chloride, benzoic acid
Massengill Vinegar & Water Extra Cleansing with Puraclean	**Douche**: Vinegar, cetylpyridinium chloride, diazolidinyl urea, EDTA
Concentrates	
ACU-dyne	**Douche**: Povidone-iodine
Operand	**Douche**: Povidone-iodine
Yeast-Gard Medicated	**Douche**: 10% povidone-iodine

VAGINAL DOUCHE PRODUCTS	
Trade name	Doseform
Liquid Concentrates	
Massengill Medicated Douche w/Cepticin	**Douche**: 12% povidone-iodine
Miscellaneous Vaginal Preparations	
Betadine Medicated	**Suppositories**: 10% povidone-iodine
Massengill Feminine Cleansing Wash	**Liquid**: Sodium laureth sulfate, sodium oleth sulfate, magnesium oleth sulfate, PEG-120, methyl glucose dioleate, parabens
Vagisil	**Powder**: Cornstarch, aloe, mineral oil, magnesium stearate, silica, benzethonium chloride, fragrance

Products listed are representative of currently available and widely distributed brands. Similar products, including regional and private label brands, may also exist.

PATIENT INFORMATION
Vaginal Douche Products

- When appropriate hygiene practices are employed, douching is usually unnecessary. Douche preparations may confound medical conditions and are best utilized under the advice of a pharmacist or physician.
- Consult manufacturer's recommendations for proper dilution and use of these products.
- Vaginal douches are **not** contraceptive agents.
- Douche no sooner than 6 hours after use of a vaginal spermicide.
- If irritation occurs, discontinue use.
- If infection or disease is suspected, consult a physician.

FEMININE DEODORANT SPRAYS

▶ **Actions**

These products are used externally and are for cosmetic use only. They are used to mask odor and are applied directly to the genital area. Good cleansing of the external genitalia with mild soap and water should minimize the perceived need for these products. Feminine deodorant sprays often contain perfumes, antimicrobials, emollients, and propellants; the actions of these ingredients are described in the table below.

Feminine Deodorant Spray Ingredients	
Ingredients	Actions
Perfumes	Mask odor. (These agents are often the primary ingredient of feminine deodorant sprays and may cause irritation in some patients.)
Antimicrobial agents	Preservatives.
Emollients	Act as a vehicle and have a soothing effect on skin.
Propellants	Expel contents from spray containers.

FEMININE DEODORANT SPRAYS	
Trade name	**Doseform**
FDS Hypo-Allergenic Feminine Deodorant with Powder	**Spray:** Isobutane, isopropyl myristate, corn starch, mineral oil, fragrance, lanolin alcohol, hydrated silica, magnesium stearate, benzyl alcohol. Talc free. Extra Strength, Baby Powder, or Shower Fresh varieties.
FDS Hypo-Allergenic Feminine Deodorant with Natural Baking Powder	**Spray:** Isobutane, isopropyl myristate, corn starch, sodium bicarbonate, mineral oil, fragrance, lanolin alcohol, hydrated silica, magnesium stearate, benzyl alcohol. Talc free.
FDS Stay Fresh Neutralizing Spray	**Spray:** Isobutane, isopropyl myristate, corn starch, sodium bicarbonate, mineral oil, fragrance, lanolin alcohol, hydrated silica, magnesium stearate, benzyl alcohol, oleyl alcohol. Hypoallergenic. *For light bladder control odors.*
Summer's Eve Feminine Deodorant	**Spray:** Isobutane, isopropyl myristate, corn starch, hydrated silica, magnesium stearate, fragrance, mineral oil, lanolin alcohol, benzyl alcohol, sodium bicarbonate. Talc free. Hypoallergenic. In Extra Strength and Baby Power Scent.

Products listed are representative of currently available and widely distributed brands. Similar products, including regional and private label brands, may also exist.

PATIENT INFORMATION

Feminine Deodorant Sprays

- Hold spray can at least 8 inches from the area to be sprayed.
- Discontinue use immediately if irritation occurs.
- Do not use on already irritated areas.
- If area is cleansed well with mild soap and water and odor persists, this may be a sign of an underlying medical condition (eg, infection, cancer). See your gynecologist or general practitioner if odor persists or worsens.

ATROPHIC VAGINITIS (POSTMENOPAUSAL)

DEFINITION

Atrophic vaginitis is the deterioration of the glycogen-rich squamous epithelium of the female genitalia during the postmenopausal period.

ETIOLOGY

Vaginal atrophy in postmenopausal women is caused by declining estrogen levels. This hormonal decrease results in thinning of epithelial mucosa in the urogenital system. Other conditions associated with estrogen loss which may result in atrophic vaginitis include the following: The postpartum state, antagonistic drug therapy, radiation therapy, oophorectomy, ovarian failure (primary and secondary), and other disease processes.

INCIDENCE

The incidence of atrophic vaginitis is difficult to predict because many older patients are reluctant to discuss the symptoms associated with vaginal atrophy with their health care providers. However, recent data indicate 20 million women in the US experience discomfort associated with urogenital aging. Studies suggest that by age 75, 2 out of 3 female patients will experience vaginal problems such as dryness, discharge, and dyspareunia.

PATHOPHYSIOLOGY

The ovaries and adrenal glands produce endogenous estrogen during the female reproductive years. The ovarian follicle produces a more potent estrogen (estradiol-17β) while the adrenal gland supplies a biologically weaker estrogen (estrone). The genital epithelium actively utilizes and metabolizes estrogen, primarily estradiol-17β. During the premenopausal phase, endogenous estrogen plays a multifactorial role in maintaining the physical, biochemical, and normal microbial integrity of the urogenital system.

Estrone is the primary estrogen produced and utilized after menopause; premenopausal estrogen levels are not maintained. The diminished steroid production by the ovary renders the estrogen-sensitive tissue of the female genitalia susceptible to many changes. Vaginal elasticity is lessened and submucosal connective tissue is increased. A gradual shortening and stenosis of the vagina is the result; a reduction in the rugose nature of the vaginal wall may also occur. Estrogen provides a trophic effect via glycogen production to the normal flora of the vagina. A decreased glycogen supply during hypoestrogen states is often disruptive to the protective microbial balance. Lactic acid production by the normal vaginal flora gives rise to an acidic pH. A decrease in normal flora may yield a less acidic pH causing the urogenital tract to be more susceptible to pathogens.

SIGNS/SYMPTOMS

The most common symptom is vaginal dryness, which results in dyspareunia. Vaginal odor associated with a watery discharge may occur. Other symptoms include pruritus, vulvar irritation, burning, and vaginal bleeding.

DIAGNOSTIC PARAMETERS/PHYSICAL ASSESSMENT

Clinical Observation: Patients should be referred to a gynecologist or general practitioner for a full pelvic examination. Diagnostic tests should be performed to distinguish atrophic vaginitis from other gynecologic disorders (eg, cancer of the female genitalia, infectious causes, inflammatory conditions).

Interview: Health professionals may recommend agents that provide symptomatic relief of the problems associated with vaginal atrophy. Proper patient assessment and history should be acquired prior to suggesting activities and products that will aid in reduction of symptoms. The interview should contain, but not be limited to, inquiries concerning the following:

• Other symptoms associated with menopause.
• Recent genitourinary examination.
• Increased vaginal infections.
• Frequency, duration, and occurrence of symptoms.
• Current medications and disease states.
• Pregnancy status.

TREATMENT

Approaches to therapy: All patients exhibiting signs and symptoms associated with menopause should be referred to a physician for evaluation and treatment. Other health care professionals can offer valuable information to the patient that may provide relief of symptoms and improve the patient's quality of life.

Nondrug therapy: Studies have shown that sexually active women generally have less problems associated with dyspareunia and other vaginal symptoms of menopause. Dilation of the vagina has also been shown to be helpful in preventing atrophic changes; this may be especially important in maintaining vaginal integrity in women lacking sexual partners. Dyspareunia, dryness, and itching may also be relieved by using vaginal lubricants.

Pharmacotherapy: Atrophic vaginitis is caused by decreased production of endogenous estrogen; thus, estrogen replacement therapy is the mainstay of treatment. Women with an intact uterus should use a progestin agent in combination with estrogen to deter the risk of endometrial hyperplasia. In women without an intact uterus, unopposed estrogen is appropriate if there are no other contraindications to its use.

> *Note –* Estrogen replacement therapy often requires 12 to 24 months to provide relief of vaginal pain and dryness. The use of vaginal lubricants should be encouraged during this interim. Not only do these agents replenish moisture, but they also protect the delicate tissue of the vaginal tract from friction, trauma, or tears during intercourse.

VAGINAL ANALGESICS AND LUBRICANTS

► **Indications**

Vaginal analgesics/lubricants act to replenish vaginal moisture, provide lubrication, and reduce irritation during sexual intercourse.

► **Drug Interactions**

Since these agents are for local vaginal use, no drug-drug interactions are expected.

► **Adverse Reactions**

Possible irritation and hypersensitivity may occur. Discontinue use if patient is hypersensitive to any product ingredient.

► **Administration and Dosage**

Most lubricants may be used intravaginally as well as externally; these products are used as needed to provide moisture and lubrication. Follow package labeling for specific guidelines.

Vaginal inserts used for prolonged lubrication during sexual intercourse should be inserted into the vaginal tract 5 to 30 minutes before intercourse. Allow 5 to 10 minutes for the insert to dissolve.

VAGINAL ANALGESICS AND LUBRICANTS	
Trade name	Doseform
Lubrin	**Inserts**: Caprylic/capric triglyceride, glycerin
Vaginex	**Cream**: Tripelennamine HCl
Vagi•Gard Maximum Strength	**Cream**: 20% benzocaine, 3% resorcinol, methylparaben, sodium sulfite, EDTA, mineral oil
Vagi•Gard Advanced Sensitive Formula	**Cream**: 5% benzocaine, 2% resorcinol, methylparaben, sodium sulfite, EDTA, mineral oil
Replens	**Gel**: Glycerin, mineral oil, methylparaben
Astroglide	**Gel**: Glycerin, propylene glycol, parabens
Surgel	**Gel**: Propylene glycol, glycerin
Moist Again	**Gel**: Aloe vera, EDTA, methylparaben, glycerin
WHF Lubricating Gel	**Gel**: Chlorhexidine gluconate, methylparaben, glycerin
Lubricating Jelly	**Jelly**: Glycerin, propylene glycol
K-Y	**Jelly**: Glycerin, hydroxyethyl cellulose, methylparaben
H-R Lubricating Jelly	**Jelly**: Hydroxypropyl methylcellulose, parabens
Maxilube	**Jelly**: Water, silicone oil, glycerin, carbomer 934, triethanolamine, sodium lauryl sulfate, parabens

Products listed are representative of currently available and widely distributed brands. Similar products, including regional and private label brands, may also exist.

PATIENT INFORMATION
Vaginal Analgesics and Lubricants

- Patient instructions accompany each product. Carefully read these instructions before use, preferably before leaving the pharmacy, in case of questions.
- Discontinue use if irritation or inflammation occurs.
- Consult a physician if infection or organic disease is suspected. Other causative factors should be considered (ie, STDs, candidiasis, bacterial vaginosis, neoplasms, inflammatory conditions).
- Routine gynecological exams should be continued after menopause.
- You and your spouse should be properly educated about menopause and therapy to relieve symptoms of atrophic vaginitis. Discussing estrogen replacement therapy, sexual activity, and vaginal lubricants with your physician is encouraged.

DYSMENORRHEA
(Painful Menstruation)

DEFINITION

Dysmenorrhea is painful menstruation. When the pain occurs in the absence of any pelvic pathology, it is called primary dysmenorrhea. When there is underlying pelvic pathology, it is called secondary dysmenorrhea.

ETIOLOGY

Primary dysmenorrhea occurs as a result of abnormal uterine activity during normal menstruation. The pain is thought to be directly related to increased intrauterine pressure and increased number of uterine contractions. Secondary dysmenorrhea is a result of the presence of pelvic pathology, such as endometriosis (ectopic endometrial tissue), pelvic inflammatory disease (PID), adenomysis (ectopic adenomatous tissue in uterine smooth muscle), the presence of an intrauterine device, or uterine fibroids.

INCIDENCE

Approximately 50% of menstruating females report experiencing dysmenorrhea and 10% report that the pain is severe enough to incapacitate them for 1 to 3 days per month. The peak incidence is during the late teen years through the early twenties.

PATHOPHYSIOLOGY

Primary dysmenorrhea occurs only in ovulatory cycles, suggesting that exposure to progesterone after estrogen priming is a critical part of the pathophysiology. Four basic abnormalities have been identified, all or some of which may contribute to pain in a particular woman. These are 1) elevation of myometrial resting tone, 2) elevation of contractile myometrial pressure, 3) increased frequency of uterine contractions, 4) dysrhythmia of contractions. These abnormalities increase oxygen demand which cannot be met by available blood flow, producing some uterine hypoxia. Critical mediators are the prostaglandins E_2 (PGE_2) and F_2-alpha ($PGF_{2\alpha}$). Increased concentrations of PGE_2 and $PGF_{2\alpha}$ are found in endometrial tissue and menstrual fluids of women with primary dysmenorrhea. The pathophysiology of secondary dysmenorrhea depends on the underlying pelvic pathology. A full discussion of these disorders is beyond the scope of this monograph.

SIGNS/SYMPTOMS

The hallmark of dysmenorrhea is cramping lower abdominal pain that may radiate to the back or thighs. Many women also experience nausea, vomiting, constipation, diarrhea, fatigue, headache, or dizziness.

DIAGNOSTIC PARAMETERS/PHYSICAL ASSESSMENT

Interview: The following suggest a diagnosis of primary dysmenorrhea:

- Painful menses began 6 to 12 months after menarche.
- Pain has previously responded to treatment with NSAIDs.
- Pain begins within 12 hours before menses begins, or on the first day of menses.
- The pain lasts for 24 to 72 hours.
- The patient has a normal gynecologic exam.
- The patient has an otherwise normal menstrual history (eg, periods are regular, of normal length, and menstrual flow is normal).

The following suggest the possibility of secondary dysmenorrhea:

- Painful menses began with the first menstrual period.
- Painful menses began after age 25.
- Pain begins more than 24 hours before menstruation starts.
- The patient has an intrauterine contraceptive device (IUD).
- The pain occurs in the absence of a menstrual period.
- The patient experiences abnormal bleeding.
- The patient has an abnormal vaginal discharge.
- The patient experiences painful intercourse.
- The patient is amenorrheic.
- There is known pelvic pathology.

TREATMENT

Approaches to therapy: All women with possible secondary dysmenorrhea should be referred to a physician for evaluation.

Approximately 80% of women with primary dysmenorrhea will respond to treatment with OTC medications. If recommended doses of OTC NSAIDs fail women with primary dysmenorrhea, they should be referred to a physician for prescription drug treatment (eg, combination oral contraceptives, NSAIDs). Women with primary dysmenorrhea are good candidates for a trial of nondrug and OTC NSAID therapy.

Nondrug therapy: There is no compelling scientific data to evaluate the value of regular aerobic exercise, a low-fat diet, and maintaining a healthy weight. However, anecdotal data suggest that some women's symptoms may be improved by these measures. All women should be encouraged to stop smoking. In addition to the reported cancer risk, smokers who have dysmenorrhea report more severe and longer pain episodes than nonsmokers.

Pharmacotherapy: Women with mild primary dysmenorrhea receive some benefit from aspirin or acetaminophen therapy. However, the NSAIDs are the drug of choice based on a large body of scientific evidence. When NSAID therapy fails patients who use estrogen-only oral contraceptives, such patients should be referred to their physician. Combination estrogen/progestin oral contraceptives are the treatment of choice in these patients, since they suppress ovulation in most cycles and are therefore the treatment of choice.

NONSTEROIDAL ANTI-INFLAMMATORY AGENTS

▶ **Actions**

Although most NSAIDs are primarily used for anti-inflammatory effects, they are effective analgesics and useful for relief of mild-to-moderate pain (eg, postextraction dental pain, postsurgical episiotomy pain, soft tissue athletic injuries, primary dysmenorrhea). They do not alter the course of the underlying disease. The following table describes pharmacokinetic parameters and recommended daily dosages of nonprescription NSAIDs.

Pharmacokinetic Parameters/Maximum Dosage Recommendations of OTC NSAIDs					
NSAID	Half-life (hrs)	Analgesic action[1]		Recommended total daily dose (mg)	Maximum recommended total daily dose (mg)
		Onset (hrs)	Duration (hrs)		
Ibuprofen	1.8 to 2.5	0.5	4 to 6	1200	3200
Ketoprofen	2 to 4	0.5 to 1.0	4 to 6	75	300
Naproxen	12 to 15	1	up to 8	600	1500
Naproxen sodium	12 to 13	1	up to 8	660	1375

[1] Food decreases the rate of absorption and may delay the time to peak levels.

▶ **Indications**

Dysmenorrhea: Excess prostaglandins may produce uterine hyperactivity. These agents reduce elevated prostaglandin levels in menstrual fluid and reduce resting and active intrauterine pressure, as well as frequency of uterine contractions. Probable mechanism of action is to inhibit prostaglandin synthesis rather than provide analgesia.

▶ **Contraindications**

NSAID hypersensitivity: Because of potential cross-sensitivity to other NSAIDs, do not give these agents to patients in whom aspirin, iodides, or other NSAIDs have induced symptoms of asthma, rhinitis, urticaria, nasal polyps, angioedema, bronchospasm, and other symptoms of allergic or anaphylactoid reactions.

▶ **Warnings**

GI effects: Serious GI toxicity such as bleeding, ulceration, and perforation can occur at any time, with or without warning symptoms, in patients treated chronically with NSAID therapy. Although minor upper GI problems (eg, dyspepsia) are common, usually developing early in therapy, remain alert for ulceration and bleeding in patients treated chronically with NSAIDs even in the absence of previous GI tract symptoms.

Renal effects: Acute renal insufficiency, interstitial nephritis, hyperkalemia, hyponatremia, and renal papillary necrosis may occur.

Platelet aggregation: NSAIDs can inhibit platelet aggregation; the effect is quantitatively less and of shorter duration than that seen with aspirin. These agents prolong bleeding time (within normal range) in healthy subjects. This may be exaggerated in patients with underlying hemostatic defects; use with caution in persons with intrinsic coagulation defects and in those on anticoagulant therapy.

Cardiovascular effects: May cause fluid retention and peripheral edema. Use caution in compromised cardiac function, hypertension, or other conditions predisposing to fluid retention.

Ophthalmologic effects: Perform ophthalmological studies in patients who develop eye complaints during therapy. Effects include blurred or diminished vision, scotomata, changes in color vision, corneal deposits and retinal disturbances, including maculas. Discontinue therapy if ocular changes are noted. Blurred vision may be significant and warrants thorough examination, including central visual fields and color vision testing.

Infection: NSAIDs may mask the usual signs of infection (eg, fever, myalgia, arthralgia). Use with extra care in the presence of existing controlled infection.

Concomitant therapy: Do not use naproxen sodium and naproxen concomitantly; both drugs circulate as naproxen anion.

Photosensitivity: Photosensitivity may occur; caution patients to take protective measures (ie, sunscreens, protective clothing) against ultraviolet light (eg, sunlight, tanning beds) until tolerance is determined.

Pregnancy: Category B; Category D in third trimester. Safety for use during pregnancy has not been established; use is not recommended. There are no adequate, well-controlled studies in pregnant women. An increased incidence of dystocia, increased post implantation loss and delayed parturition occurred in animals. Agents that inhibit prostaglandin synthesis may cause closure in the ductus arteriosus and other untoward effects to the fetus. GI tract toxicity increased in pregnant women in the last trimester. Some NSAIDs may prolong pregnancy if given before the onset of labor. Avoid use during pregnancy, especially during the third trimester.

Lactation: Most NSAIDs are excreted in breast milk in low concentrations. The American Academy of Pediatrics considers ibuprofen and naproxen to be compatible with breastfeeding.

▶ **Drug Interactions**

NSAID Drug Interactions		
Precipitant drug	**Object drug***	**Description**
NSAIDS	ACE Inhibitors ↓	Reduced antihypertensive effects of ACEIs (captopril and enalapril) have been reported with indomethacin. More prominent in low-renin or volume-dependent hypertensive patients. Consider this reaction when administering NSAIDs or anti-inflammatory doses of aspirin.
NSAIDs	Anticoagulants ↑	Coadministration may prolong prothrombin time (PT). Also consider the effects NSAIDs have on platelet function and gastric mucosa. Monitor PT and patients closely, and instruct patients to watch for signs and symptoms of bleeding.
NSAIDs	Beta-blockers ↓	The antihypertensive effect of the beta blockers may be impaired. Sulindac and naproxen did not affect atenolol.
NSAIDs	Cyclosporine ↑	Nephrotoxicity of both agents may be increased.
NSAIDs	Digoxin ↑	Ibuprofen and indomethacin may increase digoxin serum levels.
NSAIDs	Hydantoins ↑	Serum phenytoin levels may be increased, resulting in an increase in pharmacologic and toxic effects of phenytoin.
NSAIDs	Lithium ↑	Serum lithium levels may be increased; however, sulindac has no effect or may decrease lithium levels.
NSAIDs	Loop diuretics ↓	Effects of the loop diuretics may be decreased.
NSAIDs	Methotrexate ↑	The risks of methotrexate toxicity (eg, stomatitis, bone marrow suppression, nephrotoxicity) may be increased.

NSAID Drug Interactions			
Precipitant drug	**Object drug***		**Description**
NSAIDs	Thiazide diuretics	↓	Decreased antihypertensive and diuretic action of thiazides may occur with concurrent naproxen.
Cimetidine	NSAIDs	↔	NSAID plasma concentrations may be increased or decreased by cimetidine; some studies report no effect. Also, indomethacin and sulindac have increased ranitidine and cimetidine bioavailability.
Probenecid	NSAIDs	↑	Probenecid may increase the concentrations and possibly the toxicity of the NSAIDs.
Salicylates	NSAIDs	↓	Plasma concentrations of NSAIDs may be decreased by salicylates. Avoid concurrent use since it offers no therapeutic advantage and may significantly increase the incidence of GI effects. Use of salicylates resulted in decreased binding of ketorolac (two-fold increase of free drug).

* ↑ = Object drug increased.   ↓ = Object drug decreased.   ↔ = Undetermined effect.

▶ **Adverse Reactions**

GI: (See Warnings.) Common GI adverse reactions are listed in the table below:

Common NSAID GI Adverse Reactions (%)[1]			
GI adverse reactions	**Ibuprofen**	**Ketoprofen**	**Naproxen**
Nausea (with or without vomiting)	3-9	> 3	3-9
Vomiting	—	> 1	< 1
Diarrhea	< 3	> 3	< 3
Constipation	< 3	> 3	3-9
Abdominal distress/cramps/pain	< 3	> 3	3-9
Dyspepsia	3-9	11.5	3-9
Flatulence	< 3	> 3	—
Anorexia	—	> 1	—
Stomatitis	—	> 1	< 3

[1] These reactions occurred in patients taking higher-dose prescription products, and may not specifically apply to patients taking OTC NSAIDs. However, it is important to be aware of these potential adverse effects.

Ulcer – Gastric or duodenal ulcer with bleeding or perforation; intestinal ulceration associated with stenosis and obstruction; ulcerative stomatitis or colitis; gingival ulcer; rectal irritation.

Bleeding – Occult blood in the stool; GI bleeding with or without peptic ulcer; melena; hematemesis; rectal bleeding.

Other – Gastritis; gastroenteritis; proctitis; eructation; salivation; glossitis; dry mouth; pyrosis; sore or dry mucous membranes.

Hepatic: Jaundice; toxic hepatitis (high doses administered chronically); abnormal liver function tests; elevated liver enzymes.

CNS: Dizziness (3% to 9%); headache (naproxen 3% to 9%; ketoprofen more than 3%); somnolence/drowsiness (naproxen 3% to 9%); light-headedness; vertigo; nervousness; excitation; aggravation of epilepsy and parkinsonism; myalgia; muscle weakness; malaise; fatigue; insomnia; inability to concentrate.

Cardiovascular: Congestive heart failure; hypertension; peripheral edema and fluid retention.

Renal: Hematuria; nocturia; increased serum creatinine; decreased creatinine clearance; polyuria; dysuria; urinary frequency; pyuria; oliguria; anuria; renal insufficiency; nephrosis.

Hematologic: Neutropenia; eosinophilia; leukopenia; thrombocytopenia; agranulocytosis; granulocytopenia; decreases in hemoglobin and hematocrit; anemia secondary to obvious or occult bleeding; hypocoagulability; epistaxis; menometrorrhagia; menorrhagia; bruising; mild hepatic toxicity.

Special senses: Visual disturbances; blurred vision; photophobia; swollen, dry, or irritated eyes; conjunctivitis; reversible loss of color vision; hearing disturbances or loss; deafness; ear pain; change in taste (metallic or bitter); diplopia; cataracts; tinnitus.

Hypersensitivity: Asthma; anaphylaxis; rapid fall in blood pressure resembling a shock-like state; angioedema; dyspnea.

Respiratory: Dyspnea; hemoptysis; pharyngitis; bronchospasm; laryngeal edema; rhinitis; shortness of breath.

Dermatologic: Rash; erythema; urticaria; angioneurotic edema; ecchymosis; petechiae; purpura; pruritus; eczema; hyperpigmentation; photosensitivity; skin irritation; peeling. Rash/dermatitis, including maculopapular type (ibuprofen 3% to 9%).

Metabolic: Decreased or increased appetite; glycosuria; hyperglycemia; hypoglycemia; hyperkalemia; hyponatremia; flushing or sweating; menstrual disorders; vaginal bleeding.

Miscellaneous: Thirst; pyrexia (fever and chills); sweating.

IBUPROFEN

▶ Indications

Treatment of primary dysmenorrhea. This agent has additional labeled indications.

▶ Administration and Dosage

Adults:

OTC use (minor aches and pains, dysmenorrhea, fever reduction) – 200 mg every 4 to 6 hours while symptoms persist. If pain or fever does not respond to 200 mg, 400 mg should be used. Do not exceed 1.2 g in 24 hours. Do not take for pain for longer than 10 days or for fever for longer than 3 days, unless directed by physician.

IBUPROFEN PRODUCTS	
Trade name	Doseform
Advil[1], Maximum Strength Midol, Motrin IB, Nuprin	**Tablets:** 200 mg
Advil Liqui-Gels, Motrin IB[2]	**Gelcaps:** 200 mg

Products listed are representative of currently available and widely distributed brands. Similar products, including regional and private label brands, may also exist.

[1] Contains sucrose.
[2] Contains parabens.

PATIENT INFORMATION
Ibuprofen

- It is important to have a normal gynecological exam before self-treating dysmenorrhea.
- All NSAIDs should be taken after a meal or a snack to minimize GI side effects. Ideally, alcoholic beverages should be avoided while taking NSAIDs since alcohol may enhance the GI side effects of the NSAIDs. If GI symptoms persist, notify a physician.
- Do not combine 2 NSAID products or an aspirin-containing product with an NSAID.
- If the pain requires drug treatment for more than 3 days, contact your physician for an evaluation.
- If you have other medical conditions or take prescription drugs, discuss these issues with your physician or pharmacist before self-treating to avoid possible drug-drug or drug-disease interactions.
- Side effects of NSAIDs can cause discomfort and, rarely, more serious side effects such as GI bleeding.
- May cause drowsiness, dizziness, or blurred vision; observe caution while driving or performing other tasks requiring alertness, coordination, or physical dexterity.
- Notify physician if rash, itching, visual disturbances, weight gain, edema, black stools, or persistent headache occurs.

KETOPROFEN

▶ Indications

Temporary relief of minor aches and pains associated with primary dysmenorrhea, the common cold, headache, toothache, muscular aches, backache, minor pain of arthritis, menstrual cramps, and reduction of fever.

▶ Administration and Dosage

Adults: 12.5 mg with a full glass of liquid every 4 to 6 hours. If pain or fever persists after 1 hour, follow with 12.5 mg. With experience, some patients may find an initial dose of 25 mg will give better relief. Do not exceed 25 mg in a 4- to 6-hour period or 75 mg in a 24-hour period. Use the smallest effective dose.

Children: Do not give to children younger than 16 years of age unless directed by physician.

KETOPROFEN PRODUCTS	
Trade name	**Doseform**
Orudis KT	**Tablets**: 12.5 mg. Tartrazine, sugar.

Products listed are representative of currently available and widely distributed brands. Similar products, including regional and private label brands, may also exist.

PATIENT INFORMATION
Ketoprofen

- It is important to have a normal gynecological exam before self-treating dysmenorrhea.
- Do not give to children younger than 16 years of age unless directed by a physician.
- Take all NSAIDs after a meal or a snack to minimize GI side effects. Ideally, avoid alcoholic beverages while taking NSAIDs because alcohol may enhance the GI side effects. If GI symptoms persist, notify a physician.
- Do not combine 2 NSAID products or an aspirin-containing product with an NSAID.
- If the pain requires drug treatment for longer than 3 days, contact your physician for an evaluation.
- If you have other medical conditions or take prescription drugs, discuss these issues with your physician or pharmacist before self-treating to avoid possible drug-drug or drug-disease interactions.
- Side effects of NSAIDs can cause discomfort and, rarely, more serious side effects such as GI bleeding.
- May cause drowsiness, dizziness, or blurred vision; observe caution while driving or performing other tasks requiring alertness, coordination, or physical dexterity.
- Notify physician if rash, itching, visual disturbances, weight gain, edema, black stools, or persistent headache occurs.

NAPROXEN

▶ **Indications**

Temporary relief of minor aches and pains associated with primary dysmenorrhea, the common cold, headache, toothache, muscular aches, backache, minor pain of arthritis, pain of menstrual cramps, and reduction of fever.

▶ **Administration and Dosage**

Adults: 200 mg with a full glass of liquid every 8 to 12 hours while symptoms persist. Some patients may find an initial dose of 400 mg followed by 200 mg 12 hours later, if necessary, will give better relief. Do not exceed 600 mg in 24 hours unless otherwise directed. Use the smallest effective dose.

Children: Do not give to children younger than 12 years of age except under the advice and supervision of a physician.

NAPROXEN PRODUCTS	
Trade name	**Doseform**
Aleve	**Tablets, Caplets, and Gelcaps**: 200 mg (220 mg naproxen sodium)

Products listed are representative of currently available and widely distributed brands. Similar products, including regional and private label brands, may also exist.

PATIENT INFORMATION
Naproxen

- It is important to have a normal gynecological exam before self-treating dysmenorrhea.
- Take all NSAIDs after a meal or a snack to minimize GI side effects. Ideally, avoid alcoholic beverages while taking NSAIDs because alcohol may enhance the GI side effects. If GI symptoms persist, notify a physician.
- Do not combine 2 NSAID products or an aspirin-containing product with an NSAID.
- If the pain requires drug treatment for more than 3 days, contact your physician for an evaluation.
- If you have other medical conditions or take prescription drugs, discuss these issues with your physician or pharmacist before self-treating to avoid possible drug-drug or drug-disease interactions.
- Side effects of NSAIDs can cause discomfort and, rarely, more serious side effects such as GI bleeding.
- May cause drowsiness, dizziness, or blurred vision; observe caution while driving or performing other tasks requiring alertness, coordination, or physical dexterity.
- Notify physician if rash, itching, visual disturbances, weight gain, edema, black stools, or persistent headache occurs.

ANALGESIC COMBINATIONS

▶ **Actions**

Acetaminophen (APAP): Acetaminophen is an analgesic; however, the site and mechanism of its analgesic effect is unclear. The agent may have a direct effect on the pain threshold. For more information on acetaminophen, refer to the Acetaminophen monograph in the Premenstrual Syndrome chapter.

Caffeine: Caffeine, a traditional component of many analgesic formulations, may be beneficial in certain vascular headaches. For more information on caffeine, refer to the Caffeine monograph in the Drowsiness/Lethargy chapter.

Pamabrom: Pamabrom is used as a diuretic to ease water retention.

Pyrilamine maleate: Pyrilamine maleate is an antihistamine.

▶ **Administration and Dosage**

Do not take acetaminophen more often than directed. Do not exceed recommended dosage without the advice of a physician. Take tablets, caplets, and gelcaps by mouth. Swallow extended-release formulations whole; do not crush or chew.

Adults: The average adult dose is 1 or 2 capsules every 2 to 6 hours as needed for pain. Check individual product labeling for guidelines. Do not exceed 4 g/day for all formulations containing acetaminophen.

ANALGESIC COMBINATION PRODUCTS	
Trade name	Doseform
Women's Tylenol Menstrual Relief	**Caplets**: 500 mg acetaminophen, 25 mg pamabrom
Midol Maximum Strength Menstrual Formula	**Caplets, Gelcaps**: 500 mg acetaminophen, 60 mg caffeine, 15 mg pyrilamine maleate
Maximum Strength Multi-Symptom Pamprin	**Caplets, Tablets**: 500 mg acetaminophen, 25 mg pamabrom, 15 mg pyrilamine maleate
Maximum Cramp Relief Pamprin	**Caplets**: 250 mg acetaminophen, 250 mg magnesium salicylate, 25 mg pamabrom

Products listed are representative of currently available and widely distributed brands. Similar products, including regional and private label brands, may also exist.

PATIENT INFORMATION

Analgesic Combination Products

- It is important to have a normal gynecological exam before self-treating dysmenorrhea.
- Carefully read product instructions before use, preferably before leaving the pharmacy, in case of questions.
- Do not exceed the recommended dosage. Do not exceed a total dose of 4 g/day of acetaminophen in all formulations consumed.
- Because of possible drug interactions, do not take any OTC or prescription medications without consulting a physician or pharmacist.
- Do not take caffeine products at bedtime.
- For pain, do not use for more than 10 days in adults without consulting a physician.
- If symptoms persist or worsen, or if new symptoms develop, contact a physician.
- Be aware of other OTC (eg, combination products for pain, cold, cough, or allergy) and prescription medications that contain acetaminophen.
- If you have severe symptoms, see a physician for proper evaluation.

PREMENSTRUAL SYNDROME
(PMS)

DEFINITION

Premenstrual syndrome, often referred to as PMS, is a broad term used to describe the array of psychological and physiological symptoms that occur cyclically and consistently during the late luteal phase of the menstrual cycle and disappear within 4 days after the onset of menstruation. There are more than 150 documented symptoms used to characterize PMS; because of this vast symptomatology, PMS has no standard definition and remains a poorly defined disorder. Premenstrual dysphoric disorder (PMDD) is a severe form of PMS that is temporarily disabling and disrupts at least one aspect of the patient's daily functioning (eg, lifestyle, relationships, occupation). Definitive criteria for PMDD are a minimum of five premenstrual symptoms, one of which must be a change in emotional response.

ETIOLOGY

PMS is a symptom complex with no proven etiology. Numerous studies have been conducted attempting to elucidate a common cause; hormonal changes, neurotransmitter dysfunction, and nutritional factors have been implicated. Proposed theories include progesterone deficiency and alterations in progesterone metabolism, estrogen excess, declining estrogen levels, decreased progesterone:estrogen ratio, increased testosterone, excess prolactin, increased renin-angiotensin-aldosterone activity, prostaglandin response, endogenous endorphin withdrawal, central changes to catecholamines, abnormal serotonin functioning, deficiency of or decrease in the availability of pyridoxine, disturbances in calcium regulation, zinc deficiency, and copper excess. Results of these trials are inconsistent and conclusive evidence is lacking. Symptoms have been shown to disappear in anovulatory females; thus, current opinion focuses on biological and psychological manifestations triggered by normal physiologic changes that occur in the luteal phase but are absent in the follicular phase of the menstrual cycle.

INCIDENCE

Millions of premenopausal females have premenstrual complaints. However, the incidence is difficult to ascertain because many women do not seek advice from health professionals and often self-treat symptoms with nonprescription drugs. Although reported in all age groups, the onset of PMS is most likely to occur in ovulating females in their late twenties to early thirties. An increased risk for premenstrual symptoms is associated with increased age and parity. Prevalence rates estimate that 70% to 90% of menstruating females experience some physical, emotional, or behavioral symptoms for a few days prior to menses. PMDD afflicts 2% to 10% of ovulating females; symptoms may last up to two weeks between ovulation and menses. After the initial onset, PMS symptoms generally occur cyclically throughout the female's reproductive years.

PATHOPHYSIOLOGY

The most likely theory contributing to the pathophysiology of PMS concerns the normal hormonal fluctuations around the time of ovulation that result in a neurotransmitter disturbance. This neuroendocrine interaction may result in related biochemical events within the central nervous system and other target tissues.

SIGNS/SYMPTOMS

Symptoms/complaints include the following:

Most common: Generalized headache, breast swelling/tenderness, bloating, fatigue, anxiety, depression, irritability, mood swings, weight gain, and fluid retention are the most commonly reported symptoms. Most symptoms are considered problematic; however, one study found that 66% of women reported at least one positive symptom (eg, increased libido, creativity, energy, industriousness). Presenting symptoms usually have an individualized pattern, with severity being stabilized across several cycles.

Behavioral/Psychological: Aggression; agitation; altered libido; anger; inability to experience pleasure; anxiety; change in appetite; confusion; crying spells; decreased feelings of well-being; decreased motivation; depression; dysphoria; emotional lability; insecure feelings; suffocation feelings; food cravings (eg, for chocolate or salty/sweet foods); forgetfulness; frustration; guilt; hopelessness; hostility; hypersomnia; insomnia; irritability; loneliness; low self-esteem; nightmares; numbness; panic attacks; phobias; poor concentration; poor coordination; psychological discomfort; reduced coping skills; restlessness; reduced judgment; sadness; sense of being out of control; shame; suicidal tendencies; tearfulness; tension; violent tendencies.

Physical: Abdominal bloating; acne; backache; breast swelling and tenderness; cold sores; cold sweats; constipation; cramps; diarrhea; dizziness; fatigue; fluid retention (of the face, feet, ankles, or hands); generalized aches and pains; headaches/migraines; hot flashes; joint pain; muscle aches/pains; nausea; oily skin; palpitations; rhinitis; styes; thirst; vomiting; weight gain.

Functional: Decreased efficiency or work impairment; increased interpersonal conflicts; social isolation.

DIAGNOSTIC PARAMETERS/PHYSICAL ASSESSMENT

Clinical Observation: Diagnosis is made via a process of exclusion. Currently, there are no laboratory tests that confirm the diagnosis of PMS. However, several psychiatric, medical, and gynecological disorders with symptoms that coincide with PMS may be eliminated by laboratory testing. Furthermore, symptoms of other underlying medical and psychiatric disorders often are exacerbated during the luteal phase of the menstrual cycle. A detailed history of complaints, review of recent physical examination, and a daily symptom log maintained over a period of two or more cycles aid in the initial diagnosis of PMS.

Interview: Patients describing symptoms that significantly impact their daily functioning warrant immediate physician referral. It may be useful to inquire about the following:

- Severity, duration, and frequency of symptoms
- Regularity of menstrual cycle
- Current medical conditions
- Current medications (prescription and nonprescription)
- Lifestyle (eg, diet, exercise, sleep patterns)
- Pregnancy status

TREATMENT

Approaches to therapy: Utilize the above diagnostic parameters to evaluate the patient. In addition, a daily symptom log maintained by the patient over a period of at least two cycles is beneficial for the physician to discern the severity and cyclic regularity of complaints. Appropriate therapy is aimed at relieving bothersome symptoms. Clinicians may recommend nondrug therapy and appropriate pharmacotherapy for mild symptoms. Complaints related to severe PMS or PMDD warrant immediate referral to a physician for medical evaluation.

Note – The treatment of PMS is often a lengthy process. Each intervention should be attempted for at least two cycles to eliminate the high placebo response associated with this syndrome and allow for cycle variability.

Nondrug therapy:

Patient education and counseling – Patient education and counseling concerning PMS has been reported to be informative and therapeutic. Patient information helps improve a women's perceptions of her symptoms; this aids in helping her cope better. PMS may be treated by lifestyle modifications, which often relieve symptoms associated with mild PMS. Appropriate lifestyle changes include dietary modifications, aerobic exercise, relaxation training, cognitive-behavioral strategies, and limiting tobacco use.

Dietary recommendations – Dietary recommendations include eliminating refined sugar, artificial sweeteners, and caffeine. Encourage women to consume more complex carbohydrates, eat smaller and more frequent meals, and decrease fat, red meat, salt, chocolate, and dairy product consumption. A healthy diet generally provides symptomatic relief for many complaints of mild PMS.

Aerobic exercise – Aerobic exercise may be helpful for reducing symptoms by increasing endorphin levels. Beneficial psychological changes also are thought to accompany increased muscle tone. Personal stress, breast tenderness/swelling, and fluid retention are the symptoms most commonly relieved via aerobic exercise. Encourage women to participate in aerobic activity (eg, jogging, fitness walking, cycling) at least four times weekly for 30-minute sessions.

Relaxation training – Relaxation training (stress-reduction strategies) and cognitive-behavioral strategies (anger-management training) also have shown beneficial results.

Pharmacotherapy: Sarafem (fluoxetine hydrochloride) was the first serotonergic antidepressant approved by the FDA for PMDD. The recommended dose of this prescription drug is 20 mg/day. Doses above 60 mg/day have not been studied systemically in patients with PMDD. Do not exceed 80 mg/day fluoxetine. The effectiveness of *Sarafem* taken longer than 6 months has not been evaluated in controlled trials. Periodically reevaluate the use of *Sarafem* for extended periods for usefulness in the individual patient.

Other prescription serotonergic agents also are used for the treatment of PMDD. Agents and doses most commonly used are 50 to 150 mg/day sertraline and 12.5 to 25 mg/day paroxetine.

Nonprescription medications often are used to treat symptoms associated with PMS. Agents that may be recommended are nonsteroidal anti-inflammatory drugs (NSAIDs), acetaminophen, and aspirin. The evidence is controversial concerning the efficacy of pyridoxine, calcium, zinc, and other nutritional/herbal supplements. Further studies are needed to support the use of these supplements for the treatment of PMS.

NONSTEROIDAL ANTI-INFLAMMATORY AGENTS

▶ **Actions**

NSAIDs have analgesic, anti-inflammatory, and antipyretic activities. The major mechanism of action of NSAIDs is believed to be inhibition of cyclooxygenase activity and prostaglandin synthesis. Other mechanisms, such as inhibition of lipoxygenase, leukotriene synthesis, lysosomal enzyme release, neutrophil aggregation, and various cell-membrane functions, may exist as well.

▶ **Indications**

NSAIDs may be used to relieve symptoms of mild to moderate premenstrual and menstrual pain. These agents have numerous other labeled indications as well.

▶ **Contraindications**

NSAID hypersensitivity: Because of potential cross-sensitivity to other NSAIDs, do not give these agents to patients in whom aspirin or other NSAIDs have induced symptoms of asthma, rhinitis, urticaria, nasal polyps, angioedema, bronchospasm, and other symptoms of allergic or anaphylactoid reactions. Severe but rarely fatal anaphylactic-like and asthmatic reactions have been reported in such patients receiving NSAIDs.

▶ **Warnings**

Acute renal insufficiency: Patients with preexisting renal disease or compromised renal perfusion are at greatest risk. A form of renal toxicity seen in patients with prerenal conditions leads to reduced renal blood flow or blood volume. NSAID use may cause a dose-dependent reduction in prostaglandin formation and precipitate renal decompensation. Patients at greatest risk are the elderly, premature infants, those with heart failure, renal or hepatic dysfunction, systemic lupus erythematosus (SLE), dehydration, diabetes mellitus, external volume depletion, chronic glomerulonephritis, and patients taking diuretics. Recovery usually follows discontinuation.

Cardiovascular effects: May cause fluid retention and peripheral edema. Use with caution in patients with compromised cardiac function and hypertension, as well as those on chronic diuretic therapy or with other conditions predisposing to fluid retention. Agents may be associated with significant deterioration of circulatory hemodynamics in severe heart failure and hyponatremia, presumably because of inhibition of prostaglandin-dependent compensatory mechanisms.

Gastrointestinal effects: With chronic use of NSAIDs, gastrointestinal (GI) toxicity (including inflammation, bleeding, ulcerations, and perforation of the stomach and the small and large intestine) may occur with or without warning. High-dose NSAIDs probably carry a greater risk of causing GI adverse effects. Patients with a history of GI lesions should consult a physician before using these products. These effects may be more pronounced in elderly patients.

Hyperkalemia: Another potentially serious NSAID-induced renal electrolyte abnormality is hyperkalemia. NSAIDs tend to blunt prostaglandin-mediated renin release, leading to diminished aldosterone formation and, hence, decreased potassium excretion. NSAIDs may augment sodium and chloride reabsorption within the renal tubule in instances of diminished glomerular filtration rate by opposing natriuretic and diuretic prostaglandins. This decreases the delivery of intraluminal sodium for sodium-potassium exchange at the distal nephron.

Hypersensitivity: Severe hypersensitivity reactions with fever, rash, abdominal pain, headache, nausea, vomiting, signs of liver damage, and meningitis have occurred in ibuprofen-treated patients, especially those with SLE or other collagen diseases. Anaphylactoid reactions have occurred in patients with aspirin hypersensitivity.

Infection: NSAIDs may mask the usual signs of infection (eg, fever, myalgia, arthralgia). Use with extra care in the presence of existing controlled infection.

Platelet aggregation: NSAIDs may inhibit platelet aggregation; the effect is reversible, quantitatively less, and of shorter duration than that seen with aspirin. These agents prolong bleeding time (within normal range) in healthy subjects; this may be exaggerated in patients with underlying hemostatic defects. Use with caution in persons with intrinsic coagulation defects and in patients on anticoagulant therapy.

Photosensitivity: Photosensitivity may occur; caution patients to take protective measures (ie, sunscreens, protective clothing) against UV light or sunlight until tolerance is determined.

Renal function impairment: NSAID metabolites are eliminated primarily by the kidneys; use with caution. Reduce dosage to avoid excessive accumulation.

Pregnancy: Category B; Category D in third trimester. Safety for use during pregnancy has not been established; use is not recommended. There are no adequate and well-controlled studies in pregnant women. An increased incidence of dystocia, increased postimplantation loss, and delayed parturition occurred in animals. Agents that inhibit prostaglandin synthesis may cause closure of the ductus arteriosus and other adverse effects on the fetus. GI tract toxicity increased in pregnant women in the last trimester. Some NSAIDs may prolong pregnancy if given before onset of labor. Avoid use during pregnancy, especially during the third trimester.

Lactation: Most NSAIDs are excreted in breast milk in low concentrations. The American Academy of Pediatrics considers ibuprofen and naproxen to be compatible with breastfeeding. Data on the use of ketoprofen during nursing are lacking.

Children: The use of ibuprofen and naproxen is not recommended in children younger than 12 years of age unless directed by a physician. Ketoprofen is not recommended for use in children younger than 16 years of age.

▶ **Drug Interactions**

NSAID Drug Interactions			
Precipitant drug	**Object drug***		**Description**
Cimetidine	NSAIDs	⟷	NSAID plasma concentrations may be increased or decreased by cimetidine; some studies report no effect.
Probenecid	NSAIDs	↑	Probenecid may increase the concentrations and possibly the toxicity of the NSAIDs.
Salicylates	NSAIDs	↓	Plasma concentrations of NSAIDs may be decreased by salicylates. Avoid concurrent use because it offers no therapeutic advantage and may increase the incidence of GI effects significantly.
NSAIDs	ACE inhibitors	↓	Antihypertensive effects of captopril may be blunted or completely abolished by indomethacin. Other reports suggest that NSAIDs may diminish the antihypertensive effect of ACE inhibitors.
NSAIDs	Anticoagulants	↑	Coadministration may prolong prothrombin time (PT). Also consider the effects of NSAIDs on platelet function and gastric mucosa. Monitor PT and patients closely, and instruct patients to watch for signs and symptoms of bleeding.
NSAIDs	Beta-blockers	↓	The antihypertensive effect of beta-blockers may be impaired. Naproxen did not affect atenolol.
NSAIDs	Cyclosporine	↑	Nephrotoxicity of both agents may be increased.
NSAIDs	Digoxin	↑	Ibuprofen may increase digoxin serum levels.
NSAIDs	Diuretics	↓	Effects of the diuretics may be decreased. Decreased antihypertensive and diuretic action of thiazides may occur with concurrent naproxen.
NSAIDs	Hydantoins	↑	Serum phenytoin levels may be increased, resulting in an increase in pharmacologic and toxic effects of phenytoin.
NSAIDs	Lithium	↑	Serum lithium levels may be increased.
NSAIDs	Methotrexate	↑	The risks of methotrexate toxicity (eg, stomatitis, bone marrow suppression, nephrotoxicity) may be increased.

* ↑ = Object drug increased.   ↓ = Object drug decreased.   ⟷ = Undetermined clinical effect.

▶ **Adverse Reactions**

GI: (See Warnings.) Common GI adverse reactions are listed in the table below:

Common NSAID GI Adverse Reactions (%)[1]			
GI adverse reactions	**Ibuprofen**	**Ketoprofen**	**Naproxen**
Abdominal distress/cramps/pain	—	3 to 9	3 to 9
Anorexia	—	< 3	—
Constipation	< 3	3 to 9	3 to 9
Diarrhea	3 to 9	3 to 9	< 3
Dyspepsia	3 to 9	11	< 3
Flatulence	< 3	3 to 9	—
Nausea (with or without vomiting)	3 to 9	3 to 9	3 to 9

Common NSAID GI Adverse Reactions (%)[1]			
GI adverse reactions	Ibuprofen	Ketoprofen	Naproxen
Stomatitis	< 1	< 3	< 3
Vomiting	< 3	< 3	< 1

[1] These reactions occurred in patients taking higher-dose prescription products, and may not apply specifically to patients taking OTC NSAIDs. However, it is important to be aware of these potential adverse effects.

Ulcer – Gastric or duodenal ulcer with bleeding or perforation; intestinal ulceration associated with stenosis and obstruction; ulcerative stomatitis or colitis; gingival ulcer; rectal irritation.

Bleeding – Occult blood in the stool; GI bleeding with or without peptic ulcer; melena; hematemesis; rectal bleeding.

Other – Gastritis; gastroenteritis; proctitis; belching; salivation; glossitis; dry mouth; pyrosis; sore or dry mucous membranes.

The following adverse effects occur infrequently when using recommended doses of OTC NSAIDs intermittently. Most adverse effects with NSAIDs are related to dose and the duration of continuous therapy.

Cardiovascular: Congestive heart failure; hypertension; peripheral edema and fluid retention.

CNS: Aggravation of epilepsy and parkinsonism; dizziness; excitation; fatigue; headache (ketoprofen more than 3%); inability to concentrate; insomnia; lightheadedness; malaise; muscle weakness; myalgia; nervousness; somnolence/drowsiness; vertigo.

Dermatologic: Angioneurotic edema; ecchymosis; eczema; erythema; hyperpigmentation; peeling; petechiae; photosensitivity; purpura; pruritus; rash/dermatitis, including maculopapular type; skin irritation; urticaria.

Hematologic: Agranulocytosis; anemia secondary to obvious or occult bleeding; bruising; decreases in hemoglobin and hematocrit; eosinophilia; epistaxis; granulocytopenia; hypocoagulability; leukopenia; menometrorrhagia; menorrhagia; mild hepatic toxicity; neutropenia; thrombocytopenia.

Hepatic: Abnormal liver function tests; elevated liver enzymes; jaundice; toxic hepatitis (high doses administered chronically).

Hypersensitivity: Angioedema; anaphylaxis; asthma; dyspnea; rapid fall in blood pressure resembling a shock-like state.

Metabolic: Decreased or increased appetite; hyperglycemia; hyperkalemia; hypoglycemia; hyponatremia; flushing; glycosuria; menstrual disorders; sweating; vaginal bleeding.

Miscellaneous: Pyrexia (fever and chills); sweating; thirst.

Renal: Anuria; decreased creatinine clearance; dysuria; hematuria; increased serum creatinine; nephrosis; nocturia; polyuria; pyuria; oliguria; renal insufficiency; urinary frequency.

Respiratory: Bronchospasm; dyspnea; hemoptysis; laryngeal edema; pharyngitis; rhinitis; shortness of breath.

Special senses: Blurred vision; cataracts; change in taste (metallic or bitter); conjunctivitis; deafness; diplopia; ear pain; hearing disturbances or loss; photophobia; reversible loss of color vision; swollen, dry, or irritated eyes; tinnitus; visual disturbances.

IBUPROFEN

▶ **Administration and Dosage**

Adults: 200 mg with a full glass of liquid every 4 to 6 hours while symptoms persist (ie, as needed). If 200 mg doses are not sufficient to relieve pain, the dose may be increased to 400 mg. Do not take OTC ibuprofen for more than 10 consecutive days for pain unless instructed by a physician; daily dose should not exceed 1.2 g. If GI upset occurs, take with meals or milk. Use the smallest effective dose.

Patients consuming more than 3 alcohol-containing drinks per day should consult a physician or pharmacist for advice on when and how to take ibuprofen and other pain relievers.

Children: Do not give the following products to children younger than 12 years of age unless instructed by a physician.

IBUPROFEN PRODUCTS	
Trade name	**Doseform**
Advil	**Tablets**: 200 mg. Parabens, sucrose.
Motrin IB, Ibuprofen	**Tablets**: 200 mg.
Nuprin, Midol Cramp & Body Aches	**Caplets**: 200 mg.
Advil	**Caplets**: 200 mg. Parabens, sucrose.
Advil Liqui-Gels	**Capsules**: 200 mg. Light mineral oil, sorbitol.
Advil	**Gelcaps**: 200 mg. Glycerin.
Motrin IB	**Gelcaps**: 200 mg. Benzyl alcohol, parabens, castor oil, EDTA.

Products listed are representative of currently available and widely distributed brands. Similar products, including regional and private label brands, may also exist.

PATIENT INFORMATION
Ibuprofen

- Patient instructions accompany each product. Carefully read these instructions before use, preferably before leaving the pharmacy, in case of questions.
- Because of possible drug interactions, do not take any other OTC or prescription medications without consulting a physician or pharmacist.
- Take with a full glass of liquid.
- Food may decrease GI upset associated with NSAID therapy. Take with food if GI upset occurs.
- Avoid alcohol as well as analgesic, fever-reducing, and anti-inflammatory doses of aspirin while using an NSAID. Patients consuming more than 3 alcohol-containing drinks per day should consult a physician or pharmacist for advice on when and how to take ibuprofen and other pain relievers.
- Notify a physician if rash, itching, visual disturbances, edema, black stools, or persistent headache occurs.
- NSAIDs should be used as short-term therapy at the lowest effective doses. Length of therapy should not exceed package labeling recommendations.
- Ibuprofen may cause drowsiness; use caution while driving or performing other tasks that require mental alertness.
- Do not take for longer than 10 days for pain. If these symptoms persist, worsen, or if new symptoms develop, notify a physician.
- If you have severe symptoms, see a physician for proper evaluation.

KETOPROFEN

▶ **Administration and Dosage**

Adults: 12.5 mg with a full glass of liquid every 4 to 6 hours while symptoms persist (ie, as needed). If pain persists after 1 hour, another 12.5 mg dose may be taken. After tolerability has been established, start with an initial dose of 25 mg. Do not exceed 75 mg daily unless instructed by a physician. Use the smallest effective dose.

Patients consuming more than 3 alcohol-containing drinks per day should consult a physician or pharmacist for advice on when and how to take ketoprofen and other pain relievers.

Children: Do not give the following product to children younger than 16 years of age unless instructed by a physician.

KETOPROFEN PRODUCTS	
Trade name	Doseform
Orudis KT	**Tablets**: 12.5 mg. Tartrazine, sugar.

Products listed are representative of currently available and widely distributed brands. Similar products, including regional and private label brands, may also exist.

PATIENT INFORMATION

Ketoprofen

- Patient instructions accompany each product. Carefully read these instructions before use, preferably before leaving the pharmacy, in case of questions.
- Because of possible drug interactions, do not take any other OTC or prescription medications without consulting a physician or pharmacist.
- Take with a full glass of liquid.
- Food may decrease GI upset associated with NSAID therapy. Take with food if GI upset occurs.
- Avoid alcohol as well as analgesic, fever-reducing, and anti-inflammatory doses of aspirin while using an NSAID. Patients consuming more than 3 alcohol-containing drinks per day should consult a physician or pharmacist for advice on when and how to take ketoprofen and other pain relievers.
- Notify a physician if rash, itching, visual disturbances, edema, black stools, or persistent headache occurs.
- NSAIDs should be used as short-term therapy at the lowest effective doses. Length of therapy should not exceed package labeling recommendations.
- Ketoprofen may cause drowsiness; use caution while driving or performing other tasks that require mental alertness.
- Do not take for longer than 10 days for pain. If these symptoms persist, worsen, or if new symptoms develop, notify a physician.
- If you have severe symptoms, see a physician for proper evaluation.

NAPROXEN

▶ **Administration and Dosage**

Adults: 200 mg with a full glass of liquid every 8 to 12 hours while symptoms persist (ie, as needed). With experience, some patients may find an initial dose of 400 mg followed by 200 mg every 12 hours will give better relief. Do not exceed 600 mg in 24 hours unless instructed by a physician. Use the smallest effective dose.

Patients consuming more than 3 alcohol-containing drinks per day should consult a physician or pharmacist for advice on when and how to take naproxen and other pain relievers.

Children: Do not give the following products to children younger than 12 years of age unless instructed by a physician.

NAPROXEN PRODUCTS	
Trade name	Doseform
Aleve	**Tablets**: 200 mg. Talc.
Aleve	**Caplets**: 200 mg. Talc.
Aleve	**Gelcaps**: 200 mg. Talc, EDTA, glycerin.

Products listed are representative of currently available and widely distributed brands. Similar products, including regional and private label brands, may also exist.

PATIENT INFORMATION

Naproxen

- Patient instructions accompany each product. Carefully read these instructions before use, preferably before leaving the pharmacy, in case of questions.
- Because of possible drug interactions, do not take any OTC or prescription medications without consulting a physician or pharmacist.
- Take with a full glass of liquid.
- Food may decrease GI upset associated with NSAID therapy. Take with food if GI upset occurs.
- Avoid alcohol as well as analgesic, fever-reducing, and anti-inflammatory doses of aspirin while using an NSAID. Patients consuming more than 3 alcohol-containing drinks per day should consult a physician or pharmacist for advice on when and how to take naproxen and other pain relievers.
- Notify a physician if rash, itching, visual disturbances, edema, black stools, or persistent headache occurs.
- NSAIDs should be used as short-term therapy at the lowest effective doses. Length of therapy should not exceed package labeling recommendations.
- Naproxen may cause drowsiness; use caution while driving or performing other tasks that require mental alertness.
- Do not take for longer than 10 days for pain. If these symptoms persist, worsen, or if new symptoms develop, notify a physician.
- If you have severe symptoms, see a physician for proper evaluation.

ACETAMINOPHEN (APAP)

▶ Actions

Acetaminophen (APAP) is an analgesic; however, the site and mechanism of its analgesic effect is unclear. The agent may have a direct effect on the pain threshold.

▶ Indications

Acetaminophen may be used to relieve PMS symptoms associated with menstrual pain (eg, headache, backache, joint pain, cramps). This agent has other labeled indications as well.

▶ Contraindications

Hypersensitivity to acetaminophen.

▶ Warnings

Concurrent medications: Many other medications, specifically multi-ingredient cough and cold products, also contain aspirin or acetaminophen. It is important to advise patients of this possibility and to inquire about other medications they may be taking before recommending an analgesic.

Hepatotoxicity: Hepatotoxicity and severe hepatic failure occurred in patients with chronic alcoholism following therapeutic doses. The hepatotoxicity is believed to be caused by induction of hepatic microsomal enzymes, resulting in an increase in toxic metabolites, or by the reduced amount of glutathione responsible for conjugating toxic metabolites. A safe dose for patients with chronic alcoholism has not been determined so acetaminophen intake should be limited to 2 g/day or less.

Pregnancy: Category B. Acetaminophen crosses the placenta; however, it is used routinely during all stages of pregnancy. When used in therapeutic doses, it appears safe for short-term or episodic use.

Lactation: Acetaminophen is excreted in low amounts, but no adverse effects have been reported. The American Academy of Pediatrics considers acetaminophen to be compatible with breastfeeding.

▶ Drug Interactions

Acetaminophen Drug Interactions			
Precipitant drug	**Object drug***		**Description**
Alcohol, ethyl	APAP	↑	Hepatotoxicity has occurred in patients with chronic alcoholism following various dose levels (moderate to excessive) of APAP.
Anticholinergics	APAP	↓	The onset of APAP effects may be delayed or decreased slightly, but the ultimate pharmacological effects are not affected significantly by anticholinergics.
Beta-blockers, propranolol	APAP	↑	Propranolol appears to inhibit the enzyme systems responsible for glucuronidation and oxidation of APAP. Therefore, the pharmacologic effects of APAP may be increased.
Charcoal, activated	APAP	↓	Reduces APAP absorption when administered as soon as possible after overdose.
Contraceptives, oral	APAP	↓	Increase in glucuronidation resulting in increased plasma clearance and a decreased half-life of APAP.
Probenecid	APAP	↑	Probenecid may increase the therapeutic effectiveness of APAP slightly.

Acetaminophen Drug Interactions			
Precipitant drug	Object drug*		Description
APAP	Lamotrigine	↓	Serum lamotrigine concentrations may be reduced, producing a decrease in therapeutic effects.
APAP	Loop diuretics	↓	The effects of the loop diuretic may be decreased because APAP may decrease renal prostaglandin excretion and decrease plasma renin activity.
APAP	Zidovudine	↓	The pharmacologic effects of zidovudine may be decreased because of enhanced nonhepatic or renal clearance of zidovudine.

* ↑ = Object drug increased. ↓ = Object drug decreased. ↔ = Undetermined clinical effect.

The potential hepatotoxicity of acetaminophen may be increased by large doses or long-term administration of barbiturates, carbamazepine, hydantoins, isoniazid, rifampin, and sulfinpyrazone. The therapeutic effects of acetaminophen also may be decreased.

▶ **Adverse Reactions**

When used as directed, acetaminophen rarely causes severe toxicity or side effects. However, the following adverse reactions have been reported: Hemolytic anemia; neutropenia; leukopenia; pancytopenia; thrombocytopenia; jaundice; hypoglycemia; rash; fever.

▶ **Overdosage**

Symptoms: Acute poisoning may be manifested by nausea, vomiting, drowsiness, confusion, liver tenderness, low blood pressure, cardiac arrhythmias, jaundice, and acute hepatic and renal failure. These occur within the first 24 hours and may persist for 1 week or longer. Death has occurred because of liver necrosis. Acute renal failure also may occur. However, there are often no specific early symptoms or signs. The course of acetaminophen poisoning is divided into 4 stages (postingestion time):

Stage 1 (12 to 24 hours) – Nausea, vomiting, diaphoresis, anorexia.

Stage 2 (24 to 48 hours) – Clinically improved; AST, ALT, bilirubin, and prothrombin levels begin to rise.

Stage 3 (72 to 96 hours) – Peak hepatotoxicity; AST of 20,000 not unusual.

Stage 4 (7 to 8 days) – Recovery.

Hepatotoxicity may result. The minimal toxic dose is 10 g (140 mg/kg), but liver damage has occurred with a single 5.85 g dose; doses 20 to 25 g or more are potentially fatal. Children appear less susceptible to toxicity than adults because they have less capacity for glucuronidation metabolism. Initial signs of toxicity may include nausea, vomiting, anorexia, malaise, diaphoresis, abdominal pain, and diarrhea. Hepatotoxicity usually is not apparent for 48 to 72 hours. If an acute dose of 150 mg/kg or more was ingested, or if the dose cannot be determined, obtain a serum acetaminophen assay after 4 hours following ingestion. If in the toxic range, obtain liver function studies and repeat at 24-hour intervals. Hepatic failure may lead to encephalopathy, coma, and death.

Plasma acetaminophen levels of more than 300 mcg/mL at 4 hours postingestion were associated with hepatic damage in 90% of patients; minimal hepatic damage is anticipated if plasma levels are less than 120 mcg/mL at 4 hours or less than 30 mcg/mL at 12 hours postingestion.

■ ■ ■

Chronic excessive use (more than 4 g/day) eventually may lead to transient hepatotoxicity. The kidneys may undergo tubular necrosis, and the myocardium may be damaged.

Treatment: Perform gastric lavage in all cases, preferably within 4 hours of ingestion. Refer also to General Management of Acute Overdosage. It is important to contact a local poison control center or emergency room if overdosage is suspected.

▶ Administration and Dosage

Do not exceed recommended dosage without the advice of a physician. Take tablets, caplets, and gelcaps by mouth. Swallow extended-release formulations whole; do not crush or chew.

Adults: 325 to 650 mg every 4 to 6 hours, or 1 g three to four times daily while symptoms persist (ie, as needed). Do not exceed 4 g/day for all formulations containing acetaminophen (2 g/day in alcoholic patients).

Children (6 to 12 years of age): The usual dose is 10 mg/kg/dose, which may be repeated 4 to 5 times daily as needed. Do not exceed 5 doses in 24 hours.

Acetaminophen Dosages for Children	
Age (years)	Dosage (mg)
9 to 10	400
11	480
12 to 14	640
> 14	650

Rectal suppositories:

Adults – 650 mg every 4 to 6 hours while symptoms persist (ie, as needed); do not exceed 4 g/day. For guidelines on inserting rectal suppositories, refer to Appendix D, Administration Techniques.

Children (6 to 12 years of age) – 325 mg every 4 to 6 hours. Do not exceed 2.6 g/day.

ACETAMINOPHEN PRODUCTS	
Trade name	Doseform
Tylenol Regular Strength, Regular Strength Maxapap	**Tablets** 325 mg:
Tylenol Extra Strength, Anacin Aspirin Free Extra Strength, Maximum Strength Maxapap	**Tablets**: 500 mg
Acetaminophen	**Tablets**: 650 mg
Tylenol Arthritis Pain Extended Relief	**Caplets**: 650 mg
Tylenol Extra Strength	**Geltabs**: 500 mg. Benzyl alcohol, parabens, EDTA, castor oil.
Tylenol Extra Strength	**Gelcaps**: 500 mg. Benzyl alcohol, parabens, EDTA, castor oil.
Acephen	**Suppositories**: 125 mg. Vegetable oil.
Acetaminophen	**Suppositories**: 300 mg
Acephen	**Suppositories**: 325 mg. Vegetable oil.
Acephen, FeverAll Adults	**Suppositories**: 650 mg. Vegetable oil.

Products listed are representative of currently available and widely distributed brands. Similar products, including regional and private label brands, may also exist.

PATIENT INFORMATION
Acetaminophen

- Patient instructions accompany each product. Carefully read these instructions before use, preferably before leaving the pharmacy, in case of questions.
- Because of possible drug interactions, do not take any other OTC or prescription medications without consulting a physician or pharmacist.
- Be aware of other OTC (eg, combination products for pain, cold, cough, or allergy) and prescription medications that contain acetaminophen.
- Do not exceed the recommended dosage. Do not exceed a total dose of 4 g/day of acetaminophen in all formulations consumed.
- Patients with chronic alcoholism should limit acetaminophen intake to 2 g/day or less.
- Do not take for pain for longer than 5 days in children and 10 days in adults. If these symptoms persist, worsen, or if new symptoms develop, notify a physician.
- If you have severe symptoms, see a physician for proper evaluation.

SALICYLATES

▶ Actions

These products produce analgesia by inhibiting prostaglandin synthesis, reduce fever (by vasodilation), and have anti-inflammatory effects. In addition, of the salicylates, only aspirin significantly inhibits platelet aggregation.

▶ Indications

Relief of mild to moderate pain, fever, various inflammatory conditions (eg, rheumatic fever). In addition, daily low-dose aspirin is indicated for reducing the risk of death or myocardial infarction in patients with previous infarction or angina pectoris and for reducing the risk of transient ischemic attacks (TIAs) or strokes in patients who have had TIAs because of platelet emboli.

▶ Contraindications

Hypersensitivity to salicylates or NSAIDs. Use with extreme caution in patients with a history of adverse reactions to salicylates. Cross-sensitivity may exist between aspirin and other NSAIDs and between aspirin and tartrazine. Aspirin cross-sensitivity does not appear to occur with sodium salicylate, salicylamide, or choline salicylate. Aspirin hypersensitivity is more prevalent in patients with asthma, nasal polyposis, or chronic urticaria. Magnesium salicylate is contraindicated in advanced chronic renal insufficiency.

Contraindicated in patients with hemophilia or bleeding ulcers or patients in hemorrhagic states.

▶ Warnings

Concurrent medications: Many other medications, specifically multi-ingredient cough and cold products, also contain aspirin or acetaminophen. It is important to advise patients of this possibility and to inquire about other medications they may be taking before recommending an analgesic.

GI effects: Use caution in patients who are intolerant to salicylates because of GI irritation, and in patients with gastric ulcers, peptic ulcers, diabetes, gout, erosive gastritis, or bleeding tendencies.

Hematologic effects: Aspirin interferes with hemostasis. Avoid use in patients with severe anemia, history of blood coagulation defects, or in patients who take anticoagulants.

Hepatic function impairment: Use caution in patients with liver damage, preexisting hypoprothrombinemia, and vitamin K deficiency.

Hypersensitivity: Do not use if there is a history of sensitivity to aspirin or NSAIDs.

Aspirin intolerance, manifested by acute bronchospasm, generalized urticaria/angioedema, severe rhinitis, or shock occurs in 4% to 19% of asthmatic patients. Symptoms occur within 3 hours after ingestion.

Foods may contribute to a reaction. Some foods with high salicylate content include curry powder, paprika, licorice, Benedictine liqueur, prunes, raisins, tea, and gherkins. A typical American diet contains 10 to 200 mg/day of salicylate.

Otic effects: Discontinue use if dizziness, ringing in ears (tinnitus), or impaired hearing occurs. Tinnitus probably represents blood salicylate levels reaching or exceeding the upper limit of the therapeutic range; therefore, it is a helpful guide to dose titration. Temporary hearing loss disappears gradually upon discontinuation of the drug.

Pregnancy: Category D (aspirin); Category C (salsalate, magnesium salicylate, other salicylates). Aspirin may produce adverse effects in the mother, such as anemia, ante- or postpartum hemorrhage, or prolonged gestation and labor. Salicylates readily cross the placenta. By inhibiting prostaglandin synthesis, salicylates may cause constriction of ductus arteriosus and possibly other adverse fetal effects. Maternal aspirin use during later stages of pregnancy may cause adverse fetal effects, such as low birth weight, increased incidence of intracranial hemorrhage in premature infants, stillbirth, or neonatal death. Salicylates may be teratogenic. Avoid use during pregnancy, especially in the third trimester.

Lactation: Salicylates are excreted in breast milk in low concentrations. Adverse effects on platelet function in nursing infants are a potential risk. The American Academy of Pediatrics recommends that aspirin be used cautiously in nursing mothers.

Children: Administration of aspirin to children (including teenagers) with acute febrile illness has been associated with the development of Reye syndrome. Do not use in children and adolescents.

▶ Drug Interactions

Salicylate Drug Interactions			
Precipitant Drug	**Object Drug***		**Description**
Charcoal, activated	Aspirin	↓	Coadministration decreases aspirin absorption, depending on charcoal dose and interval between ingestion.
Aspirin	Heparin	↑	Aspirin can increase the risk of bleeding in heparin-anticoagulated patients.
Aspirin	Nitroglycerin	↑	Nitroglycerin, when taken with aspirin, may result in unexpected hypotension. Data are limited. If hypotension occurs, reduce the nitroglycerin dose.
Aspirin	NSAIDs	↓	Aspirin may decrease NSAID serum concentrations. Avoid concomitant use; it offers no therapeutic advantage and may increase incidence of GI effects significantly.

Salicylate Drug Interactions			
Precipitant Drug	**Object Drug***		**Description**
Aspirin	Valproic acid	↑	Aspirin displaces valproic acid from its protein-binding sites and may decrease its total body clearance, thus increasing the pharmacological effects.
Aspirin	Warfarin	↑	The adverse effects of aspirin on the gastric mucosa and platelet function also may enhance the possibility of hemorrhage.
Antacids, urinary alkalinizers	Salicylates	↓	Decreased pharmacologic effects of salicylates. The magnitude of the antacid interaction depends on the agent, dose, and pretreatment urine pH.
Carbonic anhydrase inhibitors	Salicylates	↑	Salicylate intoxication has occurred after coadministration of these agents. However, salicylic acid renal elimination may be increased by these drugs if urine is kept alkaline. Conversely, salicylates may displace acetazolamide from protein-binding sites, resulting in toxicity. Further study is needed.
Corticosteroids	Salicylates	↓	Corticosteroids increase salicylate clearance and decrease salicylate serum levels.
Nizatidine	Salicylates	↑	Increased serum salicylate levels have occurred in patients receiving high doses (3.9 g/day) of aspirin and concurrent nizatidine.
Urinary acidifiers	Salicylates	↑	Ammonium chloride, ascorbic acid, and methionine decrease salicylate excretion.
Salicylates	ACE inhibitors	↓	The antihypertensive effect of these agents may be decreased by concurrent salicylate administration, possibly because of prostaglandin inhibition. Consider discontinuing salicylates if problems occur.
Salicylates	Alcohol	↑	The risk of GI ulceration increases when salicylates are given concomitantly. Ingestion of alcohol during salicylate therapy also may prolong bleeding time.
Salicylates	Loop diuretics	↓	Loop diuretics may be less effective when given with salicylates in patients with compromised renal function or with cirrhosis with ascites; however, data conflict.
Salicylates	Methotrexate	↑	Salicylates increase drug levels, causing toxicity by interfering with protein binding and renal elimination of the antimetabolite.
Salicylates	Probenecid, sulfinpyrazone	↓	Salicylates antagonize the uricosuric effect. While salicylates in large doses (more than 3 g/day) have a uricosuric effect, smaller amounts may reduce the uricosuric effect of these agents.
Salicylates	Spironolactone	↓	Salicylates may inhibit diuretic effects; antihypertensive action does not appear altered. Effects depend on the dose of spironolactone.
Salicylates	Sulfonylureas, exogenous insulin	↑	Salicylates in doses more than 2 g/day have a hypoglycemic action, perhaps by altering pancreatic beta-cell function. They may potentiate the glucose-lowering effect of these drugs.

* ↑ = Object drug increased. ↓ = Object drug decreased. ↔ = Undetermined clinical effect.

▶ **Adverse Reactions**

Dermatologic: Angioedema, hives, and rash may occur, especially in patients suffering from chronic urticaria.

GI: Dyspepsia; epigastric discomfort; heartburn; nausea.

Hematologic: Decreased plasma iron concentration; leukopenia; prolonged bleeding time; purpura; thrombocytopenia; shortened erythrocyte survival time.

Miscellaneous: Dimness of vision; fever; thirst.

Allergic and anaphylactic reactions have been noted when hypersensitive individuals took aspirin. Fatal anaphylactic shock, while not common, has been reported.

Aspirin has a reversible effect on platelet aggregation.

▶ **Overdosage**

Symptoms: The approximate acute lethal dose is 10 to 30 g for adults and 4 g for children. Respiratory alkalosis is seen initially in acute salicylate ingestion. Hyperpnea and tachypnea occur as a result of increased CO_2 production and a direct stimulatory effect of salicylate on the respiratory center. Other symptoms may include nausea, vomiting, hypokalemia, tinnitus, neurologic abnormalities (eg, disorientation, irritability, hallucinations, lethargy, stupor, coma, seizures), dehydration, hyperthermia, hyperventilation, hyperactivity, thrombocytopenia, platelet dysfunction, hypoprothrombinemia, increased capillary fragility, and other hematologic abnormalities. Symptoms may progress quickly to depression, coma, respiratory failure, and collapse. Chronic salicylate toxicity may occur when more than 100 mg/kg/day is ingested for at least 2 days. It is more difficult to recognize and is associated with increased morbidity and mortality. Hyperventilation, dehydration, systemic acidosis, and severe CNS manifestations occur more frequently compared with acute poisoning.

Treatment: Initial treatment includes induction of emesis or gastric lavage to remove any unabsorbed drug from the stomach. Activated charcoal diminishes salicylate absorption most effectively if given within 2 hours after ingestion. It is important to contact a local poison control center or emergency room if overdosage is suspected.

ASPIRIN

▶ **Administration and Dosage**

Adults: 325 to 650 mg every 4 hours while symptoms persist (ie, as needed). Some extra-strength products recommend dosages of 500 mg every 3 hours or 1,000 mg every 6 hours.

Children: The analgesic/antipyretic dosage is 10 to 15 mg/kg/dose every 4 hours (see table), up to 60 to 80 mg/kg/day. Do not use in children or teenagers with chicken pox or "flu" symptoms because of the possibility of Reye syndrome. Dosage recommendations by age and weight are as follows:

Recommended Aspirin Dosage in Children					
Age (years)	Weight		Dosage (mg every 4 hours)	No. of 81 mg tablets (every 4 hours)	No. of 325 mg tablets (every 4 hours)
	lbs	kg			
9 to 10	60 to 71	26.9 to 32.3	405	5	N/A
11	72 to 95	32.4 to 43.2	486	6	1½
12 to 14	≥ 96	≥ 43.3	648	8	2

ASPIRIN PRODUCTS

Trade name	Doseform
Low Dose EC Aspirin	**Tablets, enteric coated**: 81 mg
Aspirin Regimen Bayer Adult Low Strength	**Tablets, enteric coated**: 81 mg. Lactose.
Adult Low Strength Ecotrin, Halfprin 81	**Tablets, enteric coated**: 81 mg. Talc.
Anacin 81	**Tablets, enteric coated**: 81 mg. Lactose, mineral oil.
Halfprin 162	**Tablets, enteric coated**: 162 mg
EC Aspirin	**Tablets, enteric coated**: 325 mg
Genuine Bayer Aspirin, Norwich Aspirin	**Tablets, enteric coated**: 325 mg. Parabens, glycerin.
Ecotrin Regular Strength	**Tablets, enteric coated**: 325 mg. Talc.
Ecotrin Maximum Strength	**Tablets, enteric coated**: 500 mg
Genuine Bayer	**Caplets, enteric coated**: 325 mg. Parabens, glycerin.
Extra Strength Bayer, Norwich Maximum Strength	**Caplets, enteric coated**: 500 mg
Genuine Bayer	**Gelcaps, enteric coated**: 325 mg. Parabens, glycerin.
Extra Strength Bayer	**Gelcaps, enteric coated**: 500 mg. Parabens, glycerin.

BUFFERED ASPIRIN PRODUCTS

Bayer Buffered Aspirin	**Tablets**: 325 mg with buffers
Extra Strength Bayer Plus	**Caplets**: 500 mg with 250 mg calcium carbonate
Maximum Strength Ascriptin	**Caplets**: 500 mg with alumina-magnesia and calcium carbonate. Mannitol, saccharin, sorbitol, talc.
Regular Strength Ascriptin	**Tablets, coated**: 325 mg with alumina-magnesium and calcium carbonate. Talc.
Bufferin	**Tablets, coated**: 325 mg with calcium carbonate, magnesium oxide, magnesium carbonate. Mineral oil.

Products listed are representative of currently available and widely distributed brands. Similar products, including regional and private label brands, may also exist.

PATIENT INFORMATION
Aspirin

- Patient instructions accompany each product. Carefully read these instructions before use, preferably before leaving the pharmacy, in case of questions.
- Because of possible drug interactions, do not take any other OTC or prescription medications without consulting a physician or pharmacist.
- May cause GI upset; take with food or after meals. Enteric-coated products may prevent or reduce stomach/GI distress.
- Take with a full glass of water.
- Do not use if allergic to NSAIDs or tartrazine dye.
- Notify a physician if persistent pain, rash, difficulty breathing, or ringing in the ears occurs.
- Avoid taking antacids within 2 hours of taking enteric-coated tablets.
- Do not use aspirin if it has a strong vinegar-like odor. This suggests deterioration of the product and loss of potency.
- Do not give to children or teenagers with flu-like symptoms or chicken pox without consulting a physician.
- Inform a physician or dentist about use before surgery or dental care.
- Be aware of other OTC (eg, combination products for pain, cold, cough, or allergy) and prescription medications that contain aspirin.
- If you have severe symptoms, see a physician for proper evaluation.

ANALGESIC COMBINATIONS

▶ Actions

Caffeine, a traditional component of many analgesic formulations, may be beneficial in certain vascular headaches.

Antacids are included as ingredients in some products to minimize gastric upset by salicylates.

▶ Administration and Dosage

The average adult dose is 1 or 2 capsules or tablets or 1 powder packet, every 2 to 6 hours while symptoms persist (ie, as needed). Check individual product labeling for guidelines.

ANALGESIC COMBINATION PRODUCTS	
Trade name	Doseform
Excedrin Migraine	**Tablets**: 250 mg acetaminophen, 250 mg aspirin, 65 mg caffeine. Mineral oil.
Excedrin Extra Strength	**Tablets**: 250 mg acetaminophen, 250 mg aspirin, 65 mg caffeine. Mineral oil, saccharin.
Anacin, Cope	**Tablets**: 400 mg aspirin, 32 mg caffeine
Anacin Extra Strength	**Tablets**: 500 mg aspirin, 32 mg caffeine
Excedrin Extra Strength	**Caplets**: 250 mg acetaminophen, 250 mg aspirin, 65 mg caffeine. Mineral oil, saccharin.
Aspirin Free Excedrin Extra Strength	**Caplets**: 500 mg acetaminophen, 65 mg caffeine. Parabens, mineral oil, saccharin.
Excedrin Extra Strength	**Geltabs**: 250 mg acetaminophen, 250 mg aspirin, 65 mg caffeine. EDTA, glycerin, mineral oil.
Aspirin Free Excedrin Extra Strength	**Geltabs**: 500 mg acetaminophen, 65 mg caffeine. Parabens, mineral oil, glycerin.

ANALGESIC COMBINATION PRODUCTS	
Trade name	Doseform
Goody's Extra Strength Headache Powders	**Powder**: 260 mg acetaminophen, 520 mg aspirin, 32.5 mg caffeine
BC Headache	**Powder**: 650 mg aspirin, 195 mg salicylamide, 33.3 mg caffeine. Lactose.
Arthritis Strength BC	**Powder**: 742 mg aspirin, 222 mg salicylamide, 38 mg caffeine. Lactose.

Products listed are representative of currently available and widely distributed brands. Similar products, including regional and private label brands, may also exist.

PATIENT INFORMATION
Analgesic Combination Products

- Patient instructions accompany each product. Carefully read these instructions before use, preferably before leaving the pharmacy, in case of questions.
- Because of possible drug interactions, do not take any other OTC or prescription medications without consulting a physician or pharmacist.
- May cause GI upset; take with food or after meals.
- Take with a full glass of water.
- Do not use if allergic to NSAIDs or tartrazine dye.
- Notify a physician if persistent pain, rash, difficulty breathing, or ringing in the ears occurs.
- Do not use these products if they have a strong vinegar-like odor. This suggests deterioration of the product and loss of potency.
- Do not give to children or teenagers with flu-like symptoms or chicken pox without consulting a physician.
- Inform a physician or dentist about use before surgery or dental care.
- Be aware of other OTC (eg, combination products for pain, cold, cough, or allergy) and prescription medications that contain aspirin.
- If you have severe symptoms, see a physician for proper evaluation.

Urinary Tract Infection (UTI)

DEFINITION

A urinary tract infection (UTI) is the presence of microorganisms in the urinary tract or urine in association with clinical symptoms. Terms commonly used to describe the location of the infection are cystitis and pyelonephritis. Cystitis is inflammation occurring in the urinary bladder or urethra (lower urinary tract), and pyelonephritis is inflammation of the kidney (upper urinary tract). A complicated infection occurs in the presence of other conditions or pathology that increases the risk for therapy failure or recalcitrant infection; uncomplicated infections occur in otherwise healthy individuals with anatomically normal urinary tracts.

ETIOLOGY

Most UTIs are caused by enteric gram-negative bacteria (GNB). *Escherichia coli* is the most prevalent pathogen associated with both uncomplicated and complicated infections of the urinary tract. *E. coli* causes 80% to 90% of all uncomplicated episodes and is responsible for approximately 50% of recurrent urinary infections. Other bacterial uropathogens include *Proteus mirabilis* (GNB), *Klebsiella pneumoniae* (GNB), *Enterococcus faecalis* (gram-positive bacteria or GPB), and *Staphylococcus saprophyticus* (GPB).

INCIDENCE

UTI is predominantly a condition associated with females 1 to 50 years of age. Studies indicate that approximately 10% to 50% of women will develop a UTI during their lifetime. Furthermore, of women who develop an initial infection, approximately 20% to 40% will experience at least 1 additional episode. UTI accounts for more than 7 million physician office visits each year in the US and is one of the infectious diseases most likely to require patients to seek medical advice.

PATHOPHYSIOLOGY

The occurrence of UTI is a complex interaction between host defenses and microbial virulence factors. There are 3 routes of invasion: Ascending, hematogenous, and lymphatic. Most commonly, invasion results from the ascending route via the urethra. Both cystitis and pyelonephritis may develop by urethral ascension. However, pyelonephritis frequently results from hematogenous (bloodstream to kidney) invasion.

Host factors that deter microbial colonization include micturition (urination), antibacterial properties of the urinary bladder epithelium, low urinary pH, high urine osmolality, and a competent ureteral valve that prevents backflow from the bladder to the kidneys. Factors predisposing patients to the development of complicated infections include male gender, advanced age, nosocomial infection, pregnancy, urinary catheterization or recent instrumentation, anatomic or functional urinary tract abnormality, presentation with symptoms for more than 7 days, diabetes mellitus, and immunosuppression. Most of these factors compromise the patient's defense mechanisms, and nosocomial infections involve more virulent pathogens.

SIGNS/SYMPTOMS

Dysuria (painful urination), frequent urination with small voids, and urgency are the most common symptoms experienced with a lower UTI (cystitis). Lower abdominal discomfort may also be present. The patient may also experience hematuria, nocturia, and fever.

Upper UTI (pyelonephritis) is characterized by severe flank pain, costovertebral angle (CVA) tenderness, and suprapubic pain. Other nonspecific complaints include fever and chills, headache, malaise, nausea, and vomiting. Signs and symptoms of lower UTI may also be present.

DIAGNOSTIC PARAMETERS/PHYSICAL ASSESSMENT

Clinical Observation: Home UTI tests are a beneficial screening tool for patients presenting with symptoms of dysuria, urgency, and frequency (see Home Urinary Tract Infection Tests monograph). These tests are especially beneficial for patients with a history of recurrent UTIs and those with risk factors associated with UTI. Both positive and negative test results provide useful information. However, it is important for the patient to obtain an appropriate medical diagnosis (which may include a urine culture and sensitivity test) to prevent the condition from causing additional complications.

Interview: Prescription antibiotic therapy is essential to eradicate a UTI. However, pharmacists may recommend products that provide temporary relief of symptoms associated with UTI. Complete a proper patient assessment and history prior to suggesting products that will aid in short-term symptomatic relief pending medical evaluation and during the initial days of antibiotic therapy. The interview should contain, but not be limited to, inquiries concerning the following:

- Past medical procedures (especially those involving the GU tract).
- Concurrent disease states.
- Concurrent vaginal symptoms to rule out vaginal infection as a source of symptoms.
- Pregnancy status.
- Recent use of contraceptive and feminine hygiene products.
- History of UTI.
- Current medications (use of antihistamines or anticholinergics).

TREATMENT

Approaches to therapy: Refer all patients exhibiting signs and symptoms associated with a UTI to a physician for evaluation and treatment. Other health professionals can offer valuable information to the patient concerning prophylaxis and short-term relief of symptoms.

Nondrug therapy: Studies confirm that there are several behavioral practices that may prevent the occurrence of UTI. The following strategies may be used as prophylaxis or as an adjunct to antimicrobial regimens:

- Ingestion of cranberry extract or cranberry juice: Cranberry substance exerts a bacteriostatic effect by inhibiting the adherence of microorganisms to the mucosal surface of the urinary bladder. Most studies conducted have been in elderly women; the same mechanism may apply to younger women as well.
- Avoid use of douche products: Use of these products may cause a change in the vaginal pH and flora. Avoiding use may decrease possible colonization of the vaginal canal with uropathogens.
- Avoid use of spermicide-diaphragm contraceptive combinations: Use of these products may cause a change in the vaginal pH and flora. Avoiding use may decrease possible colonization of the vaginal canal with uropathogens.
- Increased fluid intake: Fluids will increase urination, which may flush bacteria from the urinary bladder and urethra.
- Voiding 30 to 60 minutes after sexual intercourse: Urination may flush bacteria from the urethra.
- Avoid use of artificial sweeteners: These products may adversely affect urinary bladder mucopolysaccharides.
- Use appropriate post-void cleaning: Cleaning in an anal-to-urethral direction contributes to vaginal and urethral colonization with enteric pathogens. Women should be encouraged to clean in a urethral-to-anal direction. Nonprescription cleansing wipes, as well as creams to relieve irritation, are available for patients with UTI.
- Avoid tub baths and soaking with bath oils: Bathing in bathtubs and using bath oils may increase the likelihood for urethral and vaginal colonization. Showering may allow for better cleansing of the urogenital area.

Pharmacotherapy: Eradication of bacteria causing UTI requires treatment with prescription antimicrobial medications. Acute urinary symptoms will often resolve after 1 to 2 days of effective antibiotic treatment, but OTC urinary tract analgesics may be useful adjunctive products to provide immediate relief of symptoms. These agents are not a substitute for medical evaluation and appropriate prescription drug therapy.

PHENAZOPYRIDINE

▶ Actions

Phenazopyridine is an azo dye that is taken orally. It exerts a topical analgesic effect on the urinary tract mucosa when excreted into the urine. The mechanism of action is unknown. Phenazopyridine does *not* have antibacterial properties.

▶ Indications

Relief of dysuria, urgency, frequency, burning, and other discomforts arising from irritation of the lower urinary tract mucosa caused by infection. Phenazopyridine may also be used to relieve discomfort associated with procedures (surgery, endoscopic procedures, urinary catheters) that may cause trauma to the urinary tract. Its analgesic action may reduce or eliminate the need for systemic analgesics or narcotics.

Phenazopyridine may be used as an adjunct to antimicrobial therapy for the relief of pain and discomfort before antimicrobial therapy controls the infection. Phenazopyridine does *not* exert antimicrobial effects on the infection. This agent only treats painful symptoms associated with UTI; it does not alter the underlying cause of pain.

► **Contraindications**

Hypersensitivity to phenazopyridine; renal insufficiency (see Overdosage).

► **Warnings**

Skin/Sclera discoloration: Phenazopyridine (an azo dye) is rapidly excreted by the kidneys; thus, development of a yellowish tinge of the skin or sclera may be indicative of impaired renal excretion. Discontinue therapy if this occurs.

Staining of fabric and contact lenses: Phenazopyridine is a red-to-orange dye. Its presence in eye fluids can stain contact lenses, but this effect is reversible upon discontinuation of the drug. When excreted in the urine, it can stain undergarments.

Length of therapy: Phenazopyridine should *not* be administered for more than 2 consecutive days. Currently, there is a lack of evidence indicating that combined administration of phenazopyridine with an antimicrobial agent provides greater benefit than administration of the antimicrobial alone after 2 days. In treating a urinary tract infection with an antimicrobial, a full course of therapy may require 7 to 10 days of antimicrobial use. Strict adherence to the prescribed regimen is essential and increases the probability of a clinical cure and decreases the risk of a relapse.

Carcinogenesis: Long-term administration of phenazopyridine has induced neoplasia of the liver in mice and of the large intestine in rats.

Pregnancy: Category B. Use during pregnancy is not advised except under the advice of a physician. There are no adequate and well-controlled studies in pregnant women.

Lactation: No information is available on the appearance of this drug or its metabolites in breast milk.

Children: Do not give to children younger than 12 years of age unless directed by a physician.

► **Drug Interactions**

None adequately documented in humans.

Drug-lab interactions: Phenazopyridine is an azo dye; it may interfere with urinary testing that is based on spectrometry or color reactions (eg, urinalysis testing, home UTI tests).

► **Adverse Reactions**

Headache, rash, pruritus, and GI disturbances are the most common adverse reactions. Anaphylactoid-like reaction, methemoglobinemia, hemolytic anemia, and renal and hepatic toxicity (usually at overdosage levels) may occur.

► **Overdosage**

If suspected overdosage occurs, refer patient to an emergency care facility or poison control center (via a toll-free number).

Symptoms: Administration of the usual dosage to patients with renal insufficiency (common in the elderly) or exceeding the recommended dosage or duration of therapy in patients with adequate renal function may lead to increased serum concentrations and produce toxic reactions. Methemoglobinemia may result from an acute overdose. In chronic overdosage, oxidative Heinz body hemolytic anemia may occur and "bite cells" (degmacytes) may be present. Hemolysis may occur in patients with red blood cell G-6-PD deficiency. Hypersensitivity to the product may result in hepatic and renal impairment and failure.

Treatment: Contact the local poison control center and refer patients suspected of overdosage to an emergency care facility. Methemoglobinemia may be treated with methylene blue administered in doses of 1 to 2 mg/kg IV. Ascorbic acid (vitamin C) in doses of 100 to 200 mg given orally should also cause prompt reduction of methemoglobinemia and disappearance of cyanosis.

▶ **Administration and Dosage**

Do *not* use chronically to treat undiagnosed urinary tract pain. Such use may lead to serious delays in appropriate diagnosis and treatment. This agent treats pain symptoms associated with UTI but does *not* treat the source or cause of the infection.

Adults (older than 12 years of age): Administer 2 tablets (190 mg) 3 times a day after meals. Do *not* use product for more than 2 days.

PHENAZOPYRIDINE PRODUCTS	
Trade name	Doseform
Azo-Standard, Prodium	**Tablets:** 95 mg
Reazo	**Tablets:** 97 mg
Baridium, Uri-med, UTI Relief	**Tablets:** 97.2 mg

Products listed are representative of currently available and widely distributed brands. Similar products, including regional and private label brands, may also exist.

PATIENT INFORMATION
Phenazopyridine

- Follow recommendations on product labeling.
- Phenazopyridine should *not* be used for more than 2 consecutive days. This product only treats the painful symptoms of UTI and does not alter the underlying infection and source of pain.
- Take after meals to avoid GI upset.
- A reddish orange discoloration of the urine is likely to occur and may stain fabric. This is a normal occurrence and represents no cause for alarm.
- Staining of contact lenses (reversible) may occur.
- If skin develops a yellowish tinge, notify a physician or pharmacist immediately.

CRANBERRY CONCENTRATE

▶ **Actions**

Studies indicate that a substance in cranberry juice may exert a bacteriostatic effect by inhibiting the adherence of microorganisms to the mucosal surface of the urinary bladder.

▶ **Indications**

Use of this agent is not intended to diagnose, treat, cure, or prevent any disease. The product is best used as an adjunct to antimicrobial regimens or as prophylactic therapy in the management of urinary tract infections. Cranberry concentrate is a nutritional supplement, and therapeutic claims made by the manufacturer have not been evaluated by the FDA.

▶ **Contraindications**

Hypersensitivity to any component of the product.

▶ **Administration and Dosage**

Take 1 to 4 capsules per day, ideally with meals.

CRANBERRY CONCENTRATE PRODUCTS	
Trade name	Doseform
Azo-Cranberry	**Capsules:** 450 mg. Natural cranberry juice concentrate powder, cellulose powder, vegetable magnesium stearate.

Products listed are representative of currently available and widely distributed brands. Similar products, including regional and private label brands, may also exist.

PATIENT INFORMATION

Cranberry Concentrate

- Follow recommendations on product labeling.
- If possible, take with meals.
- Products containing cranberry concentrate have not been evaluated by the FDA.

VAGINAL CANDIDIASIS
(Yeast Infection; Moniliasis)

DEFINITION

Vaginal candidiasis, also referred to as a yeast infection or moniliasis, is a relatively common fungal infection of the vagina that may be recurrent or chronic.

ETIOLOGY

The most common organism associated with vaginal candidiasis is *Candida albicans* (approximately 80% of all candidiasis cases). Other less common causative organisms include *C. glabrata* and *C. tropicalis*. Possible risk factors in the occurrence of vaginal candidiasis include wearing tight-fitting clothing or nylon undergarments, pregnancy, menstruation, diabetes mellitus, immunosuppression, and use of certain drugs including broad-spectrum antibiotics (eg, ampicillin, amoxicillin, tetracyclines, cephalosporins), oral contraceptives with high estrogen content, and corticosteroids.

INCIDENCE

Candidiasis accounts for approximately 20% to 30% of all episodes of vaginal infections. More than 12 million cases of vaginal candidiasis occur each year in the US. The frequency of yeast infections is increasing, with a higher incidence noted in patients receiving chronic broad-spectrum antibiotic therapy or high-estrogen and progestin-dominant oral contraceptives, those who perform excessive douching, pregnant women, immunocompromised patients, and patients with diabetes mellitus. Approximately 75% of women will develop at least 1 episode of candidiasis, and approximately 50% of this group will have at least 1 additional episode.

PATHOPHYSIOLOGY

Generally, the fungal infection is spread from the patient's normal skin or intestinal flora; sexual transmission is an unlikely cause.

SIGNS/SYMPTOMS

Vulvar and vaginal pruritus (itching) is the most common symptom. The vulva may be red, swollen, and irritated. A vaginal discharge sometimes occurs that may appear as a white, cheesy material, often referred to as cottage cheese-like or curd-like in nature. Urination and sexual intercourse may be painful. For a comparison of the features of various vaginal infections, refer to the table in the Diagnostic Parameters/Physical Assessment section.

DIAGNOSTIC PARAMETERS/PHYSICAL ASSESSMENT

Clinical Observation: Because of the nature of the condition, clinical observation will occur only by the patient. If the woman has previously been diagnosed by a physician, she will easily recognize the signs and symptoms of vaginal candidiasis.

The following table may help in differentiating the symptoms of various other vaginal infections from vaginal candidiasis:

Vaginal Discharge Characteristics in Common Vaginal Infections				
Parameter	Normal	Candidiasis	Trichomoniasis	Bacterial Vaginosis
Color	white or clear	white or whitish	yellow-green or brown	yellow to gray
Odor	nonodorous	nonodorous	fishy smell	fishy smell
Consistency	flocculent	flocculent	homogenous	homogenous
Viscosity	high	high	low (watery)	low (watery)
pH	≤ 4.5	≤ 4.5	≥ 4.5	≥ 5
Other	-	curd-like	frothy	thin

Interview: To help the patient determine if physician referral or self-treatment is warranted, it may be beneficial to ask about the following:

- Patient age (do not recommend self-treatment in females 12 years of age or younger).
- Previous experience with symptoms, especially within the last 2 months.
- Vaginal discharge with a bad or unpleasant odor (ask patient to describe the odor).
- Color, consistency, and viscosity of vaginal discharge.
- Abdominal or back pain; fever.
- Pregnancy status.
- Medications currently using (eg, medicated douches, antibiotics, steroids, oral contraceptives).

TREATMENT

Approaches to therapy: Evaluate patients using the previous diagnostic parameters. Depending on various factors (eg, symptoms, duration, recurrence), health care providers may recommend either (1) a nondrug approach; (2) appropriate pharmacotherapy; or (3) immediate referral to a physician for medical evaluation.

Nondrug therapy: Currently there is no effective nondrug therapy available for vaginal candidiasis. Use of home remedies such as vinegar, saline, or yogurt douches is strongly discouraged. The value of dietary yogurt in preventing vaginal fungal infection is not proven. There are some measures to help prevent recurrence, including not wearing tight-fitting clothing or nylon undergarments (including pantyhose), wiping front to back after bowel movements, and not douching.

Pharmacotherapy: Self-treatment with an OTC topical antifungal is most appropriate when vaginal symptoms occur less frequently than 2 to 3 times per year, 1 or more previous episodes of vaginal candidiasis were medically evaluated, and symptoms are mild to moderate and consistent with diagnostic parameters included in this monograph. Self treatment is inappropriate in females 12 years of age or younger and during pregnancy. Once it is determined that treatment is necessary, several OTC vaginal antifungal agents are available. Imidazole products (eg, clotrimazole, miconazole, butoconazole, tioconazole) mostly have replaced nystatin therapy; they are more convenient to use, require shorter treatment time, and are well tolerated.

VAGINAL ANTIFUNGAL AGENTS

▶ **Actions**

All OTC antifungal agents are fungicidal against *Candida* species. Nystatin and clotrimazole are fungistatic and fungicidal. Nystatin binds to sterols in the cell membrane of the fungus with a resultant change in membrane permeability allowing leakage of intracellular components. The primary action of imidazoles appears to be alteration of the permeability of the fungus cell membrane, which allows leakage of essential intracellular components and cell death.

▶ **Indications**

Candidiasis: Local treatment of mild to moderately severe, nonrecurrent (less than 4 episodes per year) vulvovaginal candidiasis (eg, moniliasis, yeast infection) and relief of external vulvar itching and irritation associated with this fungal (yeast) infection.

▶ **Contraindications**

Hypersensitivity to any product component.

▶ **Warnings**

Vaginal itch/discomfort: The patient should consult a physician before using these products if it is her first experience with vaginal itching and discomfort.

Other conditions: If abdominal pain, fever, or foul-smelling, frothy or thin and/or watery vaginal discharge is present, do not use these products. If the patient does not improve in 3 days or is not cured in 7 days, stop using these products. A condition more serious than fungal candidiasis may exist, and the patient should consult her physician.

Recurrent infections: If symptoms return within 2 months, the patient could be pregnant or there could be a serious underlying medical cause for the infection, including diabetes or a damaged immune system (including HIV infection). If the patient has been exposed to HIV and is having recurrent vaginal infections, especially infections that do not clear up easily with proper antifungal treatment, consult a physician to determine the cause of the symptoms.

For vaginal use only: Do not use in mouth or eyes. Do not ingest tablets or suppositories.

Irritation: If irritation or sensitization occurs, discontinue use.

Tampons: Do not use tampons while using this medication.

Pregnancy: Some products are appropriate for use during the second and third trimesters of pregnancy; refer to labeling of individual products. Avoid use of vaginal antifungals in the first trimester of pregnancy, if possible. Vaginal applicators may not be appropriate for use in pregnancy; manual insertion of vaginal tablets or suppositories may be preferable. Pregnant women should consult a physician before using these products.

Children: Do not use in children younger than 12 years of age.

▶ **Drug Interactions**

Because these agents are for local vaginal use only, no drug-drug or drug-food interactions are expected.

▶ **Adverse Reactions**

Irritation; sensitization; vulvovaginal burning.

CLOTRIMAZOLE

▶ **Administration and Dosage**

Tablets: Refer to individual product labeling. For most products, insert 1 tablet intravaginally at bedtime for 7 consecutive days (or the number of days specified in manufacturer instructions).

Cream:

> *Intravaginal* – Refer to individual product labeling. For most intravaginal creams, insert 1 applicatorful a day, preferably at bedtime, for 7 consecutive days (or the number of days specified in manufacturer instructions).

> *Topical* – For most products, the cream can be applied to the external genitalia (vulva) twice daily (morning and evening) for 7 consecutive days (or the number of days specified in manufacturer instructions) to control itching. Check individual product labeling for specific instructions.

For guidelines on inserting intravaginal creams and tablets/suppositories, refer to Appendix D, Administration Techniques.

CLOTRIMAZOLE PRODUCTS	
Trade name	**Doseform**
Gyne-Lotrimin 3	**Vaginal Tablets:** 200 mg
Clotrimazole Three-Day Cream, 2%	**Vaginal Cream:** 2%. Benzyl alcohol, cetostearyl alcohol.
Gyne-Lotrimin 3	**Vaginal Cream:** 2%
Mycelex-7	**Vaginal Cream:** 1%. Benzyl alcohol, cetostearyl alcohol.
Gyne-Lotrimin 7	**Vaginal Cream:** 1%. Benzyl alcohol, cetearyl alcohol.
Mycelex-7 Combination Pack	**Vaginal Tablets:** 100 mg
	Topical Cream: 1% Benzyl alcohol, cetostearyl alcohol.
Gyne-Lotrimin 3 Combination Pack	**Vaginal Tablets:** 200 mg
	Topical Cream: 1%

Products listed are representative of currently available and widely distributed brands. Similar products, including regional and private label brands, may also exist.

PATIENT INFORMATION
Clotrimazole

- Patient instructions are enclosed with each product, including the proper way to prepare and insert the applicator. Read these instructions carefully before use, preferably before leaving the pharmacy, in case of any questions.
- Open applicator just prior to use to prevent contamination. If only 1 applicator is supplied, clean after use with mild soap solution and rinse thoroughly with water. If more than 1 applicator is included in the package, dispose of each applicator after use.
- Insert tablet or cream high into the vagina, except during pregnancy. Complete the full course of therapy (3 or 7 days, depending on the product) and use on consecutive days, even during menstruation, preferably at bedtime. Notify the physician if improvement is not noticed after 3 days or relief of symptoms is not noted by the end of therapy.
- Notify the physician if burning or irritation occurs or worsens.
- This product may damage condoms and diaphragms; do not rely on these devices to prevent sexually transmitted diseases or pregnancy while using clotrimazole.
- Do not use a tampon during therapy. Use a sanitary napkin or minipad if needed.
- If symptoms recur within 2 months, consult a physician.

MICONAZOLE

► Administration and Dosage

Tablets: Insert 1 suppository intravaginally once daily at bedtime for 7 consecutive days (100 mg) or 3 consecutive days (200 mg).

Cream:

Intravaginal – Insert 1 applicatorful intravaginally once daily at bedtime for 3 or 7 days, depending on the product.

Topical – Apply to affected vulvar areas twice daily (morning and evening) for 7 days.

Repeat course if necessary, after ruling out other pathogens.

For guidelines on inserting vaginal creams and suppositories, refer to Appendix D, Administration Techniques.

Storage: Store at room temperature (15° to 30°C [59° to 86°F]). Avoid heat over 30°C (86°F).

MICONAZOLE PRODUCTS	
Trade name	Doseform
Monistat 7	**Vaginal Suppositories**: 100 mg
Femizol-M	**Vaginal Cream**: 2%
Monistat 7	**Vaginal Cream**: 2%
Monistat 3	**Vaginal Cream**: 4%
Monistat 7 Combination Pack, M-Zole 7 Combination Pack	**Vaginal Suppositories**: 100 mg
	Topical Cream: 2%
Monistat 3 Combination Pack, M-Zole 3 Combination Pack	**Vaginal Suppositories**: 200 mg
	Topical Cream: 2%

MICONAZOLE PRODUCTS	
Trade name	Doseform
Monistat 1 Combination Pack	**Vaginal Suppositories**: 1200 mg
	Topical Cream: 2%

Products listed are representative of currently available and widely distributed brands. Similar products, including regional and private label brands, may also exist.

PATIENT INFORMATION
Miconazole

- Patient instructions are enclosed with each product, including the proper way to prepare and insert the applicator. Read these instructions carefully before use, preferably before leaving the pharmacy, in case of questions.
- Open applicator just prior to use to prevent contamination. If only 1 applicator is supplied, clean after use with mild soap solution and rinse thoroughly with water. If more than 1 applicator is included in the package, dispose of each applicator after use.
- Insert tablet or cream high into the vagina, except during pregnancy. Complete the full course of therapy (either 3 or 7 days depending on product), and use on consecutive days, even during menstruation, preferably at bedtime. Notify physician if improvement is not noticed after 3 days or relief of symptoms is not noted by the end of therapy.
- Notify physician if burning or irritation occurs or worsens.
- This product may damage condoms and diaphragms; do not rely on these devices to prevent sexually transmitted diseases or pregnancy while using miconazole.
- Do not use a tampon during therapy. Use a sanitary napkin or minipad if needed.

TIOCONAZOLE

▶ **Administration and Dosage**

Single dose: Insert 1 applicatorful (approximately 4.6 g) intravaginally just prior to bedtime 1 time only.

For guidelines on inserting vaginal creams/ointments, refer to Appendix D, Administration Techniques.

TIOCONAZOLE PRODUCTS	
Trade name	Doseform
Monistat-1, Vagistat-1	**Vaginal Ointment:** 6.5%

Products listed are representative of currently available and widely distributed brands. Similar products, including regional and private label brands, may also exist.

PATIENT INFORMATION
Tioconazole

- Patient instructions are enclosed with each product, including the proper way to prepare and insert the applicator. Read these instructions carefully before use, preferably before leaving the pharmacy, in case of questions.
- Open applicator just prior to use to prevent contamination.
- Insert ointment high into the vagina, except during pregnancy. This product is to be used as a 1-time dose. Use this product even during menstruation, and preferably at bedtime. Notify physician if improvement is not noticed within 3 days of application, or if relief of symptoms is not noted within 7 days after application.
- Notify physician if burning or irritation occurs or worsens.
- This product may damage condoms and diaphragms; do not rely on these devices to prevent sexually transmitted diseases or pregnancy while using tioconazole.
- Do not use a tampon during therapy. Use a sanitary napkin or minipad if needed.

BUTOCONAZOLE NITRATE

▶ **Administration and Dosage**

For guidelines on inserting vaginal creams, refer to Appendix D, Administration Techniques.

Pregnant patients: (Second and third trimesters only) - 1 applicatorful (approximately 5 g) intravaginally at bedtime for 6 days (see Warnings).

Nonpregnant patients: 1 applicatorful (approximately 5 g) intravaginally at bedtime for 3 days. May be extended to 6 days, if necessary.

Storage: Do not store at higher than 40°C (104°F). Avoid freezing.

BUTOCONAZOLE PRODUCTS	
Trade name	Doseform
Mycelex-3	**Vaginal Cream:** 2%. Parabens, cetyl alcohol, stearyl alcohol.

Products listed are representative of currently available and widely distributed brands. Similar products, including regional and private label brands, may also exist.

PATIENT INFORMATION

Butoconazole Nitrate

- Patient instructions are enclosed with each product, including the proper way to prepare and insert the applicator. Read these instructions carefully before use, preferably before leaving the pharmacy, in case of questions.
- Open applicator just prior to use to prevent contamination. If only 1 applicator is supplied, clean after use with mild soap solution and rinse thoroughly with water. If more than 1 applicator is included in the package, dispose of each applicator after use.
- Insert tablet or cream high into the vagina, except during pregnancy. Complete the full course of therapy (3 days), and use on consecutive days, even during menstruation, preferably at bedtime. Notify physician if relief of symptoms is not noticed after 3 days.
- Notify physician if burning or irritation occurs or worsens.
- This product may damage condoms and diaphragms; do not rely on these devices to prevent sexually transmitted diseases or pregnancy while using butoconazole nitrate.
- Do not use a tampon during therapy. Use a sanitary napkin or minipad if needed.

DIABETES
MANAGEMENT

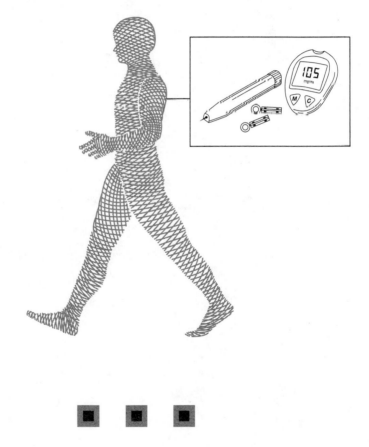

NONPRESCRIPTION DRUG THERAPY
TABLE OF CONTENTS
■ ■ ■

DIABETES MANAGEMENT

INTRODUCTION

Data indicates that approximately 16.5 million people in the US have diabetes (11 million diagnosed, 5.5 million still undiagnosed). Approximately 800,000 people are diagnosed with diabetes annually. Diabetes becomes more prevalent with aging; prevalence jumps from 0.16% for people younger than 20 years of age, to 8.2% for people who are 20 years of age or older, to 18.4% for people older than 65 years of age.

Death rates are twice as high among middle-aged people with diabetes as with middle-aged people without diabetes. Diabetes was the seventh leading cause of death listed on US death certificates in 1995, contributing to over 187,000 deaths. Many believe that diabetes as a condition and cause of death is underreported. New data from the Diabetes Control and Complications trial, the Kumamoto Type 2 study, the Wisconsin Epidemiology study, and the United Kingdom Prospective Diabetes study demonstrate the value of prompt and continuous normalization of the patient's blood glucose. This information has resulted in a call for strict guidelines for controlling diabetes. Secondary to the information that diabetes management slows the progression of complications of the disorder, nationally-based standards of diabetes care have been endorsed by the American Diabetes Association. Included in these standards are recommendations for a routine population screening program to identify people with diabetes earlier in the progression of their disease. This recommendation is based on the recognition of the toll that chronic complications can have on the patient's health.

The studies mentioned above also demonstrated and confirmed another valuable bit of information for health care providers: The only primary care provider for a person with diabetes is the *patient*, or for children, their parents. The day-to-day self-care steps for diabetes care and control really do deliver the message that self-management matters. Moreover, a set of national self-management program standards have been developed by the National Diabetes Advisory Board. These standards were tested for validity and demonstrate that, when adhered to in an educational program, they provide the information for patients to achieve better control of their diabetes. However, one should keep in mind that diabetes is a long-term endeavor and requires continual follow-up for achieving and maintaining good disease control. Pharmacists have the highest level of patient accessibility to provide this follow-up or continual care. Though a diabetic patient may learn a particular technique and perform it well (eg, self blood glucose monitoring), in time they may develop different habits or not perform the test as often as is optimal. Pharmacists can provide a review service, for example, by using short appointment times for reminders of proper technique. The pharmacist should also network with the patient's other caregivers (eg, physicians).

Because of the nature of diabetes, the patient is asked to monitor glucose levels and work to achieve a balance between nutritional intake, physical activity, and medication to maintain normal glucose levels for basic survival. These steps and other issues of diabetes care (eg, treatment of hypoglycemia, skin care, foot care, oral hygiene, nonprescription product choices, insulin syringe choice) mandate that the patient learn how to use products properly. Compared with other chronic disorders, diabetes requires the patient to use more products and devices for good management. Most people with diabetes must be instructed to use the materials and products for diabetes control. Moreover, once the patient learns the technical steps for use of the product, he or she must become capable of applying the results to his/her own care. This step moves the patient's focus from survival skills to lifestyle change and modification.

As with any group of products, correct practice is mandatory for good diabetes control. Selecting the proper insulin syringe and teaching correct administration technique (see "Insulin Injection" in Appendix D, Administration Techniques) and syringe disposal will limit the potential for incorrect dosing or accidental sticks. Self-monitoring of blood glucose requires that the patient demonstrate the ability to obtain a valid result at the time of initial training and periodically throughout their monitoring (every 3 to 6 months). Patients must know their blood glucose, blood pressure, and blood lipid goals, and become diligent in applying this information. Each blood glucose monitoring system has unique troubleshooting steps to take if a problem with the monitor is suspected. The patient must learn how to perform these controls and other tests, rather than potentially adjusting therapy with incorrect data. Significant problems can be induced from use of incorrect data. Training patients who request urine ketone test strips to know how and when to perform this test is important. The studies mentioned earlier and changes in Medicare coverage provide strong support for sales growth in diabetes care products. Pharmacists may want to include inquiries about the patient's eye care habits because diabetes is the leading cause of blindness. Networking with eye clinicians in the community to serve as a referral source for people with diabetes who have no regular eye caregiver and have not had an annual dilated eye exam is a very valuable service. Networking and communicating with a patient's other caregivers, especially physicians, is vital. This will allow the patient to reap the highest dividends from the pharmacist's service, and the physician will be able to use this information to improve the patient's care.

DIABETES MELLITUS

DEFINITION

Diabetes mellitus is a metabolic disease, usually chronic in nature, characterized by elevated blood glucose concentrations (hyperglycemia) caused by abnormalities in endogenous insulin secretion or insulin action. There are three primary diabetes classifications: type 1 (formerly called insulin-dependent diabetes mellitus), type 2 (formerly called noninsulin-dependent diabetes mellitus), and gestational diabetes mellitus (GDM). Type 1 diabetes is characterized by a total or near-total lack of endogenous insulin. The clinical onset of the disease generally occurs in childhood or adolescence, but also may occur in adulthood. Type 2 diabetes usually occurs after 40 years of age. Improper glucose utilization and hyperglycemia may occur because of the lack of endogenous insulin production or because of insulin resistance with overproduction of insulin. GDM only occurs in pregnant women with no previous history of diabetes and generally resolves after delivery of the neonate. However, women who experience GDM have an approximately 40% increased risk for developing type 2 diabetes within 15 years after the first episode of GDM.

ETIOLOGY

The etiology of diabetes is unknown. A genetic component has been implicated in all three classifications of diabetes. Other factors associated with type 1 diabetes are environmental (eg, viruses, certain chemicals, drugs) and immune mediation. Pancreatic toxins and viruses may play a role in causing the disease by triggering a reaction that produces a loss in insulin production. The immune system may be involved by causing an autoimmune destruction of the pancreatic beta cells. This destruction usually occurs several years before symptoms develop.

Major factors believed to contribute to the hyperglycemia associated with type 2 diabetes are insulin resistance, impaired pancreatic insulin secretion, and hepatic overproduction of glucose in the fasting and fed states. Genetics may play a role in type 2 diabetes, but the method of inheritance is not clear and is probably multifactorial. However, it is known that the concordance rate among identical twins is nearly 100%. Environmental and lifestyle factors also are strongly associated with the development of type 2 diabetes (eg, sedentary lifestyle, obesity, high-fat diet).

Hormonal changes and genetics may cause GDM in pregnant women. During the second and third trimesters of pregnancy, insulin-antagonist hormones increase. Pregnant women generally experience some degree of insulin resistance, and patients who are unable to compensate for the insulin resistance develop GDM. Researchers suspect the genetic basis causing insulin resistance in type 2 diabetes is the same for GDM; however, its development is not fully understood (further discussion of GDM is beyond the scope of this monograph).

Other etiologies exist. Certain genetic syndromes (eg, genetic defects of beta cell function or insulin action), medications (eg, corticosteroids), and medical complications or disorders (eg, surgery, infection, endocrinopathies) may contribute as well (further discussion of diabetes resulting from these etiologic factors is beyond the scope of this monograph).

INCIDENCE

Diabetes is a common disease in America; of the estimated 19 million people with diabetes, approximately 13 million people have been diagnosed, and approximately 1.3 million new cases occur each year. Type 1 diabetes accounts for 5% to 10% and type 2 diabetes accounts for approximately 90% of all diagnosed cases of diabetes in the United States. Most estimates indicate approximately 5.2 million additional Americans with diabetes remain undiagnosed. Between diagnosed and undiagnosed diabetes patients, there are an estimated 800,000 cases of type 1 diabetes and more than 17 million cases of type 2 diabetes. Approximately 4% of all pregnant women develop diabetes during gestation.

The prevalence of diabetes increases with age: 0.25% of all people younger than 20 years of age, 8.7% of all people 20 years of age or older, and 18.3% of all people 60 years of age and older are afflicted. Prevalence among men and women is the same: 8.7% of women and 8.7% of men ultimately develop diabetes mellitus.

PATHOPHYSIOLOGY

Normally, several metabolic processes act to maintain normoglycemia (normal blood glucose concentrations). Meal-derived nutrients (ie, carbohydrates, fats, protein) are necessary for general metabolic, growth, and repair functions. These nutrients are metabolized and absorbed as glucose, free fatty acids, glycerol, and amino acids. Glucose that is not used immediately by the body is stored in the liver and muscles in the form of glycogen, or is stored in adipose (fatty) tissue as triglyceride for use when glucose is not available readily.

Glucagon and insulin are antagonistic hormones secreted by the pancreas and act to maintain metabolic homeostasis. Glucagon primarily functions in the fasting state to supply the body's energy needs by releasing stored nutrients. In the event that glucose is not readily available to cells, glucagon is released to stimulate hepatic glycogenolysis and increase blood glucose. Secreted insulin allows cells to utilize meal-derived nutrients; it increases transport of glucose into adipocytes and myocytes and stimulates glycogen synthesis. Insulin suppresses hepatic glucose production, lipolysis, and proteolysis.

Insulin secretion is biphasic: Phase I occurs soon after stimulation (eg, ingestion of a large meal). In this phase, production and release of glucose from the liver is decreased. Phase II is a continued response to glucose stimulation, allowing glucose to enter peripheral cells. Muscle cells, hepatocytes, and adipocytes require insulin for glucose use, but several tissues (eg, brain, nerves, cornea, lens, retina, intestines, kidney tubules and medulla, pancreatic beta cells, erythrocytes) do not require insulin to absorb and use glucose.

In type 1 diabetes, because insulin is low or absent, glucose cannot be transported into muscle, liver, and fat cells. This starvation of tissues leads to further glucose production by the liver and breakdown of fat and protein stores to create additional energy sources. This abnormal metabolism of fat, protein, and carbohydrates leads to the metabolic complications of diabetes, and the long-term multiorgan problems. In type 2 diabetes, the patient is producing insulin, but the body is resistant to its actions; thus, despite apparent normal or high insulin concentrations, the liver continues to produce glucose, which is unable to be taken up by the peripheral tissues. This resistance to insulin's action by the liver and tissues results in hyperglycemia and the complications of abnormal nutrient metabolism similar to that of type 1 diabetes. Obesity in type 2 diabetes increases insulin resistance and significantly aggravates the problem.

SIGNS/SYMPTOMS

Patients with diabetes mellitus may experience a variety of signs and symptoms that result from glucose intolerance. Classic signs and symptoms are hyperglycemia (increased blood glucose concentrations), ketoacidosis, polyuria (frequent urination), glucosuria (glucose in the urine), polydipsia (increased thirst), polyphagia (increased hunger), frequent infections, fatigue, weight loss, and, in some cases, weight gain.

Disease onset generally is more profound in patients with type 1 diabetes. The patient may experience extreme weight loss along with various symptoms a few days to weeks prior to diagnosis. Diagnosis often occurs following a life-threatening episode of ketoacidosis. Onset of type 2 diabetes is insidious, and symptoms generally are not as noticeable as in type 1 diabetes. Diagnosis of type 2 diabetes often occurs after the patient experiences chronic complications from diabetes (eg, blurred vision resulting from retinopathy, tingling in the extremities resulting from peripheral neuropathy). Patients with type 2 diabetes are often hyperinsulinemic (ie, they have increased endogenous insulin concentrations) and are more likely to gain weight as a result of hyperinsulinemia. These patients also are less likely to experience ketoacidosis.

Diabetic ketoacidosis: Diabetic ketoacidosis, a potentially life-threatening condition, requires prompt diagnosis and treatment. Hyperglucagonemia, hyperglycemia, and ketoacidosis may result. Diabetic ketoacidosis may result from stress, illness, or insulin omission or may develop slowly after a long period of insulin control. Treat with fluids, correction of acidosis and hypotension, and low-dose regular insulin IM or via IV infusion. See Warnings, Insulin for a comparison with hypoglycemic reaction.

DIAGNOSTIC PARAMETERS/PHYSICAL ASSESSMENT

Clinical Observation: Definitive criteria have been established for the diagnosis of diabetes mellitus. Any of the following tests can be used for establishing a diagnosis of diabetes: random or nonfasting plasma glucose (performed anytime without regard to meals), fasting plasma glucose (FPG; no caloric intake for 8 hours prior to testing), or an oral glucose tolerance test (OGTT) in which the patient is given a glucose load containing the equivalent of 75 g anhydrous glucose dissolved in water. Regardless of the method used, a result indicative of diabetes mellitus should be confirmed subsequently on a different day by the same test or either of the remaining two tests. The following table summarizes the three diagnostic methods:

Diagnosing Diabetes Mellitus		
Test methodology	Normal result*	Result indicative of diabetes mellitus
Random/Nonfasting plasma glucose	< 200 mg/dL plus no history of signs or symptoms of diabetes mellitus	≥ 200 mg/dL plus history of classic signs and symptoms of diabetes mellitus
Fasting plasma glucose (FPG)	< 100 mg/dL	≥ 126 mg/dL
Oral glucose tolerance test (OGTT) 2-hour plasma glucose	< 140 mg/dL	≥ 200 mg/dL

* An FPG value of 100 to 125 mg/dL is considered impaired fasting glucose (IFG). In the OGTT, a 2-hour plasma glucose value of 140 to 199 mg/dL is considered impaired glucose tolerance (IGT). Both IFG and IGT results are risk factors for future development of diabetes mellitus.

The FPG is the preferred test methodology for diagnosis for the following reasons:

- Ease of administration and rapid results
- Patient convenience and acceptability
- Reproducibility of results
- Comparatively low cost

Because of the high prevalence of undiagnosed diabetes mellitus, all individuals should be tested for the disorder at age 45; if results are normal, repeat testing should be done at 3-year intervals. The presence of the following risk factors for diabetes necessitates testing at more frequent intervals or in patients younger than 45 years of age.

Diabetes Mellitus Risk Factors
•Overweight: Body mass index (BMI) 25 to 29.9 kg/m²
•Obesity: BMI ≥ 30 kg/m²
•Familial history: Immediate family members with diabetes mellitus
•Habitual physical inactivity
•Ethnicity: High-risk ethnic populations include African-Americans, Hispanic-Americans, Native Americans, Asian-Americans, Pacific Islanders
•Gestational history: Previous history of GDM or giving birth to a neonate weighing > 9 lb
•Hypertension: Blood pressure ≥ 140/90 mm Hg
•Hypertriglyceridemia: Serum triglyceride concentration ≥ 250 mg/dL
•Low high density lipoprotein (HDL) cholesterol concentration: Serum HDL concentration ≤ 35 mg/dL
•Prior diagnosis of impaired glucose tolerance (IGT or IFG)
•Polycystic ovary syndrome
•History of vascular disease

Interview: During the interview, assess the patient's disease status, symptomatology, and risk factors. The interview should contain, but not be limited to, inquiries concerning the following topics:

- Chief complaint and other symptoms
- Family history
- Gestational history
- Weight/Nutrition
- Exercise regimen
- Prescription and nonprescription medications
- Symptoms of acute and chronic complications
- Results of prior diabetes testing

TREATMENT

Approaches to therapy: All patients exhibiting signs and symptoms associated with diabetes should be referred to a physician for immediate evaluation and treatment. However, other health care professionals may provide valuable information and services to the diabetic patient that empowers the patient to achieve better glycemic control, improve quality of life, and reduce the risk of developing long-term complications.

Treatment of diabetes will vary depending on classification of the disease, the level of desired glycemic control, and the extent of patient knowledge about diabetes mellitus. Therapy generally consists of a combination of diet, exercise, and medications (ie, exogenous insulin, oral antidiabetic agents). Each component of therapy relates with the other and has a profound effect on glycemic control. Modification and assessment of one component of therapy should not be made without assessing the effect on the other components. Treatment of diabetes is most successful if therapy is a continual process that is planned and regularly evaluated by the health care team, the patient, and the patient's family. Patient and family education are important parts of the process.

Type 1 diabetes – Because the pancreas is no longer able to produce insulin, exogenous insulin is required. Strict insulin administration regimens offer little patient variability and require complete adherence to a carefully calculated diet and planned physical exercise. Intensive insulin therapy (eg, multiple daily injections, insulin administration via an insulin pump) offers greater flexibility in the patient's lifestyle (ie, dietary considerations, exercise level) but requires extensive knowledge about glycemic control and self-monitoring of blood glucose (SMBG) several times daily.

Type 2 diabetes – Exogenous insulin may or may not be required to achieve glycemic control in patients with type 2 diabetes. Some patients achieve their treatment goal(s) without pharmacologic intervention and maintain glycemic control with diet and physical activity. However, most patients with type 2 diabetes use exogenous insulin, oral antidiabetic agents, or a combination of these pharmacologic interventions (40%, 49%, and 10%, respectively).

Goals of therapy – The primary therapeutic goals are to achieve and maintain normal glycemic control and to prevent acute and chronic complications. Therapy should be individualized to eliminate symptoms, improve cardiovascular risk factors, achieve and maintain a reasonable body weight, and achieve a state of overall well-being. Areas of focus include weight management, proper nutrition and exercise, smoking cessation (refer to CNS Conditions; Tobacco Use and Smoking Cessation for product information), prevention and treatment of nephropathy and neuropathy, foot and eye examinations, aspirin therapy or other antiplatelet therapies in patients with hypertension, routine blood pressure monitoring, and control of cholesterol and blood pressure. The goal for optimal blood pressure control is less than 130/80 mm Hg. For prudent cholesterol management, the primary goal in adult patients with diabetes is to lower the low density lipoprotein (LDL) value to 100 mg/dL or below; the secondary goal is to increase the HDL value to more than 40 mg/dL in men and more than 50 mg/dL in women. Triglycerides also should be monitored and managed, if elevated.

Nondrug therapy: Regular patient education and assessment are important to attain and maintain good glycemic control and to minimize the risk of complications. The following guidelines may assist in attaining these results:

Educate diabetic patients to perform the following activities **daily**:
• Monitor blood glucose levels as prescribed by health care team
• Inspect feet for any abnormalities or changes
• Practice good dental hygiene
• Eat healthy foods
• Adhere to a prescribed medication schedule
• Engage in physical activity that provides relaxation

Have the diabetic patient make an appointment with a health care provider to accomplish the following on a **quarterly** basis:
• Have laboratory testing for glycosylated hemoglobin (eg, hemoglobin A_{1c})
• Discuss frequency, symptoms, and prevention of abnormal glucose results
• Have feet examined
• Have current diabetes management strategies assessed and evaluated
• Monitor blood pressure
• Discuss changes in activities and behaviors that may improve overall health
• Assess and review goals for glycemic control with health care provider

The patient should have the following appointments and evaluations at least **yearly**:
• Dental examination
• Eye examination for retinal changes, etc.
• Evaluation of renal function
• Assessment of blood cholesterol (LDL, HDL and total cholesterol, triglyceride concentrations)
• Assessment of factors that influence future acute and chronic complications of diabetes

INSULIN

▶ Actions

Insulin is the primary hormone required for proper glucose use in normal metabolic processes.

Insulin preparations are divided into four general categories according to their time course of action: rapid-, short-, intermediate-, and long-acting. Lispro insulin and insulin aspart, which are rapid-acting and have a rapid onset, are available by prescription only. Insulin glargine is long-acting and also available by prescription only. All other insulin preparations are available without a prescription and sold over-the-counter. The variety of preparations available provide for several different dosing regimens to accommodate the needs of the diabetic patient.

Individual response to insulin varies and is affected by diet, exercise, concomitant drug therapy, and other factors. Characteristics of various insulins administered subcutaneously are compared below:

Pharmacokinetics and Compatibility of Various Insulins				
Insulin preparations		Onset (h)	Peak (h)	Duration (h)	Compatible with
Rapid-acting	Lispro insulin solution (NPH)	0.25	0.5 to 1.5	6 to 8	Ultralente, NPH
	Insulin aspart solution	0.25	1 to 3	3 to 5	*
Short-acting	Insulin injection (regular)	0.5 to 1	2.5 to 5	8 to 12	All
	Prompt insulin zinc suspension (semilente)	1 to 1.5	5 to 10	12 to 16	Lente
Intermediate-acting	Isophane insulin suspension (NPH)	1 to 1.5	4 to 12	24	Regular
	Insulin zinc suspension (lente)	1 to 2.5	7 to 15	24	Regular, semilente
Long-acting	Protamine zinc insulin suspension (PZI)	4 to 8	14 to 24	36	Regular
	Extended insulin zinc suspension (ultralente)	4 to 8	10 to 30	> 36	Regular, semilente
	Insulin glargine solution	1.1	5	> 24	None

* Refer to product labeling for information on compatibility.

▶ Indications

Insulin preparations are used to control hyperglycemia in the diabetic patient.

▶ Contraindications

Insulin is contraindicated during hypoglycemic episodes and in patients with hypersensitivity to any of the components of the formulations.

Note: Mild hypoglycemic episodes usually can be treated with oral glucose. Adjustments in insulin therapy, diet, and exercise may be warranted. More severe hypoglycemic episodes (ie, those resulting in insulin shock or coma, or CNS or neurological impairment) require administration of glucagon (SC, IM, or IV) or concentrated IV glucose.

▶ Warnings

Change in insulin: Changes in insulin therapy should be made with caution and under medical supervision. Changes in insulin strength, brand, type, or species source may require dosage adjustment and more frequent monitoring of blood glucose levels.

Hypoglycemia: Hypoglycemia may result from excessive insulin dose or any of the following: increased work or exercise without eating; food not being absorbed in the usual manner because of postponement or omission of a meal or in illness with vomiting, fever, or diarrhea; and when insulin requirements decline.

Symptoms of Hypoglycemia vs Ketoacidosis							
Reaction	Onset	Urine glucose/ acetone	Symptoms				
			CNS	Respiration	Mouth/GI	Skin	Miscellaneous
Hypo- glycemic reaction (insulin reaction)	Sudden	0/0	Fatigue, weakness, nervousness, confusion, headache, diplopia, convulsions, psychoses, dizziness, unconsciousness	Rapid, shallow	Numb, tingling, hunger, nausea	Pallor, moist, shallow, or dry	Normal or noncharacter- istic pulse, eyeballs normal
Keto- acidosis (diabetic coma)	Gradual (hours or days)	+/+	Drowsiness, dim vision	Air hunger	Thirst, acetone breath, nausea, vomiting, abdominal pain, loss of appetite	Dry, flushed	Rapid pulse, soft eyeballs

Injection-site reactions: Lipohypertrophy, the accumulation of fatty tissue, may occur when insulin is injected repeatedly into the same site. It may interfere with insulin absorption. This condition may be avoided by rotating the injection site.

Renal or hepatic impairment: Patients who develop renal or hepatic impairment may require a dosage adjustment in insulin. Carefully monitor glucose in these patients.

Pregnancy: Category B. Insulin is the drug of choice for diabetes control during pregnancy. Patients should be kept under close medical supervision and maintain strict adherence to glucose monitoring. Dosage requirements generally are decreased during the first trimester and increased during the second and third trimesters.

▶ **Drug Interactions**

Insulin may interact with the following:

Drugs that decrease the hypoglycemic effects of insulin: acetazolamide, asparaginase, calcitonin, oral contraceptives, corticosteroids, cyclophosphamide, diltiazem, diuretics, dobutamine, epinephrine, estrogens, isoniazid, lithium carbonate, morphine sulfate, niacin, nicotine, phenothiazines, phenytoin, thiazide diuretics, thyroid hormones.

Drugs that increase the hypoglycemic effects of insulin: ACE inhibitors, alcohol, anabolic steroids, beta-blockers, calcium, chloroquine, clofibrate, lithium carbonate, MAOIs, mebendazole, pentamidine, pyridoxine, salicylates, sulfonamides, tetracyclines.

▶ **Administration and Dosage**

Individualize insulin therapy regimens according to the patient's needs. Many health care providers will prescribe an intensive regimen consisting of several daily injections in an attempt to mimic physiologic insulin secretion. Intensive management requires the patient to have a firm understanding of the principles of treatment and lifestyle factors that may affect glycemic control. For an overview of insulin injection procedures, refer to Appendix D: Insulin Injection Administration Techniques.

The number and size of daily doses, the time of administration, and diet and exercise require continuous medical supervision. Dosage adjustment may be necessary when changing types of insulin, particularly when changing from single-peak to the more purified animal or human insulins.

For insulin suspensions, ensure uniform dispersion by rolling the vial gently between hands. Avoid vigorous shaking that may result in the formation of air bubbles or foam. Regular insulin should be a clear solution.

Administer maintenance doses subcutaneously. Rotate administration sites to prevent lipodystrophy. A general rule is not to administer within 1 inch of the same site for 1 month. The rate of absorption is more rapid when the injection is in the abdomen (possibly more than 50% faster) followed by the upper arm, thigh, and buttocks. Therefore, it may be best to rotate sites within an area rather than rotating areas. Give regular insulin IV or IM in severe ketoacidosis or diabetic coma.

Dosage guidelines: Individualize dosages and closely monitor patients with diabetes mellitus; consider the following dosage guidelines:

> *Adults and children* – 0.5 to 1 unit/kg/day. Adjust doses to achieve premeal and bedtime blood glucose levels of 80 to 140 mg/dL (children younger than 5 years of age, 100 to 200 mg/dL).

> *Timing* – Give insulin aspart immediately before a meal, and give insulin lispro within 15 minutes before a meal. Human regular insulin is best given 30 to 60 minutes before a meal.

Insulin mixtures: See the Pharmacokinetics and Compatibility table in the Actions section. When mixing two types of insulin, always draw clear regular insulin into the syringe first. Patients stabilized on mixtures should have a consistent response if the mixing is standardized. An unexpected response is most likely to occur when switching from separate injections to use of a mixture or vice versa. To avoid dosage error, do not alter the order of mixing insulins or change the type or brand of syringe or needle. Each different type of insulin used must be of the same concentration (units/mL).

NPH/Regular mixtures of insulin are available from the manufacturer in premixed formulations of 70% NPH and 30% regular. A 50/50 combination also is available. NPH/Regular combinations of insulin are stable and are absorbed as if injected separately. In mixtures of regular and lente insulins, binding is detectable 5 minutes to 24 hours after mixing. If the regular/lente mixtures are not administered within the first 5 minutes after mixing, the effect of the regular insulin is diminished. The excess zinc binds with the regular insulin and forms a lente-type insulin. Thus, it is critical that mixtures of regular with the lente insulins be mixed and injected immediately.

These mixtures remain stable for 1 month at room temperature or for 3 months under refrigeration. These mixtures also can be stored in prefilled plastic or glass syringes for 1 week to possibly 14 days under refrigeration. Keep filled syringes in a vertical or oblique position with the needle pointing upward to avoid plugging problems. Prior to injection, pull back the plunger and tip the syringe back and forth, slightly agitating to remix the insulins. Check for normal appearance.

Semilente, ultralente, and lente insulins may be mixed in any ratio; they are chemically identical and differ only in size and structure of insulin particles. These mixtures are stable for 1 month at room temperature or for 3 months under refrigeration.

INSULIN PRODUCTS	
Trade name	Doseform
SHORT-ACTING: Regular Insulin Injections	
Humulin R	**Injection**: 100 units/mL human insulin (rDNA)
Novolin R	**Injection**: 100 units/mL human insulin (rDNA)
Novolin R InnoLet	**Injection**: 100 units/mL human insulin (rDNA) in a disposable pen insulin syringe
Novolin R PenFill	**Cartridges**: 100 units/mL human insulin (rDNA); for use with NovoPen
Regular Iletin II	**Injection**: 100 units/mL purified pork
INTERMEDIATE-ACTING: Isophane Insulin Suspension (NPH) (insulin combined with protamine and zinc)	
Humulin N	**Injection**: 100 units/mL human insulin (rDNA)
Novolin N	**Injection**: 100 units/mL human insulin (rDNA)
Humulin N Pen	**Injection**: 100 units/mL human insulin (rDNA) in a disposable pen insulin delivery device
Novolin N InnoLet	**Injection**: 100 units/mL human insulin (rDNA) in a disposable pen insulin syringe
Novolin N PenFill	**Cartridges**: 100 units/mL human insulin (rDNA); for use with NovoPen
NPH Iletin II	**Injection**: 100 units/mL purified pork
70% Isophane Insulin Suspension (NPH) and 30% Insulin (Regular) Injection	
Humulin 70/30	**Injection**: 100 units/mL human insulin (rDNA)
Novolin 70/30	**Injection**: 100 units/mL human insulin (rDNA)
Novolin 70/30 InnoLet	**Injection**: 100 units/mL human insulin (rDNA) in a disposable pen insulin syringe
Novolin 70/30 PenFill	**Cartridges**: 100 units/mL human insulin (rDNA); for use with NovoPen
50% Isophane Insulin Suspension (NPH) and 50% Insulin (Regular) Injection	
Humulin 50/50	**Injection**: 100 units/mL human insulin (rDNA)
Insulin Zinc Suspension (Lente) (70% crystalline and 30% amorphous insulin suspension)	
Humulin L	**Injection**: 100 units/mL human insulin (rDNA)
Iletin II Lente	**Injection**: 100 units/mL purified pork
LONG-ACTING: Insulin Zinc Suspension, Extended (Ultralente)	
Humulin U Ultralente	**Injection**: 100 units/mL human insulin (rDNA)

Products listed are representative of currently available and widely distributed brands. Similar products, including regional and private label brands, may also exist.

PATIENT INFORMATION
Insulin

- Patient information inserts are available for specific products; read and understand all aspects of insulin use. Patients must receive complete instructions about the nature of diabetes. Strict adherence to prescribed diet, exercise program, and personal hygiene are essential.
- Inject insulin preparations as instructed by your health care provider(s). Rotate subcutaneous injection sites to prevent lipodystrophy. Also refer to Appendix D: Insulin Injection Administration Techniques.
- Insulin stored at room temperature will be less painful to inject compared with that stored in the refrigerator. Allow refrigerator-stored insulin to come to room temperature prior to injecting it.
- Gently roll suspension preparations between palms of the hand before withdrawing an insulin dosage.
- Follow instructions provided if using a pen-filled device.
- Do not change the order of mixing insulins (if applicable) or change the brand, strength, type, species, or dose without your physician's knowledge.
- Insulin requirements may change in patients who become ill, especially with vomiting or fever, during stress or emotional disturbances, or during a severe infection or dietary disruption. Consult a physician.
- Use the same type and brand of syringe to avoid dosage errors
- See your dentist twice yearly; see your ophthalmologist yearly.
- Patients should wear diabetic identification (*Medic-Alert*) so appropriate emergency treatment can be given if complications occur away from home.
- Monitor blood glucose and urine for glucose and ketones as prescribed; regularly monitor blood pressure and serum lipids.
- Store unopened preparations in the refrigerator; do not freeze. Insulin in unopened, prefilled plastic or glass syringes is stable for 1 month under refrigeration. Opened preparations may be stored at room temperature for 1 month.
- Carry a snack or glucose source at all times in case of hypoglycemia.

BLOOD GLUCOSE MONITORING PRODUCTS

BLOOD GLUCOSE METERS

▶ **Actions**

Self-monitoring of blood glucose is crucial in managing diabetes and achieving glycemic control. Monitoring provides the patient and health care provider with the necessary information to individualize therapy and reduce the risks of long-term complications of diabetes. SMBG empowers the patient to become the predominant member of the health care team. Understanding results provides the patient with valuable information, such as how ingestion of certain foods will affect blood glucose levels and how stressful situations and periods of illness may adversely affect glycemic control. However, SMBG is a futile and costly practice if the results are not used to make necessary adjustments in pharmacologic, diet, and exercise regimens.

▶ **Product Selection**

Meter selection: The ability to accurately perform SMBG is one of the most important factors in determining meter selection. Ease of use also is an important consideration and may vary among individuals. The patient's manual dexterity and visual acuity can be important determinants in selecting the appropriate meter. Several meters are available with large digital readouts and other features to assist the visually impaired.

Memory and data management are important to many individuals. Patients often prefer meters that allow them to download SMBG data into their personal computer or their health care professional's computer. However, these features often make use of the meter more complicated and may not be appropriate for certain patients.

The volume of blood required to obtain an accurate reading has continued to decrease with technological advances. Currently, meters are available that require as little as 0.3 mcL of blood. Because the blood volume in 1 drop of blood varies significantly depending on the patient and lancing technique, it is difficult to determine how many drops of blood approximate the required amount for various products. However, blood glucose meter products alert the patient when a sufficient volume of blood has been obtained to receive accurate results. Meters requiring small blood volumes may be preferred by patients who perform SMBG several times daily. Patients with decreased peripheral circulation also may prefer these meters.

The cost of SMBG is often an obstacle for patients with diabetes. Many manufacturers offer incentives such as free meters or coupons that will substantially discount the price of the meter. However, the price of one package of glucose test strips required by the meter may be equivalent to the price of the meter.

Meter maintenance may be a consideration in meter selection. Generally, meters use sensor (amperometric) technology or color reflectance (photometric) technology. Meters using amperometric technology require less maintenance and do not require cleaning after use. Meters that use photometric technology are not as maintenance-friendly and must be cleaned after each use. Carefully follow the manufacturer's recommendations and take care to avoid scratching the optic window of the device.

Accuracy and precision of blood glucose monitoring: An appropriate volume of blood is required to obtain accurate results. Health care professionals should demonstrate the appropriate use of the lancet device and the proper testing techniques. Have the patient thoroughly read all instructions for proper use of the device.

BLOOD GLUCOSE METER PRODUCTS	
Trade name	Description
Accu-Chek Active	**Meter:** Photometric **Data port:** Yes **Required blood volume:** 1 mcL **Alternate test sites:** Yes
Accu-Chek Advantage	**Meter:** Biosensor **Data port:** Yes **Required blood volume:** 4 mcL **Alternate test sites:** No
Accu-Chek Compact[1]	**Meter:** Photometric **Data port:** Yes (wireless download to PC) **Required blood volume:** 1.5 mcL **Alternate test sites:** Yes
Accu-Chek Complete	**Meter:** Amperometric **Data port:** Yes **Required blood volume:** 4 mcL **Alternate test sites:** No
Accu-Chek Voicemate[2]	**Meter:** Amperometric **Data port:** Yes **Required blood volume:** 4 mcL **Alternate test sites:** No

BLOOD GLUCOSE METER PRODUCTS

Trade name	Description
Ascensia BREEZE[3]	**Meter:** Amperometric **Data port:** Yes **Required blood volume:** 2.5 to 3.5 mcL **Alternate test sites:** Yes
Ascensia CONTOUR	**Meter:** Biosensor **Data port:** Yes **Required blood volume:** 0.6 mcL **Alternate test sites:** Yes
Ascensia DEX 2[3]	**Meter:** Biosensor **Data port:** Yes **Required blood volume:** 2.5 to 3.5 mcL **Alternate test sites:** Yes
Ascensia ELITE	**Meter:** Biosensor **Data port:** No **Required blood volume:** 2 mcL **Alternate test sites:** Yes
Ascensia ELITE XL	**Meter:** Biosensor **Data port:** Yes **Required blood volume:** 2 mcL **Alternate test sites:** Yes
BD Logic	**Meter:** Biosensor **Data port:** Yes **Required blood volume:** 0.3 mcL **Alternate test sites:** No
Diascan Partner[2]	**Meter:** Photometric **Data port:** No **Required blood volume:** 10 mcL **Alternate test sites:** No
FreeStyle	**Meter:** Coulometric **Data port:** Yes **Required blood volume:** 0.3 mcL **Alternate test sites:** Yes
FreeStyle Flash	**Meter:** Coulometric **Data port:** Yes **Required blood volume:** 0.3 mcL **Alternate test sites:** Yes
InDuo[4]	**Meter:** Biosensor **Data port:** Yes **Required blood volume:** 1 mcL **Alternate test sites:** Yes
OneTouch Basic	**Meter:** Photometric **Data port:** Yes **Required blood volume:** 10 mcL **Alternate test sites:** No
OneTouch FastTake[5]	**Meter:** Biosensor **Data port:** Yes **Required blood volume:** 1.5 mcL **Alternate test sites:** Yes
OneTouch SureStep	**Meter:** Photometric **Data port:** Yes **Required blood volume:** 10 mcL **Alternate test sites:** No
OneTouch Ultra	**Meter:** Biosensor **Data port:** Yes **Required blood volume:** 1 mcL **Alternate test sites:** Yes

BLOOD GLUCOSE METER PRODUCTS

Trade name	Description
OneTouch UltraSmart	**Meter:** Biosensor **Data port:** Yes **Required blood volume:** 1 mcL **Alternate test sites:** Yes
Precision Q•I•D	**Meter:** Biosensor **Data port:** Yes **Required blood volume:** 3.5 mcL **Alternate test sites:** No
Precision Sof-Tact	**Meter:** Biosensor **Data port:** Yes **Required blood volume:** 2 to 3 mcL **Alternate test sites:** Yes
Precision Xtra[6]	**Meter:** Biosensor **Data port:** Yes **Required blood volume:** 3.5 mcL **Alternate test sites:** No
Prestige IQ	**Meter:** Photometric **Data port:** Yes **Required blood volume:** 7 mcL **Alternate test sites:** No
Prestige LX	**Meter:** Photometric **Data port:** No **Required blood volume:** 7 mcL **Alternate test sites:** No
Prestige TrueTrack Smart System	**Meter:** Electrochemical **Data port:** No **Required blood volume:** 1 mcL **Alternate test sites:** No

Products listed are representative of currently available and widely distributed brands. Similar products, including regional and private label brands, may also exist.

[1] Uses drum instead of individual test strips.
[2] Audio features for people with visual impairments.
[3] Uses disc, not strips.
[4] Also an insulin delivery system.
[5] Available through mail order only.
[6] Also measures ketones.

LANCET DEVICES

▶ Product Selection

Selection of lancet devices varies depending upon patient needs. Lancet devices approved for alternate site testing offer the option to collect blood samples from places other than the fingertip (eg, forearm, thigh). Because these areas can be less sensitive, this may be an advantage for patients who test several times per day. However, patients should be aware that these blood sugar results may differ from those with blood taken from the fingertip. Children and patients with poor coordination or tremors may prefer spring-loaded devices because they are easier to reset for the next use. Lancet devices that require removal of the cover to reset the device are generally more difficult to use than the spring-loaded devices. Devices with dials offer variability in depth of penetration. While more superficial insertions are preferred, patients may need varying depths of penetration for different fingers or when finger temperature affects blood flow. Manufacturers of blood glucose meters frequently provide lancet devices and a sample package of lancets with the purchase of a blood glucose meter.

LANCET DEVICE PRODUCTS	
Trade name	Description
Ascensia MICROLET VACULANCE[1]	**Device**: 4 depth settings, vacuum action
Gentle-Lance	**Device**: 5 depth settings
Ascensia MICROLET	**Device**: 5 depth settings, spring-loaded
Accu-Chek SoftTouch	**Device**: 5 depth settings, dial
auto-Lancet	**Device**: 5 depth settings, dial
auto-Lancet Mini	**Device**: 5 depth settings, dial
BD Lancet Device	**Device**: 6 depth settings, spring-loaded
OneTouch UltraSoft[1]	**Device**: 7 depth settings, dial
Penlet Plus	**Device**: 7 depth settings, dial
Autolet Impression[1]	**Device**: 7 depth settings, dial, force adjustment
Accu-Chek Softclix[1]	**Device**: 11 depth settings (0.8 mm to 2.3 mm), spring-loaded, dial
Single-time use lancets	
Accu-Chek Safe-T-Pro	**Device**: 1.8 mm; 21-gauge needle
Safe-T-Lance Plus	**Device**: 1.8 mm; 18-, 21-, and 25-gauge needle
Unistik 2	**Device**: 2.4 and 3 mm; 26-gauge needle
Vitalet Pro	**Device**: 2.4 and 3 mm

Products listed are representative of currently available and widely distributed brands. Similar products, including regional and private label brands, may also exist.

[1] Can be used on alternate test sites.

LANCET NEEDLES

▶ Product Selection

Lancet device compatibility, cost, and needle gauge (eg, diameter) vary. Higher-gauge (smaller diameter) needles are thinner and less painful to insert. Patients with delicate skin, children, and first-time users may prefer higher-gauge lancet needles. Also, blood glucose meters that require smaller volumes of blood might allow for use of higher-gauge lancet needles. Patients with poor circulation or calloused or tough skin may require lower-gauge (larger diameter) needles to obtain the appropriate blood volume required for their meter.

LANCET NEEDLE PRODUCTS	
Trade name	Description
BD Ultra-Fine 33	**Needle**: 33-gauge
BD Ultra-Fine II	**Needle**: 30-gauge
Sunmark Super Thin Lancets	
Accu-Chek Softclix	**Needle**: 28-gauge
Accu-Chek SoftTouch	
Ascensia MICROLET	
Cleanlet	
EZ-Lets Thin	
Gentle-Let (general purpose)	
MediSense Thin Lancets	
OneTouch UltraSoft	
Unilet ComforTouch	
Unilet GP Ultralite	

LANCET NEEDLE PRODUCTS	
Trade name	**Description**
EZ-Lets Thin	**Needle**: 26-gauge
Gentle-Let (general purpose)	
Vitalet	
Cleanlet	**Needle**: 25-gauge
OneTouch FinePoint	
EZ-Lets	**Needle**: 23-gauge
Gentle-Let (general purpose)	
Gentle-Let (safety style)	
Unilet GP Superlite	
Unilet Superlite	
Vitalet	
EZ-Lets	**Needle**: 21-gauge
Gentle-Let (general purpose)	
Gentle-Let (safety style)	
Unilet	
Unilet GP	

Products listed are representative of currently available and widely distributed brands. Similar products, including regional and private label brands, may also exist.

PATIENT INFORMATION
Blood Glucose Monitoring Products

- Follow instructions accompanying the product exactly.
- Monitor blood glucose as prescribed. Monitor urine ketones if your blood glucose level has been greater than 300 mg/dL for two consecutive blood glucose determinations.
- Blood glucose monitoring is recommended to achieve normal blood sugar levels. Keep track of your blood glucose results so that adjustments in your treatment program can be made more easily.
- Participate in a thorough diabetes education program so that you understand diabetes and all aspects of its treatment, including diet, exercise, personal hygiene, and how to self-monitor blood glucose.
- Perform the test the same way each time.
- Periodically demonstrate your SMBG technique to your health care provider, including finger lancing technique.
- Monitor glucose when you have a cold, the flu, or any other kind of illness; when you feel the signs of low or high blood sugar (greater than 240 mg/dL); when your blood sugar is well over the range your doctor has set for you; when you are under unusual physical or emotional stress; during pregnancy; or after a testing pattern has been established with your doctor or educator.
- Have all the materials you need before beginning the test: test strips, timer (stopwatch or watch with a second hand), sterile lancet, cotton or rayon balls, alcohol wipes, glucose meter.
- Color vision is needed to properly read visual, but not meter, test results. Have someone else confirm the visual test results if in doubt.
- Quality control and sample tests may be required before testing.
- If test results seem questionable, check expiration date on the test strip labeling, repeat the test using a new test strip, run controls, check glucose meter, and check procedure (timing).
- If you are unable to identify the cause of a low or high test result, contact your doctor or diabetes educator. Know the symptoms of hyperglycemia (high blood sugar), which include thirst, hunger, and frequent and excessive urination, and those of hypoglycemia (low blood sugar), which include trembling, sweating, blurred vision, rapid heartbeat, and tingling or numbness around the mouth or fingertips.
- If you experience stomach pain, vomiting, or difficulty breathing, contact your doctor immediately.
- Individuals with high uric acid, bilirubin, cholesterol, triglyceride, or hematocrit levels may have lowered glucose levels.
- Diabetes education may be obtained through your local chapter of the American Diabetes Association (http://www.diabetes.org).
- Follow the cleaning and maintenance instructions that come with the meter. Failure to follow these instructions may lead to meter errors.
- Store meter and test strips at room temperature. Avoid extreme fluctuations in climate and humidity.

HEMOGLOBIN A₁c HOME TEST

▶ **Actions**

The Hemoglobin A_{1c} (HbA_{1c}) test measures the percent of glycated hemoglobin levels in whole blood. The amount of HbA_{1c} in the blood reflects blood sugar control for the last 120 days (lifespan of a red blood cell). In healthy individuals, 5% of all hemoglobin is glycated; in patients with diabetes and high blood glucose levels, HbA_{1c} ranges from below 7% (normal) to 25%, if diabetes is poorly controlled over a long period of time.

▶ **Indications**

FDA-approved for use by diabetes patients to obtain HbA_{1c} test results at home and monitor their progress between visits.

▶ **Warnings**

People with hemophilia or on anticoagulant therapy should consult their doctor or health care provider before using this kit.

▶ **Administration and Dosage**

If blood sugar target ranges are stable, measure HbA_{1c} levels at least twice a year. If the patient is taking insulin, the patient's treatment changes (eg, new medicine), or if the patient's blood sugar is too high, measure HbA_{1c} more frequently (approximately every 3 months). This test is *not* a substitute for glucose monitoring.

Blood sample and test may be done at any time of day. No special diet is necessary. Patients should not adjust their medication unless instructed to do so by their physician.

Do not open the pouches until ready to use. If refrigerated, allow all parts of the test kit to come to room temperature (64° to 82°F; 18° to 28°C) for at least 1 hour before using. Avoid testing in direct sunlight, on hot or cold surfaces, or near sources of heat or cold. Patients should read instructions thoroughly before performing the test.

Prick finger to gather a drop of blood with supplied pipette, mix blood with reagent, and apply sample to monitor. Result will appear within 8 minutes. Record result, test date, and kit's lot number on the supplied log sheet. Patients should fill in the name and address of their health care provider on the patient result card, along with the result, and phone or mail it to their health care provider.

HEMOGLOBIN A₁c HOME TEST KIT	
Trade name	**Description**
A1cNow	**Kit**: Single-use, disposable test. Box includes monitor, Quick Start Guide with A1C Result Log, single-use lancet, sample dilution kit (tube and tube holder), blood collector, sample dropper, patient result card, and patient registration card.

Products listed are representative of currently available and widely distributed brands. Similar products, including regional and private label brands, may also exist.

PATIENT INFORMATION
Hemoglobin A$_{1c}$ Home Test

- Patient instructions accompany the product. Read instructions carefully before use, preferably before leaving the pharmacy, in case you have questions.
- The American Diabetes Association (ADA) recommends you test HbA$_{1c}$ at least twice per year.
- The ADA recommends an HbA$_{1c}$ goal of 7% or lower, and suggests action when the HbA$_{1c}$ level is above 8%. Your health care provider can tell you what level is right for you.
- Do not adjust medication unless instructed by your doctor.
- Do *not* substitute this test for glucose monitoring.
- Use only your fingerstick blood sample. Do not use any other body fluids to perform this test.
- Do not add your blood directly to the monitor. It must be added to the tube first.
- Blood sample and test may be done at any time of day. No special diet is necessary.
- Allow all parts of the test kit to come to room temperature for at least 1 hour before testing. Avoid running the test in direct sunlight, on hot or cold surfaces, or near sources of heat or cold. Do not open the test until ready to use.
- Record results as soon as possible to prevent loss of information.
- If yellow solution touches the eyes, flush with water.

HOME
DIAGNOSTICS / DEVICES

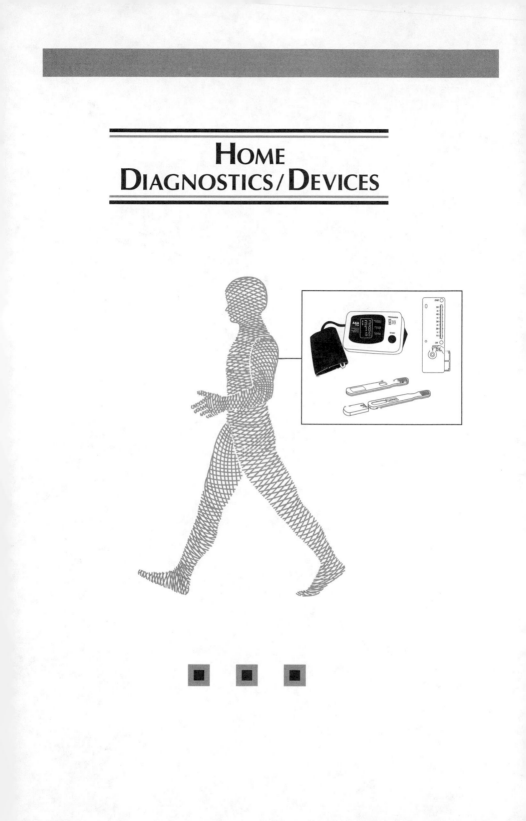

NONPRESCRIPTION DRUG THERAPY
TABLE OF CONTENTS

■ ■ ■

HOME DIAGNOSTICS/DEVICES

Home testing products serve two basic purposes: Early detection of illness (eg, UTIs, illnesses associated with fecal occult blood) or some condition (eg, pregnancy, ovulation), and monitoring of disease control (eg, blood pressure, cholesterol levels). Early detection is advantageous in alerting patients to seek medical attention in a timely fashion, while routine self-monitoring can help patients improve, or at least maintain, their health. Self-monitoring allows patients make day-to-day decisions regarding drug and non-drug therapy and can alert patients to abnormal levels more quickly. Some products are designed to be administered by the patient, who also interprets the results. Several kits have patients collect required specimens and send them to diagnostic centers for analysis. Patients then access the results by calling a toll-free number. Various contraceptive aids and devices are also available to patients, allowing them to make personal decisions that best fit their lifestyles. It is important for health care professionals to be aware of these choices to help the patient make informed decisions.

The home diagnostic industry has experienced strong growth. In July of 1998, industry revenues were predicted to double over the next 4 years to reach $2.8 billion. This growth correlates with advances in biotechnology that have greatly simplified testing procedures. Technological advances have transformed many home testing kits from mini-laboratories into easy-to-use, highly accurate products that produce rapid results at an affordable price.

Several other products are driving growth in this market. Increasing health care costs have prompted patients to try to reduce their expenditures. Home diagnostics assist in that goal by helping patients avoid unnecessary physician visits and seek earlier treatment. It is often more convenient and less expensive to perform a test at home and then follow up with a physician if needed. In addition, more patients are assuming a greater degree of personal responsibility for their health. As a result, patients are becoming increasingly committed to self-testing and monitoring on a regular basis. This provides them with feedback between physician appointments to keep them aware of their progress toward health care goals and promote their empowerment concerning their health.

Several general recommendations should be followed when using home diagnostic products. Testing must adhere strictly to the manufacturer's instructions to ensure accurate results. Patients should read instructions before performing tests and clarify any points not clearly understood. If errors are made, treatment may not be sought when it should be. False results or improper reading of tests could lead patients to seek treatment when there is no actual problem.

When recommending products, help patients select those that involve the fewest number of steps and are simplest to use. The more user-friendly versions are generally preferred because they reduce the potential for human error. It is important that patients understand that these products are not a substitute for medical care. If patients receive positive results, they must follow up with a physician for proper diagnosis and treatment. Regardless of the results, medical care should be sought if the patient experiences signs or symptoms of disease.

Patients need unbiased and complete information when evaluating the appropriateness of home diagnostics or contraceptive devices for their situation. Pharmacists can assist patients in selection and use of these products, as well as understanding their application and limitations.

Home Blood Pressure Monitors

INTRODUCTION

The increasing availability of OTC blood pressure devices has led to greater use by the public. Despite this increase, there is little guidance on product selection and use from the medical community.

The National High Blood Pressure Education Program advocated the use of home blood pressure monitoring (HBPM) in two groups of individuals, delineating the following potential advantages for each:

For the general public:

- HBPM may detect hypertension in previously undiagnosed people. This would include those having a mildly elevated reading in the past, and those concerned about the possibility of developing hypertension (ie, family history of hypertension).
- Serial blood pressure readings taken over time by individuals may help document blood pressure patterns that may be used to select proper treatment.

For patients diagnosed with hypertension:

- HBPM encourages patients and families to actively participate in the management of their hypertension.
- HBPM may increase patient compliance with prescribed lifestyle changes and pharmacotherapies.
- HBPM supplies health professionals with more objective measures to aid in making therapeutic decisions.
- HBPM may result in simplification of the treatment regimen.
- HBPM may reduce the frequency of physician office visits.

These potential advantages associated with HBPM need to be weighed against potential disadvantages. Misinterpretation or overreaction to the blood pressure readings may result in psychological distress or inappropriate self-adjustment of treatment regimens. This may lead to treatment errors or medication side effects. In addition, inadequate instruction on how to use a blood pressure measurement device may lead to inaccurate readings. Purchase of equipment that includes a cuff of improper size may yield inaccurate readings, and a hectic or noisy environment may result in increased blood pressure. However, these and other potential problems can be avoided with proper patient education and follow-up.

DEFINITION

The table below details the classification of blood pressure and blood pressure treatment goals according to the Joint National Committee on the Prevention, Detection, Evaluation, and Treatment of high blood pressure (JNC) guidelines published in 1997.

Classification of Blood Pressure for Adults ≥ 18 Years Old		
Category	Systolic (mm Hg)	Diastolic (mm Hg)
Normal Ranges		
Optimal	< 120	< 80
Normal	< 130	< 85
High-Normal	130-139	85-89
Hypertension		
Stage 1	140-159	90-99
Stage 2	160-179	100-109
Stage 3	≥ 180	≥ 110

The general treatment goal is to reduce blood pressure to below 140/ 90 mm Hg. Because of the increased risk of cardiovascular disease or complications, more aggressive goals are recommended for patients with diabetes, target organ damage, or clinical cardiovascular disease and those with renal insufficiency with proteinuria more than 1 g per 24 hours. Specific endpoints should be determined by the patient's physician.

JNC VI Treatment Goals	
General Goal	< 140/90 mm Hg
Patients with diabetes, TOD[1], or CCD[2]	< 135/85 mm Hg
Patients with renal damage + proteinuria> 1 g/24 hours	< 125/75 mm Hg

[1] Target organ disease.
[2] Clinical cardiovascular disease.

ETIOLOGY

Hypertension is classified as either primary or secondary, based on the cause. In 90% to 95% of patients with hypertension, the underlying cause is unknown. These individuals are said to have primary hypertension. Hypertension resulting from a specific identifiable cause is known as secondary hypertension. Occurring in 5% to 10% of hypertensive patients, secondary hypertension is usually caused by renal or endocrine system disease such as renovascular disease, Cushing's syndrome, etc.

The following factors increase one's risk of high blood pressure:

- Heredity.
- Race (eg, high blood pressure is more commonly seen in black patients).
- Male sex.
- Age.
- Sodium sensitivity.
- Obesity/overweight.
- Heavy alcohol consumption.
- Use of oral contraceptives (and some other medications [eg, steroids, NSAIDs, nasal decongestants, diet pills, MAOIs, tricyclic antidepressants]).
- Sedentary/Inactive lifestyle.

INCIDENCE

According to statistics provided by the American Heart Association, more than 50,000,000 Americans have high blood pressure. The estimated prevalence of hypertension for American adults aged 20 and older is 24.4% for non-

Hispanic white males and 19.3% for females; 35% for non-Hispanic black males and 34.2% for females; and 25.2% for Hispanic males and 22% for females.

SIGNS/SYMPTOMS

In general, hypertension is considered an asymptomatic disease. Although some patients with hypertension may complain of headaches, most patients will not have symptoms until target organ damage has occurred. The main organ systems affected by the disease include the heart, central nervous system, eyes, and kidney.

DIAGNOSTIC PARAMETERS/PHYSICAL ASSESSMENT

Interview: To aid patients in the selection and proper use of home blood pressure monitors, it may be beneficial to ask about the following:

- Conditions that would preclude the use of one system over another (vision/hearing impairment, physical coordination, mental acuity).
- Established diagnosis of high blood pressure. If not, has a physician recommended use or does the patient suspect they have a problem (if so, urge a physician visit)?
- Current medication profile (prescription and OTC).
- History of illness.
- Alcohol intake.
- Smoking.
- Diet.
- Family history.
- Exercise and lifestyle.

HOME BLOOD PRESSURE MONITORS

▶ **Indications**

Home blood pressure monitors help patients and health care providers distinguish true hypertension from "white coat" hypertension. These products can aid in assessing the response of antihypertensive therapy prescribed by a physician. They may also improve patient compliance and reduce costs.

▶ **Warnings**

Patients with irregular heart rhythms are generally not suitable candidates for HBPM. Arrhythmias cause beat-to-beat cardiac output to vary substantially, making blood pressure determinations difficult.

Patients with marked obesity are generally not suitable candidates for HBPM. Severely overweight patients may have difficulty obtaining an appropriately sized cuff.

Recheck monitor's accuracy every 6 months. Usually this can be done by connecting the device to a mercury column using a Y-tube. If an error of more than 4 mm Hg is detected, recalibrate the device. Calibration equipment and instructions can be obtained from the manufacturer.

Impaired hearing or vision and reduced mental acuity or poor physical coordination may interfere with the appropriate measurement technique. Patients with these conditions may find the fully automatic devices a suitable selection.

▶ Drug Interactions

The patient should not consume caffeine or nicotine during the 30 minutes prior to blood pressure measurement. Caffeine and nicotine trigger the body to release adrenalin, causing an increased heart rate and blood vessel constriction. A cup of coffee or a cigarette may increase systolic blood pressure by 15 mm Hg.

Pseudoephedrine and phenylpropanolamine may cause elevations in blood pressure secondary to vasoconstriction. These drugs are present in many OTC cold and diet preparations.

Because of inhibition of prostaglandin synthesis in the kidney, nonsteroidal anti-inflammatory drugs may cause increases in blood pressure secondary to sodium and fluid retention.

▶ Guidelines for Use

The accuracy and reliability of blood pressure measurements are enhanced by following the manufacturer's directions and the widely accepted procedures recommended by the American Heart Association.

Any clothing that restricts blood flow in the arms must be removed before measurement. Restrictive clothing, including rolled or pushed up shirt sleeves, can falsely elevate blood pressure.

The patient should be seated comfortably for at least 5 to 10 minutes before measurement. Recent stressful activity or exertion may falsely elevate blood pressure.

The patient should have his/her arm relaxed and at about heart level. Tense arm muscles may falsely elevate blood pressure. The patient should have legs uncrossed with both feet on the floor.

Two or more measurements separated by at least 2 minutes should be obtained and averaged.

Results should be recorded with the time and date of the measurement and the time of the last dose of antihypertensive medications. This information should be supplied to the physician.

▶ Product Selection

There are two basic types of HBPM devices, aneroid meters, and electronic devices. Aneroid meters rely on auscultation (measurement of sound) using a stethoscope to detect Korotkoff sounds (the sounds heard with the stethoscope during the auscultatory determination of blood pressure) as an indirect measure of blood pressure. The first audible sound represents the systolic blood pressure. As the cuff begins to deflate, the sounds change in quality and intensity until they finally disappear. The disappearance of the sound represents the diastolic blood pressure. The electronic devices rely on oscillometric (measurement of vibration) sensors to measure blood pressure by detecting blood surges. The electronic products measure blood pressure readings by detecting changes in pressure in the cuff, rather than detecting sounds with a microphone as in the aneroid meters.

Aneroid devices: The aneroid devices are generally more accurate and less expensive than the electronic models. However, they do require a certain degree of manual dexterity and hearing acuity. Most of the aneroid products come with a stethoscope attached to the cuff, making it easier to manipulate the equipment. A d-ring on the cuff allows the user to easily place the cuff properly on the arm. Aneroid devices must be checked against a mercury sphygmomanometer for accuracy at least once a year.

Electronic devices: Generally, patients find the electronic devices easier to use. Electronic home blood pressure monitors are more expensive, and many of the devices on the market lack accuracy and reliability data, although in most instances they are considered sufficiently accurate for home use if the patient has been instructed in the proper technique. These devices include manually inflating, auto-inflating, and wrist monitors. Many only require placement of the cuff, turning the device on and pressing the start button for use, requiring minimal skill. Patients with hearing difficulties or physical limitations may find these devices more useful.

There are many features available on the monitors including self-inflation, memory, extra-large displays, and print-outs of results. Selection depends on personal preference.

Finger cuff devices are not generally recommended. Because the finger is smaller than the arm and farther away from the heart, more factors can interfere with the measuring technique leading to erroneous results. However, these monitors are easiest to use.

HOME BLOOD PRESSURE MONITORS

Manufacturer	Trade name	Description
A & D Medical	UA-702 Manual Inflation	Digital; manual inflation
	UA-767 One Step Auto-Inflation	Digital; automatic inflation
	UA-777 One Step Auto-Inflation/Fuzzy Logic	Digital; automatic inflation (with micropump)
	UB-322 HealthWatch Wrist Blood Pressure Monitor	Digital; automatic inflation (with micropump)
	UB-302 Compact Wrist Blood Pressure Monitor	Digital; automatic inflation (with micropump)
	UB-325 Wrist Blood Pressure Monitor	Digital; automatic inflation (with micropump)
	Self-Storing Monitor	Digital; automatic inflation
HealthTeam	Manual Home Blood Pressure Kit	Aneroid. Includes stethoscope, blood pressure diary.
Marshall	One Person Home Blood Pressure Unit	Aneroid. Includes stethoscope, blood pressure log book.
Micronta	BP-1 Home Blood Pressure Tester	Digital
Omron	Automatic Inflation Monitor with Fuzzy Logic	Digital; automatic inflation
	Automatic Inflation Monitor	Digital; automatic inflation
	Fuzzy Logic Monitor	Digital; automatic inflation
	Compact Wrist Monitor	Digital; automatic inflation. With or without flip-up panel.
	Wrist Monitor with Graph and Memory	Digital; inflation preset switch
	Wrist Monitor	Digital; inflation preset switch
	Memory, Print-Out and Graph Monitor	Digital
	Automatic Inflation Monitor with Printer	Digital; automatic inflation
	Manual Inflation Monitor	Digital; manual inflation
Sunmark	175 Sensor Cuff Electronic/Digital Blood Pressure and Pulse Monitor	Digital; automatic inflation
Tycos	Home Blood Pressure Kit with Stethoscope	Aneroid; trigger-release inflation. Includes stethoscope and heart sounds training tape.

Products listed are representative of currently available and widely distributed brands. Similar products, including regional and private label brands, may also exist.

PATIENT INFORMATION
Home Blood Pressure Monitors

- If you suspect that you have high blood pressure but have not consulted a physician, do so before using a home blood pressure monitor.
- Ensure that you are carefully instructed on and fully understand the proper use of the device selected.
- Take readings in the morning and the evening on both work and non-work days. The frequency of readings should be based on the clinical situation; be aware that a hectic or noisy environment may lead to increased blood pressure. Patients newly diagnosed with high blood pressure or having recent changes in their medication regimen should monitor their blood pressure several days per week. Stable patients require less frequent readings.
- Obtaining accurate results depends on using a proper cuff size. Using a cuff that is too small can yield falsely elevated results.
- Wait 10 to 15 minutes after a bath and 30 minutes after eating before using these devices.
- There is no universally accepted upper limit of normal blood pressure. A generally accepted reading is 135/85 mm Hg. Patients with repeated elevated readings should contact a physician for evaluation.
- Blood pressure varies minute-to-minute and day-to-day. This variability is expected and should not cause alarm. A single elevated reading does not constitute a diagnosis of hypertension, but indicates that further observation is necessary.
- Do not self-adjust your blood pressure medications unless specifically instructed to do so by your physician.
- The mechanical devices tend to be sensitive to arm movements. The arm should remain stationary during the measuring procedure.
- A trained medical professional should routinely check your technique.
- Equipment should be calibrated at least once a year.
- Home blood pressure monitoring is not a substitute for routine physician evaluations.

FECAL OCCULT BLOOD KITS

DEFINITION

Fecal occult blood test kits are screening devices used to assist in identifying medical disorders that cause lower intestinal bleeding. A positive test result indicates the patient needs a thorough medical examination to determine the cause of bleeding, thus serving as an early warning signal of gastrointestinal disorders needing medical attention.

The most publicized use of these products is to aid in detecting colorectal cancer. The advantage of these products is that they may be used at the patient's convenience and in the privacy of the home. They are convenient to use, relatively inexpensive, and noninvasive.

ETIOLOGY

A number of conditions, including ulcers, regional enteritis (Crohn disease), colitis, anal fissures, diverticulitis, hemorrhoids, and cancer of the colon and rectum, can cause blood in the stool.

INCIDENCE

There is evidence that fecal occult blood screening and early detection can reduce mortality from colorectal cancer, which is the second most common form of cancer in the US, accounting for 15% of all cancers. Early detection, which may be aided by fecal occult blood tests, and treatment are significant factors in the management of diseases of the GI tract.

DIAGNOSTIC PARAMETERS/PHYSICAL ASSESSMENT

Interview: To aid in the selection and proper use of fecal occult blood testing kits, it may be beneficial to ask patients about the following:

- If blood has already been noticed in the stool, how long has the patient noticed this?
- Appearance of the stool (eg, blood-tinged, black, tarry).
- Appearance of blood (eg, color on surface of stool or mixed in stool).
- History of abdominal pain and the nature, intensity, and frequency of the pain.
- History of bowel disorders.
- History of familial polyposis syndrome (multiple adenomatous polyps with high malignant potential, lining the mucous membrane of the intestine), other adenomatous polyps or a family history of colorectal cancer.
- Prior use of fecal occult blood tests.
- Problems with vision or color recognition.
- Medication profile (some medications [eg, aspirin, NSAIDs] may increase the risk of GI bleeding).
- Patient's awareness of the chance of false-positive/-negative results (which may occur due to ingestion of certain foods such as rare beef).

FECAL OCCULT BLOOD TESTS

▶ Actions

The products designed for in-home use detect occult blood in the feces with a colorimetric assay for hemoglobin. A chromogenic dye, tetramethylbenzidine, and peroxide are sandwiched between two layers of biodegradable paper forming the testing device that is floated in the toilet bowl following a bowel movement. These kits are based on the premise that a significant amount of surface blood present on the stool will dislodge and float on the surface of the toilet bowl water after defecation. Hemoglobin from any blood present liberates oxygen from the peroxide, which in turn oxidizes the tetramethylbenzidine, resulting in the formation of a blue-green color on the designated area of the test pad. The tests will detect at least 2 mg of hemoglobin per 100 mL of water.

▶ Indications

Fecal occult blood kits are used to detect lower intestinal bleeding that may be associated with a medical disorder.

▶ Warnings

Occult blood may be located on the surface of the stool or within the stool matrix, depending on the source of GI bleeding.

Blood due to lower GI abnormalities is more likely to be on the stool surface than in the stool matrix. Tests designed for in-home use are limited to detecting bleeding occurring as a result of disorders of the lower GI tract.

Color vision is necessary to properly read test results. Visually impaired persons may need assistance.

Toilet bowl cleaners, disinfectants and deodorizers can interfere with the tests. Such products should be removed from the toilet bowl and tank prior to conducting the test. The toilet should be flushed twice, thus removing any foreign chemicals before the bowel movement.

With some tests, a false-positive result may occur from recent ingestion of red, rare beef. Check individual products for information.

▶ Drug Interactions

Medications known to cause GI irritation should be avoided for 2 days prior to testing and during testing. The microscopic bleeding that may result from the use of these drugs may cause false-positive test results. Specific products to be avoided include aspirin, iron, nonsteroidal anti-inflammatory agents, corticosteroids, and dipyridamole.

Vitamin C (ascorbic acid) in doses more than 250 mg/day can block the peroxidase activity of hemoglobin, resulting in a false-negative test.

The use of rectally administered medications (eg, suppositories, ointments, creams, enemas) should be avoided during the testing period.

▶ Guidelines for Use

Based on American Cancer Society recommendations for colorectal cancer screening, fecal occult blood tests should be repeated yearly for men and women over age 50, while sigmoidoscopies should be repeated every 3 to 5 years in this age group. An annual rectal exam should be performed yearly for patients over 40 years of age.

Fecal occult blood test kits include 3 separate tests which are to be conducted on 3 consecutive bowel movements. Because all intestinal abnormalities do not bleed continuously, testing on 3 occasions increases the likelihood of detecting any occult blood that may be present in the stool.

These tests involve dropping a test pad into the toilet bowl following a bowel movement and observing the pad for a color change. The test should be performed within 5 minutes after the bowel movement. The results should be read at the time specified by the manufacturer as the color reaction may fade quickly. The presence of any trace of blue-green color in the indicated test area denotes a positive test result.

The kits contain a quality control mechanism to determine if the test pad is functioning properly. The manufacturer's directions should be followed to conduct the quality control test.

The patient should record the results of each test on the postcard provided and mail the completed card to his/her physician.

▶ Product Selection

The two fecal occult blood test kit products available over-the-counter are very similar. The primary advantage of *EZ Detect* is that it does not require the patient to refrain from ingesting red/rare meats or vitamin C before and during the testing period. *ColoCare* advises against consuming both.

FECAL OCCULT BLOOD KITS	
Trade name	Description
ColoCare	**Kit**: 3 test pads and reply card.
EZ Detect	**Kit**: 5 test tissues, positive control package, and test result postcard.

Products listed are representative of currently available and widely distributed brands. Similar products, including regional and private label brands, may also exist.

PATIENT INFORMATION
Fecal Occult Blood Kits

- The tests should be performed exactly according to the manufacturer's instructions in the package labeling to ensure accurate results. Patients should carefully read these instructions before use and clarify any points not clearly understood with their pharmacist or physician.
- Increasing fiber in the diet 2 to 3 days before using the tests may aid the passage of stool and facilitate detection of lesions that bleed intermittently.
- Eating red/rare meat may cause false-positive results due to the possible presence of blood (hemoglobin). The kits vary in their instruction about ingesting dietary products before and during the testing period.
- Certain foods and medications may interfere with test results.
- Avoid drinking alcohol for 2 days before and during testing because it can cause GI irritation and bleeding.
- Consult physician before discontinuing any prescribed medications that may interfere with test results.
- These tests should not be performed during times of known bleeding such as menstrual or hemorrhoidal bleeding.
- The patient should urinate prior to each bowel movement to be tested and flush. Large amounts of urine may interfere with the accurate reading of test results.
- Toilet paper should not be thrown into the toilet bowl until after the test results are read.
- Handle the test pads by the corners only. Avoid touching the middle of the pad.
- Complete the series of 3 tests even if the first 2 produce negative results.
- These tests do not take the place of a regular physical and rectal exam by a physician. They only serve as supplemental screening tools.
- All positive results need physician follow-up in a timely manner to determine the cause of bleeding and define proper management. The test does not replace established diagnostic procedures.
- Negative tests do not necessarily eliminate the possibility of an intestinal disorder. Since lesions may bleed intermittently, report any persistent changes in bowel habits regardless of the fecal occult blood testing results. These tests are not conclusive for the absence or presence of a pathological condition.

HOME HEPATITIS C TEST

INTRODUCTION

Home hepatitis C testing kits are intended to aid in the convenient detection of the hepatitis C virus (HCV) in individuals. The kit consists of a blood specimen collection and transportation device for home use that allow consumers to obtain a blood sample they can mail away to be tested for antibodies to HCV at a laboratory site.

ETIOLOGY

HCV, 1 of 6 hepatitis viruses that have been identified (A, B, C, D, E, and G), is a blood-borne virus that is transmitted primarily through direct percutaneous exposure.

INCIDENCE

According to the Centers for Disease Control and Prevention, an estimated 4 million Americans, approximately 1.8% of the population, are infected with HCV. The highest incidence of acute hepatitis is found among people 20 to 39 years of age and is slightly more common in males than in females. Approximately 85% of HCV-infected individuals fail to clear the virus by 6 months and develop chronic viral hepatitis. HCV is the most common cause of chronic viral hepatitis in the US. Chronic liver disease evolves gradually, with cirrhosis developing in 10% to 20% of patients within 20 to 30 years after the initial infection. Hepatocellular carcinoma develops in 1% to 5% of patients with chronic hepatitis C, but the rate increases to 1% to 4% per year in those who have cirrhosis. The reasons for the variation in the severity and outcomes of chronic hepatitis C are unclear. HCV-associated liver disease is the most common reason for liver transplantation in adults. Approximately 40% of cases of chronic liver disease are due to HCV, and chronic liver disease is the tenth most common cause of death in adults in the US. The National Institutes of Health estimate that the current annual death toll from HCV (currently 8000 to 10,000) will triple within the next 20 to 30 years.

SIGNS/SYMPTOMS

The incubation period for HCV is approximately 2 months, but clinical symptoms manifest in only approximately 33% of people after viral exposure. The symptoms of acute infection are nonspecific malaise, weakness, and anorexia. Jaundice develops in approximately 25% of acutely infected patients. Most infected patients have no symptoms for 20 to 30 years, at which time signs of liver disease, such as jaundice and persistent abnormal liver enzyme tests, may become evident. Encephalopathy occurs with severe liver disease.

DIAGNOSTIC PARAMETERS/PHYSICAL ASSESSMENT

The diagnosis of HCV is made by HCV antibody testing or direct detection of HCV RNA in serum. There are currently 2 types of tests for the presence of antibodies to HCV: Enzyme immunoassay (EIA) and recombinant immunoblot supplemental assay (RIBA). EIA is used primarily for screening people at risk for the disease and for screening blood donors. RIBA is more specific than EIA. Both assays are used when blood spot samples are collected by home testing kits and sent to laboratories. The assays are more than 99% accurate, as demonstrated in multicenter trials, when properly collected.

Interview: Because HCV infection can be asymptomatic for many years, patients may be concerned that they have been exposed. To aid patients in determining if they are candidates for a home hepatitis C test, it may be beneficial to ask about the following:

- Has the patient received transfusions of blood or blood components, or an organ transplant, especially before July 1992? (Since 1992, routine testing of blood and organ donors, and viral inactivation of clotting factors and plasma derivatives have virtually eliminated the risk of contamination of blood products and transplant organs; however, patients who received these products before 1992 may have been exposed to the virus.)
- Has the patient ever injected non-prescribed drugs, such as illegal drug substances? Illegal-drug injections account for approximately 60% of HCV transmission in the US. Even a single occasion, regardless of how long ago, may have placed a person at risk for infection. Non-injected illegal drug use and intranasal cocaine use have not been associated with risk.
- Has the patient been a health care worker or worked in an occupation where inadvertent needlestick or mucosal exposure to infected blood might have occurred?
- Has the patient been on long-term hemodialysis? Risk in this group has been associated with an environment of poor infection control and cross-contamination of injectable medication supplies.
- Does the patient have tattoos or body piercings? Although the risk of these procedures as a causative factor in HCV infection is unknown, receiving these procedures in an unregulated setting or with non-sterile equipment may pose a significant health risk.
- Has the patient had sexual contact with a person known to be HCV positive?

HOME HEPATITIS C TESTS

▶ **Warnings**

The test shows whether a person has ever contracted HCV, unless exposure occurred in the previous 6 months, which may be too early for the assay to detect antibodies to HCV. A positive test indicates exposure; it does not reflect active disease or degree of disease severity.

These testing products do not yield instant results. They are designed so that the user collects the blood sample and sends it to a laboratory for the actual testing process. Results are available by calling a toll-free telephone number and providing the Personal Identification Number (PIN), which comes with each testing kit.

▶ Guidelines for Use

Each test kit is assigned a PIN, which the user registers via a toll-free telephone number before collecting his or her blood sample. Educational messages are given when the user registers; counseling is also available during this phone call.

Collecting a blood sample

1.) Date the Blood Sample Card.
2.) Wash hands with warm, soapy water.
3.) Clean the side of the fingertip of a middle or ring finger with the alcohol swab.
4.) Push down on the lancet to puncture the fingertip.
5.) Allow a large hanging drop of blood to form.
6.) Let the blood drop touch the circle on the Blood Sample Card.
7.) Apply drops of blood until it completely fills the circle and soaks through to the back of the card.

Shipping the sample

1.) Allow the blood to air-dry for 30 minutes.
2.) Place the Blood Sample Card in the Blood Sample Return Pouch and place the pouch in the pre-addressed, prepaid envelope. Mail as soon as possible.

Getting results

1.) Results are available within 10 business days. Call the toll-free number included with the kit and enter your PIN.
2.) Results will be provided by an automated system or a health care counselor.
3.) A written copy of the results is available upon request.

Product selection: Currently there is only 1 home hepatitis C test kit on the market (*Home Access Hepatitis C Check*). Home Access Health provides a telemedicine service which offers education and counseling about HCV and optional referral to a physician. These services are available 24 hours a day except during holidays.

HOME HEPATITIS C TEST KITS	
Trade name	Description
Home Access Hepatitis C Check	**Kit**: Single-use sample collection kit (includes alcohol swab, lancet, blood sample card, and return pouch), a pre-addressed, prepaid envelope, a PIN, a toll-free telephone number to call for results, and information on HCV.

Products listed are representative of currently available and widely distributed brands. Similar products, including regional and private label brands, may also exist.

PATIENT INFORMATION
Home Hepatitis C Test Kits

- The following individuals should be tested for HCV:
- Anyone who may have been exposed to HCV through a blood transfusion or organ transplant before 1992.
- Anyone who has had occupational exposure to HCV, including health care workers and military personnel.
- Anyone who may have been exposed through sexual contact with an HCV-infected individual.
- Anyone taking illegal drugs by needle.
- The test should be performed exactly according to the manufacturer's instructions to ensure accurate results. Users should read the instructions carefully before use and clarify any points not clearly understood with a pharmacist.

Home HIV Tests

DEFINITION

Home HIV tests enable users to deal anonymously with a clinical laboratory to obtain results of tests to determine the presence of HIV-1 antibodies (these tests probably do not detect the presence of HIV-2 and HIV-3 antibodies). They afford privacy, yet still provide necessary anonymous counseling and support.

The following people should consider being tested:

- Those having shared needles or syringes for the purposes of injecting abusable drugs, including steroids.
- Those having sex with an HIV-infected person.
- Those having sex with someone who injects abusable drugs.
- Those having a blood transfusion anytime between 1978 and May 1985.
- Those having sex with 2 or more partners.

HOME HIV TESTS

▶ Actions

All samples are tested in a certified laboratory using the Enzyme Linked Immunosorbent Assay (ELISA). All positive samples are rescreened twice using ELISA. Repeatedly positive samples are then confirmed using an immunofluorescent assay (IFA). These are the standard testing and confirmation methods employed by hospitals and clinics.

▶ Indications

Detection of the presence of HIV-1 antibodies.

▶ Warnings

Some home-use HIV test kits may give users false information about their HIV status, according to the Federal Trade Commission (FTC). In tests performed by the FTC, several HIV kits advertised and sold on the Internet produced false-negative results. The only FDA-approved home collection test systems for detection of HIV are *Home Access* and *Home Access Express* home-use HIV tests. Using other home-use HIV test kits could give a person who might be infected with HIV the false impression that he or she is not infected.

These products do not yield instant results. They are designed so that the consumer collects a blood sample and sends it to a laboratory for the actual testing. The consumer can then access the results in 3 or 7 business days.

The test detects the presence of HIV-1 antibodies. From the time of exposure to the HIV virus, it can take anywhere from 3 weeks to 6 months for the individual to develop enough of these antibodies to be detected. Therefore, these tests cannot detect recent infections. This time sequence must be considered when determining when to have the test performed.

► **Guidelines for Use**

Call the company's toll-free service line to register the anonymous code number for the particular test kit and complete pretest counseling. This counseling is designed to gather general demographic information and help assess the possible HIV exposure.

Using the lancet provided, prick a fingertip on a clean hand and place a few drops of blood on the blood specimen card. Generally, 2 to 4 hanging drops of blood are required to fill the designated space on the card.

Package the specimen card in the provided weather-resistant pouch and addressed, pre-paid shipping mailer.

Either 3 or 7 business days (depending on the type of kit) after shipping the specimen card, the consumer can access test results and anonymous post-test counseling by calling the toll-free service line and entering the code number included in the kit. Positive results are always communicated directly by company counselors.

► **Product Selection**

Currently there are only two home HIV test kits available on the market: *Home Access* and *Home Access Express*. The only difference between them is the length of time the user must wait before receiving the test results. Consumers using *Home Access* may retrieve results in 7 days, and those using *Home Access Express* may retrieve results in 3 business days.

HOME HIV TESTS	
Trade name	**Description**
Home Access, Home Access Express	**Kit**: Contains directional insert, blood specimen collection card with *Home Access* code number, alcohol prep pad, gauze pad, 2 safety lancets, adhesive bandage, specimen return pouch, lancet disposal container, cardboard envelope (US mail for regular, express shipping for express) and *Things You Should Know About HIV and AIDS* booklet.

Products listed are representative of currently available and widely distributed brands. Similar products, including regional and private label brands, may also exist.

PATIENT INFORMATION

Home HIV Tests

- HIV is a virus that attacks the immune system and causes AIDS. If infected by HIV, the body creates HIV antibodies. The home HIV kits test the blood specimen for antibodies to HIV.

- HIV home collection kits can provide a safe and effective alternative to conventional venous HIV antibody testing.

- Perform the test exactly according to the manufacture's instructions to ensure accurate results. Users should carefully read these instructions before use and clarify any points not clearly understood.

- According to the manufacturer's literature, in clinical trials conducted at 9 US medical centers, test results from participants using the *Home Access* HIV test product were compared with professionally collected venous blood samples from the same participants. The 2 groups of test results correlated completely for an overall test accuracy of more than 99.99%. *Home Access* and *Home Access Express* are the only FDA-approved home collection test products for detection of HIV. Other home-use test kits may yield false-negative results.

HOME DRUG TESTING KITS

DEFINITION

Home drug testing kits are intended to be an aid in determining illegal drug use. These products are marketed primarily to parents who have reasonable cause to suspect drug abuse in their children. Home drug testing kits should not be considered a substitute for maintaining proper and open parent-child communication regarding drug abuse.

These kits enable one to deal anonymously with a clinical laboratory to obtain test results and determine the presence of drugs of abuse in urine or hair samples. Samples are collected at home and mailed to the laboratory for testing. Some testing kits include phone numbers for drug testing services that provide further counseling and information.

Urine testing kits: Urinalysis detects drug use that occurred within the last 2 to 3 days. This method of testing, however, may be susceptible to evasive maneuvers and false-positive results caused by passive drug exposure (eg, poppy seed ingestion). The sample is tested to determine if it was altered in an attempt to "beat the test." The pH level of the sample is measured to check for common household chemicals that may have been added to mask the presence of drugs. Then the level of creatinine is measured. Unusually dilute levels of creatinine may indicate that water was added to the sample in an effort to lower drug concentrations. Enzyme Multiplied Immunoassay Technique (EMIT) is run as an initial screening test to detect the presence of a foreign substance. Gas Chromatography-Mass Spectrometry (GC-MS) testing then determines the specific substances present.

Results of a urine test may not be quantitatively indicative of the severity of a patient's drug use. The amount of drug found in a sample is determined by the time elapsed since drug use, the dose of the drug taken, and the amount of water the subject consumed prior to urine sampling.

Hair testing kits: These tests detect the trace amounts of ingested drugs that become trapped in the core of the hair shaft as it grows. These drug residues are stable over time and are only released when the hair fiber is destroyed. A 1½ inch hair sample records one's drug use during the past 90 days (based on a human hair growth rate of about ½ inch per month). The testing procedure involves two tests. The first test uses radioimmunoassay techniques to detect the presence of drugs. All positives are then confirmed using GC-MS analysis.

INCIDENCE

Drug use among children is not uncommon and of great concern to most parents. It has been shown that approximately 45% of children try marijuana before they graduate high school. One in 4 children in the 9-to 12-year-old range has reported being offered drugs of abuse in the past year.

SIGNS/SYMPTOMS

The signs and symptoms of drug use vary with the particular substances used. In addition, it may be difficult to separate typical adolescent behavior from drug-induced behavior. In general, the following changes may be indicative of drug abuse: Withdrawal and isolation, decline in school performance, giving up previously important activities, persistent fatigue, change in eating or sleeping patterns, persistent coughing, red eyes.

DIAGNOSTIC PARAMETERS/PHYSICAL ASSESSMENT

Clinical Observation: Monitor for signs and symptoms presented above.

Interview: To aid patients in the selection and proper use of home drug testing kits, it may be beneficial to ask about the following:

- Professional advice already sought by the parent/guardian if drug abuse is suspected in a child.
- If test results confirm suspected drug abuse, is the parent prepared to seek further counseling as necessary?
- Suspected drug(s) of abuse. Is casual or chronic drug use suspected?
- Likelihood that the patient will cooperate in the drug screening procedure.
- General understanding by purchaser/test administrator of the potential for false-negative or false-positive results.

HOME DRUG TESTING KITS

▶ **Warnings**

Unless used as a screening tool (eg, for recovering drug users or as a method of employment screening) these tests should be used only when there is a reasonable cause to suspect drug abuse.

It is not recommended that these tests be administered in a secretive manner (eg, by taking samples from hair brushes). The best use of drug testing kits is with the full knowledge and consent of the person being tested.

Some medications and foods, such as codeine-containing cough medicines, decongestants, antidiarrheals, and poppy seeds (eg, substances structurally related to certain illegal drugs), may cause positive test results with urine testing because they contain chemicals similar to those found in drugs of abuse. Inquire about all prescription and nonprescription drugs (including herbal products) in the person's current medication profile.

These testing products do not yield instant results. They are designed so that the user collects the sample (urine or hair) and sends it to a laboratory for the actual testing process. Results are available by calling a toll-free telephone number and giving the kit's identification number.

When a person takes a drug, it generally takes a few hours for the drug to appear in the urine, and then it will only be present for a few days. If a urine sample is collected too early or too late, the sample may test negative even if drug use has occurred.

After taking a drug, it takes 5 to 7 days for the hair to grow out sufficiently to test. If the sample is collected too early; the sample may test negative even if drug use has occurred.

There is some evidence that people with black hair tend to accumulate larger quantities of certain drugs (eg, cocaine) than fair-haired people.

Drinking large quantities of liquids within several hours of giving a urine sample may dilute samples, creating a false-negative result.

Do not leave urine samples in direct sunlight or in an unusually hot environment (eg, a hot car).

In an informal evaluation of the PDT-90 test, the test failed to detect low-level marijuana use in 2 of the 3 subjects.

► **Guidelines for Use**

Urine tests: Kits contain all supplies necessary for urine collection, storage, and mailing.

Collect the urine sample as directed.

If the kit contains a temperature strip on the bottle, this is to be checked immediately to ensure the sample is between 90° and 100°F. If not in this temperature range, the sample may have been altered.

Pack and mail the urine as directed.

Approximately 2 to 3 days after receipt of a sample, results are available by calling a toll-free telephone number and giving the identification number accompanying the kit.

Hair tests: Collect the hair sample as directed. From the crown of the head, cut a sample 1/2 inch wide and about one strand deep, as close to the scalp as possible.

Keeping the cut ends aligned, place the hair in the collection package according to the directions.

Mail the stored sample in the addressed prepaid shipping mailer.

Approximately 5 business days after receipt at the laboratory, the parent can access test results by calling a toll-free telephone number and relaying the code number accompanying the kit.

► **Product Selection**

The following variables should be considered when helping patients select a home drug testing kit:

The panel of drugs tested: The list of drugs that may be identified with each kit varies. Select a kit that tests for the substance(s) of concern.

Characteristics of results: The results of urine tests will indicate that the sample tested positive or negative for a drug. No additional details, such as the quantity of drug ingested or the route of administration, are known. The results of positive hair testing are reported as a number indicating low, medium, or high levels of use for all the drugs tested except for marijuana.

Characteristics of home drug testing kits are described in the table below.

Characteristics of Home Drug Testing Kits		
Product	**Test type**	**Substances detected**
Dr. Brown's Home Drug Testing System	urine	marijuana, cocaine, amphetamine, phencyclidine (PCP), codeine, morphine, heroin
Parent's Alert Home Drug Testing Service	urine	marijuana, cocaine, opiates, methamphetamine, ecstasy, barbiturates, benzodiazepines, lysergic acid diethylamide (LSD)
PDT-90 Personal Drug Testing Service	hair	marijuana, cocaine, opiates, methamphetamine, PCP

Testing window: Urine testing will detect use during the previous 2 to 3 days for most drugs. Substances can generally be detected in the urine within hours after drug use. Hair testing can test for drug use within a 90-day period or more; however, it takes 5 to 7 days from the point of ingestion for the hair to grow out of the follicle sufficiently to be clipped for testing purposes.

Ability to tamper with the sample: People may try to tamper with a urine sample in a variety of ways in an effort to "beat the test." This includes adding chemicals to the sample, using someone else's sample, and diluting the sample. Hair is not subject to adulteration or sample substitution. Illicit drug users cannot evade detection by treating their hair with chemical hair treatments (eg, bleaching, straightening or getting a permanent). In general, hair tests are considered less accurate than urine tests in detecting low-level, casual drug use.

HOME DRUG TESTING KITS	
Trade name	**Description**
Dr. Brown's Home Drug Testing System	**Kit**: Urine collection tubes, tube holder, absorbent pad and pouch, prepaid mailing pouch
Parent's Alert Home Drug Testing Service	**Kit**: Collection bottle, specimen bag, prepaid shipping pouch and label
PDT-90 Personal Drug Testing Service	**Kit**: Hair sample collection package with acquisition card and prepaid return envelope

Products listed are representative of currently available and widely distributed brands. Similar products, including regional and private label brands, may also exist.

PATIENT INFORMATION
Home Drug Testing Kits

- Before considering home drug testing, carefully consider all ethical issues as well as alternative interventions, such as counseling.
- Perform the test strictly according to the manufacturer's instructions to ensure accurate results. Users should carefully read instructions before use and clarify any points not clearly understood with a pharmacist or the test manufacturer.
- Use the collection device provided to collect the urine sample. Do not take urine from the toilet.
- Samples for hair testing should not generally be obtained from hair brushes because there is no guarantee that the hair sample is actually from the person to be tested.
- If positive test results are obtained, consider potential problems with the test itself (eg, false positives, poor sample collection) before drawing any firm conclusions. Conversely, do not assume a negative result is accurate.
- Some medications and foods, such as codeine-containing cough medicines, decongestants, antidiarrheals, and poppy seeds (eg, substances structurally related to certain illegal drugs), may cause positive test results with urine testing because they contain chemicals similar to those found in drugs of abuse.

OVULATION DETECTION KITS

DEFINITION

Ovulation detection test kits utilize diagnostic technology that provide women with an accurate method of identifying the time of ovulation in a given menstrual cycle as a means of enhancing chances of conception. These products are designed for use by couples who are having trouble conceiving. These products are *not* intended to help patients predict ovulation for the purpose of contraception.

DIAGNOSTIC PARAMETERS/PHYSICAL ASSESSMENT

Interview: To assist patients in the selection and correct use of ovulation detection kits, it may be beneficial to ask about the following:

- The desirability of pregnancy (patients should know that these products are not to be used as a form of birth control).
- Any fertility medication the patient is taking currently. Patients should consult a physician before using these products.
- Any concurrent medications that may interfere with test results (eg, antiparkinson, antipsychotic, and anticonvulsant agents). Patients should consult a physician before using these products.
- Any problems with vision or recognition of color (the tests use color to indicate results). Someone must be present who does not have color-defective vision or other visual impairment in order to interpret test results correctly.

OVULATION DETECTION KITS

▶ **Actions**

These kits use monoclonal or polyclonal antibodies specific for luteinizing hormone (LH) in the urine. LH is present throughout the menstrual cycle and rises rapidly and sharply just prior to ovulation to produce what is termed the "LH surge" (see the "Ovulatory phase" in Figure 1).

This increase in LH causes an ovarian follicle to rupture and release a mature egg. Ovulation generally occurs 24 to 36 hours after the LH surge is observed in the urine. Predicting ovulation in advance is important because fertilization of an egg only can occur 6 to 24 hours after ovulation. Sperm, however, can survive up to 72 hours; therefore, if a woman has intercourse before her LH surge is detected, the egg still may be fertilized. The LH surge is an accurate predictor of ovulation. Once a patient knows that she is about to ovulate by detecting the LH surge, she is at the start of the most fertile time in her monthly cycle. By having intercourse during the 24 to 36 hours after detection of the LH surge, the chances of becoming pregnant are maximized. Through a change in color intensity on the test detection device (eg, stick, cassette), ovulation detection kits indicate the amount of LH bound to the monoclonal or polyclonal antibodies. The intensity of the resulting color is directly proportional to the amount of LH in the urine sample. A test result yielding a color darker than the reference color indicates an increase in LH level.

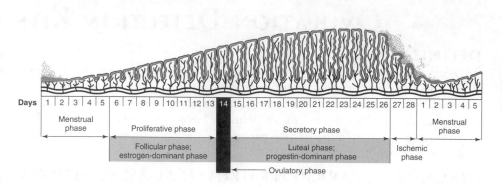

Figure 1. The Menstrual Cycle

Saliva-based ovulation predictors test for estrogen increases in saliva. Biochemical and hormonal changes that occur 24 to 72 hours before ovulation, causing dried saliva to form in a "ferning" pattern, are seen on a lens with a microscope. This "ferning" or "crystal" pattern indicates that ovulation is about to occur.

▶ **Warnings**

None of these products is intended to be used as a method of birth control.

Color vision is necessary to read test results utilizing urine properly. Visually impaired persons may need assistance in observing increases in color intensity.

Some women do not ovulate every cycle, and, therefore, will not detect any increase in the urine level of LH during nonovulating cycles.

Some women do not ovulate mid-cycle, and, therefore, may not detect the LH surge in urine with the number of tests included in 1 kit. They may continue testing with an additional test kit.

Conditions that may cause high urine LH levels that are not caused by ovulation may alter test results. The structural similarity between LH and thyroid-stimulating hormone, human chorionic gonadotropin, and follicle-stimulating hormone also may interfere with test accuracy. Conditions in which these circumstances may occur include endometriosis, ovarian cysts, menopause, recent pregnancy, and hyperthyroidism. Consult a physician for guidance.

Proteinuria or hematuria may interfere with urine test results. The red color of blood in the urine may interfere with accurately reading the color change indicating test results.

Because the start of ovulation may be delayed 1 month or more after discontinuing oral contraceptives (OCs), women who have discontinued OC use recently should delay use of any ovulation detection kits until several months have passed.

Use saliva-based ovulation predictors first thing in the morning before eating, drinking, brushing one's teeth, or smoking. These activities may interfere with test results. A saliva sample obtained from underneath the tongue will provide the most reliable results.

Do not use products after their expiration dates.

▶ **Drug Interactions**

Women receiving fertility medications should consult their physician before using these tests. Drugs that promote ovulation, such as danazol (eg, *Danocrine*) and menotropins (eg, *Humegon, Pergonal*), interfere with test results. Although clomiphene (eg, *Clomid*) elevates LH levels during administration, the levels generally decrease before ovulation detection testing is scheduled to begin. An interaction is not expected to occur; however, it is best to advise patients taking fertility drugs to consult their physician before use.

Some antiparkinson, antipsychotic, and anticonvulsant agents may increase baseline LH secretion, thus interfering with test accuracy.

▶ Guidelines for Use

Most urine kits contain 5 or more tests, enough to detect the LH surge in most ovulating women with regular cycles.

The first day of testing should be 2 to 3 days before ovulation is expected. The most difficult aspect of using these products is determining the cycle day on which to begin testing. Each kit contains a method for determining this date based on the average length of the woman's menstrual cycle. Carefully follow the manufacturer's directions.

During the identified testing period, conduct a urine test once daily. Most tests may be conducted at any time of day. Check first with manufacturer's directions; **however, administer tests at approximately the same time each day**.

The exact testing procedure varies with each product. Most commonly, a test stick or test cassette is used. Urine is introduced by holding the stick in the urine stream or placing a specified number of drops of urine into a well on the cassette. Test results are read after a specific amount of time by comparing the color intensity of the resulting test line to a reference line.

Continue testing once a day until the first noticeable increase in color intensity, indicating the LH surge. At this point, discontinue testing for this cycle, saving any unused tests for later use if the procedure is to be repeated.

Saliva tests involve putting a saliva sample on a lens and allowing it to dry for 5 to 10 minutes. Then, view the lens under a microscope. "Ferning", or a "crystal" pattern, indicates fertility. Compare results with pictures in the package insert literature.

Ovulation should occur 24 to 36 hours after the LH surge is detected in the urine. Intercourse should occur within 24 to 36 hours of detecting the LH surge. Because sperm can survive for 72 hours, and an egg is viable for up to 24 hours, a woman's most fertile time is the 2 days prior to ovulation, the day of ovulation, and the day after ovulation.

▶ Product Selection

Ovulation detection kits vary in the complexity of the test procedure, the length of time to complete the test, and the number of individual tests provided. With the simplest urine testing product, the woman urinates onto the test stick and reads the results in 3 minutes. The more complicated products require a series of timed steps involving test solutions and droppers. Each step required is a potential opportunity for human error; therefore, the simpler tests are generally more desirable.

OVULATION DETECTION KITS	
Trade name	**Description**
Answer Quick & Simple, First Response	**5-Day Test Kit**: Test sticks
Assure Ovulation Predictor	**6- or 9-Day Test Kit**: Test cassette, dropper, plastic cup

OVULATION DETECTION KITS	
Trade name	**Description**
Clearblue Easy Digital Ovulation Test	**7-Day Test Kit**: Digital test sticks
Clearblue Easy Ovulation Test Pack	**7-Day Test Kit**: Test sticks
Lady Q Ovulation Predictor Test System	**Unlimited Testing**: Magnification microscope, reusable lens
Fertile Focus	**Unlimited Testing**: Saliva ovulation fertility test microscope, reusable magnification ocular lens (warranty for 1 year)
OvuLite	**Unlimited Testing**: Microscope with ocular lens, slide (reusable), carrying case
OvuLook Saliva Ovulation Test	**Ovulation Tester**: Two tracking disks (with 31 glass slides each), applicator brush, storage purse
OvuQuick One-Step	**6-Day Test Kit**: Test cassette, plastic cup, dropper

Products listed are representative of currently available and widely distributed brands. Similar products, including regional and private label brands, may also exist.

PATIENT INFORMATION
Ovulation Detection Kits

- Perform ovulation detection testing exactly according to the manufacturer's instructions to ensure accurate results. Carefully read these instructions before use and clarify any points not clearly understood with a physician or pharmacist.
- If the testing procedure involves the collection of a urine sample, use the container provided. Household containers may have soap or detergent residue that may interfere with test results.
- If the patient has sexual intercourse at any time during the 1 to 3 days after detection of the LH surge, the chances of becoming pregnant will be maximized. There is no need to wait until ovulation before having intercourse.
- Reduce liquid intake for 2 to 4 hours before testing, per manufacturer's instructions, to avoid diluting the urine concentration of LH. Avoid urination for approximately 4 hours prior to testing.
- Use saliva-based ovulation predictors first thing in the morning before eating, drinking, brushing one's teeth, or smoking for the most reliable test results. Saliva samples obtained from underneath the tongue give the most reliable results.
- These products are 94% to 99% accurate.
- Couples having difficulty conceiving after using these kits for several months should consult a physician.

PREGNANCY TESTING

DEFINITION

Pregnancy testing products provide a convenient, reliable, and economical method to self-test for pregnancy. Early detection of pregnancy enables the woman to make decisions and choices regarding prenatal care, nutritional care, and lifestyle changes that may help ensure a healthy pregnancy and optimal fetal growth and development.

INCIDENCE

Pregnancy tests are reported to be used by approximately one third of women who think they may be pregnant.

DIAGNOSTIC PARAMETERS/PHYSICAL ASSESSMENT

During pregnancy, human chorionic gonadotropin (hCG) is present in the plasma and urine. Levels of hCG begin to increase immediately after fertilization, peak at 60 to 70 days after fertilization, and then decline to steady state during pregnancy.

With the first-generation home pregnancy tests, hemagglutination-inhibition (HI) or monoclonal antibodies were used to detect the presence of hCG in the urine. For the HI method, a urine sample was added to a test tube containing red blood cells (RBCs) coated with hCG-antiserum and hCG-antigen. The hCG bound with the antiserum, uncoating the RBCs. The RBCs settled to the bottom of the test tube in a ring configuration, indicating a positive test for pregnancy. If hCG was not present, the antiserum and antibodies bound, forming a clump at the bottom of the test tube.

Current pregnancy tests are more advanced, convenient, and reliable, and involve the use of monoclonal antibodies (MCAs) that bind to hCG present in the urine during pregnancy. When the monoclonal antibodies bind to the hCG, a distinctive color change occurs in the test material. If hCG is not present, no color change occurs or a color change occurs only in the control test area. When used correctly, these diagnostic tests are more than 95% accurate.

Interview: To help individuals select and administer the most appropriate home pregnancy test, it may be beneficial to ask about the following:

- Number of days that have elapsed since the missed onset of menstruation.
- Limitations interpreting colors (eg, color blindness or vision impairment).
- Preference regarding time of day the sample is taken.
- Preference between collecting urine sample for testing versus urination onto a test strip.
- Preference for having test done by a laboratory. Most patients will be best served by the current OTC tests.

TREATMENT

Approaches to testing – If pregnancy testing is being considered, women may have the test performed either by a clinical laboratory or do the test themselves, using one of many available home pregnancy tests. When carefully conducted, in accordance with the instructions that accompany the product, home pregnancy testing approaches 99% accuracy.

The simplest and most reliable technique involves detection of hCG in the urine by a color change resulting from binding of hCG to monoclonal antibodies. Procedures for analysis differ between dipping a test strip into a urine sample versus urination onto the test strip. Some tests are so sensitive most women will have detectable amounts of hCG in their urine within a day or two after fertilization and certainly by the first day of their missed menses. Most test results can be read in 1 to 5 minutes and involve only two steps. To assist the patient in interpreting test results correctly, some pregnancy tests contain a control that illustrates the appearance of a negative test.

HOME PREGNANCY TEST KITS

▶ **Actions**

Home pregnancy tests detect hCG, a hormone produced by the placenta shortly after fertilization and implantation. This hormone is present in the plasma and urine of pregnant women and can be utilized as a marker to confirm pregnancy.

▶ **Indications**

Confirmation of pregnancy.

▶ **Drug Interactions**

The tests should not be affected by hormone therapies containing clomiphene citrate (eg, *Clomid, Serophene*), alcohol, analgesics (painkillers), antibiotics, or the contraceptive pill.

Drugs that contain luteinizing hormone or hCG or stimulate increases in these hormones may cause false-positive results. Examples of drugs or conditions that may alter pregnancy test results include the following:

- Medications containing the pregnancy hormone hCG (eg, *Humegon, Pregnyl, Profasi*); these can yield false-positive results.
- Ovarian cysts or an ectopic pregnancy (ie, pregnancy outside the uterus).
- Using within 8 weeks of giving birth or having a miscarriage or abortion may yield a false-positive result because hCG may still be in the system.

▶ **Guidelines for Use**

Instructions and guidelines for proper use accompany individual products. These should be followed very carefully to ensure accuracy.

Most tests can be used on the first day of expected menstruation. Women who do not have a regular period or who are breastfeeding can test as early as 14 days after unprotected sex if they think they became pregnant.

HOME PREGNANCY TEST KITS	
Trade name	Description
Answer	**Kit**: Test stick. Results after 3 minutes.
Answer Early Result[1]	**Kit**: Test stick. Results in 3 minutes.

HOME PREGNANCY TEST KITS

Trade name	Description
Answer Quick & Simple One-Step	**Kit**: Test stick. Results after 2 minutes.
ClearBlue	**Kit**: Test stick. Results after 1 minute.
e.p.t.	**Kit**: Test stick. Results after 3 minutes.
Fact Plus Pro	**Kit**: Test cassette, urine cup, dropper. Results after 5 minutes.
Fact Plus Select	**Kit**: Test stick. Results after 3 minutes.
First Response 1-Step	**Kit**: Test stick. Results after 3 minutes.
First Response Early Result[1]	**Kit**: Test stick. Results after 3 minutes.

Products listed are representative of currently available and widely distributed brands. Similar products, including regional and private label brands, may also exist.

[1] May be used 3 days before expected period.

PATIENT INFORMATION
Home Pregnancy Tests

- Instructions accompany each product. Read these instructions carefully, preferably before leaving the pharmacy, in case there are any questions. Follow the instructions exactly.
- Performing the test too early may produce a false-negative test result.
- Check the pregnancy test expiration date. Do not use if the pregnancy test is out of date.
- Follow the manufacturer's storage instructions exactly. Heat and cold extremes should be avoided.
- The first morning urine contains the highest concentration of hCG and may be recommended for testing.
- Test sticks should be used immediately after opening and should not be reused.
- If urine collection is required, use the urine collection device supplied with the kit in order to prevent inaccurate test results. Waxed cups and containers that have been washed with detergents can interfere with test results.
- Test instructions may indicate that if the urine sample is not used immediately after collection, it may be stored in the refrigerator. However, the urine must be at room temperature before performing the test. Chilled urine may yield a false-negative pregnancy result.
- Assume you are pregnant if the pregnancy test is positive and schedule an appointment with a obstetrician/gynecologist at the earliest possible opportunity. This referral is essential to optimal maternal and prenatal care.
- Repeat a negative test after the recommended number of days if menstruation has not begun. If the results are negative again and if menstruation has not started, a physician should be contacted to determine the cause of amenorrhea.
- Not for internal use.
- Keep out of reach of children.

Home Cholesterol Tests

DEFINITION

Home cholesterol tests allow patients to measure their total blood cholesterol level at their convenience in their own home. The single-use products contain all the components necessary to run the test so that fingerstick whole-blood specimens can be analyzed by the non-technically trained consumer. The National Cholesterol Education Program recommends that all adults 20 years or older have their cholesterol measured at least every 5 years.

HOME CHOLESTEROL TESTS

► **Actions**

The hand-held test cassette contains a blood filtration system and the enzymatic assay. The filtration device separates plasma from the whole blood and delivers the necessary sample volume. The test reaction is then initiated once the consumer pulls a tab on the side of the cassette. The assay consists of two separate processes. The first process involves a solid-phase enzymatic method releasing hydrogen peroxide from the cholesterol present in the blood sample. In the second process, the hydrogen peroxide interacts with another enzyme and a dye substrate to form a chromogenic complex which is proportional to the cholesterol concentration in the specimen.

► **Warnings**

Cholesterol values can change from day to day. An individual's cholesterol measurement can vary about 2% to 3% within the same day. Seasonal variations can also occur with levels tending to be lower in the summer and higher in the winter.

According to product literature, *CholesTrak* (see product listing) has been shown to be 97% accurate on average.

Patient variables such as weight loss, illness, and stress may influence cholesterol results. It is important to understand and control these factors as much as possible to obtain accurate results.

Since cholesterol values vary and patient variables affect results, the National Cholesterol Education Program recommends that at least 2 results be averaged rather than relying on a single result.

This product should not be used by patients taking anticoagulants or hemophiliacs because of the risk of excessive bleeding from the fingerstick. These individuals should have their cholesterol tested while under the direct care of a physician.

These tests only measure total cholesterol (TC). They do not provide a breakdown of LDL, HDL, and triglycerides.

Performing this test in direct sunlight may cause inaccurate results due to fading of the purple bar on the cassette or the color pad on the test strip.

Proper finger sticking technique is regained to avoid erroneous results. Excessive squeezing of the finger affects the quality of the blood sample. A falsely low cholesterol value may result if the blood sample is too small or if it takes greater than 5 minutes to fill the well of the test cassette or strip.

Each kit comes with a chart to be used to interpret test results. Each chart is specific for that test cassette or strip and should not be used for interpretation of other cassettes.

▶ Drug Interactions

Vitamin C in doses greater than 500 mg or standard doses of acetaminophen should be avoided for at least 4 hours before using the test. If this interaction is not avoided, the results could be falsely low.

▶ Guidelines for Use

Using the device supplied, prick a clean finger to obtain the blood sample necessary to perform the test. Wipe off the first sign of blood from the finger and then fill the well of the test cassette as indicated as quickly as possible.

Once the well is filled, wait 2 to 4 minutes and then pull the tab on the side of the cassette to activate the test.

In 5 minutes a purple dot will appear in the "test working" window located on one end of the cassette. Approximately 10 minutes later, a green dot will appear in the window located at the opposite end of the cassette indicating the test has been completed.

The length of the resultant purple bar is read like a thermometer against the printed scale on the cassette, and this value is converted to mg/dL of cholesterol using the conversion chart provided.

Read the results within 30 minutes. If the results are not interpreted within this time period, the results will be inaccurate.

Controls: The test cassette contains indicator windows to alert the user that the test is working properly and that the test is complete.

Reporting results: CholesTrak is calibrated to measure total cholesterol (TC) levels within a range of 3 to 5 mg/dL.

HOME CHOLESTEROL TEST KITS	
Trade name	Description
CholesTrak	**Kit:** Test cassette containing a blood filtration system and enzymatic assay, gauze, push-button fingerprick device, and bandage

Products listed are representative of currently available and widely distributed brands. Similar products, including regional and private label brands, may also exist.

PATIENT INFORMATION
Home Cholesterol Tests

- The tests should be performed exactly according to the manufacturer's instructions to ensure accurate results. Patients should carefully read these instructions before use and clarify any points not clearly understood.
- Each kit comes with everything needed: Gauze, fingerstick device, bandage, and test cassette or strip, except a watch or clock to time the necessary steps of the testing procedure.
- Sit and relax 5 minutes before beginning the test to stabilize cholesterol level.
- The test can be conducted at anytime during the day. Recent food intake does not affect total cholesterol values.
- Results should be interpreted as follows:
  - Less than 200 mg/dL = desirable
  - 200 to 239 mg/dL = borderline high; see physician for complete medical evaluation
  - 240 mg/dL and greater = high; see physician for complete medical evaluation
- Patients should not adjust their cholesterol-lowering medications based on the results of this test without consulting their physician.

HOME URINARY TRACT INFECTION TESTS

DEFINITION

Urinary tract infections (UTIs) are caused by bacteria in the urethra, bladder, or kidneys. The majority of UTIs are caused by gram-negative bacteria, with *Escherichia coli* being responsible for approximately 80% of these infections. Quantitative urine cultures are the most reliable method for diagnosing UTIs. Limitations of the routine use of this diagnostic procedure include the following: need for trained personnel, cost, inconvenience of collecting clean-voided specimens, and the need to treat symptomatic patients before the results are available. Home UTI tests can serve as simple screenings for bacteriuria to identify patients requiring further work-up. The home UTI tests have two primary uses:

- As a follow-up to drug therapy. The test is administered following a course of antibiotic therapy to confirm the infection has been cured. Used in this manner, these tests can detect treatment failure due to bacterial resistance, inappropriate drug selection, or patient noncompliance.
- As a screening tool in patients at risk for or with a history of UTIs. This patient population includes females with a history of multiple UTIs, pregnant women, diabetic patients, men older than 50 years of age, and patients with catheters. This use facilitates early detection of UTIs.

HOME URINARY TRACT INFECTION TESTS

▶ **Actions**

The *UTI Home Screening Test Kit* is a screen for bacterial reduction of urinary nitrate to nitrite. Urinary nitrite is often associated with urinary tract infections.

The *First Response* test detects catalase activity. Catalase is a substance produced by white blood cells and bacteria. There normally should not be any bacteria or white blood cells in the urine.

▶ **Warnings**

These tests cannot be used by themselves to diagnose a UTI. They are designed to alert the patient to the need for further evaluation. Additional testing is required to confirm possible infection and aid in proper therapy selection.

These products do not identify the specific pathogen or indicate which antibiotic is indicated for treatment.

UTIs caused by pathogens that do not convert nitrate to nitrite, such as enterococci and streptococci, will not be detected.

Color vision is necessary to properly read test results for the *UTI Home Screening* test. Visually impaired persons may need assistance.

► **Drug Interactions**

High doses (greater than 250 mg) of ascorbic acid may block the test reaction producing false-negative results. Avoid doses in this range for 10 hours prior to testing. Antibiotic use may also produce false-negative results.

UTI Home Screening Test: False-positive results may be caused by the presence of dietary or therapeutic dyes or drugs, such as phenazopyridine, which could give the appearance of a positive test result by changing the sensor pad to a pink color.

► **Guidelines for Use**

UTI Home Screening Test: Dip the test area of the strip in the urine and remove immediately. Tap the test strip on the edge of toilet bowl or cup to remove any excess urine. Wait 1 minute and examine (in good lighting) the strip for any color change. Carefully match the color of the strip, if any, to the color blocks on the vial label. The appearance of a pink color on the test strip indicates a positive result.

If the user prefers not to collect the urine sample, the test strips may be passed directly through the urine stream.

Read the results within 2 minutes of conducting the test. Ignore any color changes that occur after this time.

Urine that cannot be tested within 1 hour should be refrigerated immediately and brought back to room temperature before testing (or retesting).

First Response Uriscreen UTI Test: Collect a urine sample in one of the collection cups. Set up one test stand and place a results tube in the stand. Use a dropper to fill the results tube with urine to the line indicated on the test stand; do not overfill. Using the dropper, slowly mix the urine sample with the tube contents. Add 4 drops from the activator vial to the results tube.

Read the result after 2 minutes. White foam on the top of the blue liquid indicates a positive result.

► **Product Selection**

Currently there are two home UTI testing products on the market: *First Response* and *UTI.*

First Response detects catalase, an enzyme produced by white blood cells and most bacteria. The product can detect infections secondary to gram-positive as well as gram-negative bacteria. Results are determined by the presence or absence of foam.

UTI screens for nitrite. Results are determined by comparing the color change on the test strip to the color printed on the vial label.

URINARY TRACT INFECTION TEST KITS	
Trade name	**Description**
UTI Home Screening Test	**Test kit**: 6 test strips, 6 collection cups, color chart on vial containing test strips. Results in 1 minute.
First Response Uriscreen Urinary Tract Infection Test	**Test kit**: 2 collection cups, 2 droppers, 2 results tubes, 1 activator vial, instructions. Results in 2 minutes.

Products listed are representative of currently available and widely distributed brands. Similar products, including regional and private label brands, may also exist.

PATIENT INFORMATION
Home Urinary Tract Infection Kits

- Perform the tests exactly according to the manufacturer's instructions to ensure accurate results. Read these instructions carefully before use and clarify any points not clearly understood.
- Conduct the test using the first-morning urine to ensure a sufficient incubation period (4 to 6 hours) of urine in the bladder to allow the reduction of the nitrates or production of catalase.
- Women should not perform tests during menstruation. Blood in urine may cause false-positive results.
- To improve the sensitivity of the tests, it is suggested that the test be conducted on 3 consecutive first-morning urine samples.
- If a positive test result is obtained, contact your physician immediately for a complete evaluation and appropriate therapy.
- These tests will detect approximately 90% of UTIs. This means about 10% will not be detected. Therefore, if a negative result is obtained, but symptoms suggestive of a UTI are present (burning or pain on urination, urinary frequency, cloudy urine, abdominal discomfort, blood in the urine, fever, lower back pain), contact your physician immediately.
- Inaccurate results can occur if tests are read too early or too late.
- Do not change or stop taking your medication based on test results.
- Do not use products past the expiration date. Do not open kits until ready to use.
- Do not touch the sensor pad on test strips. Skin oils can interfere with the test reaction.
- Store strips in their original vial and replace cap immediately after opening. Do not use test strips more than once. Discard after use.
- *First Response* contains ingredients that may irritate or stain the skin. Avoid contact with eyes, skin, or clothing. In case of contact, wash affected area immediately with water.
- Store at room temperature (59° to 86°F). Do not freeze. Avoid exposure to moisture (such as in a steamy bathroom). Avoid exposure to sunlight.
- Not for internal use.
- For adult use only. Keep out of reach of children.

COMPLEMENTARY THERAPIES

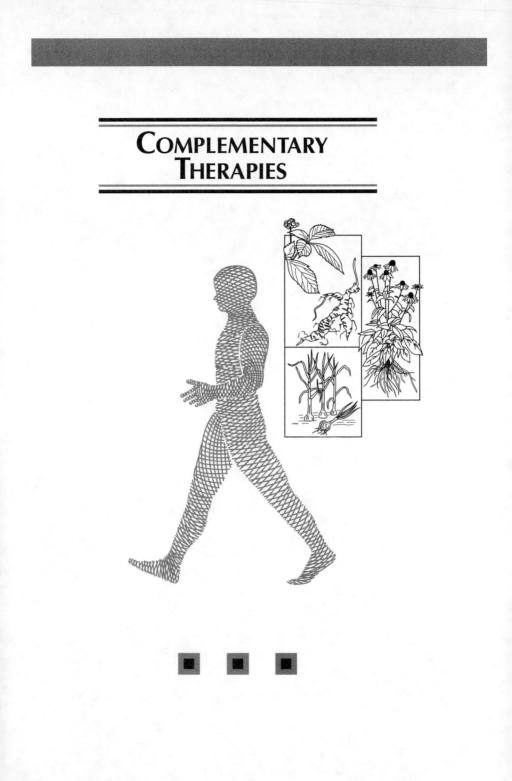

COMPLEMENTARY THERAPIES

■ ■ ■

INTRODUCTION

The last decade has witnessed an acceleration in the purchase and use of alternative/complementary medicine in the Western world, particularly in the United States. Alternative/complementary therapy, which complements conventional health care, is defined as the diagnosis, treatment, or prevention of diseases. This practice encompasses such techniques as acupuncture, Ayurvedic medicine, herbal formulas, homeopathy, massage, manipulation, and rolfing and offers patients many alternative caregivers (ie, acupuncturists, chiropractors, herbalists, homeopaths, naturopaths).

Most conventional health care professionals have not been educated in the heterogeneous group of alternative/complementary theories and practices. Yet, consumers and patients would like to turn to their providers for advice and guidance.

Approximately 25% to 50% of American adults consult alternative/complementary practitioners annually. Of all forms of alternative/complementary therapies, herbal products are the most commonly employed; more than 60 million Americans consume 1 or more herbal products in a given year. In addition, more than 80% of those who use alternative/complementary therapies combine that practice with conventional medicine. Some reported reasons for using alternative/complementary therapies have included dissatisfaction with mainstream medicine and the desire to try the untried. One study revealed that most patients using alternative/complementary medicine tend to be educated, in poor health, and find these therapies to be more compatible with their values, philosophies, and beliefs regarding their health and life.

Viable drug discoveries from plant sources often create a confidence in many consumers that all natural or plant sources of potential therapeutic agents are both effective and safe for general use. Only limited evidence from randomized controlled trials (RCT) exists to help answer questions regarding effectiveness of and safety of specific alternative/complementary therapies. Many users of these therapies perceive "natural" to imply no side effects. In general, most therapies have the potential to produce adverse events and interact with conventional and alternative medicines and with certain conditions (ie, pregnancy, pediatrics, organ dysfunction). Some of these alternative/complementary products contain powerful pharmacological substances that may be toxic alone or in combination with other agents. Unfortunately, the frequency of such events cannot be reliably defined and is poorly documented.

According to the Dietary Supplement Health and Education Act (DSHEA) passed in 1994, dietary supplements are defined to include herbs, vitamins, minerals, and amino acids. With the enactment of the DSHEA, Congress has liberated dietary supplement manufacturers from being regulated by the same FDA guidelines used in pharmaceuticals. Therefore, many of these products lack comprehensive data regarding safety and efficacy. According to the DSHEA, supplements cannot be promoted for traditional pharmaceutical claims relating to the diagnosis, treatment, cure, or prevention of any disease. Only "structure and function" claims relating to the dietary supplement's effect on the structure or a function of the body can be presented on labeling and advertisements.

Approximately 70% of patients who use alternative/complementary therapies do not inform their conventional health care providers of such use. The role of health care providers is to discuss permanent issues intelligently and nonjudgementally so patients will more likely be truthful regarding the use of adjuvant treatments in use. This will help patients incorporate more scientific evidence into their health care decisions.

Most indicative of the escalating interest in these practices is the willingness of conventional agencies to acknowledge the public's unconventional inclinations. The Office of Alternative Medicine (OAM) was established in 1992 by Congress as a part of the National Institute of Health (NIH). The OAM and NIH collaborate of the identification and support in alternative and complementary medicine research applications and new program developments. In addition, more than 40 medical schools in the United States have incorporated complementary courses into their curriculum.

The Complementary Therapies chapter of *Nonprescription Drug Therapy: Guiding Patient Self-Care* is designed to present data on selected herbal products possessing the greatest quantity and quality of data supporting clinical use in the complementary management of medical conditions. The individual monographs are designed to provide decision support information to conventional health care providers. Health care professionals given appropriate information, can assist patients greatly in selecting, using, and monitoring herbal therapies. The prudent integration of conventional and alternative/complementary health care is in the public interest.

Because more patients are taking herbal preparations, clinicians should have some basic knowledge and understanding of herbal therapies even if there is a lack of clinical and scientific study. The following list offers key issues to be discussed with any patient taking or contemplating using herbal products.

1.) Ask patients about herbal therapy use and dietary supplements. Document uses in medical record.
2.) "Natural" does not necessarily mean safe.
3.) Herbal-pharmaceutical interactions do occur; avoid combined use.
4.) Lack of standardization of herbal agents may result in variability in herbal content and efficacy among manufacturers.
5.) Lack of quality control and regulation may result in contamination during manufacturing and potential misidentification of plant species.
6.) Do not use herbal treatments if the patient is contemplating pregnancy or during pregnancy or lactation because of lack of long-term clinical trials proving safety. Some herbal products may cause premature uterine contractions and cross the placental barrier.
7.) Do not use herbal treatments in larger-than-recommended dosages.

8.) Do not use herbal treatments for more than several weeks because of a lack of studies proving long-term safety.

9.) Avoid herbal treatments with known adverse effects and toxic effects (eg, germander, life root, comfrey, pennyroyal).

10.) Do not use herbal treatments in infants, children, or the elderly without professional advice. These patients are more prone to adverse effects because of a decrease in metabolism.

11.) Accurate diagnosis and discussion or proven treatment options are essential prior to the patient's consideration of herbal treatments.

12.) Document adverse effects in the patient's chart, and discontinue therapy.

Because of the lack of adequate efficacy and toxicity information, patients and clinicians should be aware that advice about herbal products is not absolute and is a matter of judgement. Base advice on available knowledge that is congruent with the patient's needs and the physician's best judgement.

These recommendations are not evidence-based; a conservative approach is warranted. More study regarding safety and efficacy is needed, but herbal products have significant potential for adding to the medicinal market already in place.

ALOE

SCIENTIFIC NAME(S)

Aloe vera L., *A. perryi* Baker (Zanzibar or Socotrine aloe), *A. barbadensis* Miller (also called *A. vera* Tournefort ex Linne or *A. vulgaris* Lamarck; Curaçao or Barbados aloe), or *A. ferox* Miller (Cape aloe). *A. vera* Miller and *A. vera* L. may or may not be the same species. Family: Liliaceae Nichols or *Sabal serruolatum* Schult. Family: Palmae

COMMON NAME(S)

Cape, Zanzibar, Socotrine, Curaçao, and Barbados aloes and aloe vera

---

PATIENT INFORMATION

- *Warnings:* Products containing aloe are considered dietary supplements and are **not** FDA-approved for medical use. Products containing this agent should be considered **complementary** therapies and not **alternative** therapies. Standard medical care and prescribed therapy should not be abandoned, nor should appropriate medical attention be delayed. Such practices can be dangerous when herbal products are being used.

  Except for dried latex, products containing aloe are **not** approved for internal use.

  Aloe-containing products should not be ingested by children or by pregnant/lactating women, because severe gastric cramping may result.

  Aloe products should not be applied to broken or abraded skin.
- *Uses:* Aloe may assist in inhibiting certain infections and promote healing of minor burns and wounds and possibly healing of skin affected by diseases such as psoriasis. Dried aloe latex is used, with caution, as a drastic laxative.
- *Side Effects:* There has been 1 report that using the gel as standard wound therapy actually delayed healing. The gel may cause contact dermatitis and a burning sensation in dermabraded skin.
- *Dosing:* As a gel, *A. vera* may be applied externally ad lib. The resin product is cathartic at doses of 250 mg and is not recommended for internal use.

BOTANY

Aloes, of which there are about 500 species, belong to the family Liliaceae. The name, meaning bitter and shiny substance, derives from the Arabic "alloeh." Indigenous to the Cape of Good Hope, these perennial succulents grow throughout most of Africa, southern Arabia, and Madagascar. Although they do not grow in rain forests or arid deserts, they are cultivated in the Caribbean, Mediterranean, Japan, and America. Their fleshy leaves are stiff and spiny along the edges and grow in a rosette. Each plant has 15 to 30 tapering leaves, each up to 0.5 m long and 8 to 10 cm wide. Beneath the thick cuticle of the epidermis lies the chlorenchyma. Between this layer and the colorless mucilaginous pulp containing the aloe gel are numerous vascular bundles and inner bundle sheath cells from which a bitter yellow sap exudes when the leaves are cut.

HISTORY

In 4th millennium B.C., aloe wall carvings were found in Egyptian temples. Called the "Plant of Immortality," it was a traditional funerary gift for the pharaohs. The *Egyptian Book of Remedies* (ca. 1500 B.C.) notes that aloe was used in curing infections, treating the skin, and preparing drugs that were chiefly used as laxatives. The Gospel of John (19:39-40) says that Nicodemus brought a mixture of myrrh and aloes for the preparation of Christ's body. In A.D. 74, the Greek physician Dioscorides recorded aloe's use in healing wounds, stopping hair loss, treating genital ulcers, and eliminating hemorrhoids. In 6th century A.D., Arab traders carried aloe to Asia, and in the 16th century, it was carried to the New World by the Spaniards. Its use in the United States began in the 1930s as a treatment for x-ray-induced dermatitis.

ACTIONS

Aloe latex has been used as a drastic cathartic. The aloinosides exert strong purgative effects by irritating the large intestine. These should be used with caution in children.

The most common use of the gel remains the treatment of minor burns and skin irritations. The activity of aloe in treating burns may stem from its moisturizing effect, which prevents air from drying the wound. Current theory suggests that healing is stimulated by the mucopolysaccharides contained in aloe in combination with sulfur derivatives and nitrogen compounds. Topical aloe treatment for burns has not been adequately documented. Two FDA advisory panels found insufficient evidence to show that *A. vera* is useful in the treatment of minor burns and cuts or vaginal irritations.

More recent studies have found preparations containing aloe to accelerate wound healing, even in frostbitten patients. In patients undergoing dermabrasion, aloe accelerated skin healing by approximately 72 hours compared with polyethylene oxide gel dressing. However, at least 1 study found that aloe delayed wound healing (83 vs 53 days).

One study using *A. vera* gel found no activity against *Staphylococcus aureus* and *Escherichia coli*. Other tests found that *A. chinensis* inhibited growth of *S. aureus*, *E. coli*, and *Mycobacterium tuberculosis*, but that *A. vera* was inactive. Further, these extracts lost their in vitro activity when mixed with blood. The latex form has shown some activity against pathogenic strains. Two commercial preparations (*Aloe gel* and *Dermaide Aloe*) exerted antimicrobial activity against gram-negative and gram-positive bacteria as well as *Candida albicans* when used in concentrations higher than 90%.

Aloe-emodin is antileukemic in vitro; other studies showed *A. vera* gel to be less cytotoxic than indomethacin (eg, *Indocin*) or prednisolone (eg, *Delta-Cortef*) in tissue cultures. The clinical impact of these observations has not been determined.

An emulsion of the gel was reported to cure 17 of 18 patients with peptic ulcers, but no control agent was used in the study.

Only the dried latex form is approved for internal use as a cathartic. In some cases, *A. vera* is sold as a food supplement. The FDA has only approved *A. perryi*, *A. vera*, *A. ferox*, and certain hybrids for use as natural food flavorings.

TOXICOLOGY

Because aloe is used extensively as a folk medicine, its adverse effects have been well documented. Except for the dried latex, aloe is not approved as an internal medication. Aloe-emodin and other anthraquinones may cause severe gastric cramping and are contraindicated in children and pregnant women. The external use of aloe usually has not been associated with severe adverse reactions. Reports of burning skin following topical application of aloe gel to dermabraded skin have been described. Contact dermatitis from the related *A. arborescens* has been reported.

References are available upon request.

L-ARGININE

COMMON NAME(S)
L-arginine

PATIENT INFORMATION

- *Warnings:* Products containing L-arginine are considered dietary supplements and are **not** FDA-approved for medical use. Products containing this agent should be considered **complementary** therapies and not **alternative** therapies. Standard medical care and prescribed therapy should not be abandoned, nor should appropriate medical attention be delayed. Such practices can be dangerous.
- *Uses:* L-arginine has been beneficial in several cardiovascular diseases. It plays an important role in healing and increases nitric oxide concentrations.
- *Side Effects:* L-arginine has few reported side effects. Nausea and diarrhea have been reported infrequently. Parenteral administration at high doses has caused metabolic acidosis or electrolyte alterations.
- *Dosing:* L-arginine has been studied at oral doses of 6 to 17 g/day for a variety of conditions.

BOTANY
Amino acids are the major components of protein. Animal and plant products contain several amino acids, including arginine. Some of these sources are meats, milk, and eggs. The physiologically active form, L-arginine, is the natural product obtained by hydrolysis of proteins. In the laboratory, arginine can be precipitated from gelatin hydrolysate. L-arginine also can be synthesized from L-ornithine and cyanamide in aqueous solution in the presence of $Ba(OH)_2$. Because L-arginine can be synthesized endogenously from L-citrulline, it is classified as a nonessential amino acid in adults. However, in children and in certain conditions (eg, trauma, infection), L-arginine synthesis may become compromised and then may be considered "semiessential."

HISTORY
L-arginine is commonly sold as a health supplement claimed to be capable of improving vascular health and enhancing sexual function in men.

ACTIONS
Nitric oxide is produced by a variety of animal and human cells and is involved in many physiological and pathophysiological processes. Nitric oxide is a free radical, generated from L-arginine by the enzyme nitric oxide synthase. L-arginine supplementation to raise nitric oxide levels has been suggested to be beneficial in many areas.

TOXICOLOGY

Parenteral administration of L-arginine in high doses has caused metabolic acidosis including elevated potassium levels due to effects on intra- and extracellular potassium balance. Oral administration of L-arginine in humans has not caused any major adverse effects. L-arginine may exacerbate sickle cell crisis. Doses up to 30 g/day are well tolerated, with infrequent reports of nausea and diarrhea. No adverse effects were reported with 9 g/day L-arginine over 6 months. Arginine may trigger onset of herpes infection, although there is no solid evidence to confirm this.

References are available upon request.

BLACK WALNUT

SCIENTIFIC NAME(S)
Juglans nigra Family: Juglandaceae

COMMON NAME(S)
Black walnut

PATIENT INFORMATION

- *Warnings:* Products containing black walnut are considered dietary supplements and are **not** FDA-approved for medical use. Products containing this agent should be considered **complementary** therapies and not **alternative** therapies. Standard medical care and prescribed therapy should not be abandoned, nor should appropriate medical attention be delayed. Such practices can be dangerous.

- *Uses:* Black walnut has been used as a wood source. It can also be beneficial in certain skin disorders, for constipation, and as an anti-infectant or vermifuge. It has nutritional value and its EFAs help protect against heart disease and reduce cholesterol. There are no human trials to support these effects.

- *Side Effects:* Do not use during pregnancy or chronic gastrointestinal tract disease. Juglone, the naphthaquinone found in black walnut and many others in the family Juglandaceae, is regarded as a toxin. Allergic reactions have occurred.

BOTANY

There are about 15 species of Juglans. "Walnut" refers to several varieties, most commonly the English or Persian walnut (*J. regia*) and the black walnut (*J. nigra*). Walnut trees have short trunks with round-topped crowns, and can grow to 45 m in height. The black walnut is native to the deciduous forests of the eastern United States (central Mississippi, Appalachian regions) and Canada. Its wood is valued for its rich beauty and yields valuable lumber, prized for furniture, cabinets, and gun stocks. The fruit is an elongated drupe, containing a 4-ribbed edible nut within a thick, hard, black shell (smaller in size than the English walnut).

HISTORY

Walnuts have been found in prehistoric deposits dating from the Iron Age in Europe. They are mentioned in the Bible; King Solomon's nut garden dates back to 940 BC. Black walnuts were an important food for American Indians and early settlers. The genus name, *Juglans*, comes from the Latin *Jovis glans*, meaning "nut of Jupiter" or nut of the gods. Many legends have been associated with the walnut. Greeks and Romans regarded it as a symbol of fertility. In the Middle Ages, walnuts were thought to ward off witchcraft, the evil eye, and epileptic fits from evil spirits lurking in the walnut branches. Medicinal uses of walnuts included treatments for swollen glands, shingles, and sores. The oil was used for intestinal discomfort.

ACTIONS

Aside from the use of its wood as a valuable lumber, black walnut has been employed in other ways; extract of black walnut was used to dye the hair, skin, and clothing. Black walnut as a food is common, including its presence in baked goods, candies, and frozen foods. Even its shells, after hulling, have been used as fillers in glues, roofing materials, and tiles. They are also employed as stuffing for toys and as abrasives. Walnut shells are even burned for energy.

The black walnut is important for its nutritional value. The nuts are high in calories, a good protein source, and rich in dietary fiber and essential fatty acids (EFAs), which protect against heart disease and reduce cholesterol. EFAs reduce platelet adhesion and may also play a role in reducing arrhythmias and cardiac arrest. Dietary fiber content not only helps reduce cholesterol but aids in relieving constipation.

Black walnut is beneficial in certain skin problems, including eczema, pruritus, psoriasis, and blistering. It has been used as an astrigent to shrink tissues and as a tonic restorative. Black walnut has been shown to kill skin parasites due to its disinfectant qualities. Constituent juglone is antimicrobial and antiparasitic. Black walnut has been used for warts. Eye irritations and styes have been relieved by black walnut as well. Internally, black walnut is beneficial for these same conditions. It is mentioned by many sources as a vermifuge. The anthelmintic properties are said to be due to high tannin content. The bark (including kernel and green hull) has been used by Asians and certain American Indian tribes to expel worms. Other fungal and parasitic infections including ringworm and tapeworm have been eliminated by black walnut. Other uses for black walnut include reduction of fluid secretion in glandular disturbances, treatment of gout and rheumatism, and for purported anti-cancer effects. The toxic nature of juglone makes it a possible candidate for chemotherapy.

No major human clinical trials regarding black walnut and its claimed uses have been found through a search of medical literature.

TOXICOLOGY

Juglone, the naphthaquinone found in black walnut and many others in the family Juglandaceae, is regarded as a toxin. Induced toxicosis in horses has been studied. Juglone 1 g orally administered in horses caused inconsistent mild signs of laminitis, in which inflammation of the feet around the hooves occurs, resulting in lameness from the pain. Other studies have confirmed this type of toxicosis from black walnut, including a detailed description in a case report. In contrast, 1 report confirms the laminitis to be from black walnut but not from the constituent juglone because the heartwood of black walnut, which is devoid of this component, was used. Black walnut's effects on equine vasculature have been evaluated. One mechanism suggested in another report is that black walnut increases capillary pressure, causing transvascular fluid movement, resulting in edema and possible eventual ischemia.

Allergic reactions to black walnut in animals and humans have occurred. Allergy studies involving skin testing with black walnut pollen (and other pollens) finds moderate allergic reactions in certain individuals. Reports on dermatitis from black walnut, and on *E. coli* in black walnut are available.

Black walnut is contraindicated in pregnancy because of possible cathartic effects at higher doses and in patients with chronic disease of the GI tract.

References are available upon request.

CHONDROITIN

SCIENTIFIC NAME(S)
Chondroitin sulfate, chondroitin sulfuric acid

COMMON NAME(S)
Chondroitin

PATIENT INFORMATION

- *Warnings:* Products containing chondroitin are considered dietary supplements and are **not** FDA-approved for medical use. Products containing this agent should be considered **complementary** therapies and not **alternative** therapies. Standard medical care and prescribed therapy should not be abandoned, nor should appropriate medical attention be delayed. Such practices can be dangerous.
- *Uses:* Chondroitin has been used to treat osteoarthritis. It has also been studied for use in drug delivery and antithrombotic and extravasation therapy.

  There is no clinical data to suggest that combining glucosamine with chondroitin is more beneficial than glucosamine alone.
- *Side Effects:* Epigastric pain and nausea have been reported, as have intra-ocular hypertension, discomfort, and corneal edema after surgery. There is little information on chondroitin's long-term effects. Most reports conclude that it possesses little toxicity.
- *Dosing:* Chondroitin sulfate has been administered orally for treatment of arthritis at a dose of 800 to 1,200 mg/day. Positive results often require several months to manifest, and a posttreatment effect has been observed.

BIOLOGY

Chondroitin is a biological polymer that acts as the flexible connecting matrix between the protein filaments in cartilage. Chondroitin can be derived from natural sources (eg, shark or bovine cartilage) or it can be manufactured in the laboratory. Danaparoid sodium, a mixture of heparin sulfate, dermatan sulfate, and chondroitin sulfate in a ratio of 21:3:1, is derived from porcine intestinal mucosa.

HISTORY

Chondroitin sulfates were first extracted and purified in 1960. Studies suggested that if enough chondroitin sulfate was available to cells manufacturing proteoglycan, stimulation of matrix synthesis could occur, leading to an accelerated healing process.

ACTIONS

One report evaluated half-lives of distribution and elimination, volumes of distribution, excretion values, urine and blood levels, and bioavailablity. Another report concluded that oral chondroitin sulfate B (dermatan sulfate) reaches significant plasma levels, with 7% bioavailability. In 22 patients with renal failure, the chondroitin sulfate half-life was prolonged.

There is considerable controversy regarding absorption of chondroitin. Absorption of glucosamine is 90% to 98%, but chondroitin absorption ranges from 0% to 13% because of its molecule size. The chondroitin molecule is 50 to 300 times larger than glucosamine. Chondroitin may be too large to be delivered to cartilage cells. There may be purification and identification problems with chondroitin products, some of which have tested subpotent.

The use of chondroitin in treating osteoarthritis has gained popularity. Articular cartilage found between joints (eg, finger, knee, hip) allows for easy, painless movement. It contains 65% to 80% water, collagen, and proteoglycans. Chondrocytes found within this matrix produce new collagen and proteoglycans from building blocks, that include chondroitin sulfate, a glycosaminoglycan (GAG). Glucosamine, another of the beneficial substances in this area, stimulates chondrocyte activity. It is also the critical building block of proteoglycans and other matrix components. Both chondroitin and glucosamine play roles in joint maintenance, which is why the combination of the two are found in many arthritic nutritional supplements.

Inflammation and repeated wear of the joint disturb chondrocyte function, altering the matrix composition, which causes breakdown. Proper supplementation with glycosaminoglycans (eg, chondroitin sulfate) may enable chondrocytes to replace proteoglycans, offering "chondroprotection." Cartilage contains biological resources that enhance repair of degenerative injuries and inflammation. It has been proposed that a certain chondroitin sulfate sequence, released from cartilage proteoglycans, can inhibit elastase, regulating the matrix.

Several studies, some of which are uncontrolled or anecdotal, in finger, knee, and hip joint therapy suggest beneficial results in osteoarthritis treatment. An overview of chondroitin sulfate use in another report concluded the product has no clear value in osteoarthritis treatment.

Chondroitin sulfate has been used as a drug delivery system for diclofenac and flurbiprofen. The polymer also has been used as a stabilization agent for iron hyperalimentation.

Chondroitin sulfate B (dermatan sulfate) has potential as an antithrombolytic agent because it inhibits venous thrombi with less effect upon bleeding than heparin. It may prove to be an effective anticoagulant in hemodialysis. Dermatan sulfate's antithrombolytic activity, compared with heparin, has been observed in acute leukemia patients.

Chondroitin sulfate has been used to treat extravasation after ifosfamide therapy, decreasing pain and inflammation. It has also been used to treat extravasation caused by vindesine, doxorubicin, and vincristine and an etoposide needlestick injury in a health care worker. Levels of chondroitin sulfate increase 10 to 100 times in tumors compared with normal tissue. This may provide a potential new marker for diagnosis and follow-up of cancer therapy. General reviews are available on chondroitin sulfate and chondroitin sulfate B.

TOXICOLOGY

Little information about long-term toxic effects of chondroitin sulfate is available. Because chondroitin is concentrated in cartilage, it is thought to produce little or no toxicity or teratogenic effects. Long-term, placebo-controlled, double-blind clinical trials with larger populations are needed to fully determine toxicity.

References are available upon request.

> ## PATIENT INFORMATION
>
> - *Warnings:* Products containing chromium are considered dietary supplements and are **not** FDA-approved for medical use. Products containing this agent should be considered **complementary** therapies and not **alternative** therapies. Standard medical care and prescribed therapy should not be abandoned, nor should appropriate medical attention be delayed. Such practices can be dangerous.
> - *Uses:* Chromium is a necessary nutrient. Deficiencies, though rare, may contribute to adult diabetes and atherosclerosis, as well as complicating aging and pregnancy. Safety of use during pregnancy has not been established.
> - *Side Effects:* Ingestion or exposure to certain forms of chromium may cause or contribute to GI irritation and ulcers, cancer, dermatitis, circulatory shock, kidney damage and hepatitis.

BIOLOGY

Chromium is abundant in the earth's crust and is found in concentrations ranging from 100 to 300 ppm. Commercially, it is obtained from chrome ore, among other sources. The organic form of chromium exists in a dinicotino-glutathionine complex in natural foods, and appears to be absorbed better than the inorganic form. Good dietary sources of chromium include brewer's yeast, liver, potatoes with skin, beef, fresh vegetables, and cheese.

HISTORY

Chromium is important as an additive in the manufacture of steel alloys (chrome-steel, chrome-nickel-steel, stainless steel) and greatly increases the durability and resistance of these metals. Synthetically produced $_{51}$Cr is used as a tracer in various hematologic disorders and in the determination of blood volume. Because chromium is a recognized element required for normal glucose metabolism, a number of OTC products promote the use of chromium, alone or in combination with niacin, glycine, glutamic acid, and cysteine (components of the glucose torerance factor, GTF) to improve carbohydrate utilization. The effectiveness of these products has not been established, although they represent nutritionally sound sources of chromium.

ACTIONS

The recommended daily allowance (RDA) for chromium in healthy adults is 50 to 200 mcg.

Trivalent chromium plays a role in a cofactor complex for insulin, and is involved in normal glucose utilization. Chromium forms part of the GTF that may facilitate binding of insulin to insulin receptors, thereby amplifying its effects on lipid and carbohydrate metabolism.

Chromium deficiency is very rare in the general US population but may play an unsubstantiated role in the development of adult diabetes mellitus and atherosclerosis. Persons who have a high intake of highly refined foods may be at risk for developing chromium deficiency, as are patients receiving total parenteral nutrition. Trace metal solutions for IV administration containing chromium alone or in combination with other metals are available. These patients may experience peripheral neuropathy or encephalopathy that can be alleviated by administration of chromium. Marginal levels of chromium have been associated with decreased glucose utilization during pregnancy and in the elderly. Administration of chromium may have improved glucose tolerance in these patients, however the risk of supplemental chromium in pregnancy has not been established. It should be noted that supplemental amounts of dietary chromium do not have a hypoglycemic effect in healthy individuals. Most absorbed chromium is eliminated through the kidneys (3 to 50 mcg/day).

TOXICOLOGY

Acute oral ingestion of chromate salts may lead to irritation of the GI tract (nausea, vomiting, ulcers), circulatory shock, or hepatitis. Renal damage (including acute tubular necrosis) has been observed following occupational exposure to chromium. Trivalent chromium compounds (the kind found in foods) show little or no toxicity.

Exposure to occupational dust contaminated with hexavalent chromium and CrO_3 or CrF_2 (which are used as corrosion inhibitor pigments, and in metallurgy and electroplating) has been associated with the development of mucous hypersecretion and respiratory (lung) cancers. The incidence of lung cancer is increased up to 15 times the normal rate in workers exposed to chromite, chromic oxide, or chromium ores. The hexavalent species of chromium appears to be most highly associated with the development of cancers.

Topical effects following exposure to chromium and chromates may lead to incapacitating eczematous dermatitis and ulceration. Ulceration and perforation of the nasal septum have also occurred. About 1% to 4% of a topically applied dose of hexavalent and trivalent chromium penetrates guinea pig skin in 24 hours. Only 2 mcg of hexavalent chromium are required to induce a topical reaction in sensitive individuals. Chromium may be chelated by the systemic administration of dimercaprol.

References are available upon request.

CRANBERRY

SCIENTIFIC NAME(S)

Vaccinium macrocarpon Ait. (cranberry, trailing swamp cranberry), *V. oxycoccos* L. (small cranberry), *V. erythrocarpum* Michx. (Southern mountain cranberry), *V. vitis* (lowbush cranberry), *V. edule* (highbush cranberry). Family: Ericaceae

COMMON NAME(S)

See above.

PATIENT INFORMATION

- *Warnings:* Products containing cranberry are considered dietary supplements and are **not** FDA-approved for medical use. Products containing this agent should be considered **complementary** therapies and not **alternative** therapies. Standard medical care and prescribed therapy should not be abandoned, nor should appropriate medical attention be delayed. Such practices can be dangerous.
- *Uses:* Cranberries and cranberry juice appear to assist in managing recurrences of urinary tract infections (UTIs). For more information, see the Urinary Tract Infection (UTI) monograph in the Women's Health chapter. If daily intake is adequate, the acids lower urine pH levels enough to slow urine degradation and odor in incontinent patients.
- *Side Effects:* Extremely large doses can produce GI symptoms such as diarrhea.
- *Dosing:* Cranberry juice, juice concentrate, and dried extract have been studied in urinary tract infections. Doses of juice studied have ranged from 120 to 4,000 mL/day; 400 mg of cranberry extract daily has been given in an effort to avoid the large volumes that seem to be required for efficacy.

BOTANY

A number of related cranberries are found in areas ranging from damp bogs to mountain forests from Alaska to Tennessee. Cranberry plants grow as small trailing evergreen shrubs. Their flowers vary from pink to purple and bloom from May to August, depending on the species. The *Vaccinium* genus also includes the blueberry (*V. angustifolium* Ait.) and bilberry (*V. myrtillus*).

HISTORY

During the mid-1800s, German physicians observed that the urinary excretion of hippuric acid (a bacteriostatic agent in high concentrations) increased after the ingestion of cranberries. It was believed that cranberries, prunes, and plums contained benzoic acid or another compound that the body metabolized and excreted as hippuric acid. This hypothesis has been disputed because the small amounts of benzoic acid present in these fruits (approximately 0.1% by weight) could not account for the excretion of the larger amounts of hippuric acid.

Despite a general lack of scientific evidence to indicate that cranberries or their juice are effective urinary acidifiers, interest persists among the public regarding the clinical use of cranberries or cranberry juice. Cranberries are used in eastern European cultures because of their folkloric, but unsubstantiated, role in the treatment of cancers and in reducing fever. Cranberries make flavorful jams and preserves.

ACTIONS

The ability of cranberries to acidify urine was discovered during an experiment with 2 healthy subjects. Following a basal diet, 1 subject was given 305 g of cooked cranberries while the other received an unspecified amount of prunes. In the first subject, urinary pH decreased from 6.4 to 5.3, with a concomitant increase in the excretion of total acids. Hippuric acid excretion increased from 0.77 to 4.74 g. Presumably, urinary hippurate came from the slow biotransformation of quinic and benzoic acids or from a glucoside that hydrolyzes to quinic acid. Because mammalian tissues cannot convert quinic to hippuric acid, intestinal bacteria may play a role in this conversion.

Despite these uncontrolled, small-scale observations, the value of cranberries or cranberry juice in preventing and treating UTIs is quite controversial. In 1 study, 3 of 4 subjects given 1.5 to 4 L/day of cranberry cocktail (⅓ juice mixed with water and sugar) showed only transient changes in urinary pH. The maximum tolerated amounts of cranberry juice (approximately 4 L/day) rarely result in enough hippuric acid excretion to achieve urinary concentrations that are bacteriostatic at the optimum activity level of pH 5. The antibiotic activity of hippuric acid decreases approximately 5-fold at pH 5.6. When 5 subjects were given 1.2 to 4 L/day of cranberry juice, urinary pH decreased only 0.2 to 0.5 units after 4 days of treatment; no urinary pH was ever lowered to pH 5. A recent placebo-controlled study assessed the effect of drinking 300 mL/day of cranberry juice on bacteria and white blood cell counts in the urine of 153 elderly women. The odds of having bacteria or white blood cells in the urine were lower in the women who ingested real cranberry juice, and their odds of remaining bacteriuric-pyuric from 1 month to the next were only 27% of the odds in the control group ($P = 0.006$). This is one of the largest and best-designed studies of its kind and suggests that there may be an indirect microbiologic basis for cranberry's activity.

It is most likely, however, that the juice does not exert a direct antibacterial effect via a compound such as hippuric acid, but that an alternate mechanism accounts for the anti-infective activity. This is supported by the observation that cranberry and blueberry juices contain a high molecular weight compound (eg, either condensed tannins or proanthocyanidins) that inhibits the common urinary pathogen *Escherichia coli* from adhering to sites within the urinary tract, thus limiting the ability of the bacteria to initiate and spread infections.

One promising use for the juice is as a "urinary deodorant." The malodor of fermenting urine from incontinent patients is a persistent aesthetic problem in hospitals and long-term care facilities. Cranberry juice appears to lower urinary pH sufficiently to retard the degradation of urine by *E. coli*, limiting the generation of the pungent "ammonia-like" odor.

Using the juice daily has been suggested for the long-term suppressive therapy of UTIs. Anecdotal reports have described the benefits of drinking 6 ounces of cranberry juice twice daily to relieve symptoms of chronic pyelonephritis and decrease recurrence of urinary stones.

TOXICOLOGY

There have been no reports of significant toxicity with the use of cranberries or their juice. The ingestion of large amounts (more than 3 to 4 L/day) of the juice often results in diarrhea and other GI symptoms.

References are available upon request.

DONG QUAI

SCIENTIFIC NAME(S)

Angelica polymorpha Maxim. var. sinensis; *A. atropurpurea; A. dahurica; A. sinensis diels.* Family: Apiaceae

COMMON NAME(S)

Dong quai, tang-kuei, dang-gui, Chinese angelica

PATIENT INFORMATION

- *Warnings:* Products containing dong quai are considered dietary supplements and are **not** FDA-approved for medical use. Products containing this agent should be considered **complementary** therapies and not **alternative** therapies. Standard medical care and prescribed therapy should not be abandoned, nor should appropriate medical attention be delayed. Such practices can be dangerous when herbal products are being used.

  Safety of dong quai use during pregnancy and lactation has not been confirmed. Pregnant and lactating women should not use this agent.

- *Uses:* Derivatives of dong quai have been used primarily for their uterine tonic and antispasmodic effects. Dong quai also may provide modest analgesic and anti-inflammatory activity.

- *Drug Interactions:* Dong quai may interact with warfarin (eg, *Coumadin*) and other anticoagulants, leading to an increased risk of bleeding complications.

- *Side Effects:* Components of dong quai can potentially cause skin problems, ranging from photosensitization to skin cancer.

- *Dosing:* Crude dong quai root has been given in doses ranging from 0.75 g/day to as much as 30 g/day. More typical doses are around 4.5 g/day.

BOTANY

Dong quai is an aromatic herb widely distributed throughout the Orient. The root of this plant is used medicinally.

HISTORY

The plant has been used for centuries in traditional Asian medicine as a decoction (ie, a boiled preparation of the plant) for treatment of a variety of gynecologic problems (eg, menstrual cramps, irregular menses). Historically, it has been used as an antispasmodic, a "blood purifier," and in the management of hypertension, rheumatism, ulcers, anemia, constipation, and various types of allergic reactions.

ACTIONS

Many coumarins of dong quai have been shown to exert vasodilatory and antispasmodic effects.

Coumarins in dried roots of *Angelica dahurica* were found to activate epinephrine- and corticotropin-induced lipolysis and inhibit insulin-induced lipogenesis.

An aqueous extract of dong quai has been found to inhibit experimentally-induced IgE titers, suggesting that components of the plant may have immunosuppressive activity. However, no therapeutic benefit has been determined clinically.

TOXICOLOGY

The furocoumarin components of dong quai, psoralen and bergapten, can induce photosensitization, resulting in potentially severe photodermatitis. These episodes have generally been confined to people collecting plants of the family Apiaceae. Psoralens induce melanization in human skin in the presence of light and have been used medicinally in the treatment of skin depigmentation and psoriasis. However, these agents are photocarcinogenic and are mutagenic even in the absence of light. There is no firm evidence that ingesting plants containing psoralens is dangerous, but the potential toxicity should be considered by the user. It should also be recognized that safrole, found in the essential oil, is carcinogenic and is not recommended for ingestion.

References are available upon request.

ECHINACEA

SCIENTIFIC NAME(S)

Echinacea angustifolia DC. The related species *E. purpurea* (L.) Moench and *E. pallida* (Nutt.) Britton have also been used in traditional medicine. Family: Compositae (Asteraceae)

COMMON NAME(S)

American coneflower, black susans, comb flower, Echinacea, hedgehog, Indian head, Kansas snakeroot, narrow-leaved purple cone flower, purple coneflower, scurvy root, snakeroot

---

PATIENT INFORMATION

- *Warnings:* Products containing echinacea are considered dietary supplements and are **not** FDA-approved for medical use. Products containing this agent should be considered **complementary** therapies and not **alternative** therapies. Standard medical care and prescribed therapy should not be abandoned, nor should appropriate medical attention be delayed. Such practices can be dangerous when herbal products are being used.

  Safety of echinacea use during pregnancy and lactation has not been confirmed. Pregnant and lactating women should avoid use of this agent.
- *Uses:* Echinacea has been used for prevention and treatment of the common cold and flu, for topical wound healing, and for internal stimulation of the immune system.
- *Side Effects:* Side effects associated with use of echinacea are poorly defined. Its extracts and components have been injected at high doses without overt toxic effects.
- *Dosing:* Echinacea clinical trials for prevention or treatment of cold symptoms have been run primarily on the frest pressed juice of the herb, which is preserved with 22% alcohol. Typical daily doses are 5 to 10 mL of the juice. *Echinacin* (Madaus, EC31) and *Echinagard* are fresh juice prepared from the herb. Extracts of the root are available, including *Echinaforce* and *Echinacea Plus.* These have been given at doses corresponding to 1 g of the crude herb or root 3 times/day.

BOTANY

Echinacea is native to Kansas, Nebraska, and Missouri. There has been significant confusion regarding the naming and identification of the *Echinacea* species. Because of this confusion, much of the early research conducted on this plant (and in particular with European *E. angustifolia*) was probably conducted on *E. pallida.* Numerous synonyms have been applied to the *Echinacea* species.

E. angustifolia is a perennial herb with narrow leaves and a stout stem that grows to approximately 3 feet in height. The plant terminates in a single colorful flower head. The plant imparts a pungent, acrid taste when chewed and causes tingling of the lips and tongue.

Echinacea products have been found to be adulterated with another member of the Compositae, *Parthenium integrifolium* L., a plant with no known pharmacologic activity.

HISTORY

Echinacea is a popular herbal product in the central United States. The plant was used by the American Indians and was quickly adopted by the settlers. During the 1800s, claims for the curative properties of the plant ranged from a "blood purifier" to a treatment for dizziness and rattlesnake bites. During the early 20th century, extracts of the plant were used as an anti-infective. However, the use of these products fell out of favor after the discovery of more effective anti-infective agents in the 1930s and beyond.

However, the plant and its extracts continue to be used topically for wound healing and internally to stimulate the immune system. Most of the research during the past 10 years has focused on the immunostimulant properties of this plant.

ACTIONS

A small body of evidence is evolving to support the use of echinacea as a wound-healing agent and immunostimulant, but not as primary anti-infective therapy.

Several caffeoyl conjugates have been isolated from *E. angustifolia* that demonstrate antihyaluronidase activity; these include chicoric acid, cynarine, chlorogenic acid, and caffaric acid. The inhibition of hyaluronidase is believed to limit the progression of certain degenerative inflammatory diseases.

Anecdotal reports and several controlled studies have suggested that echinacea may have beneficial effects in the prevention and treatment of the common cold and flu. However, evidence remains insufficient to support therapeutic recommendations. Most studies have indicated that the lipophilic fraction of the root and leaves contains the most potent immunostimulating components. Although a number of pharmacologically active components have been isolated, no single compound appears to be responsible for the plant's activity. Much of the relevant literature focuses on the immune stimulating action of the high molecular weight polysaccharides. There is some indication that the alkamide fraction stimulates phagocytosis, and there is also some evidence that these 2 groups of compounds operate synergistically.

The suggested, but inadequately documented, ability of echinacea extracts to enhance the immune response is perhaps the plant's most intriguing activity. A number of in vitro and animal studies have documented the activation of immunologic activity. These extracts appear to stimulate phagocytosis, increase cellular respiratory activity, and increase the mobility of leukocytes.

Extracts of *E. purpurea* have been found to increase the phagocytosis of *Candida albicans* by granulocytes and monocytes in vitro, although the extract had no effect on the intracellular killing of bacteria or yeasts. The clinical value of these effects in patients is unknown.

The root oil inhibits certain types of leukemia cells in vitro and in vivo. The compound (Z)-1,8-pentadecadiene appears to be the active principle and can account for up to 44% of the root oil in some species. Its trans isomer is less active.

The purified polysaccharide arabinogalactan, isolated from *E. purpurea*, was effective in activating macrophages to become cytotoxic against certain types of tumor cells and selected microorganisms following intraperitoneal injection in mice. This polysaccharide appears to induce macrophages to produce tumor necrosis factor, interleukin-1, and interferon beta-2.

One study found that the administration of echinacea extracts in humans stimulated cell-mediated immunity following a single dose, but that repeated daily doses produced the undesirable effect of suppressing the immune response. In a study conducted in a small number of patients (n = 15) with advanced metastasized colorectal cancer, *E. purpurea* extracts were added to cyclophosphamide and thymostimulin treatment; the mean survival time was 4 months, and 2 patients survived for more than 8 months. The cause-and-effect relationship of adding these extracts to the regimen is not clear but warrants further study. This form of immunotherapy may have some value in treating certain types of cancer.

Although some study results are encouraging, they are too preliminary to draw conclusions about the appropriate therapeutic uses of echinacea extracts. There are no well-controlled studies that have evaluated the clinical effects of nonprescription echinacea dietary supplements in the management of disease. Dosages are not well defined.

TOXICOLOGY

Little is known about the toxicity of this plant despite echinacea's widespread use in many countries. It has been used in American folk medicine for more than a century and generally has not been associated with debilitating acute or chronic toxicity. Purified echinacea polysaccharide is relatively nontoxic in amounts consumed in OTC products.

References are available upon request.

SCIENTIFIC NAME(S)

Many members of the genus *Ephedra* have been used medicinally. The most common of these include *E. altissima*, *E. sinica* Stapf., *E. intermedia* Schrenk and Meyer, and *E. nevadensis* Watson. Family: Ephedraceae (Gnetaceae).

COMMON NAME(S)

Sea grape, ma-huang, yellow horse, yellow astringent, joint fir, squaw tea, Mormon tea, popotillo, teamster's tea.

PATIENT INFORMATION

- *Warnings:* Products containing ephedras are considered dietary supplements and are **not** FDA-approved for medical use. Products containing this agent should be considered **complementary** therapies and not **alternative** therapies. Standard medical care and prescribed therapy should not be abandoned, nor should appropriate medical attention be delayed. Such practices can be dangerous.
- *Uses:* Ephedra preparations are traditionally used to relieve colds, improve respiratory function, lose weight, and treat a range of ills from headaches to venereal diseases. Evidence shows that plant parts of various species exert hypoglycemic, hypertensive, diuretic, and anti-inflammatory effects.
- *Side Effects:* Large doses may cause a variety of ill effects from skin reactions to toxic psychosis and mutagenic effects. Those with high blood pressure and diabetes should exercise caution before using ephedra.
- *Dosing:* Levels of ephedrine vary markedly in the crude herb, making standardization on ephedrine content crucial for safe use. Doses of the herb range from 1 to 6 g/day, with doses in clinical trials for weight loss ranging from 50 to 150 mg ephedrine. The potential for drug interactions with several types of agents mandates caution in use.

BOTANY

Ephedra species have a worldwide distribution. They are generally erect evergreen plants, often resembling small shrubs. The plants resemble a bunch of jointed branches covered with minute leaves. These plants usually have a strong pine odor and astringent taste.

HISTORY

The Ephedras have a long history of use as stimulants and for the management of bronchial disorders. It is believed that these plants were used more than 5,000 years ago by the Chinese to treat asthma. Ephedra has been used in Asian medicine to treat colds, flu, fevers, chills, headaches, edema, lack of perspiration, nasal congestion, aching joints and bones, coughing, and wheezing. Today, Ephedra continues to find a place in herbal preparations designed to relieve cold symptoms and improve respiratory function. However, the use of standardized ephedrine/pseudoephedrine preparations has supplanted the use of the crude drug in most developed countries.

North American species, which are alkaloid-free (eg, *E. nevadensis*), have been made into refreshing, non-stimulating beverages. The fruits of some species are eaten, while ashes of *E. intermedia* are mixed with chewing tobacco in Pakistan.

ACTIONS

Ephedrine and its related alkaloids are CNS stimulants. Ephedrine is active when given orally, parenterally, or ophthalmically. It stimulates the heart, causing increased blood pressure and heart rate and is a bronchodilator. It can stimulate contraction of the uterus and has diuretic properties. Because it constricts peripheral blood vessels, it can relieve congestion in mucous tissues. Pseudoephedrine has a weaker cardiac effect but a greater diuretic activity. Administration of the fluid extract and decoction of Mormon tea has resulted in diuresis, most likely caused by compounds other than ephedrine. Teas of these plants can cause constipation as a result of their tannin content.

Crude aerial parts of Ephedra (known in Chinese as mao) cause hyperglycemia, most likely induced by the ephedrine alkaloids. However, investigations into the crude drug found a fraction that exhibited repeated hypoglycemic effects.

Although crude Ephedra aerial parts (mao) can induce hypertension, crude ephedra root (mao-kon) causes hypotension. This effect is caused by several related macrocyclic spermine alkaloids that are designated ephedradines.

Others studies of the hypotensive effect of the root preparation have isolated L-tyrosine betaine (maokonine), a compound that induces hypertension, suggesting that, depending on the species, a variable effect on blood pressure may be observed.

TOXICOLOGY

In large doses, ephedrine causes nervousness, irritability, headache, insomnia, dizziness, palpitations, skin flushing, tingling, vomiting, anxiety, and restlessness. Toxic psychosis may be induced by ephedrine. Skin reactions have been observed in sensitive patients. Patients with high blood pressure and diabetes should exercise caution when using these plants.

E. altissima yields several mutagenic n-nitrosamines under simulated gastric conditions. For example, N-nitrosephedrine causes metastasizing liver-cell carcinomas, as well as cancer of the lung and forestomach in animals. However, investigators noted that the potential for endogenous formation of these compounds following ingestion of the tea is small.

The FDA warns consumers not to purchase or consume ephedrine-containing dietary supplements with labels that often portray the products as apparent alternatives to illegal street drugs such as "ecstacy," because these products can pose serious health risks to consumers.

References are available upon request.

EVENING PRIMROSE OIL

SCIENTIFIC NAME(S)
Oenothera biennis L. Family: Onagraceae

COMMON NAME(S)
Evening primrose, EPO, OEP

PATIENT INFORMATION

- *Warnings:* Products containing evening primose oil are considered dietary supplements and are **not** FDA-approved for medical use. Products containing this agent should be considered **complementary** therapies and not **alternative** therapies. Standard medical care and prescribed therapy should not be abandoned, nor should appropriate medical attention be delayed. Such practices can be dangerous when herbal products are being used.
- *Uses:* OEP has been used to treat cardiovascular disease, breast disorders, premenstrual syndrome, mastalgia, rheumatoid arthritis, multiple sclerosis, atopic eczema, dermatological disorders and other illnesses.
- *Side effects:* There have been no adverse effects attributed to oil of evening primrose.
- *Dosing:* Evening primrose oil has been administered orally in clinical trials for arthritis, atopic dermatitis, PMS, and diabetic neuropathy at doses between 3 and 6 g/day. The typical content of gamma-linolenic acid is 8% to 10% in the oil.

BOTANY

The evening primrose is a large, delicate wildflower native to North America and is not a true primrose. The blooms usually last only 1 evening. Primrose is an annual or biennial and can grow in height from 1 to 3 meters. The flowers are yellow in color and the fruit is a dry pod about 5 cm long that contains many small seeds.[3] The small seeds contain an oil characterized by its high content of gamma-linolenic acid (GLA). Wild varieties of O. biennis contain highly variable amounts of linoleic acid and GLA; however, extensive cross-breeding has produced a commercial variety that consistently yields an oil with 72% cis-linoleic acid and 9% GLA. This is perhaps the richest plant source of GLA. A commercially grown mold has been reported to produce an oil containing 20% GLA, and newer strains may produce even greater yields.

The oil from evening primrose (OEP) seeds is cultivated in at least 15 countries and is available in more than 30 countries as a nutritional supplement or as a constituent in specialty foods. US and Canadian production total more than 300 to 400 tons of seeds yearly. US production centers are in California, North Carolina, South Carolina, Oregon and Texas.

TOXICOLOGY

As a nutritional supplement, the maximum label-recommended daily dose of OEP is approximately 4 g. This dose contains 300 to 360 mg GLA, which contributes: (1) 6 to 7 mg GLA/kg/day likely to be produced from linoleic acid in the normal adult female, (2) 23 to 65 mg GLA/kg/day consumed by a breastfed baby or (3) 70 to 400 mg/kg/day of all the metabolites of linoleic acid consumed by a breastfed infant. According to these estimates, the amounts of GLA in the recommended doses of OEP are in the same range as the amounts of GLA and other related EFAs present in widely consumed foods. Thus, there is little concern about the safety of OEP as a dietary supplement in the recommended dosage range. There are considerable data on the safety of OEP from Efamol, Ltd., a major commercial supplier of oil derived from specially selected and hybridized forms of Oenothera species. In toxicological studies carried out for 1 year, OEP at doses up to 2.5 mL/kg/day in rats and 5 mL/kg/day in dogs was found to possess no toxic properties. Similar results were obtained in 2-year carcinogenicity and teratological investigations. With approximately 1,000 tons of OEP sold in several countries as a nutritional supplement since the 1970s, there have been no complaints concerning the safety of the product.

References are available upon request.

FEVERFEW

SCIENTIFIC NAME(S)

Tanacetum parthenium (L.) Schulz-Bip. synonymous with *Chrysanthemum parthenium* (L.) Bernh., *Leucanthemum parthenium* (L.) Gren and Godron, and *Pyrethrum parthenium* (L.) Sm. Alternately described as a member of the genus *Matricaria*. Family: Asteraceae

COMMON NAME(S)

Feverfew, featherfew, altamisa, bachelor's button, featherfoil, febrifuge plant, midsummer daisy, nosebleed, Santa Maria, wild chamomile, wild quinine

---

PATIENT INFORMATION

- *Warnings:* Products containing feverfew are considered dietary supplements and are **not** FDA-approved for medical use. Products containing this agent should be considered **complementary** therapies and not **alternative** therapies. Standard medical care and prescribed therapy should not be abandoned, nor should appropriate medical attention be delayed. Such practices can be dangerous.

  Feverfew should not be used by pregnant or lactating women or children younger than 2 years of age.

  Patients with headache should seek medical treatment **before** starting feverfew Headache is a prominent symptom in a variety of CNS disorders. It is essential that a proper diagnosis be made and the cause of headache be determined **before** initiating self-treatment.

- *Uses:* Traditionally an antipyretic, feverfew has been used in recent times to avert migraines and relieve menstrual pain, asthma, dermatitis, and arthritis.

- *Drug Interactions:* Possible interactions with anticoagulants and nonsteroidal anti-inflammatory drugs (NSAIDs).

- *Side Effects:* Patients withdrawn from feverfew experienced nervous system reactions (eg, rebound of migraine symptoms, anxiety, poor sleep patterns) and muscle/joint stiffness. Most adverse effects of treatment with feverfew are mild, although some patients experience increased heart rate.

- *Dosing:* Feverfew generally is given for migraine at a daily dose of 50 to 150 mg of dried leaves. While some products have been standardized for parthenolide content (0.2 to 0.6 mg/dose), this compound has not been confirmed as a major active principle for migraine.

BOTANY

A short bushy perennial that grows from 6 inches to 2 feet tall along fields and roadsides, the feverfew's yellow-green leaves and yellow flowers resemble those of chamomile (*Matricaria chamomilla*). The flowers bloom from July to October.

HISTORY

Feverfew has had a long history of use in traditional and folk medicine, especially among Greek and early European herbalists. During the last few hundred years feverfew had fallen into general disuse. However, it has recently become popular as a prophylactic treatment for migraine headaches, and its extracts have been claimed to relieve menstrual pain, asthma, dermatitis, and arthritis. Traditionally, the herb has been used as an antipyretic, from which its common name is derived. The leaves are ingested, fresh or dried, with a typical daily dose of 2 to 3 leaves. These are bitter and are often sweetened before ingestion. Because of its strong, lasting odor, it has also been planted around houses to enhance the aroma of the air. A tincture of its blossoms has been used as an insect repellent and balm for insect bites. It was once used as an antidote for opium overindulgence.

ACTIONS

Feverfew extracts affect a wide variety of physiologic pathways.

In vitro: Feverfew may inhibit prostaglandin synthesis. Extracts of the above-ground portions of the plant suppress prostaglandin production; however, this effect is not moderated by cyclooxygenase.

Aqueous extracts prevent the release of arachidonic acid and inhibit in vitro aggregation of platelets stimulated by adenosine diphosphate (ADP) or thrombin. It is controversial whether these extracts block the synthesis of thromboxane, a prostaglandin involved in platelet aggregation. Data suggest that feverfew's mechanism of prostaglandin synthesis inhibition differs from that of salicylates and NSAIDs. Extracts may inhibit platelet behavior via effects on platelet sulfhydryl groups.

Feverfew extracts are potent inhibitors of serotonin release from platelets and polymorphonuclear leucocyte granules, providing a plausible connection between the claimed benefit of feverfew in migraines and arthritis. Feverfew may produce an antimigraine effect similar to methysergide maleate (*Sansert*), a known serotonin antagonist. Extracts of the plant also inhibit the release of enzymes from white cells found in inflamed joints (a similar anti-inflammatory effect may occur in the skin), providing a theoretical basis for the use of feverfew in managing psoriasis.

In addition, feverfew extracts inhibit phagocytosis, the deposition of platelets on collagen surfaces, and mast cell release of histamine. Feverfew also exhibits antithrombotic potential and cytotoxic activity and has in vitro antibacterial activity. Monoterpenes in the plant may exert insecticidal activity, and alpha-pinene derivatives may possess sedative and mild tranquilizing effects.

Clinical Uses: Much interest has been focused on the activity of feverfew in the treatment and prevention of migraine headaches. The first account of its use as a preventative for migraine appeared in 1978 and described a woman who had suffered from severe migraines since 16 years of age. At the age of 68, she began using 3 leaves of feverfew daily, and after 10 months, her headaches ceased altogether. This case prompted further studies.

A study in 8 feverfew-treated patients and 9 placebo-controlled patients found that fewer headaches were reported by patients taking feverfew for up to 6 months of treatment. Patients in both groups had self-medicated with feverfew for several years before enrolling in the study. The incidence of headaches remained constant in those patients taking feverfew but increased almost 3-fold in those switched to placebo during the trial ($P < 0.02$). Abrupt discontinuation of feverfew in patients switched to placebo caused incapacitating headaches in some patients. Nausea and vomiting were reduced in patients taking feverfew. The statistical analysis of this study has been questioned, but the results provide a unique insight into the activity of feverfew. These results were confirmed in a more recent placebo-controlled study. More controlled clinical trials are needed to confirm that feverfew will be useful not only for the classical migraine and cluster headache, but also for premenstrual, menstrual, and other headaches as well.

Some studies reveal that experimental observations may not be clinically relevant to migraine patients taking feverfew. Ten patients who had taken extracts of the plant for up to 8 years to control migraine headaches were evaluated for physiologic changes. The platelets of all treated patients aggregated characteristically to ADP and thrombin and were similar to those of control patients. However, aggregation in response to serotonin was greatly attenuated in the feverfew users.

Canada's Health Protection Branch has granted a Drug Identification Number (DIN) for a British feverfew (*Tanacetum parthenium*) product. This allows the manufacturer, Herbal Laboratories, Ltd., to claim the product's effectiveness as a nonprescription drug in the prevention of migraine headache. Canada's Health Protection Branch recommends a daily dose of 125 mg of a dried feverfew leaf preparation, from authenticated *Tanacetum parthenium* containing 0.2% or more parthenolide for the prevention of migraine.

TOXICOLOGY

In 1 study, patients received 50 mg/day, roughly equivalent to 2 leaves. Adverse effects during 6 months of continued feverfew treatment were mild and did not result in discontinuation. Four of the 8 patients taking the plant had no adverse effects. Heart rate increased by up to 26 bpm in 2 treated patients. There were no differences between treatment groups in laboratory test results.

Patients who were switched to placebo after taking feverfew for several years experienced a cluster of nervous system reactions (eg, rebound of migraine symptoms, anxiety, poor sleep patterns) along with muscle and joint stiffness, which was referred to as "postfeverfew syndrome."

In a larger group of feverfew users, 18% reported adverse effects, the most troublesome being mouth ulceration (11%). Feverfew can induce more widespread inflammation of the oral mucosa and tongue, often with lip swelling and loss of taste. Dermatitis has been associated with ingestion of this plant.

The leaves of the plant have been shown to possess potential emmenagogue (abortifacient) activity, and feverfew is not recommended for pregnant or lactating mothers or children younger than 2 years of age. Although an interaction with anticoagulants is undocumented, this may be clinically important in sensitive patients.

Analysis of the frequency of chromosomal aberrations and sister chromatid exchanges in circulating lymphocytes in patients who ingested feverfew for 11 months did not reveal any aberrations, which suggested that the plant does not induce chromosomal abnormalities.

References are available upon request.

SCIENTIFIC NAME(S)
Allium sativum L. Family: Liliacea.

COMMON NAME(S)
Garlic, allium, stinking rose, rustic treacle, nectar of the gods, camphor of the poor, poor man's treacle.

PATIENT INFORMATION

- *Warnings:* Products containing garlic are considered dietary supplements and are **not** FDA-approved for medical use. Products containing this agent should be considered **complementary** therapies and not **alternative** therapies. Standard medical care and prescribed therapy should not be abandoned, nor should appropriate medical attention be delayed. Such practices can be dangerous.
- *Uses:* Evidence suggests garlic lowers blood sugar, cholesterol, and lipids. Among its historical uses, it has been used for its antiseptic and antibacterial properties.
- *Side Effects:* Garlic may adversely affect those requiring stringent blood glucose control or those being treated with anticoagulants (eg, blood thinness).
- *Dosing:* Garlic dosage is complicated by the volatility and instability of important constituents and by such products as "deodorized garlic," "aged" extracts, and distilled oils. Doses of fresh bulbs studied in clinical trials for hyperlipidemia or atherosclerosis range from 2 to 4 g/day and a daily intake of 2 to 12 mg allicin has been proposed. Because garlic is a widely consumed foodstuff, dosage will remain a matter of personal tolerance.

BOTANY
A perennial, odiferous bulb with a tall, erect flowering stem growing from 60 to 90 cm in height, garlic produces pink-to-purple flowers that bloom from July to September.

HISTORY
The name *Allium* comes from the Celtic word "all" meaning "burning or smarting." Garlic was valued as an exchange medium in ancient Egypt and described in Cheops pyramid inscriptions. The folk uses of garlic have ranged from the treatment of leprosy in humans to managing clotting disorders in horses. During the Middle Ages, physicians prescribed the herb to cure deafness, while the American Indians used garlic as a remedy for earaches, flatulence, and scurvy.

ACTIONS
Researchers at the Shandong Academy of Medical Science reported that allicin, a compound in garlic, increased the levels of 2 important antioxidant enzymes in the blood, catalase and glutathione peroxidase.

Garlic has been reviewed for its potential ability to slow the process of athero-sclerosis. In one study, 10 healthy subjects received a fatty meal containing 100 g of butter either alone or with 50 g of garlic juice. After 3 hours, the garlic-treated group showed mean serum cholesterol levels 7% lower than baseline compared to the untreated group, which was 7% above baseline ($P < 0.001$ for both groups). Furthermore, the garlic-treated group had a 15% increase in fibrinolytic activity compared to controls (49% decrease) ($P < 0.001$ for both groups). In 1 study, 20 healthy subjects were fed garlic (0.25 mg/kg per day of oil in 2 divided doses) for 6 months. The oil lowered mean serum cholesterol and triglyceride levels while raising high-density lipoprotein (HDL) levels. Sixty-two patients with coronary artery disease and elevated cholesterol levels were randomly assigned to 2 subgroups; 1 group was fed garlic for 10 months and the second group served as the untreated con-trols. Garlic decreased the serum cholesterol, triglyceride, and low-density lipoprotein (LDL) levels ($P < 0.05$) while increasing the HDL fraction ($P < 0.001$).

Garlic oil appears to inhibit platelet function, probably by interfering with thromboxane synthesis. Ariga, et al isolated a component of garlic oil that inhibits platelet aggregation and identified it as methylallyltrisulphide (MATS).

Further studies indicate that the most potent antithrombotic compound in garlic is ajoene, which is formed by an acid-catalyzed reaction of 2 allicin mol-ecules followed by rearrangement. Unlike other antithrombotics, ajoene appears to inhibit platelet aggregation regardless of the mechanism of induc-tion.

Scientists have demonstrated the effect of ajoene in preventing clot forma-tion caused by vascular damage. The experiment mimicked the conditions of blood flow in small- and medium-sized arteries by varying the velocity of the blood; the compound proved to be effective in both conditions.

The inhibition of platelet aggregation is also observed in people who ingest fresh garlic. In 1 study, the platelets from subjects who had eaten garlic cloves (100 to 150 mg/kg) showed complete inhibition to aggregation induced by 5-hydroxytryptamine. The effect was no longer detectable 2.5 hours after ingestion.

Although an earlier study concluded that dried garlic, administered in the form of sugar-coated tablets, had no effect on blood lipids, apolipoproteins, and blood coagulation parameters in patients with primary hyperlipoprotein-emia, more recent studies have found that garlic tablets produce a signifi-cantly greater reduction in total cholesterol and LDL-C than with placebo.

Another study stated that total cholesterol levels in those taking garlic tablets dropped by 6% and LDL cholesterol was reduced by 11%. Researchers have discovered that garlic tablets reduced the susceptibility of LDL oxidation by 34% vs the placebo group.

Garlic has reduced blood-sugar levels. Researchers noted an increase in serum insulin and improvement in liver glycogen storage after garlic administration.

As recently as World War II, garlic extracts were used to disinfect wounds. During the 1800s, physicians routinely prescribed garlic inhalation for the treatment of tuberculosis. Garlic extracts inhibit the growth of numerous strains of Mycobacterium, but at concentrations that may be difficult to achieve in human tissues.

TOXICOLOGY

Although garlic is used extensively for culinary purposes with essentially no ill effects, the long-term safety of concentrated extracts is unclear.

A single 25 mL dose of fresh garlic extract has caused burning of the mouth, esophagus, and stomach, nausea, sweating, and lightheadedness, and the safety of repeated doses of this amount has not been defined. Repeated exposure to garlic dust can induce asthmatic reactions.

There are no studies that evaluate the effect of garlic and its extracts in patients who require stringent blood glucose control or in those being treated with anticoagulants (coumarins, salicylates, "antiplatelet" drugs), but the potential for serious interactions should be kept in mind.

References are available upon request.

■ ■ ■

GINGER

SCIENTIFIC NAME(S)
Zingiber officinale Roscoe; occasionally *Z. capitatum* and *Z. zerumbet* Smith are used. Family: Zingiberaceae

COMMON NAME(S)
Ginger

PATIENT INFORMATION

- *Warnings:* Products containing ginger are considered dietary supplements and are **not** FDA-approved for medical use. Products containing this agent should be considered **complementary** therapies and not **alternative** therapies. Standard medical care and prescribed therapy should not be abandoned, nor should appropriate medical attention be delayed. Such practices can be dangerous when herbal products are being used.
- *Uses:* Ginger roots and rhizomes are used as a seasoning. In traditional medicine, ginger has been used as a carminative, stimulant, a diuretic, and antiemetic. It also has been used as an insecticide and fungicide.
- *Side Effects:* Excessive amounts may cause CNS depression and cardiac arrhythmias.
- *Dosing:* Ginger root has been given for nausea in clinical trials in 1 g doses, repeated as necessary.

BOTANY
This perennial grows in warm climates such as India, Jamaica, and China, and is native to southeast Asia. The plant carries a green-purple flower in terminal spikes; the flowers are similar to orchids. The rhizome is aromatic and the source of the dried powdered spice.

HISTORY
The roots and rhizomes of ginger have been used as a seasoning and have played an important role in Chinese, Indian, and Japanese medicine. Ginger is thought to possess carminative, stimulant, diuretic, and antiemetic properties. Fluid extracts of ginger have been used since the 1500s for the treatment of GI distress. In China, ginger root and stem are used as pesticides against aphids and fungal spores.

ACTIONS
The gingerols and the related compound shogaol have been found to possess cardiotonic activity. Crude methanol extracts of ginger are known to have a powerful and positive inotropic effect on animal hearts. The gingerols exert a dose-dependent positive inotropic action at doses as low as 10^{-4}g/mL when applied to isolated atrial tissue.

Administration of [6]-gingerol and [6]-shogaol (1.75 to 3.5 mg/kg IV and 70 to 140 mg/kg orally) inhibited spontaneous motor activity, produced antipyretic and analgesic effects and prolonged hexobarbital-induced sleeping time in laboratory animals. The [6]-shogaol was generally more potent than [6]-gingerol and exhibited an intense antitussive effect when compared to dihydrocodeine phosphate. Interestingly, [6]-shogaol inhibited intestinal motility when given IV, but facilitated GI motility after oral administration. Both compounds were cardiodepressant at low doses and cardiotonic at higher doses. [6]-gingerol, the dehydrogingerdiones, and the gingerdiones are potent inhibitors of prostaglandin biosynthesis through the inhibition of prostaglandin synthetase.

The volatile oil of ginger root was capable of inhibiting the growth of bacteria in a closed chamber, and commercial applications of this activity are being investigated.

The cytotoxic compound zerumbone and its epoxide have been isolated from the rhizomes of *Z. zerumbet*. This plant, also a member of the family Zingiberaceae, has been used traditionally in China as an antineoplastic. The isolates inhibited the growth of a hepatoma tissue culture. In addition, juice prepared from ginger root inactivates the mutagenicity of tryptophan pyrolysis products in vitro.

The root stock of the related *Z. capitatum* contains a heat-stable interferon that possesses some immune-stimulating activity. It has no direct virucidal or antitumor action.

Little is known about the human pharmacology of ginger. One widely publicized double-blind study was conducted to compare the effect of 940 mg powdered ginger root, 100 mg dimenhydrinate (eg, *Dramamine*, an antihistamine), and placebo (chickweed herb) in the prevention of motion sickness. Thirty-six subjects were given the preparations and placed blindfolded in a rotating chair. Subjects who received ginger root remained in the chair an average of 5.5 minutes, compared to 3.5 minutes for the dimenhydrinate group and 1.5 minutes for the placebo group. Half of the ginger-treated subjects remained in the chair for the full 6 minutes of the test; none of the subjects in the other groups completed the test. In general, it took longer for the ginger group to begin feeling sick, but once the vomiting center was activated, sensations of nausea and vomiting progressed at the same rate in all groups. The authors postulated that, unlike antihistamines which act on the CNS, the aromatic, carminative, and possibly absorbent properties of ginger, ameliorate the effects of motion sickness in the GI tract itself. It may increase gastric motility, blocking GI reactions and subsequent nausea feedback.

More recently, pregnant women suffering from hyperemesis gravidarum received ginger (250 mg 4 times daily) or placebo for 4 days. A significant ($P = 0.003$) percentage of women (70.4%) subjectively preferred ginger treatment, with greater symptomatic relief being observed compared to placebo.

TOXICOLOGY

There are no reports of severe toxicity in humans from the ingestion of ginger root. In culinary quantities, the root is generally devoid of activity. Large overdoses carry the potential for causing CNS depression and cardiac arrhythmias. Reports that ginger extracts may be mutagenic or antimutagenic in experimental test models require confirmation. There is no good evidence regarding the safety of ingesting large amounts of this material by pregnant women.

References are available upon request.

GINKGO

SCIENTIFIC NAME(S)
Ginkgo biloba L. Family: Ginkgoaceae

COMMON NAME(S)
Ginkgo, maidenhair tree, kew tree, ginkyo, yinhsing (Silver Apricot-Japanese)

PATIENT INFORMATION

- *Warnings:* Products containing ginkgo are considered dietary supplements and are **not** FDA-approved for medical use. Products containing this agent should be considered **complementary** therapies and not **alternative** therapies. Standard medical care and prescribed therapy should not be abandoned, nor should appropriate medical attention be delayed. Such practices can be very dangerous when herbal products are being used.

  Because no human data are available concerning pregnancy and lactation, ginkgo use should be avoided by pregnant and lactating women.

  Contact your physician before taking ginkgo if you are also taking aspirin, warfarin, or other blood-thinning agents.

- *Uses:* Ginkgo has been used in nontraditional medicine to treat Raynaud disease, cerebral insufficiency, anxiety/stress, tinnitus, dementias, circulatory disorders, and asthma. It is thought to have positive effects on memory.

- *Side Effects:* Severe side effects are rare; documented effects include headache, dizziness, heart palpitations, and GI and dermatologic reactions. Ginkgo pollen can be strongly allergenic. Contact with the fleshy fruit pulp may cause allergic dermatitis, similar to poison ivy.

- *Dosing:* Standardized gingko leaf extracts such as EGb761 (*Tebonin forte*, Schwabe) have been used in clinical trials for dementia, memory, and circulatory disorders at daily doses of 120 to 720 mg of extract. Extracts usually are standardized to 24% flavones and 6% terpene lactones.

BOTANY
The ginkgo is the world's oldest living tree species and can be traced back more than 200 million years to fossils of the Permian period. It is the sole survivor of the family Ginkgoaceae. Individual trees may live as long as 1,000 years. They grow to a height of approximately 120 feet and have fan-shaped leaves. The species is dioecious; male trees more than 20 years old blossom in the spring. Adult female trees produce a plum-like gray-tan fruit that falls in late autumn. Its fleshy pulp has a foul, offensive odor and may cause contact dermatitis. The edible inner seed resembles an almond and is sold in Asian markets.

HISTORY

In China, where the species survived the ice age, ginkgo was cultivated as a sacred tree, and is still found decorating Buddhist temples throughout Asia. It has not been found in the wild. Preparations have been used for medicinal purposes for more than 1,000 years. Chinese physicians used ginkgo leaves to treat asthma and chillblains, which is the swelling of the hands and feet from exposure to damp cold. The ancient Chinese and Japanese ate roasted ginkgo seeds, and considered them a digestive aid and a preventive against drunkenness. The flavonoids act as free radical scavengers and the terpenes (ginkgolides) inhibit platelet activating factor. Currently, oral and IV forms are available in Europe. Neither form has been approved for medical use in the United States, where ginkgo is sold as a nutritional supplement only.

ACTIONS

Numerous studies on the pharmacological actions of ginkgo have been reported, including treatment of cerebral insufficiency, dementia, circulatory disorders, and asthma. The plant is known for its antioxidant and neuroprotective effects. In addition, ginkgolides competively inhibit the binding of platelet-activating factor (PAF) to its membrane receptor.

Cerebral insufficiency: Cerebral insufficiency may cause anxiety and stress; memory, concentration, and mood impairment; and hearing disorders. Cerebral insufficiency in 112 patients (average age 70.5 years) treated with ginkgo leaf extract (120 mg/day) for 1 year, resulted in reduced symptoms such as headache, dizziness, short-term memory loss, and vigilance. Electroencephalographic effects of different preparations of GBE have been measured. A review of 40 clinical trials (most evaluating 120 mg GBE/day for 4 to 6 weeks) revealed that only 8 of these studies were of high quality, and 7 of the 8 showed improvement in cognition and symptoms. The studies suggested that long-term treatment (more than 6 weeks) is required and that any effect is similar to that observed following treatment with ergoloids. A meta-analysis of 11 placebo-controlled, randomized, double-blinded studies, concluded GBE (150 mg/day) was superior to placebo in patients with cerebrovascular insufficiency.

Stress: MAO inhibition in rats was induced by extracts of ginkgo (dried and fresh leaves) was detected, which suggested a mechanism by which the plant exerts an antistress action. Glucocorticoid synthesis, which is regulated by ACTH (adrenocorticotropic hormone), accelerates cholesterol transport, and can lead to neurotoxicity. Ginkgolides A and B decrease cholesterol transport, resulting in decreased corticosteroid synthesis. The anti-stress and neuroprotective effects of GBE may also be caused by this mechanism.

Memory improvement: In elderly men with slight age-related memory loss, ginkgo supplementation reduced the time required to process visual information. Effects of GBE on event-related potentials in 48 patients with age-associated memory impairment has been measured. Memory improvement (as measured by a series of psychological tests) in 8 patients (average age, 32 years) was found 1 hour after administration of 600 mg GBE vs placebo, again confirming the possible usefulness of GBE in memory improvement. Yet overall, studies of ginkgo for memory improvement have been inconclusive; only small-scale trials have been performed. The reported improvements in memory were seen with high doses, and benefits were limited to 1 of many assessment categories.

Tinnitus/Hearing disorder therapy: Because of the diverse etiology of tinnitus and a lack of objective measurement methodology, results using GBE for treatment of this condition are contradictory. GBE may have positive effects in some individuals.

In patients with hearing disorders secondary to vascular insufficiency in the ear, approximately 40% of those treated orally with a leaf extract for 2 to 6 months showed improvement in auditory measurements. The extract was also effective in relieving vertigo associated with vestibular dysfunction.

Dementias: Therapeutic effectiveness of *Ginkgo biloba* in dementia syndromes has been demonstrated. Effects of 240 mg/day GBE in approximately 200 patients with mild-to-moderate Alzheimer-type dementia and multi-infarct dementia, have been investigated in a randomized, double-blind, placebo-controlled, multi-center study. Parameters such as psychopathological assessment, attention, memory, and behavior were monitored, with results demonstrating clinical efficacy of the extract in dementias of both types. In a 52-week, randomized, double-blinded, placebo-controlled, multi-center study, mild-to-severe Alzheimer or multi-infarct dementia patients received 120 mg/day GBE vs placebo. However, only 44% of the patients completed the study, and the first 6 months of results were extrapolated to 12 months, which did not completely account for disease progression. Thus, results are inconclusive.

Circulatory disorders/Asthma: Ginkgolides competively inhibit the binding of platelet-activating factor (PAF) to its membrane receptor. Effects of this action may be useful in the treatment of allergic reaction and inflammation (asthma and bronchospasm) and also in circulatory diseases.

In one double-blinded, randomized, crossover study in asthma patients, ginkgolides were effective in early and late phases of airway hyperactivity.

A meta-analysis evaluating GBE in peripheral arterial disease suggested a therapeutic benefit. Numerous studies are available concerning GBE use and circulatory disorders, including its ability to adjust fibrinolytic activity, and, in combination with aspirin, to treat thrombosis. It also appears useful in management of peripheral vascular disorders such as Raynaud disease, acrocyanosis, and postphlebitis syndrome.

A 6-month, double-blind trial suggested some efficacy in treating obliterative arterial disease of the lower limbs. Patients who received extract showed a clinically and statistically significant improvement in pain-free walking distance, maximum walking distance, and plethysmographic recordings of peripheral blood flow. GBE improved walking performance in 60 patients with intermittent claudication, with good tolerance to the drug. However, another report concluded that GBE 120 mg/day has no effect on walking distance or leg pain in intermittent claudication patients (but found other cognitive functions to be improved). A review of 10 controlled trials evaluating treatment of the plant for this condition, found poor methodological quality, but did note the studies revealed clinical effectiveness of GBE in treating intermittent claudication.

Antioxidant/Neuroprotective effects: GBE is known to improve diseases associated with free radical generation, such as Alzheimer disease. Both the ginkgolides and flavonoids contribute to neuroprotective effects. The flavonoids are free radical scavengers, while the ginkolides facilitate blood flow. Both classes of components are important in alleviating hypoxia, seizure activity, and peripheral nerve damage.

GBE exerts protective action on the neuronal membrane in aged rats. It was also shown to protect rat cerebellar neurons from oxidative stress induced by hydrogen peroxide. GBE may be a potent inhibitor of nitric oxide production under tissue-damaging inflammatory conditions in murine macrophage cell lines. GBE was found to be more effective than water-soluble antioxidants and as effective as lipid-soluble antioxidants, in an in vitro model using human erythrocyte suspensions.

In Chernobyl accident recovery workers, GBE's antioxidant effects were also studied. Clastogenic factors (risk factors for development of late effects of irradiation) were thought to be successfully reduced by GBE.

A number of other potentially beneficial effects have been observed for ginkgo, including its ability to prevent the deterioration of lipid profiles when subjects were challenged with high-fat meals over an extended holiday season, improvement in the symptoms of PMS. Its scavenging abilities appeared to reduce functional and morphological retina impairments. When GBE extract was given, peripheral blood flow increased by 40% to 45%, compared with an increase of 35% after administration of nicotinic acid. Other reports suggest GBE may be of some value in arresting fibrosis development (in 86 chronic hepatitis patients), promoting hair regrowth in mice, and relaxing penile tissue in vitro, suggesting a possible use as a drug for impotence. Seed extracts of the plant possess antibacterial and antifungal activity of various types, but the clinical value of these effects has not been determined in human trials.

TOXICOLOGY

Adverse events from doses of up to 160 mg/day for 4 to 6 weeks did not differ from the placebo group. German literature lists possible side effects as headache, dizziness, heart palpitations, GI disturbances, and dermatologic reactions.

A toxic syndrome, ("Gin-nan" food poisoning) has been recognized in Asia in children who have ingested ginkgo seeds. Approximately 50 seeds produce tonic/clonic seizures and loss of consciousness. Seventy reports (between

1930 and 1960) collectively showed 27% lethality, with infants being most vulnerable. Ginkgotoxin (4-O-methylpyridoxine), found only in the seeds, was responsible for this toxicity.

Contact with the fleshy fruit pulp has been known since ancient times to be a skin irritant. Constituents alkylbenzoic acid, alkylphenol, and their derivatives cause reactions of this type. Allergic dermatitis such as erythema, edema, blisters, and itching have all been reported. A cross-allergenicity exists between ginkgo fruit pulp and poison ivy. Ginkgolic acid and bilobin are structurally similar to the allergens of poison ivy, mango rind, and cashew nut shell oil. Contact with the fruit pulp causes erythema and edema, with the rapid formation of vesicles accompanied by severe itching. Symptoms last 7 to 10 days. Ingestion of two pieces of pulp has been reported to cause perioral erythema, rectal burning, and painful spasms of the anal sphincter.

Ginkgols and ginkgolic acids can cause contact reactions of mucous membranes, resulting in cheilitis and GI irritation. However, oral ginkgo preparations are not allergenic because the ginkgols and ginkgolic acids have been removed. Ginkgo pollen can be strongly allergenic.

In one report, spontaneous bilateral subdural hematomas have been associated with ingestion of ginkgo. Careful monitoring is warranted in patients taking aspirin, warfarin, or other similar agents.

Because no human data are available about pregnancy and lactation, ginkgo should be avoided by these populations.

References are available upon request.

GINSENG

SCIENTIFIC NAME(S)

Scientific Name	Common Name	Distribution
P. quinquefolium L.	American ginseng	United States
P. ginseng C.A. Meyer	Korean ginseng	Northeast China, Korea, East Siberia, Japan
P. pseudoginseng Wall. var. notoginseng	Sanchi ginseng	Southwest China
P. pseudoginseng var. major	Zhuzishen	China
P. pseudoginseng (Will.) subsp. japonicus	Chikusetsu ginseng	Japan
P. pseudoginseng subsp. himalaicus	Himalayan ginseng	Japan
P. trifolius L.	Dwarf ginseng	United States

PATIENT INFORMATION

- *Warnings:* Products containing ginseng are considered dietary supplements and are **not** FDA-approved for medical use. Products containing this agent should be considered **complementary** therapies and not **alternative** therapies. Standard medical care and prescribed therapy should not be abandoned, nor should appropriate medical attention be delayed. Such practices can be dangerous when herbal products are being used.

   Ginko use should be avoided by pregnant and lactating women.

   Diabetic patients taking ginseng should monitor their blood glucose levels regularly; hypoglycemic effects have been reported.

- *Uses:* Ginseng is widely used in various ingestible forms and in cosmetics. Limited evidence lends some support to its value as an antistress treatment. It seems to lower cholesterol and blood sugar, may help resist infection, and has a modest estrogen-like effect on women. It is claimed to increase strength, endurance, and mental acuity. Ginseng may depress or stimulate the CNS.

- *Drug Interactions:* Patients on anticoagulant therapy should consult a physician before taking ginseng.

- *Side Effects:* Nervous excitation induced by ginseng use reportedly diminishes over time or with downward dose adjustment. Difficulty concentrating has been reported following long-term use. Diabetic patients should use ginseng with caution because of the hypoglycemic effects and associated difficulty in managing blood sugar levels.

- *Dosing:* Ginseng root is standardized on content of ginsenosides, which should be greater than 1.5%. Extracts typically contain from 4% to 7% ginsenosides. Note that the profile of particular ginsenosides differs between American and Asian ginseng; however, the total ginsenoside content is similar. In numerous clinical trials, dosage of crude root has been from 0.5 to 3 g/day and dosage of extracts generally from 100 to 400 mg.

BOTANY

Ginseng commonly refers to *Panax quinquefolium* L. or *P. ginseng* C.A. Meyer. A number of *Panax* species grow in various areas of the world and are used in local traditional medicine. The roots or rhizomes of these plants are used medicinally.

In the United States, ginseng is found in rich, cool woods; a significant crop is also grown commercially. The short plant grows from 3 to 7 compound leaves that drop in the fall. It bears a cluster of red or yellowish fruits from June to July. The roots mature slowly and usually are harvested only after the first 3 years of growth. The shape of the root can vary between species and has been used to distinguish types of ginseng.

HISTORY

For more than 2000 years, various forms of ginseng have been used in medicine. The genus name *Panax* is derived from the Greek word "panacea" meaning "all healing." Ginseng root's man-shaped figure (shen-seng means "man-root") led proponents of the "Doctrine of Signatures," the concept that the key to humanity's use of various plants is indicated by the form of the plant, to believe that the root could strengthen any part of the body. Through the ages, the root has been used in the treatment of asthenia, atherosclerosis, blood and bleeding disorders, colitis, and for the relief of symptoms of aging, cancer, and senility.

Claims that the root possesses a general strengthening effect, raises mental and physical capacity, and exerts a protective effect against experimental diabetes, neurosis, radiation sickness, and some cancers have been made. Today, its popularity is due largely to the modest "adaptogenic" (stress-protective) effect of the triterpenoid saponin glycoside content, although this effect does not occur consistently.

ACTIONS

It has been claimed subjectively that ginseng exerts a strengthening effect while raising physical and mental capacity for work. These properties have been defined as an "adaptogenic effect" or a nonspecific increase in resistance to the noxious effects of physical, chemical, or biological stress. The panaxosides, or ginsenosides, a group of triterpenoid saponin glycosides, may alter the activity of hormones produced by the pituitary, adrenal, or gonadal tissue. The beneficial or adverse consequences of these effects are not known.

Despite the shortcomings of many animal studies, limited evidence subjectively describes some of the pharmacologic effects of the panaxosides. For example, ginsenoside Rb-1 demonstrates CNS activity, may protect against the development of stress ulcers, and accelerates glycolysis and nuclear RNA synthesis. Ginseng may potentiate the normal function of the adrenal gland, possibly having some "antistress" activity.

Five glycans, collectively called panaxans, show strong hypoglycemic activity and have been isolated from the root. Ginsenoside Rg-1 given to postoperative gynecologic patients caused a greater increase in hemoglobin and hematocrit levels among treated women than among placebo-treated controls. Serum protein and body weight also increased to a greater degree in the treatment group. The adaptogenic effect has not been well documented in humans, although there is a body of evidence from folk and foreign medicine.

TOXICOLOGY

Through its extensive history of use in popular herbal products, ginseng has established a reasonable safety record. It is estimated that more than 6 million people regularly ingest ginseng in the United States. There have been a few reports of severe adverse reactions. One controversial report described a "ginseng-abuse syndrome" among 133 patients who ingested relatively large doses of the root (more than 3 g/day) for up to 2 years. Patients reported a feeling of stimulation, well-being, and increased motor and cognitive efficiency, but also noted frequent diarrhea, skin eruptions, nervousness, sleeplessness, and hypertension. This was an open, uncontrolled study, and the simultaneous intake of other drugs (eg, caffeine) confounded interpretation of the data.

Other reports have suggested that ginseng has an estrogen-like effect in women. One case of diffuse mammary nodularity has been reported, as well as a case of vaginal bleeding in a 72-year-old woman.

The most common side effects of ginseng are nervousness and excitation, which usually diminish after the first few days of use or with dosage reduction. Inability to concentrate has also been reported following long-term use.

The hypoglycemic effect of the whole root and individual root components has been reported. Diabetic patients should contact a physician before taking ginseng and monitor their blood glucose regularly.

A patient receiving warfarin experienced a decrease in the international normalized ratio (INR) 2 weeks after starting ginseng, which reversed within 2 weeks of stopping ginseng. Patients on anticoagulant therapy should consult a physician before taking ginseng.

References are available upon request.

GLUCOSAMINE SULFATE

SCIENTIFIC NAME(S)

2-Amino-2-deoxyglucose. Glucosamine sulfate, glucosamine hydrochloride, and N-acetyl-D-glucosamine are all available commercially, but studies have only been performed on glucosamine sulfate.

COMMON NAME(S)

Chitosamine

PATIENT INFORMATION

- *Warnings:* Products containing glucosamine are considered dietary supplements and are **not** FDA-approved for medical use. Products containing this agent should be considered **complementary** therapies and not **alternative** therapies. Standard medical care and prescribed therapy should not be abandoned, nor should appropriate medical attention be delayed. Such practices can be dangerous.

  Safety of glucosamine use during pregnancy and lactation has not been confirmed. Pregnant and lactating women should avoid use of this agent.

  Diabetic patients should consult a physician before taking glucosamine and monitor blood sugar levels frequently if glucosamine is taken. Some studies indicate that this agent increases blood sugar levels.

  Some glucosamine products are derived from marine exoskeletons and may cause reactions in people allergic to shellfish. If you are allergic to shellfish, consult a physician before taking this agent.

  Glucosamine sulfate may cause allergic-type reactions (eg, hives, itching, wheezing, or difficulty breathing) in people sensitive to sulfites. If any of these symptoms occur, contact your physician immediately. If you know you are allergic to sulfites, do not take this agent.

- *Uses:* Glucosamine is being investigated extensively as an antiarthritic in osteoarthritis. Combining glucosamine with chondroitin does not appear to increase the value of either agent given alone.

- *Side Effects:* Possible side effects include nausea, dyspepsia, heartburn, diarrhea, and constipation. Headache can also occur.

BIOLOGY

Glucosamine is found in mucopolysaccharides, mucoproteins, and chitin. Chitin is found in yeasts, fungi, arthropods, and marine invertebrates as a major component of the exoskeleton. It also occurs in other lower animals and certain plants.

ACTIONS

Glucosamine has been referred to as a pharmaceutical aid that may assist in the management of osteoarthritis. There is a progressive degeneration of cartilage glycosaminoglycans (GAGs) in osteoarthritis. The idea of using glucosamine orally is to provide a "building block" for cartilage regeneration. Glucosamine is part of the rate-limiting step in GAG biosynthesis. It is formed in vivo from the glycolytic intermediate fructose-6-phosphate by way of glutamine amination to yield glucosamine-6-phosphate. This is subsequently converted to galactosamine before being incorporated into growing GAG. Theoretically, this will stimulate production of cartilage components and bring about joint repair. Several double-blind studies indicate that glucosamine sulfate may be superior to some nonsteroidal anti-inflammatory drugs (NSAIDs) and placebo in relieving pain and inflammation caused by osteoarthritis. The efficacy and safety of IM glucosamine sulfate in osteoarthritis of the knee was studied in a randomized, placebo-controlled, double-blind study that revealed that the treatment was well tolerated and effective. Other double-blind clinical studies of intra-articular glucosamine injection were conducted and showed reduced pain, increased angle of joint flexion, and restored articular function compared with placebo. The relative efficacy of ibuprofen and glucosamine sulfate was compared in the management of osteoarthritis of the knee. At 8 weeks, glucosamine 1.5 g/day orally was more effective in reducing pain than ibuprofen 1.2 g/day. Oral glucosamine sulfate therapy vs placebo in osteoarthritis was studied; researchers found that glucosamine 1.5 g/day orally decreased symptoms and improved autonomous motility in a group of 80 patients. These investigators also employed in vitro electron microscopy studies on cartilage and found that patients who had received placebo showed a typical picture of established osteoarthrosis, while those receiving glucosamine showed a picture similar to healthy cartilage. They inferred that glucosamine appears to assist in rebuilding damaged cartilage, thus contributing to improved articular function in most patients with osteoarthritis.

Studies have shown that glucosamine can be safe and effective in the treatment of various forms of osteoarthritis. Standard drug therapy has only palliative benefits. Glucosamine is an intermediate in mucopolysaccharide synthesis and has been shown in cartilage tissue culture to be a rate-limiting intermediate in proteoglycan production. Reviews of related literature also reveal glucosamine's effectiveness in decreasing pain and improving mobility in osteoarthritis patients. By mechanisms still unknown, the natural methyl donor S-adenosylmethionine also promotes production of cartilage proteoglycans and is likewise therapeutically beneficial in osteoarthritis at well-tolerated oral doses. One researcher promotes the use of glucosamine and other safe nutritional measures that support proteoglycan synthesis; these may offer a practical method of preventing or postponing the onset of osteoarthritis in athletes and the elderly.

Other studies have focused on pharmacokinetics (radiolabeled glucosamine was quickly and completely absorbed orally and IV); an attempt to synthesize glucosamine derivatives with immunomodulating activity; glucosamine's ability to inhibit viral cytopathic effects and production of infective viral particles; and D-glucosamine's inhibitory effects on a carcinoma relative to protein, RNA, and DNA synthesis.

Some studies indicate that glucosamine increases blood sugar levels. Therefore, diabetic patients should consult a physician before taking this agent and monitor blood sugar levels frequently if glucosamine is taken.

Glucosamine sulfate may cause sulfite sensitivity in susceptible individuals. This may involve allergic-type reactions (eg, hives, itching, wheezing, anaphylaxis). Although the prevalence of sulfite sensitivity in the general population is probably low, it is more frequent in asthmatics or atopic nonasthmatics.

TOXICOLOGY

No direct toxic effects of glucosamine could be found in scientific literature; however, one study, which included glucosamine, showed potential bronchopulmonary complications. Glucosamine in large doses may also be associated with headache and GI problems (eg, nausea, dyspepsia, heartburn, diarrhea, constipation) in some patients.

References are available upon request.

GOLDENSEAL

SCIENTIFIC NAME(S)
Hydrastis canadensis L. Family: Ranunculaceae

COMMON NAME(S)
Eye balm, eye root, goldenseal, ground raspberry, Indian dye, jaundice root, orange root, turmeric root, yellow Indian paint, yellow puccoon, yellow root.

PATIENT INFORMATION

- *Warnings:* Products containing goldenseal are considered dietary supplements and are **not**FDA-approved for medical use. Products containing this agents should not be considered **complementary** therapies and not **alternative** therapies. Standard medical care and prescribed therapy should not be abandoned, nor should appropriate medical attention be delayed. Such practices can be dangerous when herbal products are being used.
- *Uses:* Goldenseal has been used as an immunostimulant, an eyewash, an antispasmodic, for the treatment for dysmenorrhea and minor sciatica, and to alleviate rheumatic and muscular pain. It is most often found in combination products for prevention and treatment of the common cold and flu.
- *Side Effects:* Large doses may be toxic, causing a variety of problems including irritation of the mouth and throat, nausea, vomiting, diarrhea, hypertension, decreased blood sugar, convulsions, and respiratory failure.
- *Dosing:* Goldenseal has not been the subject of any formal clinical trials for external antiseptic or antiherpes properties. Extracts standardized to 5% hydrastine are available; however, the berberine content may be more important for goldenseal's medicinal uses. Doses of 100 mg hydrastine and 2 g crude root have been proposed.

BOTANY
Goldenseal is a stout perennial found in deep, rich woods from Vermont to Arkansas. The 5- to 9-lobed palmate leaves can grow to approximately 10 inches. It produces dark red berries from green-white flowers in April and May. The rhizomes are golden-yellow and knotted.

HISTORY
North American settlers learned of its use from the American Indians who used goldenseal as a dye for its medicinal properties. It has been used as a bitter stomachic for the relief of catarrhal conditions and as an eye wash. After the Civil War, goldenseal was an ingredient in many patent medicines. It was collected to the point of near extinction. Today, it is farmed but is till costly, and in many places it has been almost exterminated by commercial wild harvesting. Preparations containing goldenseal have been marketed for the treatment of menstrual disorders, pain of minor sciatica, rheumatic or muscu-

lar pain, and as an antispasmodic. Goldenseal may be found as an ingredient on some commercial sterile eye washes.

Earlier in the century, goldenseal has gained the reputation of being able to prevent the detection of morphine in urine samples. This notion arose from a plot in John Uri Lloyd's novel *Stringtown on the Pike* (Dodd Mead, 1990), and was given further credence by the fact that Lloyd was an internationally known plant pharmacist. However, studies have found no basis for this belief.

ACTIONS

The activity of goldenseal is due largely to the presence of the alkaloid hydrastine and to a lesser extent from berberine. Goldenseal has been used as a uterine hemostatic but was found to be unreliable in its action; its activity was inferior to that of the ergot alkaloids in the treatment of postpartum hemorrhage. Berberine stimulates bile secretion. It has weak antibiotic activity and some antineoplastic activity, but no documented clinical value in either instance.

Hydrastine constricts peripheral blood vessels and has been investigated for the treatment of gastric inflammation. Hydrastine administered internally can result in a rise in blood pressure, whereas berberine can induce hypotension. The plant has been associated with a hypoglycemic effect. Diabetic patients should not consume this product without consulting a physician. Empirical evidence and experience suggest goldenseal may be useful in helping to "cleanse" the liver or blood and restore digestive function in alcoholics.

TOXICOLOGY

In higher doses, hydrastine can cause exaggerated reflexes, hypertension, convulsions, and death from respiratory failure. Large doses of the plant irritate the mouth and throat and cause nausea, vomiting, diarrhea, and paresthesias. CNS stimulation and respiratory failure induced by the plant can be fatal. Moderate doses of the alkaloid hydrastine causes peripheral vasoconstriction and may increase cardiac output. A 10% solution of hydrastine causes pupillary dilation.

References are available upon request.

GREEN TEA

SCIENTIFIC NAME(S)
Camellia sinensis L. Kuntze. Family: Theaceae

COMMON NAME(S)
Tea, green tea

PATIENT INFORMATION

- *Warnings:* Products containing green tea are considered dietary supplements and are **not** FDA-approved for medical use. Products containing this agent should be considered **complementary** therapies and not **alternative** therpaies. Standard medical care and prescribed therapy should not be abandoned, nor should appropriate medical attention be delayed. Such practices can be dangerous.
- *Uses:* Green tea retains many chemicals of the fresh leaf. It is thought to reduce cancer, lower lipid levels, help prevent dental caries, and possess antimicrobial, antimutagenic, and antioxidative effects.
- *Side Effects:* The FDA advises those who are or may become pregnant to avoid caffeine. Tea may impair iron metabolism.
- *Dosing:* Green tea has been studied as a component of diet for its cancer preventative and caries preventative properties. A typical tea bag contains 2 g of leaf. Doses of 4 to 5 cups/day (corresponding to ca. 300 mg caffeine) are considered high, depending on the patient's caffeine tolerance. The content of polyphenols increases with extended brewing time. Green tea extracts are available standardized to 25%, 60%, and 80% total polyphenols, compared with a content of 8% to 12% in the leaf. Use of this extract can avoid the inconvenience of drinking large volumes of liquids.

BOTANY
C. sinensis is a large shrub with evergreen leaves native to eastern Asia. The plant has leathery, dark green leaves and fragrant, white flowers with 6 to 9 petals.

HISTORY
The dried, cured leaves of *C. sinensis* have been used to prepare beverages for more than 4000 years. The method of curing determines the nature of the tea to be used for infusion. Green tea is prepared from the steamed and dried leaves; by comparison, black tea leaves are withered, rolled, fermented, and then dried. Oolong tea is semifermented and considered to be intermediate in composition between green and black teas. The Chinese regarded the drink as a cure for cancer, although the tannin component is believed to be carcinogenic. The polyphenol presence in tea may play a role in lowering heart disease and cancer risk.

ACTIONS

Blood and urine levels have been investigated Drinking green tea daily may maintain significant plasma catechin levels that may exert antioxidant activity against lipoproteins in blood circulation. High performance liquid chromatography (HPLC) determination of catechins and polyphenol components have been performed.

TOXICOLOGY

The FDA has advised that women who are or may become pregnant should avoid caffeine-containing products. Drinking moderate amounts of caffeine has shown inconsistent results, with more recent studies not demonstrating adverse effects on the fetus. Caffeine-containing beverages may also alter female hormone levels, including estradiol.

There is evidence that condensed catechin tannin of tea is linked to a high rate of esophageal cancer in regions of heavy tea consumption. This effect may be overcome by adding milk, which binds the tannin, possibly preventing its detrimental effects. Catechins have also been linked to tea-induced asthma. One study reports that catechins may have antiallergic effects, inhibiting type I allergic reactions. Green tea workers experienced shortness of breath, stiffness, pain in neck and arms, and other occupation-related problems.

The daily consumption of an average of 250 mL of tea by infants has been shown to impair iron metabolism, resulting in a high incidence of microcytic anemia.

References are available upon request.

GUAR GUM

SCIENTIFIC NAME(S)
Cyamopsis tetragonolobus (L.) Taub. synonymous with *C. psoralioides* DC. Family: Fabaceae or Leguminosae.

COMMON NAME(S)
Guar, guar flour, jaguar gum

PATIENT INFORMATION

- *Warnings:* Products containing guar gum are considered dietary supplements and are **not** FDA-approved for medical use. Products containing this agent should be considered **complementary** therapies and not **alternative** therapies. Standard medical care and prescribed therapy should not be abandoned, nor should appropriate medical attention be delayed. Such practices can be dangerous.
- *Uses:* Guar gum is a food additive shown to reduce serum cholesterol with prolonged use. It appears useful for managing blood glucose. It has been used to promote weight loss.
- *Side Effects:* Guar gum may cause GI obstruction. It should be used cautiously with diabetics. Flatulence and other forms of GI distress are common during initial use.

BOTANY
The guar plant is a small nitrogen-fixing annual that bears pods, each containing a number of seeds. Native to tropical Asia, the plant grows throughout India and Pakistan and has been grown in the southern United States since the beginning of the twentieth century.

HISTORY
Guar gum has been used for centuries as a thickening agent for foods and pharmaceuticals. It continues to find extensive use for these applications and also is used by the paper, textile and oil drilling industries.

Guar gum is a dietary fiber obtained from the endosperm of the Indian cluster bean. The endosperm can account for more than 40% of the seed weight and is separated and ground to form commercial guar gum.

ACTIONS
Guar gum forms a mucilaginous mass when hydrated. This material has been shown to reduce total serum cholesterol and LDL-cholesterol levels by approximately 10% to 15% when taken for 3 months. In addition, guar has been found to reduce post-prandial insulin and glucose levels and appears to be a useful adjunct in the management of non-insulin-dependent diabetes mellitus. Guar is used as a common food additive and is not associated with

adverse effects in the low quantities generally used in foods. Severe gastrointestinal obstructions have been reported with the use of some guar-containing dietary supplements.

TOXICOLOGY

In the colon, guar gum is fermented to short-chain fatty acids. Both guar and its resultant by-products do not appear to be absorbed by the gut. The most common adverse effects, therefore, are gastrointestinal, including gastrointestinal pain, nausea, diarrhea, and flatulence. Approximately half of those taking guar experience flatulence; this usually occurs early in treatment and resolves with continued use. Starting with doses of about 3 g three times a day, not to exceed 15 g per day, can minimize gastrointestinal effects.

Guar gum may affect the absorption of concomitantly administered drugs. Bezafibrate, acetaminophen (eg, *Tylenol*), digoxin (eg, *Lanoxin*), glipizide (eg, *Glucotrol*) or glyburide (eg, *DiaBeta, Micronase*) are generally unaffected by concomitant administration. The ingestion of more than 30 g guar per day by diabetic patients did not adversely affect mineral balances after 6 months.

Guar gum in a weight-loss product has been implicated in esophageal obstruction in a patient who exceeded the recommended dosage. In a recent review, 18 cases of esophageal obstruction, seven cases of small bowel obstruction, and possibly one death were associated with the use of *Cal-Ban 3000*, a guar gum-containing diet pill. The water-retaining capacity of the gum permits it to swell to 10- to 20-fold and may lead to luminal obstruction, particularly when an anatomic predisposition exists. Guar always should be taken with large amounts of liquid. Occupational asthma has been observed among those working with guar gum.

Because of its potential to affect glycemic control, guar gum should be used cautiously by diabetic patients. Guar gum is not teratogenic nor does it significantly affect reproduction in rats.

References are available upon request.

GUARANA

SCIENTIFIC NAME(S)

Paullinia cupana Kunth var. sorbilis (Mart.) Ducke or P. sorbilis (L.) Mart.
Family: Sapindaceae

COMMON NAME(S)

Guarana, guarana paste or gum, Brazilian cocoa, Zoom

PATIENT INFORMATION

- *Warnings:* Products containing guarana are considered dietary supplements and are **not** FDA-approved for medical use. Products containing this agents should not be considered **complementary** therapies and not **alternative** therapies. Standard medical care and prescribed therapy should not be abandoned, nor should appropriate medical attention be delayed. Such practices can be dangerous when herbal products are being used.
- *Uses:* Guarana is a source of flavoring and caffeine. It has been used as a folk remedy and appetite suppressant.
- *Side Effects:* Severe toxicity has not been reported, but the usual cautions regarding caffeine apply.
- *Dosing:* Guarana paste is used as a stimulant at a dose of 1 g, usually dissolved in water or juice. The caffeine content is between 3.6% and 5.8%.

BOTANY

Guarana is the dried paste made from the crushed seeds of *P. cupana* or *P. sorbilis*. A fast-growing woody perennial shrub native to Brazil and other regions of the Amazon, guarana bears orange-yellow fruit that contains up to 3 seeds each. The seeds are collected and dry-roasted over fires. The kernels are ground to a paste with cassava, molded into cylindrical sticks, and then sun-dried. The most common forms of guarana include syrups, extracts, and distillates used as flavorings and a source of caffeine by the soft drink industry.

HISTORY

Guarana is often taken during periods of fasting to tolerate dietary restrictions in the Amazon. In certain regions, the extract is believed to be an aphrodisiac and provide protection from malaria and dysentery. Guarana is used by the Brazilian Indians in a stimulating beverage, which is sometimes mixed with alcohol to become more intoxicating. It was popular in France at the beginning of the 19th century. Natural diet aids, which rely on daily doses of tablets containing guarana, have been advertised in the lay press. Guarana is occasionally combined with glucomannan in natural weight loss tablets. The advertisements incorrectly indicate that the ingredients in guarana have the same chemical makeup as caffeine and cocaine but can be used for weight reduction without any of the side effects of these drugs.

ACTIONS

Guarana contains a high level of caffeine, ranging from 3% to more than 5% by dry weight. Coffee beans contain approximately 1% to 2% caffeine and dried tea leaves vary from 1% to 4% caffeine content. Guarana is also high in tannins, present in a concentration of 5% to 6% dry weight; these impart an astringent taste to the product. Guarana does not contain cocaine. The appetite-suppressant effect is related to the caffeine content. The increase in energy that guarana tablets are reported to give is also due to caffeine. Guarana extracts have been shown to inhibit platelet aggregation following either parenteral or oral administration.

TOXICOLOGY

There are no published reports describing severe toxicity from guarana, but people sensitive to caffeine should use guarana with caution. The expected side effects of caffeine should be considered in a person who has ingested guarana.

References are available upon request.

SCIENTIFIC NAME(S)
Piper methysticum Frost Family: Piperaceae

COMMON NAME(S)
Awa, kava-kava, tonga

PATIENT INFORMATION

- *Warnings:* Products containing kava are considered dietary supplements and are **not** FDA-approved for medical use. Products containing this agent should be considered **complementary** therapies and not **alternative** therapies. Standard medical care and prescribed therapy should not be abandoned, nor should appropriate medical attention be delayed. Such practices can be dangerous when herbal products are being used.

  Kava should be avoided by pregnant/lactating women.

  Consult your doctor before taking kava if you have liver problems. Kava users should notify their doctor immediately if they experience symptoms of liver disease (eg, yellowing of skin or eyes, dark urine).

- *Uses:* Kava has been used as a sedative, an antianxiety agent, and a sleep aid.

- *Drug Interactions:* Alcohol consumption increases kava toxicity.

- *Side Effects:* Dry, flaking, discolored skin; scaly rash; red eyes; visual disturbance; blood cell abnormalities; liver damage (mild to severe); blood in urine; pulmonary hypotension; puffy face; muscle weakness.

- *Dosing:* Dosage of kava lactones in clinical studies has been in the range of 100 to 200 mg/day, corresponding to 1.5 to 3 g of ground root.

BOTANY

Kava is the dried rhizome and roots of *P. methysticum*, a large shrub widely cultivated in the islands of the South Pacific (eg, Fiji). It has pale yellow-green cordate leaf blades that grow up to 12 inches long. The flower spikes grow up to 4 inches long.

More than 60 varieties of the kava plant have been recognized, the black and white grades having the greatest commercial importance. The black grades are preferred by growers because the shorter growing season yields a quick return on their investment. However, the white grades are generally considered of higher value.

HISTORY

Kava drink is prepared from the rhizome of *P. methysticum*. The pulverized roots are steeped in water; extraction of the root is sometimes hastened by pounding or mastication. The cloudy mixture is then filtered and served at room temperature, often combined with coconut milk.

The kava plant is indigenous to the islands of the South Pacific where it is most commonly used as a beverage to induce relaxation. The ceremonial preparation and consumption of kava is common to these Pacific islands. Traces of kava lactones can be found on artifacts in this region, linking the ancient culture of kava drinking to the archeological record. Kava drink has been compared to a Western cocktail, aiding in the establishment of a relaxed, socially cooperative atmosphere.

Folk uses of kava have included the treatment of inflammation of the uterus, headaches, colds, rheumatism, and venereal diseases; promotion of wound healing; and as an aphrodisiac. These uses lack confirmation of effectiveness.

ACTIONS

Seven major and several minor kava lactones have been identified in human urine following kava ingestion.

Masticated kava causes numbness of the mouth. Kawain has local anesthetic activity comparable to that of cocaine, with a longer duration of action than benzocaine. Hawaiians have used kava for asthma.

Naloxone inhibits morphine-induced analgesia but is ineffective in reversing kava's antinociceptive activities, showing that the analgesia produced by kava occurs via a nonopiate pathway. Kava may possess other CNS pharmacologic properties that affect sleep and anxiety.

Kava reduced nonpsychotic-type anxiety in patients with minimal adverse effects. A significant level of efficacy of kava extract is suggested in neurovegetative and psychosomatic dysfunction in the climacteric.

Kava produces mild euphoric changes characterized by happiness, fluent and lively speech, and increased sensitivity to sounds. High doses may also lead to muscle weakness. Visual or auditory changes may occur, as shown by reduced near point of accommodation and convergence, an increase in pupil diameter, and oculomotor balance disturbances.

TOXICOLOGY

Two yellow pigments, flavokawain A and B, have been isolated from the kava plant, and their presence provides a possible explanation for the skin discoloration that is observed following the chronic ingestion of kava drink. Chronic ingestion may lead to "kawaism," characterized by dry, flaking, discolored skin and reddened eyes. This scaly eruption is reversible, but the cause is unknown. It may be related to interference with cholesterol metabolism.

Ethanol markedly increases the toxicity of kava. This interaction may be of important clinical and social consequence if the two are taken concomitantly.

Heavy kava users are more likely to complain of poor health: 20% are underweight, have reduced protein levels, "puffy faces," scaly rashes, increased HDL cholesterol counts, hematuria, blood cell abnormalities (increased red blood cells, decreased platelets and lymphocytes), and some evidence of pulmonary hypertension.

Chronic kava use has been linked to severe liver damage. Some of these reported cases required liver transplantion.

References are available upon request.

SCIENTIFIC NAME(S)

Trifolium pratense Family: Leguminosae

COMMON NAME(S)

Cow clover, meadow clover, purple clover, trefoil

PATIENT INFORMATION

- *Warnings:* Products containing red clover are considered dietary supplements and are **not** FDA-approved for medical use. Products containing this agent should be considered **complementary** therapies and not **alternative** therapies. Standard medical care and prescribed therapy should not be abandoned, nor should appropriate medical attention be delayed. Such practices can be dangerous when herbal products are being used.

  Do not take during pregnancy, lactation, or in patients with a history of breast cancer, particularly those with estrogen-positive receptors in their breast tumor(s).

  Avoid large doses. Coumarin activity may be problematic at high doses.

- *Uses:* Red clover has been used as estrogen replacement therapy and in arterial compliance, and as a chemoprotective agent and expectorant, although objective and conclusive evidence of value is lacking.

- *Drug Interactions:* Isoflavonoid properties may interfere with hormonal therapies. Do not take red clover with oral contraceptives, estrogen, progesterone compounds, anticoagulants, or aspirin.

- *Dosing:* Formerly used as a sedative at doses of 4 g of blossoms, red clover is now used primarily as a source of estrogenic and antioxidant isoflavones. Extracts standardized on isoflavone content (*Menoflavon, Rimostil*) have been given to perimenopausal women in several clinical studies at daily doses of 25 to 90 mg isoflavones.

BOTANY

The plant's medicinal value is found in its red and purple fragrant blossoms, dried for utilization. It is a perennial that flowers for a short duration. Several hairy-looking stems grow 0.3 to 0.6 m high from a single base. The leaves are ovate, nearly smooth, and end in a long point; the center is usually lighter in color. It is found most commonly in meadows of a light sandy nature in Britain and throughout Europe and Asia from the Mediterranean to the Arctic Circle. It also has been found in the mountains. Red clover is now naturalized in North America and Australia for hay and as a nitrogen-fixing crop.

HISTORY

The flowers possess antispasmodic, estrogenic, and expectorant properties. Chinese medicine has used red clover in teas as an expectorant. The herb is recommended in Russia for bronchial asthma. Traditionally, the herb has been used in treating breast cancer. Topically, it has been used to accelerate wound healing and treat psoriasis. Research has indicated increased compliance of arterial vessels. In Australia, *Promensil* has been marketed for estrogen replacement and *Trinivin* for benign prostatic hyperplasia.

ACTIONS

Hormone replacement: Isoflavones mimic estrogen effects in the body. If an estrogen supplement is given, it binds to intracellular receptors and acts as an agonist to natural estrogen. Through negative feedback, production of gonadotropin-releasing hormone (GnRH), follide-stimulating hormone (FSH), and leutenizing hormone (LH) is slowed or stopped, resulting in a decline or cessation of the production of estrogen.

Arterial compliance: In a placebo-controlled study of 17 women, arterial compliance, an index of elasticity of large arteries (eg, thoracic aorta) in which compliance diminishes with age and menopause, increased 23% when 40 mg red clover was given daily for 5 weeks followed by 80 mg twice daily for 5 more weeks. The hormonal effects of the isoflavonoids appear to aid in arterial compliance. Larger controlled studies are needed to adequately evaluate the effect in arterial compliance.

Chemoprotective: Biochanin A, a composite of isoflavones, has been reported to inhibit carcinogenic activity in cell cultures, but not in human cancer.

TOXICOLOGY

Avoid doses greater than 40 to 80 mg daily. Do not take during pregnancy or lactation. Coumarin activity may also be problematic at high doses.

Avoid use in patients with a history of breast cancer, particularly in breast cancer survivors who had estrogen-positive receptors in their breast tumor(s).

References are available upon request.

ROSE HIPS

SCIENTIFIC NAME(S)
Commonly derived from *Rosa canina* L., *R. rugosa* Thunb., *R. acicularis* Lindl. or *R. cinnamomea* L. Numerous other species of rose have been used for the preparation of rose hips. Family: Rosaceae

COMMON NAME(S)
Rose hips, "heps"

PATIENT INFORMATION

- *Warnings:* Products containing rose hips are considered dietary supplements and are **not** FDA-approved for medical use. Products containing this agent should be considered **complementary** therapies and not **alternative** therapies. Standard medical care and prescribed therapy should not be abandoned, nor should appropriate medical attention be delayed. Such practices can be dangerous when herbal products are being used.
- *Uses:* Rose hips provide a source of vitamin C for natural vitamin supplements.
- *Side Effects:* There have been no reported side effects except in those exposed to rose hips dust who have developed severe respiratory allergies.

BOTANY
Rose hips are the ripe ovaries or seeded fruit of roses forming on branches after the flower.

HISTORY
Rose hips are a natural source of vitamin C, which has led to their widespread use in natural vitamin supplements, teas, and various other preparations including soups and marmalades. Although these products have been used historically as nutritional supplements, they also have been used as mild laxatives and diuretics.

ACTIONS
Vitamin C is used as a nutritional supplement for its antiscorbutic properties. Because a significant amount of the natural vitamin C in rose hips may be destroyed during drying and processing, many "natural vitamin supplements" have some form of vitamin C added to them. One must read the label carefully to determine what proportion of the vitamin C is derived from rose hips vs other sources. Unfortunately, this information is not always available on the package label.

The laxative activity of rose hips may be related to the presence of malic and citric acids or to purgative glycosides (multiflorin A and B).

TOXICOLOGY

Rose hips ingestion generally is not associated with toxicity. More than 100 g of plant material would have to be ingested to obtain a 1,200 mg dose of vitamin C, an impractical amount to ingest. Most people do not have any side effects from ingesting small gram quantities of the plant. Adverse effects associated with the long-term ingestion of multi-gram doses of vitamin C (ie, oxalate stone formation) have not been reported with rose hips. Production workers exposed to rose hips dust have developed severe respiratory allergies, with mild-to-moderate anaphylaxis.

References are available upon request.

SARSAPARILLA

SCIENTIFIC NAME(S)

Smilax species including *Smilax aristolochiifolia* Mill. (Mexican sarsaparilla), *S. officinalis* Kunth (Honduras sarsaparilla), *Smilax regelii* Killip et Morton (Honduras, Jamaican sarsaparilla), *Smilax febrifuga* (Ecuadorian sarsaparilla), *Smilax sarsaparilla, Smilax ornata.* Family: Liliaceae

COMMON NAME(S)

Sarsaparilla, smilax, smilace, sarsa, khao yen

PATIENT INFORMATION

- *Warnings:* Products containing sarsaparilla are considered dietary supplements and are **not** FDA-approved for medical use. Products containing this agent should be considered **complementary** therapies and not **alternative** therapies. Standard medical care and prescribed therapy should not be abandoned, nor should appropriate medical attention be delayed. Such practices can be dangerous.
- *Uses:* Sarsaparilla has been used for treating syphilis, leprosy, psoriasis, and other ailments.
- *Side Effects:* No major contraindications, warnings, or side effects have been documented; avoid excessive ingestion. In unusually high doses, the plant possibly could be harmful, including gastrointestinal (GI) irritation.
- *Dosing:* Typical doses of sarsaparilla for a variety of uses range from 0.3 to 2 g/day of the powdered root.

BOTANY

Sarsaparilla is a woody, trailing vine that can grow to 50 m in length. It is grown in Mexico, Honduras, Jamaica, and Ecuador. Many *Smilax* species are similar in appearance regardless of origin. The part of the plant used for medicinal purposes is the root. Although this root has a pleasant fragrance and spicy sweet taste, and has been used as a natural flavoring agent in medicines, foods, and nonalcoholic beverages.

HISTORY

The French physician Monardes described using sarsaparilla to treat syphilis in 1574. In 1812, Portuguese soldiers suffering from syphilis recovered faster if sarsaparilla was taken to treat the disease vs mercury, the standard treatment at the time. Sarsaparilla has been used by many cultures for ailments including skin problems, arthritis, fever, digestive disorders, leprosy, and cancer. Late 15th century accounts explaining the identification and the first descriptions of American drugs include sarsaparilla. Sarsaparilla's role as a medicinal plant in American and European remedies in the 16th century is also evident.

ACTIONS

Sarsaparilla has been used for treating syphilis and other sexually transmitted diseases (STDs) throughout the world for 40 years and was documented as an adjuvant for leprosy treatment in 1959.

The ability of sarsaparilla to bind to endotoxins may be a probable mechanism of action as to how the plant exerts its effects. Problems associated with high endotoxin levels circulating in the blood stream such as liver disease, psoriasis, fevers, and inflammatory processes, all seem to improve with sarsaparilla.

Antibiotic actions of sarsaparilla also are seen but are probably secondary to its endotoxin-binding effects. Antibiotic properties of the plant are shown by its treatment of leprosy and its actions against leptosirosis, a rare disease transmitted by rats.

Other positive effects of sarsaparilla on the skin have been demonstrated. The endotoxin-binding sarsaponin from the plant has improved psoriasis in 62% of patients and has completely cleared the disease in 18%. Antidermatophyte activity from the species *S. regelii* has been demonstrated in a later report. In addition, sarsaparilla has been used as an herbal or folk remedy for other skin conditions including eczema, pruritus, rashes, and wound care.

Sarsaparilla's anti-inflammatory actions are useful for treating arthritis, rheumatism, and gout. *S. sarsaparilla* inhibited carrageenan-induced paw inflammation in rats, as well as cotton pellet-induced exudation.

Advertising claims of sarsaparilla being a "rich source of testosterone," are unsubstantiated as there is no testosterone present in the plant. However, some sources state that sarsaparilla exhibits testosterogenic actions on the body, increasing muscle bulk and estrogenic actions as well to help alleviate female problems. In Mexico, the root is used for its alleged aphrodisiac properties. A recent review addresses *Smilax* compounds (among others) present in bodybuilding supplements said to "enhance performance." Results of the study of over 600 commercial supplements determined that there was no research to validate these claims.

Other documented uses of sarsaparilla include the following: improvement in appetite and digestion, adaptogenic effects from *S. regelii*, sarsaparilla in combination as an herbal remedy and mineral supplement, and haemolytic activity of steroidic saponins from *S. officinalis*. An overview of medicinal uses of sarsaparilla is available. One report evaluating fracture healing finds sarsaparilla to have insignificant effects on tensile strength and collagen deposition. Other species of smilax have been evaluated for antimutagenic actions (*S. china*) and GI disorders (*S. lundelii*). The species *S. glabra* exhibits wormicidal effects, improves hepatitis B in combination, had marked therapeutic effects (in combination) in the treatment of intestinal metaplasia and atypical hyperplasia, and has hepatoprotective effects.

TOXICOLOGY

No major contraindications, warnings, or toxicity data have been documented with sarsaparilla use. No known problems exist regarding its use in pregnancy or lactation either; however, avoid excessive ingestion. In unusually high doses, the saponins present in the plant could possibly be harmful, resulting in GI irritation. The fact that sarsaparilla binds bacterial endotoxins in the gut, making them unabsorbable, greatly reduces stress on the liver and other organs.

One report describing occupational asthma caused by sarsaparilla root dust exists in the literature.

References are available upon request.

SAW PALMETTO

SCIENTIFIC NAME(S)

Serenoa repens (Bartr.) Small. This plant is sometimes referred to as *S. serrulata* (Michx.) Nichols or *Sabal serrulatum* Schult. Family: Arecaciae

COMMON NAME(S)

Saw palmetto, sabal, American dwarf palm tree, cabbage palm

PATIENT INFORMATION

- *Warnings:* Products containing saw palmetto are considered dietary supplements and are **not** FDA-approved for medical use. Products containing this agent should be considered **complementary** therapies and not **alternative** therapies. Standard medical care and prescribed therapy should not be abandoned, nor should appropriate medical attention be delayed. Such practices can be dangerous.

  Saw palmetto should **not** be used for prostate cancer.

  Saw palmetto should **not** be used by pregnant women or those of childbearing potential.

- *Uses:* Recent studies suggest that extracts of saw palmetto may be beneficial in the management of benign prostate enlargement (benign prostatic hypertrophy [BPH]).

- *Side Effects:* No significant adverse effects are reported with saw palmetto use, although 1 case report noted cholestatic hepatitis with use. It may cause headaches and, if taken in large amounts, diarrhea.

- *Dosing:* The crude saw palmetto berries usually are administered at 1 to 2 g/day; however, lipophilic extracts standardized to 85% to 95% fatty acids in soft native extract or 25% fatty acids in a dry extract are more common. Some of the brand name products include *Permixon* (Pierre Fabre Medicament), *Prostaserene* (Indena) SCF extract, *Prostagutt* (WS 1473, Schwabe), *Remigeron* (Schaper & Brummer), *IDS 89* (Strathmann AG), *Quanterra Prostate* (Warner Lambert), and *LG 166/S* (Lab. Guidotti). Typical doses of standardized extracts range from 100 to 400 mg given twice daily for benign prostatic hypertrophy.

BOTANY

The saw palmetto plant is a fan palm that grows to approximately 10 feet with leaf clusters that can each attain a length of 2 feet or more. The plant is found from the Carolinas to Texas. Saw palmetto produces a brownish-black berry that is harvested commercially from wild sources.

HISTORY

Saw palmetto berry tea has been used for years for the management of various GU problems, to increase sperm production, to increase breast size, and to increase sexual vigor. In the early twentieth century, it was used as a mild diuretic and as a treatment for prostatic enlargement. The therapeutic value of the tea eventually came under question and saw palmetto was dropped from the National Formulary as an official drug.

ACTIONS

Although assessments based on earlier research indicate that the plant was of no therapeutic value, a number of more recent studies suggest that extracts of the plant may be beneficial in the management of prostatic enlargement (BPH). However, it should be noted that saw palmetto tea has no effect on BPH, as none of the active components of the plant are water soluble (the active components reside in the lipid-soluble fractions).

A hexane extract of the berries has been shown to have antiandrogenic properties through inhibition of the enzyme 5-alpha-reductase. Saw palmetto extract has been shown to inhibit dihydrotestosterone (DHT) binding to cellular and nuclear receptor sites, thereby increasing the metabolism and excretion of DHT. A double-blind, placebo-controlled study evaluated the hormonal effects of saw palmetto extract given to men with BPH for 3 months prior to surgery. The study found that saw palmetto had an estrogenic and antiprogesterone effect as determined by estrogen receptor activity.

The results from numerous double-blind trials and open trials on the effects of saw palmetto extract in BPH have been reported. Typically, these studies have been small and of approximately 3 months' duration.

In one of the larger trials, 110 patients each received either a hexane extract of saw palmetto or placebo under double-blind conditions for 30 days. Active treatment consisted of 320 mg/day of a commercially available 80 mg tablet preparation. Treatment was assessed based on objective measures such as nocturia, intensity of dysuria, flow rate, postmicturation residue, and subjective patient and physician assessments. *S. repens* extracts were statistically superior to placebo for every parameter after 30 days of treatment. In a study of 45 patients with BPH, prazosin (eg, *Minipress*) was found to be only marginally more effective than saw palmetto extract when given for 12 weeks, as measured by flowmetry and subjective assessments of irritation.

S. repens extracts have been shown to inhibit both cyclooxygenase and 5-lipoxygenase, thereby contributing to its anti-inflammatory and antiedematous effect. The plant has also been shown to have spasmolytic activity.

TOXICOLOGY

In most controlled trials, the incidence of side effects was low and consisted mainly of headache. No changes in blood chemistry parameters have been noted during therapy. Large amounts of the berry are reported to cause diarrhea. Although the plant has been classified as an "Herb of Undefined Safety," no severe adverse events have been reported. Because of its potential hormonal effects, the product should not be used by pregnant women or those of childbearing potential. Similarly, little is known of its effects on children or patients suffering from hormonal-dependent illnesses other than BPH (ie, prostate or breast cancers).

References are available upon request.

SOY

SCIENTIFIC NAME(S)
Glycine max L. Leguminosae/Fabaceae

COMMON NAME(S)
Soy, soybean, soya

PATIENT INFORMATION

- *Warnings:* Products containing soy are considered dietary supplements and are **not** FDA-approved for medical use. Products containing this agent should be considered **complementary** therapies and not **alternative** therapies. Standard medical care and prescribed therapy should not be abandoned, nor should appropriate medical attention be delayed. Such practices can be dangerous.
- *Uses:* Soy is commonly used as a source of fiber, protein, and minerals. The isoflavone compounds in soybeans may have anticancer effects, alleviate menopausal symptoms, prevent osteoporosis, and combat cardiovascular and GI problems.
- *Side Effects:* Overall tolerance to soybeans is good to excellent for most patients. Although there are no strong studies, the effects on infant development by phytoestrogens in soy-based formulas is of concern. Soy dust has caused an asthma epidemic.

BOTANY

The soybean is an annual plant that grows approximately 0.3 to 1.5 m tall. Bean pods, stems, and leaves are covered with short, fine hairs. The pods contain up to 4 yellow-to-brownish oval seeds. The cotyledons account for most of the seed's weight and contain most of the oil and protein.

HISTORY

Soybeans were cultivated in China as far back as the 11th century BC. Described by Chinese Emperor Shung Nang in 2838 BC, they were said to have been China's most important crop. Cultivation of the plant went to Japan, then Europe, and eventually to the United States in the early 1800s. The United States now produces half of the world's soybeans. Soybeans possess several benefits, including anticarcinogenic effects, improvement in cardiovascular and intestinal problems, and relief of menopausal symptoms. Soybeans are also an important source of nutrition.

Soy is an important food source and has been used in Asian cultures for thousands of years. These cultures consume 2 to 3 ounces of soy per day, as compared with Western diets that contain approximately 1/10 of that amount. Soybean products include soybean milk, soybean flour, soybean curd, sufu, tofu (cheese-like cake high in protein and calcium), tempeh (Indonesian main dish), fermented soybean paste (miso), soybeans sprouts, soy sauce, soybean oil, textured soy proteins (in meat extenders), soy protein drinks, and livestock feeds. Because of its low cost, good nutritional value, and versatility, soy protein is also used as part of food programs in less-developed countries. It is also used in infant formulas (most often if milk protein allergy exists).

ACTIONS

Isoflavones from the soybean have hormonal and nonhormonal actions. Hydrolysis of isoflavone glycosides by intestinal glucosidases yields genistein, daidzein, and glycitein. These may also become further metabolized to additional metabolites including equol and p-ethyl phenol. This metabolism is highly individualistic and can vary, for example, with carbohydrate intake altering intestinal fermentation. Isoflavones undergo enterohepatic circulation and are secreted into bile. Plasma half-life of genistein and daidzein is approximately 8 hours, with peak concentration being achieved in 6 to 8 hours in adults. Elimination is via urine, primarily as glucuronide conjugates. Phytoestrogens may play important roles in cancer prevention, menopausal symptoms, osteoporosis, cardiovascular disease, and GI disorders. Proposed mechanisms of the phytoestrogens include estrogenic and antiestrogenic effects, induction of cancer cell differentiation, inhibition of tyrosine kinase and DNA topoisomerase activity, angiogenesis suppression, and antioxidant effects.

TOXICOLOGY

Tolerance to soy preparations in a 164-patient study was good to excellent for most patients. The effects of phytoestrogens in soy-based infant formulas is of concern and may have some biological impact. Daily exposure of infants to the isoflavones in soy-based formula, in one report, was found to be 13,000 to 22,000 times higher than estradiol concentrations in early life. Effects of these soy isoflavones on steroid-dependent developmental processes in babies should be studied. Carefully controlled, large-scale clinical trials in this infant population should be a priority. Inhalation of soy dust caused an asthma epidemic in 26 patients exposed to an unloading of the product in Barcelona. Skin prick tests confirmed exposure to soy in all cases. Specific immunoglobulins such as IgE, are associated with this type of "soy bean asthma." Soybeans can be treated with proteases to reduce allergenicity.

References are available upon request.

St. John's Wort

SCIENTIFIC NAME(S)
Hypericum perforatum L. Family: Hypericaceae

COMMON NAME(S)
St. John's wort, klamath weed, John's wort, amber touch-and-heal, goat-weed, rosin rose, millepertuis

---

PATIENT INFORMATION

- *Warnings:* Products containing St. John's wort are considered dietary supplements and are **not** FDA-approved for medical use. Products containing this agent should be considered **complementary** therapies and not **alternative** therapies. Standard medical care and prescribed therapy should not be abandoned nor should appropriate medical attention be delayed. Such practices can be dangerous when herbal products are being used.

  If you have suicidal symptoms, do **not** take St. John's wort. See a physician immediately.

  Safety of St. John's wort use during pregnancy and lactation has not been confirmed. Pregnant and lactating women should avoid use of this agent.

  St. John's wort may cause photosensitivity. Wear protective clothing and use sunscreen while taking St. John's wort, especially if you will be spending time outdoors.

  Long-term use (more than 3 to 6 months) of St. John's wort should be avoided because no long-term safety data are available.

- *Uses:* St. John's wort has been used to treat depression and anxiety. It has also been employed as an antiviral and topical wound-healing agent.

- *Drug Interactions:* Do **not** take prescription antidepressants with St. John's wort. Wait several weeks prior to starting a new antidepressant after stopping St. John's wort.

- *Side Effects:* Side effects have included rash caused by photosensitivity, stomach upset, fatigue, sedation, dizziness, anxiety, and dry mouth.

  Some studies have indicated that St. John's wort may have adverse effects on sperm cells, possibly causing decreased fertility.

- *Dosing:* Traditional use of St. John's wort herb indicated 2 to 4 g/day doses. However, most clinical studies have been conducted on extracts, with hypericin content of 0.3% the earliest form of standardization. With the discovery of hyperforin's bioactivity, a content of 3% to 5% hyperforin has been used as a new standard. Some of the many products include *LI 160* (Lichtwer, 0.3% hypericin), *Kira* (Lichtwer, 300 mcg hypericin in 125 to 225 mg extract tablets), *Hyperiforce* (Bioforce, 0.33 mg hypericin in 60 mg extract/tablet), *Ze 117*, *WS 5573* (300 mg extract, 0.5% hyperforin), *WS 5572* (300 mg, 5% hyperforin), *STEI 300* (Steiner, 0.2% to 0.3% hypericin and 2% to 3% hyperforin), *Psychotonin*, *Esbericum*, *Neuroplant*, *Sedariston*, and *Hyperforat*. Doses of the extracts have ranged from 500 to 1,800 mg/day.

BOTANY

St. John's wort is an aromatic perennial native to Europe but is now found throughout the United States and parts of Canada. The plant is an aggressive weed growing in the dry ground of roadsides, meadows, woods, and hedges. It generally attains a height of 12 to 24 inches, except on the Pacific coast where it has reached heights of nearly 5 feet. The plant has oval leaves and yields golden-yellow flowers, which bloom from June to September. The petals contain black or yellow glandular dots and lines. Harvest of the leaves and flowers for medicinal purposes must occur during July and August, and the plant must be dried immediately to avoid loss of potency.

HISTORY

This plant has been used as an herbal remedy because of its anti-inflammatory and healing properties since the Middle Ages. Interest in St. John's wort has heightened during the past decade. It is now a component of numerous herbal preparations and is claimed to have value in the treatment of a variety of anxiety disorders and depression. The plant has been used as an antidepressant, a diuretic, and for treatment of gastritis and insomnia. An olive oil extract of the fresh flowers acquires a reddish color after standing in the sunlight for several weeks. This "red oil" has been taken internally for the treatment of anxiety but has also been applied topically to relieve inflammation and to promote healing. Topical application is said to be useful in the management of hemorrhoids. Although it is often listed as a folk treatment for cancer, there is no scientific evidence to document an anticancer effect.

ACTIONS

While the exact mechanism of action of St. John's wort remains unknown, most of the research associated with this plant has focused on the pharmacologic activity of hypericin, the best known component of St. John's wort. This compound was thought to exert a tranquilizing effect by increasing capillary blood flow. One study postulated that the action of the plant actually may be due to a combination of pharmacologic mechanisms too weak to individually produce the observed effects.

It has been suggested that the observed MAO inhibition seen with hypericin could be caused by a photo-catalyzed reaction in vitro, which would probably not be operative in the CNS. One study examined *Hypericum* fractions in vitro and ex vivo and reported no evidence of MAO inhibition except at 1 mM, probably an unrealistic concentration.

An extract of St. John's wort (*Psychotonin M*) elicited responses in experimental animal studies that were characteristic of antidepressant activity. This observed antidepressant effect was further evaluated in 6 women with clinically evident depressive symptoms. After 4 to 6 weeks of treatment with only *Psychotonin M* in a small group of patients in an uncontrolled study environment, all 6 patients showed a quantitative improvement in anxiety, dysphoric mood, loss of interest, and other psychometric measurements.

Many reports (1994 to present), including 1 study using the Hamilton depression scale, evaluated the clinical efficacy of St. John's wort in the treatment of mild-to-moderate depression. A meta-analysis that evaluated 23 randomized trials, including 1757 mild-to-moderate severely depressed patients, was conducted to investigate St. John's wort vs placebo and other conventional antidepressants. St. John's wort was superior to placebo; however, many limitations were seen in this report (eg, non-standard assessment criteria were used, information on comorbid conditions was not provided, and prescription antidepressant doses may have been inadequate for comparison). Adverse effects occurred in nearly 20% of patients on *Hypericum* and 53% of patients on standard antidepressants. Other reviews have yielded similar outcomes.

The pharmacokinetics of hypericin and pseudohypericin have been evaluated in humans, and although similar in structure, they possess substantial pharmacokinetic differences. Single-dose and steady-state pharmacokinetics have also been evaluated. A daily dose of *Hypericum*, as determined by trials and studies, is 200 to 900 mg in an alcohol extract. Other unidentified components appear to inhibit catechol-o-methyltransferase and reduce interleukin-6 expression. The latter suppression may affect mood through neurohormonal pathways. The inhibition of benzodiazepine-binding in vitro by amentoflavone, another constituent of *Hypericum* species, has been reported.

Hypericin and pseudohypericin may exert unknown clinical effects against a wide spectrum of viruses. The mechanisms by which the 2 components exert their antiviral effects do not seem to involve interruption of transcription, translation, or viral protein transport. *Hypericum* is discussed as a photodynamic agent and may be helpful in future therapeutics and diagnostics.

Extracts of the plant have been active against certain gram-negative and gram-positive bacteria in vitro. St. John's wort has been used in some countries to treat otitis externa in a 20% tincture form. Tannins probably exert a mild astringent action that contributes to the plant's traditional use as a topical wound-healing agent. However, otitis externa, otitis media, and other bacterial infections should not be "treated" with St. John's wort alone. Confirmation of antibacterial activity and value in treating various infectious diseases is lacking.

Other claimed uses include the following: Oral and topical administration of hypericin for treatment of vitiligo (failure of skin to form melanin); anti-inflammatory and anti-ulcerogenic properties from amentoflavone (a biapigenin derivative); and folk uses such as hemorrhoid and burn treatment. These "uses" have not been adequately confirmed by objective, controlled clinical trials.

TOXICOLOGY

Frequent side effects have included GI symptoms, dizziness, sedation, and dry mouth. Until further study, avoid long-term use (more than 3 to

6 months) because no long-term safety data are available. Health care providers should reassess antidepressant therapy regularly, whether it be a synthetic or botanical agent.

In controlled human studies, no changes in EEG, ECG, or laboratory test parameters were observed following treatment for up to 6 weeks.

A reaction resembling sedative-hypnotic intoxication occurred in a patient following ingestion of St. John's wort and paroxetine (*Paxil*). The reaction did not occur when the patient took the herbal product alone.

When ingested, hypericin can induce photosensitization, characterized by inflammation of the skin and mucous membranes following exposure to light. Until more is known about this agent, advise patients to wear protective clothing and to use sunscreen while using St. John's wort, especially if they plan to spend time outdoors. A case report of photosensitivity occurring in a 61-year-old female discusses "recurring, elevated, itching, erythematous lesions" during 3 years of St. John's wort therapy for depression. The rash was reversible after discontinuation of the medication.

Slight in vitro uterotonic (eg, giving muscle tone to the uterus) activity from St. John's wort has been reported in animals, suggesting use should be avoided during pregnancy.

The volatile oil from St. John's wort is an irritant.

References are available upon request.

SCIENTIFIC NAME(S)

Curcuma longa L. Synonymous with *C. domestica* Vahl. Family: Zingiberaceae

COMMON NAME(S)

Turmeric, curcuma, Indian saffron

PATIENT INFORMATION

- *Warnings:* Products containing turmeric are considered dietary supplements and are **not** FDA-approved for medical use. Products containing this agent should be considered **complementary** therapies and not **alternative** therapies. Standard medical care and prescribed therapy should not be abandoned, nor should appropriate medical attention be delayed. Such practices can be dangerous.
- *Uses:* Turmeric is used as a spice. Recent investigations indicate that the strong antioxidant effects of several components of turmeric result in an inhibiton of carcinogenesis and may play a role in limiting the development of cancers.
- *Side Effects:* There are no known side effects.
- *Dosing:* Powdered turmeric root has been used as a stimulant and carminative at doses of 0.5 to 3 g/day. Higher doses of 6 g/day were investigated for protective effects against ulcer.

BOTANY

Turmeric is a perennial member of the ginger family characterized by a thick rhizome. The plant grows to a height of about 0.9 to 1.5 m and has large oblong leaves. It bears funnel-shaped yellow flowers. The plant is cultivated widely throughout Asia, India, China, and tropical countries. The primary (bulb) and secondary (lateral) rhizomes are collected, cleaned, boiled, and dried; and lateral rhizomes contain more yellow coloring material than the bulb. The dried rhizome forms the basis for the culinary spice.

HISTORY

Turmeric has a warm, bitter taste and is a primary component of curry pow-
ders and some mustards. The powder and its oleoresins are used extensively as food flavorings in the culinary industry. The spice has a long history of use in Asian medicine. In Chinese medicine, it has been used to treat problems as diverse as flatulence and hemorrhage. It also has been used topically as a poultice, an analgesic, and to treat ringworms. The spice has been used for the management of jaundice and hepatitis. The oil is sometimes used as a perfume component.

ACTIONS

Several soluble fractions of turmeric, including curcumin, have been reported to have antioxidant properties. Turmeric inhibits the degradation of polyunsaturated fatty acids. The curcumins inhibit cancer at initiation, promotion, and progression stages of development.

In smokers, turmeric given at a daily dose of 1.5 g for 30 days significantly reduced the urinary excretion of mutagens compared with controls; turmeric had no effect on hepatic enzyme levels or lipid profiles suggesting that the spice may be an effective antimutagen useful in chemoprevention.

Ukonan-A, a polysaccharide with phagocytosis-activating activity has been isolated from *C. longa,* and ukonan-D has demonstrated strong reticuloendothelial system-potentiating activity. Aqueous extract of *C. longa* has been shown to have cytoprotective effects that inhibit chemically induced carcinogenesis, forming a basis for the traditional use of turmeric as an anticancer treatment.

A combination of turmeric and neem (*Azadirachta indica*) applied topically has been shown to effectively eradicate scabies in 97% of 814 people treated within 3 to 15 days. Other pharmacologic properties of turmeric include choleretic, hypotensive, antibacterial, and insecticidal activity.

The choleretic (bile-stimulating) activity of curcumin has been recognized for almost 40 years, and these compounds have been shown to possess strong antihepatotoxic properties.

TOXICOLOGY

No reports of toxicity have been reported following the ingestion of turmeric. No change in weight was observed following chronic treatment, although changes in heart and lung weights were observed; a decrease in white and red blood cell levels were observed. Although a gain in weight of sexual organs and an increase in sperm motility was observed, no spermatotoxic effects were found.

References are available upon request.

UBIQUINONE

SCIENTIFIC NAME(S)
Coenzyme Q-10, ubidecarenone, mitoquinone

COMMON NAME(S)
Adelir, heartcin, inokiton, neuquinone, taidecanone, udekinon, ubiquinone

---

PATIENT INFORMATION

- *Warnings:* Products containing ubiquinone are considered dietary supplements and are **not** FDA-approved for medical use. Products containing this agent should be considered **complementary** therapies and not **alternative** therapies. Standard medical care and prescribed therapy should not be abandoned, nor should appropriate medical attention be delayed. Such practices can be dangerous when herbal products are being used.

  Use is not recommended in pregnancy and lactation and in people with demonstrated hypersensitivity.

- *Uses:* Ubiquinone may have applications in treating ischemic heart disease, congestive heart failure (CHF), toxin-induced cardiopathy and hypertension, and may protect ischemic myocardium during surgery.

- *Side effects:* Rare side effects include epigastric discomfort, loss of appetite, nausea, and diarrhea.

- *Dosing:* Ubiquinone has been studied in clinical trials at doses of 90 to 200 mg/day for heart failure, cirrhosis, and antioxidant properties.

BIOLOGY

HISTORY
The first ubiquinone was isolated in 1957. Since that time, ubiquinones have been extensively studied in Japan, Russia, and Europe. Research in the United States began more recently. Lay press accounts claim that roughly 12 million Japanese use ubiquinones for the management of cardiovascular diseases. Ubiquinone is touted as an effective treatment of CHF, cardiac arrhythmias, hypertension, and in the reduction of hypoxic injury to the myocardium. Other health claims include the increase of exercise tolerance, stimulation of the immune system, and slowing the aging process. Clinical uses include the treatment of diabetes, obesity, and periodontal disease. Ubiquinone is not approved for therapeutic use in the United States, but it is available as a food supplement.

ACTIONS
Biomedical evidence provides the rationale for the use of ubiquinone in cardiovascular diseases. Endogenous forms function as essential cofactors in several metabolic pathways, especially in oxidative respiration. Supraphysiologic doses of ubiquinone may benefit tissues that have been rendered ische-

mic and then reperfused. Ubiquinone appears to function in such tissues as a free-radical scavenger, membrane stabilizer, or both. Ubiquinone as a mobile component in mitochondrial membrane and its role in electron transfer has been reported. It may have applications in treating ischemic heart disease, CHF, toxin-induced cardiopathy, and possibly hypertension. It protects ischemic myocardium during surgery.

Ubiquinone use for treatment of cardiac conditions is promising. In geriatric patients, ubiquinone treatment improved both symptoms and clinical conditions of all 34 cardiac patients with CHF. It also was effective for symptomatic mitral valve prolapse and improved stress-induced cardiac dysfunction in 400 pediatric patients. Activity tolerance improvements were observed in a double-blind study of 19 patients with chronic myocardial disease given oral ubiquinone-10. In an open, controlled study of 12 patients with advanced heart failure given 100 mg daily, 8 patients showed definite clinical improvement. Heart rate fell significantly and the heart volume decreased.

Ubiquinone's effects on lipids (eg, phospholipid digestion by phospholipase A2 and C) have also been studied. The mechanism may be membrane phospholipid protection against phospholipase attack. In its reduced form, ubiquinone's presence in all cellular membrane, blood serum, and serum lipoproteins allows protection from lipid peroxidation. Its ability to remain stable in hypercholesterolemia patients has been studied. Ubiquinol can also sustain vitamin E's antioxidant effects by regenerating the vitamin from its oxidized form.

TOXICOLOGY

No serious side effects have been associated with the use of ubiquinone. Use of the substance is contraindicated in people with demonstrated hypersensitivity. Use during pregnancy or lactation is not recommended because studies have not demonstrated the safety of ubiquinone for fetuses and infants. Rare side effects have included epigastric discomfort, loss of appetite, nausea, and diarrhea.

References are available upon request.

VALERIAN

SCIENTIFIC NAME(S)

Valeriana officinalis L. Family: Valerianaceae. A number of other members of the species have been used medicinally, including *V. wallichii* DC, *V. sambucifolia* Mik., and the related *Centranthus ruber* L.

COMMON NAME(S)

Valerian, baldrian, radix valerianae, Indian valerian (*V. wallichii*), red valerian (*C. ruber*)

PATIENT INFORMATION

- *Warnings:* Products containing valerian are considered dietary supplements and are **not** FDA-approved for medical use. Products containing this agent should be considered **complementary** therapies and not **alternative** therapies. Standard medical care and prescribed therapy should not be abandoned, nor should appropriate medical attention be delayed. Such practices can be dangerous. Valerian should not be used by pregnant or lactating women or by children younger than 2 years of age.

- *Uses:* Valerian has been used for the treatment of restlessness and sleep disorders. Valerian is classified as GRAS (generally recognized as safe) in the United States for food use.

- *Drug Interactions:* Valerian may interact adversely with a variety of prescribed and nonprescription drugs having sedation as a side effect. Excessive sedation may result from concomitant use.

- *Side Effects:* Studies have generally found valerian to have fewer side effects than other control drugs (eg, diazepam). However, morning drowsiness, headache, or excitability may occur.

- *Dosing:* Valerian root (fresh or dried) has been used at doses of 2 to 3 g given 1 to 3 times/day for nervousness or as an antispasmodic, and at bedtime for insomnia. Several types of extracts have been tested; an aqueous extract has shown activity in sleep studies at doses of 270 to 900 mg, while an ethanolic extract has been recommended at 600 mg for sleep. Combinations with extracts of hops (eg, *ReDormin, Ze 91019*) or with lemon balm (*EuVegal Forte*) are quite common as sleep aids and the valerian extract dose in combinations is 320 to 500 mg. Lipophilic extracts such as *Baldrian-Dispert* have fallen out of favor because of toxicity concerns and the failure to identify active principles in them.

BOTANY

Members of the genus *Valeriana* are herbaceous perennials widely distributed in the temperate regions of North America, Europe, and Asia. Of the approximately 200 known species, the Eurasian *V. officinalis* is the species most often cultivated for medicinal uses. The dried rhizome contains a volatile oil with a distinctive, offensive odor. The fresh drug has no appreciable smell; however, drying liberates the odiferous constituent isovaleric acid.

HISTORY

Despite its odor, valerian was considered a perfume in 16th century Europe. The tincture has been used for its sedative properties for centuries; it is still widely used in France, Germany, and Switzerland as a sleep aid. Approximately 50 tons of valerian are sold each year in France.

ACTIONS

While there is substantial debate over the constituents responsible for valerian's sedative activity, it is undeniable that valerian preparations have sedative effects. Human studies have documented valerian's effectiveness as a sleep aid.

Aqueous and hydroalcoholic extracts of valerian induce the release of [3H]GABA from rat brain synaptic vesicles, which has been interpreted as an effect on the GABA transporter. The in vitro effect was correlated with the content of GABA itself in the extract. Thus GABA may be responsible for some of the peripheral effects of valerian, while glutamine, another free amino acid in the extract, can cross the blood-brain barrier and be metabolized to GABA in situ, thereby producing central sedation.

An ethanol extract containing no valepotriates antagonized picrotoxin convulsions in mice but had no effect on metrazol- or harman-induced convulsions. The same extract prolonged barbiturate sleeping time but did not affect spontaneous motility, pain perception, or body temperature. The effects were traced to valerenic acid. A commercial aqueous alkaline extract of valerian (*Valdispert*), standardized on valerenic acid given orally to mice, reduced spontaneous motility and increased barbiturate sleeping time, but had no effect on metrazol-induced convulsions. Cerebral metabolism was examined in rats with positron emission tomography (PET) scanning, and an effect consistent with a GABAergic mechanism was reported with the methylene chloride extract of valerian; however, valepotriates and valerenic acids were not responsible for the effect. The active compounds were not identified.

Valerenic acid has been found to inhibit GABA transaminase (GABA-T), the principle enzyme that catabolizes GABA. GABA-T inhibition increases the inhibitory effect of GABA in the CNS and therefore contributes to valerian's sedative properties. Valerenic acid given intraperitoneally had CNS depressant effects in mice, including potentiating barbiturate sleeping time and decreasing spontaneous motor activity. The valepotriates isovaltrate and valtrate, along with valerenone, were found to have antispasmodic effects in isolated guinea pig ileum, as well as other smooth muscle preparations.

Clinical trials: There is evidence that valerian is effective in improving sleep quality and reducing latency to fall asleep. An aqueous extract of the root (400 mg extract) improved sleep quality in a number of subjective parameters in 128 healthy volunteers using a crossover design. Sleep latency was decreased in a group of 8 poor sleepers given an aqueous extract of valerian in a double-blind, placebo-controlled study. An uncontrolled multicenter study of more than 11,000 patients suffering from sleep-related disorders found subjective improvements in 94% of those treated. Another multicenter trial of the same preparation in a younger study population found progressive symptomatic improvement over 10 days of treatment. Valerian was found to increase slow-wave sleep in a pilot study of poor sleepers. In contrast to previous studies that demonstrated a prompt decrease in symptoms, 1 study found that 2 to 4 weeks was required to see improvement in 121 patients with serious insomnia. It also may have a mild antianxiety agent, although the effect appears to be weaker in healthy subjects than in poor sleepers. Elderly patients with nervous disorders responded positively to a commercial valerian preparation in a placebo-controlled study, as measured by both subjective and objective parameters. A sleep laboratory study found minor sedative effects in healthy volunteers.

Combination studies: Valerian is often combined with other herbs such as hops, St. John's wort, or lemon balm (*Melissa officinalis*) in commercial products. A number of these combinations have been evaluated in clinical studies. A combination of St. John's wort and valerian was evaluated for antidepressant activity in a double-blind study of 93 patients treated for 6 weeks. All psychometric scales showed statistically significant improvement. A second study of the same combination in the treatment of anxiety reached similar positive conclusions. A valerian combination preparation containing valerenic acid sesquiterpenes, but not valepotriates, improved sleep quality in a small crossover study of poor sleepers. Valerian and lemon balm were effective in combination in a study (20 patients) of poor sleepers. The same combination was found to be tolerated in healthy volunteers and increased the quality of sleep. A complex product made up of 6 herbs (*Crataegus, Ballota, Passiflora, Valeriana, Cola,* and *Paullinia*) was used to treat generalized anxiety (n = 91), producing progressive decreases in the Hamilton Anxiety Scale that were significantly greater than with placebo.

TOXICOLOGY

Concern was raised over the discovery that valepotriates are mutagenic in the Ames assay; however, their poor bioavailability makes them a dubious source of toxicity for patients. Mice have tolerated more than 1 g/kg doses of valerian by oral and intraperitoneal routes, showing ataxia, muscle relaxation, and hypothermia.

Clinical studies have generally found valerian to have fewer side effects than control drugs such as diazepam, producing little hangover effect when used as a sleep aid. However, morning drowsiness, headache, or excitability may occur with use. An intentional overdose has been reported in which 20 times the recommended dose was ingested; the patient experienced fatigue, abdominal cramps, chest tightness, tremor of the hands and feet, and lightheadedness; these symptoms resolved within 24 hours. A case of withdrawal after chronic use of valerian has been reported; however, the complex nature of the patient's medical history provides weak evidence for valerian's role.

Valerian has been classified as GRAS in the United States for food use; extracts and the root oil are used as flavorings in foods and beverages.

References are available upon request.

WITCH HAZEL

SCIENTIFIC NAME(S)
Hamamelis virginiana L. Family: Hamamelidaceae.

COMMON NAME(S)
Witch hazel, hamamelis, snapping hazel, winter bloom, spotted alder, tobacco wood, hamamelis water.

PATIENT INFORMATION

- *Warnings:* Products containing witch hazel are considered dietary supplements and are **not** FDA-approved for medical use. Products containing this agent should be considered **complementary** therapies and not **alternative** therapies. Standard medical care and prescribed therapy should not be abandoned, nor should appropriate medical attention be delayed. Such practices can be dangerous. Orally ingested witch hazel is on the US safety alert list. Any use other than topical application is strongly discouraged.
- *Uses:* Witch hazel has astringent and hemostatic properties, making it useful as a skin astringent to promote healing.
- *Side Effects:* Internal use is **not** recommended. A dose of 1 g will cause nausea, vomiting, or constipation, possibly leading to impactions. Severe liver damage may occur if the tannins are absorbed to a detectable extent.
- *Dosing:* Witch hazel leaves or bark have been used traditionally at daily oral doses of 2 to 3 g. Suppositories containing witch hazel contain from 0.1 to 1 g/dose.

BOTANY
Witch hazel grows as a deciduous bush, often reaching approximately 6 m in height. The plant is found throughout most of North America. Its broad, toothed leaves are ovate, and the golden yellow flowers bloom in the fall. Brown fruit capsules appear after the flowers, and when ripe, eject their 2 seeds away from the tree. The dried leaves, bark, and twigs are used medicinally.

HISTORY
Witch hazel is a widely known plant with a long history of use in the Americas. One reference lists more than 30 "traditional uses" for witch hazel, including the treatment of hemorrhoids, burns, cancers, tuberculosis, colds, and fever. Preparations have been used topically for symptomatic treatment of itching and other skin inflammations and in ophthalmic preparations for ocular irritations.

The plant is used in a variety of forms, including the crude leaf and bark, fluid extracts, a poultice, and most commonly as witch hazel water. The latter, also known as hamamelis water or distilled witch hazel extract, is obtained from the recently cut and partially dormant twigs of the plant. This plant material is soaked in warm water, followed by distillation and the addition of alcohol to the distillate.

Traditionally, witch hazel was known to native North American people as a treatment for tumors and eye inflammations. It was used internally for hemorrhaging. Eighteenth-century European settlers came to value the plant for its astringent effect.

ACTIONS

Witch hazel leaves, bark, and extracts have been reported to have astringent and hemostatic properties. These effects have been ascribed to the presence of a relatively high concentration of tannins in the leaf, bark, and extracts. Tannins are protein precipitants in appropriate concentrations.

Witch hazel water is devoid of tannins but still retains its astringency, suggesting that other constituents possess astringent qualities.

The mechanism of witch hazel astringency involves the "tightening" of skin proteins, which come together to form a "protective covering" that promotes skin healing. This quality is desirable in the treatment of hemorrhoids (including preventive measures for recurring hemorroids).

Some problems can be treated with witch hazel. Its drying and astringent effects help treat skin inflammations such as eczema. Witch hazel's action on skin lesions may provide modest protection against infection. Skin lotions may also contain witch hazel for these purposes. Inflammation of mucous membranes, including the mouth, throat, and gums may be treated with witch hazel in the form of a gargle.

Its ability to "tighten" distended veins and restore vessel tone is employed in varicose vein treatment. The hemostatic property of witch hazel is said to help stop minor bleeding and, if used as an enema, offers a rapid coagulant effect for inwardly bleeding piles.

TOXICOLOGY

The volatile oil of witch hazel contains the carcinogen safrole. This is found in much smaller quantities than in plants such as sassafras. Although extracts of witch hazel are available commercially, it is not recommended that these extracts be taken internally because of the toxicity of the tannins. Although tannins are not usually absorbed following oral administration, a dose of 1 g witch hazel will cause nausea, vomiting, or constipation, possibly leading to impactions; liver damage may occur if the tannins are absorbed to a detectable extent. Witch hazel water is not intended for internal use. Teas can be brewed from leaves and twigs available commercially in some health-food stores, but safety risks exist from such use.

At least 1 report is available discussing contact allergy to witch hazel.

References are available upon request.

NONPRESCRIPTION DRUG THERAPY
TABLE OF CONTENTS
■ ■ ■

APPENDIX

FDA PREGNANCY CATEGORIES

The rational use of any medication requires a risk vs benefit assessment. Among the myriad of risk factors which complicate this assessment, pregnancy is one of the most perplexing.

The FDA has established 5 categories to indicate the potential of a systemically absorbed drug for causing birth defects. The key differentiation among the categories is the degree (reliability) of documentation and the risk vs benefit ratio. Pregnancy Category X is particularly notable in that if any data exists that may implicate a drug as a teratogen and the risk vs benefit ratio does not support use of the drug, the drug is contraindicated during pregnancy. These categories are summarized below:

FDA Pregnancy Categories	
Pregnancy Category	**Definition**
A	Controlled studies show no risk. Adequate, well-controlled studies in pregnant women have failed to demonstrate risk to the fetus.
B	No evidence of risk in humans. Either animal findings show risk, but human findings do not; or if no adequate human studies have been done, animal findings are negative.
C	Risk cannot be ruled out. Human studies are lacking, and animal studies are either positive for fetal risk or lacking. However, potential benefits may justify the potential risks.
D	Positive evidence of risk. Investigational or postmarketing data show risk to the fetus. Nevertheless, potential benefits may outweigh the potential risks. If needed in a life-threatening situation or a serious disease, the drug may be acceptable if safer drugs cannot be used or are ineffective.
X	Contraindicated in pregnancy. Studies in animals or human, or investigational or post-marketing reports have shown fetal risk which clearly outweighs any possible benefit to the patients.

Regardless of the designated pregnancy category or presumed safety, no drug should be administered during pregnancy unless it is clearly needed and potential benefits outweigh potential hazards to the fetus.

CALCULATIONS

To calculate milliequivalent weight : $mEq = \dfrac{\text{gram molecular weight/valence}}{1000}$

$mEq = \dfrac{mg}{eq\ wt}$ equivalent weight or $eq\ wt = \dfrac{\text{gram molecular weight}}{\text{valence}}$

Commonly Used mEq Weights			
Chloride	35.5 mg = 1 mEq	Magnesium	12 mg = 1 mEq
Sodium	23 mg = 1 mEq	Potassium	39 mg = 1 mEq
Calcium	20 mg = 1 mEq		

To convert temperature: °C ↔ °F: $\dfrac{°C}{°F - 32} = \dfrac{5}{9}$ or $°C = \dfrac{5}{9}\ (°F - 32)$ $°F = 32 + \dfrac{9}{5}\,°C$

To calculate creatinine clearance (Ccr) from serum creatinine (mL/min):

Male: $Ccr = \dfrac{\text{weight (kg)} \times (140 - age)}{72 \times \text{serum creatinine (mg/dL)}}$ Female: Ccr = 0.85 × calculation for males

---

To calculate ideal body weight (IBW) (kg) in adults:

IBW (kg) (Males) = 50 + (2.3 × Height in inches over 60 inches)

IBW (kg) (Females) = 45.5 + (2.3 × Height in inches over 60 inches)

To calculate body surface area (BSA) in adults and children:

1) Dubois method:

$SA\ (cm^2) = wt\ (kg)^{0.425} \times ht\ (cm)^{0.725} \times 71.84$

$SA\ (m^2) = K \times \sqrt[3]{wt^2\ (kg)}$ (common K value
0.1 for toddlers, 0.103 for neonates)

2) Simplified method:

$BSA\ (m^2) = \sqrt{\dfrac{ht\ (cm) \times wt\ (kg)}{3{,}600}}$

To approximate surface area (m^2) of children from weight (kg):

Weight range (kg)	≈ Surface area (m^2)
1 to 5	(0.05 × kg) + 0.05
6 to 10	(0.04 × kg) + 0.10
11 to 20	(0.03 × kg) + 0.20
21 to 40	(0.02 × kg) + 0.40

Suggested Weights for Adults			
Height*	Weight in pounds†	Height*	Weight in pounds†
4'10"	91 to 115	5'7"	121 to 153
4'11"	94 to 119	5'8"	125 to 158
5'0"	97 to 123	5'9"	128 to 162
5'1"	101 to 127	5'10"	132 to 167
5'2"	104 to 131	5'11"	136 to 172
5'3"	107 to 135	6'0"	140 to 177
5'4"	111 to 140	6'1"	144 to 182
5'5"	114 to 144	6'2"	148 to 186
5'6"	118 to 148	6'3"	152 to 192

* Without shoes.
† Without clothes.

The higher weights in the ranges generally apply to people with more muscle and bone. Source: *Nutrition and Your Health: Dietary Guidelines for Americans*, 6th ed, 2005. US Department of Agriculture, US Department of Health and Human Services.

INTERNATIONAL SYSTEM OF UNITS

The *Système international d'unités* (International System of Units) or *SI* is a modernized version of the metric system. The primary goal of the conversion to SI units is to revise the present confused measurement system and to improve test-result communications.

The SI has 7 basic units from which other units are derived:

Base Units of SI		
Physical quantity	**Base unit**	**SI symbol**
length	meter	m
mass	kilogram	kg
time	second	s
amount of substance	mole	mol
thermodynamic temperature	kelvin	K
electric current	ampere	A
luminous intensity	candela	cd

Combinations of these base units can express any property, although, for simplicity, special names are given to some of these derived units.

Representative Derived Units		
Derived unit	**Name and symbol**	**Derivation from base units**
area	square meter	m^2
volume	cubic meter	m^3
force	newton (N)	$kg \bullet m \bullet s^{2}$
pressure	pascal (Pa)	$kg \bullet m^{-1} \bullet s^{-2} (N/m^2)$
work, energy	joule (J)	$kg \bullet m^2 \bullet s^{-2}$ (N$\bullet$m)
mass density	kilogram per cubic meter	kg/m^3
frequency	hertz (Hz)	1 cycles/s^{-1}
temperature degree	Celsius (°C)	$°C = °K - 273.15$
concentration		
mass	kilogram/liter	kg/L
substance	mole/liter	mol/L
molality	mole/kilogram	mol/kg
density	kilogram/liter	kg/L

Prefixes to the base unit are used in this system to form decimal multiples and submultiples. The preferred multiples and submultiples listed below change the quantity by increments of 10^3 or 10^{-3}. The exceptions to these recommended factors are within the middle rectangle.

Prefixes and Symbols for Decimal Multiples and Submultiples		
Factor	Prefix	Symbol
10^{18}	exa	E
10^{15}	peta	P
10^{12}	tera	T
10^9	giga	G
10^6	mega	M
10^3	kilo	k
10^2	hecto	h
10^1	deka	da
10^{-1}	deci	d
10^{-2}	centi	c
10^{-3}	milli	m
10^{-6}	micro	μ
10^{-9}	nano	n
10^{-12}	pico	p
10^{-15}	femto	f
10^{-18}	atto	a

To convert drug concentrations to or from SI units:

Conversion factor (CF) = 1,000/mol wt
Conversion *to* SI units: mcg/mL × CF = mcmol/L
Conversion *from* SI units: mcmol/L ÷ CF = mcg/mL

NORMAL LABORATORY VALUES

In the following tables, normal reference values for commonly requested laboratory tests are listed in traditional units and in SI units. The tables are a guideline only. Values are method dependent and "normal values" may vary between laboratories.

Blood, Plasma or Serum		
	Reference Value	
Determination	Conventional units	SI units
Alpha-fetoprotein	*Adult:* < 15 ng/mL *Pregnant (16 to 18 weeks):* 38 to 45 ng/mL	*Adult:* < 15 mcg/L *Pregnant (16 to 18 weeks):* 38 to 45 mcg/L
Ammonia (NH_3) - diffusion	20 to 120 mcg/dL	12 to 70 mcmol/L
Ammonia Nitrogen	15 to 45 mcg/dL	11 to 32 mcmol/L
Amylase	35 to 118 units/L	0.58 to 1.97 mckat/L
Anion gap (Na^+-[Cl^- + HCO_3^-]) (P)	7 to 16 mEq/L	7 to 16 mmol/L
Antithrombin III (AT III)	80 to 120 units/dL	800 to 1,200 units/L
Bicarbonate: Arterial	21 to 28 mEq/L	21 to 28 mmol/L
Venous	22 to 29 mEq/L	22 to 29 mmol/L
Bilirubin: Conjugated (direct)	≤ 0.2 mg/dL	≤ 4 mcmol/L
Total	0.1 to 1 mg/dL	2 to 18 mcmol/L
Calcitonin	< 100 pg/mL	< 100 ng/L
Calcium: Total	8.6 to 10.3 mg/dL	2.2 to 2.74 mmol/L
Ionized	4.4 to 5.1 mg/dL	1 to 1.3 mmol/l
Carbon dioxide content (plasma)	21 to 32 mmol/L	21 to 32 mmol/L
Carcinoembryonic antigen	< 3 ng/mL	< 3 mcg/L
Chloride	95 to 110 mEq/L	95 to 110 mmol/L
Coagulation screen:		
Bleeding time	3 to 9.5 min	180 to 570 sec
Prothrombin time	10 to 13 sec	10 to 13 sec
Partial thromboplastin time (activated)	22 to 37 sec	22 to 37 sec
Protein C	0.7 to 1.4 microunits/mL	700 to 1,400 units/mL
Protein S	0.7 to 1.4 microunits/mL	700 to 1,400 units/mL
Copper, total	70 to 160 mcg/dL	11 to 25 mcmol/L
Corticotropin (ACTH adrenocorticotropic hormone) - 0800 hr	< 60 pg/mL	< 13.2 pmol/L
Cortisol: 0800 h	5 to 30 mcg/dL	138 to 810 nmol/L
1800 h	2 to 15 mcg/dL	50 to 410 nmol/L
2000 h	≤ 50% of 0800 h	≤ 50% of 0800 h
Creatine kinase: Female	20 to 170 units/L	0.33 to 2.83 mckat/L
Male	30 to 220 units/L	0.5 to 3.67 mckat/L
Creatinine kinase isoenzymes, MB fraction	0 to 12 units/L	0 to 0.2 mckat/L
Creatinine	0.5 to 1.7 mg/dL	44 to 150 mcmol/L
Fibrinogen (coagulation factor I)	150 to 360 mg/dL	1.5 to 3.6 g/L
Follicle-stimulating hormone (FSH):		
Female	2 to 13 milliunits/mL	2 to 13 units/L
Midcycle	5 to 22 milliunits/mL	5 to 22 units/L
Male	1 to 8 milliunits/mL	1 to 8 units/L

Blood, Plasma or Serum				
Determination	**Reference Value**			
	Conventional units		**SI units**	
Glucose, fasting	65 to 115 mg/dL		3.6 to 6.3 mmol/L	
Glucose Tolerance Test (Oral)	mg/dL		mmol/L	
	Normal	*Diabetic*	*Normal*	*Diabetic*
Fasting	70 to 105	> 140	3.9 to 5.8	> 7.8
60 min	120 to 170	≥ 200	6.7 to 9.4	≥ 11.1
90 min	100 to 140	≥ 200	5.6 to 7.8	≥ 11.1
120 min	70 to 120	≥ 140	3.9 to 6.7	≥ 7.8
(γ) -Glutamyltransferase (GGT): Male	9 to 50 units/L		9 to 50 units/L	
Female	8 to 40 units/L		8 to 40 units/L	
Haptoglobin	44 to 303 mg/dL		0.44 to 3.03 g/L	
Hematologic tests:				
Fibrinogen	200 to 400 mg/dL		2 to 4 g/L	
Hematocrit (Hct):				
Female	36% to 44.6%		0.36 to 0.446 fraction of 1	
Male	40.7% to 50.3%		0.4 to 0.503 fraction of 1	
Hemoglobin A_{1c}	5.3% to 7.5% of total Hgb		0.053 to 0.075	
Hemoglobin (Hb):				
Female	12.1 to 15.3 g/dL		121 to 153 g/L	
Male	13.8 to 17.5 g/dL		138 to 175 g/L	
Leukocyte count (WBC)	3,800 to 9,800/mcL		3.8 to 9.8 $\times$ 10^9/L	
Erythrocyte count (RBC):				
Female	3.5 to 5 $\times$ 10^6/mcL		3.5 to 5 $\times$ 10^{12}/L	
Male	4.3 to 5.9 $\times$ 10^6/mcL		4.3 to 5.9 $\times$ 10^{12}/L	
Mean corpuscular volume (MCV)	80 to 97.6 mcm^3		80 to 97.6 fl	
Mean corpuscular hemoglobin (MCH)	27 to 33 pg/cell		1.66 to 2.09 fmol/cell	
Mean corpuscular hemoglobin concentrate (MCHC)	33 to 36 g/dL		20.3 to 22 mmol/L	
Erythrocyte sedimentation rate (sedrate, ESR)	≤ 30 mm/h		≤ 30 mm/h	
Erythrocyte enzymes:				
Glucose-6-phosphate dehydrognase (G-6-PD)	250 to 5,000 units/10^6 cells		250 to 5,000 microunits/cell	
Ferritin	10 to 383 ng/mL		23 to 862 pmol/L	
Folic acid: normal	> 3.1 to 12.4 ng/mL		7 to 28.1 nmol/L	
Platelet count	150 to 450 $\times$ 10^3/mcL		150 to 450 $\times$ 10^9/L	
Reticulocytes	0.5% to 1.5% of erythrocytes		0.005 to 0.015	
Vitamin B_{12}	223 to 1,132 pg/mL		165 to 835 pmol/L	
Iron: Female	30 to 160 mcg/dL		5.4 to 31.3 mcmol/L	
Male	45 to 160 mcg/dL		8.1 to 31.3 mcmol/L	
Iron-binding capacity	220 to 420 mcg/dL		39.4 to 75.2 mcmol/L	
Isocitrate dehydrogenase	1.2 to 7 units/L		1.2 to 7 units/L	

Blood, Plasma or Serum		
	Reference Value	
Determination	Conventional units	SI units
Isoenzymes		
Fraction 1	14% to 26% of total	0.14 to 0.26 fraction of total
Fraction 2	29% to 39% of total	0.29 to 0.39 fraction of total
Fraction 3	20% to 26% of total	0.20 to 0.26 fraction of total
Fraction 4	8% to 16% of total	0.08 to 0.16 fraction of total
Fraction 5	6% to 16% of total	0.06 to 0.16 fraction of total
Lactate dehydrogenase	100 to 250 units/L	1.67 to 4.17 mckat/L
Lactic acid (lactate)	6 to 19 mg/dL	0.7 to 2.1 mmol/L
Lead	≤ 50 mcg/dL	≤ 2.41 mcmol/L
Lipase	10 to 150 units/L	10 to 150 units/L
Lipids:		
Total Cholesterol		
Desirable	< 200 mg/dL	< 5.2 mmol/L
Borderline-high	200 to 239 mg/dL	< 5.2 to 6.2 mmol/L
High	> 239 mg/dL	> 6.2 mmol/L
LDL		
Desirable	< 130 mg/dL	< 3.36 mmol/L
Borderline-high	130 to 159 mg/dL	3.36 to 4.11 mmol/L
High	> 159 mg/dL	> 4.11 mmol/L
HDL (low)	< 35 mg/dL	< 0.91 mmol/L
Triglycerides		
Desirable	< 200 mg/dL	< 2.26 mmol/L
Borderline-high	200 to 400 mg/dL	2.26 to 4.52 mmol/L
High	400 to 1,000 mg/dL	4.52 to 11.3 mmol/L
Very high	> 1,000 mg/dL	> 11.3 mmol/L
Magnesium	1.3 to 2.2 mEq/L	0.65 to 1.1 mmol/L
Osmolality	280 to 300 mOsm/kg	280 to 300 mmol/kg
Oxygen saturation (arterial)	94% to 100%	0.94 to fraction of 1
PCO_2, arterial	35 to 45 mm Hg	4.7 to 6 kPa
pH, arterial	7.35 to 7.45	7.35 to 7.45
PO_2, arterial: Breathing room air[*]	80 to 105 mm Hg	10.6 to 14 kPa
On 100% O_2	> 500 mm Hg	
Phosphatase (acid), total at 37°C	0.13 to 0.63 units/L	2.2 to 10.5 units/L or 2.2 to 10.5 mckat/L
Phosphatase alkaline[+]	20 to 130 units/L	20 to 130 units/L or 0.33 to 2.17 mckat/L
Phosphorus, inorganic,[‡] (phosphate)	2.5 to 5 mg/dL	0.8 to 1.6 mmol/L
Potassium	3.5 to 5 mEq/L	3.5 to 5 mmol/L
Progesterone		
Female	0.1 to 1.5 ng/mL	0.32 to 4.8 nmol/L
Follicular phase	0.1 to 1.5 ng/mL	0.32 to 4.8 nmol/L
Luteal phase	2.5 to 28 ng/mL	8 to 89 nmol/L
Male	< 0.5 ng/mL	< 1.6 nmol/L

Blood, Plasma or Serum		
	Reference Value	
Determination	Conventional units	SI units
Prolactin	1.4 to 24.2 ng/mL	1.4 to 24.2 mcg/L
Prostate specific antigen	0 to 4 ng/mL	0 to 4 ng/mL
Protein: Total	6 to 8 g/dL	60 to 80 g/L
Albumin	3.6 to 5 g/dL	36 to 50 g/L
Globulin	2.3 to 3.5 g/dL	23 to 35 g/L
Rheumatoid factor	< 60 units/mL	< 60 kunits/L
Sodium	135 to 147 mEq/L	135 to 147 mmol/L
Testosterone: Female	6 to 86 ng/dL	0.21 to 3 nmol/L
Male	270 to 1070 ng/dL	9.3 to 37 nmol/L
Thyroid Hormone Function Tests:		
Thyroid-stimulating hormone (TSH)	0.35 to 6.2 microunits/mL	0.35 to 6.2 microunits/L
Thyroxine-binding globulin capacity	10 to 26 mcg/dL	100 to 260 mcg/L
Total triiodothyronine (T_3)	75 to 220 ng/dL	1.2 to 3.4 nmol/L
Total thyroxine by RIA (T_4)	4 to 11 mcg/dL	51 to 142 nmol/L
T_3 resin uptake	25% to 38%	0.25 to 0.38 fraction of 1
Transaminase, AST (aspartate amino-transferase, SGOT)	11 to 47 units/L	0.18 to 0.78 mckat/L
Transaminase, ALT (alanine aminotrans-ferase, SGPT)	7 to 53 units/L	0.12 to 0.88 mckat/L
Transferrin	220 to 400 mg/dL	2.20 to 4.00 g/L
Urea nitrogen (BUN)	8 to 25 mg/dL	2.9 to 8.9 mmol/L
Uric acid	3 to 8 mg/dL	179 to 476 mcmol/L
Vitamin A (retinol)	15 to 60 mcg/dL	0.52 to 2.09 mcmol/L
Zinc	50 to 150 mcg/dL	7.7 to 23 mcmol/L

* Age dependent.
† Infants and adolescents up to 104 units/L.
‡ Infants in the first year up to 6 mg/dL.

Urine		
	Reference value	
Determination	**Conventional units**	**SI units**
Calcium*	50 to 250 mcg/day	1.25 to 6.25 mmol/day
Catecholamines:		
Epinephrine	< 20 mcg/day	< 109 nmol/day
Norepinephrine	< 100 mcg/day	< 590 nmol/day
Catecholamines, 24-h	< 110 mcg	< 650 nmol
Copper*	15 to 60 mcg/day	0.24 to 0.95 mcmol/day
Creatinine: Child	8 to 22 mg/kg	71 to 195 mcmol/kg
Adolescent	8 to 30 mg/kg	71 to 265 mcmol/kg
Female	0.6 to 1.5 g/day	5.3 to 13.3 mmol/day
Male	0.8 to 1.8 g/day	7.1 to 15.9 mmol/day
pH	4.5 to 8	4.5 to 8
Phosphate*	0.9 to 1.3 g/day	29 to 42 mmol/day
Potassium*	25 to 100 mEq/day	25 to 100 mmol/day
Protein		
Total	1 to 14 mg/dL	10 to 140 mg/L
At rest	50 to 80 mg/day	50 to 80 mg/day
Protein, quantitative	< 150 mg/day	< 0.15 g/day
Sodium*	100 to 250 mEq/day	100 to 250 mmol/day
Specific gravity, random	1.002 to 1.03	1.002 to 1.03
Uric acid, 24-h	250 to 750 mg	1.48 to 4.43 mmol

* Diet Dependent

Drug Levels*		
	Reference value	
Drug determination	Conventional units	SI units
Aminoglycosides		
Amikacin		
(trough)	1 to 8 mcg/mL	1.7 to 13.7 mcmol/L
(peak)	20 to 30 mcg/mL	34 to 51 mcmol/L
Gentamicin		
(trough)	0.5 to 2 mcg/mL	1 to 4.2 mcmol/L
(peak)	6 to 10 mcg/mL	12.5 to 20.9 mcmol/L
Kanamycin		
(trough)	5 to 10 mcg/mL	nd[†]
(peak)	20 to 25 mcg/mL	nd
Netilimicin		
(trough)	0.5 to 2 mcg/mL	nd
(peak)	6 to 10 mcg/mL	nd
Streptomycin		
(trough)	< 5 mcg/mL	nd
(peak)	5 to 20 mcg/mL	nd
Tobramycin		
(trough)	0.5 to 2 mcg/mL	1.1 to 4.3 mcmol/L
(peak)	5 to 20 mcg/mL	12.8 to 21.8 mcmol/L
Antiarrhythmics		
Amiodarone	0.5 to 2.5 mcg/mL	1.5 to 4 mcmol/L
Bretylium	0.5 to 1.5 mcg/mL	nd
Digitoxin	9 to 25 mcg/L	11.8 to 32.8 nmol/L
Digoxin	0.8 to 2 ng/mL	0.9 to 2.5 nmol/L
Disopyramide	2 to 8 mcg/mL	6 to 18 mcmol/L
Flecainide	0.2 to 1 mcg/mL	nd
Lidocaine	1.5 to 6 mcg/mL	4.5 to 21.5 mcmol/L
Mexiletine	0.5 to 2 mcg/mL	nd
Procainamide	4 to 8 mcg/mL	17 to 34 mcmol/mL
Propranolol	50 to 200 ng/mL	190 to 770 nmol/L
Quinidine	2 to 6 mcg/mL	4.6 to 9.2 mcmol/L
Tocainide	4 to 10 mcg/mL	nd
Verapamil	0.08 to 0.3 mcg/mL	nd
Anticonvulsants		
Carbamazepine	4 to 12 mcg/mL	17 to 51 mcmol/L
Phenobarbital	10 to 40 mcg/mL	43 to 172 mcmol/L
Phenytoin	10 to 20 mcg/mL	40 to 80 mcmol/L
Primidone	4 to 12 mcg/mL	18 to 55 mcmol/L
Valproic Acid	40 to 100 mcg/mL	280 to 700 mcmol/L

Drug Levels*		
	Reference value	
Drug determination	Conventional units	SI units
Antidepressants		
Amitriptyline	110 to 250 ng/mL‡	500 to 900 nmol/L
Amoxapine	200 to 500 ng/mL	nd
Bupropion	25 to 100 ng/mL	nd
Clomipramine	80 to 100 ng/mL	nd
Desipramine	115 to 300 ng/mL	nd
Doxepin	110 to 250 ng/mL‡	nd
Imipramine	225 to 350 ng/mL‡	nd
Maprotiline	200 to 300 ng/mL	nd
Nortriptyline	50 to 150 ng/mL	nd
Protriptyline	70 to 250 ng/mL	nd
Trazodone	800 to 1600 ng/mL	nd
Antipsychotics		
Chlorpromazine	50 to 300 ng/mL	150 to 950 nmol/L
Fluphenazine	0.13 to 2.8 ng/mL	nd
Haloperidol	5 to 20 ng/mL	nd
Perphenazine	0.8 to 1.2 ng/mL	nd
Thiothixene	2 to 57 ng/mL	nd
Miscellaneous		
Amantadine	300 ng/mL	nd
Amrinone	3.7 mcg/mL	nd
Chloramphenicol	10 to 20 mcg/mL	31 to 62 mcmol/L
Cyclosporine§	250 to 800 ng/mL (whole blood, RIA) 50 to 300 ng/mL (plasma, RIA)	nd nd
Ethanol‖	0 mg/dL	0 mmol/L
Hydralazine	100 ng/mL	nd
Lithium	0.6 to 1.2 mEq/L	0.6 to 1.2 mmol/L
Salicylate	100 to 300 mg/L	724 to 2172 mcmol/L
Sulfonamide	5 to 15 mg/dL	nd
Terbutaline	0.5 to 4.1 ng/mL	nd
Theophylline	10 to 20 mcg/mL	55 to 110 mcmol/L
Vancomycin		
(trough)	5 to 15 ng/mL	nd
(peak)	20 to 40 mcg/mL	nd

* The values given are generally accepted as desirable for treatment without toxicity for most patients. However, exceptions are not uncommon.
+ nd = No data available.
‡ Parent drug plus N-desmethyl metabolite.
§ 24-hour trough values.
‖ Toxic: 50 to 100 mg/dL (10.9 to 21.7 mmol/L).

The following table is adopted from the Sixth Report of the Joint National Committee on Prevention, Detection, Evaluation, and Treatment of High Blood Pressure, National Institutes of Health.

Classification of Blood Pressure*			
Reference value			
Category	Systolic (mm Hg)		Diastolic (mm Hg)
Optimal[1]	< 120	and	< 80
Normal	< 130	and	< 85
High-normal	130 to 139	or	85 to 89
Hypertension[2]			
Stage 1	140 to 159	or	90 to 99
Stage 2	160 to 179	or	100 to 109
Stage 3	≥ 180	or	≥ 110

* For adults age 18 and older who are not taking antihypertensive drugs and not acutely ill. When systolic and diastolic blood pressures fall into different categories, the higher category should be selected to classify the individual's blood pressure status. In addition to classifying stages of hypertension on the basis of average blood pressure levels, clinicians should specify presence or absence of target organ disease and additional risk factors.

[1] Optimal blood pressure with respect to cardiovascular risk is below 120/88 mm Hg. However, unusually low readings should be evaluated for clinical significance.

[2] Based on the average of two or more readings taken at each of two or more visits after an initial screening.

STANDARD ABBREVIATIONS

AIDS	acquired immunodeficiency syndrome	gal	gallon
ALT	alanine aminotransferase	GI	gastrointestinal
ARC	AIDS-related complex	GU	genitourinary
AST	aspartate aminotransferase, SGOT	h or hr	hour
		HCl	hydrochloric acid, hydrochloride
AUC	area under the plasma concentration-time curve	HIV	human immunodeficiency virus
APTT	activated partial thromboplastin time	hs	at bedtime
		I	iodine
AV	atrioventricular	IM	intramuscular
ac	before meals	Inh	inhaled
bid	twice daily	IU	international unit
BP	blood pressure	IV	intravenous
bpm	beats per minute	K	potassium
BUN	blood urea nitrogen	kg	kilogram
°C	degrees Celsius	L	liter
Ca	calcium	lb	pound
Cal	Calorie (kilocalorie)	LDH	lactate dehydrogenase
CBC	complete blood count	m	meter
Ccr	creatinine clearance	M	molar
CD4	T-helper lymphocyte	m^2	square meter
CDC	Centers for Disease Control and Prevention	mcg	microgram
		mCi	millicurie
CHF	congestive heart failure	mEq	milliequivalent
CK	creatinine kinase	mg	milligram
Cl	chloride	Mg	magnesium
C_{max}	maximum effective plasma concentration	MIC	minimum inhibitory concentration
C_{min}	minimum effective plasma concentration	min	minute
		mL	milliliter
CNS	central nervous system	mm	millimeter
CPK	creatine phosphokinase	mm^3	cubic millimeter
Cr	chromium	mm Hg	millimeter(s) of mercury
CSF	cerebrospinal fluid	mmol	millimole
cu	cubic	Mn	manganese
Cu	copper	Mo	molybdenum
dL	deciliter (100 mL)	mOsm	milliosmole
DNA	Deoxyribonucleic acid	MRI	Magnetic resonance imaging
D5W	Dextrose 5% in Water Solution	Na	sodium
ECG or EKG	electrocardiogram	NF	National Formulary
EEG	electroencephalogram	ng	nanogram
F	fluoride	NS	normal saline solution
°F	degrees Fahrenheit	OTC	over the counter (nonprescription)
FA	folic acid		
FDA	Food and Drug Administration	oz	ounce
Fe	iron	P	phosphorus
g	gram	$PaCO_2$	arterial plasma partial pressure of carbon dioxide
G-6-PD	glucose-6-phosphate dehydrogenase		

PCO_2	plasma partial pressure of carbon dioxide
pKa	the negative logarithm of the dissociation constant
pc	after meals
pH	the hydrogen ion concentration or activity of a solution to that of a given standard solution
po	by mouth
PO_2	plasma partial pressure of oxygen
ppm	parts per million
prn	as needed
PT	prothrombin time
pt	pint
qid	four times daily
qd	every day
qt	quart
RBC	red blood cells
RDA	Recommended Dietary Allowance
RNA	ribonucleic acid
Rx	prescription only
SC	subcutaneous
Se	selenium
sec	second
sf	sugar free
T_3	triiodothyronine
T_4	thyroxine
$t^{1/2}$	half-life
tid	three times daily
tbsp	tablespoon
T_{max}	time to maximum concentration
TSH	thyroid-stimulating hormone
tsp	teaspoon
U	unit
UD	unit dose package
USP	United States Pharmacopeia
Vd	Volume of distribution
WBC	white blood cells
WHO	World Health Organization
Zn	zinc
$\approx$	approximately
$>$	greater than
$<$	less than
$\geq$	greater than or equal to
$\leq$	less than or equal to

APPENDIX B

GENERAL MANAGEMENT OF ACUTE OVERDOSAGE

Rapid intervention is essential to minimize morbidity and mortality in an acute toxic ingestion. Institute measures to prevent absorption and hasten elimination as soon as possible; however, symptomatic and supportive care takes precedence over other therapy. It is assumed that basic life support measures (eg, cardiopulmonary resuscitation [CPR]) have been instituted. Specific antidotes are discussed in the overdosage section of individual or group monographs. The discussion below outlines procedures used in the management of acute overdosage of orally ingested systemic drugs.

Advanced Life Support Measures

Adequate Airway: Adequate airway must be established and maintained, generally via oropharyngeal or endotracheal airways, cricothyrotomy, or tracheostomy.

Ventilation: Ventilation may then be performed via mouth-to-mouth insufflation, hand-operated bag (ambu bag), or a mechanical ventilator.

Circulation: Circulation must be maintained.

• *Hypotension:* If hypotension/hypoperfusion occurs, place the patient in shock position (head lowered, feet elevated); specific therapy may include:

Establish intravenous (IV) access and initiate IV fluids (eg, 0.9% or 0.45% saline, lactated Ringer's, dextrose). A maintenance flow rate is generally 100 to 200 mL/hour; individualize as necessary.

Plasma, plasma protein fractions, whole blood, or plasma expanders may be required.

Severe hypotension may require judicious use of cardiovascular active agents. The most commonly recommended agents are dopamine, dobutamine, and norepinephrine.

• *Arrhythmia:* Arrhythmia treatment is dictated by the offending drug.

• *Hypertension:* Hypertension, sometimes severe, may occur.

Seizures: Simple isolated seizures may require only observation and supportive care. Repetitive seizures or status epilepticus require therapy. Give IV diazepam or lorazepam followed by fosphenytoin and/or phenobarbital. Pancuronium also may be considered.

Reduction of Drug Absorption

Gastric emptying: Generally, gastric emptying is recommended as soon as possible; however, this is not very effective unless employed within the first 1 to 2 hours after ingestion. Ipecac syrup and gastric lavage are the 2 most commonly employed methods for gastric emptying.

• *Ipecac syrup:* Ipecac is the method of choice outside the hospital. Do not induce vomiting if the medication is caustic or a petroleum or if the patient is in a coma or having seizures. Ipecac takes 20 to 30 minutes to work. Consider gastric lavage if response is needed immediately.

6 months to 1 year: 10 mL
1 year to 12 years: 15 mL
older than 12 years: 30 mL

May be followed by a glass of water. A second dose may be given if results do not occur within 20 to 30 minutes.

- *Gastric lavage:* Gastric lavage is indicated in the comatose patient or for those in whom ipecac fails to produce emesis. Gastric lavage is immediate, does not have a delayed reaction, and is preferred over forced emesis. Airway protection via endotracheal intubation is appropriate for the patient without a gag reflex or for comatose patients. Position the patient left side, face down, and use a large bore tube. Instill warm water or saline 300 to 360 mL for adults. Avoid water for infants and children, use warm saline or 5% to 6% polyethylene glycol solution. Give until lavage solution returns clear. Give charcoal before removing the tube.

Adsorption: Adsorption, using activated charcoal alone or after completion of emesis or lavage, is indicated for virtually all significant toxic ingestions. It adsorbs a wide variety of toxins, and there are no contraindications. However, it adsorbs many orally administered antidotes as well, so space dosage properly. Give an adult 50 to 100 g of activated charcoal mixed in 240 mL of water; the pediatric dose is 1 g/kg, or 25 to 50 g in 120 mL of water.

Cathartics: Cathartics increase the elimination of charcoal-poison complex. Generally, using a saline or osmotic cathartic (eg, magnesium sulfate or citrate, sorbitol) to 3 mL/kg of a 35% to 75% solution of sorbitol has the most rapid effect.

Whole bowel irrigation: Whole bowel irrigation utilizes rapid administration of large volumes of lavage solutions, such as PEG. The dose is 4 to 6 L over 1 to 2 hours for adults and 0.5 L/hour for children. It may be most useful for removal of iron tablets, sustained-release capsules, or cocaine-containing condoms or balloons.

Elimination of Absorbed Drug

Interruption of enterohepatic circulation: Interruption of enterohepatic circulation by "gastric dialysis" uses scheduled doses of activated charcoal for 1 to 2 days. Gastric dialysis interrupts the enterohepatic cycle of some drugs and also creates an osmotic gradient, drawing drug from the plasma back into the gastrointestinal lumen where it is bound by the charcoal and excreted in the feces.

Diuresis: Diuresis may be effective as identified in the individual drug monographs.

- *Forced diuresis:* Forced diuresis is occasionally useful. It may cause volume overload or electrolyte disturbances. Forced diuresis is useful for phenobarbital, bromide, lithium, salicylate, or amphetamine overdoses. Do not use for tricyclic antidepressants, sedative-hypnotics, or highly protein-bound medications. The most common agents employed are furosemide and osmotic diuretics with mannitol.

- *Alkaline diuresis:* Alkaline diuresis promotes elimination of weak acids (eg, barbiturates, salicylates) and is accomplished by the administration of IV sodium bicarbonate.
- *Acid diuresis:* Acid diuresis may be indicated in overdoses with weak bases (eg, amphetamines, quinine) but use with caution in patients with renal or liver disease. It is usually accomplished with oral or IV ascorbic acid or ammonium chloride.

Dialysis: Dialysis is indicated in a minority of severe overdose cases. Drug factors that alter dialysis effectiveness include volume of distribution, drug compartmentalization, protein binding, and lipid/water solubility.

- *Hemodialysis:* Hemodialysis may be used after an overdose and when the patient is having complications (eg, severe metabolic acidosis, electrolyte imbalances, renal failure).
- *Peritoneal dialysis:* Peritoneal dialysis is even less effective than hemodialysis.
- *Charcoal hemoperfusion:* Charcoal hemoperfusion is useful when a drug can be adsorbed by charcoal (eg, theophylline, barbiturates).

Poison Control Center

Consultation with a regional poison control center is highly recommended.

MANAGEMENT OF ACUTE HYPERSENSITIVITY REACTIONS

Type I hypersensitivity reactions (immediate hypersensitivity or anaphylaxis) are immunologic responses to a foreign antigen to which a patient has been sensitized previously. Anaphylactoid reactions are not mediated immunologically; however, symptoms and treatment are similar.

Signs and Symptoms

Acute hypersensitivity reactions typically begin within 1 to 30 minutes of exposure to the offending antigen. Tingling sensations and a generalized flush may proceed to a fullness in the throat, chest tightness, or a "feeling of impending doom." Generalized urticaria and sweating are common. *Severe* reactions include life-threatening involvement of the airway and cardiovascular system.

Treatment

Appropriate and immediate treatment is imperative. The following general measures are employed commonly:

Epinephrine: Epinephrine 1:1000, 0.2 to 0.5 mg (0.2 to 0.5 mL) subcutaneously is the primary treatment. In children, administer 0.01 mg/kg or 0.1 mg. Doses may be repeated every 5 to 15 minutes, if needed. A succession of small doses is more effective and less dangerous than a single large dose. Additionally, 0.1 mg may be introduced into an injection site where the offending drug was administered. If appropriate, the use of a tourniquet above the site of injection of the causative agent may slow its absorption and distribution. However, remove or loosen the tourniquet every 10 to 15 minutes to maintain circulation.

Epinephrine IV (generally indicated in the presence of hypotension) is often recommended in a 1:10,000 dilution, 0.3 to 0.5 mg over 5 minutes; repeat every 15 minutes, if necessary. In children, inject 0.1 to 0.2 mg or 0.01 mg/kg/dose over 5 minutes; repeat every 30 minutes.

A conservative IV epinephrine protocol includes 0.1 mg of a 1:100,000 dilution (0.1 mg of a 1:1000 dilution mixed in 10 mL normal saline) given over 5 to 10 minutes. If an IV infusion is necessary, administer at a rate of 1 to 4 mcg/min. In children, infuse 0.1 to 1.5 (maximum) mcg/kg/min.

Dilute epinephrine 1:10,000 may be administered through an endotracheal tube, if no other parenteral access is available, directly into the bronchial tree. It is absorbed rapidly there from the capillary bed of the lung.

Airway: Ensure a patent airway via endotracheal intubation or cricothyrotomy (ie, inferior laryngotomy, used prior to tracheotomy), and administer oxygen. Severe respiratory difficulty may respond to IV aminophylline or to other bronchodilators.

Hypotension: The patient should be recumbent with feet elevated. Depending upon the severity, consider the following measures:

• Establish a patent IV catheter in a suitable vein.
• Administer IV fluids (eg, normal saline, lactated Ringer's).
• Administer plasma expanders.
• Administer cardioactive agents (see group and individual monographs). Commonly recommended agents include dopamine, dobutamine, norepinephrine, and phenylephrine.

Adjunctive therapy : Adjunctive therapy does not alter acute reactions, but may modify an ongoing or slow-onset process and shorten the course of the reaction.

• *Antihistamines:* Diphenhydramine 50 to 100 mg intramuscular or IV, continued orally at 5 mg/kg/day or 50 mg every 6 hours for 1 to 2 days. For children, give 5 mg/kg/day, maximum 300 mg/day.

  Chlorpheniramine (adults, 10 to 20 mg; children, 5 to 10 mg) intramuscular or slowly IV.

  Hydroxyzine 10 to 25 mg orally or 25 to 50 mg intramuscular 3 to 4 times/day.

• *Corticosteroids:* Corticosteroids (eg, hydrocortisone IV) 100 to 1,000 mg or equivalent followed by 7 mg/kg/day IV or oral for 1 to 2 days. The role of corticosteroids is controversial.

• *H_2 antagonists:* Cimetidine 300 mg every 6 hours. For children, 25 to 30 mg/kg/day IV in 6 divided doses.

  Ranitidine 50 mg IV over 3 to 5 minutes. Ranitidine may be valuable in addition to H_1 antihistamines, although this opinion is not shared universally.

APPENDIX C

THE HOME MEDICINE CABINET

The cost associated with office visits to doctors for diagnosis and treatment of minor conditions caused by accidental injury or illness amounts to hundreds of millions of dollars annually. In many instances, the time and money spent visiting the doctor can be avoided if you have a properly stocked home medicine cabinet and a basic knowledge of first aid and self care.

A properly stocked home medicine cabinet must include, but not be limited to, typical first-aid items. Having key drugs and devices available and knowing how to use them may prevent delays in treating discomforting symptoms. However, if significant relief is not achieved or the condition worsens during the first 24 hours after the accident or onset of symptoms, do not hesitate to contact a pharmacist or doctor.

When we refer to the home medicine cabinet, the tendency is to think of a bathroom cabinet or drawer. However, the humidity and temperature fluctuations of the bathroom may accelerate the deterioration of certain drugs. The bathroom is a less than ideal place to store these health care items. Also, some items are bulky (eg, cool mist vaporizer, heating pad, ice pack) and it may not be practical to store them with other items. Store the items for the home medicine cabinet in a cool, dry area out of the reach of children. The upper portion of a hall or bedroom closet are good storage areas. Consolidation of many of the items in a locked fishing tackle box or plastic tub is a good idea.

Basic Inventory

The ideal inventory for a home medicine cabinet varies widely. Contents should reflect the nature, size, lifestyle, location, age, and health status of the individual or family. The basic inventory for a household that includes one or more children is included in the following table. These items may prevent costly and unnecessary trips to the emergency room or doctor's office but must not be used as substitutes for appropriate medical attention.

First-aid items: First-aid items are employed most frequently to manage cuts, scrapes, bites, stings, sprains, and strains. Thoroughly clean all wounds involving broken skin. Mild soap and warm water are very effective. Hydrogen peroxide (3%) may be used if the wound is dirty and very sensitive. The bubbling action of the peroxide helps to remove debris physically. The antiseptic/antibacterial action of hydrogen peroxide is limited, however, and should not be overestimated. If the wound is painful, a local anesthetic spray may be applied. If no allergies to the drug exist, a thin layer of multiple antibiotic ointment or cream may be applied to a superficial wound each time the dressing is changed. Cover all wounds involving broken skin with a loose, protective dressing for a few days and change the dressing at least once daily.

Hydrocortisone ointment or cream (0.5% or 1%) is useful in treating local pain, irritation, itching, and inflammation associated with bites, stings, sunburn, and contact dermatitis associated with poison ivy, oak, or sumac. If the allergic reaction is severe, oral diphenhydramine (eg, *Benadryl*) capsules or tablets may be required to provide relief. Oatmeal baths and calamine lotion may be useful if local inflammation is widespread (eg, chickenpox). Isopropyl alcohol is included as an agent to rub on sprains and strains. If used as an antiseptic on a fresh wound, it will burn for several seconds.

An ice pack is recommended to control inflammation, pain, and swelling of bites, stings, sprains, and strains. Apply it as soon after the injury as possible. Generally, heat should not be applied to a sprain or strain for 24 to 48 hours after the acute injury.

Cold and allergy items: Antihistamines, decongestants or both will provide symptomatic relief of seasonal allergic rhinitis and the common cold. Antihistamines work best in relieving allergic symptoms and are sometimes overvalued in treating the common cold.

Gastrointestinal products: Stomach upset, heartburn, and acid indigestion may be relieved with gastrointestinal products. Simple uncomplicated diarrhea should respond to *Kaopectate, Donnagel,* or *Imodium A-D.*

Analgesic items: Fever-reducing drugs and pain relievers are essential components of the home medicine cabinet. Standard fever-reducing drugs are aspirin and acetaminophen. Pain is the most common medical symptom. More than 30 million Americans suffer from headaches each week. Because of the suspected link between aspirin use and Reye syndrome, do not give aspirin to children experiencing pain or fever. Acetaminophen is as effective as aspirin as an analgesic and fever-reducing drug. Therefore, treat children with symptoms of neuralgia, arthralgia, myalgia, headache, fever, or general discomfort associated with viral conditions (eg, chickenpox, influenza) with acetaminophen. Liquid or chewable acetaminophen may be preferable for children. Nonsteroidal anti-inflammatory drugs (eg, ibuprofen, naproxen) are alternatives to aspirin or acetaminophen as analgesics and fever-reducing agents in a variety of clinical situations.

Sunscreens: The association of excessive exposure to ultraviolet (UV) light and skin cancers of various types is real. Sunscreens are strongly recommended, regardless of skin type, if exposure to sunlight is to be lengthy.

Miscellaneous items: Tweezers are useful for removing splinters and other foreign objects embedded in the skin.

A cool mist humidifier, properly maintained and cleaned after use, helps to provide symptomatic relief from dry mucous membranes of the nasal passages and throat associated with colds and flu.

Finally, one ounce of ipecac syrup is an emergency drug that should be in every home in the event of childhood poisoning. Doses for children are smaller than adult doses. Call the nearest poison control center before administering ipecac to determine the proper dose or whether it should be used at all. Ipecac must not be used to treat some types of poisoning.

```
┌─────────────────────────────────────────────────────────────────────┐
│              Home Medicine Cabinet — Basic Inventory                  │
├─────────────────────────────────────────────────────────────────────┤
```

First Aid Items

> Assorted adhesive bandages (eg, *Band-Aids*) — 1 box
> Sterile gauze pads (2" × 2") — 1 box
> Waterproof adhesive tape (½" to 5 yards) — 1 roll
> Blunt scissors
> Elastic bandage (2" to 3" wide)
> Ice pack (6" to 9" diameter)
> Heating pad (dry or moist heat)
> Hydrogen peroxide (3%) — 8 oz
> Triple antibiotic ointment (eg, *Neosporin, Mycitracin*)
> Local anesthetic spray (eg, *Bactine, Medi-Quick*) — 1 aerosol can
> Isopropyl (rubbing) alcohol (70%) — 16 oz
> Hydrocortisone ointment or cream (0.5% or 1%) — ½ oz tube

Cold and Allergy Items

> Diphenhydramine (eg, *Benadryl*) 25 mg capsule or tablet — 24 count
> Chlorpheniramine maleate (eg, *Chlor-Trimeton*) 4 mg tablet — 24 count
> Pseudoephedrine (30 or 60 mg) tablet — 24 count

Gastrointestinal items

> Antacid (eg, *Maalox, Mylanta*) — 12 oz
> H_2 antagonist (eg, *Pepcid AC*)
> Antidiarrheal (eg, *Kaopectate, Donnagel, Imodium A-D*) — 8 oz

Analgesic items

> Aspirin (325 mg) tablet — 50 count
> Nonsteroidal anti-inflammatory drug (eg, *Advil, Motrin, Aleve*)
> Acetaminophen (325 mg) tablet, capsule, or gelcap — 50 count

Sunscreen

> Waterproof or water-resistant sunscreen with an SPF rating of at least 15

Miscellaneous Items

> Oral fever thermometer
> Rectal fever thermometer (for small children)
> Tweezers
> Cool mist humidifier
> Ipecac syrup — 1 oz
> Phone number of nearest poison control center

Conclusion

A host of other items may be appropriate additions to the home medicine cabinet. These often include foot powder; antifungal ointments, solutions, creams, or sprays; laxatives; vitamins; minerals; eye drops; and lotions. The core items recommended should serve most families well. Other items may be added as need.

Do not neglect your home medicine cabinet. At times, medicine cabinets need first aid themselves. Remove and discard old, outdated, and deteriorated items periodically. Throw away any product that has changed its color, consistency, or odor, as it has probably "gone bad." Keep remaining items orderly so they may be found when needed. If symptoms do not respond to treatment or worsen rapidly after being treated with appropriate items in the home, do not hesitate to contact a pharmacist or doctor.

TEMPERATURE-TAKING TECHNIQUES

When to Take Children's Temperatures

- Take a child's temperature if he or she appears sick, flushed, lethargic, or has been ill for a few days.
- Take the temperature in the morning or late afternoon and intermittently as needed.
- Do not give the child anything hot or cold to drink for at least half an hour before taking the temperature orally.
- Stay with the child while you are taking his or her temperature.

Call the Doctor if

- The child's temperature is higher than 101°F orally for longer than 24 hours or is 103°F or higher after giving the child medicine to lower fever (eg, acetaminophen, ibuprofen).
- Fever has been present more than 3 days.
- Behavior changes have been observed (eg, the child is fussy, lethargic, irritable).
- Convulsions are present.
- The child is unable to move or has a stiff neck.
- The child is confused or hallucinating.

Thermometers		
Type	**Advantages**	**Disadvantages**
Glass (*Oral* — Thin tip, *Rectal* — Rounder tip)	Least expensive Reliable	Record temperature slowly Hard to read Breakable
Digital	More convenient than glass thermometers Accurate Registers temperature in ≈ 30 seconds Beeps when finished Can be used orally, rectally, or axillary	More expensive than glass thermometers Runs on batteries Hazardous if ingested
Tympanic	Convenient Measures temperature in < 2 seconds Causes no discomfort Requires minimal cooperation from child	Expensive Controversial among health care providers because of questions regarding accuracy Must be used correctly
Tapes/Pacifiers	Inexpensive Convenient	Inaccurate

Methods and Instructions for Use

There are four methods of taking a child's temperature: Rectal, oral, axillary (underarm), and tympanic.

Rectal: The rectal route correlates well to the core body temperature and is more accurate than the oral or axillary methods. The child has a fever if the rectal temperature is 101.8°F (38.8°C) or higher. This method is preferred in infants and children younger than 5 years of age. The disadvantages include apprehension in the child and parent, struggling of the child, the slowness of the reading (requires 2 full minutes in the rectum), and the lag time in measurement following changes in core body temperature.

Instructions – First, lubricate the end of the rectal thermometer with petroleum jelly. Next, lay the child either on his or her back with the legs held together or stomach down across your lap. Lubricate the opening of the anus with petroleum jelly and insert the round bulb approximately an inch. **Do not force it.** Press the buttocks together to hold the thermometer in place. Glass thermometers should be left in for approximately 2 minutes; digital thermometers should remain inserted until a beep is heard (approximately 30 seconds).

Oral: The oral route underestimates the core body temperature by approximately 1°F. The child has a fever if the oral temperature is 100°F (37.8°C) or higher. A disadvantage of the oral route is that tachypnea cools the intraoral mucosa. Children younger than 5 years of age should not have temperatures taken orally.

Instructions – Shake down the glass thermometer until its reading is less than 98.6°F and rotate it slightly until the mercury line appears. Place the bulb end of the oral thermometer under the tongue toward the back of the mouth. Have the child close his mouth to keep it in place. Tell the child not to bite the thermometer because it may break. Leave it for at least 3 minutes. If using the digital thermometer, leave it under the tongue until a beep is heard (approximately 30 seconds).

Axillary: Axillary (armpit) temperatures can be measured either by a rectal, oral, or digital thermometer. The normal armpit temperature is 97.6°F. The child has a fever if the reading is 99°F (37.2°C) or higher. This is the least accurate measurement because of the high sensitivity to ambient temperatures. Readings are at least 1°F below core body temperature and the time to register is 4 to 7 minutes.

Instructions – Make sure the armpit is dry and place the tip of the thermometer in the armpit. Hold the elbow to the child's side to keep in place. Leave it in place for 4 to 7 minutes (glass) or until a beep is heard (digital).

Tympanic: Tympanic temperatures measure heat from the eardrum. Digital thermometers are used in this method; a rectal and an oral indicator correlate to the respective temperatures. The results are usually available within 2 seconds. The ear canal is well insulated from the ambient environment and is unaffected by rapid breathing, eating, drinking, and smoking. Temperatures taken in the right ear may be slightly different from those of the left ear; therefore, use the same ear repeatedly when checking for a fever. Also, sleeping on the ear may increase the temperature so wait a few minutes after the child awakens before taking a temperature. This method causes no discomfort and requires minimal cooperation from the child. However, this method is viewed with suspicion regarding accuracy among some health care providers and it must be used correctly.

Instructions – When handling the thermometer, do not touch the tip of the lens or lens filter. Do not use the thermometer without a lens filter, and store the thermometer with a new filter after each use. Practice taking the child's temperature to help ensure accuracy. Select either the oral (for adults and children older than 3 years of age) or rectal (for infants and children 3 years of age and younger) indicator. Push the on button. If using on an infant, lay the infant flat and make sure the ear is up. If right-handed, hold the thermometer with the right hand and place the thermometer in the right ear. Use free hand to grasp the outer edge of the top half of the ear and gently pull up and out to straighten the ear canal. This provides a clear view of the eardrum. If taking a temperature on a child 1 to 3 years of age, approach the ear from behind. Place the lens at the opening of the ear canal and insert the thermometer. Point toward the opposite eye and insert the lens as far as possible until the ear canal is fully sealed off. For children 4 years of age and older, follow the same procedure but point the lens slightly in front of the opposite ear. If taking a self temperature, place the free hand around the back of the head and tug. Activate the button by holding it down for 1 second. Continue pulling ear until finished taking temperature.

Other: Tapes and pacifiers are inexpensive and convenient but they are inaccurate.

OTIC ADMINISTRATION TECHNIQUES

Instilling Ear Drops

1.) Wash hands thoroughly with warm, soapy water, then dry hands.
2.) Clean and dry the external or outer ear thoroughly.
3.) Warm the ear drops to room temperature or near body temperature by placing the container in the hands and holding tightly for several minutes. Do *not* place the container in hot water or in the microwave.
4.) Lie down and tilt head sideways with the affected ear upward. For adults, gently pull the ear lobe up and back. For children, gently pull the ear lobe down and back.
5.) If the drops are in a suspension form, shake well for 10 seconds before using.
6.) Place the prescribed volume of drops into the ear without the dropper touching the ear or any other surface to prevent contamination. Remain reclined for a few minutes.
7.) Do not rinse the dropper or applicator tip after use. Wipe off the tip of the dropper or applicator tip with a clean tissue. Keep the container tightly closed.
8.) If cotton is placed into the ears after drops have been added, smear a small amount of petroleum jelly on the cotton to prevent the cotton from soaking up the ear drops. Take care not to shove the cotton deeply into the ear canal.
9.) Call a physician if symptoms persist or worsen within 2 days.

Note: It is helpful to have another person assist with this process. For safety reasons, small children should be restrained when cleaning the ear(s) or applying ear drops. The child should be placed sideways on the lap and restrained across the head and shoulders to prevent movement. Another adult should clean the ear and apply the ear drops.

Using an Ear Syringe

1.) Wash hands thoroughly with warm, soapy water, then dry hands.
2.) Clean and dry the external or outer ear thoroughly.
3.) The solution in the syringe should be at or near body temperature to avoid discomfort and dizziness.
4.) While sitting upright, tilt head slightly sideways with the affected ear upward.
5.) For adults, gently pull the earlobe up and back. For children, gently pull the earlobe down and back.

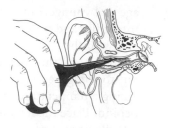

6.) Fill the syringe with irrigation solution and place the syringe into the upper part of the ear without the syringe touching the ear or any other surface to prevent contamination. To prevent a watery mess, the patient should hold a small container at the base of the ear to catch the irrigating solution and removed debris as it is flushed out of the ear.
7.) The syringe should be angled so that it is pointing at the top of the ear canal. Gently compress the syringe, allowing the irrigation solution to enter the ear and then drain at the same time to allow the contents of the ear to drain naturally downward and out the ear. Never occlude the ear canal with the tip of the syringe while placing the irrigation solution into the ear.
8.) Remove any wax or other debris remaining in the outer ear area by gently flushing the ear with a syringe using only a warm irrigation solution.
9.) Rinse the ear canal twice daily for up to 4 days, if needed, or as directed by a physician.
10.) If excessive earwax or other debris still remains, consult a physician.

Note: It is helpful to have another person assist with this process. Excessive, frequent cleaning of the ears can worsen inflammation and actually lead to an ear infection.

RESPIRATORY DRUG ADMINISTRATION TECHNIQUES

Nasal Sprays

1.) Clear nasal passageways before administering a dose by gently blowing nose.
2.) Remove cap.
3.) Insert tip into one nostril. Occlude the opposite nostril by pressing the index finger against the nose.
4.) With head upright, sniff deeply while squeezing the bottle. Direct spray away from nasal septum.
5.) Repeat with other nostril.
6.) Rinse bottle tip with warm water and replace cap.

Nasal Drops

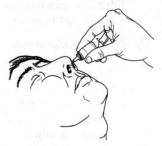

1.) Clear nasal passageways before administering a dose by gently blowing nose.
2.) Recline on a bed or hang head over the edge of the bed; remain in this position for several minutes after using the drops, turning the head from side to side.
3.) Insert dropper tip into one nostril.
4.) Squeeze dropper bulb gently to discharge contents of dropper.
5.) Repeat with other nostril.
6.) Rinse dropper with warm water and let air dry.

Metered Dose Pumps

1.) Prime the pump the first time it is used.
2.) Clear the nasal passageways before administering a dose by gently blowing nose.
3.) Insert tip of pump into one nostril. Occlude the opposite nostril by pressing the index finger against the nose.
4.) Hold head upright; sniff deeply while depressing the pump.
5.) Repeat with other nostril.
6.) Rinse tip with warm water and replace cap.

Nasal Inhalers

1.) Clear nasal passageways before administering a dose.
2.) Insert tip of inhaler into one nostril. Occlude the opposite nostril by pressing the index finger against the nose.
3.) Sniff deeply.
4.) Repeat with other nostril.
5.) Replace cap after use and keep inhalers tightly closed.
6.) Do not use propylhexedrine for longer than 3 days or l-desoxyephedrine for longer than 7 days.
7.) May cause burning, stinging, sneezing, or increased nasal discharge.
8.) Patients should not use these products if they have a history of heart disease, high blood pressure, thyroid disease, diabetes, or prostatic hypertrophy, unless directed by a physician.

OPHTHALMIC DRUG ADMINISTRATION TECHNIQUES

Ophthalmic Drops

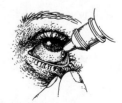

1.) Wash hands with soap and water.
2.) Remove glasses (or contacts if applicable and advised by your eyecare practitioner).
3.) Gently pinch the lower eyelid and pull downward to form a pouch.
4.) With head tilted back, place the recommended number of drops in the pouch.
5.) Close eye and press on the inner corner of the eye for a few minutes to decrease systemic absorption.
6.) Wipe excess solution from eyes or face with a clean tissue.
7.) Do not wipe or rinse the dropper before replacing the cap.
8.) Do not use eye drops that have changed color or contain a precipitate.

9.) If more than one type of ophthalmic drop is used, wait at least 5 minutes before administering the second agent.

Ophthalmic Ointments

1.) Wash hands thoroughly with soap and water.
2.) Tilt head backward or lie down and gaze upward.
3.) Gently pull down the lower lid to form a pouch.
4.) Place a 0.25 to 0.5 inch ribbon of ointment with a sweeping motion inside the lower lid by squeezing the tube gently. Slowly release the eyelid.
5.) Blink gently a few times then close the eye for 1 to 2 minutes.
6.) Temporary blurring of vision may occur. Avoid activities requiring visual acuity until blurring clears.
7.) Remove excessive ointment around the eye or ointment tube tip with a tissue. Replace cap.
8.) If using more than one kind of ointment, wait at least 10 minutes before applying the second agent.

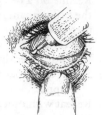

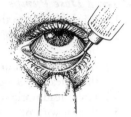

Lid Scrubs

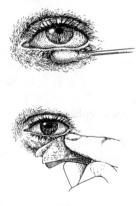

Commercially available eyelid cleansers or antibiotic solutions or ointments can be applied directly to the lid margin for the treatment of noninfectious blepharitis. This is best accomplished by applying the medication to the end of a cotton-tipped applicator and then scrubbing the eyelid margin several times daily. The gauze pads supplied with commercially available eyelid cleansers are also convenient.

INSULIN INJECTION

These guidelines are intended to help health care providers instruct diabetic patients in the proper techniques for insulin injection.

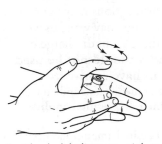
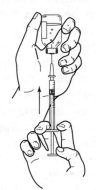
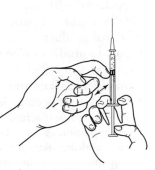

1. Check labeling on vial to ensure that the insulin is the correct strength and the expiration date has not passed. Most insulin products should not be used more than 30 days after first use of the vial. Follow manufacturer guidelines. Roll the vial between your palms to warm and mix the insulin. **Never shake the vial.** Using an alcohol swab, clean the vial's rubber stopper.

2. Inject air into the vial in an amount equal to the desired insulin volume, to prevent creating a vacuum. Draw up the insulin in the syringe.

3. If bubbles appear in the filled syringe, tap it lightly. Then, draw up more insulin if necessary. Return the plunger to the amount of the dose to push the air bubble(s) into the vial. Set syringe down and avoid needle contamination.

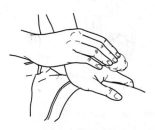
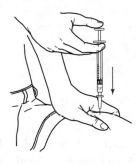

4. Select an appropriate injection site. Pull skin taut, then wipe it clean with a cotton ball or swab soaked in alcohol.

5. Use thumb and forefinger to pinch skin at injection site. Quickly plunge needle, up to its hub, into the skin fold at a 90° angle. Hold syringe with one hand. Pull back on plunger slightly with other hand (many health providers consider this step optional). Check for blood backflow. If blood appears in syringe, discard all supplies and begin process again. If no blood backflow appears, inject insulin slowly.

6. Place alcohol-soaked cotton ball over the injection site, apply light pressure while withdrawing the needle. Snap needle off syringe with a needle snipper or drop needle and syringe into a solid plastic container, and dispose of all materials properly.

VAGINAL ADMINISTRATION TECHNIQUES

Inserting Vaginal Creams

Some vaginal creams are spread externally onto irritated areas of the vulva, while others are inserted into the vagina. The following guidelines apply to creams that are to be inserted into the vagina. Most of these types of creams are packaged with applicators. Consider the directions below to be general guidelines; instruct patients to carefully follow directions provided with individual products, as administration and dosing instructions may vary from product to product. When using vaginal creams, patients may want to wear deodorant panty shields or minipads to protect clothing from discharge or cream leakage. **Tampons, douches, and spermicides should not be used until treatment is complete and vaginal symptoms have resolved.**

1.) Following manufacturer instructions, open the tube of medication and attach the applicator to the tube. (**Note: Some products include prefilled applicators, making steps 1 and 2 unnecessary.**)

2.) Carefully squeeze the cream into the applicator until desired amount has been inserted (many applicators have a plunger line marked "Full"). Replace the cap on the tube of medicated cream.

3.) Hold the applicator barrel between your thumb and third and fourth fingers of one hand, with your index finger placed at the end of the tube to push the plunger into the barrel.

4.) Insert the applicator into the vaginal canal as if you were inserting a tampon. The applicator should be inserted as far as it can comfortably go. For easier insertion, stand with feet spread apart and knees bent, or, preferably, lay on back with knees bent.

5.) Still holding the applicator between your thumb and third and fourth fingers as described above, use your index finger to gently push the plunger into the barrel of the applicator as far as possible (see illustration). After discharging contents, remove the entire applicator from the vagina.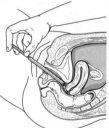

6.) If applicator is disposable, throw it away after use (do not flush applicator down the toilet). If applicator is reusable, clean it thoroughly after use by pulling the plunger and barrel apart and washing them with mild soap and warm water; rinse thoroughly and dry. Gently push the plunger back into the barrel to reassemble before next use.

7.) Lie down immediately to prevent cream from leaking from vagina.

8.) If product information recommends, repeat application at designated intervals.

Inserting Vaginal Suppositories

Most vaginal suppositories are sold with applicators. Consider the directions below to be general guidelines; instruct patients to carefully follow directions provided with individual products, as administration and dosing instructions may vary from product to product. When using vaginal suppositories, patients may want to wear deodorant panty shields or minipads to protect clothing from discharge. **Tampons, douches, and spermicides should not be used until treatment is complete and vaginal symptoms have resolved.**

1.) Following manufacturer instructions, remove the vaginal suppository from its packaging and wrapping and place it in applicator.

2.) Hold the applicator barrel between your thumb and third and fourth fingers of one hand, with your index finger placed at the end of the tube to push the plunger into the barrel.

3.) Insert the applicator into the vaginal canal as if you were inserting a tampon. The applicator should be inserted as far as it can comfortably go. For easier insertion, stand with feet spread apart and knees bent, or, preferably, lay on back with knees bent.

4.) Still holding the applicator between your thumb and third and fourth fingers as described above, use your index finger to gently push the plunger into the barrel of the applicator as far as possible. After discharging the suppository, remove the entire applicator from the vagina.

5.) If applicator is disposable, throw it away after use (do not flush applicator down the toilet). If applicator is reusable, clean it thoroughly after use by pulling the plunger and barrel apart and washing them with mild soap and warm water; rinse thoroughly and dry. Gently push the plunger back into the barrel to reassemble before next use.

6.) Lie down immediately to prevent discharge of the vaginal suppository before it dissolves.

7.) If product information recommends, repeat application at designated intervals.

RECTAL SUPPOSITORY ADMINISTRATION

1.) If a suppository has softened because of improper storage, it should be chilled in a refrigerator approximately 30 minutes prior to insertion, *or*, with wrapper intact, hold suppository under cold, running water.

2.) Gather items needed for administration of suppository (ie, suppository, water-soluble lubricant, finger cot, or disposable latex glove).

3.) Cleanse hands thoroughly with soap (preferably antibacterial) and water. Hand sanitizing agents may be used if soap and water are unavailable.

4.) The latex glove should be worn on the dominant hand. If a finger cot is used, place it on the index finger of dominant hand.

5.) If present, wrapper (usually foil) should be removed. Inspect suppository to ensure remnants of wrapper do not remain on the suppository.

6.) For ease of administration, moisten the tip or pointed end of the suppository with the lubricant. Cool water may be used to moisten the anal opening if lubricant is unavailable. Do not use petroleum jelly (*Vaseline*).

7.) The proper body positioning prior to insertion is as follows:
- Lie down on side with lower arm outstretched.
- Raise both knees toward chest or abdominal area, *or* keep lower leg straight and move upper leg toward abdomen (knee should be slightly bent).

8.) Using gloved hand, completely insert suppository into rectum.

9.) Immediately contract anal sphincter to keep the suppository in place. Buttocks of children should be held together firmly for several seconds.

10.) To avoid suppository movement, remain lying down for approximately 15 to 20 minutes.

11.) Discard used materials into appropriate waste receptacle.

12.) Wash or sanitize hands thoroughly.

ENEMA ADMINISTRATION

Consider the directions for administration of enemas to be general guidelines.

Instruct patients to carefully follow directions provided with individual premixed products as administration and dosage may vary from product to product.

1.) Shake the enema container well.

2.) Hold unit upright, grasping the flexible bulb of unit with fingers.

3.) Remove protective shield from the tip.

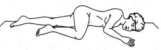

Figure 1. Left Side Position

4.) Assume the left side position (lie on left side with right knee bent and arms resting comfortably [see Figure 1]) or knee-chest position (kneel, then lower head and chest forward until left side of face is resting on surface with left arm folded comfortably [see Figure 2]).

5.) With steady pressure, gently insert tip (pointing toward navel) into the rectum with slight side-to-side movement. *Warning:* Stop insertion of enema tip if resistance is encountered. Forcing the tip can cause injury.

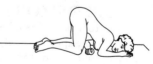

Figure 2. Knee-Chest Position

6.) Insertion may be easier if the person bears down as if having a bowel movement.

7.) Squeeze the bulb or flexible enema container until nearly all the liquid is expelled.

8.) Continue to squeeze the bottle. Remove from the rectum and discard the empty unit.

9.) Hold the enema contents in place for as long as possible by constricting the anal sphincter.

Administering Large-Volume Cleansing Enemas

1.) Close off the tubing by sliding the clamp to squeeze the tubing together.

2.) Use lukewarm water to fill the bag to the 1,500 mL mark, unless otherwise directed by your doctor.

3.) Check to see that the bag opening is closed securely by pressing 2 sides of the seal together.

4.) Remove the protective shield from the enema tip. Open the clamp and allow a small amount of liquid to flow through the tubing to eliminate insertion of air, which could cause cramping. Close the clamp.

5.) The tubing to be inserted is marked with a black line to indicate the generally accepted length of insertion. Do not insert past the mark unless otherwise instructed by your doctor.

6.) The enema must be administered while lying down.

7.) Hang or hold the bag so that the bottom of the bag is approximately 2 feet above you.

8.) Lie on your left side (see Figure 1 above) and insert the enema tip into your rectum slowly. Stop when you reach the black line, or if resistance is encountered. Forcing the tip can cause injury.

9.) Release the clamp to allow approximately one third of liquid to flow slowly into the rectum. Stop flow with clamp. Do not remove tip.

10.) Turn onto your back or stomach, whichever is more comfortable. Repeat above procedure.

11.) If you feel cramping, stop the flow for a few minutes. Do not remove tip from the rectum. Gently massage abdomen until the cramps subside, then resume.

12.) Turn onto your right side and open clamp to allow another one third of liquid to flow in slowly. Close the clamp and remove the tip from the rectum.

13.) When the urge to evacuate occurs, move to the toilet and expel as much of the liquid as you can.

14.) If you have been instructed to take tap water enemas until clear, repeat the above procedures until liquid expelled is clear.

APPENDIX E

POISON CONTROL CENTER HOTLINE

The American Association of Poison Control Centers (AAPCC) has established a national toll-free poison center hotline. Now everyone in the United States can call:

1-800-222-1222

to reach the local poison center. Poison Control Center services are available 24 hours a day, 7 days a week.

The phone number can be used for a poison emergency or questions about poisons and poison prevention.

Regardless of where the call is placed, the hotline automatically connects callers to the closest poison control center. Existing local poison center numbers will still connect callers to their poison centers.

Callers who use a TTY/TDD and non-English speaking callers can also use this hotline.

The index lists all condition names, generic drug names, drug class names, and trade names included in *Nonprescription Drug Therapy™*. For ease of reading, monograph titles are printed in **bold type** and product trade names are italicized.

We have made every effort to create an index that is comprehensive and easy to use, allowing you to find the information you need as quickly as possible.

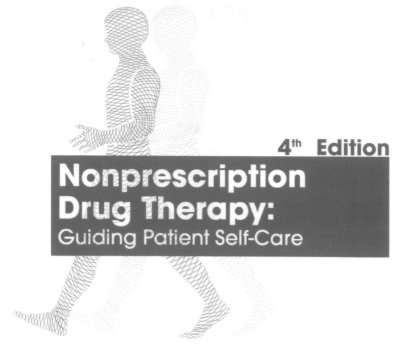

4th Edition

Nonprescription Drug Therapy:
Guiding Patient Self-Care

Designed to serve the informational needs of pharmacists, physicians, other health care providers, and self-medicating consumers, **Nonprescription Drug Therapy: Guiding Patient Self-Care (NDT)** is an easy-to-use reference for OTC drug information. Logically organized by medical condition, **NDT** presents comprehensive and current information on more than 100 commonly occurring conditions and their OTC therapy options.

Features:
- Organized by condition
- Patient interview section
- Patient information boxes
- Assists in determining if nonprescription agents, nondrug therapy, or physician referral is appropriate for individual patients

Monographs Include:
- Definition
- Etiology
- Incidence
- Pathophysiology
- Signs/Symptoms
- Diagnostic parameters
- Treatment options
- Product information

Chapters:
- CNS Conditions
- Complementary Therapies
- Dermatological Conditions
- Diabetes Management
- GI/GU Conditions
- Home Diagnostics/Devices
- Musculoskeletal Conditions
- Nutrition
- Ophthalmic Conditions
- Oral Cavity Care
- Otic Conditions
- Podiatric Conditions
- Respiratory Conditions
- Women's Health

ISBN 1-57439-223-9

90000 >

EAN

9 781574 392234

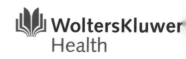

WoltersKluwer
Health